WHO Classification of Tumours • 5th Edition

Eye and Orbit Tumours

WHO Classification of Tumours Editorial Board

International Agency for Research on Cancer

World Health Organization

Suggested citation
WHO Classification of Tumours Editorial Board. Eye and orbit tumours.
Lyon (France): International Agency for Research on Cancer; 2025.
(WHO classification of tumours series, 5th ed.; vol. 13).
https://publications.iarc.who.int/660.

Sales, rights, and permissions
Print copies are distributed by WHO Press, World Health Organization, 20 Avenue Appia, 1211 Geneva 27, Switzerland
Tel.: +41 22 791 3264; Fax: +41 22 791 4857; email: bookorders@who.int; website: https://whobluebooks.iarc.who.int/

To purchase IARC publications in electronic format, see the IARC Publications website (https://publications.iarc.who.int).

Requests for permission to reproduce or translate IARC publications – whether for sale or for non-commercial distribution – should be submitted through the IARC Publications website (https://publications.iarc.who.int/Rights-And-Permissions).

Third-party materials
If you wish to reuse material from this work that is attributed to a third party, such as figures, tables, or boxes, it is your responsibility to determine whether permission is needed for that reuse and to obtain permission from the copyright holder. See *Sources*, pages 521–526. The risk of claims resulting from infringement of any third-party-owned component in the work rests solely with the user.

The contributors of all images in which the patient may be identifiable have affirmed that the appropriate informed consent has been obtained for the use of said images in this publication.

General disclaimers
The designations employed and the presentation of the material in this publication do not imply the expression of any opinion whatsoever on the part of WHO or contributing agencies concerning the legal status of any country, territory, city, or area, or of its authorities, or concerning the delimitation of its frontiers or boundaries. Dotted and dashed lines on maps represent approximate border lines for which there may not yet be full agreement.

The mention of specific companies or of certain manufacturers' products does not imply that they are endorsed or recommended by WHO or contributing agencies in preference to others of a similar nature that are not mentioned. Errors and omissions excepted, the names of proprietary products are distinguished by initial capital letters.

All reasonable precautions have been taken by WHO to verify the information contained in this publication. However, the published material is being distributed without warranty of any kind, either expressed or implied. The responsibility for the interpretation and use of the material lies with the reader. In no event shall WHO or contributing agencies be liable for damages arising from its use.

First print run (2500 copies)

Updated corrigenda can be found at https://publications.iarc.who.int

IARC Library Cataloguing-in-Publication Data
Names: WHO Classification of Tumours Editorial Board.
Title: Eye and orbit tumours / edited by WHO Classification of Tumours Editorial Board.
Description: Fifth edition. | Lyon: International Agency for Research on Cancer, 2025. | Series: World Health Organization classification of tumours. | Includes bibliographical references and index.
Identifiers: ISBN: 9789283245469 (pbk.)
Subjects: MESH: Eye Neoplasms – pathology. | Eye Neoplasms – genetics. | Orbital Neoplasms – pathology. | Orbital Neoplasms – genetics.
Classification: NLM WW 149

The WHO classification of eye and orbit tumours presented in this book reflects the views of the WHO Classification of Tumours Editorial Board that convened via video conference 25–27 April 2022, as well as subsequent consultation.

The WHO Classification of Tumours Editorial Board

Expert members: Eye and orbit tumours

For the complete list of all contributors and their affiliations, see pages 513–518.

The WHO Classification of Tumours Editorial Board (continued)

* Standing members marked with an asterisk also served as expert members for this volume.

For the complete list of all contributors and their affiliations, see pages 513–518.

WHO Classification of Tumours
Eye and Orbit Tumours

Edited by	The WHO Classification of Tumours Editorial Board
IARC Editors	Ian A. Cree Gabrielle Goldman-Lévy Dilani Lokuhetty Pavitratha Puspanathan Harshima Wijesinghe
Project Assistant	Asiedua Asante
Assistants	Camille Bou Anne-Sophie Bres
Technical Editing Production Editing	Karen O'Donnell Sharon Paul Julia Slone-Murphy
Principal Information Assistant Information Assistants	Alberto Machado Ramon Cierco Jimenez Catarina Marques
Layout	Meaghan Fortune
Printed by	Imprimerie CHIRAT 42540 Saint-Just-la-Pendue, France
Publisher	International Agency for Research on Cancer (IARC) 25 Av. Tony Garnier, CS 90627 69366 Lyon, CEDEX 07, France

Contents

List of abbreviations

ABC	activated B cell
AIDS	acquired immunodeficiency syndrome
AJCC	American Joint Committee on Cancer
AR	androgen receptor
A-scan	amplitude scan
bp	base pair
B-scan	brightness scan
cDNA	complementary DNA
CI	confidence interval
cIg	cytoplasmic immunoglobulin
CNS	central nervous system
CT	computed tomography
DNA	deoxyribonucleic acid
EBRT	external beam radiation therapy
EBV	Epstein–Barr virus
ER	estrogen receptor
FDG PET	18F-fluorodeoxyglucose positron emission tomography
FISH	fluorescence in situ hybridization
FNA	fine-needle aspiration
FNAB	fine-needle aspiration biopsy
FNAC	fine-needle aspiration cytology
GCB	germinal-centre B cell
GFAP	glial fibrillary acidic protein
H&E	haematoxylin and eosin stain
HIV	human immunodeficiency virus
HPF	high-power field
HPV	human papillomavirus
HTLV-1	human T-lymphotropic virus type 1
IARC	International Agency for Research on Cancer
ICD-11	International Classification of Diseases, 11th revision
ICD-O	International Classification of Diseases for Oncology
IIRC	International Intraocular Retinoblastoma Classification
LDS	lacrimal drainage system
M:F ratio	male-to-female ratio
Mb	megabase
MCPyV	Merkel cell polyomavirus
MIM number	Mendelian Inheritance in Man number
MITF	microphthalmia-associated transcription factor
MMR	mismatch repair
MRI	magnetic resonance imaging
mRNA	messenger ribonucleic acid
MSI	microsatellite instability
N:C ratio	nuclear-to-cytoplasmic ratio
NK cell	natural killer cell
NOS	not otherwise specified
NSE	neuron-specific enolase
Pap	Papanicolaou stain
PAS	periodic acid–Schiff
PASD	periodic acid–Schiff with diastase
PCR	polymerase chain reaction
PET-CT	positron emission tomography–computed tomography
PR	progesterone receptor
RNA	ribonucleic acid
RPE	retinal pigment epithelium
RT-PCR	reverse transcription polymerase chain reaction
sIg	surface immunoglobulin
SNP	single-nucleotide polymorphism
SNV	single-nucleotide variant
SPM	second primary malignancy
Th2	T helper 2
TNM	tumour, node, metastasis
UICC	Union for International Cancer Control
UV	ultraviolet

Foreword

The WHO Classification of Tumours is a taxonomy of cancer, published as a series of books (also known as the WHO Blue Books) and now as a website (https://tumourclassification.iarc.who.int). It is an essential tool for standardizing diagnostic practice worldwide. It also serves as a vehicle for the translation of cancer research into practice. The diagnostic criteria and standards that make up the classification are underpinned by evidence evaluated and debated by experts in the field. About 200 authors and editors participate in the production of each volume, and they give their time freely to this task. We are very grateful for their help; it is a remarkable international team effort of great significance to both patients and their doctors.

This volume, like the rest of the fifth edition, has been led by the WHO Classification of Tumours Editorial Board, composed of standing and expert members. The standing members, who have been nominated by pathology organizations, are the equivalent of the series editors of previous editions. The expert members for each volume, equivalent to the volume editors of previous editions, are selected on the basis of informed bibliometric analysis and advice from the standing members. The diagnostic process is increasingly multidisciplinary, and we are delighted that several radiology and clinical experts have joined us to address specific needs.

The most conspicuous change to the format of the books in the fifth edition is that tumour types common to multiple systems are dealt with together – so there are separate chapters on mesenchymal tumours and haematolymphoid tumours. There is also a chapter on genetic tumour syndromes associated with eye and orbit malignancies.

In this volume, orbital tumours are included for the first time in the history of the classification. With additional volumes on genetic tumour syndromes and paediatric tumours, this makes the fifth edition the first to be comprehensive: all tumour types and sites of the body are now included.

We have attempted to take a more systematic approach to the multifaceted nature of tumour classification; each tumour type is described on the basis of its localization, clinical features, epidemiology, etiology, pathogenesis, histopathology, diagnostic molecular pathology, staging, and prognosis and prediction. We have also included information on macroscopic appearance and cytology, as well as essential and desirable diagnostic criteria. This standardized, modular approach makes it easier for the books to be accessible online, and it also enables us to call attention to areas in which there is little information, and where serious gaps in our knowledge remain to be addressed. Genetic disorders are of increasing importance to diagnosis in individual patients, and the study of these disorders has undoubtedly informed our understanding of tumour biology and behaviour over the past decade.

The organization of the WHO Blue Books content now follows the normal progression from benign to malignant – a break with the fourth edition, but one we hope has been welcome.

Table A Approximate number of fields per 1 mm^2 based on the field diameter and its corresponding area

Field diameter (mm)	Field area (mm^2)	Approximate number of fields per 1 mm^2
0.40	0.126	8
0.41	0.132	8
0.42	0.138	7
0.43	0.145	7
0.44	0.152	7
0.45	0.159	6
0.46	0.166	6
0.47	0.173	6
0.48	0.181	6
0.49	0.188	5
0.50	0.196	5
0.51	0.204	5
0.52	0.212	5
0.53	0.221	5
0.54	0.229	4
0.55	0.237	4
0.56	0.246	4
0.57	0.255	4
0.58	0.264	4
0.59	0.273	4
0.60	0.283	4
0.61	0.292	3
0.62	0.302	3
0.63	0.312	3
0.64	0.322	3
0.65	0.332	3
0.66	0.342	3
0.67	0.352	3
0.68	0.363	3
0.69	0.374	3

Most volumes are still organized by anatomical site (digestive system, breast, soft tissue and bone, etc.), and each tumour type is listed within a taxonomic classification that follows the format below, which helps to structure the books in a systematic manner:

Site: e.g. eyelid

Category: e.g. epithelial tumours

Family (class): e.g. malignant epithelial tumours

Type: e.g. basal cell carcinoma

Subtype: e.g. superficial basal cell carcinoma

The issue of whether a given tumour type represents a distinct entity rather than a subtype continues to exercise pathologists, and it is the topic of many publications in the literature. We continue to deal with this issue on a case-by-case basis, but we believe there are inherent rules that can be applied. For example, tumours in which multiple histological patterns contain shared truncal mutations are clearly of the same type, despite the differences in their appearance. Equally, genetic heterogeneity within the same tumour type may have implications for treatment. A small shift in terminology in the fifth edition is that the term "variant" in reference to a specific kind of tumour has been wholly superseded by "subtype", in an effort to more clearly differentiate this meaning from that of "variant" in reference to a genetic alteration. Genetic tumour syndromes associated with eye and orbit malignancies are addressed in a dedicated chapter at the end of the volume.

Another important change in this edition of the WHO Classification of Tumours series is the conversion of mitotic count from the traditional denominator of 10 HPF to a defined area expressed in mm^2 {691A}. This serves to standardize the true area over which mitoses are enumerated, because different microscopes have high-power fields of different sizes. This change will also be helpful for anyone reporting using digital systems. The approximate number of fields per 1 mm^2 based on the field diameter and its corresponding area is presented in Table A.

We are continually working to improve the consistency and standards within the classification. In addition to having moved to the International System of Units (SI) for all mitotic counts, we have standardized genomic nomenclature by using Human Genome Variation Society (HGVS) notation. This includes the recent move in fusion gene notation to the separation of involved genes by a double colon (e.g. *BCR*::ABL1) {432A}. We have also further standardized our use of units of length, adopting the convention used by the International Collaboration on Cancer Reporting (https://www.iccr-cancer.org/) and the UK Royal College of Pathologists (https://www.rcpath.org/), so that the size of tumours is now given exclusively in millimetres (mm) rather than centimetres (cm). This is clearer, in our view, and avoids the use of decimal points – a common source of medical errors.

The WHO Blue Books are much appreciated by pathologists of all types, and they are of increasing importance to practitioners of other clinical disciplines involved in cancer management, as well as to researchers. We, along with the entire editorial board, certainly hope that the series will continue to meet the need for standards in diagnosis and to facilitate the translation of diagnostic research into practice worldwide. It is particularly important that cancers continue to be classified and diagnosed according to the same standards internationally so that patients can benefit from multicentre clinical trials, as well as from the results of local trials conducted on different continents.

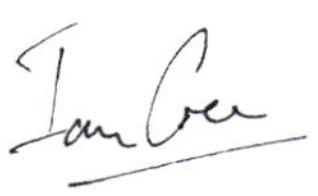

Dr Ian A. Cree

Former Head, WHO Classification of Tumours Programme
International Agency for Research on Cancer

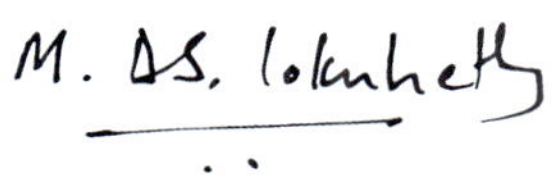

Dr Dilani Lokuhetty

Head, WHO Classification of Tumours Programme
International Agency for Research on Cancer

ICD-O topographical coding of eye and orbit tumours

The ICD-O topography codes for the main anatomical sites covered in this volume are as follows {1041A}:

C41 Bones, joints, and articular cartilage of other and unspecified sites
C41.0 Bones of skull and face and associated joints

C44 Skin
C44.1 Eyelid

C47 Peripheral nerves and autonomic nervous system
C47.0 Peripheral nerves and autonomic nervous system of head, face, and neck

C49 Connective, subcutaneous, and other soft tissues
C49.0 Connective, subcutaneous, and other soft tissues of head, face, and neck

C69 Eye and adnexa
C69.0 Conjunctiva
C69.1 Cornea, NOS
C69.2 Retina
C69.3 Choroid
C69.4 Ciliary body
C69.5 Lacrimal gland
C69.6 Orbit, NOS
C69.8 Overlapping lesion of eye and adnexa
C69.9 Eye, NOS

C70 Meninges
C70.9 Meninges, NOS

C72 Spinal cord, cranial nerves, and other parts of central nervous system
C72.3 Optic nerve

ICD-O morphological coding: Introduction

The ICD-O coding system uses a topography (T) code and a morphology (M) code together, but these are presented in separate lists for ease of use. Behaviour is coded /0 for benign tumours; /1 for unspecified, borderline, or uncertain behaviour; /2 for carcinoma in situ and grade III intraepithelial neoplasia; /3 for malignant tumours, primary site; and /6 for malignant tumours, metastatic site. Behaviour code /6 is not generally used by cancer registries. For various reasons, the ICD-O morphology terms may not always be identical to the entity names used in the WHO classification, but they should be sufficiently similar to avoid confusion. The designation "NOS" ("not otherwise specified") is provided to make coding possible when subtypes exist but exact classification may not be possible in small biopsies or certain other scenarios. Therefore, it is usual to have "NOS" even when a more specific alternative term is listed in ICD-O.

ICD-O coding of eye and orbit tumours

ICD-O-3.2	ICD-O label (subtypes are indicated in grey text, with the label indented); Please note that the WHO classification of tumour types is more readily reflected in the table of contents

Tumours of the conjunctiva and caruncle

Tumour-like lesions and choristomas of the conjunctiva

Cysts of the conjunctiva and caruncle

	Epithelial conjunctival inclusion cyst

Reactive, epithelial, and degenerative conjunctival lesions

	Reactive epithelial hyperplasia of the conjunctiva
	Papillary and follicular conjunctivitis
	Acute papillary conjunctivitis
	Chronic papillary conjunctivitis
	Giant papillary conjunctivitis
	Acute follicular conjunctivitis
	Chronic follicular conjunctivitis
	Pterygium and pinguecula

Choristomas of the conjunctiva

	Epibulbar choristoma
	Epibulbar dermoid
	Dermolipoma
	Complex choristoma
	Epibulbar osseous choristoma

Epithelial tumours of the conjunctiva

Benign epithelial conjunctival tumours

8052/0	Conjunctival squamous papilloma
8052/0	Exophytic conjunctival squamous papilloma
8053/0	Inverted (endophytic) conjunctival squamous papilloma
8052/0	Mixed conjunctival squamous papilloma†
8290/0	Conjunctival oncocytoma
	Hereditary benign intraepithelial dyskeratosis

Premalignant and malignant epithelial conjunctival tumours

	Conjunctival squamous intraepithelial neoplasia
8077/0	Conjunctival squamous intraepithelial neoplasia, mild dysplasia
8077/2	Conjunctival squamous intraepithelial neoplasia, moderate dysplasia
8077/2	Conjunctival squamous intraepithelial neoplasia, severe dysplasia
8070/3	Conjunctival squamous cell carcinoma
8560/3	Adenosquamous carcinoma

Melanocytic tumours of the conjunctiva

Benign melanocytic conjunctival tumours

	Benign epithelial melanosis of the conjunctiva
	Junctional, compound, and subepithelial conjunctival naevi
8740/0	Junctional naevus
8760/0	Compound naevus
8750/0	Subepithelial (stromal) naevus
8722/0	Balloon cell naevus
8770/0	Inflamed juvenile conjunctival naevus
8780/0	Blue naevus of the conjunctiva
8780/0	Dendritic blue naevus
8790/0	Cellular blue naevus
8720/1	WNT-activated deep penetrating / plexiform melanocytoma (naevus)
8720/0	Combined naevus
8780/0	Combined conventional and blue melanocytic naevus†
8720/1	Combined conventional melanocytic naevus and WNT-activated deep penetrating / plexiform melanocytoma (naevus)†
8720/0	Combined conventional and granular cell melanocytic naevus†
8722/0	Combined conventional and balloon cell melanocytic naevus†

ICD-O-3.2	ICD-O label (subtypes are indicated in grey text with the label indented); Please note that the WHO classification of tumour types is more readily reflected in the table of contents

Premalignant and malignant melanocytic conjunctival tumours	
	Conjunctival melanocytic intraepithelial lesions
8720/0	Low-grade conjunctival melanocytic intraepithelial lesion
8720/2	High-grade conjunctival melanocytic intraepithelial lesion
8720/3	Conjunctival melanoma
Tumours of the eyelid	
Tumour-like lesions, hamartomas, and choristomas of the eyelid	
Cysts of the eyelid	
	Epidermal inclusion cyst
	Intratarsal cyst
Choristomas of the eyelid	
	Phakomatous choristoma
Epithelial tumours of the eyelid	
Benign and premalignant epithelial eyelid tumours	
	Molluscum contagiosum
	Verruca vulgaris
8052/0	Squamous papilloma
8052/0	Seborrhoeic keratosis
8052/0	Irritated seborrhoeic keratosis
8052/0	Stucco keratosis
	Inverted follicular keratosis
8070/0	Actinic keratosis
8070/0	Proliferative actinic keratosis
8070/0	Hypertrophic actinic keratosis
8070/0	Lichenoid actinic keratosis
8070/0	Pigmented actinic keratosis
Malignant epithelial eyelid tumours	
8090/3	Basal cell carcinoma, NOS
8091/3	Superficial basal cell carcinoma
8097/3	Nodular basal cell carcinoma
8097/3	Micronodular basal cell carcinoma
8092/3	Infiltrating basal cell carcinoma
8092/3	Sclerosing/morphoeic basal cell carcinoma
8094/3	Basosquamous carcinoma
8070/3	Squamous cell carcinoma
8070/2	Squamous cell carcinoma in situ (Bowen disease)
8071/1	Keratoacanthoma
8247/3	Merkel cell carcinoma
Adnexal tumours of the eyelid	
Benign adnexal eyelid tumours	
8404/0	Ductal hidrocystoma[†]
8404/0	Apocrine hidrocystoma
8404/0	Eccrine hidrocystoma
	Sebaceous hyperplasia, sebaceous adenoma, and sebaceoma
	Sebaceous hyperplasia
8410/0	Sebaceous adenoma
8410/0	Sebaceoma

ICD-O-3.2	ICD-O label (subtypes are indicated in grey text, with the label indented); Please note that the WHO classification of tumour types is more readily reflected in the table of contents
8407/0	Syringoma
8940/0	Mixed tumour
8940/0	Apocrine mixed tumour†
8940/0	Eccrine mixed tumour†
8211/0	Tubular adenoma
8406/0	Syringocystadenoma papilliferum
8110/0	Pilomatricoma
8102/0	Trichilemmoma
8102/0	Desmoplastic trichilemmoma
Malignant adnexal eyelid tumours	
8410/3	Sebaceous carcinoma
8200/3	Adenoid cystic carcinoma
8490/3	Signet-ring cell / histiocytoid carcinoma
8480/3	Mucinous carcinoma
8509/3	Endocrine mucin-producing sweat gland carcinoma
8407/3	Microcystic adnexal carcinoma
8401/3	Apocrine carcinoma
Melanocytic tumours of the eyelid	
Benign and premalignant melanocytic eyelid tumours	
	Naevi of the eyelid
8740/0	Junctional naevus
8760/0	Compound naevus
8750/0	Dermal naevus
8770/0	Spitz naevus
8770/0	Spitz naevus with *ALK* fusion
8770/0	Spitz naevus with *ROS1* fusion
8770/0	Spitz naevus with *NTRK1* fusion
8770/0	Spitz naevus with *NTRK3* fusion
8770/0	Spitz naevus with *BRAF* fusion
8770/0	Spitz naevus with *HRAS* mutation
8770/0	Spitz naevus with *PRKAR1A* inactivation as a secondary event
8770/0	Spitz naevus with *MAP3K8* fusion
8770/0	Spitz naevus with *RET* fusion
	Cutaneous melanoma in situ
8742/2	Lentigo maligna
8743/2	Low-CSD melanoma in situ
Malignant melanocytic eyelid tumours	
	Invasive cutaneous melanoma
8743/3	Low-CSD melanoma (superficial spreading melanoma)
8742/3	Lentigo maligna melanoma
8721/3	Nodular melanoma
Tumours of the uveal tract	
Tumours of the iris	
Benign lesions and hamartomas of the iris	
	Ectopic tissue
	Ectopic lacrimal tissue
	Ectopic thyroid tissue
	Implantation cyst
	Pigmented epithelial cyst
	Lisch nodule
Melanocytic tumours of the iris	
	Ocular melanocytosis
8720/0	Iris naevus
8720/0	Circumscribed iris naevus†
8720/1	Diffuse iris naevus†
8720/3	Iris melanoma
8720/3	Ring melanoma†
8720/3	Diffuse iris melanoma†

ICD-O-3.2	ICD-O label (subtypes are indicated in grey text, with the label indented); Please note that the WHO classification of tumour types is more readily reflected in the table of contents
	Tumours of the choroid and ciliary body
	Benign melanocytic lesions of the choroid and ciliary body
	Choroidal and ciliary body naevi
8720/0	Pigmented naevus
8723/0	Halo naevus
8761/1	Giant pigmented naevus
8726/0	Uveal melanocytoma
	Bilateral diffuse uveal melanocytic proliferation
	Malignant melanocytic tumours of the choroid and ciliary body
	Choroidal and ciliary body melanomas
8772/3	Spindle cell uveal melanoma, NOS
8773/3	Spindle cell uveal melanoma, type A
8774/3	Spindle cell uveal melanoma, type B
8770/3	Mixed epithelioid and spindle cell uveal melanoma
8771/3	Epithelioid cell uveal melanoma
8720/3	Retinoinvasive melanoma†
8720/3	Ring melanoma†
8720/3	Diffuse melanoma†
	Tumours of the retina and neuroepithelium
	Tumours of the neurosensory retina
	Benign retinal tumours
	Astrocytic tumours
9384/1	Giant cell astrocytoma of the retina†
9384/1	Retinal astrocytic hamartoma†
	Nodular and massive retinal gliosis
	Premalignant and malignant retinal tumours
9510/0	Retinocytoma
9514/1	Retinoblastoma, spontaneously regressed
9510/3	Retinoblastoma
9510/3	Unilateral retinoblastoma
9510/3	Bilateral retinoblastoma
9510/3	Trilateral retinoblastoma
	Tumours of the retinal pigment epithelium
	Reactive and hamartomatous lesions of the retinal pigment epithelium
	Hamartoma of the retinal pigment epithelium
	Congenital hypertrophy of the retinal pigment epithelium
	Reactive hyperplasia of the retinal pigment epithelium
	Benign and malignant tumours of the retinal pigment epithelium
	Adenoma and adenocarcinoma of the retinal pigment epithelium
8140/0	Retinal pigment epithelial adenoma
8140/3	Retinal pigment epithelial adenocarcinoma
	Tumours of the iris and ciliary body neuroepithelium
	Reactive and cystic lesions of the iris and ciliary body pigment epithelium
	Reactive epithelial hyperplasia of the ciliary epithelium
	Nodular hyperplasia of the ciliary epithelium
	Glioneuronal hamartoma of the ciliary body
	Benign and malignant tumours of the iris and ciliary body pigment epithelium
	Adenoma and adenocarcinoma of the ciliary body
8140/0	Ciliary body adenoma
8140/3	Ciliary body adenocarcinoma
	Medulloepithelioma of the ciliary body
9501/0	Medulloepithelioma, benign
9501/3	Medulloepithelioma, malignant
9502/0	Teratoid medulloepithelioma, benign
9502/3	Teratoid medulloepithelioma, malignant

ICD-O-3.2 ICD-O label (subtypes are indicated in grey text, with the label indented);
Please note that the WHO classification of tumour types is more readily reflected in the table of contents

Tumours of the optic disc and optic nerve

Primary tumours of the optic disc and optic nerve

Malformations of the optic disc and optic nerve

Optic nerve choristoma

Primary neural tumours of the optic disc and optic nerve

Gliomas of the optic nerve

9421/1	Pilocytic astrocytoma
9425/3	Pilomyxoid astrocytoma
9400/3	Astrocytoma, IDH-mutant, grade 2
9440/3	Glioblastoma, IDH-wildtype

Pigment epithelial tumours of the optic disc and optic nerve

Medulloepithelioma of the optic disc and optic nerve

9501/0	Medulloepithelioma, benign
9501/3	Medulloepithelioma, malignant
9502/0	Teratoid medulloepithelioma, benign
9502/3	Teratoid medulloepithelioma, malignant

Meningeal tumours of the optic nerve

9530/0	Meningioma of the optic nerve

Melanocytic tumours of the optic disc and optic nerve

8726/0	Melanocytoma of the optic disc and optic nerve

Tumours of the lacrimal gland

Epithelial tumours of the lacrimal gland

Cysts of the lacrimal gland

Dacryops cyst

Benign and premalignant epithelial lacrimal gland tumours

8940/0	Pleomorphic adenoma
8290/0	Oncocytoma
8290/3	Oncocytic carcinoma
8982/0	Myoepithelioma
8982/3	Myoepithelial carcinoma
8500/2	Intraductal carcinoma

Malignant epithelial lacrimal gland tumours

8941/3	Carcinoma ex pleomorphic adenoma
8200/3	Adenoid cystic carcinoma
8500/3	Primary ductal adenocarcinoma of the lacrimal gland†
8502/3	Secretory carcinoma
8430/3	Mucoepidermoid carcinoma
8562/3	Epithelial-myoepithelial carcinoma
8550/3	Acinic cell carcinoma
8140/3	Adenocarcinoma, NOS

Tumours of the lacrimal drainage system

Epithelial tumours of the lacrimal drainage system

Benign and premalignant epithelial lacrimal drainage system tumours

Papillomas (squamous and inverted)

8052/0	Squamous papilloma, exophytic†
8053/0	Squamous papilloma, inverted
8052/0	Squamous papilloma, mixed†

Malignant epithelial lacrimal drainage system tumours

8070/3	Squamous cell carcinoma
8071/3	Squamous cell carcinoma, keratinizing, NOS
8072/3	Squamous cell carcinoma, non-keratinizing, NOS
8082/3	Lymphoepithelial carcinoma
8430/3	Mucoepidermoid carcinoma

ICD-O-3.2	ICD-O label (subtypes are indicated in grey text, with the label indented); Please note that the WHO classification of tumour types is more readily reflected in the table of contents

	Other salivary gland–type carcinomas of the lacrimal drainage system
8290/3	Oncocytic carcinoma
8200/3	Adenoid cystic carcinoma
8562/3	Epithelial-myoepithelial carcinoma
8941/3	Carcinoma ex pleomorphic adenoma
8410/3	Sebaceous carcinoma
8140/3	Adenocarcinoma, NOS, of the lacrimal drainage system
8147/3	Basaloid / basal cell adenocarcinoma
Melanocytic tumours of the lacrimal drainage system	
8720/3	Melanoma involving the lacrimal drainage system

Tumours of the orbit

Teratomas, hamartomas, and choristomas of the orbit

Choristomas and cysts	
	Orbital dermoid cyst and other orbital cysts
Vascular malformations	
9121/0	Cavernous vascular malformation
9170/0	Combined lymphatic-venous malformation of the orbit†
9122/0	Orbital venous malformation
9123/0	Arteriovenous malformation
Hamartomas	
	Orbital glial heterotopia
	Mesenchymal hamartoma of the orbit
Germ cell tumours	
	Teratoma
9080/0	Mature teratoma
9080/3	Immature teratoma
9080/3	Malignant teratoma
9071/3	Yolk sac tumour
Melanocytic tumours of the orbit	
8720/3	Primary orbital melanoma

Haematolymphoid tumours

Reactive lymphoid lesions

Reactive lymphoid lesions	
	Reactive lymphoid hyperplasia
9760/1	IgG4-related disease
Intraocular haematolymphoid proliferations	
9699/3	Primary choroidal lymphoma
9680/3	Primary vitreoretinal large B-cell lymphoma

ICD-O-3.2	ICD-O label (subtypes are indicated in grey text, with the label indented); Please note that the WHO classification of tumour types is more readily reflected in the table of contents
Ocular adnexal lymphomas	
B-cell lymphomas	
9699/3	Extranodal marginal zone lymphoma
9690/3	Follicular lymphoma
9673/3	Mantle cell lymphoma
9673/3	Cyclin D1–positive mantle cell lymphoma
9673/3	Cyclin D1–negative mantle cell lymphoma
9823/3	Chronic lymphocytic leukaemia / small lymphocytic lymphoma
9680/3	Diffuse large B-cell lymphoma
9680/3	Diffuse large B-cell lymphoma, centroblastic subtype
9684/3	Diffuse large B-cell lymphoma, immunoblastic subtype
9680/3	Diffuse large B-cell lymphoma, anaplastic subtype
9680/3	Diffuse large B-cell lymphoma, germinal-centre B-cell subtype
9680/3	Diffuse large B-cell lymphoma, activated B-cell subtype
9680/3	Diffuse large B-cell lymphoma with *MYC* and *BCL6* rearrangements
9731/3	Plasmacytoma
9734/3	Extramedullary plasmacytoma
9731/3	Solitary plasmacytoma of bone
T/NK-cell lymphomas	
	CD30-positive lymphoproliferative disorders
9718/1	Lymphomatoid papulosis
9718/3	Primary cutaneous anaplastic large cell lymphoma
9719/3	Extranodal NK/T-cell lymphoma
Myeloid tumours	
Myeloid sarcoma	
9930/3	Myeloid sarcoma
Histiocytic and dendritic cell tumours	
Histiocytic tumours	
9749/1	Juvenile xanthogranuloma
9749/3	Rosai–Dorfman disease
9749/3	Erdheim–Chester disease
9751/1	Langerhans cell histiocytosis, NOS
9751/3	Langerhans cell histiocytosis, disseminated
9756/3	Primary Langerhans cell sarcoma
9756/3	Secondary Langerhans cell sarcoma (following or associated with another haematological neoplasm)
	Xanthelasma
	Xanthoma
	Adult orbital xanthogranulomatous disease

ICD-O-3.2	ICD-O label (subtypes are indicated in grey text, with the label indented); Please note that the WHO classification of tumour types is more readily reflected in the table of contents
Soft tissue and bone tumours	
Soft tissue tumours	
Fibrous and fibroblastic tumours	
	Conjunctival stromal tumour and ocular surface fibroma
8830/0	Fibrous histiocytoma
8831/0	Deep fibrous histiocytoma
8832/0	Classic dermatofibroma
8832/0	Cellular dermatofibroma
8832/0	Aneurysmal dermatofibroma
8832/0	Atypical dermatofibroma
	Nodular and proliferative fasciitis, proliferative myositis
8828/0	Nodular fasciitis
8828/0	Proliferative fasciitis
8828/0	Proliferative myositis
	Intravascular and cranial fasciitis
8815/1	Solitary fibrous tumour, NOS
8815/0	Solitary fibrous tumour, benign
8815/3	Solitary fibrous tumour, malignant
8815/1	Fat-forming (lipomatous) solitary fibrous tumour
8815/1	Giant cell–rich solitary fibrous tumour
8815/3	Dedifferentiated solitary fibrous tumour
8825/1	Inflammatory myofibroblastic tumour
8832/1	Dermatofibrosarcoma protuberans
8833/1	Pigmented dermatofibrosarcoma protuberans
8832/3	Fibrosarcomatous dermatofibrosarcoma protuberans
8832/1	Myxoid dermatofibrosarcoma protuberans
8832/1	Dermatofibrosarcoma protuberans with myoid differentiation
8832/1	Plaque-like dermatofibrosarcoma protuberans
8841/0	Angiomyxoma
8841/0	Cutaneous myxoma (superficial angiomyxoma)
8841/0	Aggressive angiomyxoma
Adipocytic tumours	
	Benign lipomatous tumours
8850/0	Lipoma, NOS
8861/0	Angiolipoma, NOS
	Malignant adipocytic tumours
8850/1	Atypical lipomatous tumour
8851/3	Liposarcoma, well-differentiated
8858/3	Dedifferentiated liposarcoma
8852/3	Myxoid liposarcoma
8854/3	Pleomorphic liposarcoma
Skeletal muscle tumours	
	Rhabdomyosarcomas
8910/3	Embryonal rhabdomyosarcoma
8920/3	Alveolar rhabdomyosarcoma
8912/3	Spindle cell rhabdomyosarcoma
8901/3	Pleomorphic rhabdomyosarcoma
8921/3	Ectomesenchymoma
Smooth muscle tumours	
8890/0	Leiomyoma
8890/0	Mesectodermal leiomyoma†
8890/3	Leiomyosarcoma

ICD-O-3.2	ICD-O label (subtypes are indicated in grey text, with the label indented); Please note that the WHO classification of tumour types is more readily reflected in the table of contents
Peripheral nerve sheath tumours	
9560/0	Schwannoma
9560/0	Cellular schwannoma
9560/0	Plexiform schwannoma
9560/0	Epithelioid schwannoma
9560/0	Microcystic/reticular schwannoma
9540/0	Neurofibroma
9550/0	Plexiform neurofibroma
9540/0	Solitary neurofibroma
9540/0	Diffuse neurofibroma
9541/0	Melanotic neurofibroma
9570/0	Solitary circumscribed neuroma
9570/0	Plexiform solitary circumscribed neuroma
9580/0	Granular cell tumour
9580/3	Granular cell tumour, malignant
9540/3	Malignant peripheral nerve sheath tumour
9542/3	Epithelioid malignant peripheral nerve sheath tumour
Vascular tumours	
	Masson tumour
	Primary (pure) Masson tumour
	Secondary (mixed) Masson tumour
	Extravascular Masson tumour
9131/0	Infantile haemangioma
9131/0	Lobular capillary haemangioma
	Lymphangiectasia
9125/0	Epithelioid haemangioma
9125/0	Cellular epithelioid haemangioma
9125/0	Atypical epithelioid haemangioma
9161/1	Haemangioblastoma
9120/3	Angiosarcoma
Perivascular tumours	
8711/0	Glomus tumour, NOS
8711/1	Glomus tumour of uncertain malignant potential
8711/3	Glomus tumour, malignant
	Myopericytoma, including myofibroma
8824/0	Myofibroma
8824/1	Multicentric myofibromatosis
8824/0	Myopericytoma
Tumours of uncertain derivation	
	PEComa
8714/0	Perivascular epithelioid tumour, benign
8714/3	Perivascular epithelioid tumour, malignant
8804/3	Epithelioid sarcoma
8804/3	Classic epithelioid sarcoma
8804/3	Proximal epithelioid sarcoma
9040/3	Synovial sarcoma, NOS
9041/3	Monophasic synovial sarcoma
9043/3	Biphasic synovial sarcoma
9040/3	Poorly differentiated synovial sarcoma
9581/3	Alveolar soft part sarcoma

ICD-O-3.2	ICD-O label (subtypes are indicated in grey text, with the label indented); Please note that the WHO classification of tumour types is more readily reflected in the table of contents

Tumours of orbital bone

Osteogenic tumours of orbital bone

9180/0	Osteoma
9200/1	Osteoblastoma
9180/3	Osteosarcoma, NOS
9183/3	Telangiectatic osteosarcoma
9185/3	Small cell osteosarcoma
9187/3	Low-grade central osteosarcoma

Chondrogenic tumours of orbital bone

9220/0	Chondroma
9240/3	Mesenchymal chondrosarcoma

Fibrous and fibroblastic tumours of orbital bone

8818/0	Fibrous dysplasia
8818/0	Monostotic fibrous dysplasia
8818/0	Polyostotic fibrous dysplasia

Vascular tumours of orbital bone

9120/0	Haemangioma
9125/0	Epithelioid haemangioma
9133/3	Epithelioid haemangioendothelioma
9133/3	Epithelioid haemangioendothelioma with *WWTR1::CAMTA1* fusion
9133/3	Epithelioid haemangioendothelioma with *YAP1::TFE3* fusion
9120/3	Angiosarcoma

Osteoclast-rich giant cell tumours of orbital bone

9260/0	Aneurysmal bone cyst
9250/1	Giant cell tumour of bone
9250/1	Conventional giant cell tumour of bone
9250/3	Malignant giant cell tumour of bone
9250/3	Dedifferentiated giant cell tumour of bone†

Other tumours of orbital bone

9364/3	Ewing sarcoma

These morphology codes are from the International Classification of Diseases for Oncology, third edition, second revision (ICD-O-3.2) {1424A}. Behaviour is coded /0 for benign tumours; /1 for unspecified, borderline, or uncertain behaviour; /2 for carcinoma in situ and grade III intraepithelial neoplasia; /3 for malignant tumours, primary site; and /6 for malignant tumours, metastatic site. Behaviour code /6 is not generally used by cancer registries.

This classification is modified from the previous WHO classification, taking into account changes in our understanding of these lesions.

n/a, not available (provisional entity or subtype).

* Codes marked with an asterisk were approved by the IARC/WHO Committee for ICD-O at its meeting in April 2022, or during subsequent consultation.

† Labels marked with a dagger have undergone a change in terminology of a previous code.

TNM staging of eye and orbit tumours

Ophthalmic Tumours

Introductory Notes

Tumours of the eye and its adnexa are a disparate group including carcinoma, melanoma, sarcomas, and retinoblastoma. For clinical convenience they are classified in one section.

The following sites are included:

- Eyelid (eyelid tumours are classified with skin tumours)
- Conjunctiva
- Uvea
- Retina
- Orbit
- Lacrimal gland

For histological nomenclature and diagnostic criteria, reference to the WHO histological classification is recommended.[1]

Each tumour type is described under the following headings:

- Rules for classification with the procedures for assessing the T, N, and M categories
- Anatomical sites where appropriate
- Definition of the regional lymph nodes
- TNM clinical classification
- pTNM pathological classification
- Stage where applicable

Reference

1. Campbell RJ. *Histological Typing of Tumours of the Eye and its Adnexa*, 2nd edn. Berlin: Springer, 1998.

TNM staging of carcinoma of the conjunctiva

Carcinoma of Conjunctiva

(ICD-O-3 C 69.0)

Rules for Classification

There should be histological confirmation of the disease and division of cases by histological type, for example, mucoepidermoid and squamous cell carcinoma.

The following are the procedures for assessing T, N, and M categories:

T categories	Physical examination
N categories	Physical examination
M categories	Physical examination and imaging

Regional Lymph Nodes

The regional lymph nodes are the preauricular, submandibular and cervical lymph nodes.

TNM Clinical Classification

T – Primary Tumour

- TX Primary tumour cannot be assessed
- T0 No evidence of primary tumour
- Tis Carcinoma in situ
- T1 Tumour 5 mm or less in greatest dimension invades through the conjuctival basement membrane
- T2 Tumour more than 5 mm in greatest dimension, invades through the conjuctival basement membrane without invasion of adjacent structures*
- T3 Tumour invades adjacent structures*
- T4 Tumour invades the orbit or beyond
  - T4a Tumour invades orbital soft tissues, without bone invasion
  - T4b Tumour invades bone
  - T4c Tumour invades adjacent paranasal sinuses
  - T4d Tumour invades brain

Note

* Adjacent structures include: the cornea (3, 6, 9, or 12 clock hours), intraocular compartments, forniceal conjunctiva (lower and/or upper), palpebral conjunctiva (lower and/or upper), tarsal conjunctiva (lower and/or upper), lacrimal punctum and canaliculi (lower and/or upper), plica, caruncle, posterior eyelid lamella, anterior eyelid lamella and/or eyelid margin (lower and/or upper).

N – Regional Lymph Nodes

- NX Regional lymph nodes cannot be assessed
- N0 No regional lymph node metastasis
- N1 Regional lymph node metastasis

M – Distant Metastasis

- M0 No distant metastasis
- M1 Distant metastasis

pTNM Pathological Classification

The pT and pN categories correspond to the T and N categories.

pM – Distant Metastasis*

- pM1 Distant metastasis microscopically confirmed

Note

* pM0 and pMX are not valid categories.

Stage

No stage is at present recommended.

TNM staging of carcinoma of the skin of the eyelid

Carcinoma of Skin of the Eyelid

(ICD-O-3 C44.1)

Rules of Classification

There should be histological confirmation of the disease and division of cases by histological type – for example, basal cell, squamous cell, sebaceous carcinoma. Melanoma of the eyelid is classified with skin tumours, see page 142 of the eighth-edition TNM classification {414}.

The following are procedures for assessing T, N, and M categories:

T categories	Physical examination
N categories	Physical examination
M categories	Physical examination and imaging

Regional Lymph Nodes

The regional lymph nodes are the preauricular, submandibular, and cervical lymph nodes.

TNM Clinical Classification

T – Primary Tumour

- TX Primary tumour cannot be assessed
- T0 No evidence of primary tumour
- Tis Carcinoma in situ
- T1 Tumour 10 mm or less in greatest dimension
  - T1a Not invading the tarsal plate or eyelid margin
  - T1b Invades tarsal plate or eyelid margin
  - T1c Involves full thickness of eyelid
- T2 Tumour > 10 mm, but 20 mm or less in greatest dimension
  - T2a Not invading the tarsal plate or eyelid margin
  - T2b Invades the tarsal plate or eyelid margin
  - T2c Involves full thickness of eyelid
- T3 Tumour > 20 mm in greatest dimension
  - T3a Not invading the tarsal plate or eyelid margin
  - T3b Invades tarsal plate or eyelid margin
  - T3c Involves full thickness of eyelid
- T4 Any eyelid tumour that invades adjacent ocular, or orbital, or facial structures
  - T4a Tumour invades ocular or intraorbital structures
  - T4b Tumour invades (or erodes through) the bony walls of orbit or extends to paranasal sinuses or invades the lacrimal sac/nasolacrimal duct or brain

N – Regional Lymph Nodes

- NX Regional lymph nodes cannot be assessed
- N0 No evidence of lymph node involvement
- N1 Metastasis in a single ipsilateral regional lymph node, 3 cm or less in greatest dimension
- N2 Metastasis in a single ipsilateral lymph node more than 3 cm in greatest dimension or in bilateral or contralateral lymph nodes

M – Distant Metastasis

- M0 No distant metastasis
- M1 Distant metastasis

pTNM Pathological Classification

The pT and pN categories correspond to the T and N categories.

pM – Distant Metastasis*

- pM1 Distant metastasis microscopically confirmed

Note

* pM0 and pMX are not valid categories.

Stage

Stage 0	Tis	N0	M0
Stage IA	T1	N0	M0
Stage IB	T2a	N0	M0
Stage IIA	T2b,T2c,T3	N0	M0
Stage IIB	T4	N0	M0
Stage IIIA	Any T	N1	M0
Stage IIIB	Any T	N2	M0
Stage IV	Any T	Any N	M1

TNM staging of melanoma of the conjunctiva

Malignant Melanoma of Conjunctiva

(ICD-O-3 C69.0)

Rules for Classification

The classification applies only to conjunctival malignant melanoma. There should be histological confirmation of the disease.

The following are the procedures for assessing T, N, and M categories:

T categories	Physical examination
N categories	Physical examination
M categories	Physical examination and imaging

Regional Lymph Nodes

The regional lymph nodes are the preauricular, submandibular, and cervical lymph nodes.

TNM Clinical Classification

T – Primary Tumour

TX Primary tumour cannot be assessed
T0 No evidence of primary tumour
Tis Melanoma confined to the conjunctival epithelium (in situ)[a]
T1 Melanoma of the bulbar conjunctiva
- T1a Tumour involves less than or equal to one quadrant[b]
- T1b Tumour involves more than one but less than or equal to two quadrants
- T1c Tumour involves more than two but less than or equal to three quadrants
- T1d Tumour involves more than three quadrants

T2 Malignant conjunctival melanoma of the non-bulbar conjunctiva involving palpebral, forniceal, and/or caruncular conjunctiva
- T2a Non-caruncular tumour involves less than or equal to one quadrant
- T2b Non-caruncular tumour involves more than one quadrant
- T2c Caruncular tumour involves less than or equal to one quadrant of conjunctiva
- T2d Caruncular tumour involves more than one quadrant of conjunctiva

T3 Tumour with local invasion into:
- T3a Globe
- T3b Eyelid
- T3c Orbit
- T3d Paranasal sinus, nasolacrimal duct, and/or lacrimal gland

T4 Tumour invades central nervous system

Notes

[a] Melanoma in situ (includes the term primary acquired melanosis) with atypia replacing greater than 75% of the normal epithelial thickness with cytological features of epithelial cells, including abundant cytoplasm, vesicular nuclei, or prominent nucleoli, and/or presence of intraepithelial nest of atypical cells.

[b] Quadrants are defined by clock hour, starting at the limbus (e.g. 6, 9, 12, 3) extending from the central cornea, to and beyond the eyelid margins. This will bisect the caruncle.

N – Regional Lymph Nodes

NX Regional lymph nodes cannot be assessed
N0 No regional lymph node metastasis
N1 Regional lymph node metastasis

M – Distant Metastasis

M0 No distant metastasis
M1 Distant metastasis

pTNM Pathological Classification

pT – Primary Tumour

pTX Primary tumour cannot be assessed
pT0 No evidence of primary tumour
pTis Melanoma confined to the conjunctival epithelium (in situ)*
pT1 Melanoma of the bulbar conjunctiva
- pT1a Tumour 2.0 mm or less in thickness with invasion of the substantia propria
- pT1b Tumour more than 2.0 mm in thickness with invasion of the substantia propria

pT2 Melanoma of the palpebral, forniceal or caruncular conjunctiva
- pT2a Tumour 2.0 mm or less in thickness with invasion of the substantia propria
- pT2b Tumour more than 2.0 mm in thickness with invasion of the substantia propria

pT3 Melanoma invades the eye, eyelid, nasolacrimal system or orbit
- pT3a Invades the globe
- pT3b Invadea the eyelid
- pT3c Invades the orbit
- pT3d Invades the paranasal sinus and/or nasolacrimal duct or lacrimal sac

pT4 Melanoma invades central nervous system

Note

* pTis Melanoma in situ (includes the term primary acquired melanosis) with atypia replacing greater than 75% of the normal epithelial thickness, with cytological features of epithelioid cells, including abundant cytoplasm, vesicular nuclei or prominent nucleoli, and/or presence of intraepithelial nests of atypical cells.

pN – Regional Lymph Nodes
The pN categories correspond to the N categories.

pM – Distant Metastasis*
pM1 Distant metastasis microscopically confirmed

Note
* pM0 and pMX are not valid categories.

G – Histopathological Grading
Histological grade represents the origin of the primary tumour.

GX	Origin cannot be assessed
G0	Primary acquired melanosis without cellular atypia
G1	Conjunctival nevus
G2	Primary acquired melanosis with cellular atypia (epithelial disease only)
G3	Primary acquired melanosis with epithelial cellular atypia and invasive melanoma
G4	De novo malignant melanoma

Stage
No stage is at present recommended.

TNM staging of melanoma of the uvea

Malignant Melanoma of Uvea

(ICD-O-3 C69.3,4)

Rules for Classification

There should be histological confirmation of the disease.

The following are the procedures for assessing T, N, and M categories:

T categories	Physical examination; additional methods such as fluorescein angiography and isotope examination may enhance the accuracy of appraisal
N categories	Physical examination
M categories	Examination and imaging

Regional Lymph Nodes

The regional lymph nodes are the preauricular, submandibular, and cervical nodes.

Anatomical Sites

1. Iris (C69.4)
2. Ciliary body (C69.4)
3. Choroid (C69.3)

TNM Clinical Classification

T – Primary Tumour

TX Primary tumour cannot be assessed

T0 No evidence of primary tumour

*Iris**

T1 Tumour limited to iris
- T1a not more than 3 clock hours in size
- T1b more than 3 clock hours in size
- T1c with secondary glaucoma

T2 Tumour confluent with or extending into the ciliary body, choroid, or both
- T2a Tumour confluent with or extending into the ciliary body without secondary glaucoma
- T2b Tumour confluent with or extending into the choroid without secondary glaucoma
- T2c Tumour confluent with or extending into the ciliary body and/or choroid with secondary glaucoma

T3 Tumour confluent with or extending into the ciliary body, choroid or both, with scleral extension

T4 Tumour with extrascleral extension
- T4a less than or equal to 5 mm in diameter
- T4b more than 5 mm in diameter

Note

* Iris melanomas originate from, and are predominantly located in, this region of the uvea. If less than half of the tumour volume is located within the iris, the tumour may have originated in the ciliary body and consideration should be given to classifying it accordingly.

Ciliary Body and Choroid

Primary ciliary body and choroidal melanomas are classified according to the four tumour size categories listed in Figure 1.[a,b]

Thickness (mm)	≤ 3.0	3.1–6.0	6.1–9.0	9.1–12.0	12.1–15.0	15.1–18.0	> 18
> 15					4	4	4
12.1–15.0				3	3	4	4
9.1–12.0		3	3	3	3	3	4
6.1–9.0	2	2	2	2	3	3	4
3.1–6.0	1	1	1	2	2	3	4
≤ 3.0	1	1	1	1	2	2	4

Largest basal diameter (mm)

Figure 1. Classification for ciliary body and choroid uveal melanoma based on thickness and diameter.

T1 Tumour size category 1
- T1a without ciliary body involvement and extraocular extension
- T1b with ciliary body involvement
- T1c without ciliary body involvement but with extraocular extension less than or equal to 5 mm in diameter
- T1d with ciliary body involvement and extraocular extension less than or equal to 5 mm in diameter

T2 Tumour size category 2
- T2a without ciliary body involvement and extraocular extension
- T2b with ciliary body involvement
- T2c without ciliary body involvement but with extraocular extension less than or equal to 5 mm in diameter
- T2d with ciliary body involvement and extraocular extension less than or equal to 5 mm in diameter

T3 Tumour size category 3
- T3a without ciliary body involvement and extraocular extension
- T3b with ciliary body involvement
- T3c without ciliary body involvement but with extraocular extension less than or equal to 5 mm in diameter
- T3d with ciliary body involvement and extraocular extension less than or equal to 5 mm in diameter

T4 Tumour size category 4
- T4a without ciliary body involvement and extraocular extension
- T4b with ciliary body involvement
- T4c without ciliary body involvement but with extraocular extension less than or equal to 5 mm in diameter
- T4d with ciliary body involvement and extraocular extension less than or equal to 5 mm in diameter
- T4e Any tumour size category with extraocular extension more than 5 mm in diameter

Notes

[a] In clinical practice, the largest tumour basal diameter may be estimated in optic disc diameters (dd, average: 1 dd = 1.5 mm). Tumour thickness may be estimated in dioptres (average: 2.5 dioptres = 1 mm). However, techniques such as ultrasonography and fundus photography are used to provide more accurate measurements. Ciliary body involvement can be evaluated by the slit-lamp, ophthalmoscopy, gonioscopy, and transillumination. However, high-frequency ultrasonography (ultrasound biomicroscopy) is used for more accurate assessment. Extension through the sclera is evaluated visually before and during surgery, and with ultrasonography, computed tomography, or magnetic resonance imaging.

[b] When histopathological measurements are recorded after fixation, tumour diameter and thickness may be underestimated because of tissue shrinkage.

N – Regional Lymph Nodes

NX Regional lymph nodes cannot be assessed
N0 No regional lymph node metastasis
N1 Regional lymph node metastasis

M – Distant Metastasis

M0 No distant metastasis
M1 Distant metastasis
- M1a Largest metastasis 3 cm or less in greatest dimension
- M1b Largest metastasis is larger than 3 cm in greatest dimension but not larger than 8 cm
- M1c Largest metastasis is larger than 8 cm in greatest dimension

pTNM Pathological Classification

The pT and pN categories correspond to the T and N categories.

pM – Distant Metastasis*

pM1 Distant metastasis microscopically confirmed

Note
* pM0 and pMX are not valid categories.

Stage*

Stage I	T1a	N0	M0
Stage IIA	T1b,T1c,T1d,T2a	N0	M0
Stage IIB	T2b,T3a	N0	M0
Stage IIIA	T2c,T2d	N0	M0
	T3b,T3c	N0	M0
	T4a	N0	M0
Stage IIIB	T3d	N0	M0
	T4b,T4c	N0	M0
Stage IIIC	T4d,T4e	N0	M0
Stage IV	Any T	N1	M0
	Any T	Any N	M1

Note
* The stage groups are for malignant melanoma of the choroid and ciliary body but not of the iris.

TNM staging of retinoblastoma

Retinoblastoma

(ICD-O-3 C69.2)

Rules for Classification

In bilateral cases, the eyes should be classified separately. The classification does not apply to complete spontaneous regression of the tumour. There should be histological confirmation of the disease in an enucleated eye.

The following are the procedures for assessing T, N, and M categories:

T categories	Physical examination and imaging
N categories	Physical examination
M categories	Physical examination and imaging; examination of bone marrow and cerebrospinal fluid may enhance the accuracy of appraisal

Regional Lymph Nodes

The regional lymph nodes are the preauricular, submandibular, and cervical lymph nodes.

TNM Clinical Classification

T – Primary Tumour

- TX Primary tumour cannot be assessed
- T0 No evidence of primary tumour
- T1 Tumour confined to the retina with subretinal fluid no more than 5 mm from the base of any tumour, without retinal detachment
  - T1a No tumour in either eye is greater than 3 mm in largest dimension or located closer than 1.5 mm to the optic nerve or fovea
  - T1b At least one tumour is greater than 3 mm in largest dimension or located closer than 1.5 mm to the optic nerve or fovea. No retinal detachment or subretinal fluid beyond 5 mm from the base of the tumour
- T2 Tumours with vitreous or subretinal seeding or retinal detachment
  - T2a Tumour with subretinal fluid more than 5 mm from the base of any tumour
  - T2b Tumour with vitreous and/or subretinal seeding
- T3 Severe intraocular disease
  - T3a Phthisis or prephthisis bulbi
  - T3b Invasion of: choroid, pars plana, ciliary body, lens, zonules, iris or anterior chamber
  - T3c Raised intraocular pressure with neovascularization and/or buphthalmos
  - T3d Hyphema and/or massive vitreous haemorrhage
  - T3e Aseptic orbital cellulitis
- T4 Extraocular tumour
  - T4a Invasion of optic nerve or orbital tissues
  - T4b Extraocular invasion with proptosis and/or orbital mass

N – Regional Lymph Nodes

- NX Regional lymph nodes cannot be assessed
- N0 No regional lymph node metastasis
- N1 Regional lymph node metastasis

M – Distant Metastasis

- M0 No distant metastasis
- M1 Distant metastasis
  - M1a Single or multiple metastasis to sites other than CNS or brain
  - M1b Metastasis to the CNS including brain

pTNM Pathological Classification

pT – Primary Tumour

- pTX Primary tumour cannot be assessed
- pT0 No evidence of primary tumour
- pT1 Tumour confined to eye with no optic nerve or choroidal invasion
- pT2 Tumour with intraocular invasion
  - pT2a Focal choroidal invasion and pre- or intralaminar invasion of the optic nerve head
  - pT2b Tumour invasion of stroma of iris and/or trabecular meshwork and/or Schlemm's canal
- pT3 Tumour with significant local invasion
  - pT3a Choroidal invasion larger than 3 mm in diameter or multiple foci of invasion totaling more than 3 mm or any full-thickness involvement
  - pT3b Retrolaminar invasion of optic nerve without invasion of transected end of optic nerve
  - pT3c Partial-thickness involvement of sclera within the inner two-thirds
  - pT3d Full-thickness invasion into outer third of the sclera and/or invasion into or around emissary channels
- pT4 Extraocular extension: Tumour invades optic nerve at transected end, in meningeal space around the optic nerve, full-thickness invasion of the sclera with invasion of the episclera, adipose tissue, extraocular muscle, bone, conjunctiva, or eyelid

The information presented here has been excerpted from the 2017 *TNM classification of malignant tumours*, eighth edition {414,3410}.
A help desk for specific questions about the TNM classification is available at https://www.uicc.org/tnm-help-desk.

pN – Regional Lymph Nodes
pNX Regional lymph nodes cannot be assessed
pN0 No regional lymph node involvement
pN1 Regional lymph node involvement

pM – Distant Metastasis
pM0 No distant metastasis
pM1 Distant metastasis
- pM1a Single or multiple metastasis to sites other than CNS
- pM1b Metastasis to CNS parenchyma or cerebrospinal fluid

Clinical Stage

Stage I	T1,T2,T3	N0	M0
Stage II	T4a	N0	M0
Stage III	T4b	N0	M0
	Any T	N1	M0
Stage IV	Any T	Any N	M1

Pathological Stage

Stage I	T1,T2,T3	N0	M0
Stage II	T4	N0	M0
Stage III	Any T	N1	M0
Stage IV	Any T	Any N	M1

TNM staging of sarcoma of the orbit

Sarcoma of Orbit

(ICD-O-3 C69.6)

Rules for Classification

The classification applies to sarcomas of soft tissue and bone. There should be histological confirmation of the disease and division of cases by histological type.

The following are the procedures for assessing T, N, and M categories:

T categories	Physical examination and imaging
N categories	Physical examination
M categories	Physical examination and imaging

Regional Lymph Nodes

The regional lymph nodes are the preauricular, submandibular, and cervical lymph nodes.

TNM Clinical Classification

T – Primary Tumour

- TX Primary tumour cannot be assessed
- T0 No evidence of primary tumour
- T1 Tumour 20 mm or less in greatest dimension
- T2 Tumour more than 20 mm in greatest dimension without invasion of globe or bony wall
- T3 Tumour of any size with invasion of orbital tissues and/or bony walls
- T4 Tumour invades globe or periorbital structure, such as eyelids, temporal fossa, nasal cavity and paranasal sinuses, and/or central nervous system

N – Regional Lymph Nodes

- NX Regional lymph nodes cannot be assessed
- N0 No regional lymph node metastasis
- N1 Regional lymph node metastasis

M – Distant Metastasis

- M0 No distant metastasis
- M1 Distant metastasis

pTNM Pathological Classification

The pT and pN categories correspond to the T and N categories.

pM – Distant Metastasis*

- pM1 Distant metastasis microscopically confirmed

Note

* pM0 and pMX are not valid categories.

Stage

No stage is at present recommended.

The information presented here has been excerpted from the 2017 *TNM classification of malignant tumours*, eighth edition {414,3410}. © 2017 UICC.
A help desk for specific questions about the TNM classification is available at https://www.uicc.org/tnm-help-desk.

TNM staging of carcinoma of the lacrimal gland

Carcinoma of Lacrimal Gland

(ICD-O-3 C69.5)

Rules for Classification

There should be histological confirmation of the disease and division of cases by histological type.

The following are the procedures for assessing T, N, and M categories:

T categories	Physical examination and imaging
N categories	Physical examination
M categories	Physical examination and imaging

Regional Lymph Nodes

The regional lymph nodes are the preauricular, submandibular, and cervical lymph nodes.

TNM Clinical Classification

T – Primary Tumour

TX Primary tumour cannot be assessed
T0 No evidence of primary tumour
T1 Tumour 2 cm or less in greatest dimension, with or without extraglandular extension into the orbital soft tissue
- T1a No periosteal or bone involvement
- T1b Periosteal involvement without bone involvement
- T1c Bone involvement

T2 Tumour more than 2 cm but not more than 4 cm in greatest dimension
- T2a No periosteal or bone involvement
- T2b Periosteal involvement without bone involvement
- T2c Bone involvement

T3 Tumour more than 4 cm or with extraglandular extension into orbital soft tissue, including optic nerve, or globe
- T3a No periosteal or bone involvement
- T3b Periosteal involvement without bone involvement
- T3c Bone involvement

T4 Tumour invades adjacent structures (sinuses, temporal fossa, pterygoid fossa, superior orbital fissure, cavernous sinus, and/or brain)
- T4a No more than 2 cm in greatest dimension
- T4b More than 2 cm but no more than 4 cm in greatest dimension
- T4c More than 4 cm in greatest dimension

N – Regional Lymph Nodes

NX Regional lymph nodes cannot be assessed
N0 No regional lymph node metastasis
N1 Regional lymph node metastasis

M – Distant Metastasis

M0 No distant metastasis
M1 Distant metastasis

pTNM Pathological Classification

The pT and pN categories correspond to the T and N categories.

pM – Distant Metastasis*

pM1 Distant metastasis microscopically confirmed

Note
* pM0 and pMX are not valid categories.

Stage

No stage is at present recommended.

The information presented here has been excerpted from the 2017 *TNM classification of malignant tumours*, eighth edition {414,3410}
A help desk for specific questions about the TNM classification is available at https://www.uicc.org/tnm-help-desk.

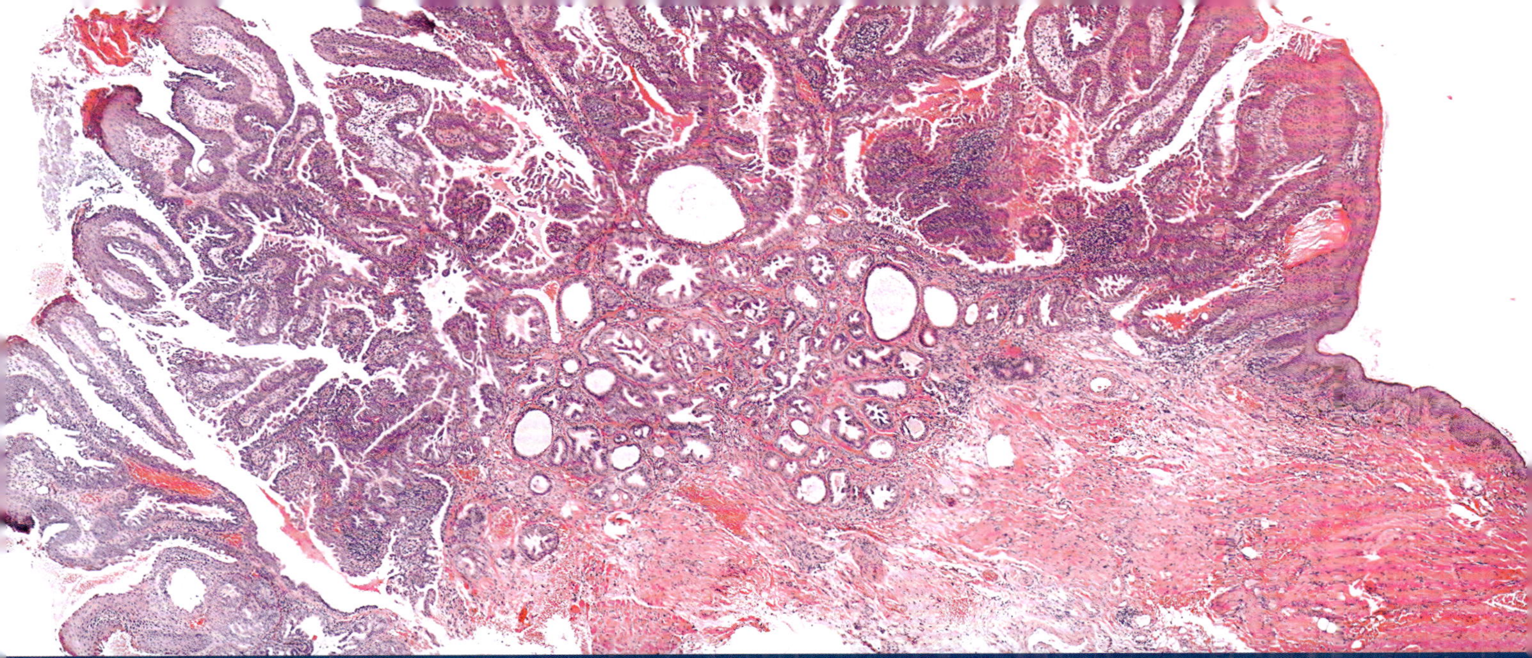

1

Introduction to eye and orbit tumours

Edited by: White VA

Introduction to eye and orbit tumours

Grossniklaus HE
Coupland SE
Eberhart CG
Esmaeli B
Heegaard S
Jager MJ
Kivelä T
Milman T
Mudhar HS
Rodríguez-Reyes AA
Vemuganti GK
Verdijk RM

Ophthalmic pathology has its roots in gross inspection of diseased ocular tissues, including when Morgagni described the gross appearance of cataracts in 1761 {1178}. Individuals have been important in advancing the field, including James Wardrop, a Scottish surgeon who described in his *Morbid anatomy of the human eye* the clinical and gross appearance of retinoblastoma, which he called "fungus haematodes". Wardrop also described the first well-documented case of metastatic uveal melanoma {1730}. A confluence of technologies, including the invention of the microscope and ophthalmoscope, and Virchow's concept of cellular pathology, enabled clinicopathological correlation of ophthalmic disease, most notably, ocular tumours. An example of this was Flexner and Wintersteiner's observation of the presence of cellular rosettes in retinoblastoma. There were many individuals who advanced the field in the 1900s, most of whom were ophthalmologists. In the mid-century, several pathologists focused their practices on ophthalmic pathology. There continued to be significant input from ophthalmology-trained ophthalmic pathologists into the interpretation of ocular and ocular adnexal tumours.

The original WHO *Histological typing of tumours of the eye and its adnexa* was published in 1980. There was a set of Kodachromes that accompanied this book, which were widely used as teaching materials. Eighteen years later, in 1998, the second edition was published. There was no third edition, and it was not until 2018 that the fourth edition was published, some 20 years after the second edition. That volume, the last in the fourth edition of the WHO Classification of Tumours series (the WHO Blue Books), brought the eye tumours volume into alignment with other volumes in the series. As in the past, clinicopathological correlation between ophthalmologists and pathologists enhanced interpretation of ocular tumour specimens.

In this, the fifth edition, we have added sections on adnexal tumours and a chapter on orbital tumours, which were not present in the fourth edition, and we have advanced the description, definition, and understanding of tumours of the eye and orbit even further. We have amalgamated sections on haematolymphoid tumours, soft tissue and bone tumours, metastases, and genetic tumour syndromes, following the format of other volumes of the fifth edition. This volume is comprehensive, accounting for almost all the tumours of the eye and ocular adnexa that an ocular oncologist and/or ophthalmic pathologist might encounter.

Specific changes and additions include:

- tumours of the eyelid
- tumours of the orbit
- cross referencing to other volumes in the WHO Classification of Tumours series for non–site-specific details.

Where possible, we have classified vascular tumours and malformations that involve the eye and its adnexa according to terminology proposed in 2014 by the International Society for the Study of Vascular Anomalies (ISSVA).

This volume was completed with the tireless efforts of many contributors and the staff at the International Agency for Research on Cancer (IARC) as we continue to strive towards our understanding of this important, and often unique, group of tumours.

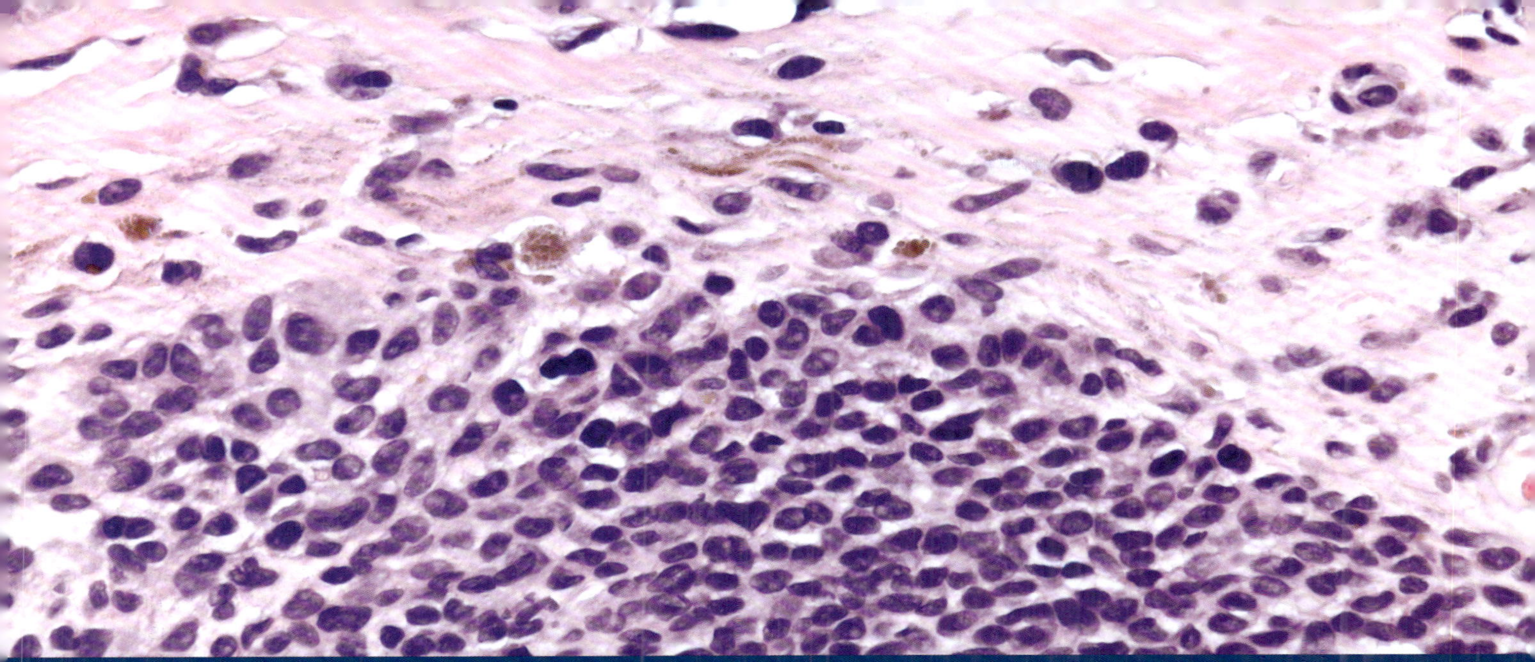

2

Tumours of the conjunctiva and caruncle

Edited by: Coupland SE, Eberhart CG, Grossniklaus HE, Milman T, Mudhar HS

Tumours of the conjunctiva and caruncle: Introduction

Coupland SE
Eberhart CG
Mudhar HS

The fifth edition of the classification of tumours of the conjunctiva and caruncle very much follows the fourth edition, with only minor organizational changes. The conjunctiva, together with the caruncle (its skin-like appendage located at the inner canthus of the eyelids), forms a protective layer that covers the anterior segment of the eye and the inner aspect of the eyelids. The conjunctiva is clinically divided into limbal, bulbar, forniceal, and palpebral parts. The epithelium is non-keratinizing and stratified columnar in type, and it harbours a population of basal melanocytes and superficial mucus-secreting goblet cells that are most abundant nasally and in crypt-like infoldings in the conjunctival fornices. The conjunctival stroma is fibrovascular and contains inflammatory cells, including lymphocytes that can form follicles and germinal centres in the fornices; it also has lymphatics and contains accessory lacrimal glands.

The chapter starts with a discussion of tumour-like lesions, including cysts, reactive epithelial lesions, and choristomas. Pseudoglandular and pseudoepitheliomatous hyperplasia are now grouped under reactive epithelial hyperplasia. Tumours more commonly found in the eyelids, such as phakomatous choristoma, keratoacanthoma, and sebaceous carcinoma, are now found under the chapter on tumours of the eyelid, which is new to this volume. Non-neoplastic epithelial conjunctival masses include epithelial inclusion cysts, as well as degenerative or inflammatory lesions, such as pingueculae, pterygia, papillary and follicular conjunctivitis, reactive epithelial hyperplasia, and various choristomas (most commonly dermoids and dermolipoma). Epithelial tumours include benign squamous papillomas and hereditary benign intraepithelial dyskeratosis, as well as premalignant and malignant conjunctival squamous intraepithelial neoplasia, squamous cell carcinoma (SCC), and adenosquamous carcinoma. New additions to the fifth edition include the inclusion of spindle SCC and of SCC with mucinous differentiation as morphological patterns within the broader group of SCCs at this site.

Benign melanocytic conjunctival tumours include benign epithelial melanosis; junctional, compound, and subepithelial conjunctival naevi; inflamed juvenile conjunctival naevus; blue naevus of the conjunctiva; and combined naevus. Spitz naevus, exceedingly rare in the conjunctiva, has moved to the new chapter on tumours of the eyelid. Premalignant and malignant melanocytic conjunctival tumours include conjunctival melanocytic intraepithelial lesions, the nomenclature for which continues to evolve, and conjunctival melanoma. A new entity in the fifth-edition volume is WNT-activated deep penetrating / plexiform melanocytoma (naevus). Use of the term "melanocytoma" has caused some discussion, but its use in the *Skin tumours* volume to identify lesions genetically intermediate between naevus and melanoma was put forward in the fourth edition and is now established. WNT-activated deep penetrating / plexiform melanocytoma (naevus) almost always presents in the conjunctiva as a combined naevus. Finally, our understanding of conjunctival melanocytic intraepithelial lesions as a spectrum from benign to preinvasive melanoma continues to advance, and the diagnostic matrix is tabulated to make this easier to use in diagnostic practice.

This chapter includes conjunctival oncocytoma, which generally arises in the accessory lacrimal glands of the caruncle. Lanugo hairs, sebaceous glands, sweat glands, and striated muscle are found only in the caruncle. Adnexal tumours, which can arise from these structures, are described primarily in the chapter on eyelids. Similarly, haematolymphoid and soft tissue tumours, which can arise in the conjunctiva and caruncle, are covered in other chapters of this volume.

Epithelial conjunctival inclusion cyst

Auw-Haedrich C
Iacob CE
Margo C

Definition
Epithelial conjunctival inclusion cysts, lined by conjunctival or caruncle-type epithelium, occur within the substantia propria of the conjunctiva and caruncle.

ICD-O coding
None

ICD-11 coding
9A61.6 Conjunctival cysts or argyrosis

Related terminology
Acceptable: conjunctival epithelial cyst.

Subtype(s)
None

Localization
Epithelial inclusion cysts reside within the substantia propria of mostly non-limbal bulbar conjunctiva or caruncle.

Clinical features
Cysts are transparent to cloudy, mostly compressible, and mobile or tethered to surrounding structures.

Epidemiology
Epithelial inclusion cysts are diagnosed at any age. There is no known sex predilection.

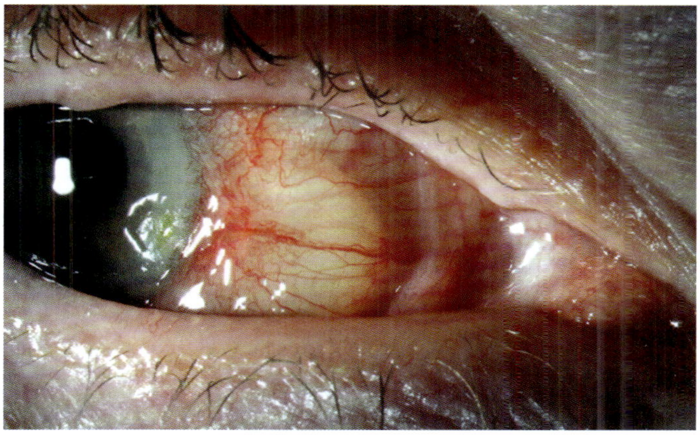

Fig. 2.01 Bulbar conjunctival cyst. A cyst between the plica semilunaris and nasal limbus with adjacent corneal dellen due to lubrication disturbance.

Etiology
Congenital inclusion cysts arise from heterotopic rests of epithelium. Acquired cysts originate from epithelial implantation after either accidental trauma or surgery {1549}. Symptoms or signs can arise years after the initiating event {1841}

Pathogenesis
Epithelial conjunctival inclusion cysts may be congenital arise spontaneously, or arise after surgical or accidental trauma {3009}.

Macroscopic appearance
Thin-walled whitish cystic structure

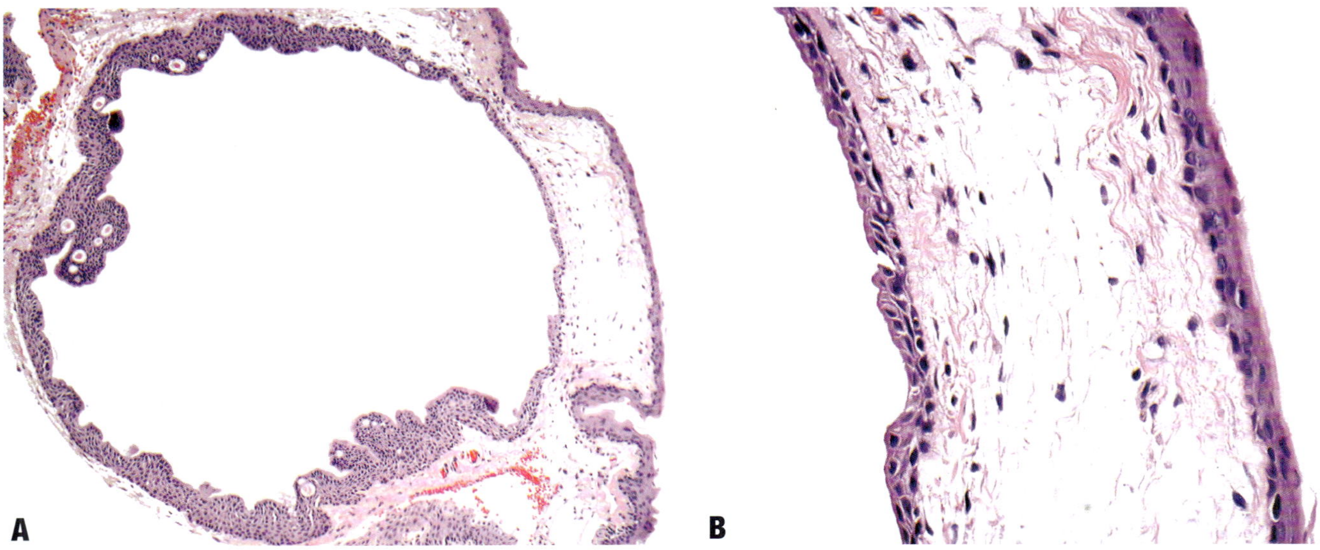

Fig. 2.02 Epithelial conjunctival inclusion cyst. **A** The normal overlying conjunctival epithelium is on the right. **B** The cyst epithelium is on the left and is composed of nonkeratinizing squamous epithelium similar in appearance to the surface conjunctival epithelium on the right.

Histopathology

Conjunctival inclusion cysts are lined by conjunctival-type, nonkeratinizing stratified squamous epithelium with or without goblet cells. The cavity can contain proteinaceous material and be surrounded by a band of stromal fibrosis and inflammation. A traumatic implantation cyst will reflect the type of surface epithelium implanted in the stroma. The caruncle is a transition zone of mucous membrane and skin and therefore can give rise to epidermal inclusion cysts, lined by skin-type epidermis or conjunctival-type epithelium {2009,3020}.

Differential diagnosis

For the conjunctiva, the differential diagnosis includes cystic crypts of Henle, dilated lymphatics (lymphangiectasia), and non–epithelial-lined lesions that can form from ocular fistulae (e.g. filtration blebs). For the caruncle, the differential diagnosis includes infundibular cyst, steatocystoma, and cystic oncocytoma {2009,3010}.

Cytology

Not applicable

Diagnostic molecular pathology

Not applicable

Essential and desirable diagnostic criteria

Essential: a cyst in the substantia propria, lined by benign conjunctival-type epithelium or benign caruncle-type epithelium.

Staging

Not applicable

Prognosis and prediction

Complete excision is curative.

Reactive epithelial hyperplasia of the conjunctiva

Margo C
Auw-Haedrich C

Definition
Reactive epithelial hyperplasia is a reactive, benign, non-neoplastic epithelial proliferation, in response to an irritating stimulus.

ICD-O coding
None

ICD-11 coding
9A6Y Other specified disorders of conjunctiva

Related terminology
Acceptable: pseudoepitheliomatous hyperplasia; pseudoadenomatous hyperplasia.
Not recommended: pseudocarcinomatous hyperplasia.

Subtype(s)
None

Localization
Pseudoepitheliomatous hyperplasia tends to affect (limbal) bulbar conjunctiva. Pseudoglandular hyperplasia preferentially occurs in the fornix and tarsal conjunctiva.

Clinical features
Pseudoepitheliomatous hyperplasia may appear as a fleshy to white mass, minimally raised or thickened {941}. Pseudoglandular hyperplasia appears as a fleshy, poorly defined mass {2072} and shares clinical features with ocular surface neoplasia.

Epidemiology
Lesions are uncommon; they have been reported in children and adults of both sexes.

Etiology
In many cases there is no known association. These lesions have been associated with granular cell tumour, blastomycosis, thermal burns, epithelial (limbal) cell transplantation, contact lens use, chemical exposure (e.g. iododerma), and previous surgery {2072,2068,962,941,1704,2919}.

Pathogenesis
Lesions arise as a result of nonspecific reactive changes in response to diverse presumed causal associations.

Macroscopic appearance
See *Clinical features*, above.

Histopathology
Pseudoepitheliomatous hyperplasia consists of acanthotic epithelium with normal keratinocyte maturation. Squamous metaplasia may be present with surface keratinization, and the superficial epithelial cells can contain keratohyaline granules. Pseudoglandular hyperplasia is composed of prominent pseudoglands of Henle, lined with stratified squamous epithelium with goblet cells. Mucin often fills the lumina of the pseudoglands, and lamellar concretions are sometimes noted.

The histological differential diagnosis for pseudoepitheliomatous hyperplasia includes papilloma, inverted papilloma, and conjunctival squamous intraepithelial neoplasia. Normal maturation of keratinocytes is lost in epithelial dysplasia, and keratinocytes display pleomorphic nuclei with variable amounts of cytoplasm and mitotic activity.

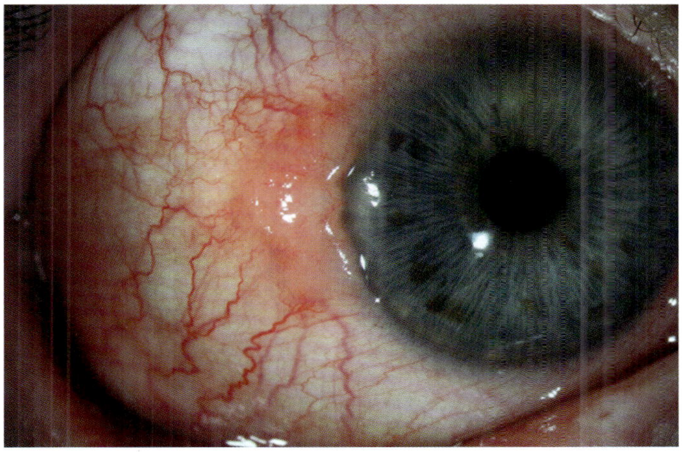

Fig. 2.03 Pseudoepitheliomatous hyperplasia. A fleshy, gelatinous mass is present from the 8 o'clock to 10 o'clock limbus, associated with vascular injection.

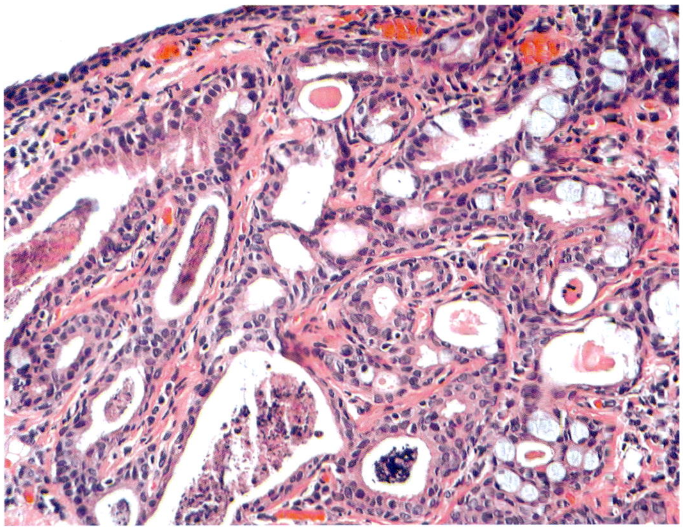

Fig. 2.04 Pseudoadenomatous hyperplasia. Hyperplastic pseudoglands of Henle without cytological atypia are seen. Note the absence of stromal desmoplasia.

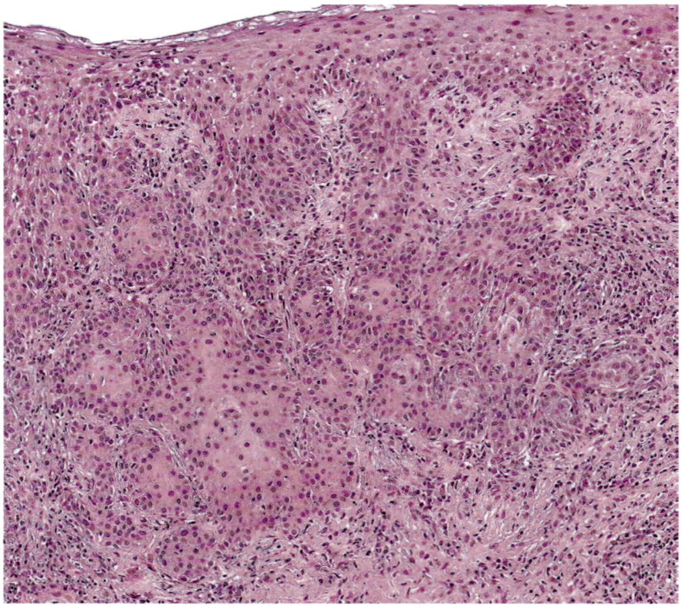

Fig. 2.05 Pseudoepitheliomatous hyperplasia. Biopsy from a limbal mass displays squamous epithelium proliferating deeply into the substantia propria. There is no cellular atypia. A dense lymphocytic infiltrate is present.

The histological differential diagnosis for pseudoglandular hyperplasia is squamous cell carcinoma with mucinous differentiation (previously known as mucoepidermoid carcinoma). This will be more cellular and the keratinocytes will display nuclear atypia with focal intracytoplasmic mucin and mitotic activity.

Cytology

Smears show benign squamous epithelium.

Diagnostic molecular pathology

There are no known genetic abnormalities.

Essential and desirable diagnostic criteria

Essential: hyperplastic epithelium with benign cytology.
Desirable: identification of an underlying causal association.

Staging

Not applicable

Prognosis and prediction

These are benign/reactive processes with a good prognosis. There are no reports about recurrences after incomplete removal or eradication of the underlying cause.

Papillary and follicular conjunctivitis

Iacob CE
Auw-Haedrich C
Margo C

Definition

Papillary conjunctivitis (PC) is an inflammatory reaction of the conjunctiva characterized by the presence of papillae, composed of oedematous, inflamed fibrovascular stromal cores, covered in non-dysplastic epithelium of variable thickness, manifesting clinically as dome-shaped or flat-topped papillae with a vascular core.

Follicular conjunctivitis (FC) is an inflammatory reaction of the conjunctiva characterized histologically by reactive lymphoid aggregates in the conjunctival substantia propria, manifesting clinically as multiple discrete, rounded elevations of the conjunctiva, with an avascular core.

ICD-O coding

None

ICD-11 coding

9A60.0 Papillary conjunctivitis
9A60.1 Follicular conjunctivitis

Related terminology

Papillary conjunctivitis

Acceptable: vernal keratoconjunctivitis; atopic keratoconjunctivitis; giant papillary conjunctivitis.

Follicular conjunctivitis

Acceptable: viral conjunctivitis; inclusion conjunctivitis.

Subtype(s)

Papillary conjunctivitis

Acute papillary conjunctivitis; chronic papillary conjunctivitis; giant papillary conjunctivitis

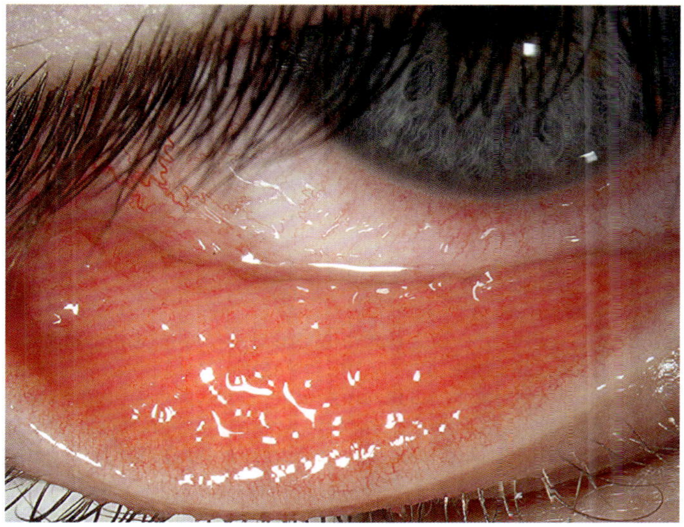

Fig. 2.06 Follicular conjunctivitis. Clinical image showing numerous follicles in the lower tarsal conjunctiva.

Follicular conjunctivitis

Acute follicular conjunctivitis; chronic follicular conjunctivitis

Localization

PC usually affects the upper tarsal conjunctiva but also the limbal conjunctiva in vernal keratoconjunctivitis {3494,1658,219, 3697,3458}.

FC usually involves the palpebral, forniceal, and bulbar conjunctiva and rarely the limbal conjunctiva {219,3697,3458}

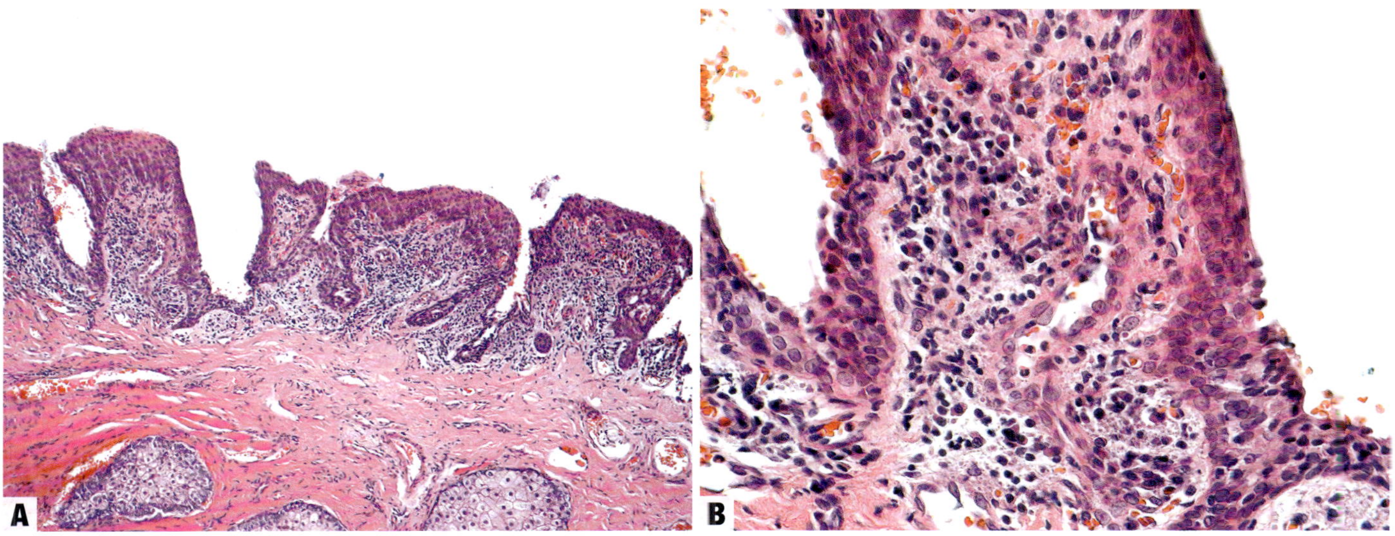

Fig. 2.07 Papillary conjunctivitis. **A** Flat-topped papillae, with fibrovascular cores, containing inflammatory cells. **B** A vessel within the core of a papilla, surrounded by stromal chronic inflammatory cells.

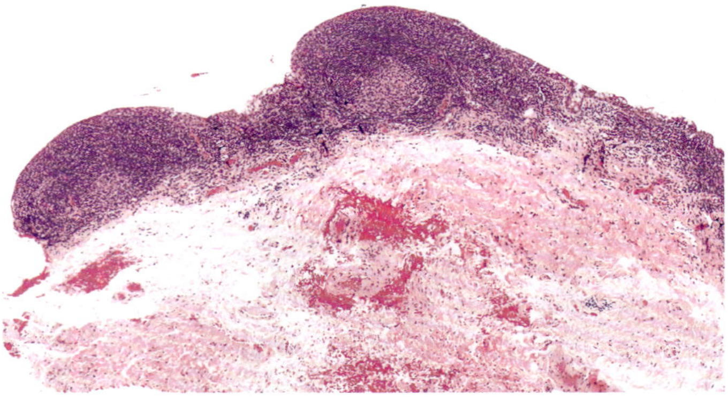

Fig. 2.08 Follicular conjunctivitis. The conjunctival substantia propria contains reactive lymphoid aggregates with lymphoid follicles causing dome-like elevation of the overlying epithelial surface.

Clinical features

PC consists of numerous dome-shaped or flat-topped papillae with a vascular core, mainly on the upper tarsal conjunctiva. The diameter of the papillae is variable. Subtypes are based on clinical criteria {222} and comprise acute papillary conjunctivitis, chronic papillary conjunctivitis, and giant papillary conjunctivitis (GPC, which is a subtype of chronic papillary conjunctivitis). In GPC, papillae can be ≥ 1 mm. Associated discharge can be purulent, mucopurulent, watery, or stringy, depending on the etiology. Associated clinical features in GPC include corneal shield ulcers, perilimbal Horner–Trantas dots (consisting of degenerate epithelial cells and eosinophils), and conjunctival scarring {1822,1658,219,3458}.

In FC, follicles are discrete hemispherical elevations of the conjunctiva. They are pink or white/yellow and have no vascular core. They are usually 0.5–2 mm in diameter and are conspicuous on the superior tarsal and inferior forniceal conjunctiva. Associated exudates can be watery or mucopurulent and can be associated with hyperaemia, photophobia, and a foreign body sensation. Depending on etiology, associated clinical features include corneal subepithelial infiltrates and corneal/conjunctival scarring {219,3458}. A clinical differential diagnosis of FC includes sarcoid granulomas that can present with multiple elevated nodules on the conjunctival surface {618}. Clinically defined subtypes are acute follicular conjunctivitis and chronic follicular conjunctivitis.

Epidemiology

PC in association with allergy occurs most often in children, with a male predominance, in warm and dry regions. The prevalence in Europe is estimated to be as high as 1.2–12.6 cases per 10 000 persons, in contrast to 2–37% in Africa {75}. Within the group of contact lens wearers, the reported prevalence of GPC varies widely between 1.5% and 47.5%, with frequency associated with several main variables. The prevalence of GPC tends to decrease with the use of rigid versus soft lenses and the availability of single-use versus non-disposable lenses {1658}.

For FC, the epidemiology varies according to etiology (e.g. chlamydia, virus, toxin, etc.) {3697}.

Etiology

Acute PC: The main cause is bacteria (*Staphylococcus aureus*, *Haemophilus influenzae*, streptococci, *Neisseria gonorrhoeae*, *Neisseria meningitidis*) {219,1137}.

Chronic PC: This can be caused by lacrimal sac infection, superior limbic keratoconjunctivitis {3201}, floppy eyelid syndrome {737,2827}, foreign bodies {2387,1533,1167}, mucus-fishing syndrome {2134}, keratoconjunctivitis sicca {2023}, and blepharoconjunctivitis {942}. GPC {1658} is usually a component of vernal and atopic keratoconjunctivitis {1628}, or a complication of exposure to contact lenses {3194,87}, ocular prostheses, or periocular devices (e.g. suture, scleral buckle, glaucoma exoplants) {1658}.

Acute FC: The main causes are viruses. These include the adenovirus {1534}, herpesvirus {3407}, picornavirus {2845,501}, orthomyxovirus {1970,690}, and togavirus families {700}; SARS-CoV-2 {562,339,2916,2362}; and the poxvirus family {2886}. It can also be caused by a few bacteria, for example *Chlamydia* (inclusion conjunctivitis) {219,3458}.

Chronic FC: The main causes include *Chlamydia trachomatis* (manifesting as trachoma or inclusion conjunctivitis based on serovars) {3161,2549,219,3458}, *Moraxella* {1827}, molluscum contagiosum {2886}, *Borrelia* (Lyme disease) {3728}, and toxic causes (eye make-up and therapeutic eye drops [antiviral, antiglaucoma, and cycloplegic agents]) {3458}.

Pathogenesis

The pathogenesis is related to the etiology and involves cellular and humoral responses to infectious agents and exposure to foreign material. Inflammatory responses are also subject to variables within the host's immune apparatus {3458,219,3697}.

Macroscopic appearance

See *Clinical features*.

Histopathology

PC: The conjunctiva forms exophytic papillae that can be dome shaped or flat topped. A papilla is made up of oedematous conjunctival stroma containing capillary-sized vessels perpendicular to the papillae, covered in conjunctival epithelium that can exhibit erosion. The stroma usually contains a variety of inflammatory cell types that can include lymphocytes, plasma cells, eosinophils, and mast cells {1665}.

FC: The conjunctival substantia propria contains reactive lymphoid aggregates with lymphoid follicles causing dome-like elevation of the overlying epithelial surface. The main histological differential diagnosis for FC includes reactive lymphoid hyperplasia (which clinically presents as a mass lesion rather than multiple follicles) and various types of lymphoma that can clinically present with a follicular conjunctivitis picture. These include follicular lymphoma {843,1824,517}, extranodal marginal zone lymphoma {1556,63,3698}, and mantle cell lymphoma {143}.

Cytology

Not relevant

Diagnostic molecular pathology
If the histology reveals a suspected lymphoma, the appropriate molecular investigations can be conducted (see *Extranodal marginal zone lymphoma*, p. 335; *Follicular lymphoma*, p. 338; and *Mantle cell lymphoma*, p. 341).

Essential and desirable diagnostic criteria
Papillary conjunctivitis
Essential: papillae that can be dome shaped or flat topped; oedematous conjunctival stroma containing capillary-sized vessels perpendicular to the papillae, covered in hyperplastic conjunctival epithelium and containing inflammatory cells.

Desirable: knowledge of the clinical setting to permit an accurate clinicopathological categorization.

Follicular conjunctivitis
Essential: reactive lymphoid aggregates with lymphoid follicles in the substantia propria causing dome-like elevation of the overlying conjunctival surface.

Desirable: knowledge of the clinical setting to permit an accurate clinicopathological categorization.

Staging
Not relevant

Prognosis and prediction
The prognosis is dependent on the elimination of the inciting agent. The outcomes in PC and FC are etiology dependent {3458,219,3697}. Keratoconjunctivitis sicca occurs after resolution of conjunctivitis in some cases, possibly owing to damage of goblet cells. Accompanying keratitis with subsequent subepithelial scars in adenovirus-associated conjunctivitis might cause longstanding visual deterioration {365}

Pterygium and pinguecula

Iacob CE
Auw-Haedrich C
Margo C

Definition
Pterygium and pinguecula are non-neoplastic, benign, degenerative, fibrovascular lesions of the bulbar conjunctiva, histologically characterized by actinic, elastotic degeneration of the substantia propria. Both arise within the interpalpebral zone, with pinguecula limited to the paralimbal conjunctiva, whereas pterygium involves the cornea as well.

ICD-O coding
None

ICD-11 coding
9A61.1 Pterygium
9A61.0 Pingueculae

Related terminology
None

Subtype(s)
None

Localization
Pinguecula is limited to the limbal bulbar conjunctiva within the interpalpebral zone. Pterygium arises within the interpalpebral zone and involves the bulbar and limbal conjunctiva and peripheral cornea, and it has a nasal predilection.

Clinical features
Pinguecula is usually located at the interpalpebral paralimbal conjunctiva, within the 3 o'clock to 9 o'clock meridian. It is often bilateral. A pinguecula is a discrete elevated nodule, sometimes wedge shaped, that has a greyish, white, or yellow mottled colour {3164}. It stops abruptly at the limbal conjunctiva and is not fixed to the underlying sclera. It usually presents as a cosmetic complaint. If inflamed (pingueculitis), it can cause ocular irritation symptoms {3164}.

Pterygium appears as a wing-like, white, fibrovascular, slightly raised plaque, extending from the conjunctiva to the cornea. A corneal Stocker iron line may be seen anterior to the leading edge. Clinical symptoms reflect the severity of the process and can include irritation, foreign body sensation, photophobia, and decreased vision due to the degradation of the refractive surface. Complications include astigmatism {2935,1242}, squamous intraepithelial neoplasia (the rate of which ranges from 1% to 11% depending on geography) {3435}, and the development of melanocytic proliferations {2535,306}.

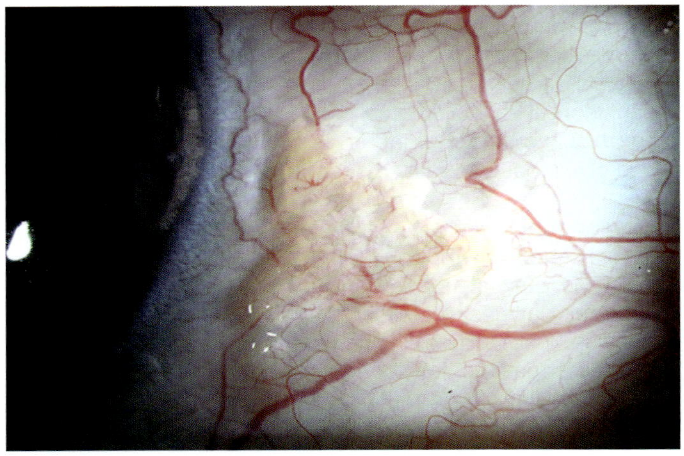

Fig. 2.09 Pinguecula. A paralimbal, yellow, wedge-shaped pinguecula is seen. The incidental corneal lesion is a limbal girdle of Vogt.

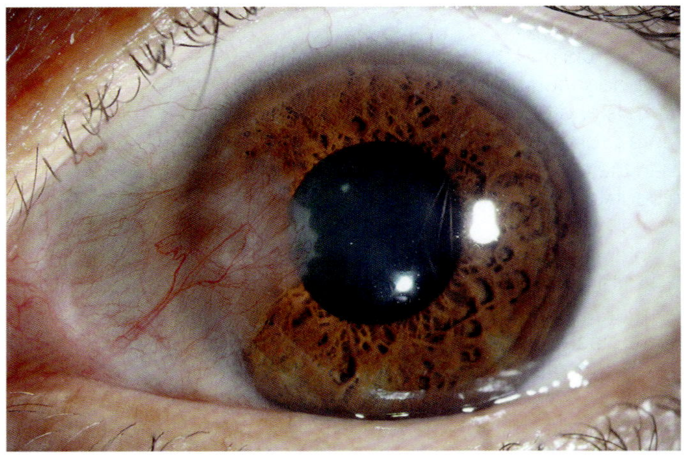

Fig. 2.10 Pterygium. Left-sided nasal pterygium encroaching on the visual axis.

Epidemiology
The prevalence of pterygium varies according to the population studied, with a range of 1–33% {2935,2010,459,3588,1019, 2016}. A meta-analysis determined the pooled prevalence to be 10% {1968}. It is most common in the tropics, within the so-called pterygium belt, where the incidence is as high as 30% {3122}. In temperate climates, the estimated incidence is 2% {2912}. Risk factors include older age {2010,459}, male sex {3270,2128}, outdoor exposure {3503,2010}, rural settings {2128}, darker skin complexion {2010}, and smoking {3588}.

Etiology
The following risk factors are associated with pingueculae and pterygia: ultraviolet A (UVA) and ultraviolet B (UVB) radiation {2265,3299}; wind, dust, and sand {667}; human papillomaviruses and herpesviruses {1063,512}; genetic predisposition {160}; and immunological {2556} and inflammatory conditions {1339}. Numerous epidemiological studies have confirmed the strong association between UVA and UVB radiation and pterygium development {3122}, especially data from the pterygium

belt. Evidence for an association with HPV16 and HPV18 {799} and with the herpes simplex virus {2935} is less robust.

Pathogenesis

The nasal proclivity for pterygium has been explained by the peripheral light focusing effect. This refers to UV light crossing through the temporal cornea, with damage to the stem cells in the nasal cornea {666}. Another hypothesis favours the temporal to nasal lacrimal flow, which refers to the concentration of dust and irritating particles from the ocular surface in the nasal aspect, locally triggering cytokine release, a causative factor for pterygium {1707}. The precise molecular pathogenesis of pterygium remains uncertain, but the progression and the recurrence in pterygium seem to have epithelial–mesenchymal transition as a common ground. A variety of studies have reported different pathways and master regulators related to epithelial–mesenchymal transition, including NOTCH, p53, WNT/β-catenin, inflammatory mediators, TGF-β, and EGFR (HER1). In addition, environmental factors like UV radiation and certain viruses have been also linked to epithelial–mesenchymal transition {2135, 1290}. As a result, mutagenicity, construction of a new vascular network, and remodelling of the extracellular mesenchymal matrix perpetuate the development of pterygium {3160}.

Macroscopic appearance

See *Clinical features*, above.

Histopathology

Pinguecula and pterygium are characterized by basophilic elastotic degeneration of the substantia propria accompanied by fibrosis and telangiectatic vessels. The elastotic degeneration is more prominent in the conjunctival portion of a pterygium rather than the corneal portion. Other stromal features include elastoid globules, dystrophic calcification, and chronic inflammation. Sometimes the latter manifests as actinic granuloma, showing granulomatous inflammation with giant cells centred on elastotic fibres {2028}. The overlying squamous epithelium can be normal or show acanthosis, squamous metaplasia, goblet cell hyperplasia, dyskeratosis, and increased melanin production {2935}. In pterygium, the peripheral Bowman layer is effaced with associated superficial corneal fibrosis. In rare cases, squamous intraepithelial neoplasia {3435} and melanocytic proliferations may be present {306,2535}.

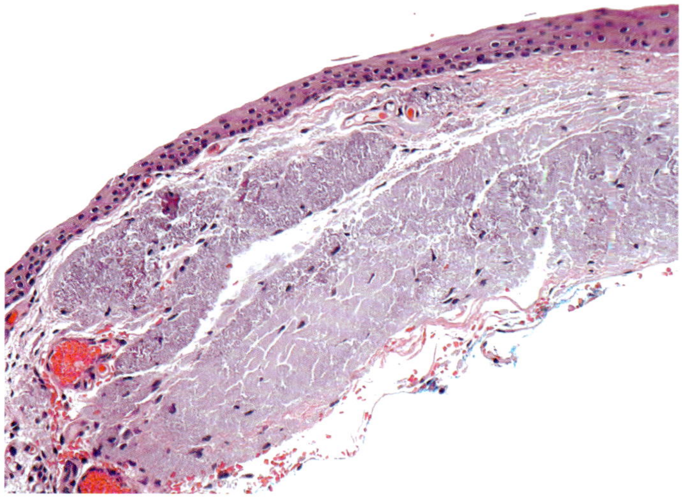

Fig. 2.11 Pterygium. There is basophilic elastotic degeneration of the substantia propria. Telangiectatic vessels are seen at the lower left.

Cytology

Exfoliative or imprint cytology from limbal lesions can be used to detect squamous epithelial dysplasia or malignancy.

Diagnostic molecular pathology

Not relevant

Essential and desirable diagnostic criteria

Essential: interpalpebral paralimbal conjunctiva (pinguecula); corneal involvement in pterygium; variable actinic elastotic degeneration in conjunctival substantia propria covered by non-dysplastic squamous epithelium.

Staging

Not relevant

Prognosis and prediction

Conventional pingueculae follow a self-limiting course. The visual prognosis for pterygia depends on the involvement of the visual axis. In the absence of squamous neoplasia, rates of recurrence vary depending on several clinical variables and method of removal {2935}.

Epibulbar choristoma

Herwig-Carl MC
Moulin A
Verdijk RM

Definition

Epibulbar choristoma is a benign congenital developmental lesion of histologically mature tissue located at conjunctival and/or corneal ectopic sites.

ICD-O coding

None

ICD-11 coding

LA14.06 Epibulbar choristoma

Related terminology

Acceptable: for epibulbar dermoid: limbal dermoid; dermoid tumour; for dermolipoma: lipodermoid; for complex choristoma: mixed dermoid.

Subtype(s)

Epibulbar dermoid; dermolipoma; complex choristoma

Localization

Epibulbar dermoids are typically located close to the inferotemporal limbus beneath the conjunctiva {2968}. If extensive, they can occupy the entire temporal quadrant. Dermoids are usually unilateral but can occur bilaterally in syndromic cases {3528}. Dermolipomas are typically located in the conjunctival superotemporal quadrant {2605}. If extensive, they can occupy the entire temporal quadrant, including the upper and lower fornices. Both types may involve the cornea.

Complex choristomas commonly extend from the superior temporal conjunctiva to the cornea. They may involve the entire temporal conjunctiva or, more rarely, the inferotemporal {844} or superior nasal conjunctiva {3060}. Occurrences in the caruncle {796} and bilaterality {844} are exceptional. Occasionally, they are buried under pterygia {3753}.

Clinical features

Epibulbar dermoids are whitish, firm lesions with hair {1354}. They are non-mobile because of their attachment to underlying sclera.

Dermolipomas are yellowish, soft, non-mobile lesions that may contain hair {1354}. The main differential diagnosis for dermolipoma is orbital fat prolapse. In dermolipoma, the conjunctiva is tethered to the underlying lesion, whereas in orbital fat prolapse, the conjunctiva is mobile over the lesion.

Complex choristomas are usually yellowish if they contain adipose tissue and pinkish with gelatinous elevations if they contain lacrimal gland {2571}. The mass can also appear whitish, harbour hair, and display fine superficial vasculature.

Epidemiology

Epibulbar choristomas are rare. As congenital lesions, they are predominantly (in 60–70% of cases) diagnosed during childhood. Together, these choristomatous lesions account for approximately 8% of all epibulbar tumours in children {2968, 3021}; in adults, this relative proportion is substantially lower (< 1%) {2968}.

All three types of epibulbar choristoma are frequently observed in patients with Goldenhar syndrome and linear naevus sebaceus syndrome (MIM number 163200), in which as many as 50% of patients are affected by ocular anomalies, most commonly epibulbar choristomas {1630,1676,2371,2571}. Epibulbar choristomas may be part of other syndromes as well {268}.

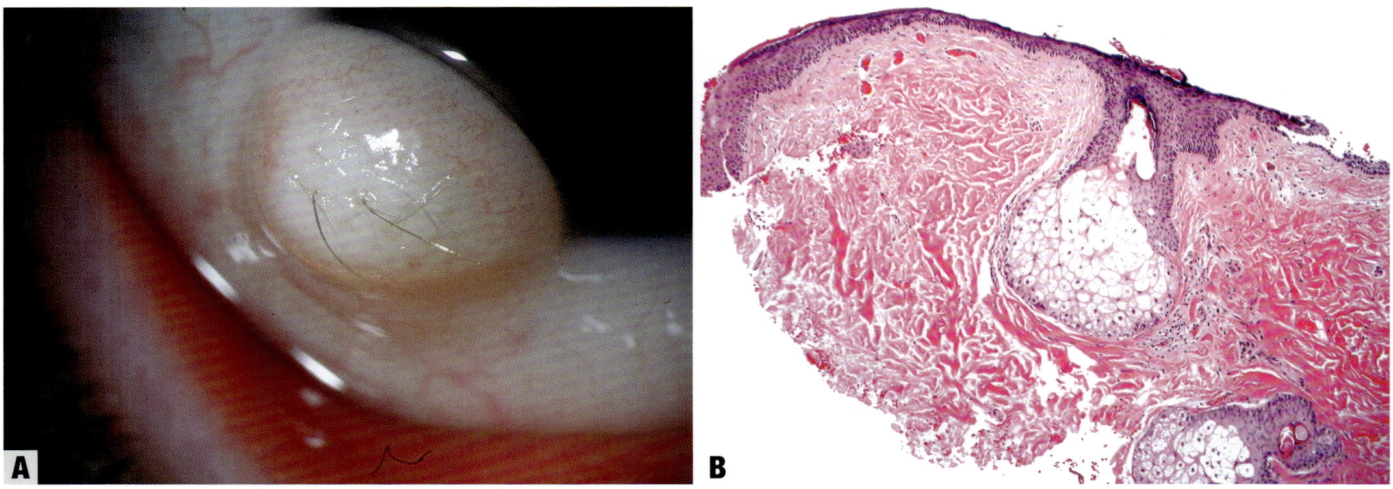

Fig. 2.12 Epibulbar dermoid. **A** An inferotemporal tumour with cilia in a 12-year-old girl. **B** A lesion comprising surface keratinizing epithelium and pilosebaceous units embedded within dermal-type stroma.

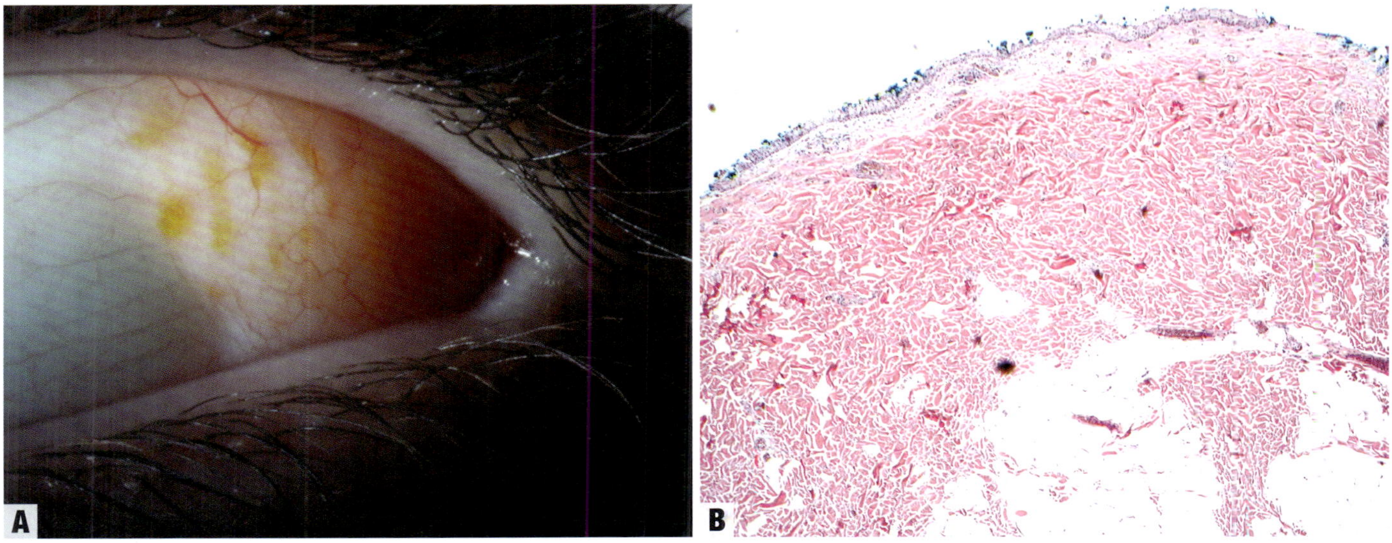

Fig. 2.13 Dermolipoma. **A** A whitish-yellowish lesion in the temporal quadrant of a 15-year-old boy. **B** A lesion with surface conjunctival-type epithelium, stromal collagen, and mature adipose tissue, resembling skin dermis and subcutis. No skin adnexal structures are present.

Etiology

Epibulbar choristoma is a developmental abnormality. The occurrence of complex choristoma has been partially attributed to early fetal altered migration of the palpebral portion of the lacrimal gland {3606}.

Pathogenesis

Epibulbar choristoma arises from tissues of dermal and mesenchymal origin.

Macroscopic appearance

See *Clinical features*, above.

Histopathology

Dermoids are composed of interweaving collagen bundles, covered by squamous epithelium (keratinized or non-keratinized with or without goblet cells). Dermal appendages, in particular pilosebaceous units and sweat glands, may be present. Variable amounts of fat can be observed.

Dermolipomas in addition contain a large amount of adipose tissue. Skin appendages, in particular pilosebaceous units and sweat glands, are found less often and are less numerous than epibulbar dermoids.

In complex choristomas, various heterotopic tissues are found. These commonly include lacrimal gland and cartilage. Further components that can be present include smooth muscle {844,2058}, peripheral nerve {844}, bone {1319}, striated muscle {2058}, immature teeth, and brain {888}. The differential diagnosis for the presence of lacrimal gland components includes conjunctival lacrimal gland hamartoma {2214}.

Cytology

Not relevant

Diagnostic molecular pathology

Not relevant

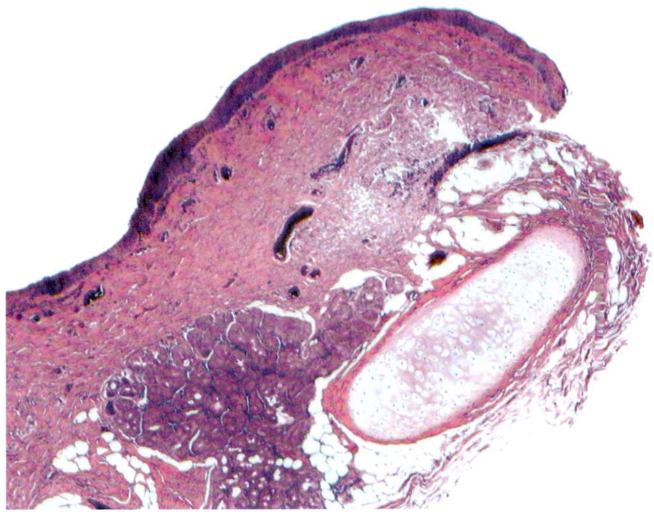

Fig. 2.14 Complex choristoma. A lesion containing cartilage and lacrimal gland tissue.

Essential and desirable diagnostic criteria

Essential: histologically mature tissue present at conjunctival and/or corneal ectopic sites.

Staging

Not relevant

Prognosis and prediction

Malignant transformation has not been described. Documented growth, possibly due to local reactive changes, has exceptionally been reported {2571,3380}. Debulking or excision is sometimes necessary to mitigate the risk of amblyopia associated with corneal lesions, inadequate lid closure, or dellen, or for cosmetic reasons {3205,1700}. Debulking may be favoured over excision to avoid complications {1700}.

Epibulbar osseous choristoma

Moulin A
Herwig-Carl MC
Verdijk RM

Definition

Epibulbar osseous choristoma is a choristoma composed of mature bone.

ICD-O coding

None

ICD-11 coding

LA14.06 Epibulbar choristoma

Related terminology

Acceptable: episcleral osseous choristoma.
Not recommended: osteoma.

Subtype(s)

None

Localization

Epibulbar osseous choristomas are typically unilateral and located in the superotemporal conjunctiva {3420,2616,3003, 372}. They can also occur temporally, and rarely they occur in the inferotemporal conjunctiva {372}.

Clinical features

Epibulbar osseous choristoma presents as a yellow, orange, pink, or white subconjunctival mass that may be multinodular and can be freely mobile or adherent to the sclera or muscles. The mass usually extends from the equator to the superotemporal fornix. Epibulbar osseous choristomas are firm, and calcifications can be seen using CT {3420}.

Epidemiology

The incidence of epibulbar osseous choristoma is unknown. It is present from birth and frequently presents in patients aged

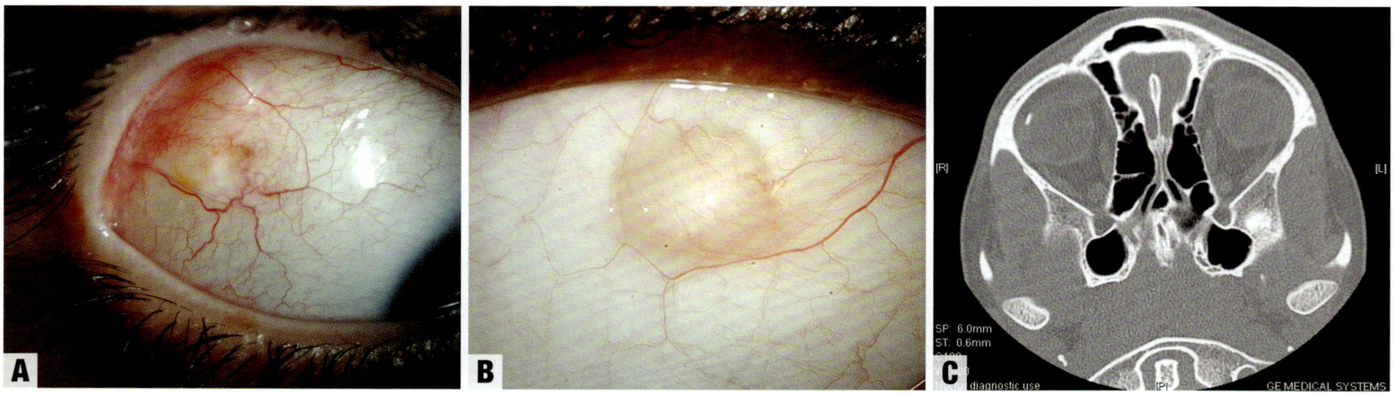

Fig. 2.15 Epibulbar osseous choristoma. **A** A multinodular whitish and firm mass can be seen in the superotemporal conjunctiva. **B** A lesion in the superotemporal conjunctiva is seen, showing a dome-shaped, yellowish mass. **C** Transverse CT shows bone in the temporal anterior episclera of the right eye.

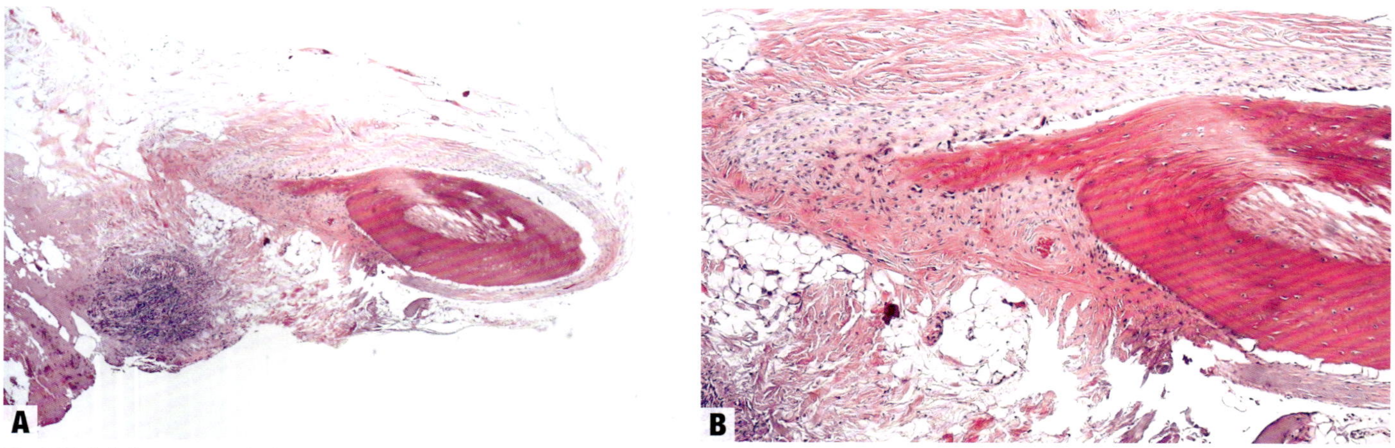

Fig. 2.16 Epibulbar osseous choristoma. **A,B** The lesion is composed of bone surrounded by fibrous and adipose tissue. There is normal compact lamellar bone with adjacent periosteum.

< 20 years {3420,1082}, but it can also be discovered later in life {3381}. There appears to be a slight female predilection {372, 1082}. Most of the reported cases have been in White people. However, a few cases have been reported in African-American patients {3003,372}.

Etiology

Epibulbar osseous choristoma is by definition a benign congenital lesion of histologically mature bone in an abnormal location.

Pathogenesis

Unknown

Macroscopic appearance

Firm whitish-yellowish mass

Histopathology

Epibulbar osseous choristomas are composed of compact lamellar bone with normal osteocytes. Haversian canals can be found. Haematopoietic bone marrow is usually absent but has been reported rarely {1082}. The bone is surrounded by periosteum and an internal osteogenic layer {372}.

Cytology

Not relevant

Diagnostic molecular pathology

Not clinically relevant

Essential and desirable diagnostic criteria

Essential: compact mature lamellar bone with normal osteocytes present at an episcleral location.

Staging

Not relevant

Prognosis and prediction

Epibulbar osseous choristomas are benign, and malignant transformation has not been described. In some exceptional cases, slight enlargement has been reported {3420,1082}.

Conjunctival squamous papilloma

Stagner AM
Dubovy SR
Grossniklaus HE
Heindl LM

Definition

Squamous papilloma is a benign epithelial proliferation composed of squamous to columnar cells, including some goblet cells, surrounding fibrovascular cores.

ICD-O coding

8052/0 Squamous cell papilloma
8052/0 Exophytic conjunctival squamous papilloma
8053/0 Inverted (endophytic) conjunctival squamous papilloma
8052/0 Mixed conjunctival squamous papilloma

ICD-11 coding

2F36.Y & XH50T2 Other specified benign neoplasm of eye or ocular adnexa & Squamous cell papilloma, NOS

Related terminology

Acceptable: conjunctival papilloma; caruncular papilloma; squamous cell papilloma.
Not recommended: mucoepidermoid papilloma.

Subtype(s)

Exophytic conjunctival squamous papilloma; inverted (endophytic) conjunctival squamous papilloma; mixed conjunctival squamous papilloma

Localization

Papillomas can arise singly or as multiple lesions on either the bulbar or the palpebral conjunctiva, but they most commonly occur on the non-limbal bulbar conjunctiva {2240}. The caruncle is often involved {3133}, and occasional corneal extension occurs.

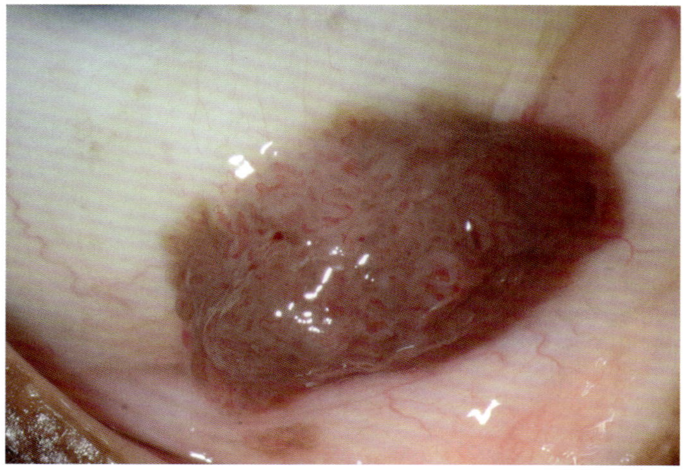

Fig. 2.17 Conjunctival squamous papilloma. Pedunculated papilloma composed of epithelial fronds with hairpin-like vascular loops, involving the inferior fornix of the conjunctiva. Note an associated secondary melanosis.

Clinical features

Tumours may display a pedunculated or sessile architecture, are often filiform, and show a variegated or cerebriform surface. They are vascular with a tan-pink to red coloration {3010}.

Epidemiology

Conjunctival papillomas are most common in men, typically aged between 21 and 40 years. Children and adolescents are also commonly affected and may have multiple lesions with extensive forniceal involvement {1570,3010,2240,3133}.

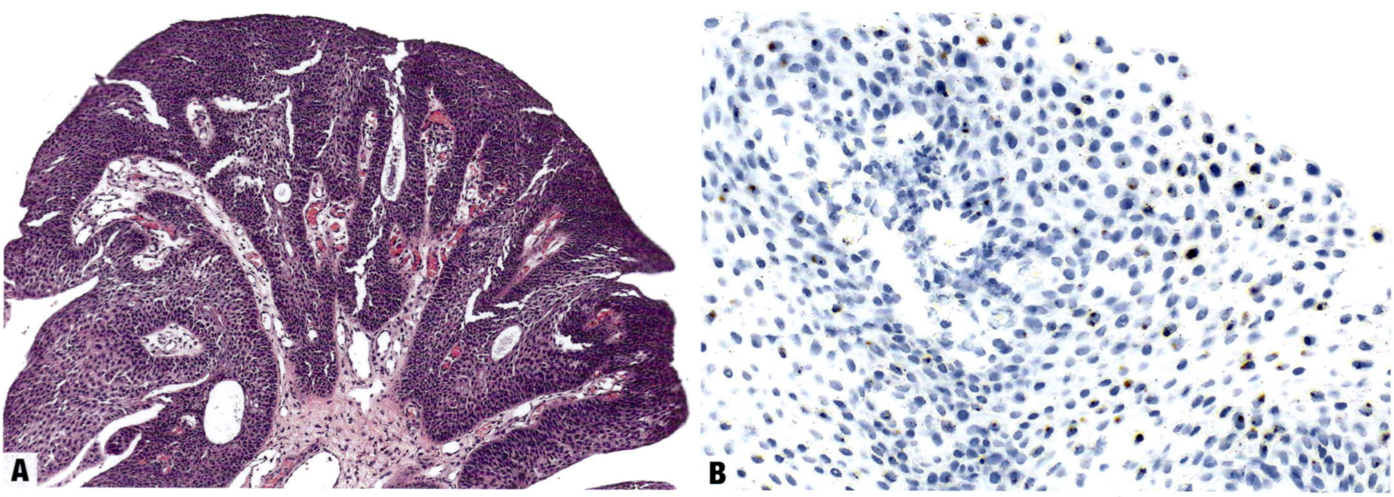

Fig. 2.18 Pedunculated conjunctival squamous papilloma. **A** Fronds of acanthotic epithelium with preserved goblet cells enclose mildly inflamed fibrovascular cores. **B** RNAScope demonstrates the presence of low-risk HPV in the lesion.

Etiology

Most conjunctival papillomas are driven by low-risk HPV subtypes, in particular HPV6 and HPV11 {2240,3486}. Occasional lesions are positive for high-risk HPV, i.e. HPV16 {2805,3134, 275,2650}. Reported rates of HPV detection vary significantly, from 44% to 92% {3325}.

Pathogenesis

HPV infection is considered to be the main stimulus of these conjunctival squamous proliferations; however, in HPV-negative lesions, the pathogenesis is unknown.

Macroscopic appearance

See *Clinical features*, above.

Histopathology

Exophytic papilloma shows a frond-like non-keratinizing squamous epithelial hyperplasia surrounding central vascular cores and containing varying numbers of goblet cells. Small intraepithelial mucous cysts or neutrophilic microabscesses may be present {540}. Surface keratinization or low-grade dysplasia / koilocytic changes may occur {2240,3133}.

Inverted papilloma appears as a well-circumscribed, endophytic squamous proliferation pushing into the substantia propria that may architecturally mimic squamous cell carcinoma (SCC) on scanning magnification {331,3124,2650,3189}.

Mixed growth patterns (i.e. both exophytic and endophytic) can also occur.

Immunohistochemistry

This is usually not required for diagnosis; however, these lesions are positive for cytokeratins (e.g. AE1/AE3, CK10/13, CK14, and CK19); Ki-67 highlights proliferating cells. Block-like expression of p16 is only seen in cases associated with high-risk HPV.

Differential diagnosis

The main differential diagnosis is SCC, particularly in inverted papilloma. An absence of cytological atypia favours inverted papilloma over SCC (see *Conjunctival squamous cell carcinoma*, p. 52). Sessile papilloma with higher-grade dysplasia is more likely to be papillary conjunctival squamous intraepithelial neoplasia / carcinoma in situ (see *Conjunctival squamous intraepithelial neoplasia*, p. 48).

Cytology

FNAB / impression cytology is not typically used to diagnose these lesions.

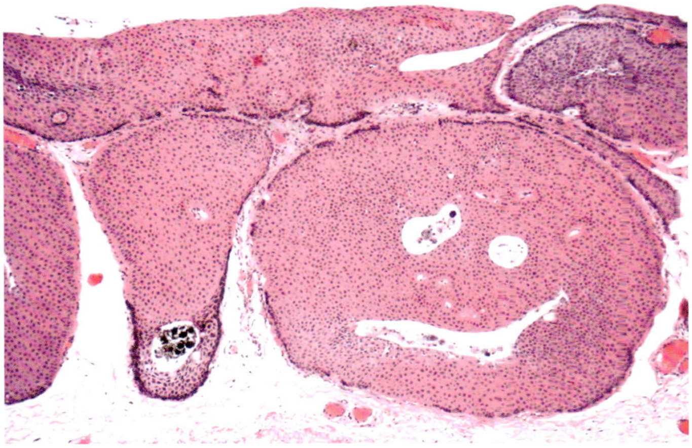

Fig. 2.19 Inverted conjunctival squamous papilloma. Endophytic squamous proliferation pushing into the substantia propria is seen, without evidence of dysplasia. Secondary melanosis is also present.

Diagnostic molecular pathology

HPV detection methods often reveal a viral etiology but are not necessary for diagnosis.

Essential and desirable diagnostic criteria

Essential: a benign, verrucous, or endophytic squamous proliferation with a variable number of goblet cells surrounding fibrovascular cores; absence of high-grade dysplasia / SCC in situ and/or invasive growth.

Desirable: demonstration of low-risk HPV infection.

Staging

Not relevant

Prognosis and prediction

Younger patients (aged ≤ 20 years) may have larger and more numerous lesions that are more likely to recur {1570}. Corneal involvement and surgical excision alone without adjuvant therapy are also documented risk factors for recurrence {1393}. Progression to SCC has been described but is rare {406}. Isolated reports suggest an increased risk of dysplasia or carcinoma in inverted (endophytic) conjunctival papillomas {275,1864}.

Conjunctival oncocytoma

Auw-Haedrich C
Heegaard S
Heindl LM

Definition

Conjunctival oncocytoma is a benign neoplasm composed of columnar eosinophilic cells with numerous mitochondria (oncocytes).

ICD-O coding

8290/0 Conjunctival oncocytoma

ICD-11 coding

2F36.Y & XH9Z86 Other specified benign neoplasm of eye or ocular adnexa & Oxyphilic adenoma

Related terminology

Acceptable: oncocytic adenoma; oxyphilic adenoma.
Not recommended: oxyphilic granular cell adenoma.

Subtype(s)

None

Localization

Periocular oncocytomas occur mostly at the caruncle, and rarely at the bulbar conjunctiva or plica semilunaris. They may also occur in the lacrimal gland (see *Lacrimal gland oncocytoma*, p. 249), lacrimal sac, or lid margin, or peripunctally {2450, 2861}.

Clinical features

Oncocytoma appears as a smooth or slightly papillomatous, circumscribed, sometimes vascularized, reddish, bluish, brownish, or (rarely) greyish or whitish nodule.

Epidemiology

Oncocytoma is diagnosed in elderly patients and represents 2–7% of benign caruncle tumours {2968,1924}. The incidence is

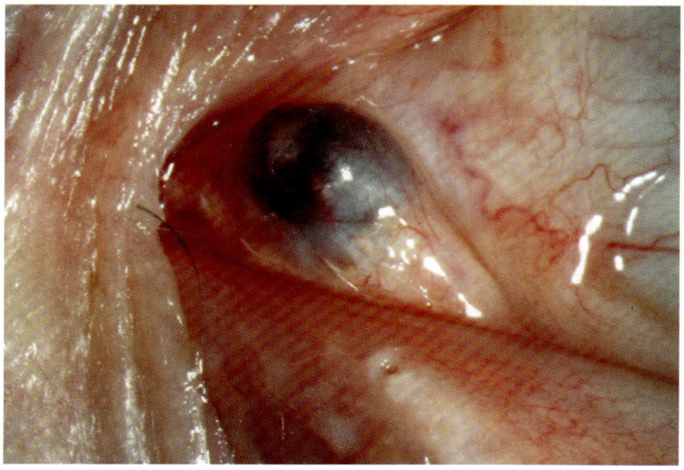

Fig. 2.20 Oncocytoma of the caruncle. Dark, almost black, ovoid subepithelial caruncular nodule in a 68-year-old male patient.

estimated to be as high as 0.3 cases per 1 million person-years. Differing results are found in the literature regarding sex predisposition: there was none in a study of 15 US cases {2861}, while in Denmark an M:F ratio of 1:2 was found in an investigation of 34 cases {2450}.

Etiology

Unknown

Pathogenesis

Oncocytomas arise as a benign proliferation of oncocytes, the cause of which is unknown. Caruncular oncocytomas most probably originate from accessory lacrimal glands of Popoff {2450} or sweat glands {1931}. Lacrimal sac oncocytomas arise in seromucinous glands. Accessory lacrimal gland

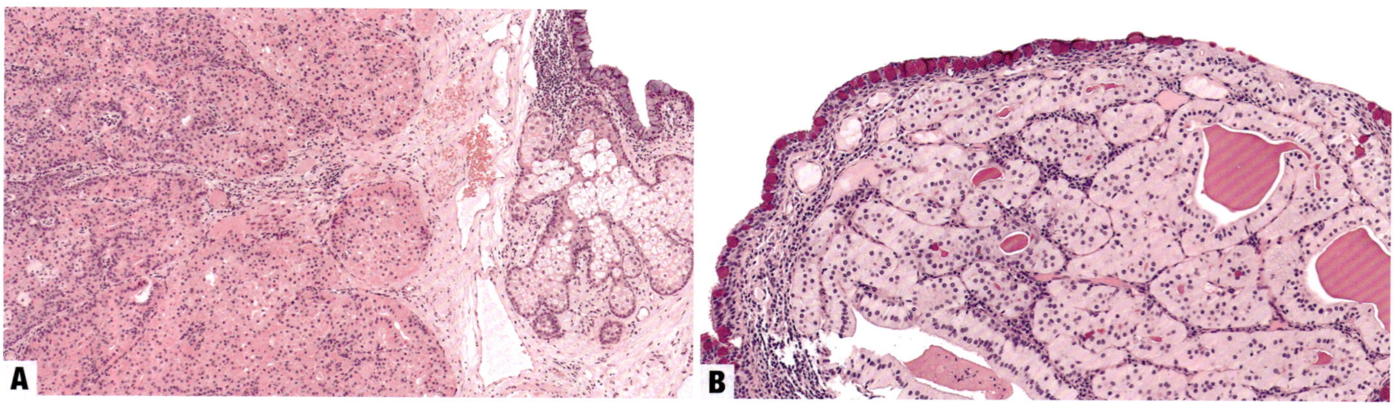

Fig. 2.21 Oncocytoma of the caruncle. **A** A circumscribed neoplasm composed of eosinophilic oncocytic cells adjacent to goblet cell–containing epithelium and sebaceous glands is seen. **B** Higher magnification of the same case shows oncocytes arranged in sheets with lumina containing proteinaceous PAS-positive fluid. Lymphoplasmacytic infiltrate is present between the tumour sheets and beneath the conjunctival epithelium.

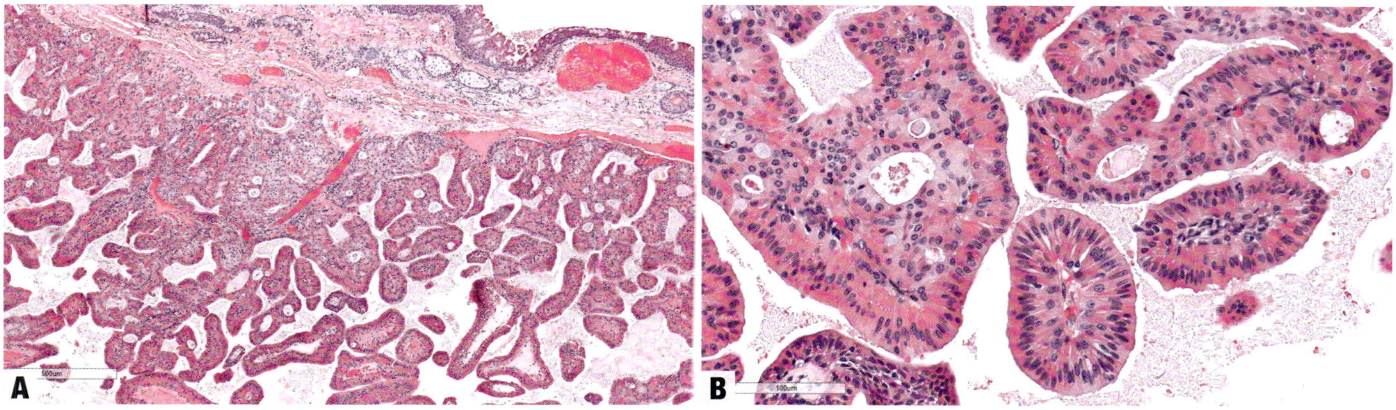

Fig. 2.22 Oncocytoma of the caruncle. **A** A circumscribed neoplasm with cystadenomatous architecture and papillary projections of oncocytic epithelium into the lumen is shown. Caruncular epithelium with goblet cells and adnexal units overlies the lesion. **B** Papillary projections of columnar oncocytic cells into a lumen filled with eosinophilic granular material can be seen.

oncocytoma was found to harbour mitochondrial DNA mutations {270}.

Macroscopic appearance

Macroscopically, oncocytoma is an ovoid, solid, sometimes cystic red-brown tumour {2861}.

Histopathology

Oncocytomas are subepithelial circumscribed neoplasms composed of oncocytes, which are columnar epithelial cells with abundant eosinophilic granular cytoplasm and monomorphic, ovoid, centrally placed nuclei with a single nucleolus. Neoplastic cells are typically arranged in sheets, nests, and microcystic patterns containing lumina with PAS-positive proteinaceous fluid. Some tumours demonstrate a cystadenomatous architecture with papillary projections into the lumen containing granular, eosinophilic, PAS-positive material. Scattered goblet cells may be present {2746}.

Immunohistochemistry

The tumour cells stain positively for antimitochondrial MU213-UC antibodies {2450}. The immunohistochemical (cytokeratin) pattern is similar to that of lacrimal and accessory lacrimal gland duct elements {2450} and also sweat glands {1931}.

Differential diagnosis

The histopathological differential diagnosis includes oncocytic mucoepidermoid carcinoma, secretory carcinoma, acinic cell carcinoma, apocrine cystadenocarcinoma/carcinoma. Characteristic oncocytic cytomorphological features combined with the absence of nuclear pleomorphism, mitotic figures, and infiltrative margin favour oncocytoma (see also *Apocrine carcinoma*, p. 138; *Secretory carcinoma*, p. 263; *Mucoepidermoid carcinoma of the lacrimal gland*, p. 265).

The clinical differential diagnosis includes melanoma {3244}, sebaceous hyperplasia {213}, papilloma, and conjunctival cyst.

Cytology

The cytology of caruncular/conjunctival oncocytoma has not been documented.

Diagnostic molecular pathology

Not relevant

Essential and desirable diagnostic criteria

Essential: a circumscribed solid/cystic tumour consisting of columnar oncocytic cells.

Staging

Not relevant

Prognosis and prediction

Oncocytoma rarely recurs despite positive tumour margins {2450}. There are no well-documented cases of malignant transformation {2450,2861}.

Hereditary benign intraepithelial dyskeratosis

Iacob CE
Cummings TJ
Eberhart CG
Heindl LM
Margo C

Definition
Hereditary benign intraepithelial dyskeratosis (HBID) is a non-neoplastic hyperkeratotic and dyskeratotic epithelial disorder of the conjunctiva and oral mucosa.

MIM numbering
127600 Hereditary benign intraepithelial dyskeratosis; HBID

ICD-11 coding
DA02.0 Genetic or developmental disorders involving lips or oral mucosa

Related terminology
Not recommended: Witkop–von Sallmann syndrome.

Subtype(s)
None

Localization
HBID presents with hyperkeratotic limbal conjunctival and/or oral mucosal lesions.

Clinical features
HBID appears as raised, leukoplakic, vascularized, and usually inflamed limbal conjunctival plaques that are frequently bilateral and change shape over time. The severity ranges from mild (erythematous) to moderate (leukoplakia limited to the conjunctiva) to severe (corneal involvement, which degrades vision because of surface irregularities and focal opacification) {439,457}. Seasonal variability exists, with exacerbation during spring and summer, followed by partial remission in autumn {695}.

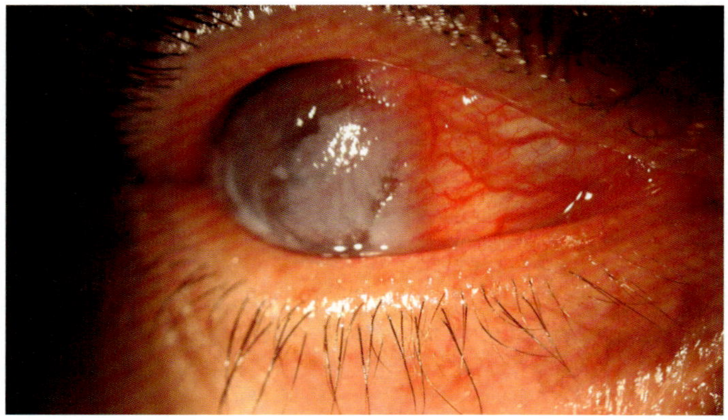

Fig. 2.23 Hereditary benign intraepithelial dyskeratosis. An elevated, plaque-like, grey, inflamed, and vascularized lesion at the limbal conjunctiva and cornea.

Epidemiology
HBID is a rare condition that is almost exclusively encountered in the Indigenous Haliwa-Saponi tribe (short for Halifax and Warren counties, their ancestral origin), native to the US state of North Carolina. There have also been isolated reports of cases in families with no relation to this tribe {439}.

Etiology
HBID is an autosomal dominant disease with high penetrance.

Pathogenesis
The HBID gene has been mapped to chromosome 4 (4q35), where copy-number duplication has been described {114,224}. No protein-coding genes have been identified at this locus

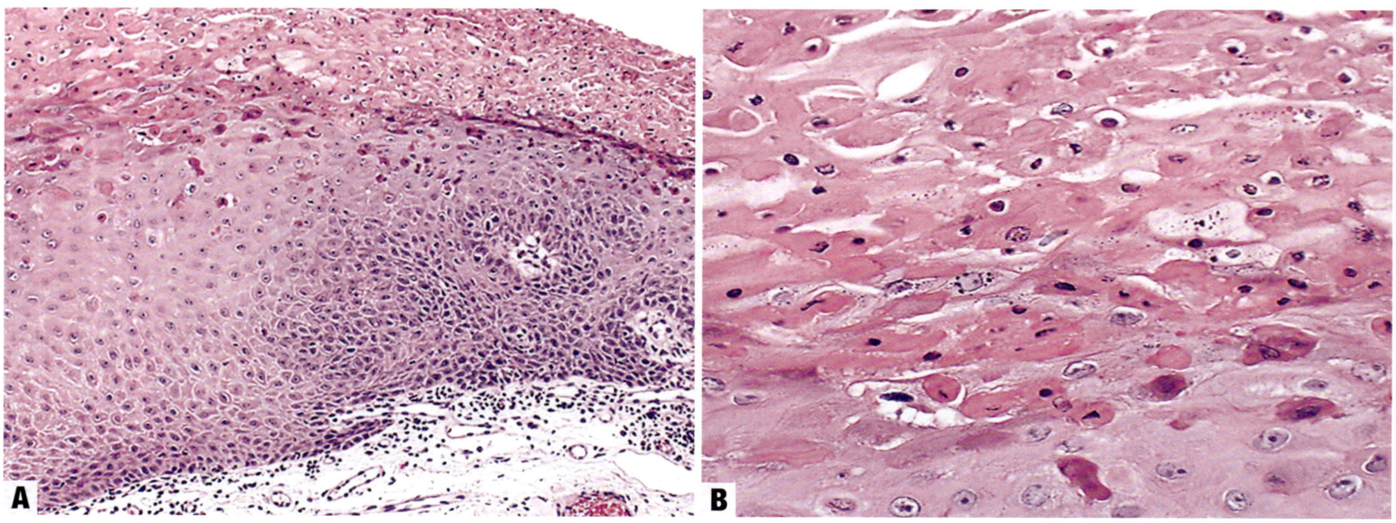

Fig. 2.24 Hereditary benign intraepithelial dyskeratosis. **A** Acanthosis with parakeratosis and intraepithelial dyskeratosis is seen. The epithelium lacks dysplasia. Chronic inflammation is present in the substantia propria. **B** Dyskeratotic squamous cells are present within the non-dysplastic epithelium.

{439}. *NLRP1* mutations have not been identified in 1 evaluated patient with HBID {439}.

Macroscopic appearance

See *Clinical features.*

Histopathology

The lesions are sharply demarcated from the surrounding conjunctiva. They show marked acanthosis with substantial multilayered parakeratosis displaying copious cytoplasmic dyskeratosis and pyknotic nuclei. Dyskeratotic cells characteristically are present within the squamous epithelium surrounded by the morphologically non-dysplastic squamous cells. No intervening granular layer is seen. Accompanying features include chronic inflammation and capillary telangiectasia in the substantia propria. The basement membrane remains intact {1229}.

Differential diagnosis

This includes conjunctival squamous intraepithelial neoplasia and squamous cell carcinoma in situ. Bilateral presentation, lack of nuclear pleomorphism, retention of the N:C ratio, and lack of atypical mitoses distinguish HBID from squamous dysplastic lesions. Patients with multiple self-healing palmoplantar carcinoma may develop conjunctival and corneal epithelial lesions histopathologically similar to HBID {2053,3759}. The skin lesions (keratoacanthomas) and germline *NLRP1* gene mutations help establish the diagnosis of multiple self-healing palmoplantar carcinoma {3157}.

Cytology

Conjunctival brushings of patients with HBID exhibit rounded squamous epithelial cells with dense homogeneous orange cytoplasm and hyperchromatic, pyknotic, or crenated nuclei {695}.

Diagnostic molecular pathology

Genetic analysis is not usually necessary as the clinical diagnosis is sufficient.

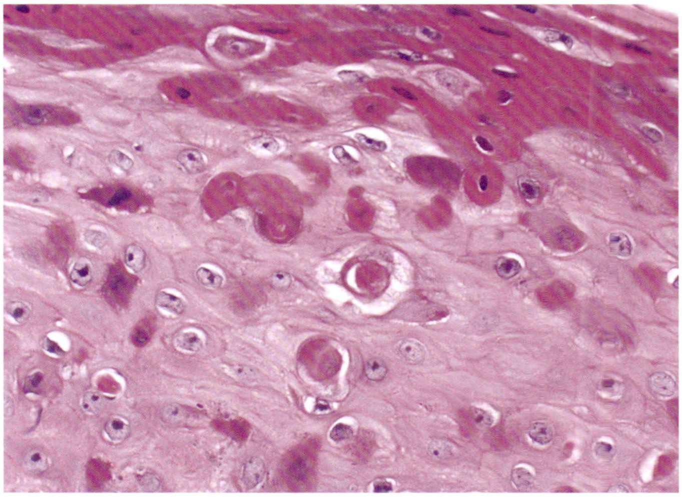

Fig. 2.25 Hereditary benign intraepithelial dyskeratosis. Dyskeratotic cells with dense eosinophilic cytoplasm and pyknotic nuclei.

Essential and desirable diagnostic criteria

Essential: sharply demarcated acanthotic limbal conjunctival lesions with prominent intraepithelial dyskeratosis; prominent inflammation in substantia propria; absence of epithelial dysplasia.

Desirable: bilateral location; family history suggestive of autosomal dominant mode of inheritance; similar-appearing lesions in oral mucosa.

Staging

Not relevant

Prognosis and prediction

While mostly self-limiting, some conjunctival lesions cause irritation and disrupt the tear film. Corneal involvement can substantially degrade vision {2903}. There is limited experience in treating vision-compromising HBID {439,457}.

Conjunctival squamous intraepithelial neoplasia

Mudhar HS
Alkatan H
Eberhart CG
Heegaard S
Heindl LM

Definition
Conjunctival squamous intraepithelial neoplasia (CSIN), also known as conjunctival intraepithelial neoplasia, is a preinvasive lesion manifesting as a range of aberrant cytological, maturational, and architectural changes, leading to varying degrees of intraepithelial squamous dysplasia, ranging from mild to severe dysplasia, and progressing ultimately to in situ squamous carcinoma.

ICD-O coding
8077/2 Conjunctival squamous intraepithelial neoplasia (conjunctival intraepithelial neoplasia and carcinoma in situ)
8077/0 Conjunctival squamous intraepithelial neoplasia, mild dysplasia
8077/2 Conjunctival squamous intraepithelial neoplasia, moderate dysplasia
8077/2 Conjunctival squamous intraepithelial neoplasia, severe dysplasia

ICD-11 coding
2F36.Y & XH4611 Other specified benign neoplasm of eye or ocular adnexa & Squamous intraepithelial neoplasia, low grade
2E6A.0 & XH3EA2 Carcinoma in situ of the conjunctiva & Squamous intraepithelial neoplasia, high grade

Related terminology
Acceptable: conjunctival intraepithelial neoplasia; intraepithelial neoplasia of the conjunctiva; conjunctival squamous dysplasia.
Not recommended: ocular surface squamous neoplasia.

Subtype(s)
None

Localization
CSIN generally occurs on the conjunctival surface that is sun exposed. The most affected sites are the limbus and the nasal and temporal bulbar conjunctiva {1680,2367,3008}. The lesions frequently show corneal invasion and occasionally involvement of the forniceal or palpebral conjunctiva {1680,2367,3008,3010}.

Clinical features
CSIN has variable clinical appearances: it can have papilliform, gelatinous, or leukoplakic (secondary to overlying hyperkeratosis) forms. The commonest type is gelatinous with feeder blood vessels and a pearly appearance, but lesions may be opaque or show loss of lustre with white plaques on the surface (leukoplakia). Most CSIN lesions are slowly growing, minimally elevated, and near the limbus, and arise within the interpalpebral fissure causing redness, irritation, and foreign body sensation. As many as 30% of cases can be asymptomatic {1506, 3010,2367}. While most lesions are typically non-pigmented, some may be melanotic in patients with more pigmented skin (Fitzpatrick skin types IV–VI) {981} and misinterpreted clinically as conjunctival melanoma {3061}. CSIN can be difficult to differentiate from invasive squamous neoplasia clinically; however, an intraepithelial lesion is usually freely mobile, in contrast to an invasive lesion, which can be fixed to the underlying episclera {2367}.

"Ocular surface squamous neoplasia" is a clinical term and should not be used to describe the histopathology of CSIN {2078}.

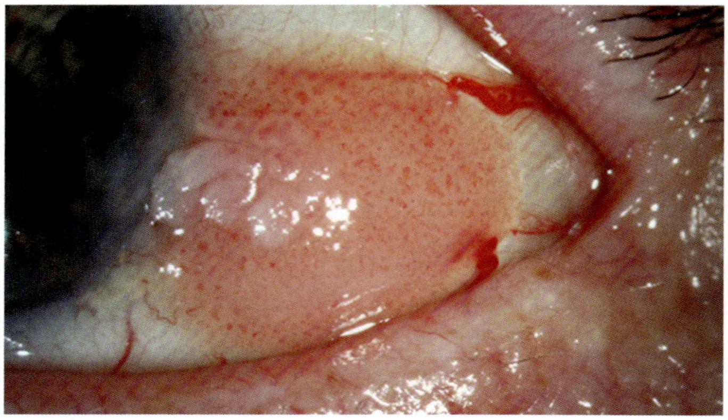

Fig. 2.26 Conjunctival squamous intraepithelial neoplasia. Clinical image of the left eye showing a raised pink lesion with feeder vessels and focal surface keratinization, located on the left lateral bulbar conjunctiva and limbus, that histologically corresponded to in situ squamous carcinoma.

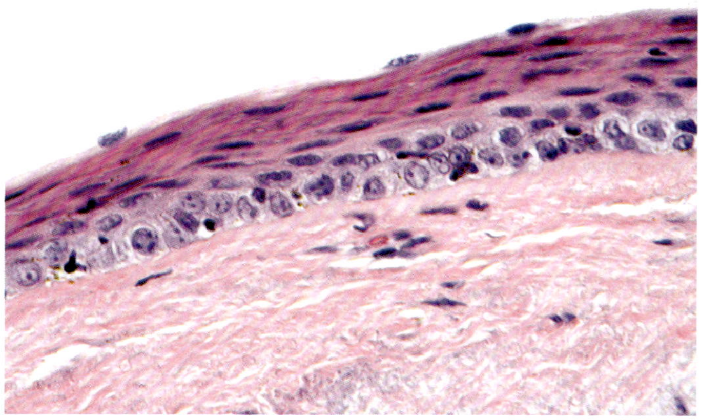

Fig. 2.27 Conjunctival squamous intraepithelial neoplasia – mild dysplasia. Note that the atypical squamous cells are confined to the lower third of the epithelium.

Epidemiology
CSIN is the most common preinvasive malignancy of the ocular surface. Its incidence varies geographically: in the United Kingdom, it is estimated at 0.4 cases per 1 million person-years,

whereas Australia shows an incidence of 19 cases per 1 million person-years {1680,1886}.

Etiology

Chronic exposure to ultraviolet B (UVB) radiation and immunosuppression are the main risk factors for CSIN, supported by ecological and mechanistic evidence {1873,2658,2373,485}. A subgroup of tumours is strongly associated with HPV {2649}, exhibiting histopathological and genomic features pathognomonic of HPV-induced disease {1170,2653}. Additional proposed risk factors include cigarette smoking, atopy, exposure to petroleum products or chemicals, DNA-repair deficiencies, chronic inflammation, and vitamin A deficiency {1113,591}.

Pathogenesis

CSIN arises from the conjunctival epithelium {3402}, and the preferred limbal location suggests that many arise from limbal stem cells. Somatic *TP53* mutations have been reported {3363}, along with chromosomal alterations involving loci encoding DNA-repair genes {204}. They have been linked to overexpression of telomerase due to *TERT* promoter mutations consistent with UV radiation–induced damage {2884}. HPV infection is present in some cases {2649,2334,1170}. However, none of these changes are pathognomonic, as they have also been reported in other conjunctival epithelial neoplasms.

Macroscopic appearance

Lesions may be flat or raised. Flat lesions are usually gelatinous cream/white epithelial thickenings. Raised lesions can be cream/white and papillomatous or verrucous. Surface keratin may be present. Some lesions can exhibit brown pigmentation, particularly in patients with more pigmented skin (Fitzpatrick skin types IV–VI).

Histopathology

Aberrant cytological, architectural, and maturation changes constitute dysplasia. At low magnification, CSIN usually shows a sharp demarcation with the background normal conjunctival epithelium, and characteristically with loss of goblet cells. At higher magnification, cytological changes comprise nuclear enlargement, hyperchromatic chromatin, nuclear pleomorphism, and an increased N:C ratio, and nuclei may show

Table 2.01 Differential diagnosis of conjunctival squamous intraepithelial neoplasia (CSIN) (continued on next page)

Diagnosis	Histological features	Immunohistochemistry	Other features	References
Conjunctival squamous intraepithelial neoplasia	See *Conjunctival squamous intraepithelial neoplasia* (p. 48) for histological details	p53+ in atypical cells CK17+ in atypical cells Loss of CK7 in atypical cells p16 block positivity in cases associated with high-risk HPV	Can be papillomatous	See *Conjunctival squamous intraepithelial neoplasia* (p. 48) {1472}
Pigmented conjunctival squamous intraepithelial neoplasia	Identical to CSIN except presence of hyperplastic dendritic melanocytes within dysplastic epithelium	Similar to CSIN in the squamous population, but no expression in the melanocytic population	Seen in patients with Fitzpatrick skin types IV–VI	{3061,2829,1785,1504}
Conjunctival intraepithelial neoplasia with mucinous differentiation	Identical to CSIN except many atypical cells contain intracytoplasmic mucin at all levels of the dysplastic epithelium	CK7+ Patchy CK17 positivity p16 block positivity in some cases	Alcian blue / PAS will stain the intracellular mucin Alternative terminology is "adenosquamous carcinoma in situ"	See *Adenosquamous carcinoma* (p. 56) {2298,2636}
Conjunctival sebaceous intraepithelial neoplasia	Atypical intraepithelial cells with variable cytoplasmic lipidization arranged in a pagetoid and/or confluent pattern; preservation of the native basal epithelial layer is very common; in some cases, loss of the epithelial cells is seen, leaving a much-attenuated epithelium	Intraepithelial sebaceous tumour cells stain for: adipophilin (vesicular cytoplasmic pattern) AR	Purely intraepithelial lesions can exist	See *Sebaceous carcinoma* (p. 124)
Conjunctival melanocytic intraepithelial lesion	Amelanotic melanocytic proliferation with varying degrees of cytological and architectural atypia; architectural patterns seen can be basal, pagetoid, nested, confluent	Melanocytic proliferation stains for: melan-A HMB45 SOX10	Not relevant	See *Conjunctival melanocytic intraepithelial lesions* (p. 72) {2220}
Squamous metaplasia / epidermalization	Maintenance of epithelial polarity; acanthotic epithelium, which can manifest a granular cell layer, surface keratin and parakeratin, rete ridges, and loss of goblet cells; gradual transition with normal epithelium, rather than a sharp cut-off; basal cell hyperplasia which appears uniform horizontally across the lesion can be present; mitotic figures may be present but usually basal and no atypical forms	Ki-67 usually confined to basal third of epithelium	Check for a history of exposure (lid ectropion, chemosis), infection, injury, allergy, autoimmune disease, topical and systemic drug reactions, and vitamin A deficiency	See *Reactive epithelial hyperplasia of the conjunctiva* (p. 31)

Table 2.01 Differential diagnosis of conjunctival squamous intraepithelial neoplasia (CSIN) (continued)

Diagnosis	Histological features	Immunohistochemistry	Other features	References
Inflammation-associated epithelial atypia	Maintenance of epithelial polarity; inflammatory cell percolation into epithelium that may be spongiotic and show basal vacuolar changes; basal cell hyperplasia which appears uniform horizontally across the lesion can be present; mitotic figures may be present but usually basal and no atypical forms	Ki-67 is usually restricted to lower third of epithelium	Check for a history of exposure (lid ectropion, chemosis), infection, injury, allergy, autoimmune disease, topical and systemic drug reactions	See *Reactive epithelial hyperplasia of the conjunctiva* (p. 31)
Topical chemotherapy–induced epithelial atypia	Random atypia of squamous cells in superficial epithelial levels with smoky/smudgy nuclear chromatin in enlarged nuclei, but retention of N:C ratio; apoptotic cells, cytoplasmic eosinophilia, and stromal chronic inflammation sometimes seen	Not relevant	Usually in response to mitomycin C	{2830,767}
Hereditary benign intraepithelial dyskeratosis	Sharply demarcated from normal conjunctiva; acanthosis, with substantial layered parakeratosis, with bright eosinophilic dyskeratotic squamous cells with pyknotic nuclei both within the epithelium and on the epithelial surface; no nuclear pleomorphism	Not relevant	Bilateral presentation; autosomal dominant condition (MIM number 127600)	See *Hereditary benign intraepithelial dyskeratosis* (p. 46)
Benign squamous papilloma	Papillomatous lesion with fibrovascular cores, draped in non-dysplastic squamous epithelium, composed of elongated cells, associated with variable numbers of goblet cells and intraepithelial neutrophils; mitotic figures can be present but no atypical forms; surface keratinization is rare and when present occurs as a reactive change at the tips of the papilloma	Not relevant	Mostly driven by HPV6 and HPV11	See *Conjunctival squamous papilloma* (p. 42)

prominent nucleoli. Dyskeratosis and apoptosis may be present with mitotic figures at varying levels of the epithelium. The epithelium shows abnormal stratification and loss of polarity and can be covered in keratin and parakeratin. The epithelium can adopt a papillomatous or verrucous configuration {1887,903,1181,2121,1597,2686,2227}.

The degrees of dysplasia can be graded as mild, moderate, or severe. Mild dysplasia is confined to the lower third of the epithelium, moderate dysplasia extends into the middle third, and severe dysplasia spreads to the upper third but retains some surface differentiation. Squamous carcinoma in situ shows full-thickness epithelial dysplasia {1887,903,1181,2121,1597,2686,2227,1235,1506}.

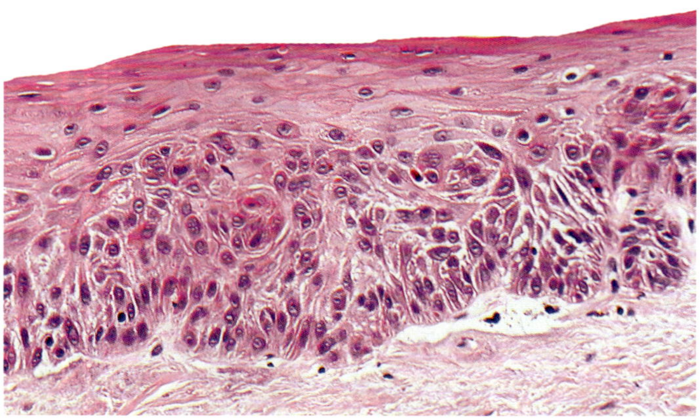

Fig. 2.28 Conjunctival squamous intraepithelial neoplasia – moderate dysplasia. Half of the thickness of the epithelium is occupied by atypical squamous cells.

Cases associated with high-risk HPV usually lack surface keratin or parakeratin, tend to exhibit full-thickness epithelial dysplasia (squamous carcinoma in situ) with hyperchromatic crowded oval nuclei without nucleoli, and have scant basophilic cytoplasm with poorly defined cell boundaries, imparting a basaloid appearance associated with apoptosis and numerous mitotic figures {1887,1170,2651}. UV radiation–associated cases can resemble skin actinic keratoses with rete-like ridges, larger eosinophilic polyhedral keratinocytes with larger hyperchromatic and pleomorphic nuclei often with prominent nucleoli, plentiful eosinophilic cytoplasm (that can contain glycogen), intercellular bridges, keratohyaline granules, squamous eddies, and variable surface keratin and parakeratin {1887,1170,2651}. Areas of elastotic degeneration are often present in the stroma, indicating chronic sun exposure, and can contain eosinophils in patients with atopy.

Pigmented CSIN pattern: Squamous intraepithelial neoplasia in patients with more pigmented skin (Fitzpatrick skin types IV–VI) can show dendritic melanocytic hyperplasia among the dysplastic squamous epithelium leading to pigmented dysplasia {3061,2829,1785,1504}.

Conjunctival intraepithelial neoplasia with mucinous differentiation pattern: This features dysplastic squamous cells and atypical cells with intracytoplasmic mucin, morphologically resembling dysplastic goblet cells and signet ring–like cells. It may be in some cases a precursor to squamous cell carcinoma with mucinous differentiation, or adenosquamous carcinoma, of the conjunctiva (see *Adenosquamous carcinoma*, p. 56).

Immunohistochemistry

p53 is expressed in atypical cells; CK17 is positive and CK7 can be lost {1472}. Cases associated with high-risk HPV can be p16-positive, but this finding is not specific in all studies {33, 2291,1170,2651}.

Differential diagnosis

CSIN can develop in pingueculae, pterygia, and viral squamous papillomas {512,1643,2735}. See Table 2.01 (p. 49).

Cytology

Exfoliative cytology {1086,3179,1887} and impression cytology {2390,3118,2391,3347,3277,2389,1674,1887} have been employed to sample the conjunctiva in suspected CSIN. Dysplastic cells show nuclear enlargement, an increased N:C ratio, irregular nuclear outlines, coarsely granular chromatin, nuclear pleomorphism, and nucleoli, with or without keratinization. Features suggestive of carcinoma in situ include syncytial sheets with poorly defined cytoplasmic borders. Impression cytology has a reported sensitivity of 70–82% for squamous dysplasia {2391,3347,3277}. A keratotic surface or deeply located intraepithelial dysplastic cells account for some false negative results {1674}. Importantly, invasive carcinoma cannot be diagnosed with these techniques.

Diagnostic molecular pathology

Not clinically relevant

Essential and desirable diagnostic criteria

Essential: dysplasia within the conjunctival epithelium characterized by atypical squamous cells with enlarged, often hyperchromatic nuclei and increased mitotic activity extending upward from the epithelial base.

Desirable: immunohistochemical proof of squamous phenotype in morphologically challenging cases; exclusion of sebaceous intraepithelial neoplasia by use of a discriminatory antibody panel, in cases where there is histological uncertainty (e.g. basaloid phenotype).

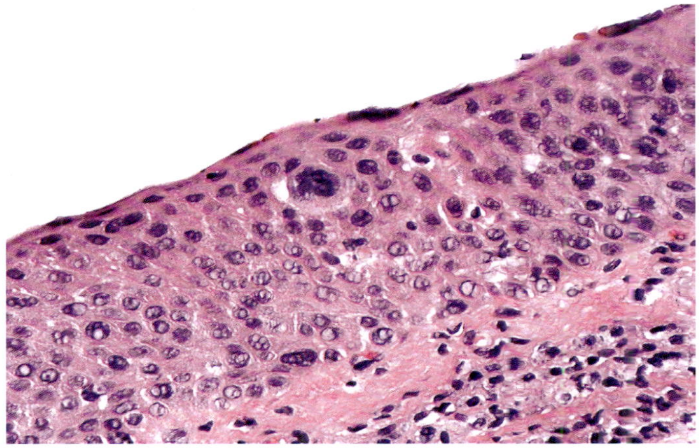

Fig. 2.29 Conjunctival squamous intraepithelial neoplasia – severe dysplasia. Almost full-thickness squamous epithelial atypia is seen.

Staging

The American Joint Committee on Cancer (AJCC) and the Union for International Cancer Control (UICC) TNM system is applied for carcinoma in situ (Tis).

Prognosis and prediction

CSIN is usually an indolent tumour but may progress to invasive squamous cell carcinoma {2518}. The underlying mechanisms for disease progression are not understood. The tumour has a high risk of recurrence, especially in cases with positive surgical margins. Immunosuppression has been documented to be a risk factor for more aggressive disease {3005}. Observational studies indicate a reduced recurrence rate with peroperative adjuvant cryotherapy of the conjunctival margins and adjuvant chemotherapy in the case of positive surgical margins {3092}.

Conjunctival squamous cell carcinoma

Heegaard S
Cherepanoff S
Eberhart CG
Ferreira TA
Heindl LM
Mudhar HS
Yamamoto H

Definition

Squamous cell carcinoma (SCC) is an invasive malignant epithelial neoplasm, arising from conjunctival epithelium that shows squamous differentiation.

ICD-O coding

8070/3 Conjunctival squamous cell carcinoma

ICD-11 coding

2D00.2 & XH0945 Squamous cell carcinoma of conjunctiva & Squamous cell carcinoma, NOS
2D00.2 & XH1U36 Squamous cell carcinoma of conjunctiva & Squamous cell carcinoma in situ with questionable stromal invasion
2D00.2 & XH4CR9 Squamous cell carcinoma of conjunctiva & Squamous cell carcinoma, keratinizing, NOS
2D00.2 & XH3GS1 Squamous cell carcinoma of conjunctiva & Basaloid squamous cell carcinoma
2D00.2 & XH6D80 Squamous cell carcinoma of conjunctiva & Squamous cell carcinoma, spindle cell

Related terminology

None

Subtype(s)

None

Localization

SCC is most commonly located in the interpalpebral conjunctiva and limbus (particularly the nasal limbus), where it frequently extends into the cornea. Less frequently, caruncular, tarsal, or forniceal conjunctiva can be involved. Tarsal and forniceal involvement by SCC is seen in immunosuppression or immunocompromised states, or in advanced, recurrent conjunctival SCC. Rarely, patients can present with glaucoma induced by intraocular invasion of SCC through the limbus. This presentation is typically seen in a setting of prior surgery {304}.

Clinical features

Conjunctival SCC most commonly appears as a unilateral, elevated, well-demarcated pearly pink to grey nodule, which can be leukoplakic, gelatinous, or papilliform. The lesions are often associated with feeder blood vessels and intrinsic vasculature. Pigmentation is variable, depending on the Fitzpatrick skin type. High-resolution optical coherence tomography, angiography, and confocal microscopy might be helpful in clinical assessment {1976,1614}. However, differentiating SCC from squamous intraepithelial neoplasia is clinically challenging, and excisional biopsy is required for definitive histopathological diagnosis. Ultrasound biomicroscopy and MRI help to assess for intraocular and orbital invasion.

High-resolution MRI allows the identification of most eyelid structures and assesses local extension of an SCC of the conjunctiva inside the eyelid {957}. It is also important to evaluate whether the nearby structures are invaded, in particular if there is orbital invasion. Furthermore, MRI aids in the differential diagnosis of eyelid masses; in particular, diffusion- and perfusion-weighted imaging help in differentiating an SCC of the conjunctiva from other benign eyelid masses.

Epidemiology

Conjunctival SCC is a very common malignancy showing an increasing incidence in recent decades. Worldwide, the mean age-standardized incidence rate is 0.18 cases per 100 000 person-years among males and 0.08 cases per

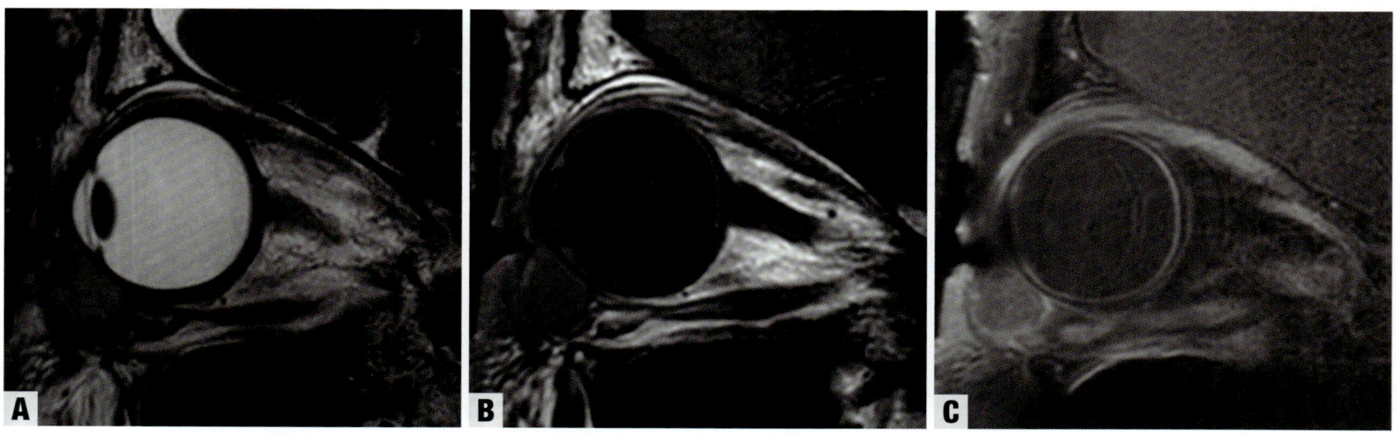

Fig. 2.30 Conjunctival squamous cell carcinoma. Sagittal T2-weighted MRI (**A**), T1-weighted MRI (**B**), and contrast-enhanced T1-weighted MRI with fat signal suppression (**C**) show a mass in the left lower eyelid, of intermediate signal intensity and enhancing. Anteriorly, it is located posterior to both the inferior tarsus and the orbicularis oculi muscle. Posteriorly, there is orbital invasion, with the tumour extending until the region of the globe attachment of the inferior rectus muscle.

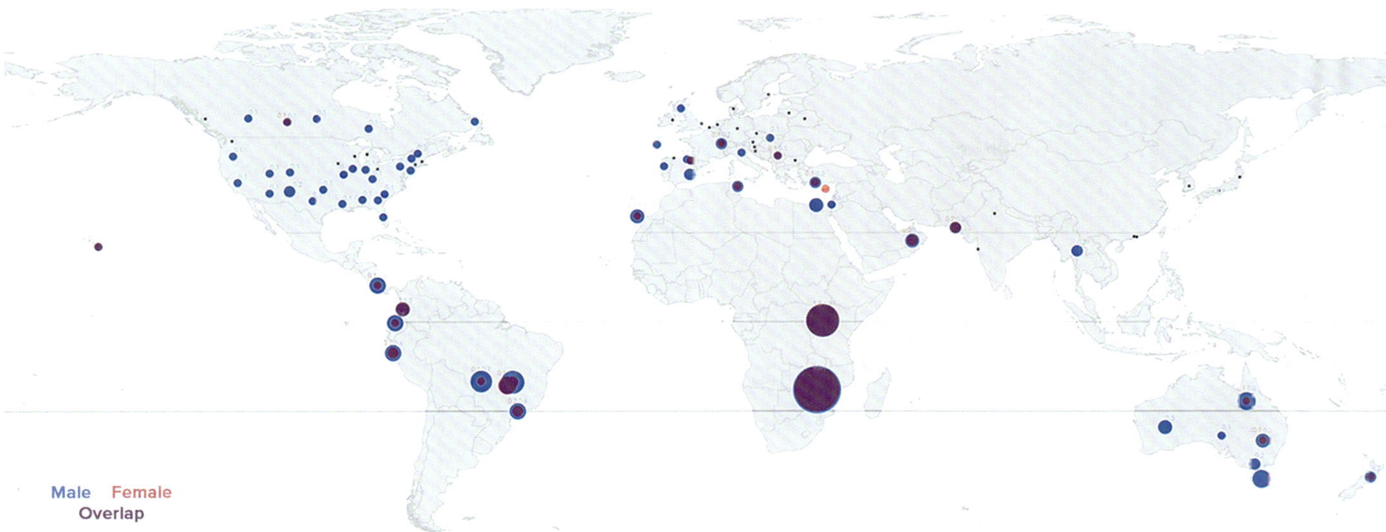

Fig. 2.31 Age-standardized incidence rates (per 100 000 person-years) of squamous cell carcinoma of the eye, by region. The data include all ocular squamous cell carcinoma cases, including those involving eyelid skin. The dot size is directly proportional to incidence. Blue, rates among males; red, rates among females; purple, overlaps between rates among males and females.

100 000 person-years among females {1113,2373,3239, 3678}. Two broad patterns of disease incidence are recognized: in immunocompetent populations in temperate countries, the incidence is higher in men and increases with age, sunlight exposure, and fairer skin {897,3239,722}, whereas on the African continent the disease mainly affects women, at a younger age, and is strongly associated with HIV infection and variably with HPV infection {1113,1238}. The incidence rate decreases by 49% with each 10° increase in latitude {2373}. Worldwide, a high incidence rate has been demonstrated among individuals with HIV {2374,2854,3345} and in other immunosuppressed populations {1189,3430}.

Etiology

Ultraviolet (UV) radiation is the strongest environmental etiological factor {2373}. Impaired immunosurveillance also plays a role and links risk factors such as UV radiation (which suppresses cell-mediated immunity) and immunosuppression (e.g. due to HIV infection or immunosuppressive therapy after organ transplantation). Reduced immunity potentiates the effect of oncogenic viruses such as HPV {1112}.

The prevalence of HPV infection in conjunctival SCC in immunocompetent populations has been controversial {799,2334}. Although no strong causal association between HPV infection and conjunctival SCC was found when the available data were

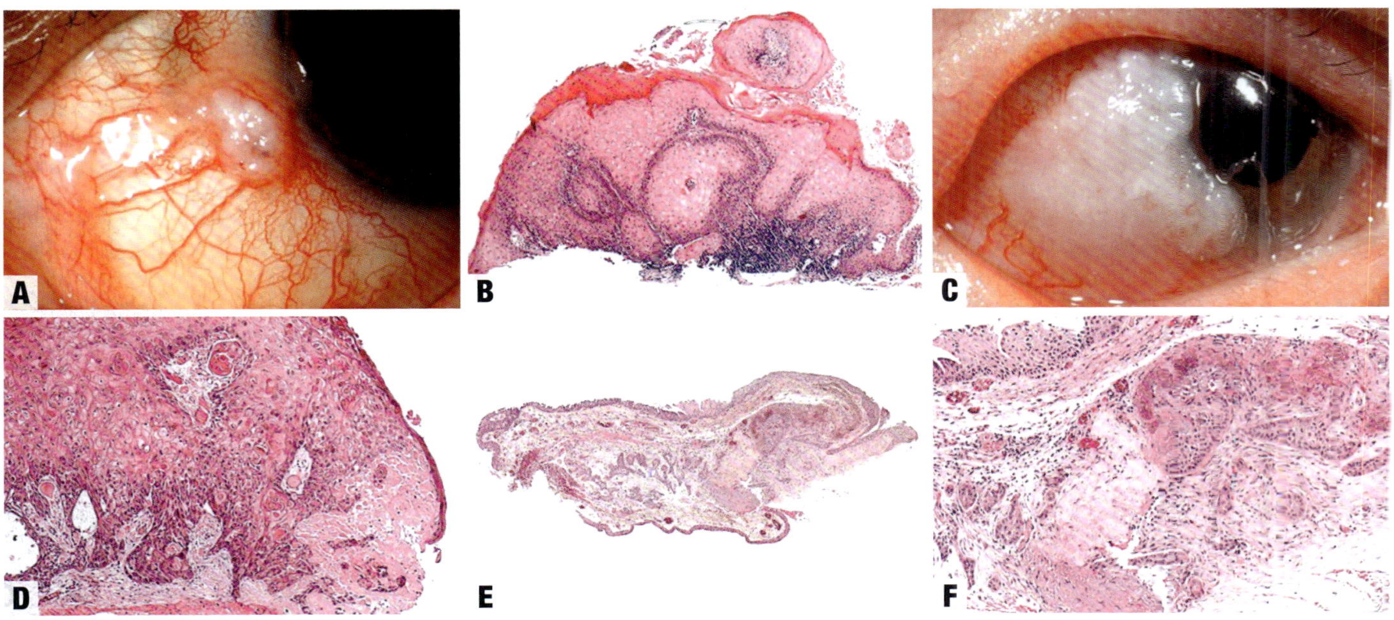

Fig. 2.32 Conjunctival invasive squamous cell carcinoma (SCC). **A** This keratotic nodule showed invasive SCC histologically. **B** The tumour has pushing, rather than infiltrative, deep borders; determining the degree of dysplasia and differentiating in situ from invasive disease can be clinically challenging. **C** The index of clinical suspicion for SCC is higher in larger lesions such as this one. **D** Histologically, this tumour has infiltrating borders. **E,F** Both in situ and invasive SCCs can occasionally involve pterygia.

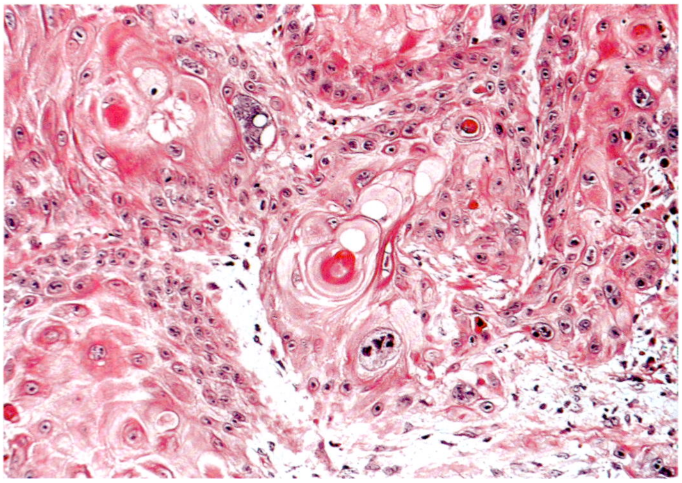

Fig. 2.33 Conjunctival well-differentiated keratinizing squamous cell carcinoma. Higher magnification showing atypical squamous cells with squamous eddy and keratin pearl formation.

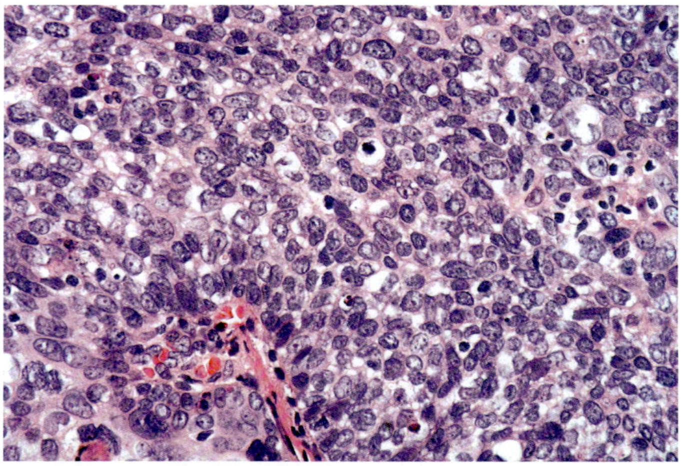

Fig. 2.34 Conjunctival invasive basaloid squamous carcinoma. A high-power view shows basaloid poorly differentiated invasive squamous cell carcinoma. Note that the basaloid cells have a high N:C ratio and do not show keratinization.

evaluated by the International Agency for Research on Cancer (IARC) in 2007 {1414}, other evidence, including a recent systematic review, suggests that the association may have been underestimated {33,2649}. In Africa, a confluence of low latitude and high prevalence of HIV and HPV infection probably explains the high incidence of conjunctival SCC. EBV has also been associated with increased risk of conjunctival neoplasia, mainly in individuals infected with HIV {1058}. Atopy is also linked to conjunctival SCC and may predispose to HPV infection {1170}. There is an association with ocular cicatricial pemphigoid and xeroderma pigmentosum {1580,591}.

Pathogenesis

The frequent limbal location suggests a vulnerability of limbal stem cells to oncogenic factors, although conjunctival SCC can also arise at other sites. It has been hypothesized that limbal stem cells are particularly vulnerable to the oncogenic effects of UV radiation and viral infection {1112}. UV radiation–induced mutations in *TP53* and the *TERT* promoter have been identified in conjunctival SCC and its precursors {3196,1951,1112}. *EGFR* mutations have also been reported {2819}. Copy-number analysis of conjunctival SCC has identified amplification of the 8p11.22 locus in some cases {204}. Gene expression analysis and more targeted studies suggest that overexpression of matrix metalloproteinases may also play a role in the pathogenesis of this disease {2030,791}. Chronic immunosuppression and antigenic stimulation are the proposed mechanisms for SCC associated with pemphigoid {591}.

Macroscopic appearance

Non-keratinizing tumours are gelatinous greyish nodular lesions, whereas keratinizing tumours are white/greyish with verrucous or papilliform architecture. Invasion of the cornea, sclera, intraocular contents, and orbit soft tissue may be apparent on gross examination, depending on the specimen type.

Histopathology

Invasive conjunctival SCC breaches the basement membrane to invade the underlying substantia propria. When the invasion is subtle and just beyond the basement membrane, the term "early stromal invasion" is permissible. The tumour usually arises from conjunctival squamous carcinoma in situ (see *Conjunctival squamous intraepithelial neoplasia*, p. 48). Invasive tumours can have infiltrative or pushing/expansive borders {1887,2234}. The tumour triggers a desmoplastic response. Perineural, vascular, or lymphatic invasion can be identified.

Morphological patterns

SCC patterns include conventional, basaloid, spindle, squamous carcinoma with mucinous differentiation, pigmented, and acantholytic {1887,2234}.

Conventional SCC shows various degrees of keratinization. Well-differentiated tumours show cells with eosinophilic polyhedral cytoplasm, intercellular prickles, single cell keratinization, and squamous pearls. The nuclei are hyperchromatic or have open chromatin with eosinophilic nucleoli. There is minimal pleomorphism. Surface keratin and parakeratin may be seen. Mitotic figures are sparse. Moderately differentiated tumours show focal keratinization with more prominent nuclear pleomorphism and mitotic activity. Poorly differentiated tumours show very little or no keratinization, higher N:C ratios, and higher degrees of nuclear pleomorphism and increased mitoses {1887,2234}.

Basaloid SCC is poorly differentiated, with scant basophilic cytoplasm, a high N:C ratio, and poorly defined cell boundaries, with oval to spindle hyperchromatic nuclei without prominent nucleoli, and shows apoptosis and tumour necrosis {1887, 2234}. Cases associated with high-risk HPV are usually basaloid {3461,1170,2651}.

Spindle SCC is poorly differentiated, comprising pleomorphic spindle-shaped cells with tapering eosinophilic cytoplasm, with poorly defined cell boundaries, arranged as solid sheets or in a storiform manner. Mitotic figures are conspicuous. Areas of conventional SCC and dysplastic epithelium may be present {1887,2234,634}.

SCC with mucinous differentiation (formerly mucoepidermoid carcinoma) shows conventional SCC with focal intracytoplasmic mucin, resembling signet-ring cells highlighted by mucin stains. There is no true gland formation. SCC in situ or conjunctival intraepithelial neoplasia with mucinous differentiation is usually

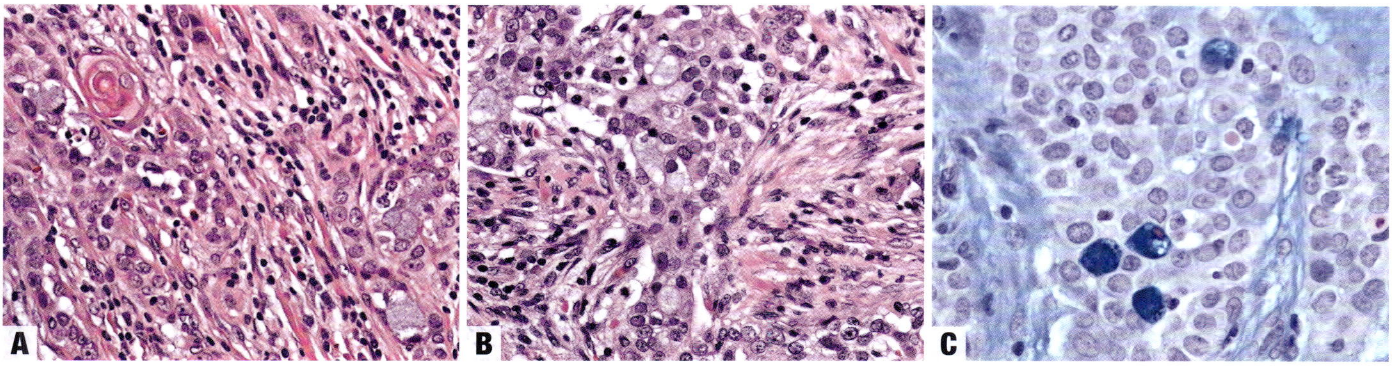

Fig. 2.35 Conjunctival squamous cell carcinoma with mucinous differentiation. **A** Bands and strands of invasive squamous cell carcinoma with focal keratin pearl formation (upper left) and bluish mucin within individual tumour cells (lower right). **B** Higher magnification of the signet ring–like or goblet cell–like cells containing cytoplasmic mucin. **C** Alcian blue stain highlighting intracytoplasmic mucin in some of the tumour cells.

present (see *Conjunctival squamous intraepithelial neoplasia*, p. 48, and *Adenosquamous carcinoma*, p. 56).

Pigmented invasive SCC is found in patients with Fitzpatrick type IV–VI skin types and shows conventional SCC with hyperplastic melanocytes and melanophages among the tumour cells, and melanosomes in some SCC cells {1504,2829}.

Acantholytic SCC is characterized by acantholytic pseudolumina that contain acantholytic and dyskeratotic cells with debris {2120}.

Immunohistochemistry

This is only required for diagnosis in poorly differentiated tumours. SCC is positive for broad-spectrum and high-molecular-weight cytokeratins {1408,2311,3461}, EMA {2311}, and p63 {215,1557}, and negative for AR {2311}. In spindle cell carcinoma, the cytokeratin positivity can be focal, with other spindle cells exhibiting SMA and calponin positivity {1408,634}. Block-like p16 positivity can be predictive of high-risk HPV infection {2298,2651} but has poor specificity for a diagnosis of SCC {2651,1360}.

Differential diagnosis

For basaloid SCC the main differentials are poorly differentiated sebaceous carcinoma, and cutaneous basal cell carcinoma invading the conjunctiva. For spindle cell carcinoma, the main differentials are spindle cell melanoma and atypical fibroxanthoma. For SCC with mucinous differentiation, the main differential is adenosquamous carcinoma (see *Adenosquamous carcinoma*, p. 56).

Cytology

Features suggestive of invasive SCC on exfoliative {1086,3179, 1887} and impression cytology {2390,3118,2391,3347,3277, 2389,1674,1887} include atypical nuclei, tadpole and spindle cells, and hyperkeratinization with a background of tumour diathesis.

Diagnostic molecular pathology

Diagnostic molecular pathology is not clinically relevant. While routine HPV-specific testing is not recommended in conjunctival SCC, it can occasionally be helpful for diagnostic purposes.

Essential and desirable diagnostic criteria

Essential: a malignant tumour arising in the conjunctiva with squamous differentiation that invades the substantia propria.

Desirable: immunohistochemistry for spindle SCC and basaloid SCC to exclude morphologically similar entities.

Staging

SCC is staged using the most recent American Joint Committee on Cancer (AJCC) and Union for International Cancer Control (UICC) TNM classification system for conjunctival carcinomas.

Prognosis and prediction

Conjunctival SCC has a relatively high rate of local recurrence (~10–40%) and the recurrence is often associated with positive surgical margins and larger tumour size {3678,2142,3715, 296,1360,1580}. The reported incidence of lymph node metastasis is up to 1–2% {3715,1360,1580}. The prognosis is generally favourable; the overall risk of tumour-related death is nearly 2% {1360,1580}. In a series of 38 cases of T3/4 conjunctival SCC, the reported rates of metastasis and death due to tumour were 13% and 5%, respectively {2205}. The significance of high-risk HPV infection for worse prognosis or higher risk of recurrence has been controversial {548,2334,2651,1360}. Spindle cell carcinoma is thought to have aggressive biological behaviour, but its rarity has not permitted accurate prognostication {100}.

Adenosquamous carcinoma

Mudhar HS
Eberhart CG
Heindl LM
Hyrcza MD

Definition

Adenosquamous carcinoma is an invasive carcinoma arising from dysplastic conjunctival epithelium, with biphenotypic differentiation comprising squamous cell carcinoma (SCC) and adenocarcinoma.

ICD-O coding

8560/3 Adenosquamous carcinoma

ICD-11 coding

2D00.Y & XH7873 Other specified malignant neoplasm of conjunctiva & Adenosquamous carcinoma

Related terminology

Not recommended: mucoepidermoid carcinoma; squamous carcinoma with mucinous differentiation.

Subtype(s)

None

Localization

Adenosquamous carcinoma can occur at the limbal, bulbar, forniceal, and palpebral conjunctiva {2662,484,1524,2298,2732,1502}.

Clinical features

Patients present with a conjunctival mass of short duration, usually several weeks to months. The tumour may be nodular, multinodular, and fleshy pink-red, and can be associated with mild irritation {2298,1751}. Other presentations include leukoplakic, infiltrative, ulcerative, or papillomatous lesions {2662,1502,2250,1618,1617,2298,484,1524,2732,1751}. Involvement of the tarsal and forniceal conjunctiva is common (~60% of cases) {2298,1751}. For SCC with mucinous differentiation, see *Conjunctival squamous cell carcinoma* (p. 52).

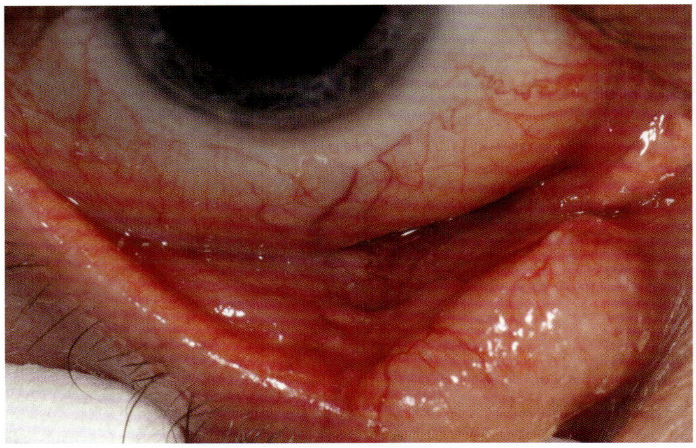

Fig. 2.36 Adenosquamous carcinoma of the conjunctiva. The tumour arises in the tarsal conjunctiva and presents as a tarsal-based mass with involvement of the eyelid margin.

Epidemiology

This tumour is rare. The mean patient age at presentation is 64 years, and there is a male predilection {484,2250,2662}.

Etiology

Chronic exposure to ultraviolet B (UVB) radiation may be a risk factor for adenosquamous carcinoma {2658,2373}, because of the described association of adenosquamous carcinoma with UV radiation–induced conjunctival intraepithelial neoplasia

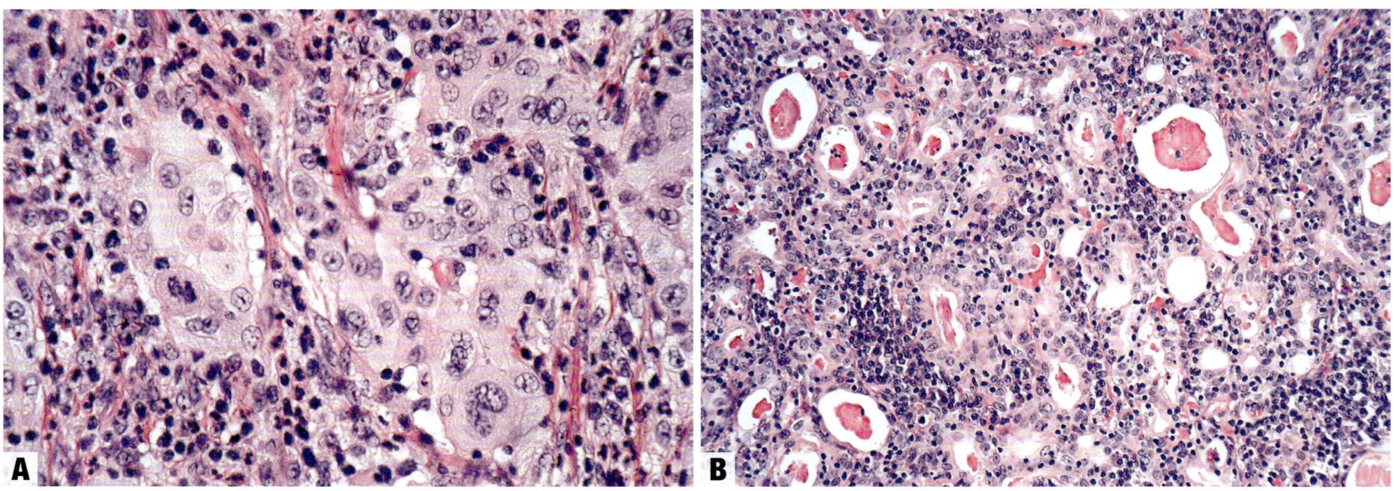

Fig. 2.37 Adenosquamous carcinoma. **A** Invasive non-keratinizing squamous carcinoma component of the adenosquamous carcinoma. **B** Higher magnification of the adenocarcinoma component of the conjunctival adenosquamous carcinoma, with eosinophilic material in the neoplastic gland lumina.

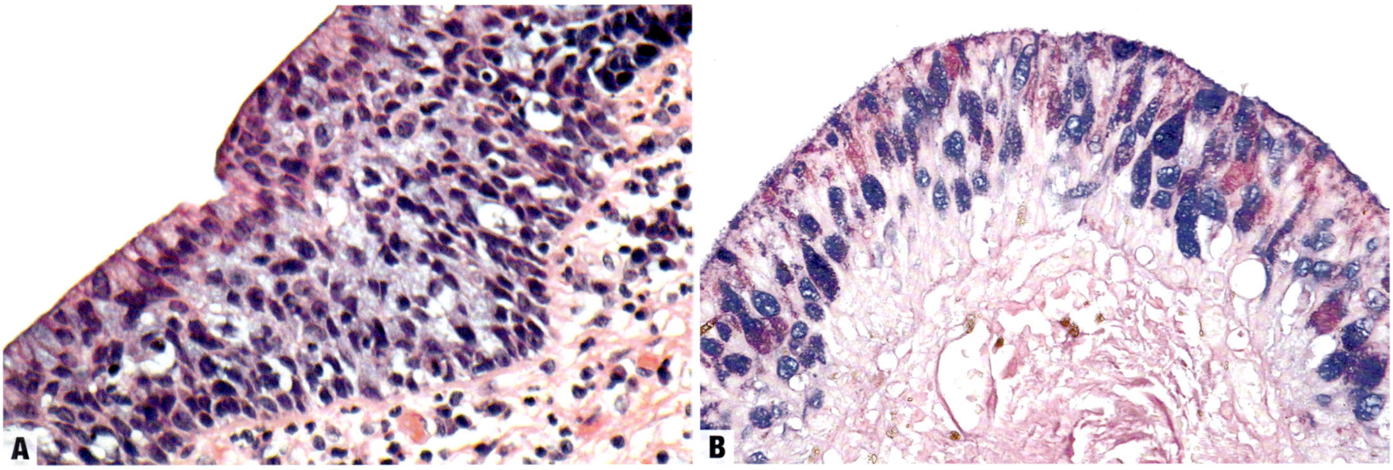

Fig. 2.38 Conjunctival intraepithelial neoplasia with mucinous differentiation. **A** Note the intracellular bluish mucin across almost the full thickness of the dysplastic epithelium. This lesion may be a precursor to invasive adenosquamous carcinoma. **B** Alcian blue / PAS staining of a conjunctival intraepithelial neoplasia with mucinous differentiation shows intracytoplasmic mucin in atypical epithelial cells.

{2298,1524,2071}. No association with HPV has been demonstrated so far {2298}.

Pathogenesis

Adenosquamous carcinoma often arises from conjunctival SCC in situ or conjunctival intraepithelial neoplasia with mucinous differentiation {1524,2071,2298}. All reported cases to date have lacked *MAML2* gene rearrangements {2298,1881}.

Macroscopic appearance

These tumours generally have both nodular and infiltrative components, with variable keratinization.

Histopathology

Adenosquamous carcinoma exhibits biphenotypic differentiation comprising SCC and adenocarcinoma. The ratio of these two components varies between cases. The SCC can be keratinizing or non-keratinizing, of variable differentiation, and arranged as infiltrative cords or sheets {2662,2732,1502,1618,1617,1881,2298}. The adenocarcinoma component can be tubuloglandular or comprise confluent sheets of atypical cells with intracytoplasmic mucin, resembling signet-ring cells and atypical goblet cells {2662,1327,2897,2732,1502,2250,2298,1617,1618}. The bordering conjunctival epithelium demonstrates SCC in situ or conjunctival intraepithelial neoplasia with mucinous differentiation {2298,1524,2071}. The mucin within the tubuloglandular areas and the confluent intracellular vacuoles is positive for mucicarmine, Alcian blue, and PAS with diastase {1502,2298}.

Immunohistochemistry

The SCC component is positive for p40, CK5/6, and CK17. The adenocarcinoma component is positive for CK7, EMA (MUC1), and CEA, and with BerEP4 {1502,1881,2298}.

Differential diagnosis

This includes pseudoglandular hyperplasia {2072} and SCC with mucinous differentiation. Pseudoglandular hyperplasia does not show cytological atypia. Squamous carcinoma with mucinous differentiation does not feature true neoplastic glands / ducts / confluent sheets of cells with intracytoplasmic mucin and, instead, shows scattered small groups or individual cells with intracytoplasmic mucin among malignant squamous cells (see *Conjunctival squamous cell carcinoma*, p. 52). Mucoepidermoid carcinoma of the accessory and main lacrimal glands can sometimes enter the differential diagnosis, particularly in tumours without a well-established in situ component (see *Mucoepidermoid carcinoma of the lacrimal gland*, p. 265).

Cytology

FNAB or impression cytology is not recommended for this entity.

Diagnostic molecular pathology

Genetic studies are limited, and no particular diagnostic molecular changes have been proposed {1881,2298}.

Essential and desirable diagnostic criteria

Essential: a conjunctival tumour with both SCC and adenocarcinoma components.

Desirable: presence of adjacent SCC in situ or conjunctival intraepithelial neoplasia with mucinous differentiation; keratinization of the squamous carcinoma component.

Staging

Adenosquamous carcinoma is staged using the most recent American Joint Committee on Cancer (AJCC) and Union for International Cancer Control (UICC) TNM classification system for conjunctival carcinomas.

Prognosis and prediction

This tumour is aggressive, with extensive local recurrence that can involve the orbit and the globe after local (or even wider) resection (i.e. enucleation or exenteration) {484,2250,2732}. Lymph node metastasis is uncommon, and death related to this tumour is rare {2298,1033,1751}.

Benign epithelial melanosis of the conjunctiva

Coupland SE
Mudhar HS

Definition
Benign epithelial melanosis of the conjunctiva is characterized by increased production of melanin without significant proliferation of conjunctival melanocytes, which remain normal in size and location, and transfer melanin into adjacent keratinocytes.

ICD-O coding
None

ICD-11 coding
9A61.6 Conjunctival or subconjunctival degenerations or deposits

Related terminology
Acceptable: constitutional melanosis; complexion-related melanosis.
Not recommended: non-proliferative melanocytic pigmentary patch; ephelis; freckle.

Subtype(s)
Congenital conjunctival epithelial melanosis; acquired conjunctival epithelial melanosis

Localization
Conjunctival epithelial melanosis is usually bilateral and can be unifocal or multifocal. It is most common in the perilimbal region, but it can also occur in the bulbar conjunctiva and extend to the palpebral conjunctiva {714,1457,1261,410}.

Clinical features
Congenital (primary) conjunctival melanosis may be visible from birth as mottled or patchy intraepithelial pigmented lesions that are not fixed to the sclera and may extend onto the peripheral corneal epithelium. The lesions can darken and may increase in size during childhood and adolescence {2743,410}.

Acquired (secondary) conjunctival epithelial melanosis occurs with increasing age and ionizing ultraviolet (UV) radiation exposure, and can be associated with underlying systemic conditions, for example, treatment with calcium blockers and/or in the setting of Addison disease {714,410}.

Epidemiology
Conjunctival epithelial melanosis is common. It is frequent in people with Fitzpatrick skin types IV–VI, occurring with lower frequency in White populations {714,410}.

Etiology
The etiology is unknown but probably multifactorial. Proposed causes include UV irradiation, hormonal changes, chemical irritation, or chronic inflammatory conjunctival disorders {1943,1657,410}.

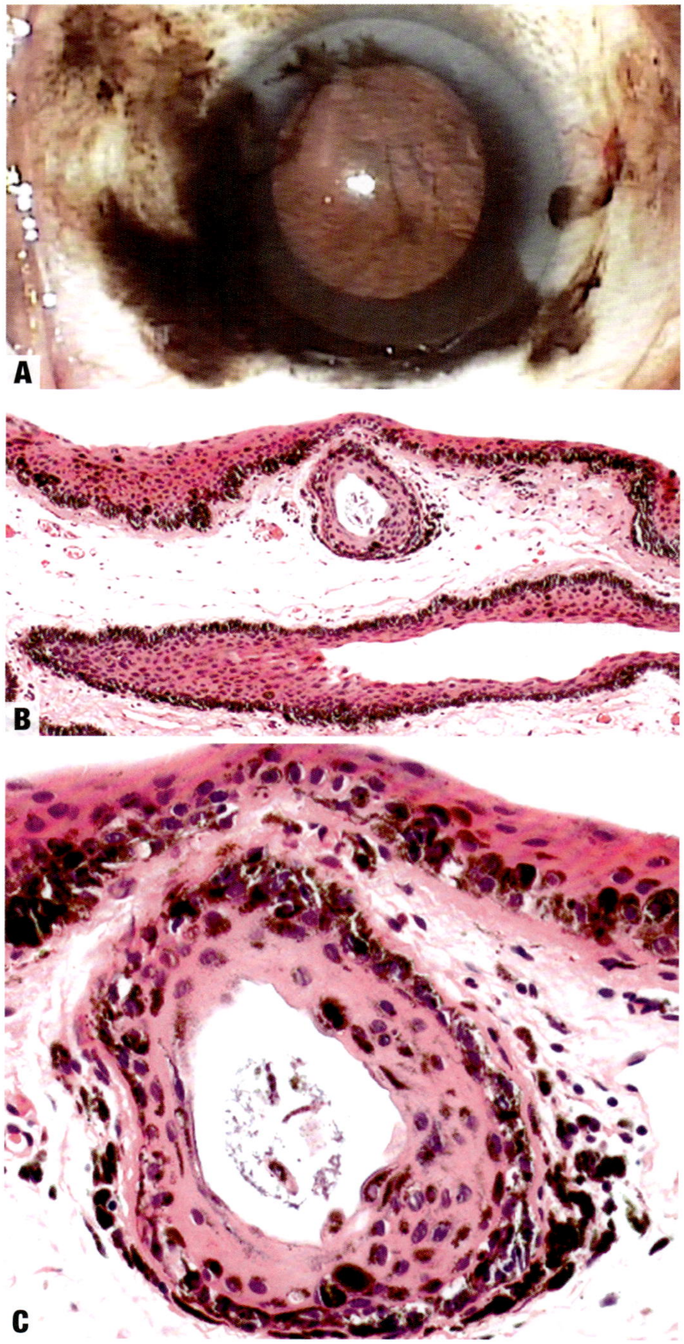

Fig. 2.39 Benign epithelial melanosis of the conjunctiva. **A** Abnormal pigmentation of the conjunctiva at the superior and temporal limbus with extension into the bulbar conjunctiva is seen. Prominent striate melanokeratosis is present throughout the cornea extending into the visual axis. **B** There is secondary pigmentation of the basilar keratinocytes and an epithelial inclusion cyst in the substantia propria. **C** There is secondary pigmentation in the basilar keratinocytes in the epithelial inclusion cyst.

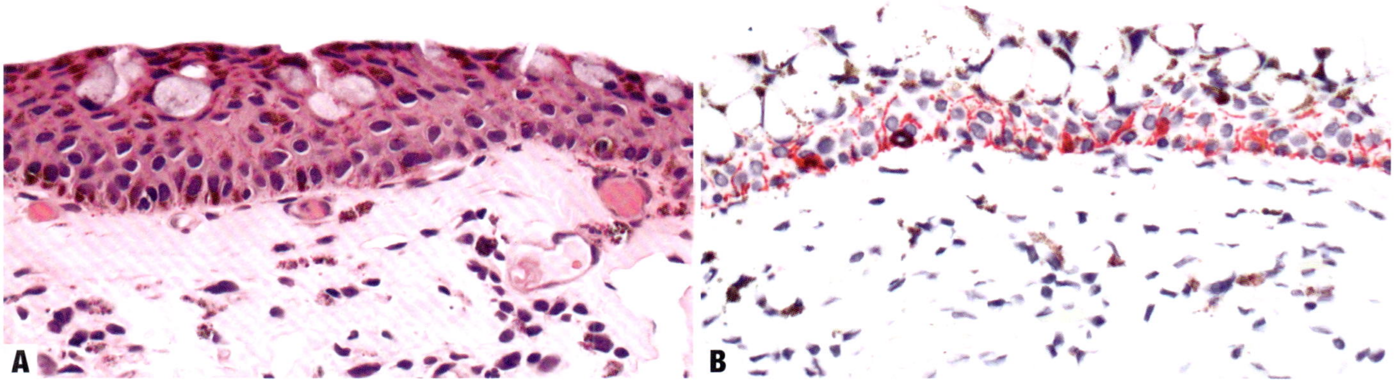

Fig. 2.40 Benign epithelial melanosis of the conjunctiva. **A** The conjunctival epithelium is pigmented, with some melanophages present in the substantia propria as well. Melanocytes, however, appear normal. **B** A melan-A (MART1) immunostain confirms normal density of dendritic-appearing melanocytes.

Pathogenesis

Like in hyperpigmentation of the skin, the eumelanin-to-pheomelanin ratio and the size of melanosomes within the conjunctival melanocytes, and how they react to external factors, have been proposed to play a role {3705}. Melanocytes transfer melanosomes to keratinocytes to such an extent that the pigmented keratinocytes can outnumber the melanocytes. Mechanisms relating to this transfer are unclear and require investigation {1464}.

Macroscopic appearance

See *Clinical features*, above.

Histopathology

Conjunctival epithelial melanosis appears microscopically as increased melanin pigmentation predominantly within keratinocytes. The melanocytes are normal in number or show only a slightly increased density and are located predominantly within basal epithelium. They retain normal dendritic morphology. Features such as nuclear enlargement, prominent nucleoli, and mitoses are not present {714,2209}. Melanophages may be present in the underlying conjunctival stroma.

Immunohistochemistry

Conjunctival melanocytes are positive for melanocytic markers, including melan-A, MITF, HMB45, and SOX10.

Differential diagnosis

This includes other conjunctival melanocytic lesions, such as naevi and conjunctival melanocytic intraepithelial neoplasia/lesions, as well as other ocular surface lesions, such as pterygia or squamous cell carcinoma in situ with hyperpigmentation {714,1261,1457,2209}.

Cytology

See *Histopathology*. FNAB or impression cytology is usually insufficient for definitive diagnosis.

Diagnostic molecular pathology

Usually not required

Essential and desirable diagnostic criteria

Essential: a mottled or patchy intraepithelial pigmented lesion not fixed to the sclera; histological features demonstrating conjunctival melanocytes without significant increase in number or atypia.

Desirable: immunohistochemistry – melan-A, MITF, HMB45, and/or SOX10 expression (preferably using a red chromogen).

Staging

Not clinically relevant

Prognosis and prediction

The prognosis is very good. Malignant transformation into conjunctival melanocytic intraepithelial neoplasia / conjunctival melanocytic intraepithelial lesions / primary acquired melanosis with atypia and/or conjunctival melanoma is exceedingly rare {1261}.

Junctional, compound, and subepithelial conjunctival naevi

Rodríguez-Reyes AA
Coupland SE
Mihic-Probst D
Mudhar HS
Stagner AM
Zembowicz A

Definition

Junctional, compound, and subepithelial conjunctival naevi are benign localized clonal proliferations of melanocytic naevus cells located (1) within the conjunctival epithelium and its invaginations, (2) at the epithelial–subepithelial junction and in the stroma, and (3) in the stroma with no junctional component, respectively.

ICD-O coding

8740/0 Junctional naevus
8760/0 Compound naevus
8750/0 Subepithelial (stromal) naevus
8722/0 Balloon cell naevus

ICD-11 coding

2F36.Y & XH1M79 Other specified benign neoplasm of eye or ocular adnexa & Junctional naevus, NOS
2F36.Y & XH27A6 Other specified benign neoplasm of eye or ocular adnexa & Compound naevus
2F36.Y & XH2MQ5 Other specified benign neoplasm of eye or ocular adnexa & Dermal naevus

Related terminology

Acceptable: conjunctival melanocytic naevus.

Subtype(s)

Junctional naevus; compound naevus; subepithelial (stromal) naevus; balloon cell naevus

Localization

Junctional melanocytic naevi are usually located at the juxtalimbal bulbar conjunctiva {2976}. Most compound and subepithelial melanocytic naevi are located in the bulbar (commonly juxtalimbal) conjunctiva, caruncle, and plica semilunaris; rarely, they occur in the palpebral and forniceal conjunctiva {993,1096, 1685,2976}.

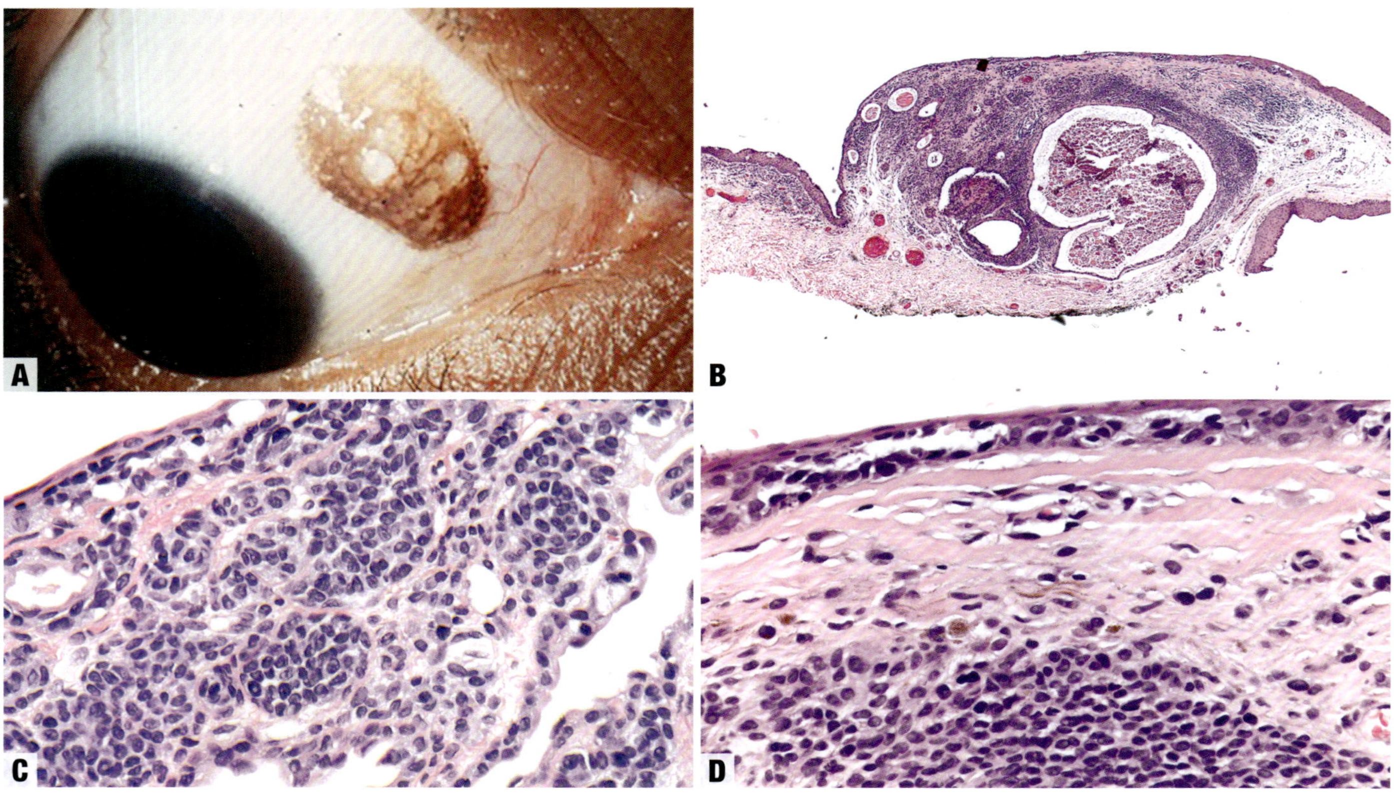

Fig. 2.41 Conjunctival naevus, compound. **A** A variably pigmented, well-circumscribed lesion is shown. **B** A lesion associated with epithelial inclusion cysts is seen. The lesion shows maturation with depth. **C** An example of a conjunctival compound naevus with prominent cysts is shown. **D** The image shows a case with a nested junctional component. In the context of thin conjunctiva, melanocytic nests appear to be confluent and show consumption of the epidermis. Such a pattern is common in conjunctival naevi and does not indicate atypia.

Clinical features

Conjunctival naevi are well-defined, variably pigmented (usually tan to brown) or amelanotic, mobile lesions, commonly arising on the bulbar conjunctiva followed by the caruncle; tarsal naevi are extremely rare {1083,3739}. As in the skin, junctional naevi are flat and compound, while subepithelial naevi show three-dimensionality. Compound naevi often show multiple small epithelial inclusion microcysts that are observed on the slit-lamp and suggest the benign nature of the lesion {993,410}.

Epidemiology

Junctional, compound, and subepithelial melanocytic naevi account for 3–6%, 70–78%, and 15–24% of biopsied conjunctival naevi, respectively {94,1096,2976,3739}. Junctional melanocytic naevi have an M:F ratio of 2:1 and occur in childhood and adolescence. Compound and subepithelial melanocytic naevi are diagnosed at a median patient age of 22 years (range: 5–74 years) and 46 years (range: 12–87 years), respectively {94,993,1096,2976}. Compound and subepithelial melanocytic naevi have an M:F ratio of 1:1 and are more common in White populations.

Etiology

Conventional conjunctival naevi are acquired melanocytic naevi that arise from neural crest–derived melanocytes that have migrated into the conjunctival epithelium (junctional naevi) {1025}. As in their cutaneous counterparts, the intraepithelial melanocytes migrate partially into the substantia propria and then ultimately into the subepithelial compartment (the equivalent of cutaneous dermal naevi) {993,3739}. Naevus melanocytes mature and become smaller and spindle shaped with descent into the substantia propria and with progressive loss of pigmentation {410}.

Pathogenesis

Very few molecular analyses of conjunctival naevi are published compared with those of skin naevi. However, these studies confirm the parallels between the two lesions {1025}.

Conjunctival naevi have mutually exclusive *BRAF* and *NRAS* mutations, which leads to constitutive activation of the MAPK pathway {1859,2592,2747,2574}. In a study investigating 25 conjunctival naevi, 9 (39%) were immunoreactive for NRAS p.Q61R and 13 (57%) for BRAF p.V600E. Next-generation sequencing identified an additional *NRAS* p.Q61K mutation in 1 immunohistochemistry-negative naevus case. *GNAQ* mutations are not typically present in junctional, compound, or subepithelial melanocytic naevi, but have been found in rarer conjunctival blue naevi {1025}. Conjunctival naevi with *NRAS* mutations appear to be larger in diameter and associated with a younger age of onset than naevi with *BRAF* mutations {1025}.

Macroscopic appearance

The naevi are discrete; flat or slightly elevated; circumscribed; pink, yellow-tan, brown, or non-pigmented; and located in the interpalpebral zone near the limbus {2976}.

Histopathology

The three main histological types of melanocytic naevi are junctional, compound, and subepithelial.

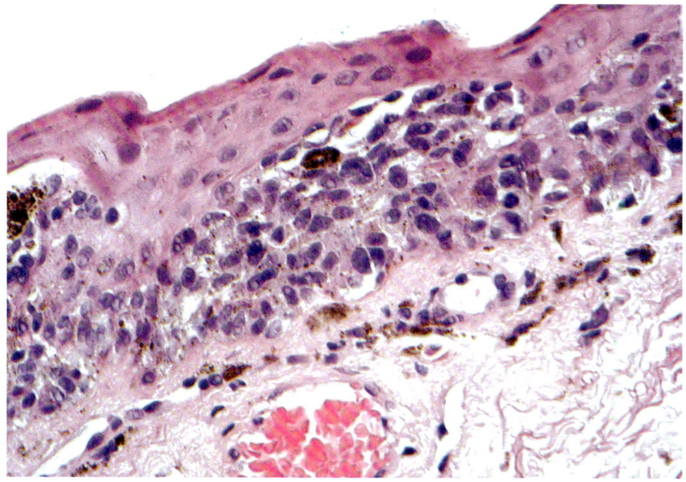

Fig. 2.42 Conjunctival naevus, junctional. Junctional naevus nests in a young teenager.

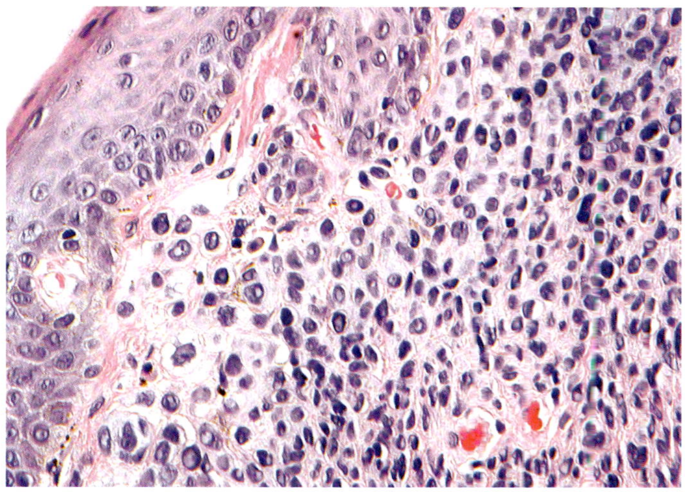

Fig. 2.43 Conjunctival naevus, subepithelial. Higher-power view of a conjunctival subepithelial melanocytic naevus, showing mature naevus cells.

Junctional naevi exhibit an intraepithelial proliferation of round to oval epithelioid cells and/or oval to cuboidal, intermediate, or lymphocyte-like naevus cells {993,3739}. The nucleoli are usually basophilic without atypia. Mitotic figures are rare {993,3739}. The naevus cells can be arranged as single, confluent or irregular nests, and extend in a lentiginous fashion, but without pagetoid spread {993,3739}.

Compound naevi contain naevus cells within the epithelium and the substantia propria, exhibiting maturation with depth. Solid and cystic surface epithelial invaginations of conjunctival epithelium (with goblet cells) are common between the naevus cells. Mitotic activity, if present, appears in the superficial layer {993,3739}.

Subepithelial naevi are located in the substantia propria and often arranged as nests. They are more likely to be amelanotic or minimally pigmented {1460}. The superficial naevus cells tend to be larger and more polygonal, whereas the deep naevus cells may display neuroid differentiation {993,1460}. Sporadic pleomorphism can be seen. Mitotic figures are generally absent

{1460}. Solid and cystic conjunctival epithelial invaginations and entrapped nests are seen in about half of cases {1460,2976}.

Uncommonly, junctional and compound naevi may show disordered architectural alterations intermediate between conventional naevi and melanoma, such as increased diameter > 5 mm, peripheral extension of the junctional component, asymmetry, poor circumscription, irregular and horizontally confluent junctional nesting, and focal pagetoid spread. Aberrant alterations in the subepithelial component may include diminished or even reversed maturation, nodule formation, and occasional mitotic activity. On occasion, naevi may be inflamed with prominent lymphocytic infiltrates resembling halo naevi in the skin. Eosinophils may be prominent in some cases.

Immunohistochemistry

Most conjunctival naevi demonstrate positivity for HMB45 in the superficial areas only {2951}, but homogeneous deeper staining for melan-A, SOX10, and MITF. They are usually negative for cyclin D1 and PRAME, whereas most conjunctival melanomas are positive for these markers {2910,1878,2301}.

Differential diagnosis

For junctional melanocytic naevi, the main differential is conjunctival melanocytic intraepithelial lesion (see *Conjunctival melanocytic intraepithelial lesions*, p. 72). Junctional melanocytic lesions in an adult should be assumed to be conjunctival melanocytic intraepithelial lesions until proven otherwise {714, 993,3739,2209}. For compound and subepithelial melanocytic naevi, the two main differentials are conjunctival melanoma and extraocular extension of uveal melanoma. Conjunctival melanoma usually exhibits a larger size, aberrant architecture (e.g. confluent and hypercellular nesting), cytological atypia, and greater mitotic activity as compared with naevi. Melanoma cells are larger than naevus cells and show conspicuous nuclear atypia {993,1656}. Adjoining melanoma in situ may be present.

Extraocular extension of a uveal melanoma will show widespread broad involvement of the biopsy base by melanoma cells with characteristic cytology and genetics {685,1450} (see *Choroidal and ciliary body melanomas*, p. 179, for details of cytology and genetics).

Cytology

Cytology shows oval cells (type A), oval to cuboidal cells (type B), and spindle-like cells (type C) {3739}.

Diagnostic molecular pathology

Not relevant

Essential and desirable diagnostic criteria

Essential: a conjunctival melanocytic lesion composed of naevus cells arranged in orderly junctional and/or subepithelial nests, cords, and individual cell patterns with maturation and general absence of architectural and cytological abnormalities.

Desirable: entrapped conjunctival epithelial cysts and nests surrounded by naevus cells.

Staging

Not relevant

Prognosis and prediction

Rarely, a junctional or compound naevus of the conjunctiva can give rise to conjunctival melanoma {993,1812,2976}. Subepithelial naevi have a low risk of progression to melanoma {993}.

Inflamed juvenile conjunctival naevus

Rodríguez-Reyes AA
Chevez-Barrios P
Peer J
Stagner AM

Definition

Inflamed juvenile conjunctival naevus (IJCN) is a compound naevus of childhood and adolescence, associated with prominent inflammation.

ICD-O coding

8770/0 Inflamed juvenile conjunctival naevus

ICD-11 coding

2F36.Y & XH8WP0 Other specified benign neoplasm of eye or ocular adnexa & Inflamed juvenile conjunctival naevus

Related terminology

Acceptable: inflamed conjunctival naevus of puberty and young adulthood; inflammatory juvenile compound conjunctival naevus.

Subtype(s)

None

Localization

Most IJCNs occur in the juxtalimbal zone of the bulbar conjunctiva {3733}.

Clinical features

IJCN presents with a well-circumscribed nodule, either amelanotic or pale flesh colour with areas of congested vessels. It may be pinkish or slightly and focally pigmented. The variation in the degree of pigmentation usually happens during growth of the IJCN and presents as an orange/red nodule secondary to both the vascularization and increase in pigmentation. One key finding is that the IJCN contains cystic structures and is freely movable, except when located in the limbus. A clinical characteristic of IJCN is the excessive concern it causes because of the rapid growth, vascularization, and congestion of the vessels {2052,3327,3733,1625,674}.

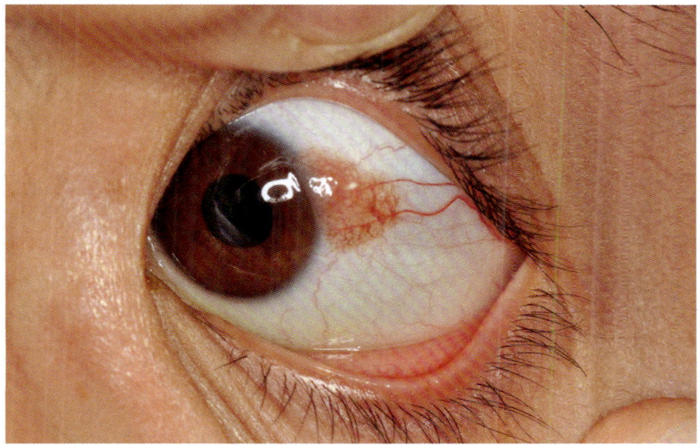

Fig. 2.44 Inflamed juvenile conjunctival naevus. An amelanotic conjunctival lesion adjacent to the temporal limbus with prominent cysts, feeder vessels, and intrinsic vascularity.

Epidemiology

The mean patient age at presentation with IJCN is 13 years. It is generally associated with puberty and arises most frequently in boys. Patients with IJCN may also have asthma, atopic dermatitis, bilateral papillary conjunctivitis, and vernal conjunctivitis {1922,2052,3327,3733,1625,3739,593}.

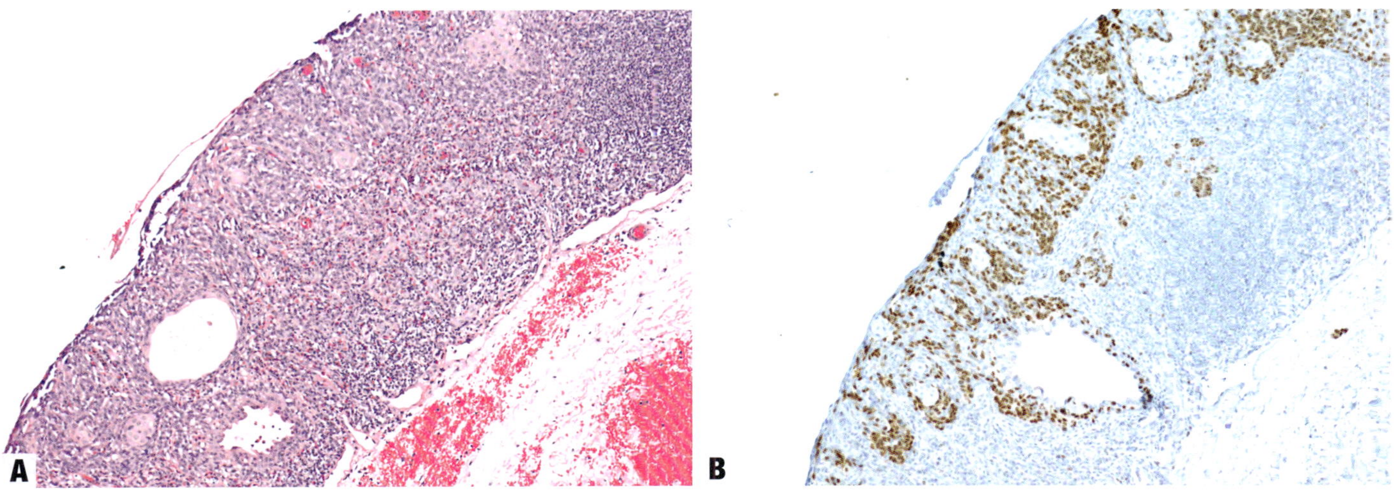

Fig. 2.45 Inflamed juvenile conjunctival naevus. **A** This was removed from a 7-year-old boy. **B** An MITF immunostain highlights the melanocytic elements, including extensive junctional activity as well as naevoid cells surrounding epithelial cysts extending into the substantia propria. Note the numerous non-staining inflammatory cells in the stroma surrounding the melanocytes.

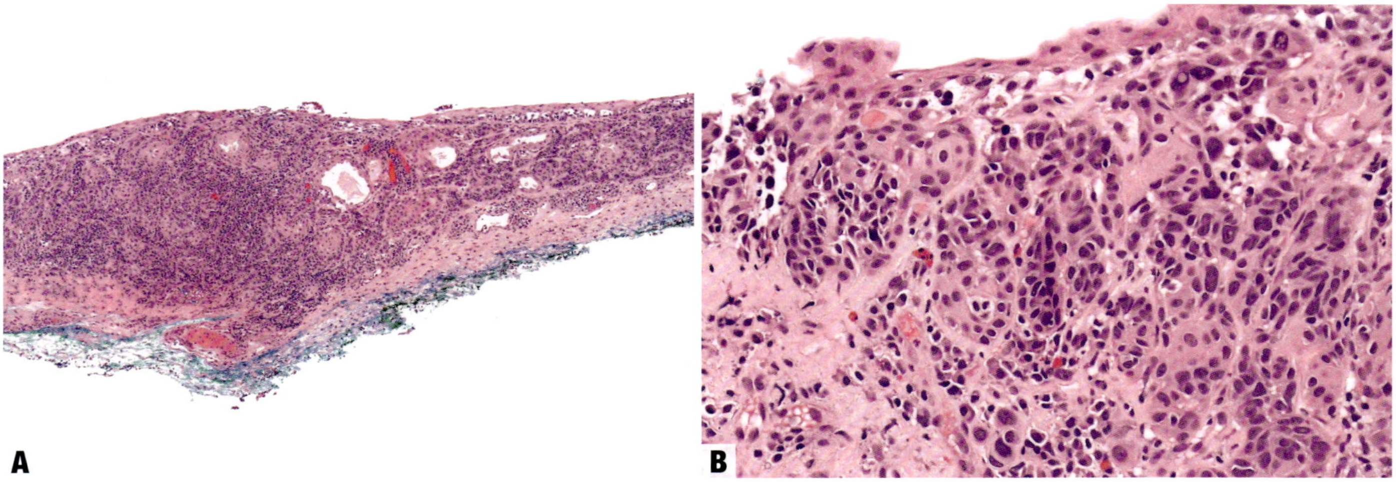

Fig. 2.46 Inflamed juvenile conjunctival naevus. **A** A low-power view of the inflamed naevus shows the combination of naevus cells and epithelium with a residual cystic component. On the left, there is more inflammatory component with lymphocytes and plasma cells. **B** Notice the eosinophils percolating into the superficial epithelium. In the background there are naevus cells, some with intranuclear inclusions, and some plasma cells.

Etiology

The etiology is unknown. There is no known genetic susceptibility, including cutaneous dysplastic naevus or melanoma syndromes {3327,3733}. However, 75% of patients have a history of allergic disease with papillary conjunctivitis and many eosinophils in the naevus-accompanying inflammatory infiltrate, leading to the presumption that IJCN occurs in those susceptible to allergy {3733}.

Pathogenesis

It is presumed that IJCN carries the same driver mutations as conventional conjunctival naevi, namely, mutually exclusive *NRAS* or *BRAF* mutations. This has been demonstrated in one of four studied IJCNs (*BRAF* c.1799T>A) {1143}. Of 12 other juvenile conjunctival naevi, 4 showed the same canonical *BRAF* mutation, and the remainder displayed *NRAS* mutations; whether or not an associated inflammatory infiltrate was present in the latter group of juvenile naevi was not specified {1025}.

IJCN is a compound naevus with predominance of the epithelial naevus component, and it is associated with eosinophilic and/or chronic inflammation. Expression of IL-17 in inflammatory cells of the naevus and VEGF in the vascular endothelium has been found in IJCN suggesting that these play a role in the pathogenesis and that they may have a potential role in treatment. The inflammatory reaction appears to be more stable; however, if the inflammation is composed predominantly of eosinophils, then the variation in size may be attributed to the inflammatory component. The eosinophilic infiltrate is more common in children with atopic and allergic conditions. Otherwise, a direct immune response induced by the naevus may be the cause of the inflammation {1922,593,1948,1441}.

Macroscopic appearance

Grossly, the lesions can be melanotic or amelanotic and flat or raised nodules {593}.

Histopathology

IJCN shares features of a conjunctival compound naevus, including the presence of cystic and solid epithelial nests in most of them. The cystic component often contains goblet cells, which give a positive PAS reaction {593}. Prominent lymphocytic inflammation is characteristic. Well-defined germinal centres may be present. Plasma cells and eosinophils are seen in about three quarters of IJCNs. Periods of rapid growth represent inflammatory infiltration and cystic enlargement by mucin production and accumulation {3733,1948,993,593}. IJCN shows apparent disordered growth such as prominent confluent junctional nests and lack of, or incomplete, maturation or paradoxical reverse maturation in which the nuclear and cytoplasmic size of naevus cells is greater in the subepithelial component than in the junctional region. This may lead to mistaken interpretation as a premalignant or malignant melanocytic lesion. The junctional component often extends horizontally beyond the subepithelial one {2052,3327,3739,674}. Mitotic figures are rare, and the Ki-67 index is low. IJCN is positive for HMB45 in the superficial layer only. Tumoural cells can show immunopositivity for melan-A and S100 {674}. Immunohistochemistry for CD45 (LCA), CD3, and CD20 shows a mixed population of B cells and T cells {2052,3327,593}.

Cytology

Not relevant

Diagnostic molecular pathology

Not relevant

Essential and desirable diagnostic criteria

Essential: childhood or adolescent presentation; features of a conjunctival compound naevus mixed with inflammatory cells (lymphocytes, plasma cells, eosinophils), and occasional lymphoid follicles.

Staging

Not relevant

Prognosis and prediction

IJCN recurs exceptionally and is rarely the source of conjunctival melanoma {3733,3327}.

Blue naevus of the conjunctiva

Mudhar HS
Rodríguez-Reyes AA
Stagner AM

Definition

Blue naevus is a stromal melanocytic tumour composed of dendritic, spindle, and/or ovoid cells associated with melanin pigment and stromal sclerosis; it has a blue tinctorial appearance clinically.

ICD-O coding

8780/0 Blue naevus of the conjunctiva
8780/0 Dendritic blue naevus
8790/0 Cellular blue naevus

ICD-11 coding

2F20.Y & XH7QJ7 Other specific types of melanocytic naevus & Blue naevus, NOS
2D00.Y & XH1G74 Other specified malignant neoplasm of conjunctiva & Blue naevus, malignant

Related terminology

None

Subtype(s)

Dendritic blue naevus; cellular blue naevus

Localization

The distribution is relatively even throughout the bulbar, forniceal, and palpebral conjunctiva and the caruncle {94,309,1479,2976}.

Clinical features

Blue naevi present as dark-brown to black, sharply demarcated, unifocal or multifocal, slightly elevated conjunctival masses, with a thickness of approximately 2 mm {309}. Unlike common acquired conjunctival naevi, blue naevi lack epithelial cysts and infrequently contain intrinsic or feeder vessels {309,2976}.

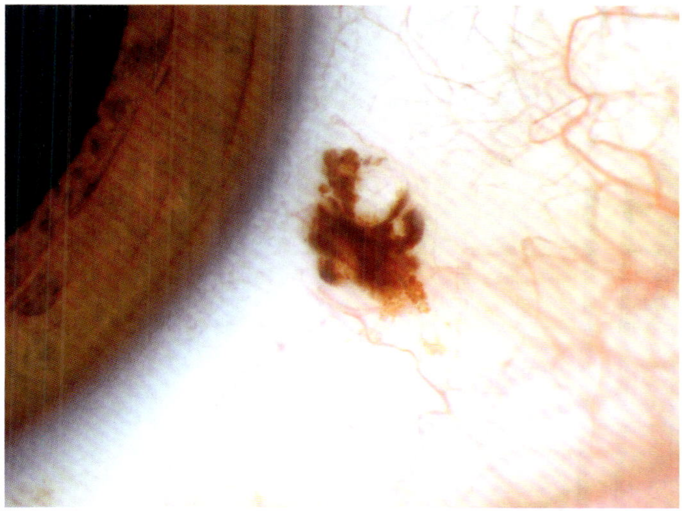

Fig. 2.47 Blue naevus of the conjunctiva. Clinical image showing a perilimbal conjunctival blue naevus.

Epidemiology

Blue naevi represent < 4% of conjunctival and caruncular naevi, occur with a slightly increased predilection in women, and are more common in White people {94,1096,2976,2862}. Conjunctival blue naevi are thought to be congenital, although most of them are diagnosed in the third to fifth decades of life {94,309,1096,2976}.

Etiology

Blue naevi are considered neural-crest lesions derived from primitive Schwann cell and melanocyte precursors. In contrast to common acquired naevi and cutaneous melanomas, ultraviolet (UV) sun light irradiation is not an important etiological factor {274}. Familial/syndromic aggregation exists, such as in

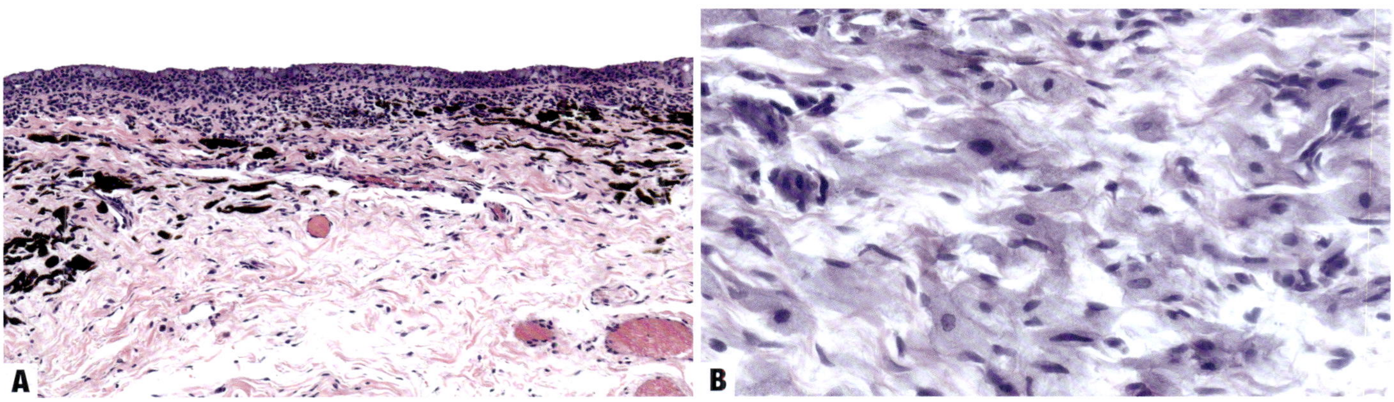

Fig. 2.48 Dendritic blue naevus of the conjunctiva. **A** Conjunctival substantia propria containing pigmented bland spindle/dendritic/stellate melanocytic cells in the conjunctival substantia propria is seen. The melanocytic cells show slender, branching networks of dendritic processes. **B** A bleach preparation reveals the bland spindle cells of dendritic (common) blue naevus.

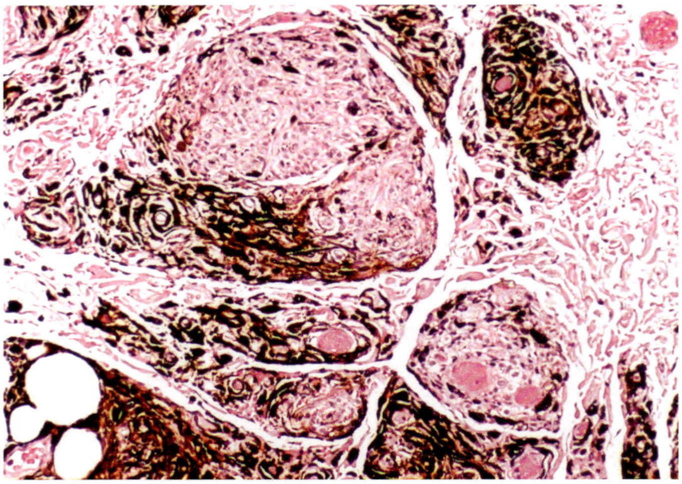

Fig. 2.49 Cellular blue naevus of the conjunctiva. This shows a combination of conjunctival conventional blue naevus and cellular blue naevus. The latter is seen as less-pigmented nests of plumper spindle/ovoid cells.

LAMB syndrome (lentigines, atrial myxomas, mucocutaneous myxomas, and blue naevi) or NAME syndrome (naevi, atrial myxomas, myxoid neurofibromas, and ephelides) of the Carney complex {3740,2320}.

Pathogenesis

Blue naevi and intradermal melanocytic proliferations (melanocytic neoplasms of the uvea and leptomeninges) probably arise from a distinct type of melanocyte that originates from the neural crest through the ventromedial developmental pathway arresting in the conjunctival substantia propria {274,2747}. Although less well described than in cutaneous blue naevi, driver mutations in G protein–coupled receptors (especially those in *GNAQ*) have also been reported in conjunctival blue naevi {1025,1148}.

Macroscopic appearance

See *Clinical features*.

Histopathology

Dendritic (common) blue naevi comprise heavily pigmented bland spindle/dendritic/stellate melanocytic cells in the conjunctival substantia propria {2862,309,886,993,1463}. The melanocytic cells show slender, branching networks of dendritic processes, frequently associated with melanophages and stromal fibrosis {2862,309,886,993}. No cellular atypia is present.

Cellular blue naevi contain dense aggregates of cytologically bland, pigmented spindle cells and/or ovoid, variably pigmented melanocytic cells, located in the substantia propria, arranged as sheets or fascicles, surrounded by collagen and melanophages, frequently set in a background of common blue naevus {2862,358,772,993}.

In both benign blue naevus subtypes, mitotic figures are absent {993}. There is no associated junctional melanocytic proliferation or entrapped epithelial cysts, except in combined or collision lesions such as combined melanocytic naevus. These show features of both conventional melanocytic and blue naevi {689,1685}. The histological differential diagnosis is covered in Table 2.02.

Immunohistochemistry

The spindle/dendritic/stellate melanocytic cells are positive for S100, melan-A, and SOX10, and they can be positive for HMB45 antigen {2862}. The melanophages are CD68 positive {2862}.

Table 2.02 Differential diagnosis of conjunctival blue naevus

Diagnosis	Main histological features	References
Conventional conjunctival blue naevus	Heavily pigmented bland spindle/dendritic/stellate melanocytic cells in the conjunctival substantia propria; melanocytic cells show slender, branching networks of dendritic processes, frequently associated with melanophages and stromal fibrosis; no cellular atypia is present; mitotic figures are absent; no associated junctional melanocytic proliferation or entrapped epithelial cysts, except in combined or collision lesions	See *Blue naevus of the conjunctiva* (p. 65) {2862,993}
Cellular blue naevus	Dense aggregates of cytologically bland pigmented spindle cells and/or ovoid variably pigmented melanocytic cells, arranged as sheets or fascicles, surrounded by collagen and melanophages, frequently set in a background of common blue naevus	See *Blue naevus of the conjunctiva* (p. 65) {2862,993}
Pigmented conventional melanocytic naevus	Do not tend to feature spindle/dendritic/stellate melanocytic cells and commonly contain epithelial cysts	See *Junctional, compound, and subepithelial conjunctival naevi* (p. 60) {2862,993}
Invasive conjunctival melanoma	Cytologically atypical melanocytic cells in the substantia propria with or without mitotic figures; conjunctival melanocytic intraepithelial lesion may be present	See *Conjunctival melanoma* (p. 75) {2862,993}
Malignant blue naevus	Less pigmented, cytologically atypical, mitotically active melanocytic cells in the context of a blue naevus background	{772,2862,993}
Extrascleral extension of uveal melanoma	Will contaminate the deep aspect of the biopsy with a broad base and will comprise atypical spindle/epithelioid melanocytic cells with prominent nucleoli, with or without mitotic figures, in the setting of an intraocular uveal mass	See *Choroidal and ciliary body melanomas* (p. 179) {2862,993}
Pigmented foreign bodies	Intrinsically acellular although may excite a foreign body histiocytic response mimicking melanophages; examples include minerals, mascara, graphite, and adrenaline pigment	{2119,3045,1219,2691}

Cytology
Not relevant

Diagnostic molecular pathology
Diagnostic molecular pathology may be helpful in occasional difficult cases (see *Pathogenesis*).

Essential and desirable diagnostic criteria
Dendritic blue naevus
Essential: heavily pigmented, loosely arranged, non-atypical spindle/stellate/dendritic cells within the conjunctival substantia propria; the melanocytic cells do not show pleomorphism, nuclear atypia, or hyperchromasia.

Desirable: sclerotic stroma with melanophages; immunohistochemical positivity with the melanocytic markers melan-A, SOX10, and S100; CD68 positivity of melanophages.

Cellular blue naevus
Essential: sheets or fascicles of variably pigmented spindle to ovoid cells surrounded by sclerotic stroma and numerous melanophages; the melanocytic cells do not show pleomorphism, nuclear atypia, or hyperchromasia.

Desirable: presence of dendritic blue naevus features surrounding cellular blue naevus; immunohistochemical positivity with the melanocytic markers melan-A, SOX10, S100; CD68 positivity of melanophages.

Staging
Not relevant

Prognosis and prediction
The prognosis for blue naevi is excellent. Blue naevi (particularly the cellular subtype) of the conjunctiva have very rarely been described to give rise to conjunctival melanoma, which has been described in just 1 case after acquisition of *BAP1* loss {772,1148}.

WNT-activated deep penetrating / plexiform melanocytoma (naevus)

Pižem J
Moulin A
Verdijk RM

Definition

WNT-activated deep penetrating / plexiform melanocytoma (naevus) (DPMN) is a melanocytic tumour composed of relatively large, finely pigmented ovoid or epithelioid melanocytes and genetically characterized by activation of the MAPK and WNT/β-catenin pathways. On the conjunctiva, almost all such lesions present as combined naevi.

ICD-O coding

8720/1 WNT-activated deep penetrating / plexiform melanocytoma (naevus)

ICD-11 coding

2F20.Y & XH81Y1 Other specific types of melanocytic naevus & Deep penetrating naevus

Related terminology

Acceptable: deep penetrating melanocytoma; plexiform spindle cell melanocytoma; deep penetrating naevus; plexiform spindle cell naevus.

Not recommended: epithelioid naevus; inverted type A naevus; clonal naevus.

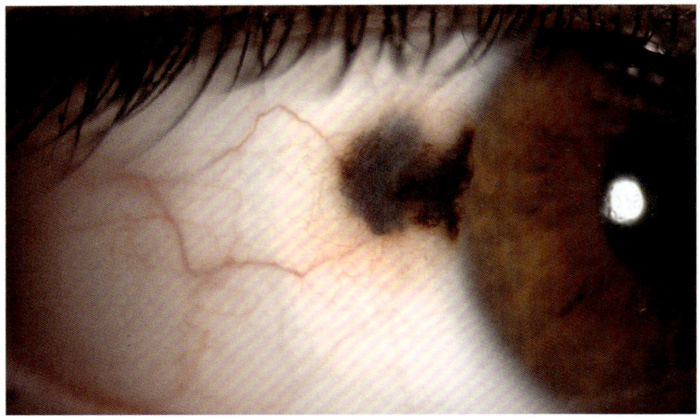

Fig. 2.50 Combined deep penetrating naevus. A variably pigmented combined conventional and deep penetrating naevus involving the bulbar conjunctiva and limbus.

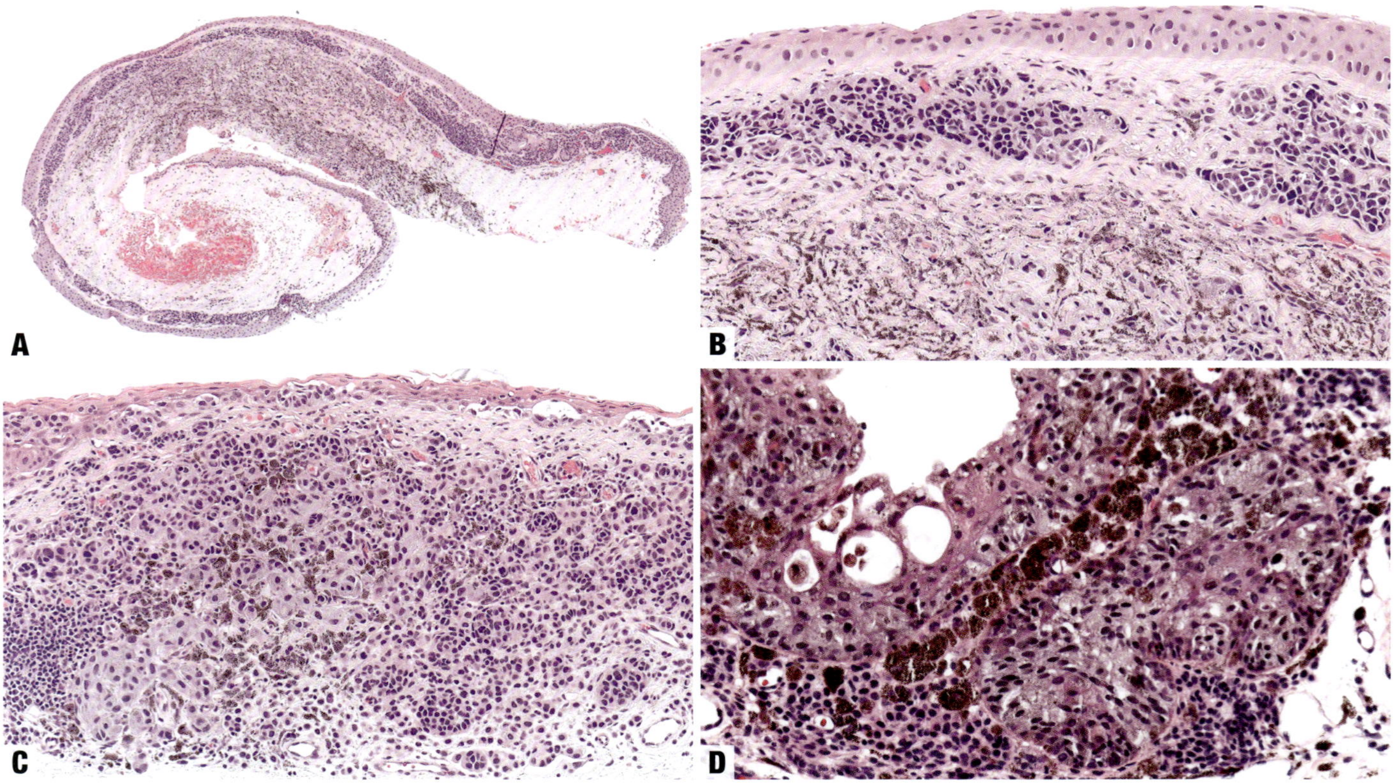

Fig. 2.51 Combined deep penetrating naevus. **A** Pigmented subepithelial deep penetrating naevus beneath a superficially located conventional naevus. **B** In the deep penetrating naevus, intensely pigmented melanophages predominate over small nests of lightly pigmented epithelioid melanocytes. **C** Subepithelial deep penetrating naevus (left) within a conventional naevus. **D** Combined deep penetrating naevus with an intraepithelial component of a deep penetrating naevus within the epithelium of inclusion cysts and an adjacent subepithelial component of a conventional naevus.

Subtype(s)
None

Localization
WNT-activated DPMNs are most frequent on the bulbar conjunctiva, followed by the plica and caruncle {2911,1463,3441}.

Clinical features
Most WNT-activated DPMNs are darkly pigmented. Changes in size and colour are noted in three quarters of cases, sometimes raising the clinical suspicion of a melanoma. An appearance of dark pigmentation within a pre-existent naevus may point to a WNT-activated DPMN {2911,1463,3441,1330}.

Epidemiology
WNT-activated DPMN of the conjunctiva shows a slight female predilection, with a wide age range (7–56 years). Combined lesions are relatively common, representing 9% of all excised conjunctival naevi in one series {2911}.

Etiology
Unknown

Pathogenesis
WNT-activated DPMN develops through combined activation of the MAPK pathway and WNT/β-catenin signalling, which is usually mediated by a *CTNNB1* gene mutation {3693}. In WNT-activated DPMN of the conjunctiva, the MAPK pathway activation seems to be exclusively mediated by the *BRAF* p.V600E mutations {2911,3441}.

Macroscopic appearance
WNT-activated DPMN is usually a dark-brown lesion, measuring from < 1 to 4 mm, sometimes in the background of a less intensively pigmented conventional naevus {2911}.

Histopathology
WNT-activated DPMN is characterized by nested or plexiform growth of relatively large ovoid or epithelioid melanocytes with a large amount of finely pigmented (dusty) cytoplasm. Maturation is absent. Mitoses are usually absent. Nests of melanocytes are practically always accompanied by melanophages {2911,3441, 1463,1330,3327}. Almost all WNT-activated DPMNs of the conjunctiva are part of a combined naevus (with either a common or an inflamed juvenile naevus) and in most cases represent its minor component. Most WNT-activated DPMNs are purely subepithelial, but they may be compound (in one third of cases) or rarely purely intraepithelial {2911}.

WNT-activated DPMNs of the conjunctiva are positive for BRAF p.V600E by immunohistochemistry and also show nuclear positivity for β-catenin and cyclin D1 {2911,3441,869}.

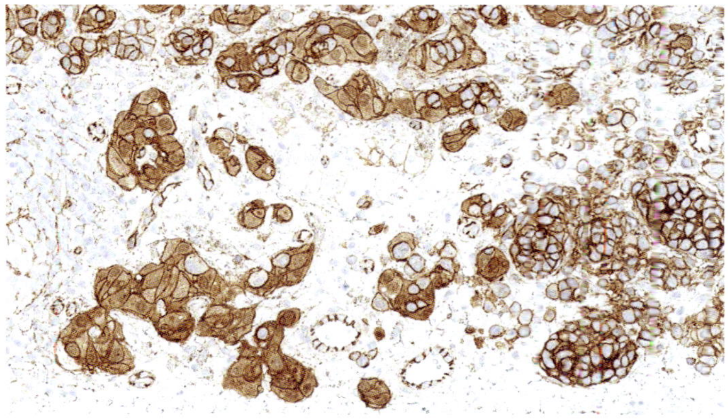

Fig. 2.52 Combined deep penetrating naevus. A diffuse nuclear positivity for β-catenin in melanocytes of deep penetrating naevus (lower left) and an absence of nuclear reaction in melanocytes of conventional naevus (right).

Retained p16 immunoreactivity and absent or only focal expression of PRAME can assist in differentiating WNT-activated melanocytoma from melanoma {859,1994,2910}

Cytology
Not clinically relevant

Diagnostic molecular pathology
In diagnostically challenging cases, molecular analysis can be performed to confirm the presence of a *CTNNB1* or *APC* mutation and to exclude additional mutations (such as *TERT* promoter mutations) and DNA copy-number changes indicative of melanoma {3441,859}.

Essential and desirable diagnostic criteria
Essential: nested or plexiform growth of large ovoid or epithelioid melanocytes with finely pigmented cytoplasm, typically accompanied by melanophages.

Desirable: nuclear positivity for β-catenin or a proven mutation in the WNT pathway.

Staging
Not clinically relevant

Prognosis and prediction
In diagnostically challenging cases, molecular analysis can be performed to confirm the presence of a *CTNNB1* or *APC* mutation and to exclude additional mutations (such as *TERT* promoter mutations) and DNA copy-number changes indicative of melanoma {3441,859}. This is a benign lesion with a very low risk of local recurrence {2911,3441,869}. While these lesions are histologically and molecularly similar to the skin equivalent, no further treatment is needed in most cases {2911,3441}.

Combined naevus

Pižem J
Mihic-Probst D
Moulin A
Verdijk RM

Definition
Combined naevus is a conjunctival compound or subepithelial melanocytic naevus with multiple histopathological phenotypes (clones) within the same lesion.

ICD-O coding
8720/0 Combined naevus
8780/0 Combined conventional and blue melanocytic naevus
8720/1 Combined conventional melanocytic naevus and WNT-activated deep penetrating / plexiform melanocytoma (naevus)
8720/0 Combined conventional and granular cell melanocytic naevus
8722/0 Combined conventional and balloon cell melanocytic naevus

ICD-11 coding
2F20.Y & XH0DU8 Other specific types of melanocytic naevus & Combined naevus

Related terminology
Acceptable: biphenotypic naevus; combined conjunctival melanocytoma.

Subtype(s)
Combined conventional and blue melanocytic naevus; combined conventional melanocytic naevus and WNT-activated deep penetrating / plexiform melanocytoma (naevus); combined conventional and granular cell melanocytic naevus; combined conventional and balloon cell melanocytic naevus

Localization
The distribution of combined naevi seems to be similar to that of conventional naevi; they are most common on the bulbar conjunctiva {688,2911,868,1463,3329}.

Clinical features
Combined naevi may show atypical features, including atypical dark coloration, irregular pigmentation, and a history of recent growth, prompting surgical excision or even raising the clinical suspicion of a melanoma {688,2911,868,1463}.

Epidemiology
Combined blue melanocytic naevi and combined WNT-activated deep penetrating / plexiform melanocytomas (naevi) (DPMNs) are relatively common {688,2976,2911}. Combined balloon cell naevi and combined granular cell naevi are rare. Age distribution seems to be similar to that of conventional naevi; they are most common in children and young adults but may affect elderly people {688,2911,868,1463,3329,869}.

Etiology
Unknown

Pathogenesis
It is currently unknown whether, similarly to combined WNT-activated DPMNs, the development of a blue, balloon cell, or granular cell component within a conventional naevus is caused by a secondary genetic event or is only a morphological spectrum of conventional naevi {688,2911,868,1463,3329,869}.

Macroscopic appearance
See *Clinical features*.

Histopathology
Combined melanocytic naevi are composed of a conventional naevus component (including inflamed juvenile naevus) and another morphologically distinct component {500}.

In combined blue naevus, a subepithelial blue naevus component is characterized by moderately to heavily pigmented fusiform and dendritic melanocytes. The extent of the blue naevus

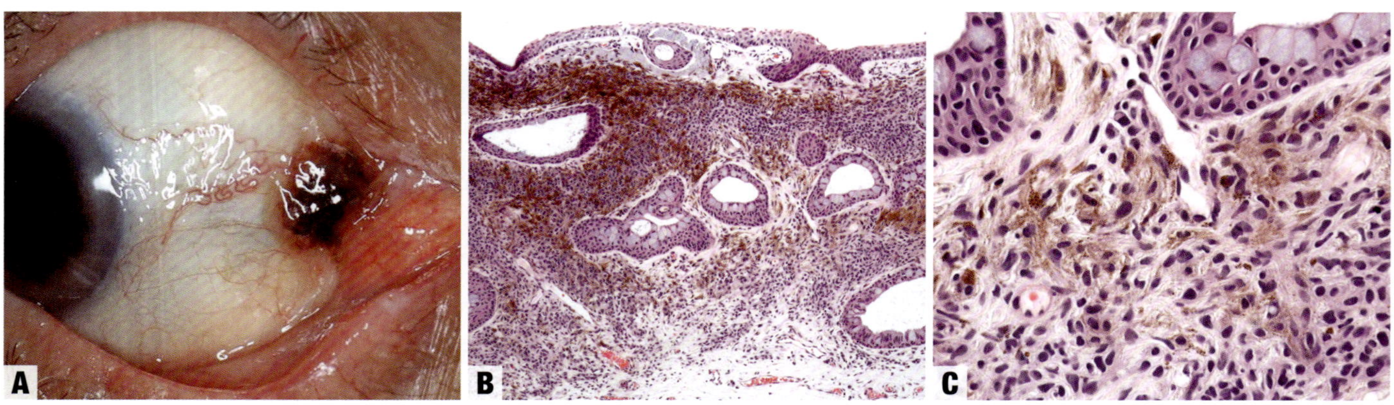

Fig. 2.53 Combined conventional and blue melanocytic naevus. **A** A raised, darkly pigmented lesion on the plica is seen. **B** The naevus is variably pigmented with entrapped epithelial cysts. **C** The blue naevus component is represented by pigmented spindled and dendritic melanocytes.

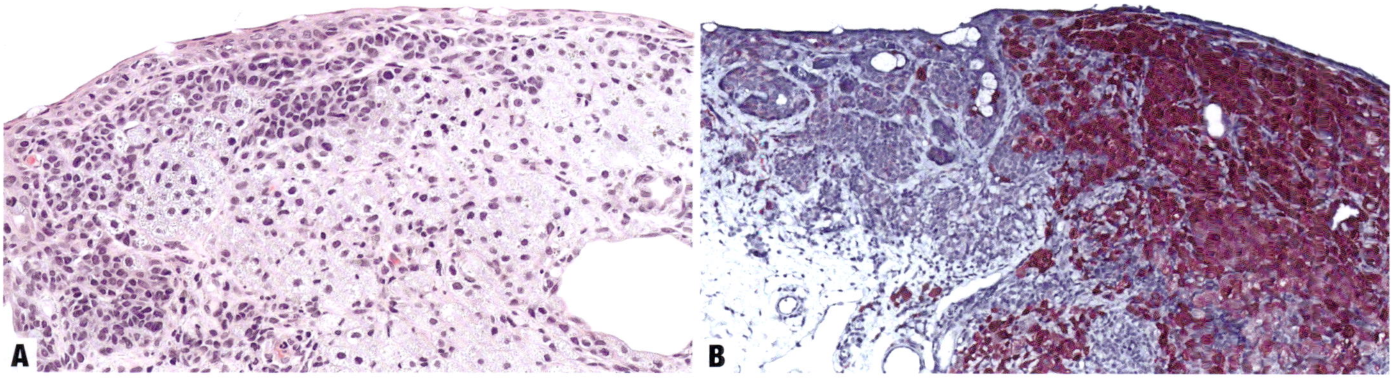

Fig. 2.54 Combined conventional and granular cell melanocytic naevus **A** The granular cell component is composed of relatively large melanocytes with lightly pigmented granular cytoplasm. **B** Diffuse positivity for HMB45 is seen in the granular cell component in contrast to the conventional naevus (left).

component varies from focal to extensive; it tends to be located in the deepest part of the naevus but may be superficial {688,1491}.

In combined WNT-activated DPMNs, a WNT-activated component is composed of nests of relatively large, finely pigmented ovoid or epithelioid melanocytes accompanied by melanophages (see *WNT-activated deep penetrating / plexiform melanocytoma (naevus)*, p. 68) {2911,3441}.

Combined granular cell naevus, characterized by large melanocytes with centrally placed nuclei, inconspicuous nucleoli, and abundant eosinophilic to lightly pigmented granular cytoplasm, has also been reported in the conjunctiva {868,1463}. The number of cases is small, and genetic changes are not yet well characterized, making it difficult to determine if these represent a distinct subtype. In contrast to those in WNT-activated DPMN, melanocytes in granular cell naevus lack nuclear expression of β-catenin {869}.

Balloon cell naevus is composed of large epithelioid melanocytes with abundant vacuolated, clear, or slightly foamy cytoplasm, usually lacking melanin pigment. There is no significant cytological atypia or mitotic activity. Balloon cells tend to lack expression of HMB45 {3329}.

Cytology

Not clinically relevant

Diagnostic molecular pathology

Not clinically relevant

Essential and desirable diagnostic criteria

Essential: the presence of two or more morphologically distinct melanocytic naevus components in a single lesion; a melanoma ex naevus must be ruled out.

Staging

Not clinically relevant

Prognosis and prediction

Combined naevi are benign lesions {688,2311,868,3329,869}.

Conjunctival melanocytic intraepithelial lesions

Coupland SE
Brouwer NJ
Milman T
Verdijk RM

Definition

Conjunctival melanocytic intraepithelial lesions (C-MILs) represent a spectrum of morphological changes ranging from melanocytic hyperplasia through degrees of melanocytic atypia to melanoma in situ.

ICD-O coding

8720/0 Low-grade conjunctival melanocytic intraepithelial lesion
8720/2 High-grade conjunctival melanocytic intraepithelial lesion

ICD-11 coding

2E63.1 Melanoma in situ of conjunctiva

Related terminology

Acceptable: conjunctival melanocytic intraepithelial neoplasia (C-MIN); primary acquired melanosis (PAM); melanoma in situ.

Not recommended: precancerous melanosis; premalignant melanosis; intraepithelial melanocytic proliferation with atypia.

Subtype(s)

None

Localization

These lesions are generally unilateral but often multifocal; they vary in size, involving a mean of three clock-hours of the conjunctiva {1859,3068,1902}. In decreasing frequency, C-MILs involve the bulbar, limbal, forniceal, and palpebral conjunctiva; they can also extend to the cornea and occur in the caruncle {3068}.

Clinical features

C-MIL is usually unilateral and appears as an acquired lesion in young to middle-aged adults. The lesions appear as flat, irregular brown discolourations of the conjunctiva, which may change (wax and wane) over time. The pigmentation is mobile over the substantia propria and Tenon fascia and episclera. In rare cases, C-MIL can be amelanotic, making it difficult to recognize clinically {714,3068}.

Imaging of conjunctival melanocytic lesions involves regular anterior segment photodocumentation (including with eversion of eyelids), slit-lamp microscopy, and potentially ultrasound biomicroscopy. Recent developments include anterior segment optical coherence tomography {3505,424} and in vivo reflectance confocal microscopy {622}.

Epidemiology

All of these lesions are most common in middle-aged and elderly people with a light complexion, but they can occasionally occur in individuals with darker pigmentation, and even in teenagers or young adults. The precise incidence of pigmented conjunctival lesions is difficult to estimate. In a North American analysis of 311 eyes with PAM (C-MIL), 96% of the cases were in White individuals and 4% were in Black, Hispanic, or Asian

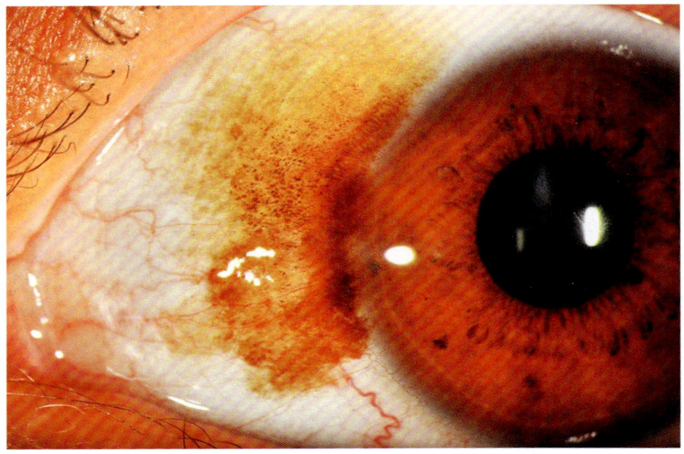

Fig. 2.55 Conjunctival melanocytic intraepithelial lesion. An example presenting as a flat, variably pigmented lesion in the bulbar conjunctiva and limbus.

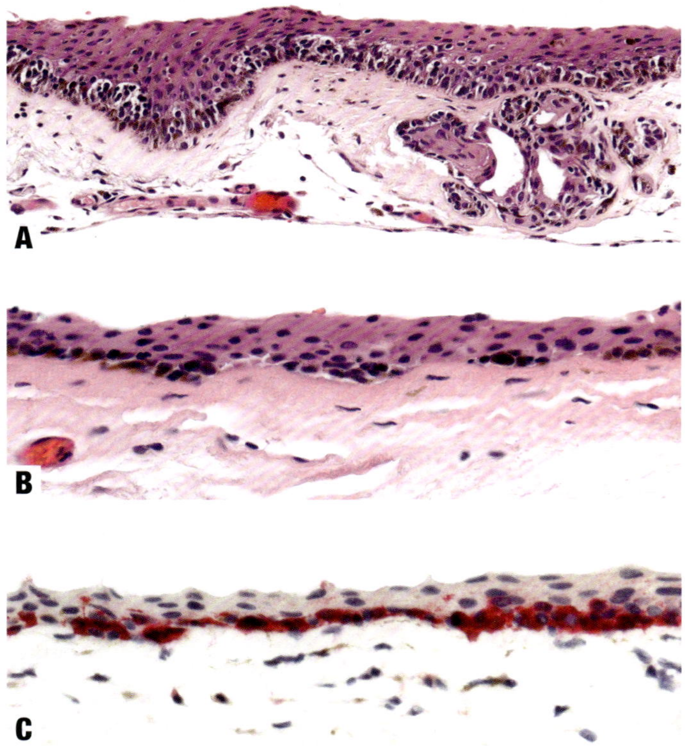

Fig. 2.56 Conjunctival melanocytic intraepithelial lesion. **A** A high-grade lesion with proliferation of neoplastic melanocytes. **B** A low-grade lesion with lentiginous proliferation of melanocytes. **C** A low-grade lesion with neoplastic cells displaying melan-A positivity.

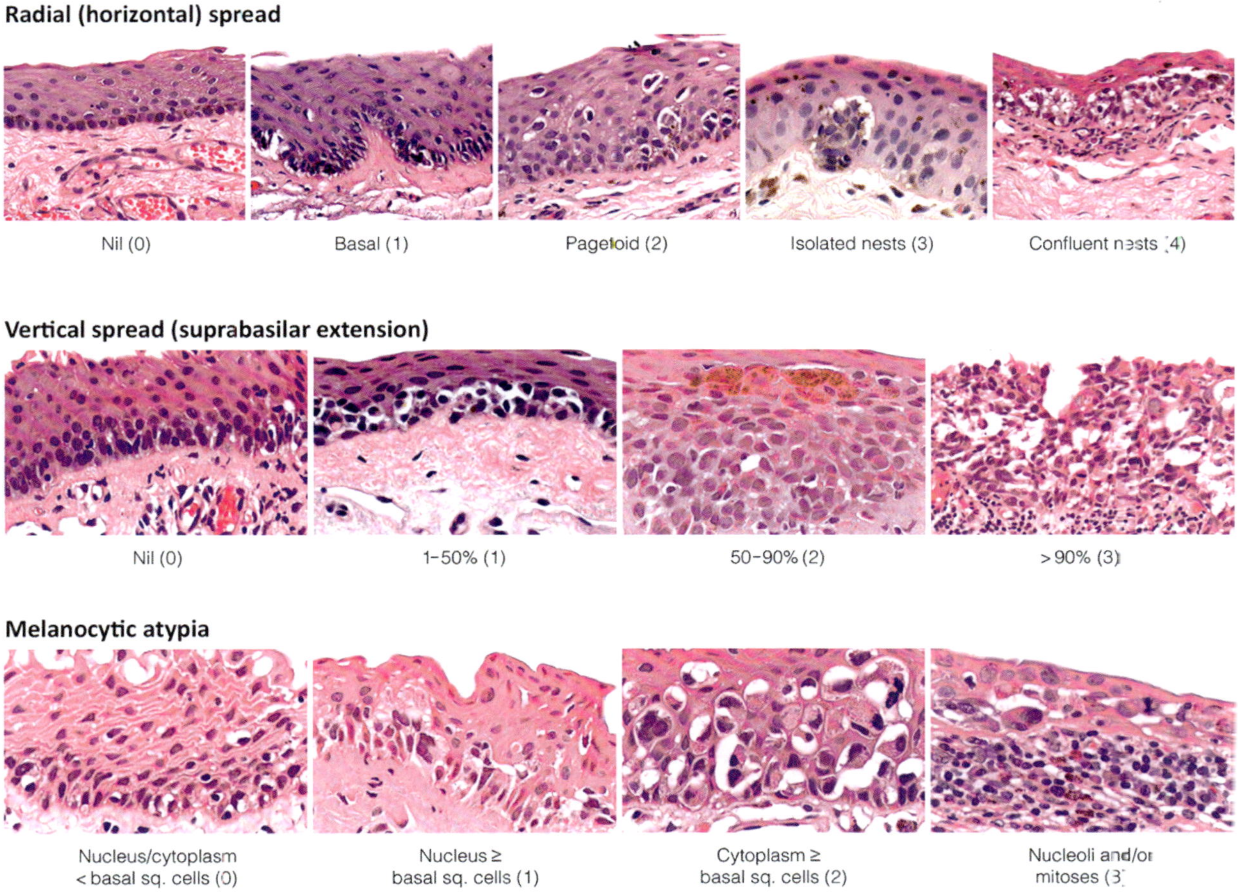

Fig. 2.57 Conjunctival melanocytic intraepithelial neoplasia scoring. Conjunctival melanocytic intraepithelial neoplasia is scored out of 10 based on the extent of horizontal (radial) spread and vertical spread (suprabasilar extension) of melanocytes, as well as the degree of atypia. sq., squamous.

individuals, with a patient age range of 15–90 years (mean: 56 years) {3068,1902}. There is no sex predilection {714,3068}.

Etiology

No environmental cause has been clearly established, but atypical C-MILs develop most frequently in the interpalpebral zone, suggesting an association with ultraviolet (UV) radiation {3719}.

Pathogenesis

C-MIL arises from basal conjunctival melanocytes {1457}. Little is known about the underlying genetic alterations, although *TERT* promoter mutations were found in 2 of 25 (8%) cases of PAM with atypia {1770}. *BRAF* p.V600E alterations occur in approximately 40% of conjunctival melanomas, but some studies suggest that these cases arise from naevi with mutations rather than from C-MIL {476,1860}.

Macroscopic appearance

See *Clinical features*.

Histopathology

The key microscopic features in C-MIL include increased cellularity of intraepithelial conjunctival melanocytes with increasing cytological atypia, while the basal membrane remains intact {3739,994,2209}. The spectrum of cytological features ranges from small melanocytes with nuclear hyperchromasia and scant cytoplasm to severely atypical large pleomorphic epithelioid cells with ample cytoplasm and prominent eosinophilic nucleoli. Atypical architectural patterns may be difficult to discern in the context of thin conjunctival epithelium. They include basilar single cell hyperplasia, basilar nesting, intraepithelial nests, pagetoid proliferation of single cells, and a confluent growth pattern at the epithelial–stromal junction {3739,994,2209}.

Terms commonly used to classify these lesions include "primary acquired melanosis (PAM) with atypia" and "conjunctival melanocytic intraepithelial neoplasia (C-MIN)", along with an emerging simplified classification into low-grade C-MIL, high-grade C-MIL, and conjunctival melanoma in situ. Various grading or scoring systems have been used for C-MIL {994,1465, 3229,714,715,1657,1457,2209}. The grading of the cytological atypia in PAM (mild, moderate, or severe) was like that used in the skin and other mucosal sites {994,2052}. The C-MIN scoring system was based on architectural features (i.e. horizontal and vertical spread) and cytological atypia with a C-MIN score of 0 representing hypermelanosis only (see *Benign epithelial melanosis of the conjunctiva*, p. 58); of 1 corresponding to PAM without atypia; of 2–4 being PAM with atypia; and of ≥ 5 equating to melanoma in situ {715}.

The fourth edition of the WHO classification of tumours of the eye proposed a simplified terminology: (1) low-grade C-MIL

Table 2.03 2022 WHO classification of conjunctival melanocytic intraepithelial lesions

WHO terminology	Acceptable alternative terminology	Increased cellularity	Histological features	Risk of association with or progression to invasive melanoma
Not applicable	Benign melanosis Primary acquired melanosis (PAM) without atypia Conjunctival melanocytic intraepithelial neoplasia (C-MIN) (grades 0–1)	No/minimal	Conjunctival hypermelanosis (increased pigment in epithelial cells without melanocytic hyperplasia or atypia); slight or focal melanocytic hyperplasia without atypia (parabasal melanocytes with condensed round nuclei, smaller than basal epithelial cells, inconspicuous nucleoli, and inconspicuous cytoplasm) may be seen	None
Low-grade conjunctival melanocytic intraepithelial lesion (C-MIL)	PAM with mild atypia C-MIN (grades 2–4)	Yes	Predominantly basilar melanocytic proliferation with low-grade atypia (dendritic or small to moderate-sized polyhedral, usually non-epithelioid melanocytes with round to irregular nuclear contours, often nuclear hyperchromasia, inconspicuous nucleoli, and inconspicuous or scant cytoplasm)	Lower
High-grade C-MIL	PAM with moderate to severe atypia C-MIN (grades 5–10)	Yes	More confluent basilar and significant non-basilar proliferation of melanocytes with high-grade atypia (moderate to severe), evidence of intraepithelial nested and/or pagetoid growth, and epithelioid cell cytomorphology	Higher
	Melanoma in situ	Yes	The term "melanoma in situ" may be used for (1) the most atypical high-grade C-MILs involving close to full thickness of the epithelium, (2) histologically obvious melanomas without documented evidence of subepithelial invasion	Highest

corresponding to PAM without atypia or with mild atypia and lesions with C-MIN score of 1–2; (2) high-grade C-MIL, corresponding to PAM with moderate to severe atypia and C-MIN scores of 3–5; and (3) conjunctival melanoma in situ, corresponding to PAM with severe atypia generally involving > 75% of the epithelium and a C-MIN score of > 5 (see Table 2.03) {2295}. This C-MIL system results in similar interobserver agreement to PAM and C-MIN terminology {2209}. The C-MIL definition of conjunctival melanoma in situ is concordant with that of the current American Joint Committee on Cancer (AJCC) TNM staging system (pTis) {414}.

Immunohistochemistry

Atypical conjunctival melanocytes are immunoreactive for melan-A, S100, HMB45, MITF, and SOX10. Cyclin D1 is also of value in highlighting the atypical melanocytes {2301}. The role of PRAME immunohistochemistry requires further examination {1878,2910}. Melanocytic proliferation can be assessed by Ki-67 staining {3169}.

Differential diagnosis

Potential mimics of C-MIL include benign epithelial melanosis of the conjunctiva (see *Benign epithelial melanosis of the conjunctiva*, p. 58); oculodermal melanocytosis; conjunctival naevi, particularly those with junctional activity (see *Junctional, compound, and subepithelial conjunctival naevi*, p. 60); invasive melanoma (see *Conjunctival melanoma*, p. 75); pigmented conjunctival squamous intraepithelial neoplasia (see *Conjunctival squamous intraepithelial neoplasia*, p. 48) {693}; systemic conditions, such as Addison disease {1657}; postinflammatory hyperpigmentation; and conjunctival tattooing {2993}. Extension of C-MIL into conjunctival epithelial invaginations in the underlying lamina propria (pseudoglands of Henle) should not be misdiagnosed as invasive conjunctival melanoma.

Cytology

Not commonly performed

Diagnostic molecular pathology

Diagnostic molecular pathology is not regularly used, although assessment of copy-number variations involving *RREB1* (6p24), *MYB* (6q23), and *CCND1* (11q13) have been found to be of value in difficult cases {452,2304}.

Essential and desirable diagnostic criteria

Essential: varying degrees of increased cellularity and atypia of conjunctival melanocytes within the epithelium extending upward from the epithelial base, displacing squamous and/or goblet cells; no evidence of invasive growth.

Desirable: immunohistochemistry to confirm melanocytic phenotype, particularly in morphologically challenging cases.

Staging

The AJCC / Union for International Cancer Control (UICC) TNM staging system is used (pTis = conjunctival melanoma in situ).

Prognosis and prediction

PAM/C-MIL is a precursor of 50–70% of all conjunctival melanomas {1657}; consequently, there is an absolute clinical need to know when to treat patients with surgery, cryotherapy, and/or topical chemotherapeutics (e.g. topical mitomycin C) {714,3068}. Epithelioid cell morphology with cytological atypia, cell nesting, and pagetoid spread is associated with an increased risk of recurrence and progression to melanoma {2052,994,3229,3739, 3068}. In contrast, C-MIL composed solely of hyperchromatic melanocytes with scant cytoplasm and nuclei devoid of discernible nucleoli is less likely to be associated with invasive melanoma {3229,3068}. For prognosis and prediction regarding conjunctival melanoma see *Conjunctival melanoma* (p. 75).

Conjunctival melanoma

Moulin A
Brouwer NJ
Ferreira TA
Jager MJ
Verdijk RM

Definition
Conjunctival melanoma is an invasive malignant melanocytic neoplasm arising in the conjunctiva.

ICD-O coding
8720/3 Conjunctival melanoma

ICD-11 coding
2D00.0 Melanoma of conjunctiva

Related terminology
None

Subtype(s)
None

Localization
Conjunctival melanoma can affect any part of the conjunctiva (i.e. bulbar, forniceal, palpebral, caruncular/plical). Most often it presents on the bulbar surface, near the limbus. Invasion of corneal tissue, eyelid margin, sclera, or orbit may occur in advanced tumours {2995}.

Clinical features
Lesions vary in size, configuration, and colour. Nodular lesions may be well circumscribed, while flat lesions with irregular margins can be difficult to delineate, particularly in cases with surrounding primary acquired melanosis / conjunctival melanocytic intraepithelial lesion. The colour of lesions may range from amelanotic (pale or pink) to darker shades of brown or black, and can be patchy or mixed within one lesion {425}. No pigmentation, or mixed tumour pigmentation, is found in 40% of cases. Lack of cysts (observed in conjunctival naevi), tumoural haemorrhage, large tumour base, tortuous feeder vessels, adherence to the sclera away from the limbus, corneal invasion, and multifocal lesions favour melanoma over conjunctival naevus {3021}.

High-resolution MRI allows the identification of most eyelid structures. Therefore, MRI has a crucial role in the assessment of the local extension of a melanoma of the conjunctiva inside the eyelid. It is also important to evaluate whether the nearby structures are invaded, in particular if there is orbital invasion. Furthermore, MRI aids in the differential diagnosis with other eyelid masses; in particular, diffusion- and perfusion-weighted imaging help in differentiating a melanoma of the conjunctiva from benign eyelid masses. Finally, in the case of a melanotic melanoma, high signal on T1-weighted images and low signal on T2-weighted images are expected, also helping in distinguishing a melanoma of the conjunctiva from other eyelid masses {957}.

Epidemiology
Conjunctival melanoma represents 5% of all ocular melanomas and is the second most prevalent malignancy of the conjunctiva {2969}. The incidence ranges from 0.3 to 0.8 cases per 1 million person-years. The incidence is highest in (northern) Europe and North America; people of Asian or African descent are less commonly affected {3400,1106,3499,1384}. The incidence of conjunctival melanoma has risen over the last five decades {1432,1859}. Conjunctival melanoma mainly affects patients from the fifth or sixth decade of life onwards and is rare in children. There is no clear sex predilection {1432,3400,1859}.

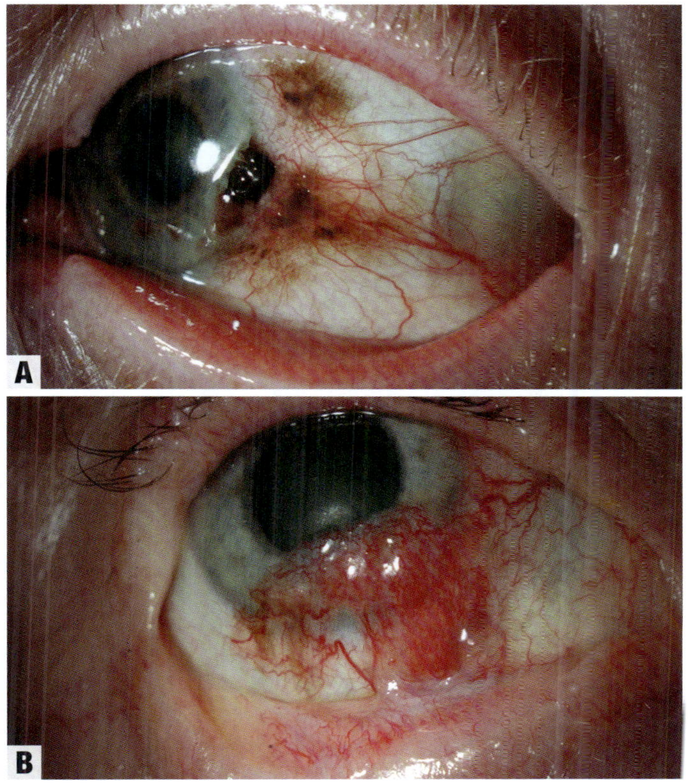

Fig. 2.58 Conjunctival melanoma. **A** Limbal masses with tortuous feeder vessels are shown. There is multifocal irregular pigmentation. **B** Aggressive recurrences can be non-pigmented.

Etiology
Several studies revealed C>T transitions suggestive of ultraviolet (UV) light exposure {624,765,2314,2722}, consistent with more frequent development in the interpalpebral fissure, which is exposed to the sun. Since conjunctival melanoma can develop in non-exposed sites, other (unknown) mechanisms are debated {427}.

Pathogenesis
Conjunctival melanoma arises in 60–70% of cases from conjunctival melanocytic intraepithelial lesions (C-MIN/PAM with

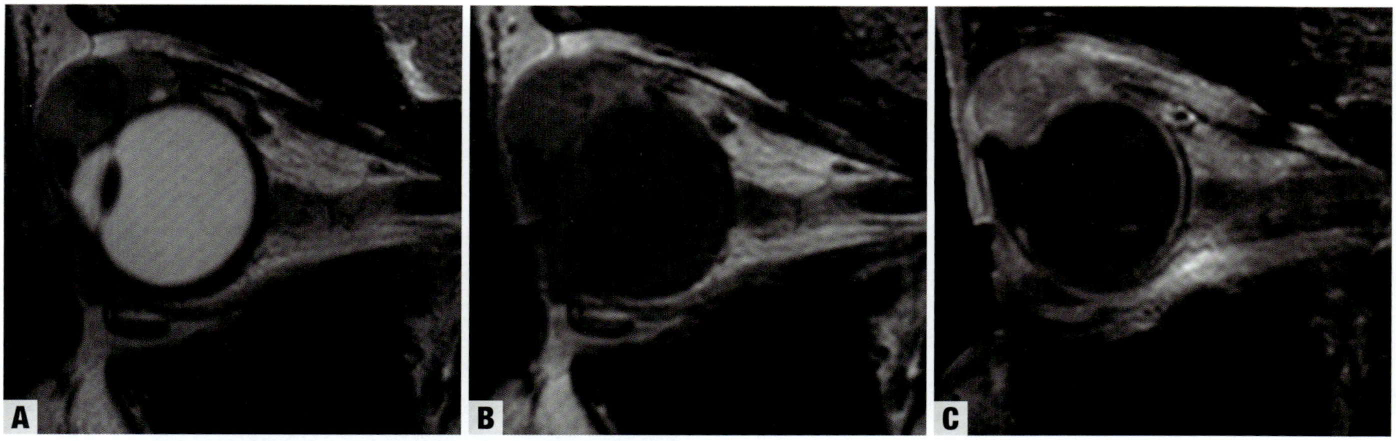

Fig. 2.59 Conjunctival melanoma. Sagittal T2-weighted MRI (**A**), T1-weighted MRI (**B**), and contrast-enhanced T1-weighted MRI with fat signal suppression (**C**) show a bilobated mass located deep in the right upper eyelid, of intermediate signal intensity on the T1- and T2-weighted images and enhancing. Anteriorly, it invades the orbital septum and almost reaches the orbicularis oculi muscle. Posteriorly, there is orbital invasion, with the tumour invading the levator palpebrae and superior rectus muscles.

atypia), while a smaller proportion develop from pre-existing naevi or are de novo {1860,2995}.

Pan-genomic studies demonstrated a high tumour mutation burden {624,765,2314,2722}. Driver mutations include *NF1* (33–50%), *BRAF* (29–46%), and *NRAS* (11–26%) mutations {624, 1859,1169,2881,1074,3446}. An *ATRX* mutation (25%) often co-occurs with an *NF1* mutation {1842}. *TERT* promoter mutations, identified in as many as 54% of cases, and *NRAS* mutations have been associated with metastatic disease {3446,1842}. Other oncogenic mutations occur in *CTNNB1* (17%) {1074}; *ACSS3* {624}; and (rarely) *RET*, *TP53*, *KIT*, *TET2*, *CDKN2A*, *MAPK21*, *RAC1*, *MET*, *SF3B1*, *GNAQ*, and *GNA11* {624,1074, 1842}. Gain of 6p is the most common aneuploidy, and 10q loss has been associated with metastatic disease {1656}. Many other copy-number alterations have been described {1656, 624}. Most tumours show cytogenetic rearrangements involving multiple chromosomes {1656,624}.

Macroscopic appearance

Lesions appear as flat to nodular conjunctival masses with variable pigmentation.

Histopathology

The histological features are similar to those of invasive melanoma in the skin or mucosa {3739}. The intraepithelial/radial component can be nested, pagetoid, lentiginous, or (rarely) absent. It can extend well beyond the invasive component and involve the skin, minor lacrimal glands, and/or cornea. The subepithelial/vertical component shows stromal invasion by nests or sheets of atypical melanocytes. Melanoma cells can show the entire spectrum of cytomorphology encountered in melanoma elsewhere, ranging from small naevoid cells to highly atypical pleomorphic melanocytes with spindle or epithelioid cytomorphology. Nuclei can be hyperchromatic with inconspicuous nucleoli or vesicular with prominent nucleoli, and sometimes giant, pleomorphic nuclei can be found. Ulceration, mitotic activity, angiotropism, satellite and in-transit metastases, and neurotropism may be seen. A residual naevus may be present. Invasive growth can be associated with melanophages as well as a predominantly lymphocytic infiltrate. Increased mitotic activity (> 5.5 mitoses/mm^2) has been associated with nodal metastasis, whereas ulceration and greater tumour thickness have been associated with increased mortality {912}. Conjunctival melanomas express melan-A (MART1), S100, SOX10, HMB45, and MITF. PDL1 may be expressed {1865}.

Conjunctival melanoma in situ and C-MIN/PAM with atypia can extend into pseudoglands of Henle, and this should be distinguished from truly invasive melanoma. The distinction from an atypical conjunctival naevus can also sometimes be

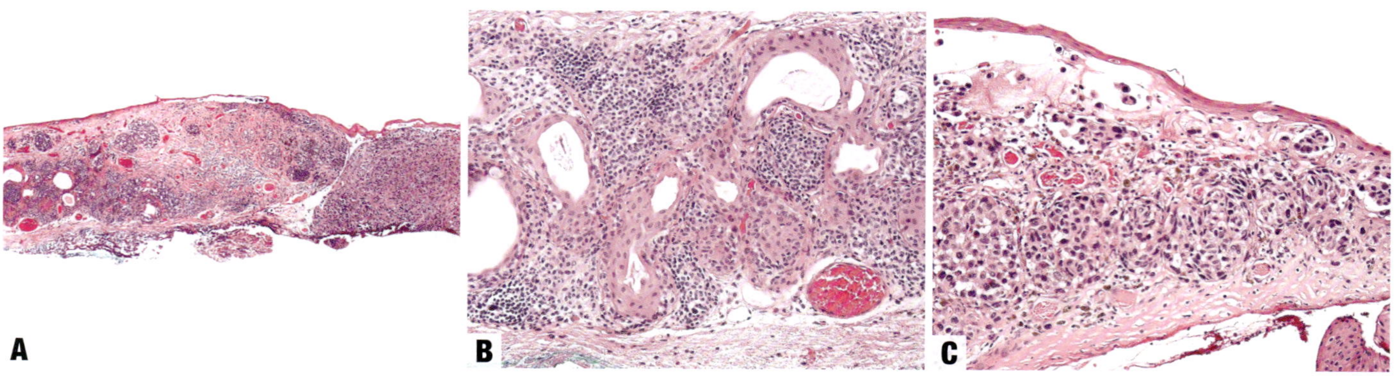

Fig. 2.60 Conjunctival melanoma. **A** Conjunctival melanoma (right) and residual naevus with pseudoglands (left). **B** Residual naevus with maturation. **C** Melanoma with intraepithelial large nests of discohesive, epithelioid cells and vertical growth phase in large nests.

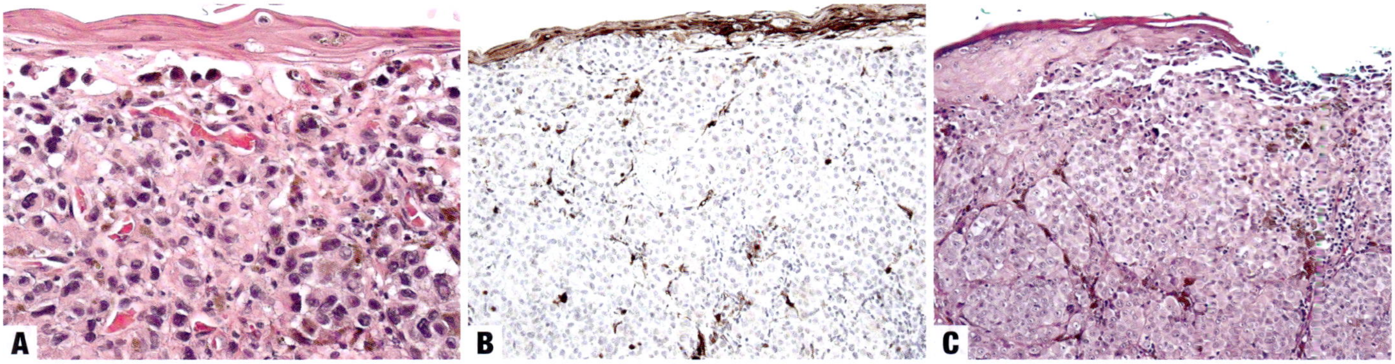

Fig. 2.61 Conjunctival melanoma. **A** Atypical cells with enlarged hyperchromatic nuclei are seen. Pagetoid spread is also present. **B** p16 nuclear loss in the radial and vertical growth phase. **C** Recurrent conjunctival melanoma with epithelioid morphology invading the eyelid.

challenging, especially at a young age, notably in inflamed juvenile naevus. Conjunctival naevi can also show lateral extension beyond the subepithelial component, large junctional nests, and pagetoid spread. Locally invasive behaviour, necrosis, and mitotic activity in the deep stromal portion of the tumour are features favouring malignancy. Immunohistochemistry can be helpful: loss of p16 nuclear expression, 5-hydroxymethylcytosine loss, PRAME nuclear expression, and pS6 activation have been described in conjunctival melanoma {3191,2910,877}.

Cytology

Not relevant

Diagnostic molecular pathology

Aneuploidy, assessed by FISH (6p gains, 11q gains, and/or 6q loss), has been used to distinguish conjunctival melanoma from atypical conjunctival naevus {2304,2080}. Nuclear expression of PRAME and loss of p16 on immunohistochemistry is more common in conjunctival melanoma than in naevi {2910, 877}.

As some tumours have actionable mutations, molecular investigation of lesions is often indicated, particularly if metastatic. Targeted therapy aimed at reported mutations (see *Pathogenesis*, above) is currently under investigation {427}.

Essential and desirable diagnostic criteria

Essential: stromal invasion; severe cytological and architectural atypia exceeding that expected in a naevus.

Desirable: demonstration of melanocytic markers by immunohistochemistry; pagetoid growth; mitotic activity; invasion into cornea or skin; ulceration; tumour necrosis.

Staging

Tumours are clinically staged by the American Joint Committee on Cancer (AJCC) / Union for International Cancer Control (UICC) TNM system, which has been validated for development of metastasis and survival {1454,1519}.

While sentinel lymph node biopsy appears promising, large comparative studies are lacking {2263}.

Prognosis and prediction

Conjunctival melanoma may extend locally into the eye or eyelid, invade the orbit, disseminate through the lacrimal drainage system, or spread through the lymphatics {913}.

Local recurrences occur in 29–45% in 5 years {2995,3400, 426}. Factors associated with local recurrence include tumour thickness ≥ 2 mm, non-bulbar location, epithelioid cell type, lack of tumour pigmentation, and lymphatic invasion {2995, 3400,1519,426}.

The 10-year disease-specific mortality rate is 25–35% {2488, 2995}. Tumour-related death has been associated with de novo origin and location in the non-bulbar conjunctiva, as well as nodular growth, multifocal location, and sentinel lymph node positivity {2969,145,2488,2995,912}. Negative microscopic features include mitoses {911} and lymphatic invasion {2995,3400, 1519}, as well as angiotropic satellite and in-transit metastases {261}. Lymphocytic infiltration may be favourable, but the findings are conflicting {427}.

Metastatic spread may occur to regional lymph nodes, or be more general, most often involving the lungs, liver, and brain {913,426}. Factors predictive of metastasis include larger size, increased tumour thickness, and orbital invasion. Incisional biopsy and excision without adjuvant therapy have also been correlated with poor outcome {1860,426}.

Conjunctival melanomas may respond to targeted therapy with tyrosine kinase inhibitors, or immunotherapy {1172,427}. PDL1 is expressed in conjunctival melanoma and relates to the presence of distant metastases and worse survival {1865,475}. Checkpoint inhibitor therapy has been reported as successful in several cases and is currently under investigation {427}.

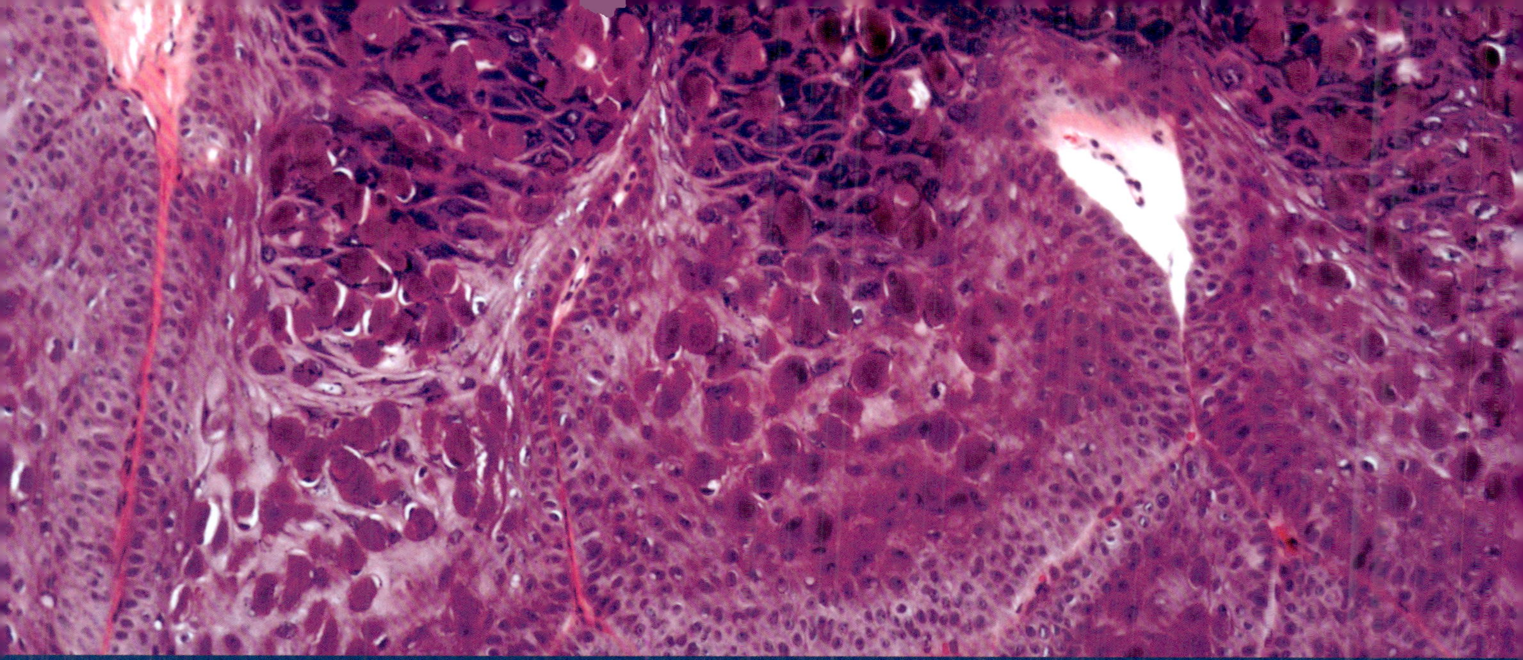

3

Tumours of the eyelid

Edited by: Coupland SE, Eberhart CG, Esmaeli B, Grossniklaus HE, Lazar AJ, Milman T, Mudhar HS, Vemuganti GK, Verdijk RM

Tumours of the eyelid: Introduction

Mudhar HS
Eberhart CG

The eyelid comprises five layers: skin, subcutis, orbicularis muscle, tarsal plate (containing the Meibomian glands), and tarsal conjunctiva. The grey line that represents the most superficial fibres of orbicularis divides the eyelid into an anterior lamella (skin and orbicularis) and a posterior lamella (tarsal plate and conjunctiva). The eyelid is replete with glandular tissue: the eccrine glands, the glands of Moll (apocrine glands), the accessory lacrimal glands of Wolfring, and the sebaceous glands (Meibomian glands and glands of Zeis).

Eyelid skin gives rise to a rich variety of epithelial and non-epithelial benign and malignant tumours. Many of these lesions are covered in this chapter with attention to site-specific characteristics. Most eyelid-skin tumours are benign, with the commonest entities being squamous papilloma, seborrhoeic keratosis, melanocytic naevus, and hidrocystoma {776}. Malignant tumours account for 5–10% of all skin cancers. There is considerable geographical, racial, and age-related variation in the incidence of various eyelid tumours. Among White people, basal cell carcinoma accounts for most cases of malignant eyelid tumours in the Western Hemisphere {776,1200}, whereas in Asia, sebaceous carcinoma is the commonest eyelid malignancy {2381, 1569,2037}.

Given the concentration of various glands in the eyelid tissues, there are a number of rare adnexal tumours that have a particular proclivity for the eyelid. These include sebaceous neoplasms (adenoma, sebaceoma, and carcinoma), endocrine mucin-producing sweat gland carcinoma {3738,2111}, mucinous carcinoma {286,43}, eccrine signet-ring cell / histiocytoid carcinoma {2701}, microcystic adnexal carcinoma {236}, and apocrine neoplasms (adenoma and adenocarcinoma). These tumours are encountered more frequently by ophthalmic pathologists than general pathologists and dermatopathologists in routine practice.

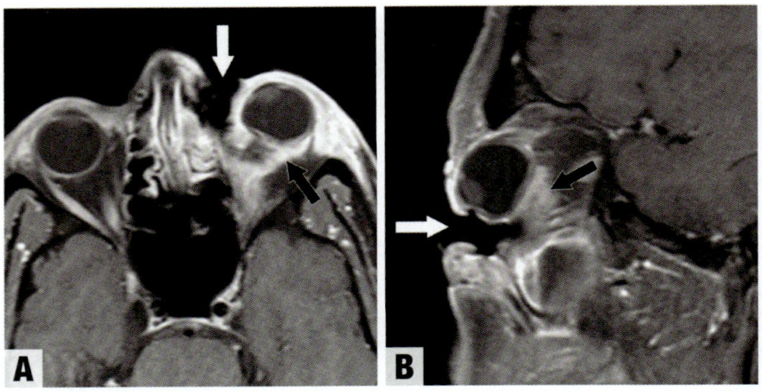

Fig. 3.01 Imaging of the eyelid. Basal cell carcinoma. **A,B** Axial and sagittal T1-weighted postcontrast MRI shows tumour involving the left eyelid and periorbital soft tissues with ulceration in the medial canthal region, left nose, and premaxillary soft tissues extending inferior to the globe (white arrows). Enhancing tumour is present posterior to and indenting upon the globe (black arrows).

There are also certain lesions that are unique to the eyelid. These include intratarsal keratinous cyst {1471}, a lesion that is derived from the Meibomian sebaceous gland duct, and phakomatous choristoma {3771,1552}, a congenital lesion of lenticular anlage that usually presents in the subcutis of the medial lower eyelid.

Looking to the future, an increasing knowledge of the molecular pathogenesis of eyelid and skin tumours will refine histological

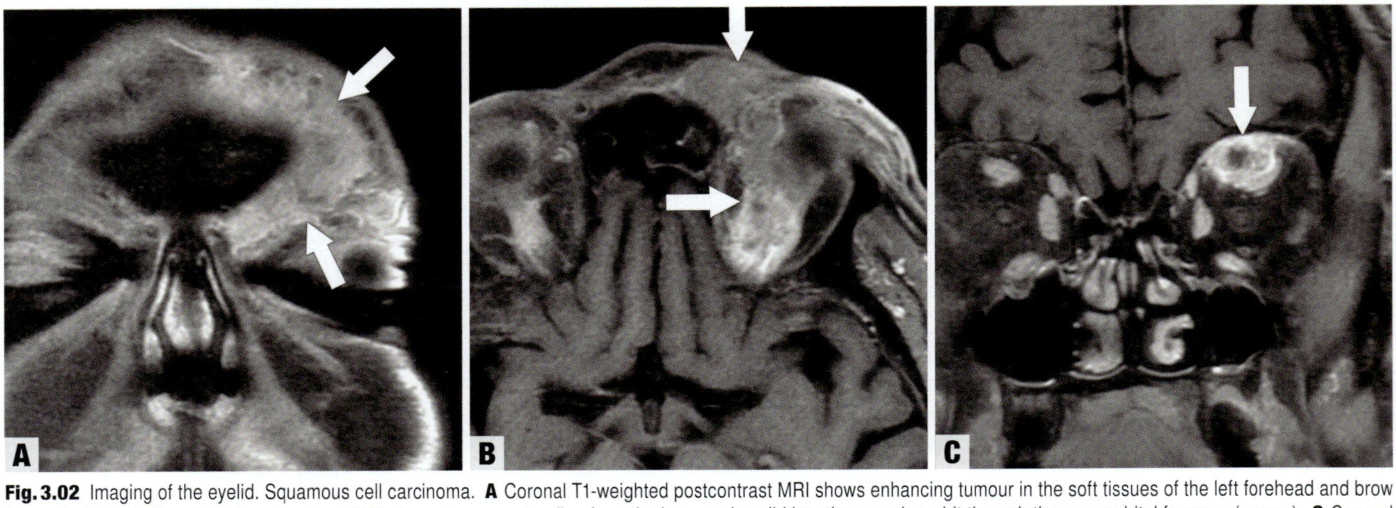

Fig. 3.02 Imaging of the eyelid. Squamous cell carcinoma. **A** Coronal T1-weighted postcontrast MRI shows enhancing tumour in the soft tissues of the left forehead and brow (arrows). **B** Axial T1-weighted postcontrast MRI shows tumour extending from the brow and eyelid into the superior orbit through the supraorbital foramen (arrows). **C** Coronal T1-weighted postcontrast MRI shows tumour in the superior left orbit spreading along the ophthalmic nerve (arrow).

diagnosis, permit accurate prognostication, and open the way for more conservative molecular therapies rather than resorting to routine surgical intervention {2215,2632,3546,2111,758,520, 3313,2397}.

For tumours of the eyelids and periorbital soft tissues, cross-sectional imaging is complementary to the physical examination as it can demonstrate the full extent of the tumour. Thin-section CT can be used to show the tumour matrix and is best suited to detect bony involvement. High-resolution MRI allows the identification of most eyelid structures and provides an assessment of soft tissue disease, perineural tumour spread, and intracranial extension {957}. Diffusion- and perfusion-weighted imaging will aid in the differentiation between the benign or malignant etiology of a lesion. PET-CT evaluates the tumour metabolic activity and detects local and distant metastases.

The ophthalmic site-specific staging system developed by the Union for International Cancer Control (UICC) and the American Joint Committee on Cancer (AJCC) is the main staging system used for eyelid carcinomas {1013,77,3660}.

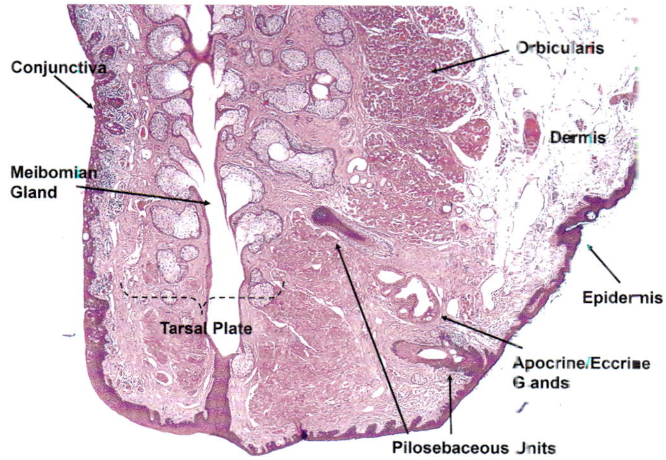

Fig. 3.03 Normal upper eyelid anatomy. Histology of the various tissue layers of the upper eyelid.

Epidermal inclusion cyst

Stagner AM
Wolkow N

Definition
Epidermal inclusion cyst (EIC) is a common, benign cyst lined by epidermis with a formed granular cell layer, containing flaky, basket-weave, or epidermal-type keratin.

ICD-O coding
None

ICD-11 coding
EK70.0Z Epidermoid cyst, unspecified

Related terminology
Acceptable: epidermal cyst; epidermoid cyst.

Subtype(s)
None

Localization
Cysts are most frequently found on the scalp and face, and they may occur along the eyelid margin in association with the cilia, along the brow, or elsewhere on the eyelid in association with the follicular units of vellus hairs.

Clinical features
EIC is typically a slow-growing, well-circumscribed, firm, and mobile dermal or subcutaneous mass. A central pore may be visible clinically {1797}. Imaging has limited value in many eyelid lesions, but CT and MRI can confirm the diagnosis and delineate the extent of large subcutaneous epidermoid cysts {1349}.

Epidemiology
EICs may occur in adolescents to elderly patients, without sex predilection. Occasional epidermoid cysts are congenital.

Etiology
EICs are believed to arise from the infundibular portion of the pilosebaceous unit or from traumatic implantation of surface epidermis into the dermis/subcutis {2491}.

Pathogenesis
Pathogenesis is typically unknown but may result from follicular occlusion. Multiple epidermal cysts may occasionally be associated with Gardner or Muir–Torre syndromes {1797}. Rarely, EICs have been associated with medications, including BRAF inhibitors (e.g. vemurafenib) {393}, cyclosporin A, and tacrolimus {3485}.

Macroscopic appearance
EICs appears as well-circumscribed, white to yellow, oval to round masses filled with caseous or paste-like keratinous contents and occasionally hair shafts.

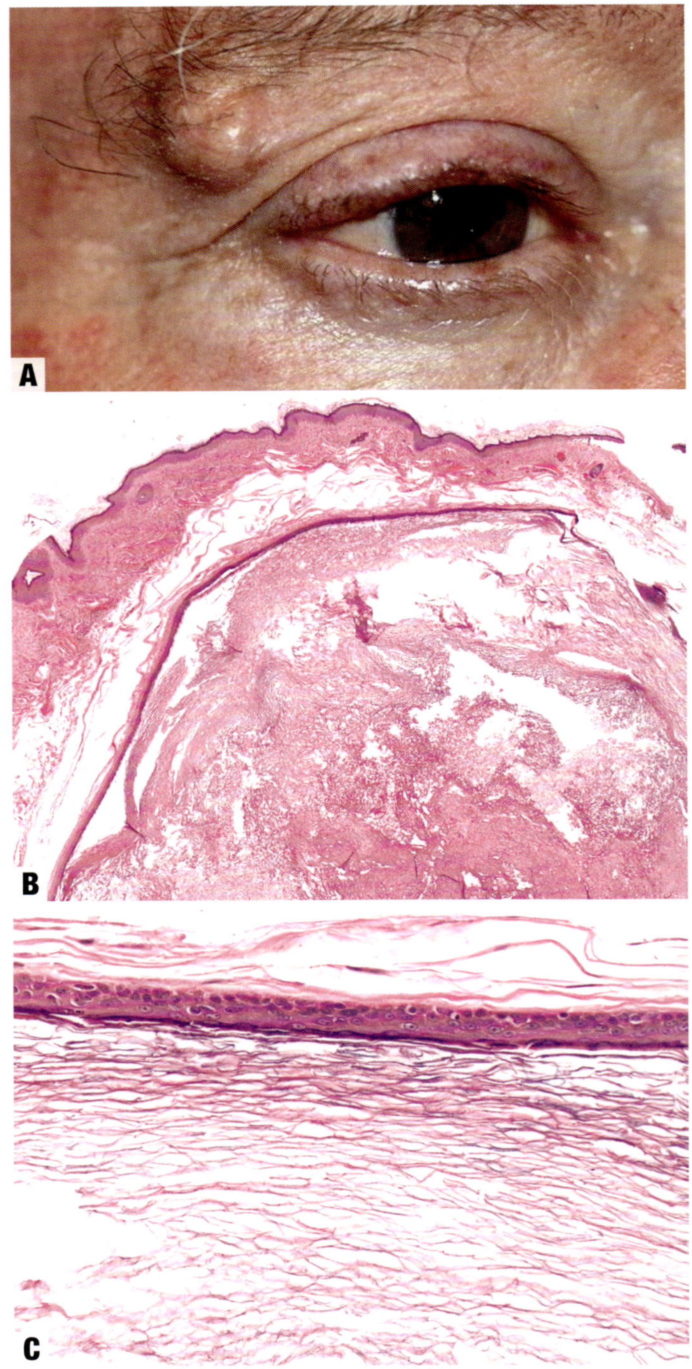

Fig. 3.04 Epidermal inclusion cyst. **A** Clinical image of a cyst close to the upper lid. **B** Dermal-based cyst without an epidermal connection containing abundant flaky orthokeratin. **C** The cyst lining recapitulates normal epidermis with a stratum granulosum.

Histopathology

EICs are lined by stratified squamous epithelium identical to that of the surface epidermis and follicular infundibulum. A well-developed stratum granulosum is present, unlike the lining of pilar cyst. Contents consist of abundant flakes of laminated orthokeratin.

The differential diagnosis includes dilated pore of Winer, dermoid cyst, pilar (trichilemmal) cyst, vellus hair cyst, comedonal cyst, milium or hybrid cyst (mixed hidrocystoma and EIC; see *Ductal hidrocystoma*, p. 107).

Cytology

FNAB or impression cytology is not typically used to make the diagnosis of this entity at this site. When performed, aspirates show many nucleate and anucleate mature squamous cells and keratinaceous debris {1244}.

Diagnostic molecular pathology

Not relevant

Essential and desirable diagnostic criteria

Essential: a cyst in the dermis or subcutis; lined by epidermis with a granular cell layer; containing epidermal-type keratin; without an associated atypical squamous proliferation.

Staging

Not relevant

Prognosis and prediction

Complete excision is typically curative. Rare cases of carcinoma (squamous or basal cell carcinoma) arising within an EIC have been reported {2202,1488}, and cysts may become secondarily infected {498}. Rupture without infection is common {2491}.

Intratarsal cyst

Wolkow N
Stagner AM

Definition
Intratarsal cysts are benign keratin-containing cysts derived from Meibomian gland ducts.

ICD-O coding
None

ICD-11 coding
2F36.4 Cysts of eyelid

Related terminology
Acceptable: intratarsal keratinous cyst; tarsal epithelial cyst; Meibomian gland ductal cyst.
Not recommended: intratarsal inclusion cyst; keratocyst; keratic cyst.

Subtype(s)
None

Localization
Intratarsal keratinous cysts arise within the tarsus of the eyelids, with a predilection for the upper eyelids.

Clinical features
Intratarsal keratinous cysts present as painless, well-defined firm nodules fixed to the tarsus, with no signs of inflammation or attachment to the skin. Eyelid eversion reveals a cream-coloured, yellowish, or sometimes blue-grey well-defined intratarsal nodule without associated inflammation {47,1471,3627,119}.

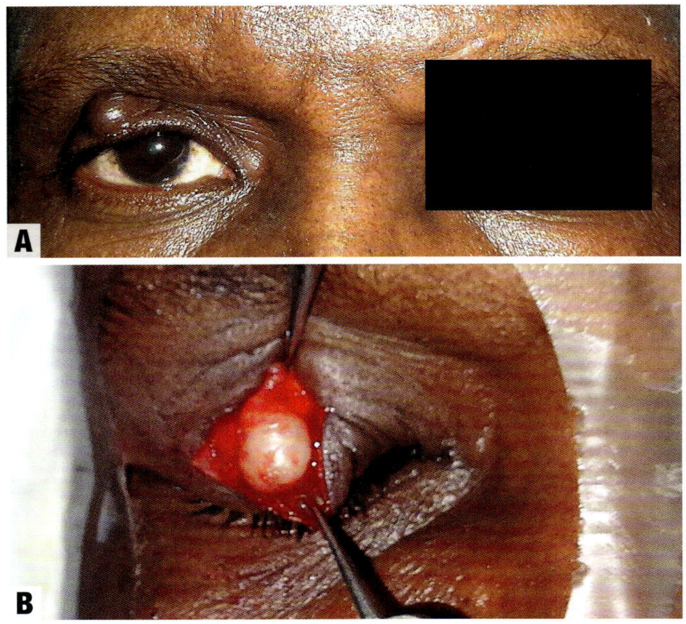

Fig. 3.05 Intratarsal keratinous cyst. **A** External photograph demonstrates a circumscribed deep-seated lesion in the right upper eyelid. **B** Intraoperatively, the lesion appears as a circumscribed pearly nodule inseparable from the tarsus.

Epidemiology
Sporadic cysts are most common and are usually isolated lesions in the upper eyelids of older individuals (aged in their fifties to seventies). Multiple cysts, cysts in the lower eyelids, or

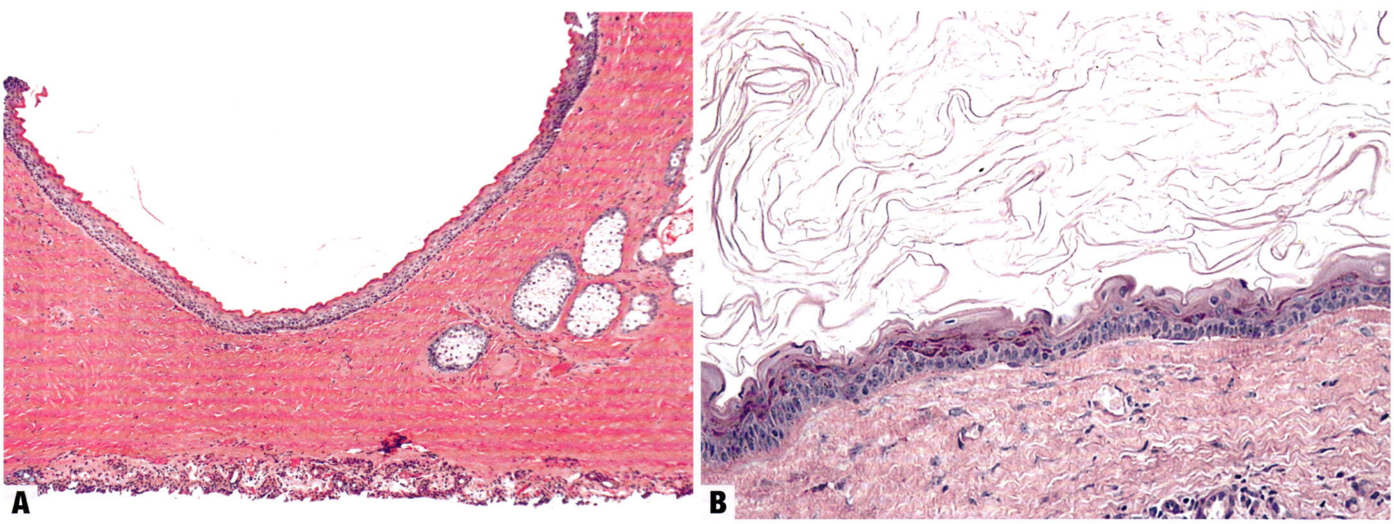

Fig. 3.06 Intratarsal keratinous cyst. **A** The posterior lamella of the eyelid, including tarsus and conjunctiva, with an intratarsal cyst is seen. The intratarsal cyst displays characteristic lining with a corrugated eosinophilic cuticle and wispy luminal keratin. Meibomian gland lobules are present in the adjacent tarsus. **B** The cyst lining features a palisaded basal layer with hyperchromatic nuclei, a corrugated surface without keratohyaline granules, and delicate lamellated luminal keratin (PAS staining).

cysts in a young patient can be associated with naevoid basal cell carcinoma syndrome (Gorlin syndrome) {3627}.

Etiology

The etiology of intratarsal keratinous cysts is not clear. Some cysts are associated with Meibomian gland blockage, trauma and naevoid basal cell carcinoma syndrome {3627,119,2641}.

Pathogenesis

Blockage of a Meibomian gland duct with secondary dilation is one of the postulated mechanisms {119,2641}. The rare association with naevoid basal cell carcinoma syndrome raises speculation that some cysts may arise from alterations in the sonic hedgehog signalling pathway genes {3627}, analogous to odontogenic keratocysts {2471}.

Macroscopic appearance

The lesions are circumscribed and grey to yellow or bluish with a milky or keratinous luminal material.

Histopathology

The cysts have a characteristic stratified squamous epithelial lining that is 4–6 cells thick, with the basal layer consisting of hyperchromatic cells with stringy eosinophilic cuticle in the lumen. The lining cells lack keratohyaline granules and display a corrugated, brightly eosinophilic cuticle similar to that in odontogenic keratocyst and steatocystoma.

Immunohistochemistry is not required for diagnosis. The lining cells and keratin are strongly positive for CK17 while the luminal portion of the lining and the contents may be positive for CEA and EMA {3286,1471}.

Cytology

Not relevant

Diagnostic molecular pathology

Not relevant

Essential and desirable diagnostic criteria

Essential: intratarsal location with a characteristic lining featuring corrugated eosinophilic cuticle without keratohyaline granules.

Staging

Not relevant

Prognosis and prediction

Treatment consists of complete excision of the cyst lining; partial excision may lead to recurrence.

Phakomatous choristoma

Verdijk RM
Herwig-Carl MC
Moulin A

Definition

Phakomatous choristoma is a benign congenital developmental lesion of lenticular anlage, composed of extraocular crystalline lens tissue and its basement membrane.

ICD-O coding

None

ICD-11 coding

LA14.0Y Other specified structural developmental anomalies of eyelids

Related terminology

Not recommended: Zimmerman tumour.

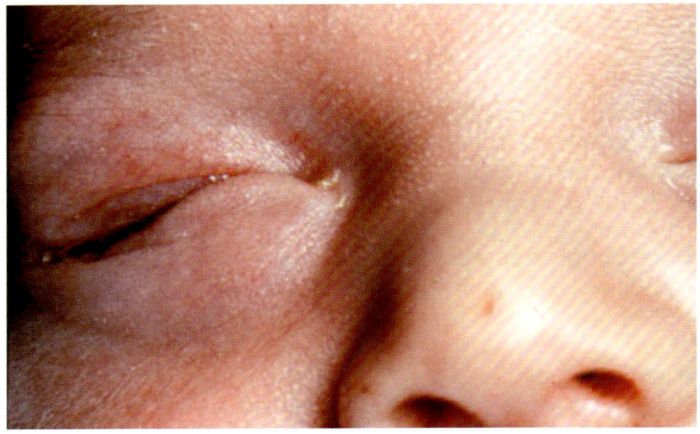

Fig. 3.07 Phakomatous choristoma. A congenital mass involves the medial lower eyelid.

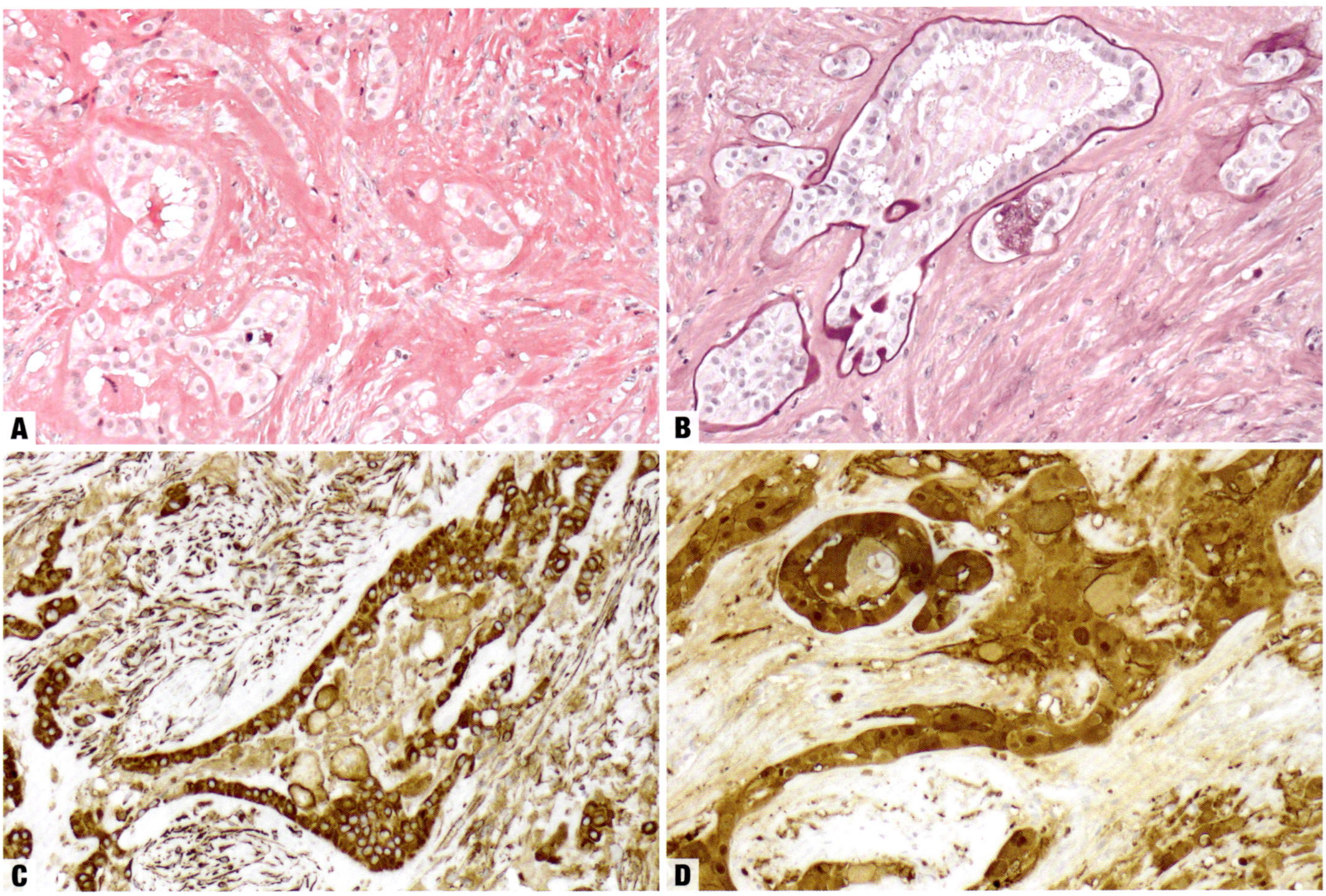

Fig. 3.08 Phakomatous choristoma. **A** Histopathologically, the lesion is composed of lens epithelial cells surrounded by acellular eosinophilic material. **B** The PAS reaction highlights PAS-positive basement membrane material surrounding the epithelial cells. **C** The epithelial cells and cells of the surrounding stroma are highlighted by a vimentin immunostain. **D** The epithelial cells are also strongly positive for S100.

Subtype(s)
None

Localization
Phakomatous choristoma generally occurs deep in the medial lower eyelid. Cases with exclusive involvement of the inferior anterior orbit, lacrimal sac, nasolacrimal duct, and extraocular muscles have been reported {1263,2923,3771,1552}.

Clinical features
Patients present in infancy with a smooth, firm, slowly growing subcutaneous mass in the medial lower eyelid, already present at birth. On imaging, the tumour is solid, well circumscribed, and contrast enhancing, without bone erosion {1552,2455}.

Epidemiology
Phakomatous choristoma is extremely rare, with < 30 cases reported worldwide. There is a slight male predominance (68%) {1552}.

Etiology
This is a developmental abnormality.

Pathogenesis
Two hypotheses have been proposed as to the origin of the lesion: formation of an additional lens vesicle locus from surface ectoderm {3771}, and displacement or migration of cells from the lens placode {2148,3149}.

Macroscopic appearance
Phakomatous choristoma macroscopically appears as an ovoid, white-grey, firm mass, measuring as large as 20 mm {1877,1552}.

Histopathology
Phakomatous choristoma has a characteristic morphological appearance and consists of islands of cuboidal to polygonal cells, reminiscent of lens epithelium, and bladder (Wedl) cells surrounded by a thick layer of eosinophilic PAS-positive material analogous to lens capsule. Psammomatous calcification can be seen. Dense collagenous stroma is present in the background {3771}.

Immunohistochemistry is not required for diagnosis. The epithelial and bladder cells stain positively for vimentin, S100, PAX8, and lens crystalline proteins, and are negative for cytokeratins {1552, 2216}. Electron microscopy demonstrates 10 nm whorled cytoplasmic microfilaments within degenerating epithelial cells {2148}.

Cytology
Not relevant

Diagnostic molecular pathology
Not relevant

Essential and desirable diagnostic criteria
Essential: extraocular crystalline lens tissue and dense collagen bundles surrounded by a PAS-positive membrane localized to the eyelid/orbit.

Staging
Not relevant

Prognosis and prediction
Phakomatous choristoma is benign. Malignant transformation has not been described. Simple resection is curative {1552}. Rare associations include myopia, colobomatous hypoplastic optic disc, and staphyloma {3320}.

Molluscum contagiosum

Van Ginderdeuren R
Fullen DR

Definition
Molluscum contagiosum is a benign and self-limited viral skin infection that presents as multiple epidermal nodular, umbilicated lesions on the skin.

ICD-O coding
None

ICD-11 coding
1E76 Molluscum contagiosum

Related terminology
None

Subtype(s)
None

Localization
Skin lesions of molluscum contagiosum may occur anywhere on the body but most commonly involve the head and neck, trunk, flexural areas of the extremities, axillae, and groin. Periocular location is evenly distributed on the upper and lower eyelids {2772}.

Clinical features
Solitary or (more commonly) multiple skin lesions usually present as discrete 2–5 mm umbilicated, waxy, flesh-coloured to erythematous papules. Giant lesions (≥ 10 mm) occasionally occur, especially in individuals with HIV, but they also may occur in immunocompetent individuals {1888}. Around the eye they can provoke a follicular conjunctivitis {2924}.

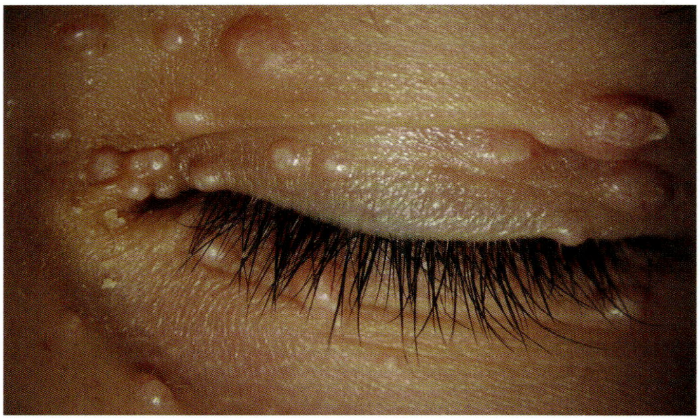

Fig. 3.09 Molluscum contagiosum. A child with multiple mollusca contagiosa on the eyelids.

Epidemiology
Molluscum contagiosum occurs worldwide and is more frequent in children, although adolescents and adults may also be affected. The overall prevalence in children is 8.3%. The prevalence among people with HIV is estimated to approach 20%. There is no sex predilection {2194}.

Etiology
Molluscum contagiosum is caused by the molluscum contagiosum virus belonging to the Poxviridae family.

Pathogenesis
The virus is transmitted by direct skin contact, autoinoculation, or contaminated fomites in children, immunocompromised

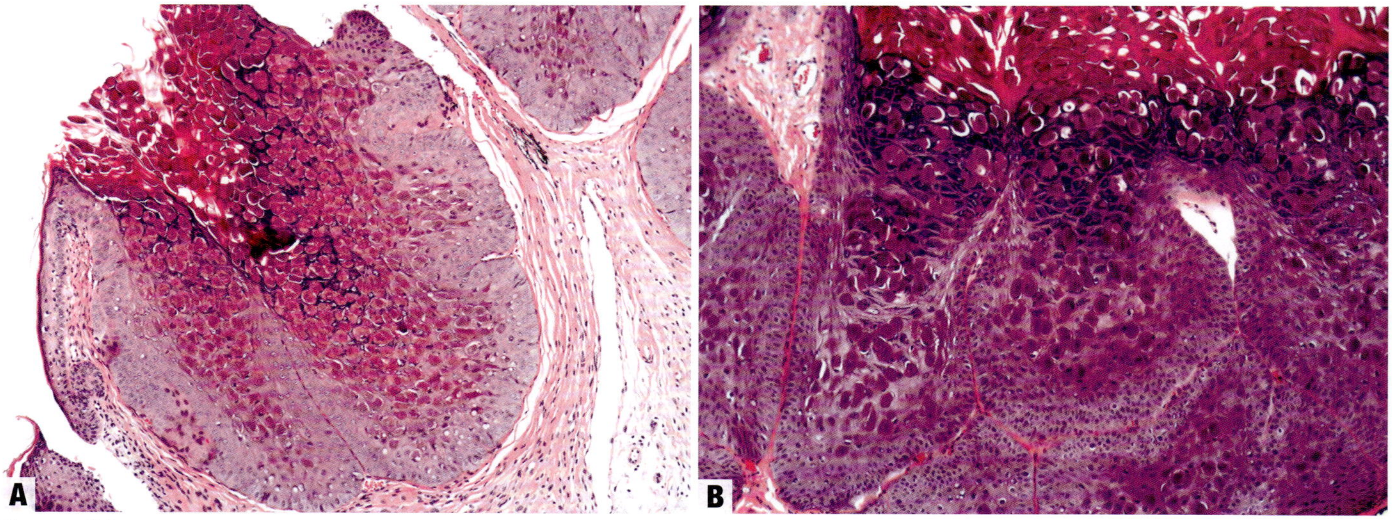

Fig. 3.10 Molluscum contagiosum. **A,B** Histopathology showing molluscum bodies.

individuals, or sexually active adults {1011,2194}. The virus then replicates within the cytoplasm of keratinocytes of the epithelium.

Macroscopic appearance

The individual papule is crateriform and contains a thick, whitish-yellow, cheesy, or curd-like material.

Histopathology

The typical elevated crateriform lesion is formed by endophytic lobules of acanthotic epidermis containing large, eosinophilic intracytoplasmic inclusion bodies, known as molluscum bodies or Henderson–Paterson bodies, that compress the nucleus to the periphery of the cell. Ruptured lesions incite an inflammatory response, which sometimes demonstrates lymphocyte atypia resembling lymphoma, including the presence of CD30-positive large cells {3581}. The surrounding stroma is often oedematous, mucinous, and/or fibrous {1435}.

Cytology

Molluscum bodies can be identified in a Tzanck smear {2786}.

Diagnostic molecular pathology

Not relevant

Essential and desirable diagnostic criteria

Essential: crateriform, acanthotic epidermis; molluscum bodies.

Staging

Not relevant

Prognosis and prediction

Spontaneous regression typically occurs within 12–18 months. A variety of treatment modalities, such as cryotherapy, curettage, topical chemical agents, immunomodulators, or pulsed dye laser, can be used for extensive disease, secondary complications such as superinfection, or aesthetic purposes {2194, 1011}. Immunocompromised individuals need more vigorous treatment to eradicate the disease {324}.

Verruca vulgaris

Van Ginderdeuren R
Mihic-Probst D
Tan KB

Definition
Verruca vulgaris is a common benign HPV-driven epidermal squamoproliferative lesion.

ICD-O coding
None

ICD-11 coding
1E80 Common warts

Related terminology
Acceptable: common viral wart.

Subtype(s)
None

Localization
The common sites of occurrence of verruca vulgaris are the fingers, hands, elbows, knees, and face {481,1681,694,2369, 2164}.

Clinical features
Verruca may present as single or multiple papules, keratotic plaques, and nodules, most ranging between 1 and 20 mm {481,1681}. Lesions may also occur on eyebrow tattoos {2369, 644}.

Epidemiology
The reported prevalence is as many as 3.5% of adults and 20–33% of adolescents {325,1861,743,433}. Immunosuppression is a significant risk factor, with multiple verrucae often occurring per patient {481,853}.

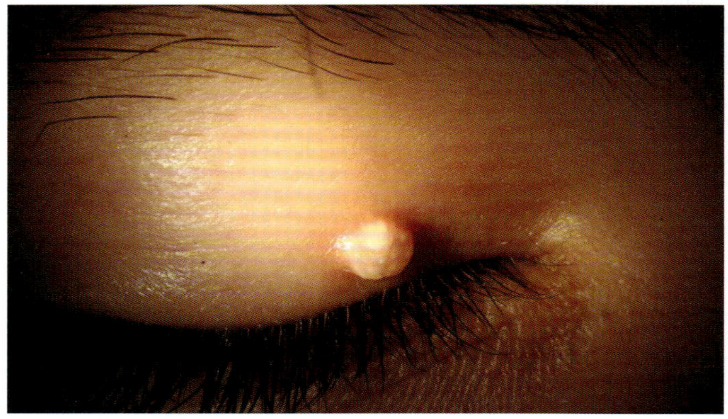

Fig. 3.11 Verruca vulgaris. Typical verruca vulgaris on the upper eyelid of a child.

Etiology
Low-risk HPV subtypes 1, 2, 4, 7, and 26–29 are well documented in common warts {481,635}. HPV subtypes 75–77 have been reported in lesions in immunocompromised patients {2035}.

Recognized ways of contracting cutaneous HPV infection include via direct physical contact, tattooing, fomites, or autoinoculation {694,644}. For the latter, hand transfer helps explain the development of facial or eyelid lesions {694}.

Pathogenesis
After inoculation of the skin via a break in the epithelial barrier, keratinocytes are infected. HPV DNA production and viral assembly occur progressively in the superficial layers of the epidermis, with the eventual release of viral particles with desquamated cells {635}.

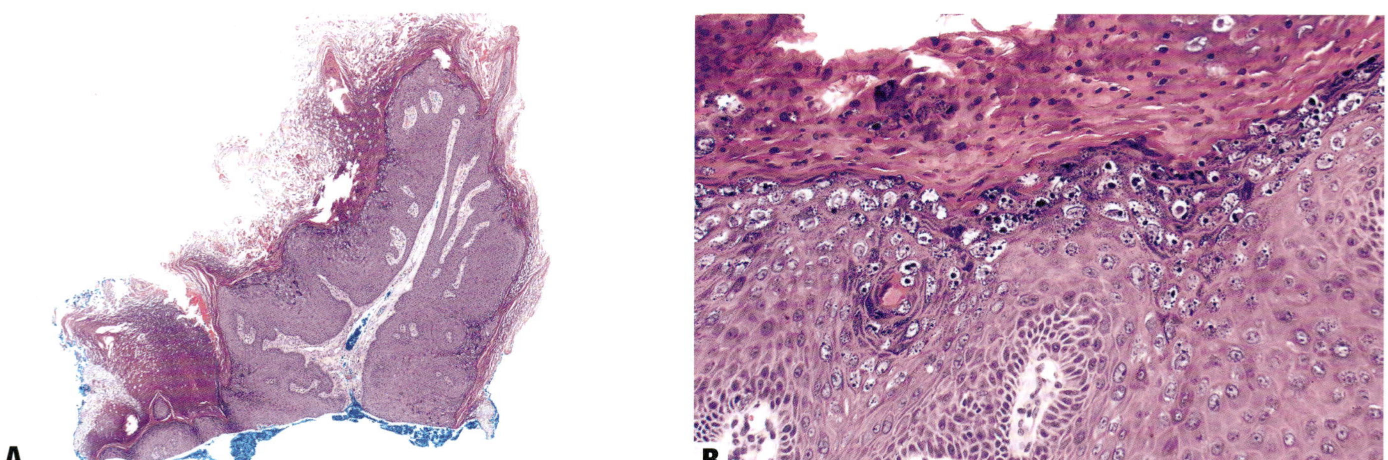

Fig. 3.12 Verruca vulgaris. **A** Epidermal lesion showing hyperkeratosis, acanthosis, and papillomatosis. **B** There is parakeratosis and koilocytosis, with some cells containing coarse keratohyaline granules.

Macroscopic appearance

Verruca vulgaris presents as a skin-coloured elevated nodule with a keratotic and papillomatous surface {15}. Facial lesions may possess a filiform configuration {2164}.

Histopathology

Verrucae are characterized by papillomatous epidermal projections tipped by columns of parakeratosis, alongside hyperkeratosis. Superficial keratinocytes feature coarse keratohyaline granules and the characteristic koilocytes are often present, frequently underneath the parakeratosis {481,1681,694}. Elongated rete ridges are oriented centrally and dermal papillae show prominent blood vessels. A lymphocytic infiltrate with basal keratinocytic degeneration may be present, typically associated with regression {308,1776}.

Seborrhoeic keratosis and trichilemmomas displaying hyperkeratosis and papillomatosis are differential diagnoses. The difficulty is compounded by koilocytes being often absent in older verrucae.

Cytology

Not relevant

Diagnostic molecular pathology

Not relevant

Essential and desirable diagnostic criteria

Essential: papillomatosis; hypergranulosis; hyperkeratosis; parakeratosis.

Desirable: koilocytosis.

Staging

Not relevant

Prognosis and prediction

Verrucae typically resolve spontaneously with time: in children, about 80% of lesions regress in 2 years {694,3206}. In immunosuppressed individuals, verrucae may be more persistent {481}. Different treatment modalities in recalcitrant cases or in immune deficiency include curettage, cryotherapy, chemical agents, and laser {15}.

Squamous papilloma of the eyelid

Mihic-Probst D
Auw-Haedrich C

Definition
Squamous papilloma is a benign exophytic verrucous or broad-based skin tumour, with or without signs of HPV infection.

ICD-O coding
8052/0 Squamous papilloma

ICD-11 coding
2F36.Y & XH50T2 Other specified benign neoplasm of eye or ocular adnexa & Squamous cell papilloma, NOS

Related terminology
Acceptable: skin tag; squamous cell papilloma.
Not recommended: acrochordon.

Subtype(s)
None

Localization
Lesions can be anywhere on the skin, including the eyelid.

Clinical features
Squamous papilloma is a sessile or pedunculated soft, smooth lesion with a similar colour to adjacent skin. The surface is more-or-less verrucous, with or without a keratin crust. Ulceration due to mechanical irritation may be present. Papillomas are often multiple {776}.

Epidemiology
Squamous papilloma is among the most common benign eyelid tumours and can occur at any age, with no sex predilection {3721,1394,26}.

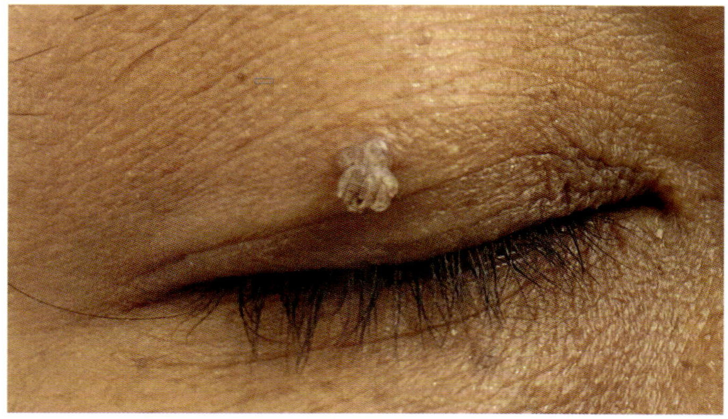

Fig. 3.13 Squamous papilloma. Clinical appearance in a 51-year-old woman with a papillomatous skin lesion on the upper right eyelid.

Etiology
Some lesions are HPV-related and may represent burned-out HPV infections {2799}.

Pathogenesis
Low-risk HPV types induce benign neoplastic epithelial proliferation.

Macroscopic appearance
Squamous papilloma is a sessile or pedunculated, small, skin-coloured lesion. The surface is more-or-less verrucous, with or without a keratin crust. It is sometimes ulcerated.

Histopathology
Squamous papilloma is a verrucous, broad-based or finger-like exophytic epithelial neoplasm with a fibrovascular core. There is an absence of dysplasia and of relevant mitotic activity, with no signs of dermal invasion. Hyperparakeratosis or ulceration due to mechanical irritation may be present. In contrast to verruca

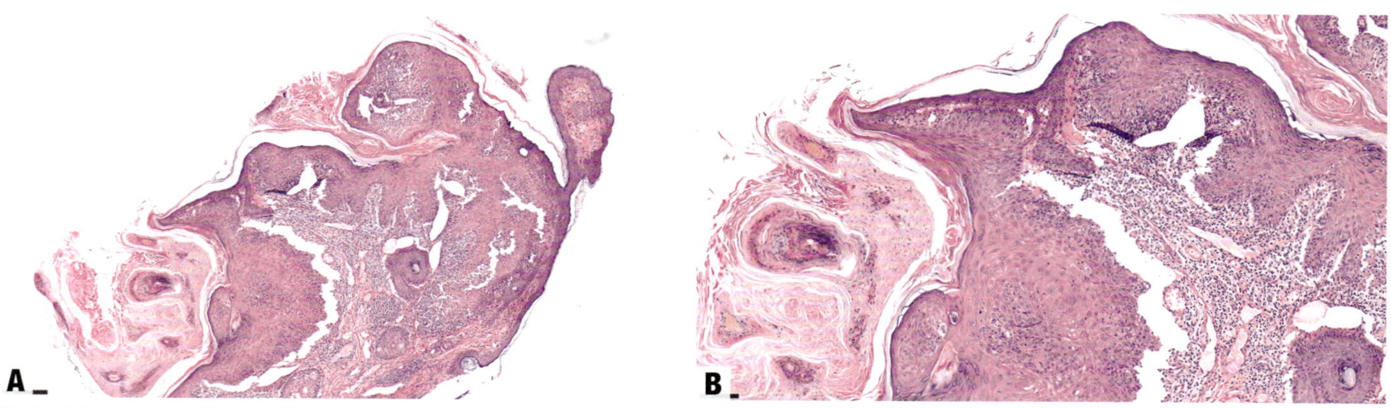

Fig. 3.14 Squamous papilloma. **A** The epidermis is hyperplastic with papillomatosis and acanthosis. **B** High magnification shows an absence of epidermal dysplasia, mitosis, or dermal invasion. This is a highly irritated lesion with hyperparakeratosis and dermal chronic lichenoid inflammation.

vulgaris, squamous cell papillomas have an exophytic, papillomatous, and less acanthomatous growth pattern. HPV cytopathic signs, such as koilocytes or double nuclei, may occur. However, some squamous cell papillomas may represent regressed verruca vulgaris.

Cytology

Not relevant

Diagnostic molecular pathology

Not relevant

Essential and desirable diagnostic criteria

Essential: finger-like projections of vascularized connective tissue covered by hyperplastic epithelium; absence of dysplasia.

Staging

Not relevant

Prognosis and prediction

Recurrences occur in cases of incomplete removal

Seborrhoeic keratosis

Auw-Haedrich C
Mihic-Probst D

Definition

Seborrhoeic keratoses are benign intraepithelial neoplastic squamous proliferations encountered on ageing skin.

ICD-O coding

8052/0 Seborrhoeic keratosis
8052/0 Irritated seborrhoeic keratosis
8052/0 Stucco keratosis

ICD-11 coding

2F21.0 Seborrhoeic keratosis

Related terminology

Not recommended: senile wart; seborrhoeic wart; basal cell papilloma.

Subtype(s)

Irritated seborrhoeic keratosis; stucco keratosis

Localization

Seborrhoeic keratoses are found on periocular skin, including the lid margin.

Clinical features

Patients with seborrhoeic keratosis present with a papillomatous, most often sessile tumour with a stuck-on appearance. The papules or plaques are tan to brown and keratotic; owing to the sometimes heavy pigmentation, they can clinically impress as naevi. An acute onset of multiple seborrhoeic keratosis can occur in the setting of internal malignancies, known as the Leser–Trélat sign {2891}.

Epidemiology

Seborrhoeic keratosis is most often diagnosed at an older age (> 50 years). There is no known sex predisposition.

Etiology

Age is a widely acknowledged risk factor for seborrhoeic keratosis. A proposed association with HPV is contested, especially for non-genital lesions {3758,2365}.

Pathogenesis

Seborrhoeic keratosis is associated with ultraviolet (UV) radiation with a typical UV radiation signature, with the majority of alterations being C>T and CC>TT base changes at dipyrimidinic sites {1305}. Somatic mutations have been reported in *FGFR3*, which may result in increased keratinocyte proliferation and reduced apoptosis {1987,314,1228,1226}. Other mutated genes include *PIK3CA*, *KRAS*, *HRAS*, *EGFR*, and *AKT1* {1227,1094,1305}.

Macroscopic appearance

Seborrhoeic keratosis is a papillomatous, sometimes pigmented tumour with a broad base.

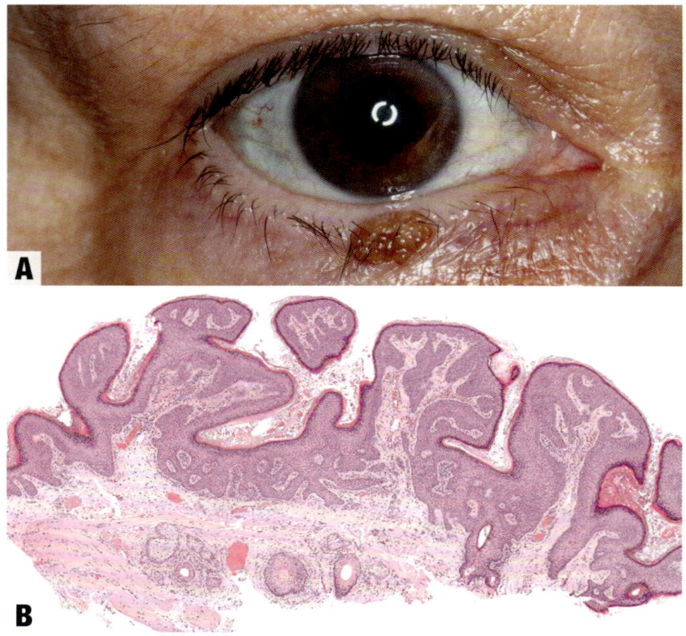

Fig. 3.15 Seborrhoeic keratosis. **A** Pigmented seborrhoeic keratosis of the lower lid with papillomatous surface and intact eyelashes. **B** Histology of the same case with acanthotic, reticulated areas, and hyperkeratosis.

Histopathology

A well-demarcated, thickened epidermal layer due to an increase in basaloid keratinocytes with a flat or reticulated base is seen. Mitoses are rare. The basal epithelial cell layer often contains intracellular pigment. Horn cysts can be found between the basal cells and at the tumour surface hyperkeratosis. There may be lymphoplasmacellular inflammation at the tumour base {1282}. Different growth patterns and subtypes may be encountered, and they are described in greater detail in the *Skin tumours* volume of this series {3597}.

Cytology

Not applicable

Diagnostic molecular pathology

Not relevant

Essential and desirable diagnostic criteria

Essential: a well-circumscribed intraepidermal squamous proliferation with a flat base, lacking squamous dysplasia.

Staging

Not relevant

Prognosis and prediction

Complete excision is curative.

Inverted follicular keratosis

Mihic-Probst D
Auw-Haedrich C
Eagle RC Jr

Definition

Inverted follicular keratosis (IFK) is characterized by a benign epithelial expansion by proliferation of squamous and basaloid cells of the follicular infundibulum.

ICD-O coding

None

ICD-11 coding

2F21.0 Seborrhoeic keratosis

Related terminology

None

Subtype(s)

None

Localization

IFK is found anywhere on the skin, including the eyelid {3178}.

Clinical features

IFKs are white-tan to pink asymptomatic papules of the eyelid; they may rarely present as cutaneous horns. Clinically they are often considered to be viral warts, and the remainder are often misdiagnosed as basal cell carcinoma {221,2855}.

Epidemiology

IFKs arise in middle-aged to elderly patients. Men are affected about twice as often as women {221,2855}.

Etiology

The etiology is unknown, although multiple IFKs can be considered an indicator of Cowden syndrome, an autosomal dominant disorder associated with a propensity for tumour formation due to a mutation in *PTEN* {2781}.

Pathogenesis

Unknown

Macroscopic appearance

Dome-shaped pinkish or skin-coloured papule

Histopathology

IFK is usually a symmetrical invaginated (inverted) proliferation of basaloid and squamoid cells deriving from the follicular infundibulum. There is a lobular endophytic and exophytic growth pattern. The lobules contain a more-or-less central longitudinal crypt with keratin and lining by squamous epithelium. Basaloid cells are located at the periphery and squamoid cells at the centre of the lobule/crypt. The crypt may open onto the surface. While basaloid cells sometimes merge with squamous cells indefinably, it is at the points of junction of these two cell

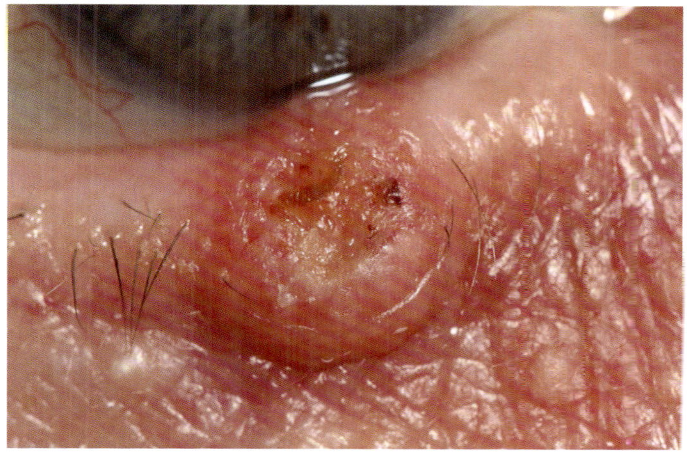

Fig. 3.16 Inverted follicular keratosis. An 84-year-old woman with inverted follicular keratosis mimicking a nodular basal cell carcinoma.

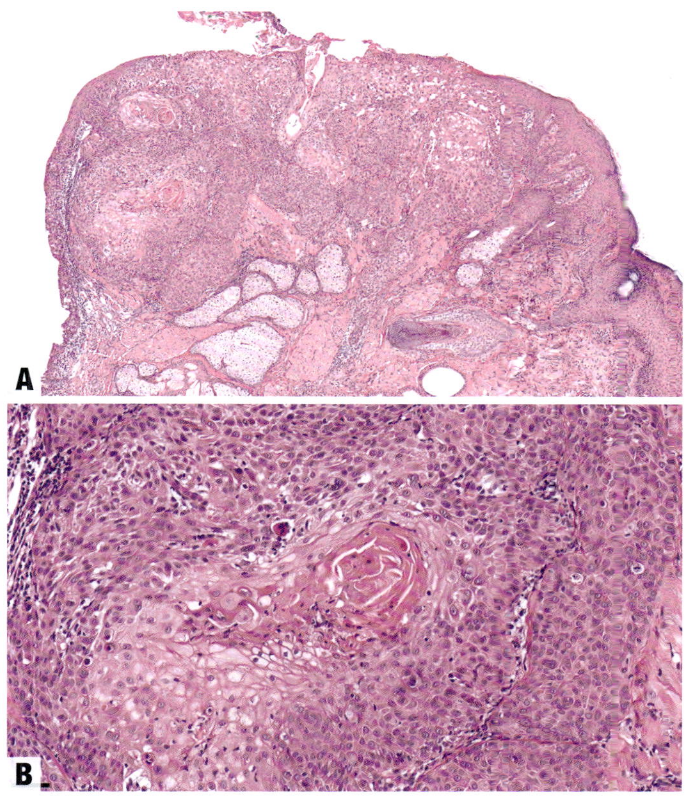

Fig. 3.17 Inverted follicular keratosis. **A** An eyelid covered by skin and conjunctiva is shown. There is nodular inverted proliferation of basaloid and squamoid cells deriving from the follicular infundibulum, with a crypt opening to the surface. There is absence of an infiltrative destructive growth pattern. Intermingled basaloid and squamoid cells are present with focal acantholysis and a squamous eddy. **B** Higher magnification of a squamous eddy with basaloid cells located at the periphery and squamoid cells at the centre of the lobule. A single mitotic figure is present.

types that squamous eddies are frequently found. This consists of a sharply demarcated, rounded group of larger, eosinophilic, polygonal cells set in a background of basaloid cells. Mitotic figures are present but not atypical. In contrast to squamous cell carcinoma, the cells lack pleomorphism or atypia. There is no dermal destructive invasion. However, there may be heavy dermal chronic inflammation and acantholysis, which can pose difficulties in excluding invasion and in distinguishing from well-differentiated squamous cell carcinoma. In those cases, absence of dysplasia of the adjacent epidermis and absence of elastoid degeneration in IFK may be helpful {221}.

Cytology

Not relevant

Diagnostic molecular pathology

Multiple IFKs can be considered an indicator of Cowden syndrome, an autosomal dominant disorder associated with a propensity for tumour formation due to a mutation in the *PTEN* gene {2781}.

Essential and desirable diagnostic criteria

Essential: symmetrical invaginated (inverted) proliferation of basaloid and squamoid cells deriving from the follicular infundibulum without atypia.

Staging

Not relevant

Prognosis and prediction

With incomplete excision IFK may recur within several weeks.

Actinic keratosis

Auw-Haedrich C
Mihic-Probst D

Definition

Actinic keratosis (AK) is a very common neoplastic intraepidermal squamous proliferative lesion associated with ultraviolet (UV) light exposure and characterized by squamous dysplasia. AK may remain stable, regress spontaneously, or progress to invasive squamous cell carcinoma.

ICD-O coding

8070/0 Actinic keratosis
8070/0 Proliferative actinic keratosis
8070/0 Hypertrophic actinic keratosis
8070/0 Lichenoid actinic keratosis
8070/0 Pigmented actinic keratosis

ICD-11 coding

EK90.0 Actinic keratosis

Related terminology

Acceptable: solar keratosis.
Not recommended: keratinocytic intraepidermal neoplasia; bowenoid solar keratosis; senile keratosis.

Subtype(s)

Proliferative actinic keratosis; hypertrophic actinic keratosis; lichenoid actinic keratosis; pigmented actinic keratosis

Localization

AK arises on sun-exposed skin, such as periocular skin, including the lid margin.

Clinical features

AKs are erythematous scaly patches and plaques, often with irregular fuzzy margins, in patients with sun-damaged skin.

Epidemiology

AK is diagnosed at older ages (> 60 years) and represents the third most often diagnosed skin disease {873}. There is no known sex predisposition.

Etiology

UV radiation exposure is the main risk factor. Other predisposing factors are fair skin (Fitzpatrick type I and type II), immunosuppression, and genetic diseases such as xeroderma pigmentosum with autosomal recessive inherited impaired DNA repairing mechanisms {794}.

Pathogenesis

AKs have a UV radiation–induced high mutation burden (43.5/Mb) and UV radiation signatures (cytosine to thymidine transition at dipyrimidine sites). Copy-number alterations, mutation signatures, and patterns of driver gene mutations are similar to those of cutaneous squamous cell carcinoma. The most common alterations are *TP53*, *NOTCH1*, *NOTCH2*, and *FAT1* mutations, and a loss of heterozygosity of p16 {455,3331,2368}.

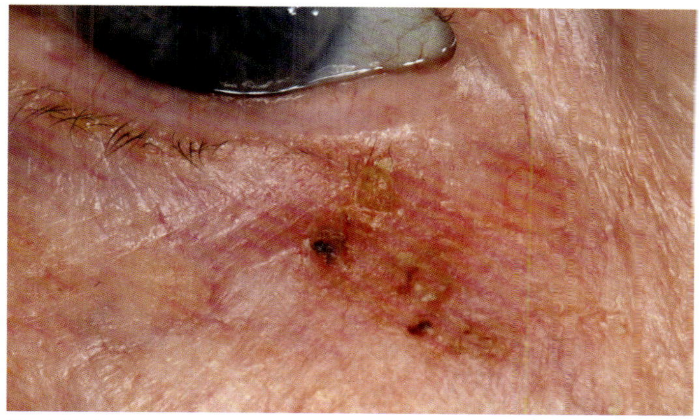

Fig. 3.18 Actinic keratosis. Erythematous, hyperkeratotic, actinic keratosis at the temporal lower lid.

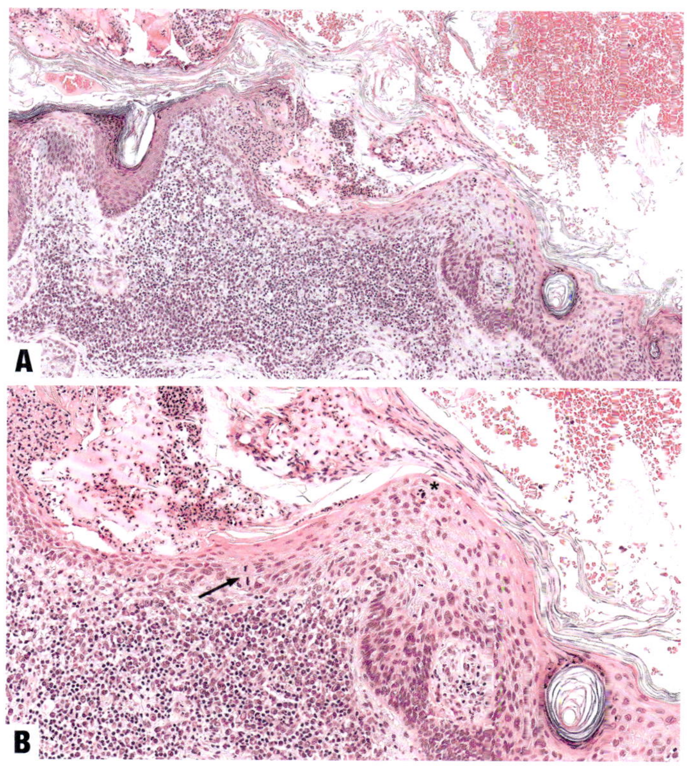

Fig. 3.19 Actinic keratosis. **A** Hyperkeratotic actinic keratosis with subepithelial chronic inflammatory infiltration. **B** Dysplasia of the epidermis including mitoses of two adjacent cells at different levels (arrow) and a superficial cell with an apoptotic nucleus (asterisk).

Macroscopic appearance

AKs appear as erythematous, scaly patches and plaques, often with irregular fuzzy margins.

Histopathology

Skin with atrophic or hyperplastic epidermis, hyperkeratosis/parakeratosis, dyskeratosis, apoptosis, and dermal elastoid degeneration is seen. There is neoplastic keratinocyte proliferation with enlarged, pleomorphic, hyperchromatic nuclei and increased mitosis. Dysplastic cells replacing the mid to upper epidermal layers and mitosis throughout the epidermis represent high-grade dysplasia in an AK and should be mentioned. Atrophic, bowenoid, and acantholytic patterns may be recognized. Moderate atypical melanocytes may be increased.

Immunohistochemistry

p53 and Ki-67 immunohistochemistry is useful proof of AK, or it can be used to assist in the grading of dysplasia, if this is difficult. p40 and SOX10 staining is recommended to avoid an incorrect diagnosis of lentigo maligna in pigmented AK.

Differential diagnosis

The differential diagnosis includes basal cell carcinoma, squamous cell carcinoma, seborrhoeic keratosis {794}, lentigo maligna, inflammatory skin disease such as discoid lupus erythematosus, and psoriasis {3471}. Squamous cell carcinoma in situ is characterized by full-thickness dysplasia (see the relevant section in the *Skin tumours* volume of this series {3597}).

Cytology

Not relevant

Diagnostic molecular pathology

Not relevant

Essential and desirable diagnostic criteria

Essential: intraepidermal squamous dysplasia that is not full thickness.

Staging

Not relevant

Prognosis and prediction

AK is a precursor of squamous cell carcinoma {3094}. At least two thirds of squamous cell carcinomas arise from AK. However, the estimated progression rate is < 0.075% per lesion per year and about 0.53% if the patient already had squamous cell carcinoma elsewhere. At the same time, single lesions have frequently been found to regress (15–53% per year), but also to recur (long-term recurrence rates > 50%) {3582}.

Basal cell carcinoma of the eyelid

Kaliki S
Eiger-Moscovich M
Mihic-Probst D
Scolyer RA

Definition

Basal cell carcinoma (BCC) is a family of carcinomas that arises from epithelial cells of either the epidermis or hair follicle stem cells. It is composed of nests of basaloid cells, variably arranged.

ICD-O coding

8090/3 Basal cell carcinoma, NOS
8091/3 Superficial basal cell carcinoma
8097/3 Nodular basal cell carcinoma
8097/3 Micronodular basal cell carcinoma
8092/3 Infiltrating basal cell carcinoma
8092/3 Sclerosing/morphoeic basal cell carcinoma
8094/3 Basosquamous carcinoma

ICD-11 coding

2C32.2 Superficial basal cell carcinoma of skin
2C32.0 Nodular basal cell carcinoma of skin
2C32.0 & XH4GJ2 Nodular basal cell carcinoma of skin & Basal cell carcinoma, micronodular
2C32 & XH5VK4 Basal cell carcinoma of skin & Infiltrating basal cell carcinoma, NOS
2C32.Y & XH4C18 Other specified basal cell carcinoma of skin & Basosquamous carcinoma
2C32.1 Sclerosing basal cell carcinoma of skin

Related terminology

Not recommended: basal cell epithelioma; basalioma; trichoblastic carcinoma.

Subtype(s)

See Box 3.01 (p. 100).

Localization

BCC is predominantly found in sun-exposed skin. Periocular BCC arises in the lower eyelid (50%), medial canthus (30%), upper eyelid (15%), and lateral canthus (5%) {1051,2964}.

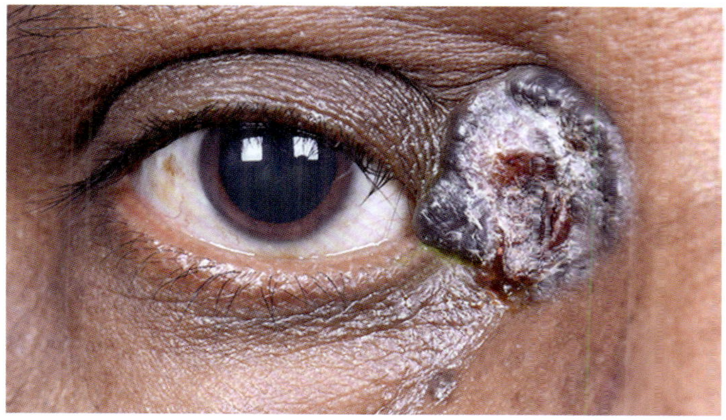

Fig. 3.20 Periocular basal cell carcinoma. A 45-year-old male patient presented with pigmented basal cell carcinoma at the medial canthus of the right eye.

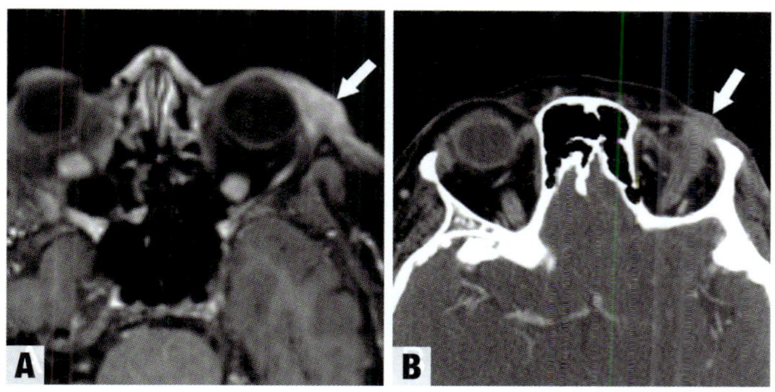

Fig. 3.21 Basal cell carcinoma. **A** Axial T1-weighted postcontrast MRI shows tumour involving the left eyelid, lateral canthus, and periorbital soft tissues (arrow). **B** Axial CT with contrast in a different patient shows recurrent tumour in the left upper eyelid (arrow).

Clinical features

BCCs located near the eyelid margin can cause madarosis. Orbital and/or perineural intracranial invasion, seen in 2–4% of cases, presents with diplopia or globe displacement {3632,

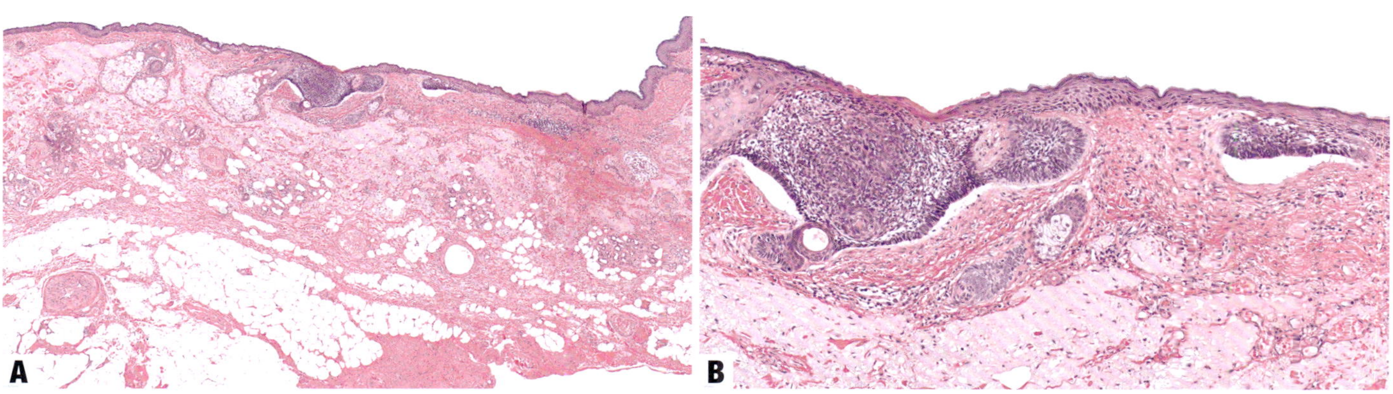

Fig. 3.22 Basal cell carcinoma, superficial. **A** Superficial basaloid small nests attached to the epidermis on actinic damaged skin with elastoid degeneration. **B** Small superficial nests of basaloid cells with peripheral palisading and contraction artefact to the dermis.

Box 3.01 Histological subtypes of basal cell carcinoma (BCC) stratified by risk of recurrence

Lower risk
Nodular BCC
Superficial BCC
Pigmented BCC
Infundibulocystic BCC
Fibroepithelial BCC

Higher risk
Basosquamous carcinoma
Sclerosing/morphoeic BCC
Infiltrating BCC
BCC with sarcomatoid differentiation
Micronodular BCC

1910}. Definite BCC typing can only be performed on an excision specimen, rather than an incisional biopsy {3241}.

Epidemiology

BCC is the most common eyelid malignancy in the White population. Owing to chronic sun exposure, climatic changes, and individual and social conditions, its incidence is increasing worldwide. Incidence rates are inversely related to geographical latitude and are higher in lighter-skinned populations. The risk of BCC steadily increases with age {625}. Exposure to indoor tanning is a risk factor for early onset {144}.

Etiology

Ultraviolet (UV) radiation exposure is the most important risk factor for BCC carcinogenesis. Ionizing radiation and systemic arsenic exposure are also known environmental insults, and immunosuppressed patients develop BCC at a rate as high as 10 times that of the general population {3484,1111}.

Naevoid BCC syndrome (Gorlin–Goltz syndrome) is an autosomal dominant disorder characterized by multiple BCCs, odontogenic keratocysts of the jaws, tarsal cysts, palmar and/or plantar pits, and skeletal abnormalities {1844}. Other genetic abnormalities that predispose individuals to BCC include xeroderma pigmentosum, Bazex–Dupré–Christol syndrome, and Rombo syndrome {492}.

Pathogenesis

BCC has one of the highest prevalence rates of somatic mutations of all cancers. Loss of heterozygosity or mutations of *PTCH1* are found in 58–69% of sporadic BCCs, as well as in all BCCs in patients with naevoid BCC syndrome. *TP53* mutations are frequent (44–65%) and *MC1R* variants are also implicated in BCC pathogenesis {2873,1508,2453}.

Macroscopic appearance

Pentagonal (eyelid margin location) or oval excision specimens show a well-circumscribed nodular tumour, often with central ulceration and rolled-up edges.

Histopathology

All types of BCC are characterized by basaloid tumour cells with hyperchromatic nuclei and scant cytoplasm. Apoptotic cells are common within the nests. Stromal changes include fibromyxoid change, retraction of tumour nests from stroma, calcification, and amyloid deposition. Tumour nests may be colonized by melanocytes and contain melanin pigment. Mature keratinization is most common in nodular BCC.

Superficial BCC: This shows lobules of basaloid cells with peripheral palisading extending from the base of the epidermis, and occasionally the adnexal epithelium, into the papillary dermis {2140,3282}. Lesions may appear multifocal but are connected in three dimensions {1854}.

Nodular BCC: Well-circumscribed, variably sized nodules of basaloid cells with peripheral palisading and retraction spaces are seen; disorganized nuclear arrangement with apoptosis is frequently observed in the centre of the nodules. The tumour is usually connected with the epidermis. Keratinizing BCC tumour nests show central mature keratinization. Nodulocystic or cystic BCC shows cystic degeneration within tumour islands.

Micronodular BCC: This is composed predominantly of rounded, ovoid, or slender groups of basaloid cells often scattered throughout the dermis and subcutis {953,2921}. These may appear as separate satellites outlined by a thin rim of stroma and separated by normal dermis. The tumours have an irregular, tentacular, and infiltrative deep or peripheral edge composed predominantly (i.e. > 50%) of rounded small discrete groups of cells (< 0.15 mm in diameter). Single nodules may be seen distant from the bulk of the main tumour. The tumours can reach a large size and may demonstrate perineural involvement.

Infiltrating BCC: Variably sized, sometimes jagged nests of basaloid tumour cells infiltrate the normal dermal collagen. The tumour has an irregular permeating pattern of invasion at the

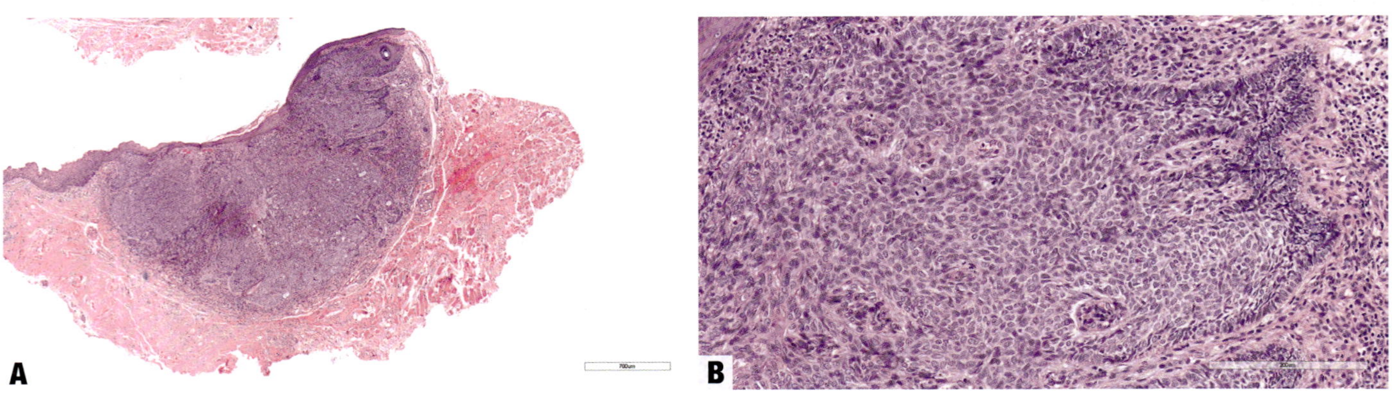

Fig. 3.23 Basal cell carcinoma, nodular. **A** Histopathology shows a nodular basaloid epithelial tumour arising from the epidermis and invading the dermis (stroma). **B** There are islands of basaloid cells with peripheral palisading from the adjacent tumour stroma.

deep tumour edge {2143}. Perineural invasion is more frequent in this subtype {1909}.

Sclerosing/morphoeic BCC: Narrow cords of tumour (1–5 cells thick) are compressed by induced sclerotic collagenous stroma, disrupting the normal dermal architecture. Peripheral palisading and retraction artefacts are uncommon. These tumours penetrate deeply and show an irregular/tentacular, deeply infiltrative border with the surrounding stroma. There is often overlap with infiltrating BCC, which lacks the prominent induced collagenous stroma.

Basosquamous BCC: Lesions show histologically and immunophenotypically distinct zones of BCC intermixed with squamous cell carcinoma, in varying proportions. There may be a zone of transition between the two growth patterns, or they may be closely intertwined. The BCC areas show the typical basaloid cell growth and are often of infiltrative histology; SCC zones show histological atypia with keratinization.

Differential diagnosis

The differential diagnosis includes basaloid follicular neoplasms (trichoepithelioma, trichoblastoma, basaloid follicular hamartoma), basaloid squamous cell carcinoma, sebaceous carcinoma, and Merkel cell carcinoma. BCC shows strong expression of p40/p63 and CK5/6, diffuse BCL2 and CD10 positivity, and focal AR expression, and is negative for EMA, CEA, and CK20. The basaloid follicular neoplasms show colonizing CK20-positive Merkel cells, stromal but not tumoural CD10 expression, and peripheral BCL2 positivity. Basaloid squamous cell carcinoma is positive for EMA and negative with BerEP4, and sebaceous carcinoma is strongly positive for EMA, AR, and adipophilin, but negative with BerEP4. Merkel cell carcinoma is diffusely CK20-positive with perinuclear dot-like positivity, and diffusely expresses neuroendocrine markers {3193}.

Cytology

Not relevant

Diagnostic molecular pathology

Molecular pathology may be performed if an inherited genetic background is suspected or if sonic hedgehog–targeting therapy is considered.

Essential and desirable diagnostic criteria

Essential: nests, nodules, and/or infiltrative cords of basaloid cells with hyperchromatic-staining nuclei and scant eosinophilic cytoplasm; peripheral palisading and retraction artefact to often mucinous stroma.

Desirable: in most cases, numerous mitotic and apoptotic figures.

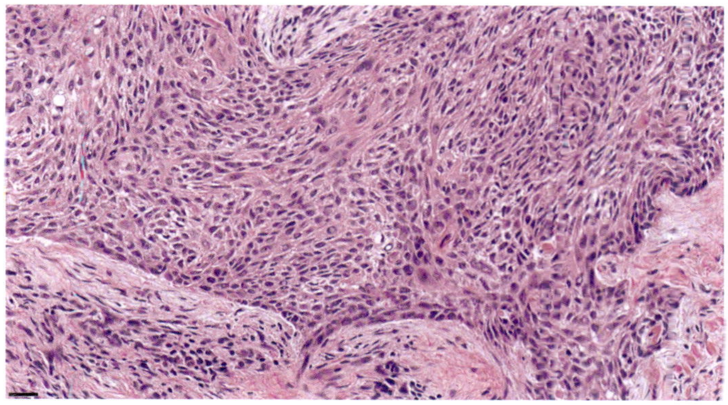

Fig. 3.24 Basal cell carcinoma, basosquamous. Basaloid cells and larger polygonal eosinophilic squamoid cells with no transition zone are seen. An absence of peripheral palisading is common, as shown here.

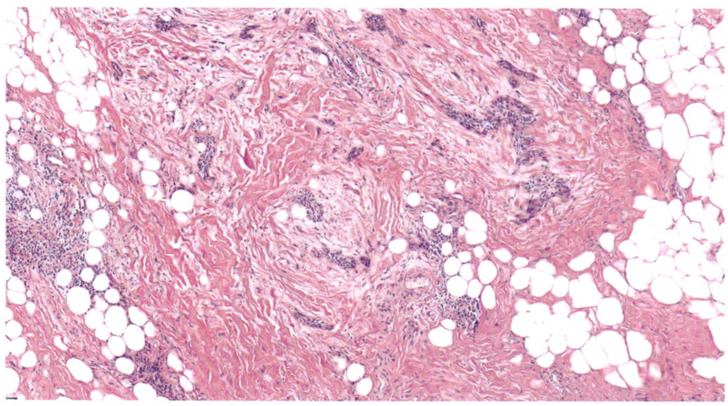

Fig. 3.25 Recurrent basal cell carcinoma, diffuse infiltrative. Small nest without palisading and single cells infiltrating the subcutaneous tissue.

For each subtype, see the related sections in the *Skin tumours* volume {3597}.

Staging

The American Joint Committee on Cancer (AJCC) and the Union for International Cancer Control (UICC) TNM system for non-melanoma eyelid carcinoma applies.

Prognosis and prediction

In order to avoid local recurrence, wide excision is crucial {1051}. Tumours in the medial canthus and sclerosing/morphoeic BCC tend to be incompletely excised resulting in a higher risk of recurrence {1346}. Locally invasive / unresectable tumours can be treated by hedgehog pathway inhibitors (vismodegib) {735, 871} before resection. BCC metastasis is extremely rare; most commonly, regional lymph nodes are involved {2282}.

Squamous cell carcinoma of the eyelid

Kaliki S
Messina JL
Mihic-Probst D
Pe'er J
Scolyer RA

Definition
Eyelid squamous cell carcinoma (SCC) is a malignancy of epidermal keratocytes that exhibit a variety of grades, from dysplasia to invasive carcinoma in situ.

ICD-O coding
8070/3 Squamous cell carcinoma
8070/2 Squamous cell carcinoma in situ (Bowen disease)
8071/1 Keratoacanthoma

ICD-11 coding
2C31.Z & XH0945 Cutaneous squamous cell carcinoma & Squamous cell carcinoma, NOS

Related terminology
Not recommended: squamous cell epithelioma; epidermoid carcinoma; epithelioma spinocellulare; prickle cell epithelioma; spinalioma.

Subtype(s)
Squamous cell carcinoma in situ (Bowen disease)

Localization
The lower eyelid is most commonly involved, followed by the medial canthus, upper eyelid, and lateral canthus {2519,3236}.

Clinical features
SCC is usually painless and presents as an indurated eyelid plaque or nodule. Lesions commonly show keratinization, central ulceration, and rolled-out irregular borders. Subtle tumours can mimic chronic blepharitis wherein eyelid architecture and integrity of eyelashes has to be carefully assessed with a high index of suspicion. A biopsy confirms the diagnosis in suspicious early lesions. Keratoacanthoma-like lesions have also been described. Other presentations include cystic or papillomatous lesions and cutaneous horns {2519,3236}. The presence of pain, paraesthesia, hypoesthesia, or extraocular motility disturbances is suggestive of perineural invasion {3174}.

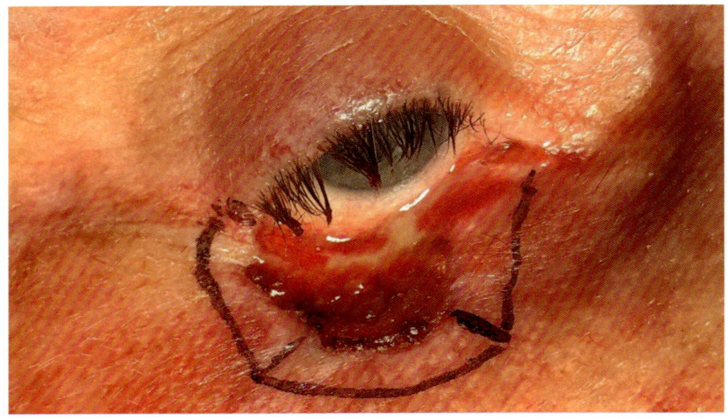

Fig. 3.26 Squamous cell carcinoma. A clinical image of an ulcerated squamous cell carcinoma of the lower eyelid.

Epidemiology
Eyelid SCC is the second most common malignancy of the eyelids after basal cell carcinoma {3236}. In Asian Indians, it is the third, with sebaceous carcinoma being the most common followed by basal cell carcinoma {1571}. It is seen in elderly fair-skinned individuals with chronic sun exposure. Children and young adults with xeroderma pigmentosum can develop SCC at a younger age {2519}. Men are 2–3 times more commonly affected than women {3236}.

Etiology
The most significant risk factor is exposure to ultraviolet A (UVA) light and actinic damage. Other factors include radiation, hydrocarbons, arsenic, and immunosuppression. Individuals with fair skin, immunosuppression, albinism, xeroderma pigmentosum, and epidermodysplasia verruciformis are prone to developing

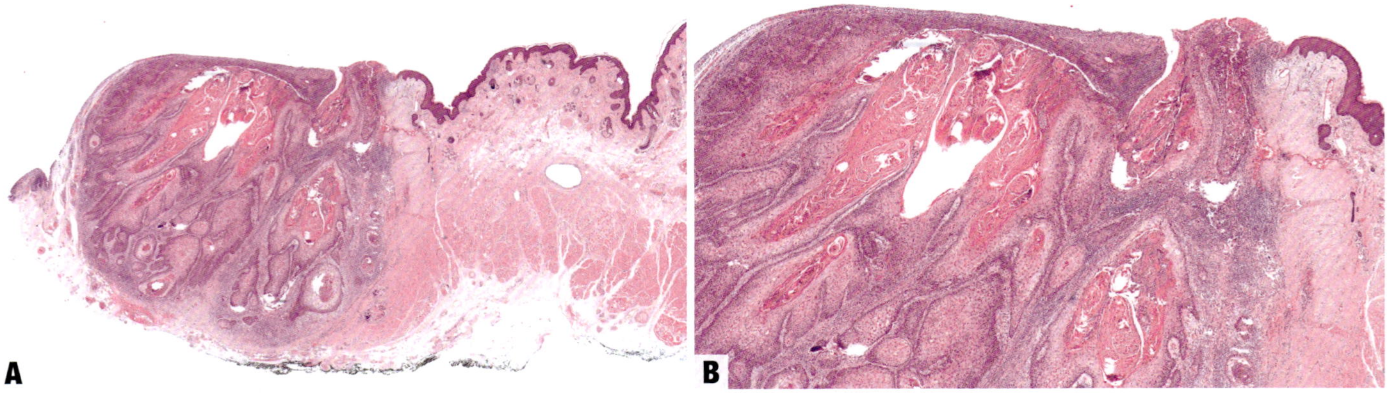

Fig. 3.27 Squamous cell carcinoma. **A,B** A well-differentiated squamous cell carcinoma arranged in solid areas with pushing borders.

Table 3.01 Histological features of keratoacanthoma and keratoacanthoma-like cutaneous squamous cell carcinoma (cSCC-KAL)

Feature	Keratoacanthoma	cSCC-KAL
Symmetry	Yes	Variable
Exoendophytic	Yes	Variable
Even, bowl-shaped base	Yes	Variable
Keratotic crater	Well formed in mature stage	Variable
Overhanging lips of epidermis	Well formed in mature stage	Variable
Width-to-thickness ratio	Typically 2–3:1	Variable, may be < 2:1 (verticality)
Borders of invasion in proliferative phase	Usually infiltrative at the periphery, can be mainly circumscribed	Variable, but often circumscribed and pushing
Depth relative to sweat gland coils	Usually at the same level; below uncommon	Variable; may be high, at the same level, or below
Predominant parakeratosis with hyperchromatic and crowded nuclei	Minimal	Often present, but variable
Infundibular keratinization: laminated with keratohyalin granules	Predominates superficially and centrally	Usually less orderly
Trichilemmal keratinization: compact with deficient keratohyalin granules	Predominates deeply and peripherally	Usually less orderly
N:C ratio in peripheral cells	Typically 1:1 and preserved in cells with large nuclei or multinucleation	Variable, often reduced
Mitotic activity beyond peripheral 1–3 cells	Minimal	Usually present
Nuclear pleomorphism beyond peripheral 1–3 cells	Minimal	Usually present, may be focal
Spontaneous acantholysis (not associated with neutrophils)	Absent	Frequent, may be focal
Intraepithelial "follicular" mucin	Absent	Frequent, may be focal
Necrosis	Absent	Uncommon
Perineural invasion	Uncommon (< 1%)	Uncommon
Venous invasion	Rare	Rare
Elastic and collagen entrapment (H&E or elastic stains)	Common, often widespread, occasionally absent	Variable, often absent
Band-like, lichenoid tissue reaction, lymphocytes predominant, variable eosinophils and neutrophils	Often prominent in mature stage but lacking in early proliferative lesions	Variable, can be prominent
Plasma cells	Minimal	Variable, may be prominent
Regression: loss of proliferative zone (squamatization), numerous Civatte and colloid bodies, peripheral fibrosis, keratin granulomas	Established regression supports diagnosis	Variable but usually lacking
Desmoplastic stroma	Peripheral to lesion in late regressing stage	Variable but often lacking
Severe solar elastosis	Uncommon	Common
Directly associated actinic keratosis	Rare	Uncommon

SCC {3236}. SCC can arise de novo or from precursor lesions such as actinic keratosis or Bowen disease {2519}. Anecdotal reports of the development of SCC in eyelid scar from thermal burns {3690} and seborrhoeic keratosis {3309} exist.

Pathogenesis

Laboratory evidence supports a stepwise fashion of evolution of SCC after exposure to UVA light. UVA-induced mutations in *TP53* lead to altered apoptosis and proliferation of keratinocytes, which either progress to actinic keratosis or papilloma or regress, subject to the presence or absence of continued UVA exposure and other risk factors. In the event of continued exposure, further mutations in *RAS*, loss of FAS ligand, and loss of apoptosis ensue, culminating in a malignant neoplasm {3236}.

Macroscopic appearance

See *Clinical features*, above.

Histopathology

Many SCCs progress from in situ lesions to progressively more deeply invasive tumours. Classic SCC in situ shows full-thickness keratinocyte atypia with absence of maturation, mitoses at all levels, and dyskeratotic cells. Invasive SCC varies from well to poorly differentiated, with most cases classified as well to moderately differentiated. Some well-differentiated forms histologically resemble keratoacanthoma and are now termed keratoacanthoma-like SCC (see the *Skin tumours* volume of this series {3597}). The main histological features distinguishing keratoacanthoma and keratoacanthoma-like SCC are outlined

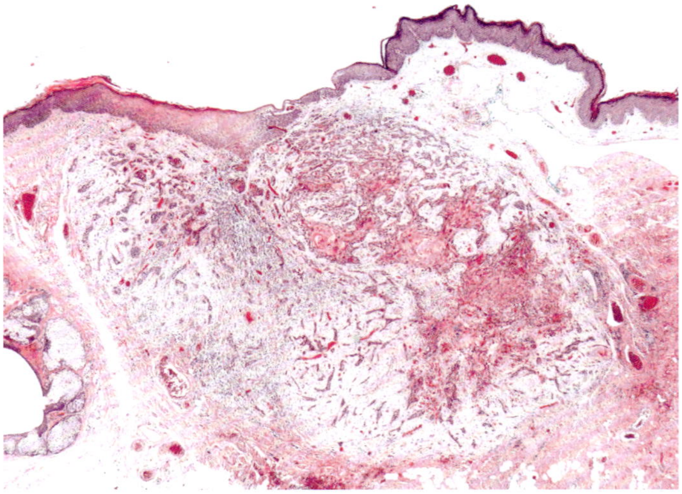

Fig. 3.28 Squamous cell carcinoma. A diffusely infiltrating tumour consisting of cells with abundant eosinophilic cytoplasm and hyperchromatic nuclei, dyskeratosis, and preserved intercellular bridges.

in Table 3.01 (p. 103). Invasive tumour shows polygonal cellular profiles, pleomorphism, and varying amounts of cytoplasmic and extracytoplasmic keratin. Immunohistochemistry is generally not required, except for some poorly differentiated SCCs.

Immunohistochemistry

The tumour cells express p63, p40, CK5/6, MNF116 keratin, and 34βE12 keratin, although immunostains are frequently not needed.

Differential diagnosis

Well-differentiated SCC may be difficult to distinguish from keratoacanthoma. Although there is still controversy, cutaneous keratoacanthoma is probably an entity separate from SCC, with different clinical behaviour, in particular its spontaneous regression {2914,483,229}. Poorly differentiated SCC can resemble sebaceous or basal cell carcinoma.

Cytology

FNAC may be used to evaluate enlarged regional lymph nodes.

Diagnostic molecular pathology

Overexpression of EGFR and PDL1 has been reported and could be of clinical relevance {2086}.

Essential and desirable diagnostic criteria

Essential: a solitary plaque, often progressing to a hyperkeratotic or ulcerated nodule; infiltration of the dermis by islands of atypical cells with variable keratinization.

Desirable: an in situ component may be present; expression of p63, p40, CK5/6, MNF116 keratin, and 34βE12 keratin in morphologically challenging cases.

Staging

The Union for International Cancer Control (UICC) TNM system for non-melanoma eyelid carcinoma applies and has been validated in several studies {3660}.

Prognosis and prediction

The prognosis for localized lesions amenable to surgical excision and with no locoregional extension or metastasis is excellent. Management of tumours that involve the lacrimal system, orbit, and intracranial cavity can be challenging {2519}. Although advanced tumours have conventionally warranted exenteration and metastatic lesions have uniformly been fatal, targeted therapy with EGFR inhibitors and immunotherapy with PD1/PDL1 inhibitors have shown promise for both local/regional control and eye preservation in cases of locally advanced orbital and periocular squamous carcinoma {890,1144,2086}.

Merkel cell carcinoma of the eyelid

Salomao DR
Rao N
Sagiv O

Definition

Merkel cell carcinoma (MCC) is the eponymous name for primary cutaneous neuroendocrine carcinoma.

ICD-O coding

8247/3 Merkel cell carcinoma

ICD-11 coding

2C34 & XH81N8 Cutaneous neuroendocrine carcinoma & Merkel cell carcinoma

Related terminology

Acceptable: primary cutaneous neuroendocrine carcinoma.
Not recommended: trabecular carcinoma; Toker tumour; primary small cell carcinoma of the skin.

Subtype(s)

None

Localization

The majority of MCCs occur on sun-damaged skin, most commonly in the head and neck region (mainly the cheek and eyelids) and less frequently on the extremities and trunk.

Clinical features

MCC is a rapidly growing, indurated, reddish-blue, non-ulcerating nodule on sun-exposed skin of elderly White patients. Lesions are usually painless, with occasional ulceration {639}. Eyelid tumours are often misdiagnosed as chalazion, delaying diagnosis and treatment {2403,1318}.

Epidemiology

The estimated incidence is 0.25–0.32 cases per 100 000 person-years {40A,2688A}. MCC is relatively more common in men, and the median age at diagnosis is 73.6 years. Incidence increases several-fold in individuals aged > 85 years, patients with AIDS, solid-organ transplant recipients, and patients with leukaemia.

Etiology

Exposure to ultraviolet (UV) radiation, immunosuppression, advanced age, and infection with Merkel cell polyomavirus (MCPyV) are risk factors.

Pathogenesis

Although the precise interaction of the risk factors in development of MCC is not clear, MCPyV is reported to be linked to development of MCC in 60–80% of tumours. Viral integration in the genome acts on T-antigen transcripts enhancing viral replication and clonal expansion of MCC cells. Viral-negative MCC reveals UV radiation damage in the form of CC to TT transition at dipyrimidine bases, and mutations in *RB1*, *TP53*, and NOTCH family genes, deregulation of p53 protein expression, and aberrations in the PI3K/AKT/mTOR pathway. Mutation tumour burdens are high in viral-negative MCC {1071,761,2230}.

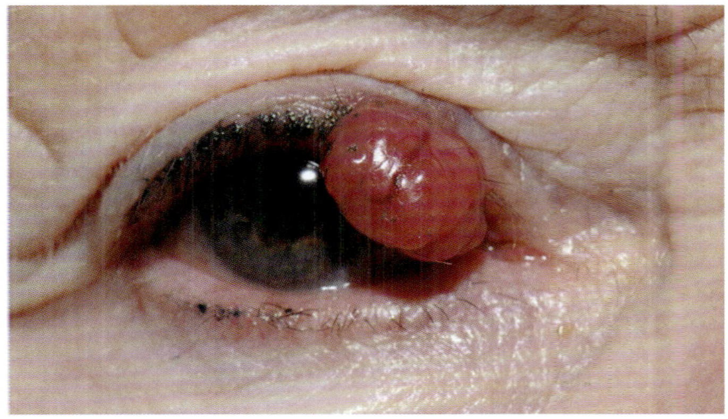

Fig. 3.29 Merkel cell carcinoma. Clinical image of a Merkel cell carcinoma.

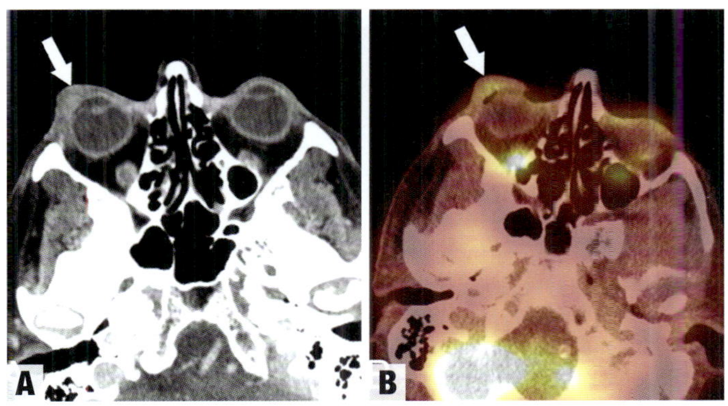

Fig. 3.30 Merkel cell carcinoma. **A** Axial CT with contrast shows a protuberant mass in the right lower eyelid (arrow). **B** 18F-FDG PET-CT shows FDG avidity of the mass (arrow).

Macroscopic appearance

Lesions usually occur as well-circumscribed dermal/subcutaneous nodules, with occasional cutaneous ulceration in larger tumours.

Histopathology

A high-grade small blue cell neoplasm is seen composed of uniform cells with round/oval nuclei, scant cytoplasm, distinct nuclear membranes, finely granular chromatin, and inconspicuous nucleoli. Sheets of tumour cells diffusely infiltrate the dermis and subcutaneous tissue. There is a trabecular growth pattern, and ribbons or festoons can be seen in the periphery of the mass {2568}. Pseudorosettes are rare. Pagetoid spread within the epidermis may be present; rarely, the tumour is entirely confined in the epidermis {428}. Mitotic figures are numerous. Large lesions may show ulceration, zonal necrosis, and angiolymphatic invasion. Areas of squamoid or adnexal differentiation,

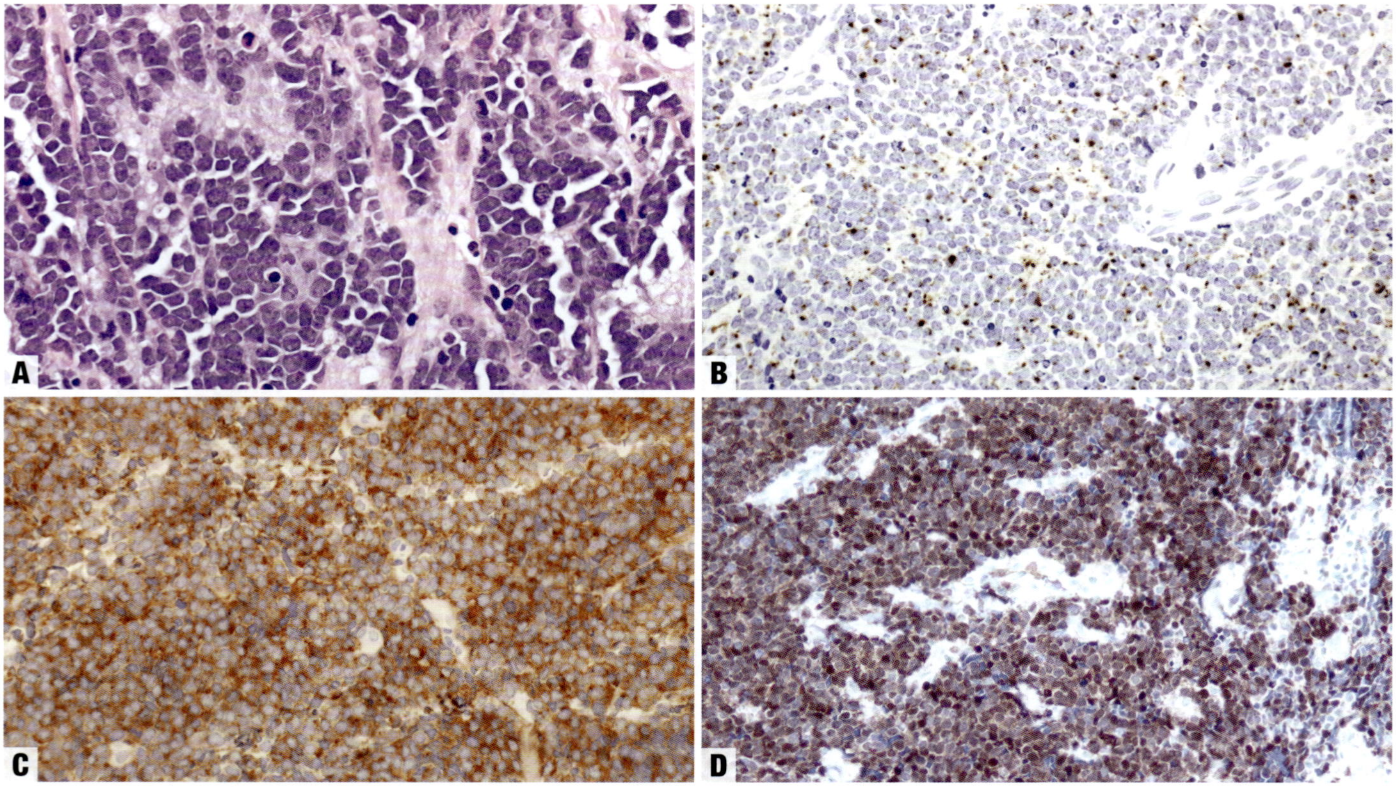

Fig. 3.31 Merkel cell carcinoma. **A** Tumour cells are characterized by scant cytoplasm and indistinct cellular membranes. Nuclei have finely dispersed chromatin and nucleoli are inconspicuous. Numerous mitotic figures and pyknotic nuclei are observed. **B** Perinuclear dot-like pattern observed with CK20 immunohistochemistry. **C** Diffuse cytoplasmic staining with synaptophysin immunohistochemistry. **D** Nuclear positivity with Merkel cell polyomavirus immunohistochemistry.

and infrequently sarcomatoid differentiation, are observed in a minority of cases {3533}.

Immunohistochemistry

Immunohistochemistry shows positivity for CK20, low-molecular-weight keratins (dot-like pattern), and neuroendocrine markers (synaptophysin, chromogranin, INSM1, CD56); and negativity for CK7, CD45, thyroid transcription factor 1 (TTF1), melanocytic markers, and CDX2. Staining with CM2B4 (MCPyV antibody, MCPyV nuclear stain) is positive in most cases {3534}.

Differential diagnosis

The differential diagnosis includes metastatic lung small cell carcinoma, other neuroendocrine tumours, lymphoma/leukaemia, melanoma, round cell sarcomas, and poorly differentiated carcinoma {2604}.

Cytology

Dispersed cells with scant cytoplasm, round nuclei, finely granular chromatin, and no nucleoli are seen. Apoptotic bodies and background necrosis may be present {2966}.

Diagnostic molecular pathology

Detection of MCPyV by PCR varies from 24% {1075} to 85% {283}. Studies have shown gains of chromosomes 1, 5, 6, 18q, and 20, and loss of 10q23; rearrangements of 1p and 3q; and trisomy 6 and 1p deletion. Mutations in *TP53* and *HRAS* have also been observed {2123}.

Essential and desirable diagnostic criteria

Essential: a blue cell tumour in the dermis with salt-and-pepper neuroendocrine cytology; immunophenotype of neuroendocrine differentiation (INSM1, chromogranin, and synaptophysin positivity; paranuclear dot-like staining for cytokeratin); negative for TTF-1.

Desirable: MCPyV positivity.

Staging

The Union for International Cancer Control (UICC) / American Joint Committee on Cancer (AJCC) eighth-edition TNM staging system is used, separating clinical and pathological staging groups and providing more accurate prognostication {1255}.

Prognosis and prediction

Prognosis in patients with MCC is mostly affected by metastasis: the 5-year overall survival rate is 50.6% for patients with local disease, 35.4% for patients with nodal metastasis, and 13.5% for patients with distant metastasis {1255}. T category, based on tumour size, has a significant impact on prognosis: the 5-year overall survival rates are 55.8% for T1, 41.1% for T2/3, and 31.8% for T4 in patients with local disease only. Additional features associated with worse prognosis are infiltrative growth pattern, lymphovascular invasion, presence of tumour-infiltrating lymphocytes, older age, male sex, tumour site, and immunosuppression {1545,72}. Sentinel lymph node biopsy is recommended by some authors {1318,910}.

Ductal hidrocystoma

Stagner AM
Wolkow N

Chapter 3

Definition

Hidrocystomas are benign, sweat gland–derived cysts lined by a dual layer of cuboidal to columnar eosinophilic cells with variable decapitation secretions.

ICD-O coding

8404/0 Ductal hidrocystoma
8404/0 Apocrine hidrocystoma
8404/0 Eccrine hidrocystoma

ICD-11 coding

EK70.3 Hidrocystoma

Related terminology

Acceptable: apocrine gland cyst; eccrine ductal cyst.
Not recommended: sudoriferous cyst.

Subtype(s)

Apocrine hidrocystoma; eccrine hidrocystoma

Localization

Hidrocystomas most commonly involve the lower eyelid (40%), followed by the lateral canthus (30%), upper eyelid (18%), and medial canthus (13%) {2027}. Apocrine hidrocystomas, derived from glands of Moll, typically involve the eyelid margin or the skin immediately adjacent to the mucocutaneous junction/cilia {1487,1480}. Eccrine hidrocystomas may arise in the pretarsal or preseptal eyelid skin.

Clinical features

Hidrocystomas are skin-coloured to blue-tinged and sometimes pigmented (brown), smooth-surfaced, soft, compressible cysts that usually transilluminate. Cysts may be multilocular, multiple, and bilateral and enlarge over months to years, typically presenting at < 5 mm in this location.

Epidemiology

Hidrocystomas typically appear in adults (mean ages of 56 years and 64 years in two large studies) {2027,1487}. There is no consistent sex or race predilection.

Etiology

Hidrocystomas are largely derived from ectasias of the apocrine or eccrine units (ductal or secretory epithelium). Some apocrine hidrocystomas may be neoplastic {258}.

Pathogenesis

Apocrine hidrocystomas do not have clear inciting factors. Some cases of bilateral, multiple apocrine hidrocystomas are associated with Schöpf–Schulz–Passarge syndrome {2027}.

Eccrine hidrocystomas may be associated with retention of sweat and development may be affected by heat and humidity.

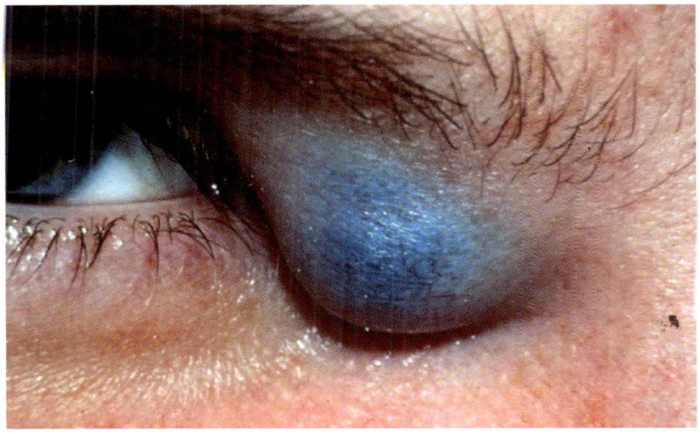

Fig. 3.32 Apocrine cyst. A blue-tinged cyst at the right canthus.

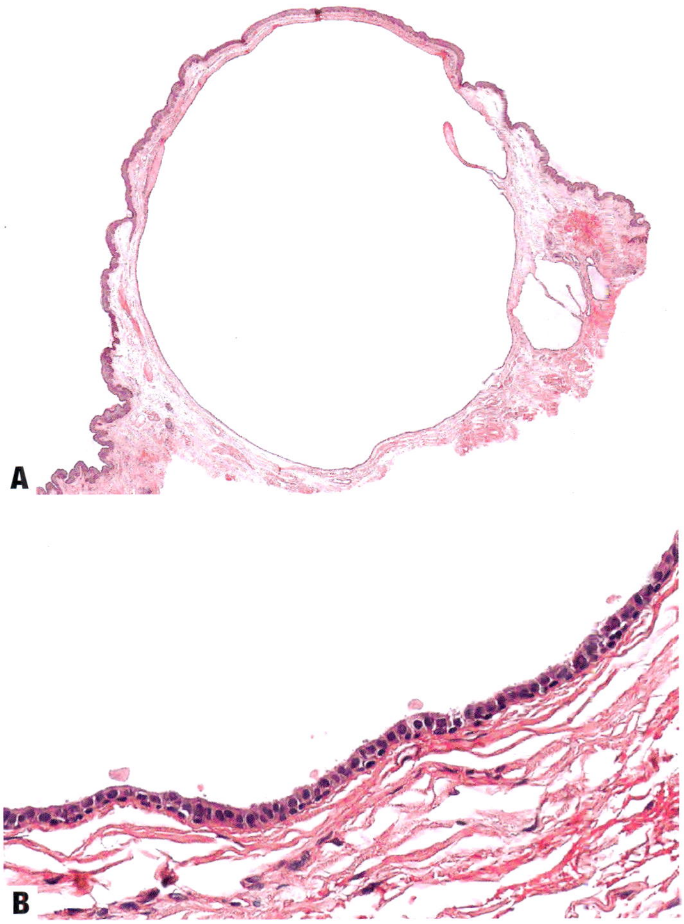

Fig. 3.33 Apocrine hidrocystoma. **A** Multilocular cyst focally filled with eosinophilic proteinaceous material. **B** The cyst is composed of an inner layer of cuboidal cells with apical decapitation secretion and an outer layer of flattened myoepithelial cells.

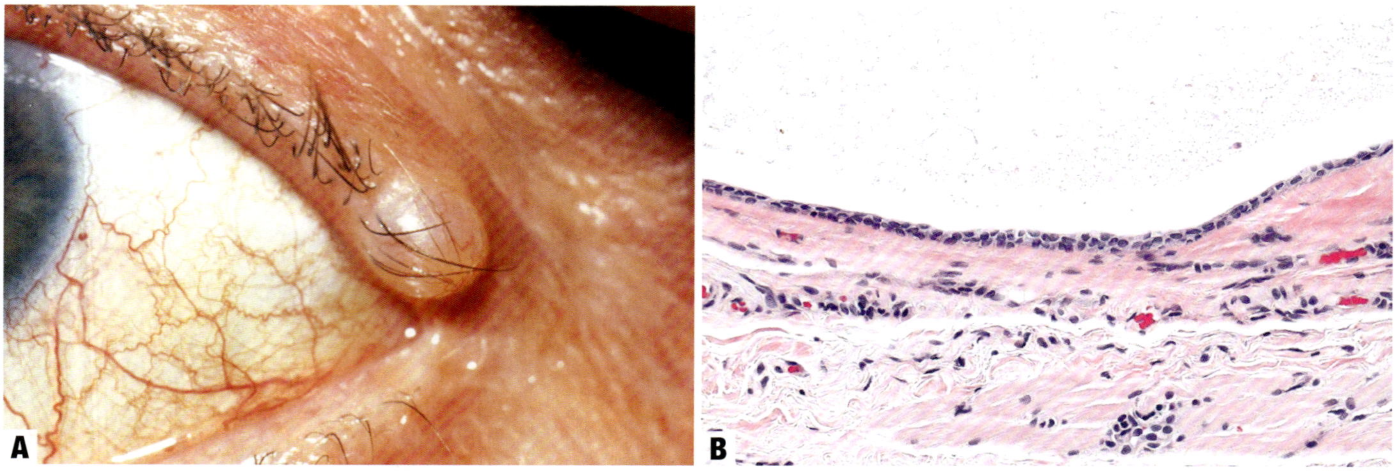

Fig. 3.34 Eccrine hidrocystoma. **A** Translucent cyst at the lateral canthus. **B** The epithelial bilayer is composed of low-cuboidal cells with pale eosinophilic cytoplasm. Eosinophilic proteinaceous material is present in the lumen.

Macroscopic appearance

Cysts are thin and smooth walled, and contain clear to occasionally milky or brownish serous fluid.

Histopathology

Apocrine hidrocystomas (most common in the eyelids) can be multiloculated and are lined by an epithelial-myoepithelial bilayer. The apocrine epithelium is high cuboidal to columnar with glassy, deeply eosinophilic cytoplasm; apical decapitation snouts are present, but may be focal. A dense fibrous wall is common. Some lesions may demonstrate oncocytic change {1480}. Focal proliferative epithelial changes may be seen, manifesting as epithelial multilayering or papillary projections without a fibrous core {539,3231}. Brown or black luminal pigment in the form of lipofuscin may be encountered {118,1480}.

Eccrine hidrocystomas are unilocular and are lined by a low-cuboidal epithelial bilayer with pale eosinophilic cytoplasm lacking apical snouts. Hybrid cysts derived from the junction of the pilosebaceous and apocrine/eccrine units are also relatively common, and these compromise the eccrine unit–type epithelial-myoepithelial layer, merging with areas of an epidermal cyst epithelial lining, containing both keratin and serous fluid {2212}.

Immunohistochemistry

Apocrine hidrocystoma expresses GCDFP-15 and CK7 in the epithelium and SMA in myoepithelial cells. Eccrine hidrocystoma lacks expression of these markers {1487}. (Immunohistochemistry is not required for diagnosis.)

Differential diagnosis

Apocrine cystadenoma, low-grade cystadenocarcinoma, and endocrine mucin-producing sweat gland carcinoma are the main diagnostic considerations and can occur in association with hidrocystoma. Goblet cells / intracytoplasmic mucin, papillae with fibrous cores, and complex cribriform lining should lead to consideration of these entities (see *Apocrine carcinoma*, p. 138, and *Endocrine mucin-producing sweat gland carcinoma*, p. 134) {3231,3738}.

Cytology

Not relevant

Diagnostic molecular pathology

Not relevant

Essential and desirable diagnostic criteria

Essential: a cyst lined by a sweat ductal bilayer containing serous secretion; lack of goblet cells or complex architecture.
Desirable: apocrine secretion in apocrine hidrocystoma.

Staging

Not relevant

Prognosis and prediction

Simple excision is typically curative (recurrence rate of 0–3%). Injection, electrodesiccation, and laser therapy have also been successfully utilized.

Sebaceous hyperplasia, sebaceous adenoma, and sebaceoma

Tetzlaff M
Alkatan H
Eiger-Moscovich M

Definition

Sebaceous hyperplasia is a benign lesion comprising hyperplastic lobules of mature sebaceous glands emanating from a central hair follicle.

Sebaceous adenoma and sebaceoma are a spectrum of benign sebaceous tumours, in which sebocytes predominate over basaloid cells in sebaceous adenoma, whereas basaloid cells predominate over sebocytes in sebaceoma.

ICD-O coding

8410/0 Sebaceous adenoma
8410/0 Sebaceoma

ICD-11 coding

ED91.1 Sebaceous gland hyperplasia
2F22 & XH0QL4 Benign neoplasms of epidermal appendages & Sebaceoma
2F22 & XH1NC5 Benign neoplasms of epidermal appendages & Sebaceous adenoma

Related terminology

Not recommended: sebaceous epithelioma.

Subtype(s)

None

Localization

Sebaceous hyperplasia, sebaceous adenoma, and sebaceoma occur most commonly on the skin of the head and neck. They only rarely occur in the ocular adnexa.

Clinical features

Sebaceous hyperplasia, sebaceous adenoma, and sebaceoma are well-circumscribed yellow-tan nodules {2397,955}. Lesions associated with Muir–Torre syndrome may be multifocal.

Epidemiology

Sebaceous hyperplasia occurs in older patients. Sebaceous adenomas develop in patients aged > 40 years and account for 0.2% of all eyelid lesions {1448}. Sebaceoma occurs in older patients (> 70 years) and is slightly more common in women {2397,2783,3379} and is very rarely reported on the eyelids {3702,2235,2223}.

Etiology

Sebaceous adenoma and sebaceoma show an association with Muir–Torre syndrome (MIM number 158320), whereas sebaceous hyperplasia does not. Muir–Torre syndrome is a rare autosomal dominant cancer predisposition syndrome, defined by the association of cutaneous lesions and Lynch syndrome–associated visceral malignancies {2397,1872}. Muir–Torre syndrome is caused by inherited germline abnormalities of DNA mismatch repair protein genes {42,1046}. Sebaceous adenomas and sebaceomas developing in this setting may show loss of mismatch repair protein expression, including MLH1, MSH2, MSH6, and PMS2 {327,1527,2246,2940}, although this may also occur sporadically, emphasizing the need to integrate clinical factors into patient assessment {2724,2725}.

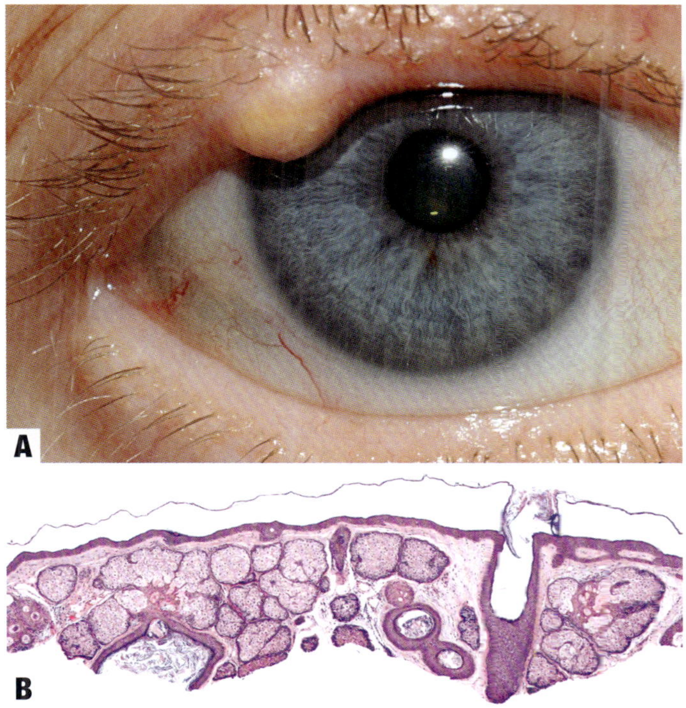

Fig. 3.35 Eyelid sebaceous hyperplasia. **A** A right upper eyelid margin lesion, histologically proven to be sebaceous hyperplasia, is shown. The lesion is yellow, dome shaped, and smooth, with no evidence of eyelash loss. **B** Sebaceous hyperplasia consists of multiple, enlarged lobules of mature sebaceous glands grouped around a central hair follicle.

Pathogenesis

Limited sequencing studies have shown mutations in *TP53*, *CDKN2A*, *EGFR*, *CTNNB1*, and *KRAS* {1258}.

Macroscopic appearance

See *Clinical features*.

Histopathology

Sebaceous hyperplasia consists of multiple, enlarged lobules of mature sebaceous glands grouped around a central hair follicle. Each hyperplastic lobule consists of mature sebocytes, with a non-atypical germinative basaloid layer at the periphery that is no more than 2 cell layers thick.

Sebaceous adenoma and sebaceoma do not show a relationship to hair follicles and are well-circumscribed nodules

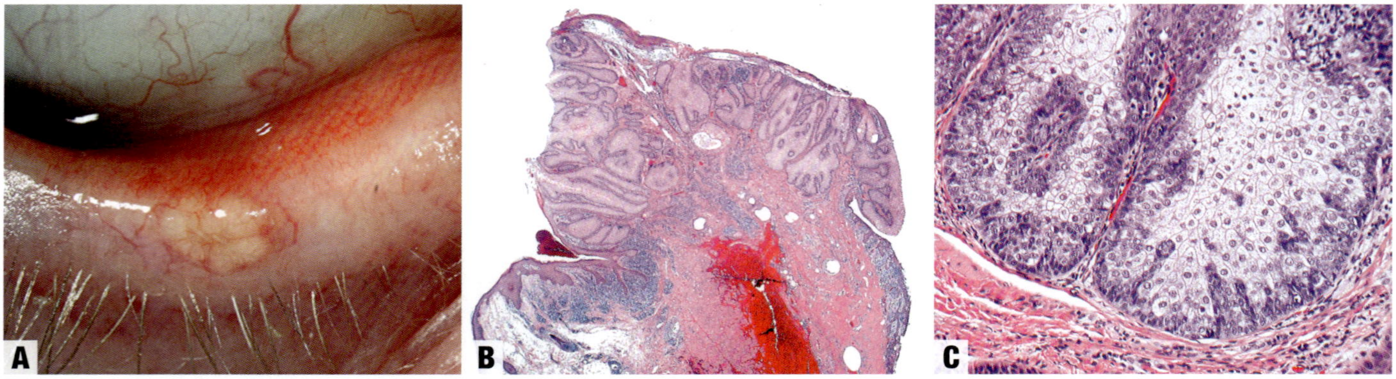

Fig. 3.36 Eyelid sebaceous adenoma. **A** A right lower eyelid lesion, histologically proven to be sebaceous adenoma. Note the yellow lobulated appearance. **B** A lesion of the eyelid margin showing sebaceous adenoma. **C** Higher-power view showing well-formed sebocytes predominating over basaloid cells, which are conspicuous in sebaceous adenoma.

that may show a direct connection to the epidermis. They consist of an admixture of basaloid cells and mature sebocytes. In sebaceous adenoma, sebocytes predominate over basaloid cells, whereas in sebaceoma, basaloid cells predominate over sebocytes. In sebaceous adenoma, the sebocytes are usually central within the lobules and the basaloid cells are sited peripherally. In sebaceoma, the sebocytes are randomly scattered (as individuals or groups) among the basaloid cells. Sebaceoma may also contain ducts and cysts containing sebaceous debris. The basaloid cells have round or oval vesicular nuclei and little cytoplasm and may show mitotic activity. Mild atypia may be seen. The sebocytes are larger in size, with frothy cytoplasm with a central, hyperchromatic, crenated nucleus.

Differential diagnosis

Whereas sebaceous hyperplasia and sebaceous adenoma are typically readily recognized, sebaceoma with many basaloid cells may be difficult to distinguish from sebaceous carcinoma and basal cell carcinoma. Sebaceous carcinomas often show intraepithelial extension, infiltrative growth, and cytological atypia. In contrast to most sebaceomas, basal cell carcinomas show peripheral palisading, retraction artefact, mucinous stroma, and isolated necrotic basaloid keratinocytes.

Cytology

None

Diagnostic molecular pathology

None

Essential and desirable diagnostic criteria

Sebaceous hyperplasia

Essential: hyperplastic lobules of mature sebaceous glands attached to a central hair follicle, with a basaloid layer no more than two cell layers thick; no cytological atypia.

Sebaceous adenoma

Essential: a well-circumscribed sebaceous tumour where sebocytes outnumber basaloid cells; the sebocytes are central and the basaloid cells are at the periphery; the sebocytes are cytologically bland.

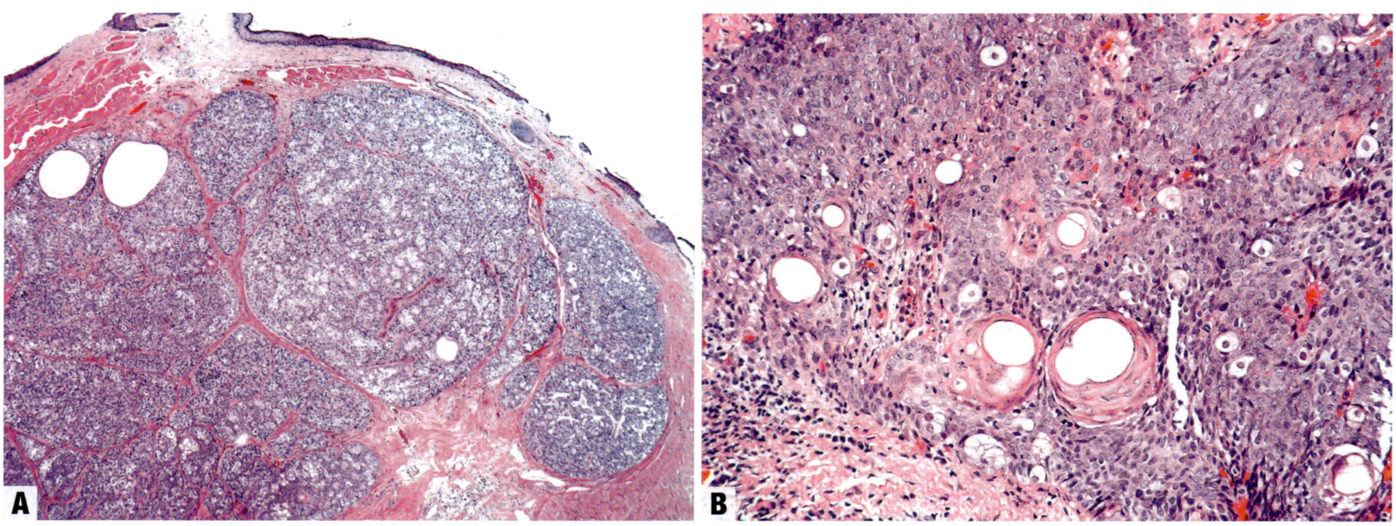

Fig. 3.37 Eyelid sebaceoma. **A** Eyelid sebaceoma with basaloid cells predominating over sebocytes. **B** Basaloid cells predominate over scattered sebocytes in sebaceoma. Note the conspicuous duct formation.

Sebaceoma

Essential: a well-circumscribed sebaceous tumour where basaloid cells outnumber sebocytes; the sebocytes are randomly scattered (individual or grouped) among the basaloid cells; the sebocytes are cytologically bland.

Desirable: presence of ducts and cysts containing sebaceous debris.

Staging

Not relevant

Prognosis and prediction

Sebaceous hyperplasia, sebaceous adenoma, and sebaceoma are benign lesions, and simple excision is typically curative. In sebaceoma, anecdotal examples have shown malignant transformation into sebaceous carcinoma {2224,3539,1884}. A subset of patients with sebaceous adenoma and sebaceoma have Muir–Torre syndrome and may experience morbidity and mortality from associated visceral malignancies {1448,2716}.

Syringoma

Sangüeza OP
Grossniklaus HE

Definition
Syringoma is a benign adnexal tumour of eccrine sweat gland origin.

ICD-O coding
8407/0 Syringoma

ICD-11 coding
2F22 & XH6325 Benign neoplasms of epidermal appendages & Syringoma, NOS

Related terminology
None

Subtype(s)
None

Localization
Most syringomas arise in the lower eyelids and periorbital area {1314}.

Clinical features
Syringoma presents as skin-coloured or slightly yellow smooth papules. Multiple syringomas may resemble milia cysts. When the lesions are pigmented, they may simulate urticaria pigmentosa or confluent and reticulated papillomatosis of Gougerot–Carteaud.

Epidemiology
Syringomas most commonly affect the lower eyelids of middle-aged to older women, but the eruptive pattern is most common in young women {3158}. Clear cell syringoma is more common in people with diabetes.

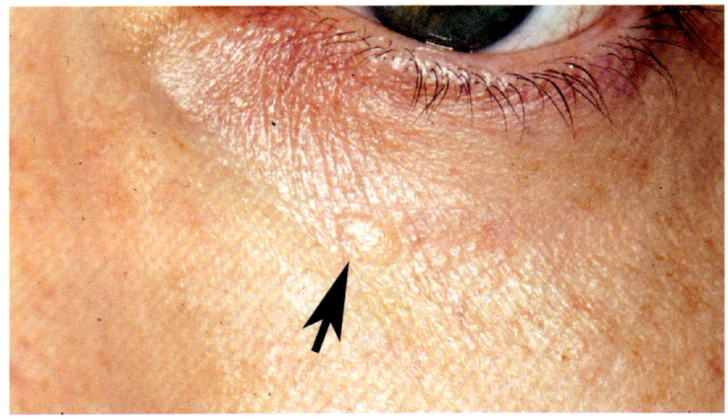

Fig. 3.38 Eyelid syringoma. Clinical photo of the typical appearance of a lower eyelid syringoma.

Etiology
Syringomas are common in patients with Down syndrome {2872}, and they have also been described in patients with hyperthyroidism, Ehlers–Danlos syndromes, Marfan syndrome, and Nicolau–Balus syndrome {845}. In familial forms, multiple syringomas affect several family members.

Pathogenesis
Syringomas resemble the ductal portion of the eccrine gland.

Macroscopic appearance
See *Clinical features*.

Histopathology
Syringomas are well-circumscribed lesions typically affecting the upper half of the dermis; occasionally they can extend into the deep dermis or even the subcutis. Syringoma has two components: epithelial cells forming ducts, cords, tubules, and cysts, and a homogeneous and sclerotic stroma. The lumina of the

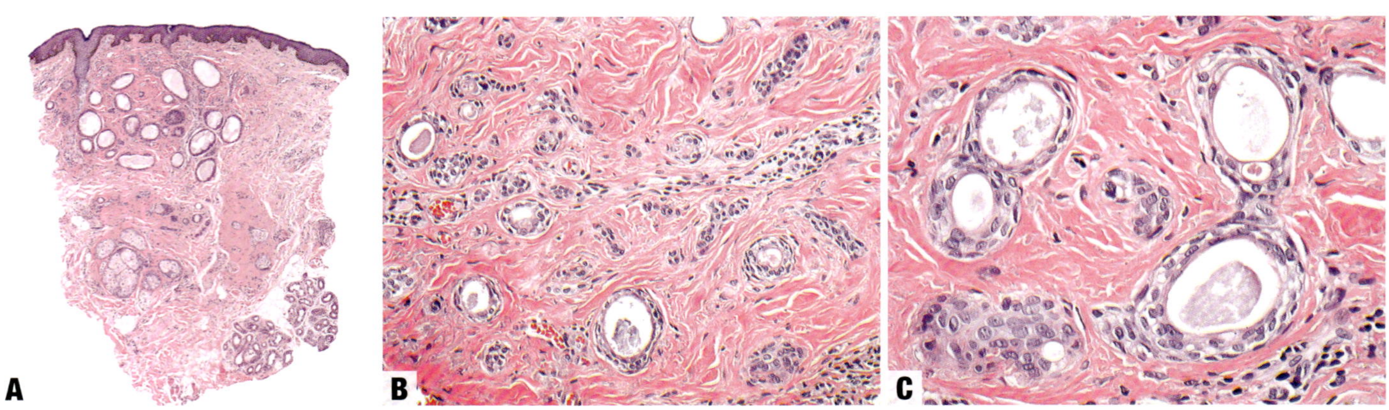

Fig. 3.39 Eyelid syringoma. **A** A neoplasm composed of cystic and tubular structures embedded in a sclerotic stroma. **B** Some ducts show tail-like structures. **C** Higher magnification showing the two layers of cuboidal epithelium lining the ductal structures.

ductal and tubular structures are lined by a double layer of cuboidal cells, sometimes containing a granular basophilic material. The ducts often show characteristic extensions resembling a tadpole tail. Solid collections of epithelial cells are also observed, often containing multiple confluent cytoplasmic vacuoles. Small cysts are often present, filled with basket-weave, basophilic, and orthokeratotic keratin and lined by squamous epithelium. The stroma consists of thick bundles of compact and sclerotic collagen. In eruptive syringoma, the stroma is less prominent.

Differential diagnosis

In superficial biopsies, the differential diagnosis includes microcystic adnexal carcinoma, sclerosing/morphoeic basal cell carcinoma, and desmoplastic trichoepithelioma / columnar trichoblastoma, from which distinction may be impossible without complete removal and clinicopathological correlation.

Cytology

Not relevant

Diagnostic molecular pathology

Not relevant

Essential and desirable diagnostic criteria

Essential: skin-coloured or slightly yellow smooth papules; tubular and cystic structures with circumscribed architecture and benign cytology, embedded in a sclerotic stroma

Staging

Not relevant

Prognosis and prediction

Syringomas are benign lesions. Low-energy radio frequency ablation and carbon dioxide laser have been used with good outcomes and are less invasive and associated with better aesthetic outcomes {1276}.

Mixed tumour

Sangüeza OP
Grossniklaus HE

Definition
Mixed tumour is a benign sweat gland neoplasm composed of epithelial, myoepithelial, and mesenchymal elements; it is the cutaneous analogue of pleomorphic adenoma.

ICD-O coding
8940/0 Mixed tumour
8940/0 Apocrine mixed tumour
8940/0 Eccrine mixed tumour

ICD-11 coding
2F22 & XH2KC1 Benign neoplasms of epidermal appendages & Mixed tumour, NOS

Related terminology
Not recommended: chondroid syringoma.

Subtype(s)
Apocrine mixed tumour; eccrine mixed tumour

Localization
Mixed tumour is more common in the upper eyelid (upper eyelid 60% of cases, lower eyelid 40% of cases) and brow area {1203}.

Clinical features
Mixed tumours are usually solitary, slow-growing, asymptomatic, well-circumscribed non-ulcerating nodules with a smooth surface. They are usually 5–30 mm {1203} and not fixed to underlying structures {1203}.

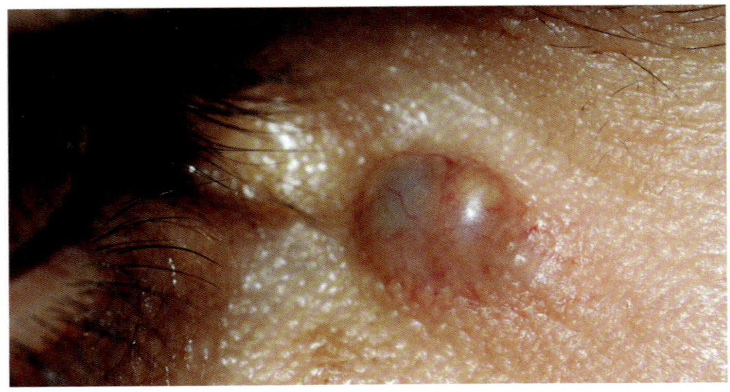

Fig. 3.40 Mixed tumour. Medial canthus mixed tumour with a smooth surface and bluish coloration.

Epidemiology
Mixed tumour of the eyelid has a male predilection, and the average patient age is 50 years (range: 22–73 years) {2056, 3452,1203}.

Etiology
Unknown

Pathogenesis
Pluripotent cells are probably the source of glandular and myoepithelial cells. *PLAG1* {230} and *EWSR1* {988} are rearranged in cutaneous mixed tumours. *PLAG1* is a developmentally regulated zinc-finger proto-oncogene. Rearrangements of *PLAG1* are detected by FISH in less than half of cutaneous mixed tumours {2474}. *PLAG1* activation through gene fusion typically occurs owing to promoter swapping from various fusion partner genes that are ubiquitously expressed, such as *CTNNB1*, *LIFR*, and *CHCHD7*.

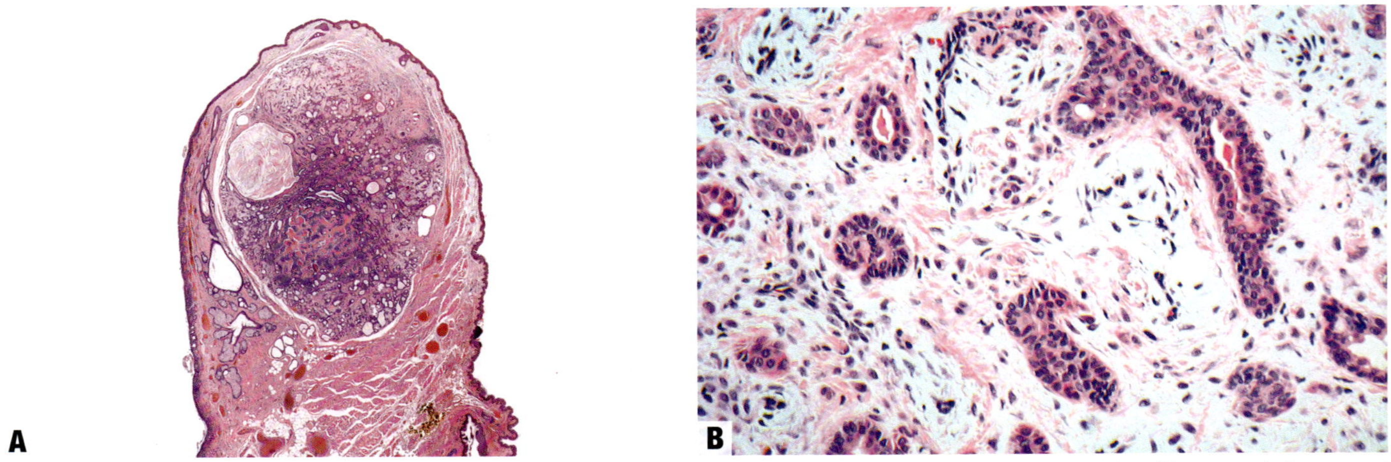

Fig. 3.41 Eyelid mixed tumour (apocrine). **A** Scanning-power images showing a well-defined, unencapsulated tumour in the upper medial eyelid, composed of stroma and epithelial ducts. **B** Fibromyxoid stroma containing benign ducts/tubules.

Macroscopic appearance

See *Clinical features.*

Histopathology

Mixed tumour has two main subtypes: apocrine and eccrine. Apocrine cases present as a well-circumscribed lesion with three components: epithelial, myoepithelial, and mesenchymal (i.e. mucinous, chondroid, osseous, adipocytic, or fibrotic). The epithelial component is composed of elongated branched tubules and cystic spaces. These epithelial structures are lined by two cell layers; the peripheral layer is composed of cuboidal myoepithelial cells, and the inner layer is formed by columnar cells. The luminal cell layer may exhibit secretion by decapitation. Cystic areas often contain homogeneous eosinophilic material. Solid aggregates of epithelial cells, as well as isolated polygonal and plasmacytoid epithelial cells, may be also seen. Tumours with a prominent myoepithelial component may show focal cytological atypia; such cases have been called hyaline cell–rich mixed tumour {1633}. Follicular and/or sebaceous differentiation can be present {3670}.

The eccrine subtype of mixed tumour is less common and lacks the *PLAG1* gene rearrangement {2793}. It is composed of numerous non-branching, round ductal elements lined by a single layer of cuboidal cells embedded in a predominantly myxoid or chondromyxoid stroma. Small solid epithelial aggregates may be seen. Unusual findings include cribriform areas, clear cell change, hyaline cells, pseudorosette-like structures, prominent osseous metaplasia, and striking intracytoplasmic vacuolization of the neoplastic cells resulting in physaliphorous-like cells {1635}.

Immunohistochemistry

Mixed tumours express SOX10, p63, S100, calponin, SMA, EMA, KIT, CEA, various cytokeratins, and PLAG1, although the eccrine subtype does not express this marker.

Differential diagnosis

Myoepithelioma is a related entity distinguished by the lack of ductal structures. When the mesenchymal component is prominent, the differential diagnosis of mixed tumour includes chondroma, but chondromas do not contain epithelial cells.

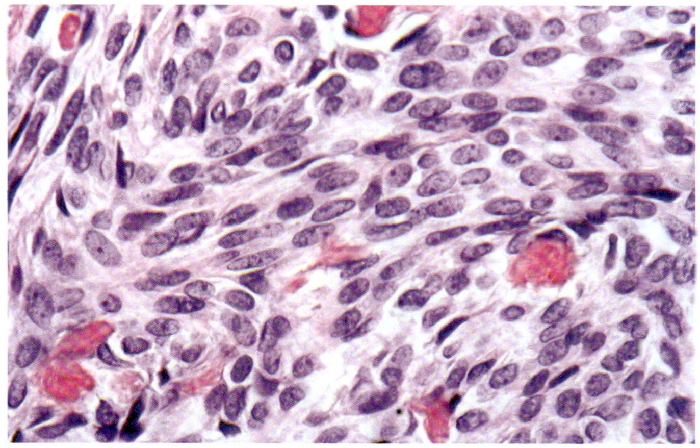

Fig. 3.42 Eyelid mixed tumour. A solid myoepithelial-rich area within the tumour.

Cytology

Although not described from the eyelid, FNAB of these tumours shows appearances reflecting their histology: fibrillary chondromyxoid material, with a prominent cellular component composed of epithelial and myoepithelial cells {836,2745,2941}.

Diagnostic molecular pathology

Not clinically relevant

Essential and desirable diagnostic criteria

Essential: a well-circumscribed smooth-surfaced nodule; tubules and cords of benign glandular epithelium embedded in a myxo-hyalinized or a cartilaginous stroma; in eccrine mixed tumours, there are no signs of decapitation secretion or of sebaceous or follicular differentiation.

Staging

Not relevant

Prognosis and prediction

Mixed tumours are benign neoplasms that grow slowly and can reach several centimetres. Complete surgical excision is curative. Incomplete excision can result in local recurrence {3238, 1203}.

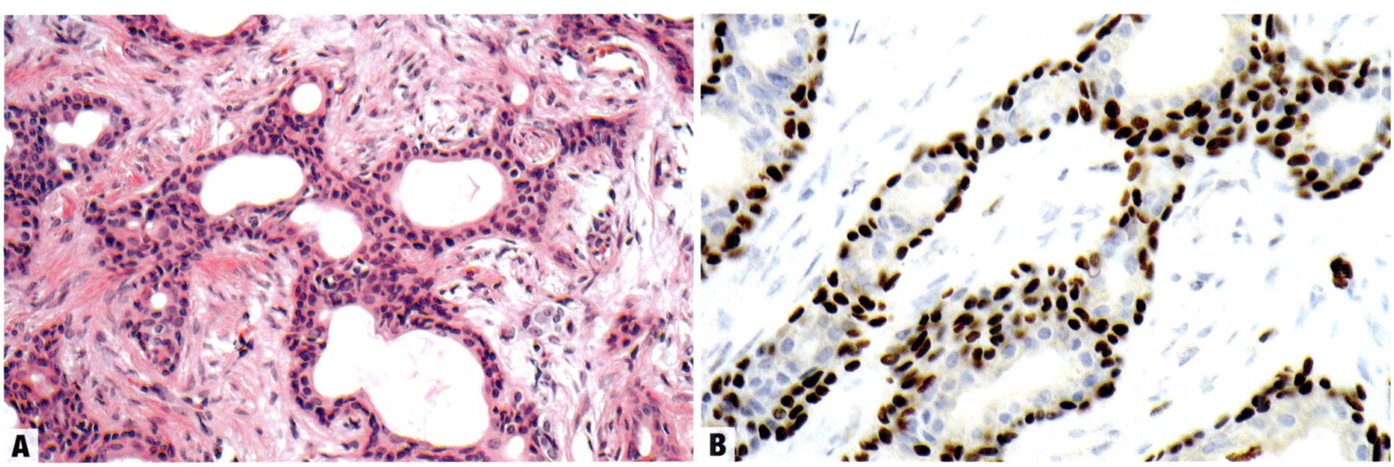

Fig. 3.43 Mixed tumour. **A** Benign ducts/tubules lined by two layers of epithelium: an inner epithelial layer and an outer myoepithelial layer. **B** p63 stains the outer myoepithelial cells of the epithelial tubules/ducts, whereas the inner epithelial cells are not stained.

Tubular adenoma

Sangüeza OP
Grossniklaus HE

Definition

Tubular adenoma is a benign apocrine neoplasm comprising lobules of multiple irregularly shaped tubular structures that have a double- to several-layered cell lining (inner epithelial and outer myoepithelial), embedded in a fibrous stroma.

ICD-O coding

8211/0 Tubular adenoma

ICD-11 coding

2F22 & XH7SY6 Benign neoplasms of epidermal appendages & Tubular adenoma, NOS

Related terminology

Acceptable: tubulopapillary adenoma; papillary eccrine adenoma; tubular apocrine adenoma.

Subtype(s)

None

Localization

Equal numbers of cases are located on the upper and lower eyelid {872}.

Clinical features

The duration of symptoms is 6–12 months. The lesion size (where the data is available) is 6–8 mm. It presents as an asymptomatic, single, round, well-circumscribed nodule with a smooth surface {872}.

Epidemiology

There are very few reported cases of pure eyelid tubular adenoma. The age range is 38–63 years (mean: 47 years). The M:F ratio is 1:1. It mostly affects White people {872}.

Etiology

Unknown

Pathogenesis

Activating mutations in the MAPK signalling pathway, affecting *BRAF*, *KRAS*, and *HRAS*, are present in syringocystadenoma papilliferum and tubular adenoma {2960,1940,2018}. These increase cell growth, differentiation, and survival. Tubular adenoma can develop sporadically or, more frequently, on the genetic background of a cutaneous mosaic RASopathy, such as naevus sebaceus of Jadassohn {3561}.

Macroscopic appearance

See *Clinical features*, above.

Histopathology

Tubular adenomas are well-circumscribed dermal neoplasms that may extend into the subcutis. They have an overall lobular architecture and are typically encased by a fibrous stroma. The lobules consist of multiple irregularly shaped tubular structures that have a double- to several-layered epithelial lining. The peripheral epithelial layer consists of cuboidal to flattened (myoepithelial) cells, and the luminal layer consists of columnar cells that sometimes demonstrate decapitation secretion. In some tubules, papillary cellular extensions that are devoid of stroma project into the lumina. Cellular debris and eosinophilic granular material are found within

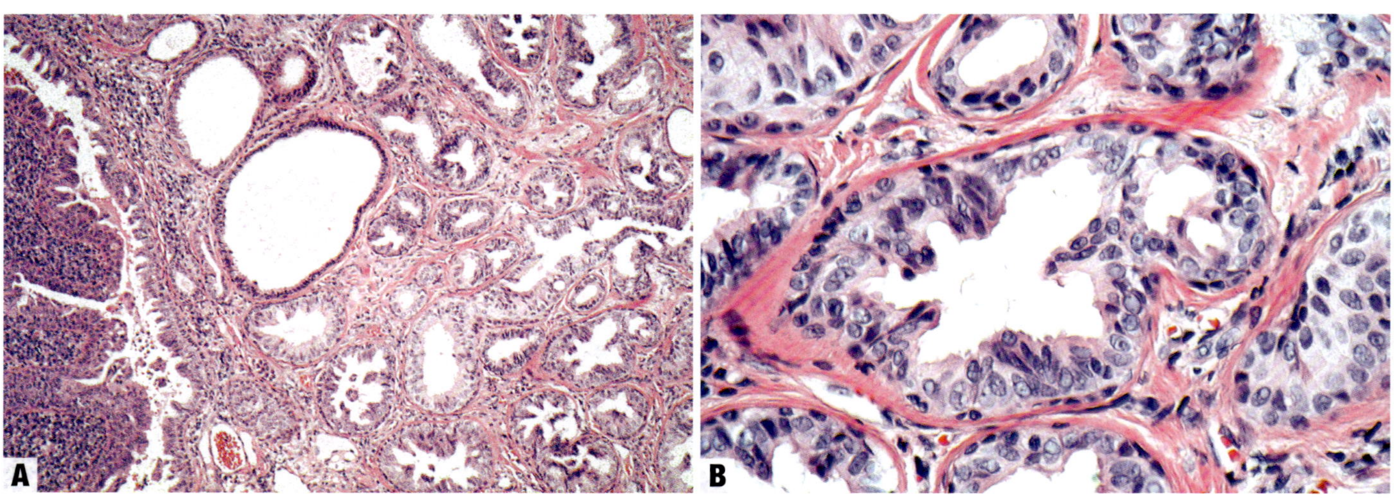

Fig. 3.44 Eyelid tubular adenoma. **A** On the left is an eyelid syringocystadenoma papilliferum and on the right is a tubular adenoma. **B** A high-power view of an eyelid tubular adenoma shows the inner epithelial layer and the outer myoepithelial layer. Note how the inner epithelial layer is papilleroid in some profiles.

some lumina {1852}. The neoplasm lacks cytological atypia and mitotic figures. Overlying epidermal hyperplasia may be present. In cases that occur in conjunction with syringocystadenoma papilliferum {165,3362}, the tubular adenoma component is typically present underlying the syringocystadenoma component.

Immunohistochemistry

BRAF p.V600E (antibody clone VE1) can be assessed by immunohistochemistry {1037} and is seen in syringocystadenoma papilliferum and tubular adenoma. The luminal cells of syringocystadenoma papilliferum and tubular adenoma are positive for CEA and EMA, whereas the outer cell layer is typically reactive for myoepithelial markers including SMA, calponin, SOX10, and p63 {2702}. A focal lack of myoepithelial cells can be seen in areas with prominent squamous metaplasia or intraluminal secretions.

Cytology

Not relevant

Diagnostic molecular pathology

BRAF p.V600E mutations are present in 66% of tubular adenomas {2018}. Naevus sebaceus–associated tubular adenomas consistently harbour *HRAS* or *KRAS* mutations {1175}. In sporadic tumours, *HRAS* p.G13R mutations are found in a few cases; *KRAS* p.G12D mutations are less frequent {2960}.

Essential and desirable diagnostic criteria

Essential: lobules consisting of multiple irregularly shaped tubular structures that have a double- to several-layered epithelial lining, embedded in a fibrous stroma.

Staging

Not relevant

Prognosis and prediction

Tubular adenomas are benign neoplasms. Excision with clear margins is curative. Incompletely excised lesions can recur {872,3387,287}. There are no cases of malignant transformation of tubular adenoma.

Syringocystadenoma papilliferum

Sangüeza OP
Grossniklaus HE

Definition
Syringocystadenoma papilliferum (SCAP) is a benign apocrine neoplasm, composed of two layers of cells (inner epithelial and outer myoepithelial layer) forming dilated papillary and cystic structures with the stroma containing abundant plasma cells.

ICD-O coding
8406/0 Syringocystadenoma papilliferum

ICD-11 coding
2F22 & XH1PY0 Benign neoplasms of epidermal appendages & Syringocystadenoma papilliferum

Related terminology
None

Subtype(s)
None

Localization
Most cases are located on the lower lid margin. Smaller numbers of cases are seen on the upper lid or canthal area {3387, 287}.

Clinical features
The duration of the lesion before presentation ranges from 2 months to 70 years (mean: 24 years). The lesion size range is 4–25 mm. The main symptoms are swelling, pruritis, and bleeding. The appearance can be nodular, papular, verrucous, cystic, ulcerated, or crusted, or an umbilicated pore that oozes fluid {3387,287}. SCAP can be misdiagnosed as basal cell carcinoma, sebaceous cyst, recurrent chalazion, and hidrocystoma {3387,287}.

Epidemiology
The age range is 8–82 years (mean: 44 years). The M:F ratio is 1:2, and the lesion mostly affects White ethnic groups {3387, 287}.

Etiology
Unknown

Pathogenesis
Activation of mutations in the MAPK signalling pathway, affecting *BRAF*, *KRAS*, and *HRAS*, are present in SCAP and tubular adenoma {2960,1940,2018}. These activating mutations increase cell growth, differentiation, and survival.

Macroscopic appearance
See *Clinical features*.

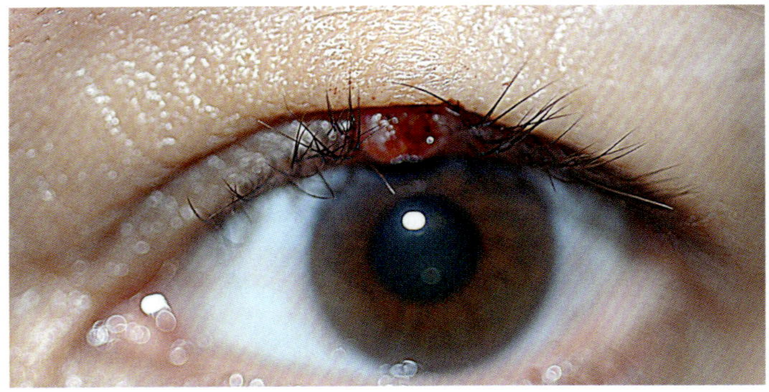

Fig. 3.45 Syringocystadenoma papilliferum. Clinical photo of an upper eyelid syringocystadenoma papilliferum.

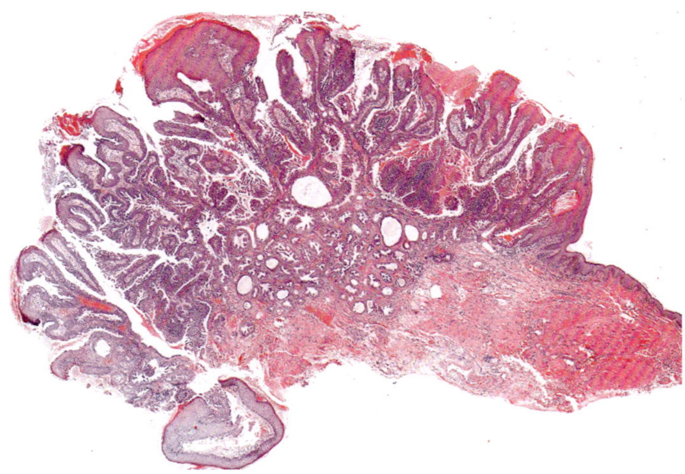

Fig. 3.46 Eyelid syringocystadenoma papilliferum. At scanning magnification, the lesion shows an exoendophytic architecture, with invaginations of epithelium, which is squamous at the surface and papilliform towards the deeper invaginations.

Histopathology
SCAP is an endophytic crateriform lesion, connected focally to the epidermis / hair follicle and composed of two layers of cells forming dilated papillary and cystic structures. The luminal cells are columnar with rounded or oval nuclei near the basal pole of the cell and abundant eosinophilic cytoplasm with decapitation secretion. Mucinous metaplasia may be observed. The outer layer consists of basal/myoepithelial cells. The overlying squamous epithelium often displays prominent hyperplasia. The epidermis surrounding SCAP is often papillomatous or wart like, particularly in cases associated with naevus sebaceus of Jadassohn. The stroma contains numerous plasma cells.

Immunohistochemistry
BRAF p.V600E (antibody clone VE1) can be assessed by immunohistochemistry {1037} and is seen in SCAP and tubular

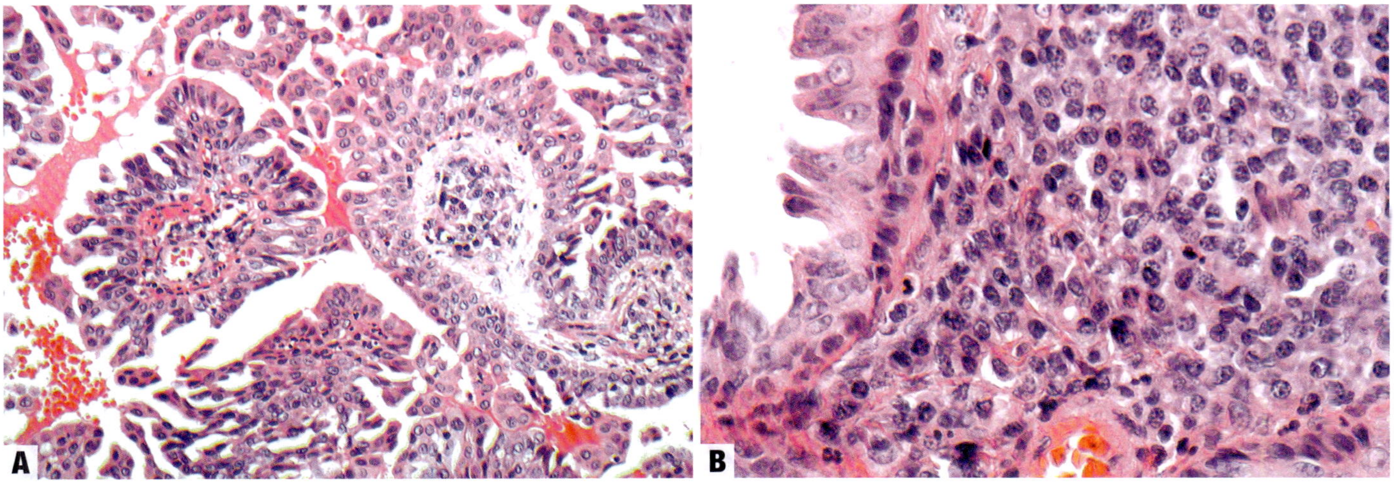

Fig. 3.47 Eyelid syringocystadenoma papilliferum. **A** Papillary cores draped in epithelial cells showing a papilliform architecture. **B** Prominent plasma cells within the cores of the papillary frond.

adenoma. The luminal cells of SCAP and tubular adenoma are positive for CEA and EMA, whereas the outer cell layer is typically reactive for myoepithelial markers, including SMA, calponin, SOX10, and p63 {2703}. A focal lack of myoepithelial cells can be seen in areas with prominent squamous metaplasia or intraluminal secretions.

Differential diagnosis

The histopathological differential diagnosis of SCAP includes hidradenoma papilliferum {1765}. Hidradenoma papilliferum has papillary formations similar to those of SCAP, and the epithelial cells lining these structures also show evidence of secretion by decapitation. However, hidradenoma papilliferum is not connected to the epidermis and lacks plasma cells.

Cytology

Not relevant

Diagnostic molecular pathology

BRAF p.V600E mutations are present in 50–64% of SCAPs {2018}.

Essential and desirable diagnostic criteria

Essential: tubular structures with papillary projections and plasma cells in the stroma.

Staging

Not relevant

Prognosis and prediction

SCAP is a benign neoplasm. Excision with clear margins is curative. Incompletely excised lesions can recur {872,3387, 287}. There is 1 reported case of malignant transformation of SCAP, harbouring invasive squamous cell carcinoma {409}.

Pilomatricoma

Alkatan H
Eberhart CG
Ferreira TA

Definition

Pilomatricoma is a benign cutaneous adnexal neoplasm that shows differentiation towards matrical cells and the hair cortex.

ICD-O coding

8110/0 Pilomatricoma

ICD-11 coding

2F22 & XH9E37 Benign neoplasms of epidermal appendages & Pilomatricoma, NOS

Related terminology

Acceptable: pilomatrixoma.
Not recommended: calcifying epithelioma of Malherbe.

Subtype(s)

None

Localization

Pilomatricoma mostly involves the upper eyelids and medial eyebrow area {3685,3775,1923,1548,80,1012}.

Clinical features

Pilomatricoma usually presents as a solitary, well-defined, painless, slowly growing, subcutaneous reddish-blue mass, which is firm and freely mobile, and has a gritty sensation due to calcification {3062,1923}. It can show rapid growth due to inflammation {1923,558}. It is usually < 10 mm in diameter. Calcification may result in the tent sign due to angulation of the tumour {2562, 1323}. Multiple lesions have been described {1548,2562,1323}.

High-resolution MRI allows the identification of most eyelid structures and can assess the precise location of pilomatricomas inside the eyelid {957}. Furthermore, MRI aids in the differential diagnosis of eyelid masses, and perfusion-weighted imaging helps in differentiating a pilomatricoma from a malignant eyelid mass. Although it is a benign lesion, a low apparent diffusion coefficient can be seen, probably due to the presence of calcifications.

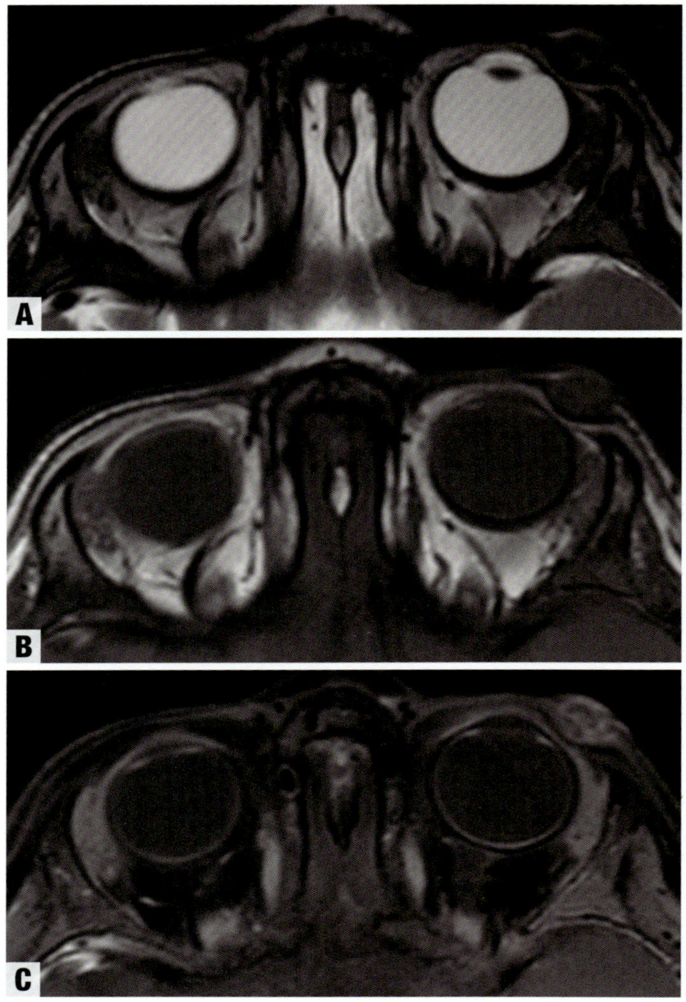

Fig. 3.48 Pilomatricoma. Images showing a mass located superficially in the left upper eyelid, in front of the orbicularis oculi muscle. **A** Axial T2-weighted MRI. The mass is mostly hypointense on T2-weighted images. **B** Axial T1-weighted MRI. **C** Axial contrast-enhanced T1-weighted MRI with fat signal suppression. The mass is heterogeneously enhancing.

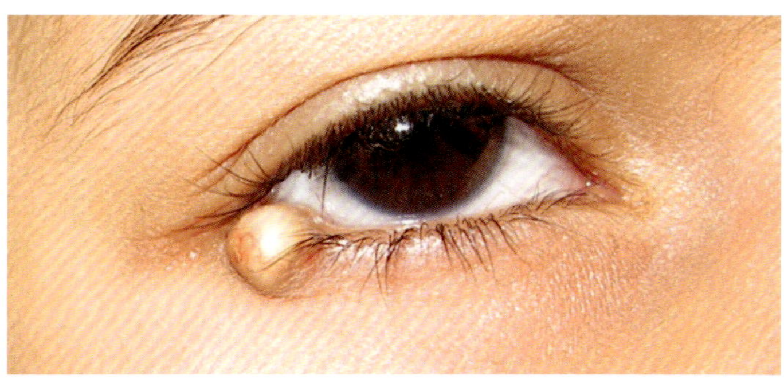

Fig. 3.49 Pilomatricoma. The clinical appearance of an eyelid pilomatricoma in a child.

Epidemiology

The M:F ratio in White people is 2:3 {1923}. It has a bimodal presentation, with one peak in children and young adults (40% in the first decade of life and 20% in the second decade of life) and another peak between 50 and 65 years of age {1923,1548, 2165}.

Etiology

Most are sporadic. Familial and multiple cases are linked to genetic conditions such as myotonic muscular dystrophy, Gardner syndrome, basal cell naevus syndrome, and xeroderma pigmentosum {2562,1262}. Associations with blunt trauma, hypercalcaemia, and sarcoidosis {3664,1923} are reported.

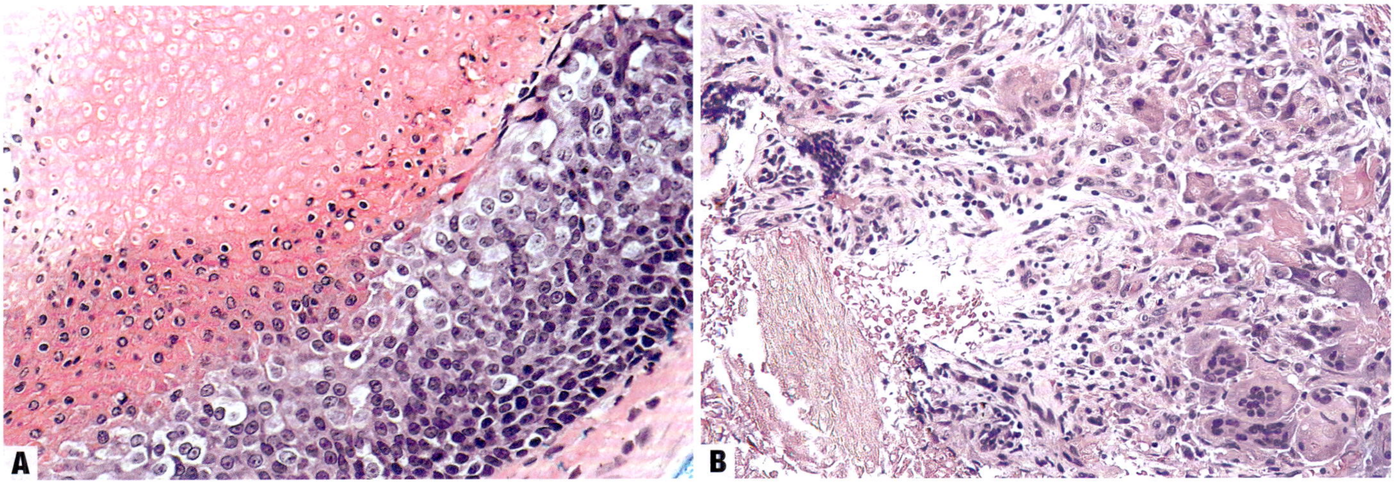

Fig. 3.50 Eyelid pilomatricoma. **A** The three classic components of a pilomatricoma comprising basaloid cells, with scant cytoplasm, an intermediate zone with smaller pyknotic basophilic nuclei with eosinophilic cytoplasm, and a central area with shadow cells with eosinophilic cytoplasm and non-staining empty nuclei. **B** Histopathological appearance of pilomatricoma with an area of numerous multinucleated foreign body–type giant cells.

Pathogenesis

Pathogenesis has been linked to disruption of the hair growth anagen phase {1923} and to the *CTNNB1* gene mutation {1567}.

Macroscopic appearance

Lesions appear as pink to tan-coloured well-circumscribed firm nodules that may be pseudoencapsulated {537,558}.

Histopathology

The tumour comprises one or several dermal nodules. The periphery of the nodules shows mitotically active basaloid cells, with scant cytoplasm. An intermediate zone shows smaller pyknotic basophilic nuclei with a paler cytoplasm and the central area shows shadow cells with eosinophilic cytoplasm and non-staining empty nuclei centrally {1221,537}. Shadow cells may calcify over time {1923}. Focal granulomatous inflammation, sheets of keratin-like material, and foreign body–type giant cells are also common {1923,373,97}.

Cytology

FNAB produces smears with recognizable clusters of basaloid cells and foreign body–type multinucleated cells {1239,197}. Ghost cells can be difficult to find {1239}.

Diagnostic molecular pathology

Not clinically relevant

Essential and desirable diagnostic criteria

Essential: the presence of basaloid cells at the periphery, an intermediate zone with smaller pyknotic basophilic nuclei, and eosinophilic shadow (ghost) cells centrally.

Staging

Not relevant

Prognosis and prediction

Recurrence has been reported in 1.4% of cases in one series within an average time of 1.6 years {2562}. Malignant transformation into pilomatrix carcinoma is rare {2087}.

Trichilemmoma

Cherepanoff S
Stagner AM

Definition
Trichilemmoma is a benign tumour that differentiates towards the outer root sheath epithelium of the hair follicle infundibulum (trichilemmal differentiation).

ICD-O coding
8102/0 Trichilemmoma
8102/0 Desmoplastic trichilemmoma

ICD-11 coding
2F22 & XH5AU2 Benign neoplasms of epidermal appendages & Trichilemmoma

Related terminology
None

Subtype(s)
Desmoplastic trichilemmoma

Localization
The central face is the most common site of involvement, including the eyebrow and eyelid {1333}. Rarely, the lid margin or inner canthus can be involved. Lesions can be solitary or multiple.

Clinical features
Trichilemmoma is typically a slow-growing flesh-coloured papule or nodule of 1–5 mm, although it rarely may be > 10 mm {1333}. Trichilemmoma can also present as a papillomatous lesion mimicking verruca vulgaris. The desmoplastic subtype may mimic invasive carcinoma {1333}.

Epidemiology
Trichilemmoma affects a wide age range, although the majority of cases are seen in adults. There is a predominance in White people and an equal sex distribution {1333}. Lesions are typically solitary. Multiple lesions or paediatric presentation raises the possibility of Cowden syndrome {2550} (a member of the *PTEN* hamartoma tumour syndrome) {2190}, in which the prevalence of trichilemmomas is 6–38% {3272,2553,1292,435}.

Etiology
The etiology of sporadic lesions is unknown. Owing to the papillomatous appearance of some trichilemmomas, a link to HPV infection has been suggested, although there is limited published evidence {2751,2869}.

Multiple lesions are associated with Cowden syndrome (a member of the *PTEN* hamartoma tumour syndrome) {2550}, an autosomal dominant disorder caused by mutations in *PTEN*.

Pathogenesis
For solitary lesions, the pathogenesis is unknown.

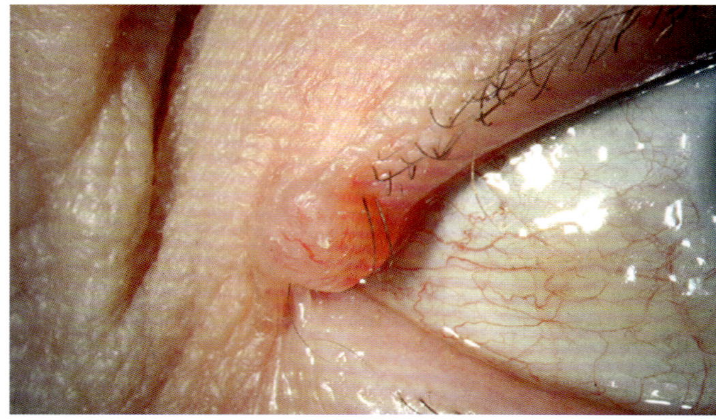

Fig. 3.51 Trichilemmoma. Clinical image showing a nodular configuration of trichilemmoma, which in this case was of the desmoplastic histological type.

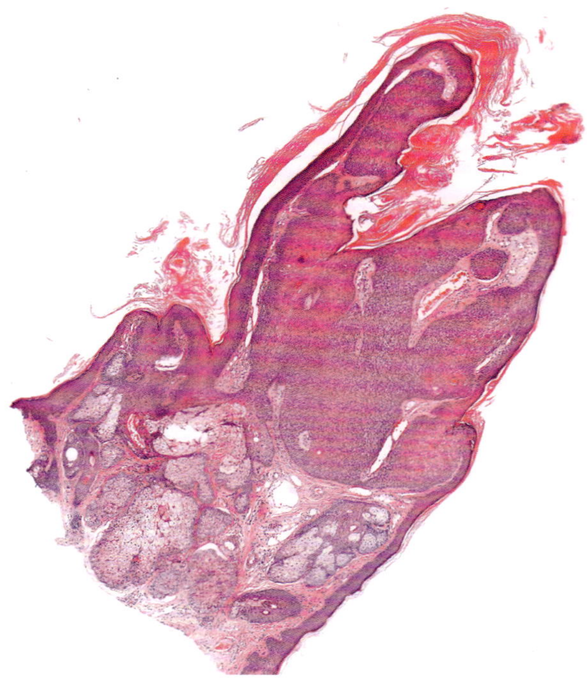

Fig. 3.52 Trichilemmoma. Low-power view showing the exophytic warty architectural configuration of a conventional trichilemmoma.

For trichilemmomas occurring in Cowden syndrome, mutations in the *PTEN* gene cause absence of PTEN inhibition, causing AKT activation, resulting in phosphorylation of proteins such as mTOR that affect cell growth, cell-cycle entry, and cell survival {473}.

Macroscopic appearance
Skin-coloured firm papule or wart-like lesion

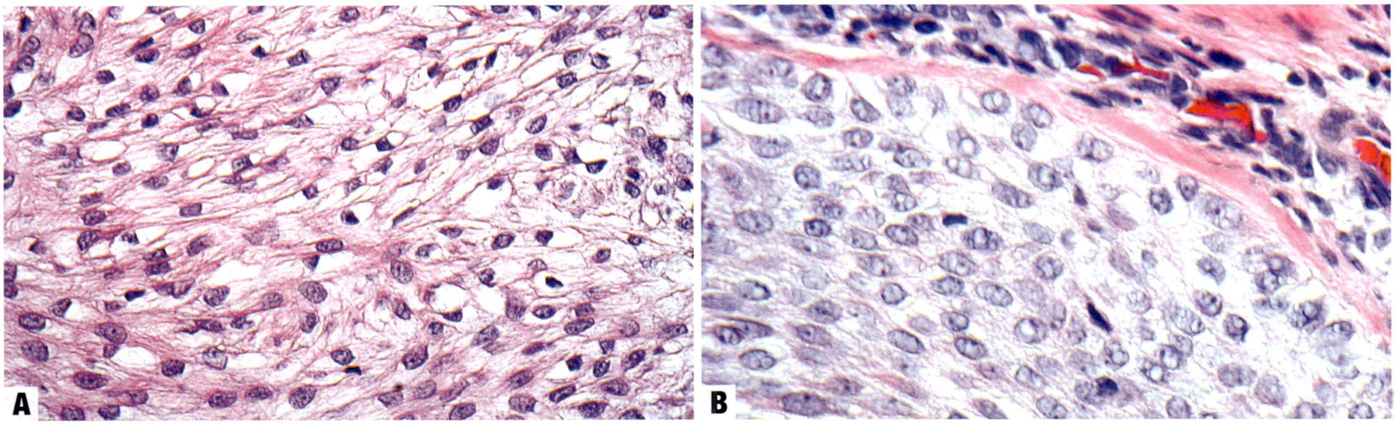

Fig. 3.53 Trichilemmoma. **A** Typical cytoplasmic glycogen vacuolation of trichilemmoma cells is seen, indicative of differentiation towards the hair outer root sheath. **B** A prominent eosinophilic basement membrane can surround the tumour lobules.

Histopathology

Conventional trichilemmoma: At low magnification, the lesion can be exophytic / wart like or bulbous, can be associated with a pre-existing hair follicle, often shows an epidermal collarette, and is connected to the epidermis. There may be hyperkeratosis and parakeratosis of the overlying epidermis. The tumour is lobulated and often surrounded by an eosinophilic, thickened basement membrane, resembling the basement membrane of the lower hair follicle. The lobules are composed of eosinophilic, bland squamoid cells, some of which exhibit trichilemmal differentiation resembling the hair follicle outer root sheath cells. This is characterized by cytoplasmic glycogen vacuolation within bland, monomorphic cells, without mitotic activity or pleomorphism. The edges of the lobules display a palisade with columnar cells that can show reverse polarity. Squamous eddies / morules are often present in the lesion {429,1333}.

Desmoplastic trichilemmoma: This has identical features to a conventional trichilemmoma except there is a central sclerotic area of excessive basement membrane–like material embedded within which are irregular epithelial strands that show little glycogen vacuolation. These strands mimic invasive carcinoma {1407,3306}.

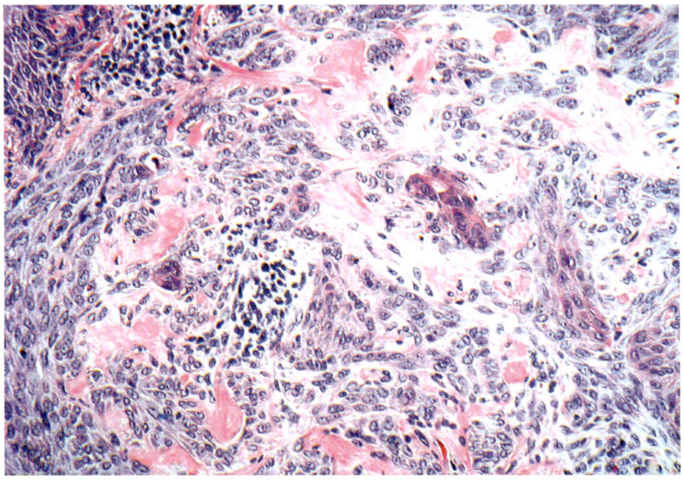

Fig. 3.54 Desmoplastic trichilemmoma. Irregular tongues of more squamoid-looking cells are seen, lacking cytoplasmic glycogen vacuolation, embedded within sclerotic stroma. This is the typical appearance of a desmoplastic focus within a desmoplastic trichilemmoma.

Immunohistochemistry

Trichilemmomas express CD34 in the tumour epithelial cells (which can be rather focal) and p16 {1340,3290}, and are negative with BerEP4.

Differential diagnosis

The differential diagnosis includes inverted follicular keratosis, viral wart, tumour of the follicular infundibulum, eccrine poroma, basal cell carcinoma with trichilemmal differentiation, invasive squamous cell carcinoma, trichilemmal carcinoma {3100}.

Cytology

Not relevant

Diagnostic molecular pathology

Diagnostic molecular pathology is not performed routinely for solitary tumours in adults. For multiple trichilemmomas or those presenting in children, germline testing for *PTEN* mutations may be indicated in the appropriate clinical context. Loss of PTEN, seen with immunohistochemistry, is more frequent in syndromic tumours and may be useful as an initial screening tool {131}.

Essential and desirable diagnostic criteria

Essential: for conventional trichilemmoma: bland squamoproliferative lesion connected to the epidermis with a palisade showing trichilemmal differentiation characterized by cytoplasmic glycogen vacuolation; for desmoplastic trichilemmoma: as for conventional trichilemmoma, with a central area of excessive basement membrane–like material containing irregular epithelial strands, mimicking invasive carcinoma.

Desirable: demonstration of CD34 immunohistochemical positivity in morphologically challenging lesions; loss of PTEN staining in suspected Cowden syndrome.

Staging

Not relevant

Prognosis and prediction

Trichilemmoma is a benign lesion. Surgical excision is curative.

Sebaceous carcinoma

Tetzlaff M
Alkatan H
Eiger-Moscovich M
Esmaeli B
Heindl LM
Rao N

Definition
Sebaceous carcinoma is a malignant neoplasm demonstrating sebaceous differentiation.

ICD-O coding
8410/3 Sebaceous carcinoma

ICD-11 coding
2C33 & XH4VR2 Adnexal carcinoma of skin & Sebaceous carcinoma

Related terminology
Acceptable: Meibomian gland carcinoma.

Subtype(s)
None

Localization
Sebaceous carcinoma occurs most commonly in and around the eyelids {2663}. Periocular sebaceous carcinoma accounts for 75% of all cases {3028,2307,2663,1355,3668,3706}.

Clinical features
Periocular sebaceous carcinoma presents as a tan-pink-yellow immobile nodular lesion (10–30 mm). It may be mistaken clinically for benign inflammatory or neoplastic conditions, leading to higher morbidity and mortality {808,1129,3626,2307,1311}. Pagetoid sebaceous carcinoma may resemble chronic blepharoconjunctivitis {2307}.

Epidemiology
Sebaceous carcinoma develops in older adults, with no sex predilection. The median age at diagnosis is 73 years. The estimated incidence (per 1 million person-years) is approximately 2 cases in White populations, 1 case in Asian and Pacific Islander populations, and 0.5 cases in Black populations {723}.

Etiology
Risk factors include prior radiotherapy, sun exposure, *TP53* mutations, viral infections (HIV and HPV), and Muir–Torre syndrome {2307,1377}.

Pathogenesis
Periocular sebaceous carcinoma can harbour mutations in *TP53*, *RB1*, the NOTCH gene family, and *ZNF750*, as well as gain of the *MYC* locus {3314,2539}. A small subset are related to high-risk HPV infection {3313,2261,2398,2397}. While some extraocular sebaceous carcinomas are related to Muir–Torre syndrome, with most showing defective mismatch repair {3314, 2400}, periocular sebaceous carcinomas rarely show defective mismatch repair {3314,2400,3,2642,327,2031,2940}.

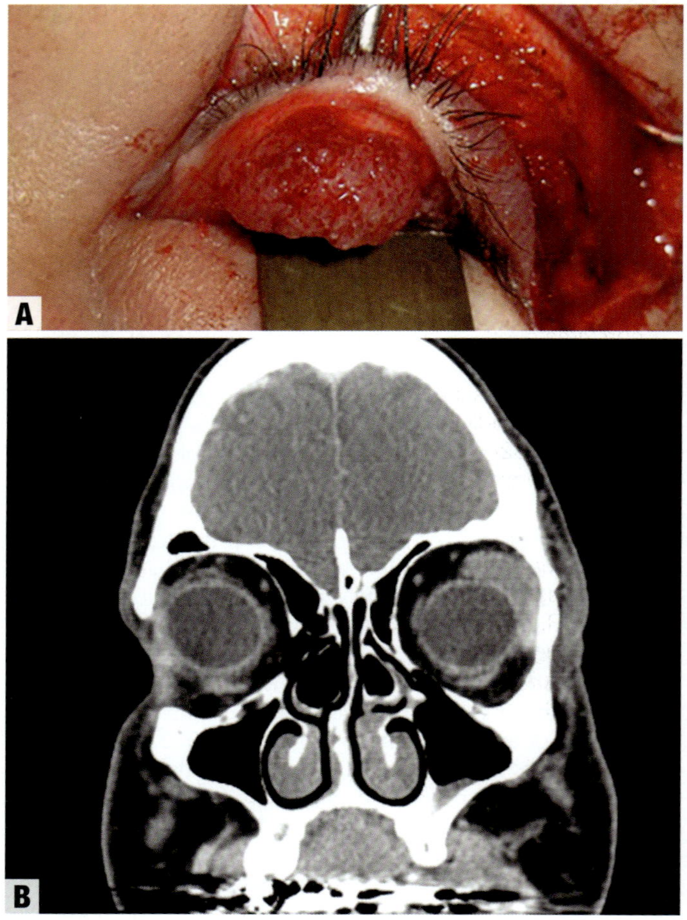

Fig. 3.55 Sebaceous carcinoma. **A** A tumour involving the upper eyelid. **B** CT shows a periocular sebaceous carcinoma forming a mass lesion in the left eye.

Macroscopic appearance
See *Clinical features.*

Histopathology
Well-differentiated sebaceous carcinoma consists of polygonal tumour cells with atypical oval vesicular nuclei and abundant intracytoplasmic vacuoles that impart a foamy appearance and impinge on the nucleus creating scalloping. More poorly differentiated tumours show a higher N:C ratio, nuclear pleomorphism, prominent nucleoli, and basophilic cytoplasm, with fewer intracellular vacuoles {417} and brisk mitotic activity. Sebaceous carcinoma may show basaloid, squamoid (often with keratin pearl formation), spindle-cell/sarcomatoid, or neuroendocrine (rippled or organoid growth) features {3626,1637,1821}.

Invasive tumours can adopt various architectural patterns, including well-circumscribed lobules with pushing borders and

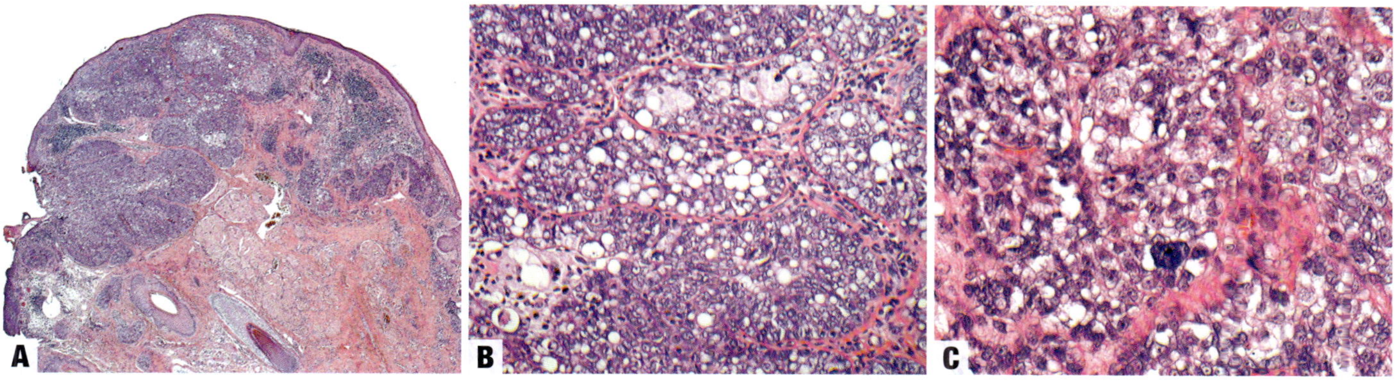

Fig. 3.56 Eyelid sebaceous carcinoma. **A** Low-power image of an eyelid showing basophilic bulbous deposits of invasive sebaceous carcinoma. **B** High-power image of an invasive eyelid sebaceous carcinoma showing intracytoplasmic lipid vacuoles. **C** Invasive eyelid-skin sebaceous carcinoma showing highly atypical nuclei and multivesicular cytoplasmic vacuoles.

variable comedonecrosis, papillary, and highly infiltrative cords. Combinations of these patterns are often observed.

Approximately 60% of cases carry an intraepithelial component (pagetoid spread) with extension along and partial replacement of the pre-existing pilosebaceous units in the skin, and the conjunctival epithelium. Notably, intraepithelial skip lesions may also occur {2532} and sebaceous carcinoma in situ (restricted to the epithelium) may be encountered {211,1638}.

Immunohistochemistry

Sebaceous carcinoma shows immunoreactivity for pancytokeratin (and also CK7). Staining is variably positive for adipophilin, EMA, AR, p40, and p63, and with BerEP4 {3312,166,2451}. EMA labelling may enhance the cytoplasmic vacuolization of the tumour cells, but it is often only positive in well-differentiated tumours and lacks specificity. Adipophilin is a more sensitive and specific marker of sebaceous differentiation {2451,3312}. Positivity for CD10, DOG1, KIT (CD117), p16, p53, perforin, and factor XIIIa has also been reported in sebaceous carcinoma {1156,1925,2231,295}.

Differential diagnosis

Sebaceous carcinoma should be excluded when examining basaloid, squamoid, and clear cell epithelial tumours in a periocular location. The differential diagnosis includes sebaceoma, balloon cell melanoma, clear cell squamous cell carcinoma, basal cell carcinoma, Merkel cell carcinoma, and metastatic clear cell carcinomas from visceral organs.

Cytology

None

Diagnostic molecular pathology

None

Essential and desirable diagnostic criteria

Essential: an invasive or intraepithelial tumour showing sebaceous differentiation, manifesting as multivesicular cytoplasmic clearing with nuclear scalloping.

Desirable: immunohistochemical confirmation of sebaceous differentiation is critical in cases lacking obvious histopathological evidence of sebaceous differentiation.

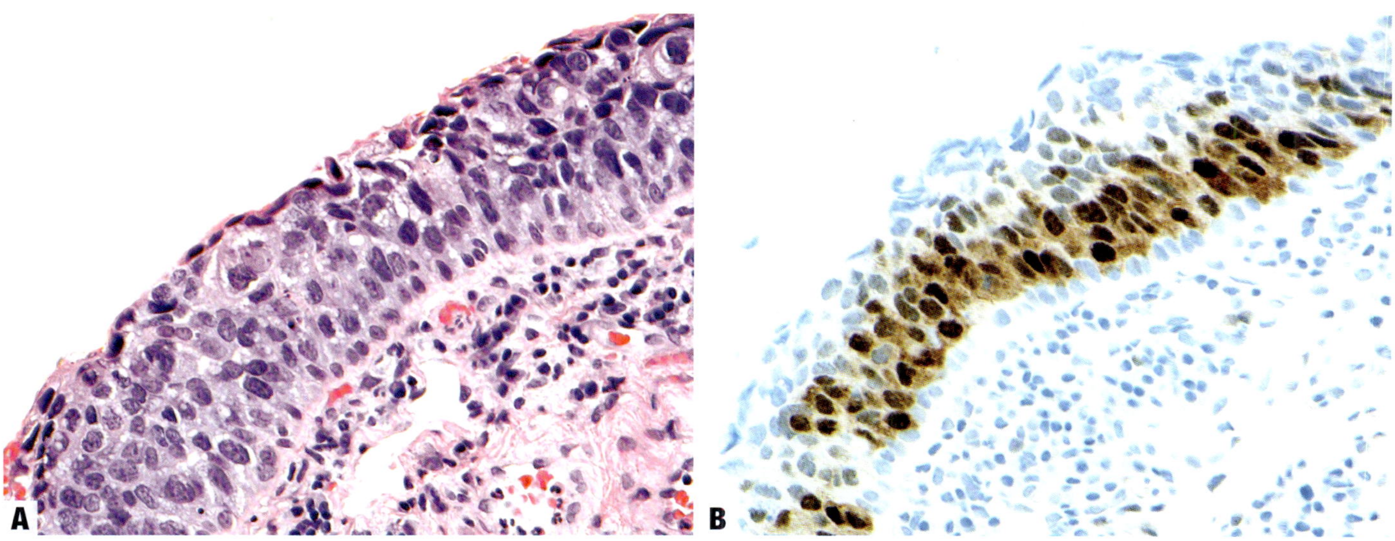

Fig. 3.57 Conjunctival intraepithelial sebaceous carcinoma. **A** Sebaceous tumour cells with multivesiculated cytoplasm replacing much of the conjunctival epithelium. Note the intact basal layer of the conjunctival epithelium. **B** AR positivity of intraepithelial sebaceous tumour cells. Note the negative staining of the surrounding conjunctival squamous epithelium, including the basal layer beneath the tumour cells.

Staging

The eighth edition of the Union for International Cancer Control (UICC) / American Joint Committee on Cancer (AJCC) TNM system forms the basis for staging. The application of the eighth edition of the AJCC staging system was found useful in predicting nodal metastasis; however, local recurrence and distant metastasis were not significantly correlated to the T classification {77}.

Prognosis and prediction

Eyelid sebaceous carcinoma has a 5–25% local tumour recurrence rate after surgery {2796}. According to the eighth edition of the UICC/AJCC TNM system, risk factors for local recurrence include stage T3b (> 20 mm) or worse disease, pagetoid spread, diffuse growth pattern, and multicentric origin. The literature review shows that surgical excision with frozen section control is the optimal modality, and any pagetoid spread is treated with topical chemotherapy and cryotherapy {2796}.

According to the eighth edition of the UICC/AJCC TNM system, the 5-year Kaplan–Meier estimate rate for regional lymph node metastasis varies between 9% (T1) and 42% (T4), the rate for systemic metastasis varies between 0% (T1) and 34% (T4), and the rate for metastasis-related death varies between 0% (T1) and 43% (T4) {2270}.

Adenoid cystic carcinoma of the eyelid

Zembowicz A
Kaliki S
Roberts F

Definition

Adenoid cystic carcinoma (AdCC) is a malignant basaloid epithelial/myoepithelial neoplasm arising in the accessory lacrimal glands or sweat glands of the periocular skin with striking propensity for perineural invasion and local infiltration.

ICD-O coding

8200/3 Adenoid cystic carcinoma

ICD-11 coding

2C33 & XH4302 Adnexal carcinoma of skin & Adenoid cystic carcinoma

Related terminology

None

Subtype(s)

None

Localization

Eyelid AdCCs arise in the accessory and ectopic lacrimal glands or sweat glands. They can involve both the upper and the lower eyelids and the periocular skin, with extension into the anterior orbital soft tissue {1155,2837,1699,81}.

Clinical features

Eyelid AdCC presents as a slow-growing, non-tender, firm, well-circumscribed nodule with or without distortion or loss of eyelashes {497,1699}. It can masquerade as chalazion {2172}, sebaceous gland carcinoma {2064}, or basal cell carcinoma {2757}.

Epidemiology

The exact incidence of eyelid AdCC is unknown but it is a rare entity. It most commonly occurs in middle-aged or elderly patients with an average age of 60 years. There is a male predilection (M:F ratio: 2.7:1) {497,633,2757}. Eyelid AdCC can also

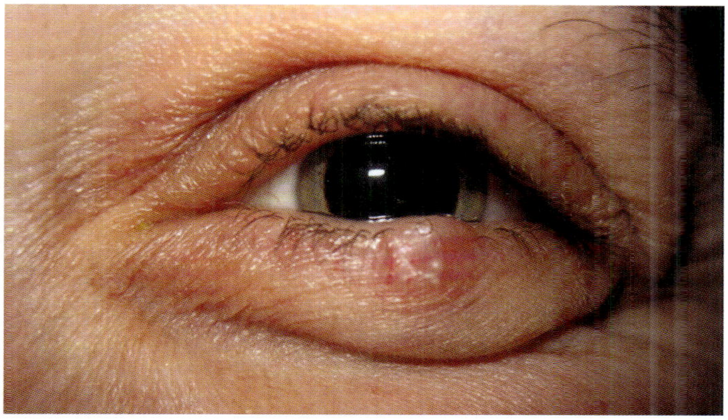

Fig. 3.58 Adenoid cystic carcinoma. Clinical photograph of a primary adenoid cystic carcinoma of the lower eyelid in an otherwise healthy 43-year-old woman.

arise from secondary spread or metastasis from the lacrimal gland or adjacent skin {2489}.

Etiology

Unknown

Pathogenesis

About 60% of AdCCs harbour *MYB* abnormalities, either mutations or structural rearrangements such as *MYB::NFIB* t(6;9)(q22-q23;p24-p23) {2596}. This fusion product activates the transcription of genes involved in apoptosis, cell-cycle control, and DNA repair {2399}. Perineural invasion is suggested to be due to activation of the PI3K/AKT signalling pathway by nerve growth factor {110}.

Macroscopic appearance

See *Clinical features.*

Histopathology

AdCC is typically an infiltrating neoplasm composed of variably sized nests of basaloid cells showing a solid, cribriform, and/or

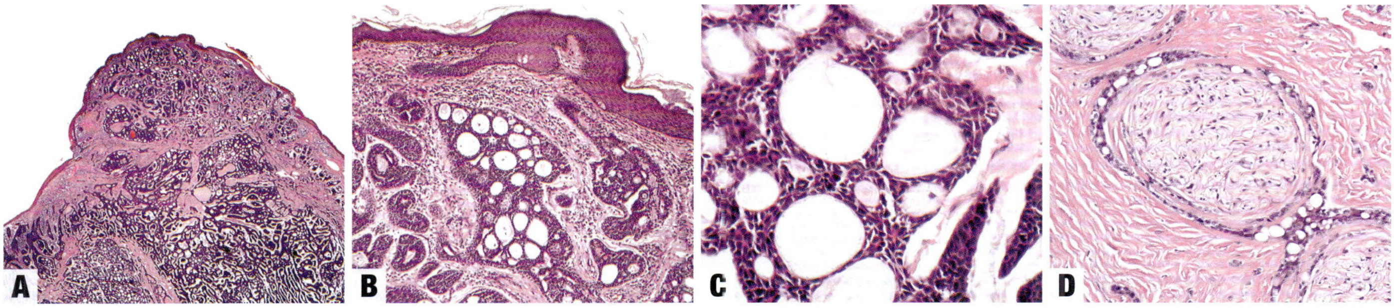

Fig. 3.59 Adenoid cystic carcinoma. **A** Low-power view shows a lower lid containing primary adenoid cystic carcinoma. **B** The typical cribriform appearance of primary eyelid-skin adenoid cystic carcinoma is seen. **C** High-power view shows the monomorphic myoepithelial cells within cribriform architecture, with myxoid globules. **D** Perineural invasion is a common feature.

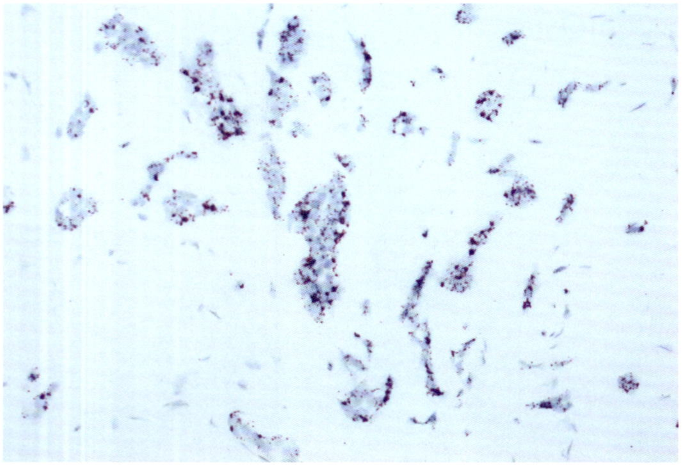

Fig. 3.60 Adenoid cystic carcinoma. RNA in situ hybridization shows increased MYB expression in a periocular adenoid cystic carcinoma.

tubular growth pattern. The solid areas are composed of small basaloid cells with hyperchromatic, slightly angulated nuclei and scant cytoplasm. The cribriform nests and pseudocystic structures are formed by decohesion of cells forming nests and contain basophilic mucinous material that stains with Alcian blue and/or hyalinized eosinophilic material that stains with PAS. Basaloid material may encapsulate nests and form lumina of pseudoglandular or pseudoductal arrangements. The true ducts are usually sparse. They have small round lumina and are composed of inner epithelial cells with uniform round nuclei with or without small nucleoli surrounded by an outer layer of basal/myoepithelial cells. Intraluminal secretion can be seen. Mitotic activity is usually low {2646}. Perineural invasion is common {2757}.

Immunohistochemistry

The neoplastic cells show diffuse cytoplasmic positivity for broad-spectrum keratins, CAM5.2, and CK7. Staining for CK5/6 and with D2-40 is variable. The basaloid and myoepithelial cells display nuclear staining for SOX10. The luminal cells surrounding the true ducts often stain positive for EMA, CEA, and CK15. The myoepithelial component is highlighted by staining for SMA, p63, and calponin. Most tumours express MYB and are positive for KIT (CD117) {918,2399}.

Differential diagnosis

In the eyelid, the major differential diagnosis is with other cribriform tumours. The solid pattern can be difficult to distinguish from basal cell carcinoma in small biopsies. See the *Skin tumours* volume {3597} for a more extensive discussion.

Cytology

None

Diagnostic molecular pathology

MYB alterations or overexpression can help to distinguish AdCC from other basaloid neoplasms with similar appearance {2759}.

Essential and desirable diagnostic criteria

Essential: hyperchromatic, angulated nuclei; mixture of tubular, cribriform, and solid patterns associated with basophilic matrix and reduplicated basement membrane material.

Desirable: perineural invasion; immunohistochemical expression of MYB and KIT (CD117).

Staging

The American Joint Committee on Cancer (AJCC) and the Union for International Cancer Control (UICC) TNM system for non-melanoma eyelid carcinoma applies.

Prognosis and prediction

Local control of AdCC is very difficult. AdCC has a propensity for local recurrence, which can occur many years after the initial presentation. Metastases are rare. Curative therapy may require wide excision and adjuvant radiotherapy if perineural invasion is identified. Radiation therapy may be associated with significant morbidity in the periocular region, but with careful planning it can be done in the lower eyelid {438}. In the upper eyelid, high dose radiation therapy is associated with significant toxicity to the ocular structures, particularly the cornea {438,497,1380}.

Signet-ring cell / histiocytoid carcinoma

Zembowicz A
Kaliki S
Roberts F

Definition
Signet-ring cell / histiocytoid carcinoma is an aggressive adnexal neoplasm composed of neoplastic cells with signet-ring or histiocytoid morphology that diffusely involves the dermis and subcutis of the eyelid.

ICD-O coding
8490/3 Signet-ring cell / histiocytoid carcinoma

ICD-11 coding
2C33 & XH0XE5 Adnexal carcinoma of skin & Signet ring cell/ histiocytoid carcinoma

Related terminology
Not recommended: monocle tumour.

Subtype(s)
None

Localization
Dermis and subcutis in the eyelid and periocular skin

Clinical features
Signet-ring cell / histiocytoid carcinoma is most common in elderly men, where it presents insidiously as painless swelling, often affecting both upper and lower eyelids, and sometimes simulating periorbital oedema {3687,2465,3209,1302}, and can lead to a monocle appearance. The nonspecific nature of the clinical features can frequently lead to delayed diagnosis.

Epidemiology
The tumour has an M:F ratio of about 4:1 {2701}. The reported age range is 42–87 years, with a median patient age of 66 years {2701}.

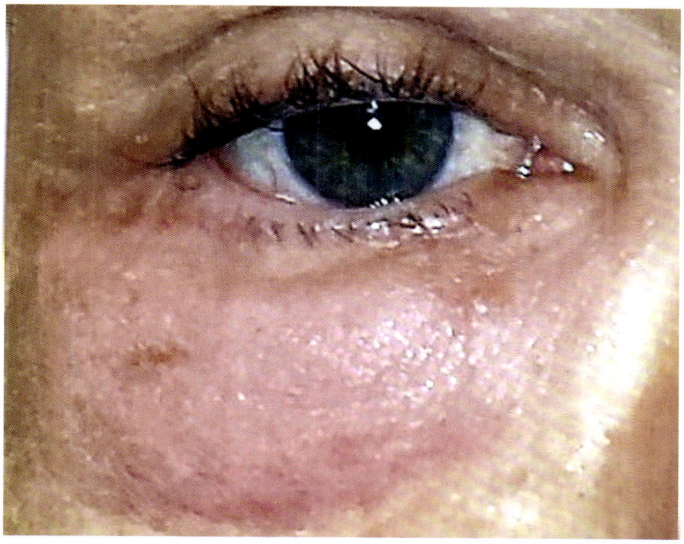

Fig. 3.61 Eccrine signet-ring cell / histiocytoid carcinoma. Patient presenting with a painless erythematous swelling of the right lower eyelid.

Etiology
Unknown

Pathogenesis
Next-generation sequencing has shown mutations in *CDH1*, the gene encoding E-cadherin {2632,3546,758}. Mutations in this gene are known to confer signet-ring morphology in other carcinomas. Mutations in *NTRK3*, *p27* (*CDKN1B*), *ERBB2*, *TP53*, and *PIK3CA* have also been detected {3546}. It is suggested that mutations particularly in *CDH1* induce E-cadherin dysfunction which may play a role in tumour progression.

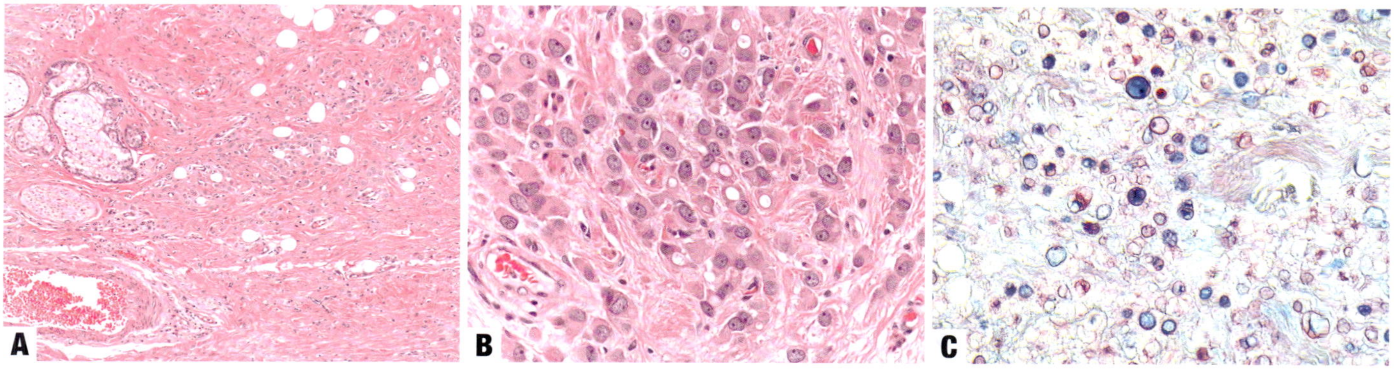

Fig. 3.62 Eccrine signet-ring cell / histiocytoid carcinoma. **A** Peripheral edge of the tumour showing single cell infiltration without stromal reaction. **B** High-magnification view illustrating the cytological features of the tumour cells, which show histiocytoid appearance with some signet-ring cells showing intracytoplasmic vacuoles and eccentric nuclei. **C** Combined Alcian blue / PAS stain showing neutral and acid mucin within the tumour signet-ring cytoplasmic vacuoles.

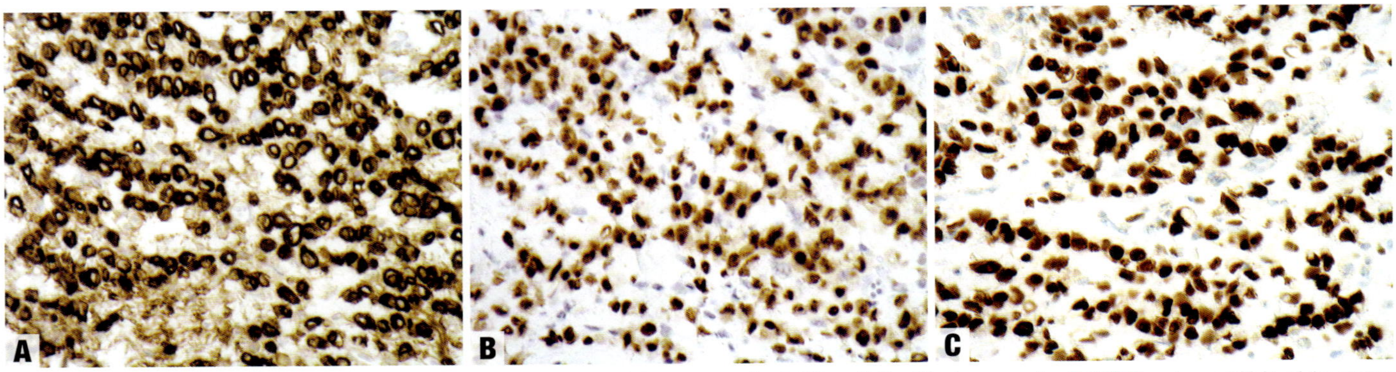

Fig. 3.63 Eccrine signet-ring cell / histiocytoid carcinoma. **A** CK7 positivity of the tumour cells. **B** ER positivity of the tumour cells. **C** GATA3 nuclear positivity of the tumour cells.

Macroscopic appearance

In exenteration specimens there may be a poorly defined periocular mass often involving both upper and lower eyelids. Complete surgical resection may be difficult to accomplish given the single-file nature of tumour cells and thus difficulty in achieving negative margins with conservative surgery.

Histopathology

The tumour is composed of signet-ring or histiocytoid epithelial cells (exhibit eosinophilic granular cytoplasm) which diffusely infiltrate the collagen bundles of the dermis with sparing of the epidermis. The tumour cells may show a single-file pattern. Immunohistochemical staining is positive for cytokeratins (pancytokeratin and CK7). Staining is positive for GATA3, EMA (MUC1), MUC5AC, and AR, and with BerEP4 {1157}. GCDFP-15 and E-cadherin stain positive in the majority of cases {2465}. ER and PR are variably expressed {3687}.

Differential diagnosis

Metastatic breast lobular carcinoma and gastrointestinal adenocarcinomas with a signet-ring cell morphology are the main differential diagnoses. Immunohistochemistry (negative staining for CDX2 and CK20) is helpful to confirm a skin primary. However, a full clinical assessment is essential to rule out breast and gastrointestinal primaries.

Cytology

There are no reports of cytology.

Diagnostic molecular pathology

CDH1 mutations are not in routine use to assist diagnosis.

Essential and desirable diagnostic criteria

Essential: diffuse infiltrate of signet-ring or histiocytoid cells; exclusion of metastatic signet ring carcinoma from other sites.

Desirable: immunohistochemical expression of cytokeratins and AR.

Staging

The American Joint Committee on Cancer (AJCC) and the Union for International Cancer Control (UICC) TNM system for non-melanoma eyelid carcinoma applies.

Prognosis and prediction

There are limited data, owing to the small number of cases. Treatment usually requires exenteration with or without adjuvant radiotherapy. About of one third of cases are reported to develop metastasis over a 10-year follow-up period {2465}.

Mucinous carcinoma

Kazakov DV
Kaliki S

Definition
Mucinous carcinoma of the eyelid is a rare adnexal carcinoma with neoplastic cells floating in lakes of extracellular mucin.

ICD-O coding
8480/3 Mucinous carcinoma

ICD-11 coding
2C33 & XH1S75 Adnexal carcinoma of skin & Mucinous adenocarcinoma

Related terminology
Acceptable: mucinous adenocarcinoma.

Subtype(s)
None

Localization
The eyelid or brow is the most common location in the periorbital area, accounting for 30–45% of all cases of primary cutaneous mucinous carcinoma {28,1587,2718}. Mucinous carcinoma affects the lower lid more than the upper {2906} and can be bilateral in a small number of cases {319,236,2906}.

Clinical features
Mucinous carcinoma is a slowly growing lesion and may be less aggressive in terms of its clinical behaviour compared with other subtypes of sweat gland carcinoma {236}. It has a variable clinical presentation. Lesions are often present for > 12 months before clinical presentation. Tumours can be firm or cystic; they can be tan, blue, red, or grey in colour; and they can assume a papillomatous, pedunculated, or fungating architecture, with a bumpy, smooth, or crusted surface {3646,2906,3170,3749, 1}. Eyelid lesions are usually no more than 25 mm {1} and can mimic a wide variety of benign and malignant eyelid tumours. These include chalazion, papilloma, myxoma, haemangioma, pyogenic granuloma, keratoacanthoma, basal cell carcinoma, squamous carcinoma, sebaceous carcinoma, melanoma, and Kaposi sarcoma {3646}.

Epidemiology
The age-adjusted incidence is 0.04 cases per 100 000 person-years. A systematic review of 159 published cases found that 122 (~77%) of the patients were White, 20 (~13%) were Asian, and 16 (~10%) were Black {1587}. Mucinous carcinoma has a male predilection and presents in the fifth to seventh decades of life (mean: 61 years) {3646}.

Etiology
Unknown

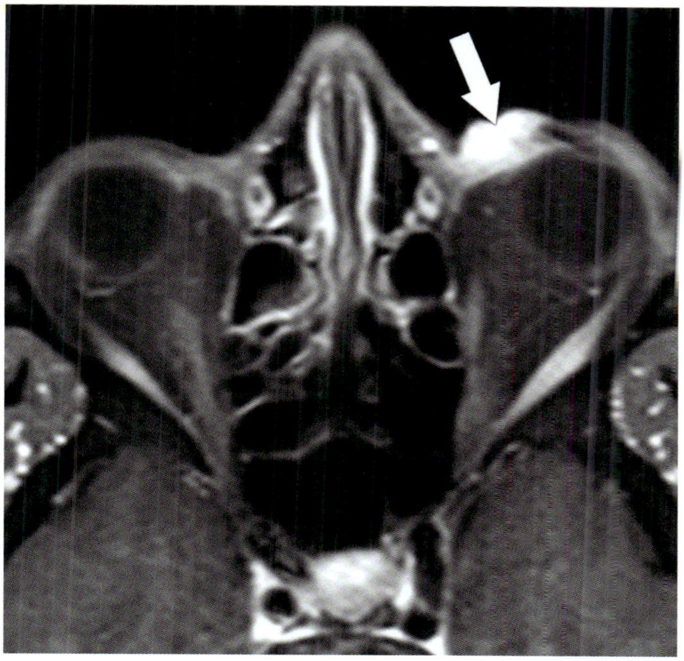

Fig. 3.64 Mucinous carcinoma. Axial T1-weighted postcontrast MRI shows an exophytic enhancing mass in the left lower eyelid and medial canthus (arrow).

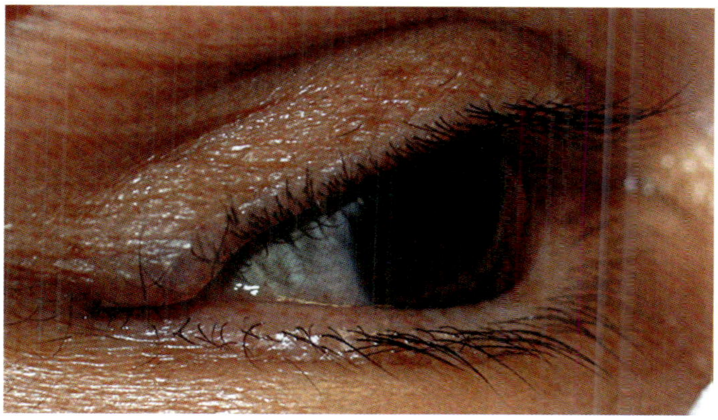

Fig. 3.65 Eyelid mucinous carcinoma. A lesion of the upper lateral eyelid. Note the bluish-brown raised nodule.

Pathogenesis
Mucinous carcinoma appears to result from progression from an in situ neoplasm. Inverse cell polarity, where tumour cells facing the stroma acquire apical secretory properties, is suggested to account for the accumulation of mucus. Although electron microscopic studies have suggested an eccrine lineage, about 50% of cases exhibit apocrine secretion, supporting apocrine differentiation. The gene *ERBB2*, encoding ERBB2 (HER2), was not found to be amplified in the few tumours in which it has been

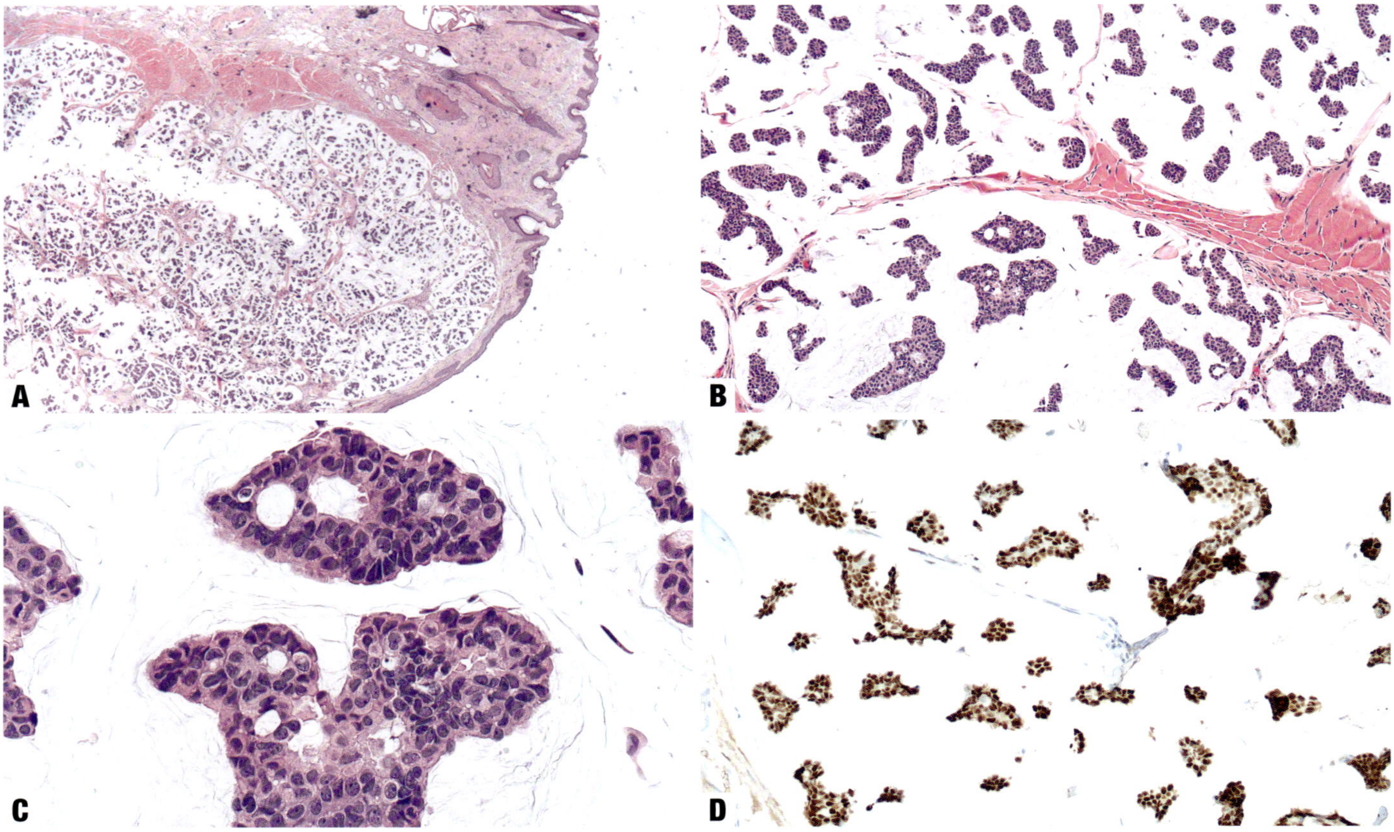

Fig. 3.66 Mucinous carcinoma. **A** A tumour extensively involves the eyelid dermis. **B** Nests of tumour cells in pools of mucin are seen. **C** Tumour nests are composed of relatively bland round to oval cells, and some form glands. **D** Immunohistochemical evidence of PR expression supports apocrine differentiation.

investigated {1639}. Endocrine mucin-producing sweat gland carcinoma in situ is also a precursor lesion {985,3738,43}.

Macroscopic appearance

The tumours are soft nodules or masses, with a gelatinous or mucinous appearance. They are unencapsulated and often poorly circumscribed and are without lobulation.

Histopathology

Tumour cells are arranged in nests, strands, or individual units and float in lakes of extracellular mucin, sometimes separated by variably thin fibrous septa. The histopathological spectrum of primary cutaneous mucinous carcinoma is wide, and analogous to that seen in its mammary counterparts, with at least two distinguishable patterns: a more-common pure tumour, in which extracellular mucin constitutes > 90%; and a rare mixed form, in which there is an invasive ductal component in addition to the mucinous element {1639,3669}. The floating neoplastic epithelial cells are usually relatively monomorphic, although some tumours may show substantial nuclear pleomorphism. Mitoses are generally scarce. A feature which should be looked for is an in situ component; it is detected in most cases (60–70%) and defines the neoplasm as primary cutaneous. In situ lesions usually constitute the minor moiety, and they include (using mammary pathology terminology) ductal hyperplasia, atypical ductal hyperplasia, and ductal carcinoma in situ (cribriform, micropapillary, papillary, and solid), occurring individually or (more rarely) in combination.

Immunohistochemistry

The in situ component can be highlighted by staining for myoepithelial markers (p63 and calponin). The epithelial cells express low-molecular-weight cytokeratin, EMA, CEA, E-cadherin, GATA3, and GCDFP-15. ER and PR are expressed in most cases. The typical CK7+/CK20− phenotype can sometimes be useful in the differential diagnosis with metastatic lesions. Neuroendocrine differentiation can be encountered in cutaneous mucinous carcinomas of both pure and mixed types, without a prominent solid component.

Differential diagnosis

Primary cutaneous mucinous carcinoma must be differentiated from a metastatic mucinous carcinoma {2485}. The presence of an in situ component qualifies the tumour as primary cutaneous; however, its absence does not necessarily imply an extracutaneous origin, because disrupted myoepithelial cells may no longer be identifiable during disease progression {1639,2627}. For such cases, a full clinical workup is needed to establish the origin.

Cytology

Not clinically relevant

Diagnostic molecular pathology

None

Essential and desirable diagnostic criteria

Essential: a periorbital slow-growing lesion; nests and strands of epithelial cells floating in lakes of extracellular mucin.

Desirable: the presence of an in situ lesion, to confirm the lesion is a skin primary; in the absence of an in situ component, metastasis should be excluded by clinical investigation.

Staging

The American Joint Committee on Cancer (AJCC) and the Union for International Cancer Control (UICC) TNM system for non-melanoma eyelid carcinoma applies.

Prognosis and prediction

Primary cutaneous mucinous carcinoma has a propensity to recur at a rate of 26–40% {2906,3646}. The recurrence rate is lower after surgery with intraoperative evaluation of surgical margins (i.e. either Mohs surgery or excision with frozen section control) {1587,2481}. Increased rates of recurrence and metastasis have been associated with White race, younger age at presentation, and large tumour size (> 15 mm) {1587}. In a large study, 67% of patients had local disease, 10.5% had regional disease, and 5.8% had distant disease {2718}. The mean overall survival is reported to be 11.4 years, with 5-year and 10-year overall survival at 85% and 78%, respectively {286}

Endocrine mucin-producing sweat gland carcinoma

Zembowicz A
Agni M
Hyrcza MD
Kaliki S
Mulay K

Definition

Endocrine mucin-producing sweat gland carcinoma (EMPSGC) is a low-grade, mucin-producing, adnexal neoplasm of sweat gland origin that shows neuroendocrine differentiation, with a predilection for the eyelid and periorbital skin.

ICD-O coding

8509/3 Endocrine mucin-producing sweat gland carcinoma

ICD-11 coding

2C33 & XH4EK4 Adnexal carcinoma of skin & Endocrine mucin-producing sweat gland carcinoma
2C33 & XH8010 Adnexal carcinoma of skin & Endocrine mucin-producing sweat gland carcinoma in situ

Related terminology

Not recommended: cutaneous analogue of solid papillary carcinoma of the breast.

Subtype(s)

None

Localization

EMPSGC has a predilection for the eyelid/periorbital skin, with rare extrafacial occurrence {3383}.

Clinical features

Lesions present as slow-growing, skin-coloured or bluish nodules, papules, or cysts. They may be multifocal {3738}.

Epidemiology

The true incidence is unknown. EMPSGC typically occurs in the sixth and seventh decades of life. Women are affected twice as often as men {43,3738}.

Etiology

No known causes or risk factors

Pathogenesis

EMPSGC is a cutaneous analogue of solid papillary carcinoma of the breast {985,43}. In some cases it is associated with adjacent mucinous carcinoma and most probably represents a precursor lesion {985,3738,43}.

Macroscopic appearance

See *Clinical features*.

Histopathology

EMPSGC grows as well-demarcated expansile nodules with cystic, solid, papillary, or cribriform architecture. Tumour cells are polygonal to round, small to intermediate-sized ductal cells with amphophilic or bluish cytoplasm and round to oval nuclei with finely stippled chromatin and inconspicuous nucleoli. Small amounts of intracellular and extracellular mucin can be demonstrated by mucicarmine or PAS staining {985,3738,43}. EMPSGC is frequently seen within dilated eccrine ducts, undermining benign ductal epithelium with a complete myoepithelial layer. At this stage the tumour represents carcinoma in situ. As it grows and the nests become large expansile nodules, the myoepithelial rim becomes incomplete or lost entirely, consistent with invasive carcinoma with pushing invasion {3738,954}. Mitotic activity is low, and the Ki-67 proliferation index is seldom greater than 5–10% {3086}. The presence of extracellular pools of stromal mucin and/or infiltrating tumour glands and nests

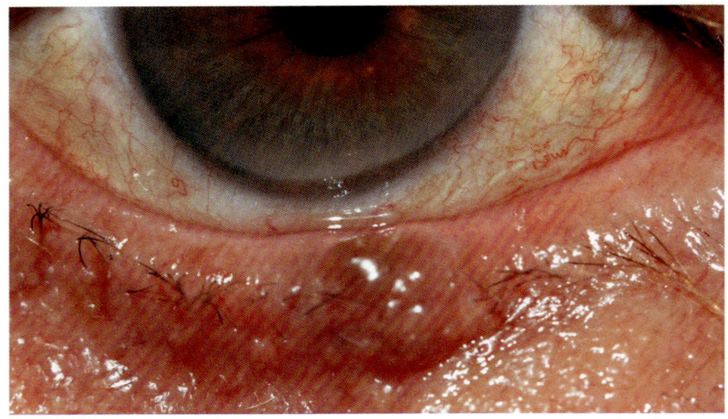

Fig. 3.67 Endocrine mucin-producing sweat gland carcinoma. Lower-eyelid endocrine mucin-producing sweat gland carcinoma, showing a brown/bluish nodule.

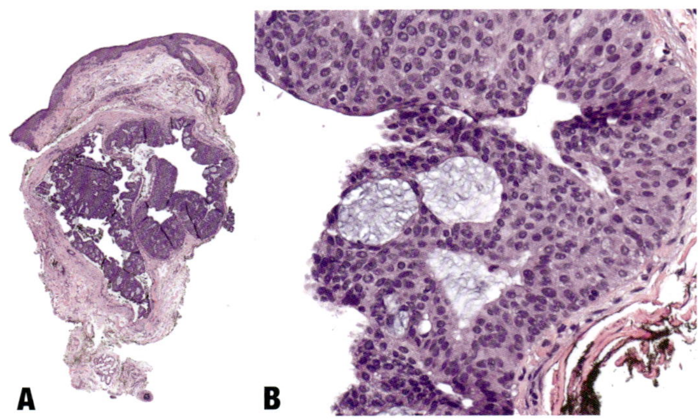

Fig. 3.68 Endocrine mucin-producing sweat gland carcinoma. **A** Architectural patterns of endocrine mucin-producing sweat gland carcinoma are shown, at low magnification. A dermal nodule with multinodular, cystic, solid, and papillary growth and scattered pools of sparse, light-blue stromal mucin is identified. The tumour cells look bland to uniform with bluish, amphophilic cytoplasm. **B** A higher magnification highlights the cyst wall mural thickenings. The tumour cells resemble bland eccrine ductal cells with moderately enlarged ovoid nuclei with stippled chromatin and inconspicuous nucleoli, bluish cytoplasm, and intracellular and extracellular mucin. Note the incomplete myoepithelial rim.

indicates progression to mucinous adenocarcinoma. Such tumours should be diagnosed as invasive mucinous carcinoma {43}.

Immunohistochemistry

INSM1 is the most sensitive neuroendocrine marker {2500}; staining with synaptophysin or chromogranin can be focal or absent {43}. EMPSGC typically strongly expresses ER, PR, and CK7. Markers such as p63 or calponin can highlight the myoepithelial layer. EMPSGC has also been shown to express CK8, CK18, AE1/AE3, CAM5.2, EMA, GATA3, GCDFP-15, WT1, and RCCm {3738,3086,954,14,167}.

Cytology

Not relevant

Diagnostic molecular pathology

Not relevant

Essential and desirable diagnostic criteria

Essential: cystic, solid, papillary, or cribriform architecture; polygonal cells with bluish cytoplasm; neuroendocrine nuclei and intracellular or extracellular mucin.

Desirable: immunohistochemical expression of neuroendocrine markers; INSM1 is currently the most sensitive neuroendocrine marker for EMPSGC.

Staging

The American Joint Committee on Cancer (AJCC) and the Union for International Cancer Control (UICC) TNM system for non-melanoma eyelid carcinoma applies.

Prognosis and prediction

EMPSGC has an excellent prognosis after excision with clear margins, recurring in up to 10% of cases {43,1043}. The recurrence rate of EMPSGC-associated mucinous sweat gland carcinoma is about 20% {43}. Rarely, metastases may arise many years after surgery {1042,1223,2850}.

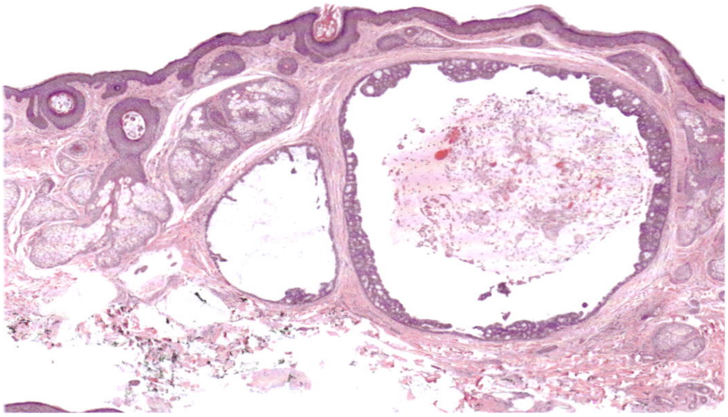

Fig. 3.69 Invasive mucinous carcinoma arising in endocrine mucin-producing sweat gland carcinoma. Endocrine mucin-producing sweat gland carcinoma with invasive mucinous component, at low magnification. An expansile nodule with cystic and papillary growth and nests of tumour cells floating in copious, central extracellular mucin, signifying transformation to invasive mucinous carcinoma.

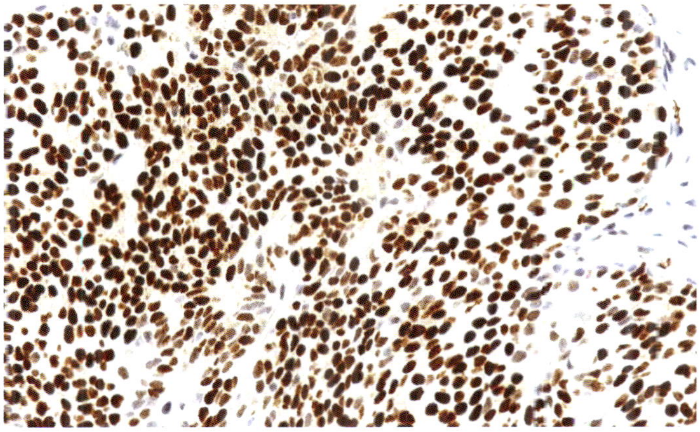

Fig. 3.70 Endocrine mucin-producing sweat gland carcinoma. Tumour cells show diffuse nuclear staining for INSM1, a highly sensitive neuroendocrine marker for endocrine mucin-producing sweat gland carcinoma.

Microcystic adnexal carcinoma

Zembowicz A
Kaliki S

Definition

Microcystic adnexal carcinoma (MAC) is a locally infiltrative adnexal carcinoma with bland cytology and focal sweat ductal / syringomatoid and/or follicular/trichoepithelial differentiation.

ICD-O coding

8407/3 Microcystic adnexal carcinoma

ICD-11 coding

2C33 & XH17P2 Adnexal carcinoma of skin & Microcystic adnexal carcinoma

Related terminology

Acceptable: sclerosing sweat duct carcinoma.

Not recommended: malignant syringoma; eccrine epithelioma; syringomatoid carcinoma.

Subtype(s)

None

Localization

MAC occurs in the upper and lower eyelids and the medial and lateral canthal areas. The lower eyelid is where most cases have been recorded {1977,1908,841,2380}.

Clinical features

MAC presents as a yellow or skin-coloured firm indurated small nodule or hard plaque which can be associated with telangiectasia and marked eyelid distortion or retraction {1977} and (rarely) ulceration and madarosis {631}. Its growth can be insidious, and the diagnosis can be delayed by years {1977}. Periocular pain or numbness indicates perineural or intraneural invasion.

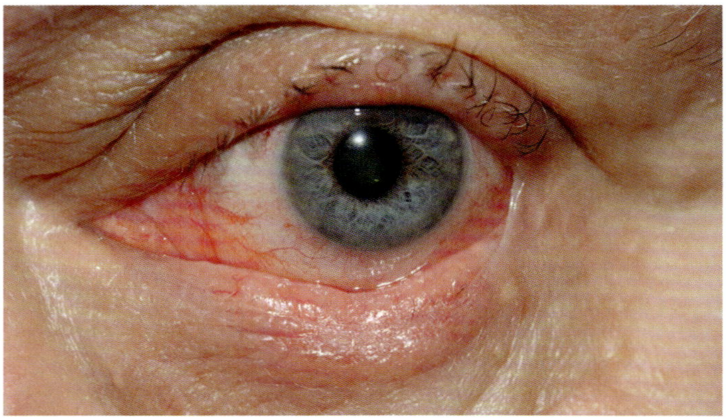

Fig. 3.71 Microcystic adnexal carcinoma. Lower-eyelid plaque-like pinkish lesion of microcystic adnexal carcinoma.

Epidemiology

Eyelid MAC occurs predominantly in White people. The age range is 18–95 years (average: 52 years). There is a female predilection {1977,1908,841,2380,1514,420,1331,1752}.

Etiology

Unknown

Pathogenesis

MAC can show sweat duct and/or follicular differentiation {1145,1624,2383,3599,1636,1879}. Next-generation sequencing revealed a low mutation burden, and p53 and JAK/STAT signalling pathway mutations, but no ultraviolet (UV) radiation signature {520}.

Macroscopic appearance

See *Clinical features*.

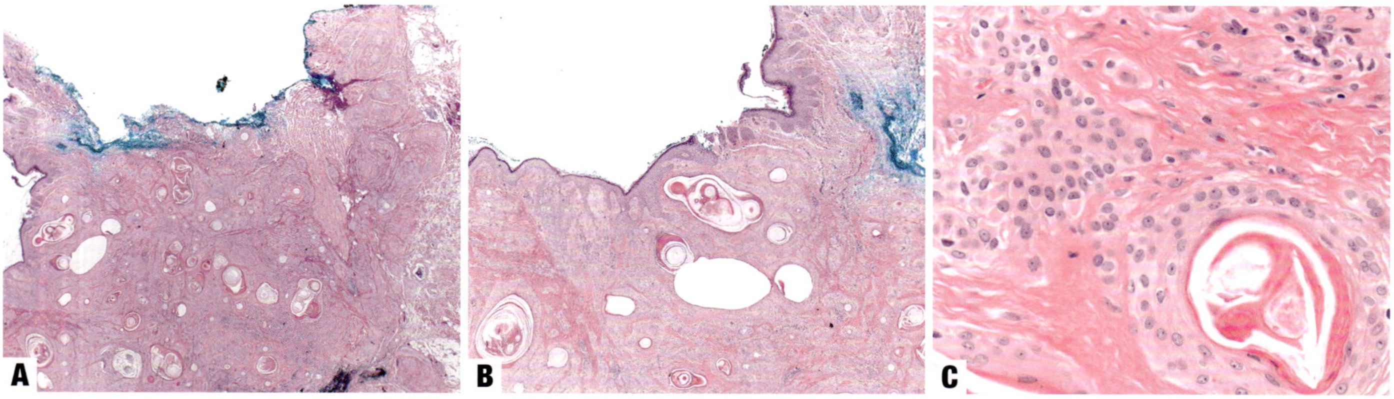

Fig. 3.72 Microcystic adnexal carcinoma. **A** Low-magnification view illustrating the infiltrative nature of the tumour with involvement of the subcutaneous tissue. **B** Superficial portion of the tumour showing trichoepitheliomatous keratocysts, essentially indistinguishable from those expected in trichoepithelioma. **C** Bland cytological features with no mitotic activity.

Histopathology

MAC is an infiltrative epithelial neoplasm that involves the deep dermis and typically extends to the subcutis. It is composed of small, bland, monomorphic epithelial cells forming small nests, strands, or columns associated with various proportions of trichoepithelioma-like keratocysts and/or syringomatoid, duct-like structures composed of two layers of small cuboidal cells (empty or filled with eosinophilic material). Clear cell differentiation can be seen.

Perineural or muscle invasion is common. Mitoses are rare or absent. The stroma can be sclerotic or tumour cells may infiltrate without much stromal alteration. MAC expresses cytokeratins (e.g. AE1/AE3, CK5/6) and p63. Ductal differentiation can be highlighted by staining for EMA or CEA {1044,3599}. Staining for GCDFP-15 and with BerEP4 is negative. CK20-positive Merkel cells typically seen in trichoepithelioma are absent {917}.

Diagnosis of MAC on a superficial biopsy can be impossible as the histological features may resemble trichoepithelioma (infundibular keratocysts), syringoma (tadpole-like ductal structures), or infiltrating basal cell carcinoma (infiltrating nests and strands) {16,1348,3150,3386,3599,1634}. In some cases diagnosis may have to be deferred to a re-excision {991}.

Cytology

Not relevant

Diagnostic molecular pathology

Not relevant

Essential and desirable diagnostic criteria

Essential: a highly infiltrative tumour composed of small, bland, monomorphic epithelial cells forming small nests, strands, or columns associated with various proportions of trichoepithelioma-like keratocysts and/or syringomatoid, duct-like structures composed of two layers of small cuboidal cells.

Desirable: perineural invasion.

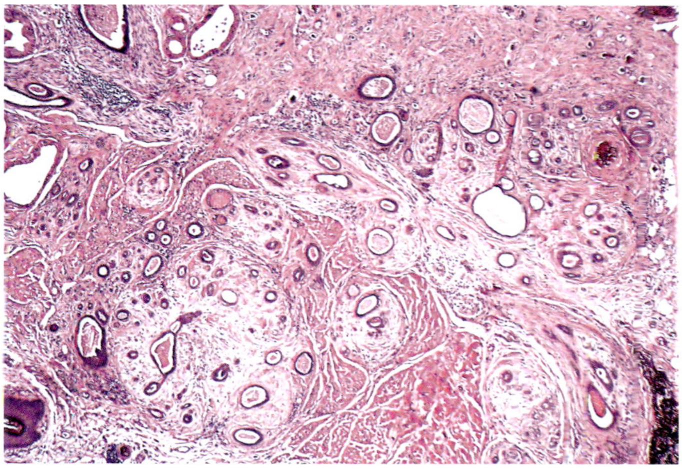

Fig. 3.73 Eyelid-skin microcystic adnexal carcinoma. Widely infiltrating microcystic adnexal carcinoma, with syringomatous duct-like structures, within the orbicularis muscle and tarsal plate. Note the loose desmoplastic reaction around the tumour nests.

Staging

The American Joint Committee on Cancer (AJCC) and the Union for International Cancer Control (UICC) TNM system for non-melanoma eyelid carcinoma applies.

Prognosis and prediction

MAC is a locally aggressive carcinoma. If treated by standard wide local excision, there is a high rate of recurrence {1908, 2266} with long-term follow-up. Mohs micrographic surgery is more effective at clearing tumour and is associated with a lower recurrence compared with standard surgical excision {1908, 236}. Exenteration may be required for orbit invasive tumours {1977}. Adjuvant radiotherapy has been used after surgery, in the presence of perineural invasion, or as a primary modality in unresectable cases {1977,2266,1362,236}. Regional lymph node and distant metastases are extremely rare {246,587,1040, 1055,2335,3153}.

Apocrine carcinoma

Kazakov DV
Kaliki S

Definition

Apocrine carcinoma is an epithelial neoplasm exhibiting apocrine differentiation, typically characterized by decapitation secretion and/or the presence of cytoplasmic zymogen granules.

ICD-O coding

8401/3 Apocrine carcinoma

ICD-11 coding

2C33 & XH9L77 Adnexal carcinoma of skin & Apocrine adenocarcinoma

Related terminology

Acceptable: apocrine adenocarcinoma; apocrine gland carcinoma.

Not recommended: Moll gland carcinoma; Moll gland adenocarcinoma.

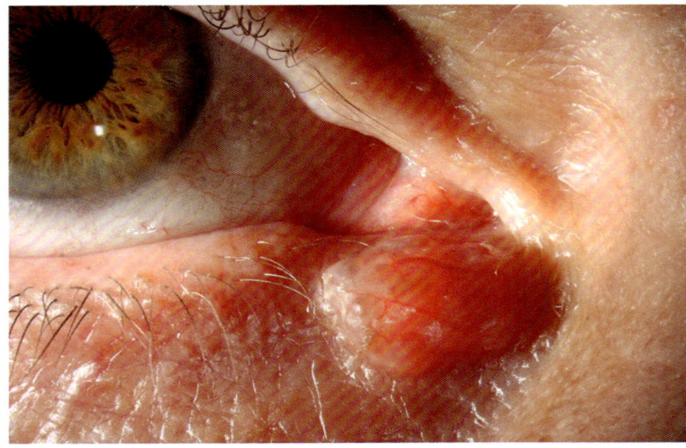

Fig. 3.74 Apocrine carcinoma. A right lower medial eyelid tumour of tan and reddish colour is seen, part solid and part cystic appearing with overlying prominent vessels. Histologically this was an apocrine cystadenoma evolving into an invasive apocrine carcinoma.

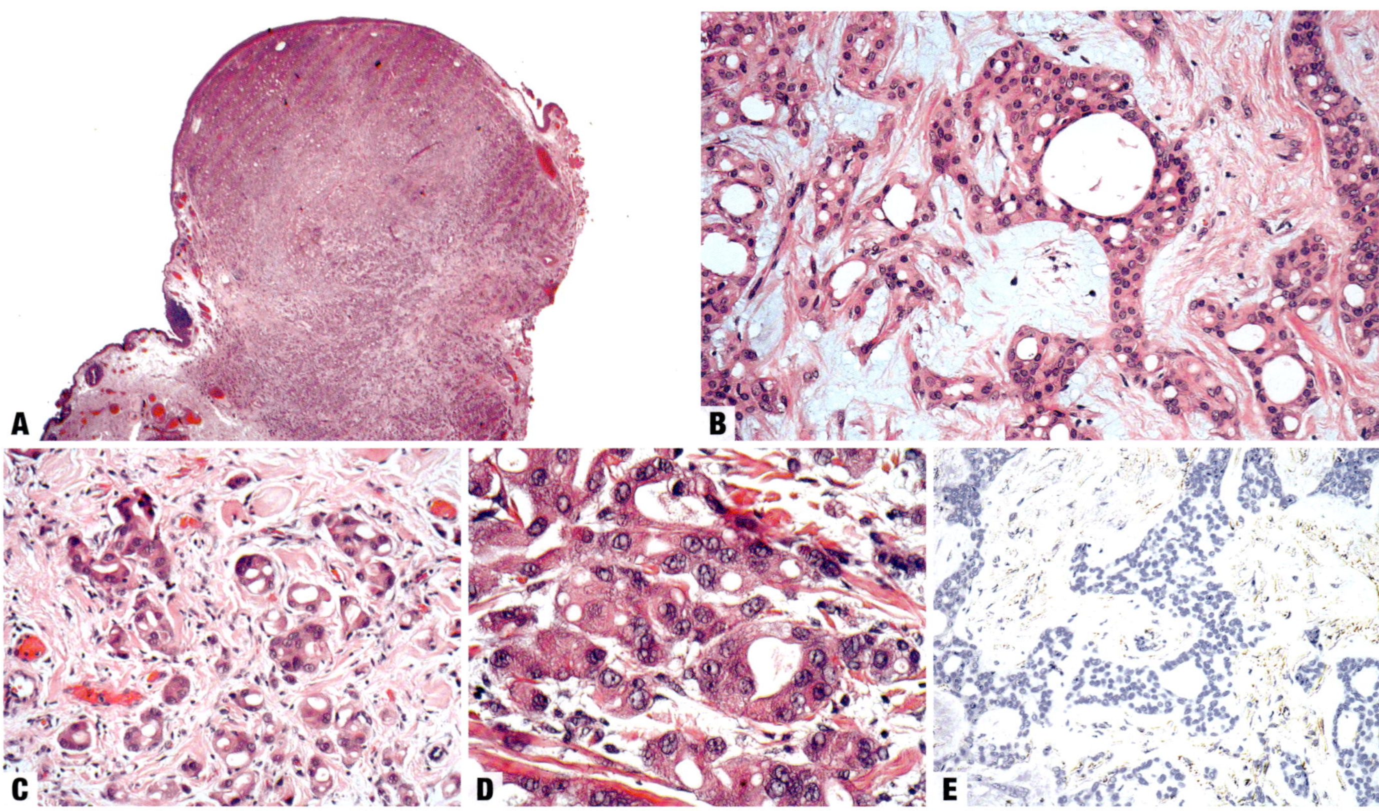

Fig. 3.75 Invasive apocrine carcinoma. **A** A low-power image of an eyelid containing a solid eosinophilic tumour is shown. **B** The tumour is composed of cytologically atypical cells with apocrine differentiation, arranged as glands and strands, surrounded by desmoplasia. **C** Invasive atypical glands infiltrating eyelid stroma with apocrine histology. **D** Invasive glandular structures are seen, lined by apocrine-type epithelium with cytological atypia, infiltrating the eyelid tissue. **E** There is loss of p63 positivity in an area of invasive apocrine carcinoma.

Subtype(s)
None

Localization
The eyelid is by far the most common location. The skin of the upper and lower eyelids is equally affected {1352,972}.

Clinical features
The tumour appears as a solitary nodule that is bluish/brown in colour. Symptoms and signs include ulceration, bleeding, excess lacrimation, lash loss, swelling, congestion and discharge, rapid growth, or bleeding {2765,2463}. Some cases can resemble a chalazion, which can delay diagnosis and treatment {3431}.

Epidemiology
There is a male predilection and an age range of 44–91 years {2765}.

Etiology
Unknown

Pathogenesis
Some cases of apocrine carcinoma with invasion are associated with a benign apocrine lesion or an apocrine carcinoma in situ, suggesting malignant evolution {258,2922}.

Macroscopic appearance
Lesions appear as a solid or solid-cystic, poorly circumscribed bluish/brown nodule.

Histopathology
Apocrine carcinoma is usually highly infiltrative with a sclerotic stroma. It can exhibit glandular, tubular, papillary, tubulopapillary, or solid growth patterns. The tumour cells have plentiful eosinophilic cytoplasm, which can be granular and sometimes partly vacuolated. The nuclei are oval and vacuolated and show prominent eosinophilic nucleoli. Decapitation secretion is seen but can be focal. Pleomorphism and mitotic figures are present and vary according to the tumour differentiation. The tumour can show perineural, blood vessel, and lymphatic invasion {972,2733}

Apocrine carcinoma can be seen in association with various precursor benign and carcinoma in situ lesions. Benign lesions include apocrine gland hyperplasia, adenoma, and cystadenoma {258,2922}. If apocrine carcinoma in situ is present, it has striking resemblance to breast ductal carcinoma in situ and is surrounded by an intact myoepithelial cell layer.

Histochemistry
Apocrine tumours contain PASD-positive cytoplasmic granules. Some cases show cytoplasmic iron.

Immunohistochemistry
The tumour cells express AE1, AE3, CAM5.2, CK7, GCDFP-15, GATA3, CEA, S100, EMA, ER, PR, AR, and lysozyme {164,1988, 2560,2733}.

Differential diagnosis
Metastatic apocrine breast carcinoma and endocrine mucin-producing sweat gland carcinoma require exclusion. The presence of eyelid apocrine precursor lesions such as an apocrine adenoma/cystadenoma or apocrine carcinoma in situ would exclude metastatic apocrine breast carcinoma. In their absence, comprehensive clinical examination is mandatory to exclude metastatic apocrine breast carcinoma. Endocrine mucin-producing sweat gland carcinoma expresses INSM1 and MUC2 and has mucinous elements, whereas apocrine carcinoma is negative for these markers and does not produce mucin {2619}.

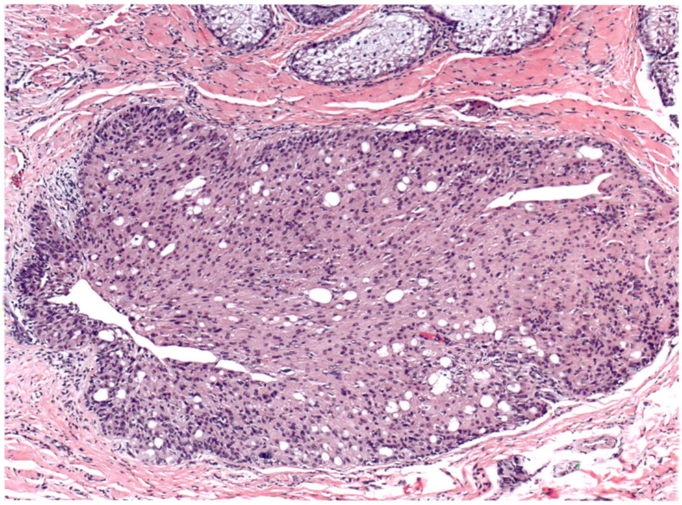

Fig. 3.76 Precursor lesion: apocrine carcinoma in situ. Apocrine carcinoma in situ showing a well-defined focus of back-to-back glands, resembling breast ductal carcinoma in situ.

Cytology
Not clinically relevant

Diagnostic molecular pathology
None

Essential and desirable diagnostic criteria
Essential: an invasive carcinoma with apocrine differentiation (histologically or immunohistochemically confirmed); exclusion of metastatic breast apocrine carcinoma.

Desirable: the presence of a benign apocrine lesion or an apocrine in situ carcinoma, to support a primary eyelid origin

Staging
Staging follows the eighth edition of the Union for International Cancer Control (UICC) TNM classification for eyelid carcinoma.

Prognosis and prediction
Cases localized to the eyelid skin can be surgically excised with adequate margins. Tumours that extend into the orbit have been treated successfully with orbital exenteration. Adjuvant postoperative radiotherapy has been used in some cases if there is concern of a high risk of local recurrence, for instance if perineural invasion is present. Rare cases of eyelid apocrine carcinoma have displayed rapid local recurrence and metastasis to regional lymph nodes or distant sites. Some of these cases have been treated successfully by chemotherapy {2765,972, 1804,2380}.

Naevi of the eyelid

Mihic-Probst D
Esmaeli B
Moulin A
van Doorn R

Definition
Junctional, compound, and dermal naevi are benign localized neoplastic proliferations of naevus melanocytic cells.

ICD-O coding
8740/0 Junctional naevus
8760/0 Compound naevus
8750/0 Dermal naevus

ICD-11 coding
2F36.Y & XH1M79 Other specified benign neoplasm of eye or ocular adnexa & Junctional naevus, NOS
2F36.Y & XH27A6 Other specified benign neoplasm of eye or ocular adnexa & Compound naevus
2F36.Y & XH2MQ5 Other specified benign neoplasm of eye or ocular adnexa & Dermal naevus

Related terminology
None

Subtype(s)
Junctional naevus; compound naevus; dermal naevus

Localization
Eyelid and periorbital skin

Clinical features
Depending on the subtype, most are well circumscribed, sharply demarcated, uniformly pigmented, light brown to dark brown or black in colour, and < 5 mm in diameter. The lesions are not ulcerated, unless they are traumatized.

Epidemiology
Most common naevi are acquired during childhood and reach maximum number in adolescence, declining in number thereafter owing to a process of senescence {2867}. Junctional, compound, and dermal naevi are the most common in the eyelid.

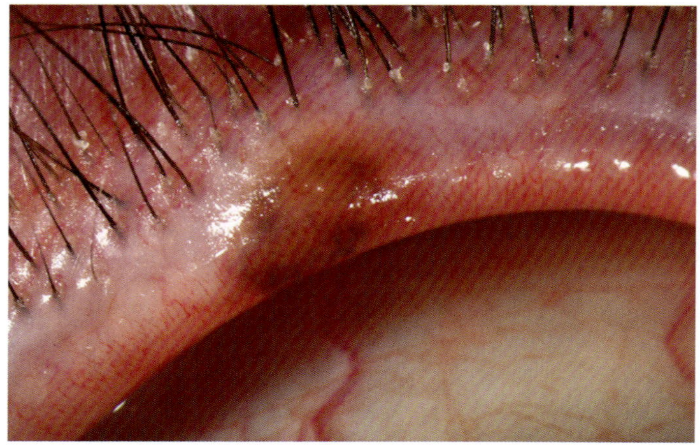

Fig. 3.77 Dermal naevus. A 68-year-old man with pigmented lesion, upper eyelid edge.

Etiology
The number of naevi in various populations depends on genetic factors and exposure to ultraviolet (UV) radiation, in particular sunburn during childhood {2375}.

Pathogenesis
Most melanocytic naevi are driven by activating the MAPK pathway. After initial clonal proliferation, melanocytes enter a stable cell-cycle arrest. *BRAF* oncogene mutation, commonly *BRAF* p.V600E, is found in > 60% of cases. A minority, especially congenital naevi, are caused by *NRAS* mutations whereas others have gene fusions {2937}. *BRAF* and *NRAS* mutations are mutually exclusive {2592,2747,2574}.

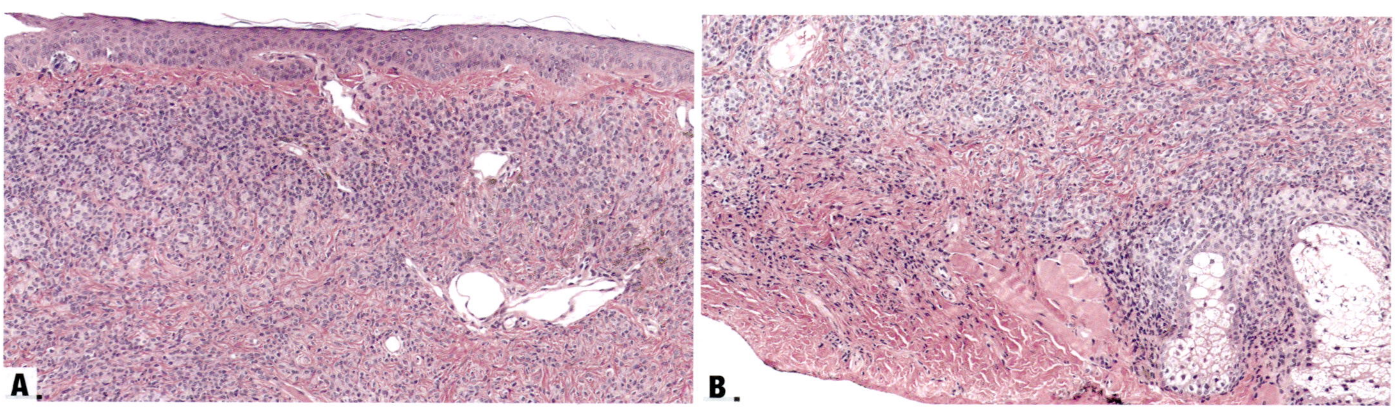

Fig. 3.78 Dermal melanocytic naevus. **A** Larger nests of melanocytes and melanocytes in the upper dermis compared with the depth. **B** Smaller nests of melanocytes and melanocytes in the depth compared with the upper dermis (maturation).

Macroscopic appearance

See *Clinical features*, above.

Histopathology

In a junctional naevus, nests are present by definition at the base of the epidermis, and often admixed with single cells. In a compound naevus, nests are also present in the dermis. In a dermal naevus, there is no junctional component. The lesions are sharply laterally demarcated and symmetrical. In compound and dermal naevi, melanocytes and nests usually decrease in size towards depth (type A cells with more cytoplasm and type B lymphocyte-like cells with maturation). Single, but not atypical, and upper dermal mitoses can be found.

Immunohistochemistry

As *CDKN2A* (*P16*) is often mutated in melanomas, but highly uncommon in naevi, p16 immunohistochemistry can be helpful to differentiate naevi from melanoma. In addition, positivity for PRAME is seen rarely in naevi {2199,1926}.

Differential diagnosis

Other types of naevi are seen more rarely and are covered in greater depth in the *Skin tumours* volume of this series {3597}. Around the eye, congenital naevi, naevus of Ota, and Spitz naevi (see *Spitz naevus*, p. 142) may be encountered. Blue naevus is intradermal and shows similar features to naevi in the conjunctiva (see *Blue naevus of the conjunctiva*, p. 65), as do WNT-activated deep penetrating / plexiform melanocytoma (naevus) (see *WNT-activated deep penetrating / plexiform melanocytoma (naevus)*, p. 68) and combined naevus (see *Combined naevus*, p. 70).

Cytology

Not relevant

Diagnostic molecular pathology

Next-generation sequencing can be helpful in cases of uncertain malignancy. Identifying the driver mutation without additional genetic alterations underlines a benign diagnosis of naevus.

Molecular testing is recommended to rule out malignancy in the diagnosis of spitzoid neoplasms {303} (see *Spitz naevus*, p. 142). WNT-activated deep penetrating / plexiform melanocytoma (naevus) (see *WNT-activated deep penetrating / plexiform melanocytoma (naevus)*, p. 68) usually has *BRAF* mutation combined with *CTNNB1* (β-catenin) mutation or loss of *APC* {3693}. and naevus of Ota commonly has *GNAQ* mutation. BAP1-inactivated naevus usually has *BRAF* mutation combined with *BAP1* loss or mutation, although combination with *NRAS* mutation can also occur.

Essential and desirable diagnostic criteria

Essential: a clinically small (< 5–6 mm), well-circumscribed, symmetrical, uniformly coloured lesion; histologically composed of naevus cells arranged in orderly junctional nests and/or in dermal nests, cords, and individual cell patterns with maturation and general absence of architectural and cytological abnormalities.

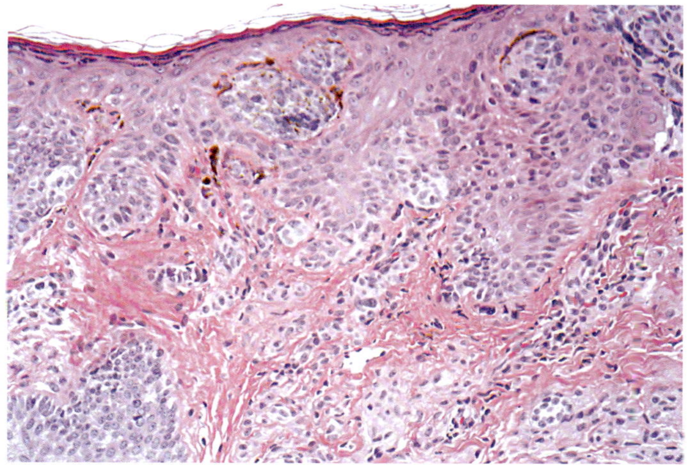

Fig. 3.79 Compound naevus. A lesion showing junctional nests and dermal naevus cells as clusters and nests of maturing cells.

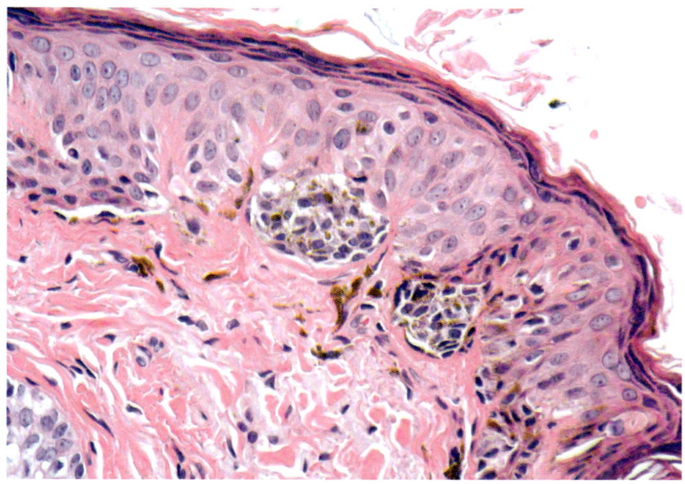

Fig. 3.80 Junctional naevus. There are variably pigmented nests of melanocytic naevus cells along the base of the epidermis.

Staging

Not relevant

Prognosis and prediction

Incompletely excised naevi may recur. Owing to disorganization and pagetoid spread over the scar, they are melanoma simulators {1706}. Individuals with an increased total number of naevi and large congenital naevi are at increased risk of melanoma. About one third of melanomas arise in compound naevi. However, the risk of progression of naevi is very low {1067,2102, 2939,2937}.

Spitz naevus

Verdijk RM
Mihic-Probst D
Moulin A
Pižem J

Definition

Spitz naevi are melanocytic neoplasms composed of large epithelioid and/or spindled melanocytes with a regular architecture, and usually *HRAS* mutations or receptor kinase fusions.

ICD-O coding

8770/0 Spitz naevus
8770/0 Spitz naevus with *ALK* fusion
8770/0 Spitz naevus with *ROS1* fusion
8770/0 Spitz naevus with *NTRK1* fusion
8770/0 Spitz naevus with *NTRK3* fusion
8770/0 Spitz naevus with *BRAF* fusion
8770/0 Spitz naevus with *HRAS* mutation
8770/0 Spitz naevus with *PRKAR1A* inactivation as a secondary event
8770/0 Spitz naevus with *MAP3K8* fusion
8770/0 Spitz naevus with *RET* fusion

ICD-11 coding

2F20.Y & XH2HG8 Other specific types of melanocytic naevus & Epithelioid and spindle cell naevus

Related terminology

Not recommended: spindle and/or epithelioid cell naevus; naevus of large spindle and/or epithelioid cells.

Subtype(s)

See Table 3.02.

Localization

Spitz naevus has rarely been described in the eyelid {1343,787, 3075,242}.

Clinical features

The clinical presentation is nonspecific: a rapidly growing, pinkish-red, vascularized, solitary lesion seen mostly in young patients {3021}. Most Spitz naevi in children are located in the head and neck {2700,3564}.

Epidemiology

Because of its extreme rarity (< 10 cases reported), the incidence of Spitz naevus is unknown {3075,1343,242,787}. Since published cases to date have not been molecularly confirmed, the diagnosis should currently be defined as provisional.

Etiology

The etiology of eyelid Spitz naevus is unknown.

Pathogenesis

Spitz naevus may evolve from junctional proliferations of melanocytes, which then extend into the stroma. Some Spitz naevi lack an intraepithelial component.

Table 3.02 Spitz naevus subtypes

Subtype	Histological patterns	Clinical subtype
Spitz naevus with *ALK* fusions {1644A,2535A}	Plexiform with elongated fascicles of spindle cells, myxoid, angiomatoid Often high mitotic counts and may have ulceration	
Spitz naevus with *ROS1* fusions {1644A,1094A,2632A}	Plexiform or plaque like, angiomatoid Highly characteristic features are floating nests in the epidermis, with transepidermal elimination of nests and pagetoid spread	Eruptive
Spitz naevus with *NTRK1* fusions {140A,3692A}	Filigree-like rete ridges, exaggerated maturation, (often) pigmentation, and predominantly spindle cell morphology are common; lobulated nesting pattern; rosettes; dysplastic naevus–like appearance	
Spitz naevus with *NTRK3* fusions {3449A,743A}	PSCN appearance	
Spitz naevus with *BRAF* fusions {1644A,140A}	Hyalinizing, dysplastic, often predominantly epithelioid	
Spitz naevus with *HRAS* mutations {2852A,3602A}	Desmoplastic	Eruptive
Spitz naevus with *PRKAR1A* inactivation as secondary event {3754A,743B}	Pigmented epithelioid cell	
Spitz naevus with *MAP3K8* fusion {2618A}	Predominantly epithelioid and often highly pleomorphic, sometimes pigmented	
Spitz naevus with *RET* fusions {1682A}	Plaque-type, sometimes with dyscohesive nesting	

PSCN, pigmented spindle cell naevus.
Note: Specific molecular anomalies, particularly fusion genes in the MAPK pathway, appear to have a correlation with various histological patterns. However, it is important to note that multiple histological patterns may occur within the same tumour, and this may not necessarily indicate an exclusive genetic alteration.

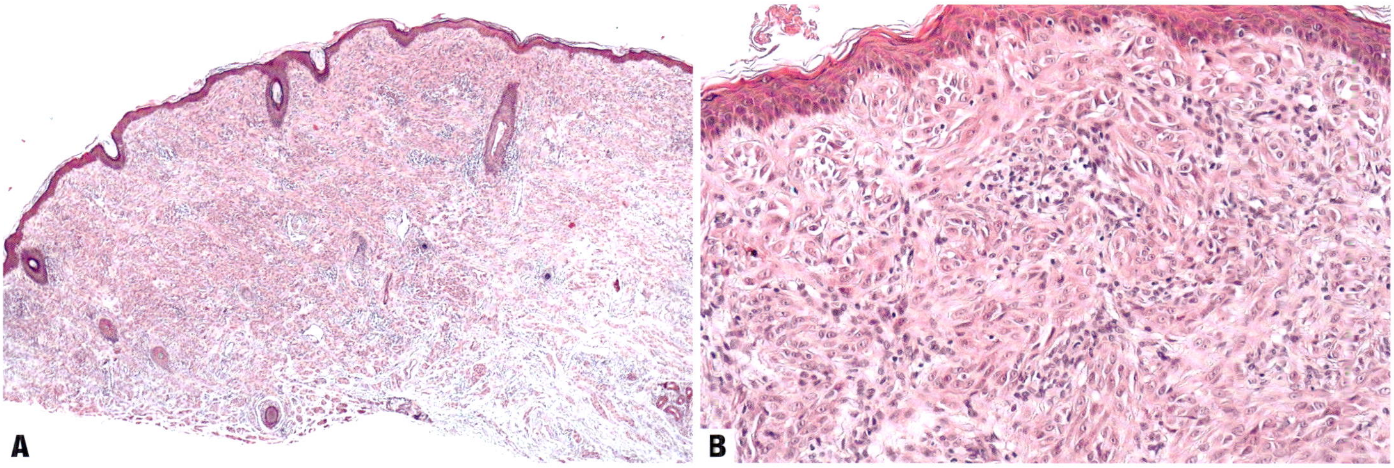

Fig. 3.81 Spitz naevus. **A** A symmetrical, well-circumscribed, dome-shaped dermal lesion with a maximum diameter of 4.9 mm. **B** Large spindle and epithelioid cells with nuclei containing prominent nucleoli arranged in fascicles.

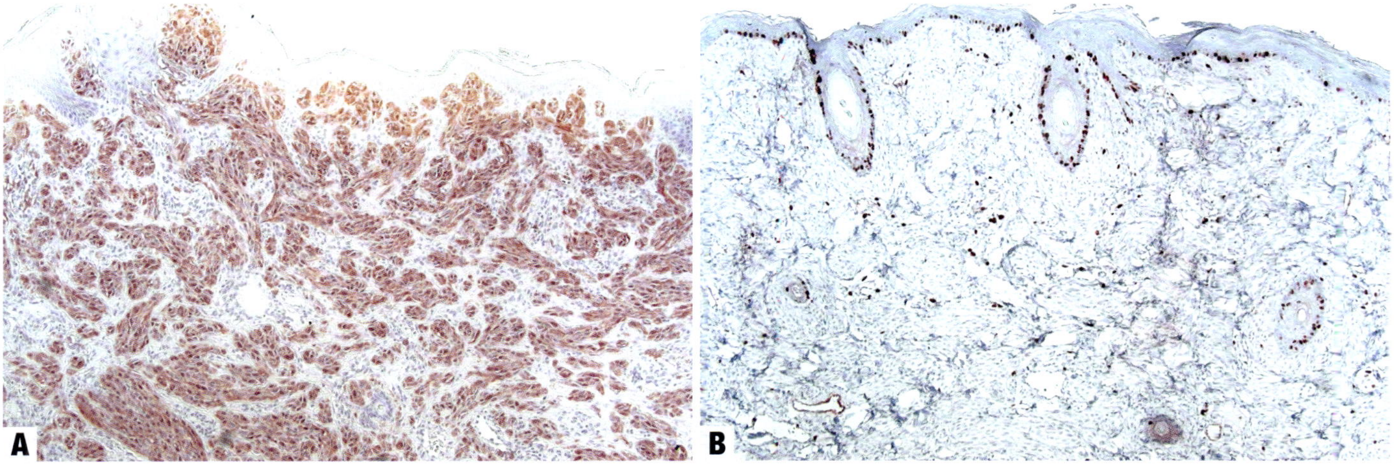

Fig. 3.82 Spitz naevus. **A** There is a diffuse expression of S100. **B** Ki-67 highlights proliferating cells within the lesion. The proliferative activity is limited and only two superficial mitoses were present in the sections.

Over 50% of Spitz naevi of the skin are the result of activating structural rearrangements such as chimeric fusions and truncations, whereas about 20% of Spitz naevi harbour activating *HRAS* mutations. Cases classified as atypical Spitz tumour may have additional mutations in other genes such as *CDKN2A* as well as some chromosomal copy-number aberrations {3689}. For details, the reader is referred to the *Skin tumours* {3597} and *Paediatric tumours* volumes {3596}.

Macroscopic appearance

Spitz naevi are typically < 6 mm but may exceed 10 mm in diameter and may be variable in colour, ranging from red/pink to tan or black {3564}. They may present as macules, papules, plaques, or nodules with a smooth or verrucous epidermal surface. Some Spitz naevi are polypoid. Compound Spitz naevi typically extend into the dermis and less commonly into the subcutis.

Histopathology

Spitz naevi are well circumscribed, with symmetrical borders. A benign lymphoplasmacytic infiltrate is present around the tumour, with multiple epithelial invaginations or cysts with goblet cells. The neoplastic cells are distributed in circumscribed nests and fascicles, oriented perpendicular to the surface. The eosinophilic cells are large and epithelioid or spindle shaped, with medium to large nuclei. Mitoses can be found in the superficial layers. The cytomorphology of the cells is uniform throughout the entire lesion. Pagetoid migration of lesional cells into the epidermis may be quite marked, especially in young children {648}. High-grade atypia must be absent. Maturation of the tumour cells can be observed. The agminated subtype has been described to occur in the eyelid {2698,441}; see the *Skin tumours* volume {3597} for further details.

Immunohistochemistry

The cells stain for S100, SOX10, and melan-A. Junctional cells are HMB45-positive. Ki-67 staining can be positive in the superficial layers, and p16 is preserved {648,3489}

Cytology

Not relevant

Diagnostic molecular pathology

The molecular features of conjunctival Spitz naevi are not known. See the *Skin tumours* {3597} and *Paediatric tumours* volumes {3596} for further details of Spitz naevi elsewhere.

Essential and desirable diagnostic criteria

Essential: a circumscribed cutaneous neoplasm usually < 5 mm in diameter; enlarged epithelioid and/or spindled melanocytes with limited or no architectural aberration, cytological atypia, or mitoses (0–2 per mm^2).

Desirable: histological features including symmetry, clefting about junctional nests, epidermal hyperplasia with a vertical raining down appearance of melanocytes, maturation of dermal melanocytes, wedge- or V-shaped dermal configuration, and absence of deep/marginal mitoses; confirmation of the melanocytic lineage with melanocytic markers such as melan-A (MART1) or SOX10 is useful for confirming the melanocytic lineage; retention of p16 expression; a single genetic alteration such as an *HRAS*-activating mutation or gene fusion involving genes such as *ALK*, *NTRK1*, *NTRK2*, or *NTRK3* confirms the Spitz lineage and the exclusion of other entities; absence of additional pathogenic genetic alterations, or copy-number aberrations other than 11p gain or those associated with kinase fusions, particularly in adults.

Staging

Not relevant

Prognosis and prediction

Spitz naevi are benign lesions. They have a low risk of recurrence and are rarely precursors to melanoma.

Cutaneous melanoma in situ

Mihic-Probst D
Esmaeli B
Moulin A
van Doorn R

Definition
Melanoma in situ is a preinvasive form of melanoma. The atypical melanocytes proliferate intraepidermally and may extend down along hair follicle epithelium or eccrine ducts.

ICD-O coding
8742/2 Lentigo maligna
8743/2 Low-CSD melanoma in situ

ICD-11 coding
2E63.0 & XH08X7 Melanoma in situ of skin & Superficial spreading melanoma
2E63.0 & XH9NL4 Melanoma in situ of skin & Lentigo maligna melanoma

Related terminology
Not recommended: Hutchinson melanocytic freckle.

Subtype(s)
Lentigo maligna (LM); low cumulative sun damage (CSD) melanoma (superficial spreading melanoma [SSM] in situ)

Localization
LM, a precursor of lentigo maligna melanoma (LMM), develops on high-CSD skin. The head and neck region, including the eyelid and periocular skin, is most commonly affected. In contrast, melanoma in situ leading to low-CSD melanoma (SSM) is related to sunburn in childhood and intermittent sun exposure, so eyelids and periocular skin are less-common locations {2054,2942}.

Clinical features
LM typically occurs on the face, scalp, and neck of elderly patients with severe chronic sun damage. The lesions may be large, are poorly defined, and often merge with other cutaneous changes of chronic sun damage {3218}. Low-CSD melanoma / SSM in situ occurs in middle-aged patients who are mostly lighter skinned (Fitzpatrick skin types I–III), and it is usually smaller and well circumscribed. Owing to their radial growth phase, both melanoma types are usually flat. They are asymmetrical in shape and structure and may have more than one colour.

Epidemiology
See *Invasive cutaneous melanoma* (p. 147).

Etiology
In situ melanocytic tumours may occur in chronically sun-damaged skin (LM), or in a low-CSD setting (SSM in situ).

Pathogenesis
See *Invasive cutaneous melanoma* (p. 147).

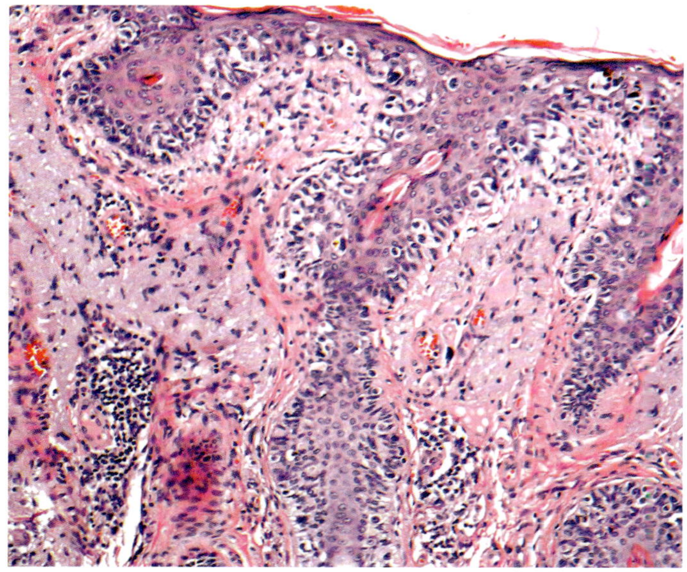

Fig. 3.83 Lentigo maligna. An example from the eyelid skin with colonization of a hair follicle is seen. Elastotic degeneration is also present in the dermis.

Macroscopic appearance
Lesions appear as pigmented, flat, asymmetrical lesions that are multicoloured, light brown, dark brown, blue-black, or black, with irregular or circumscribed borders.

Histopathology
LM occurs in chronic actinic damaged skin with elastoid degeneration and epidermal atrophy. There is proliferation of atypical melanocytes involving the (supra)basal epidermis. Hair follicle epithelium or eccrine ducts may be involved. Nuclei are atypical, enlarged or small with perinuclear halo, hyperchromatic, and pleomorphic. Scattered mitosis may be present {3500}. Two major growth patterns exist: classic LM and dysplastic naevus–like LM {939}. The classic-pattern type has epidermal atrophy, loss of rete ridges, and few irregularly distributed nests, which hang down from the junction in a droplet-like pattern; in contrast, the dysplastic LM type has a stronger tendency of nest formation, and some nests bridge elongated rete ridges. The distinction from junctional dysplastic naevus can be difficult, particularly in partial biopsy specimens. Owing to an extensive longstanding radial growth phase, LM may be large and spread on the conjunctiva.

In low-CSD melanoma in situ (SSM in situ), usually there is a proliferation of atypical melanocytes at many levels of a normal or even hyperplastic epidermis. There are variably sized nests along the dermoepidermal junction. A confluence of intraepidermal nests and prominent buckshot pagetoid spread is seen. The tumour cells may extend down hair follicle epithelium or eccrine ducts. The atypical melanocytes have large nuclei, irregular clumped or dense chromatin, prominent nucleoli, and eosinophilic or pigmented cytoplasm. In contrast to melanoma, LM actinic damage is not a dominating feature.

Immunohistochemistry

Atypical melanocytes can be highlighted with SOX10 immunohistochemistry. Caution is advised with melan-A or HMB45 staining, which can have a nonspecific reaction in keratinocytes of heavily pigmented actinic keratosis {1309}. Positive immunostaining for PRAME or loss of p16 can support melanoma in situ diagnosis. Since lentigo solaris can also be positive, caution is also required here {1926}.

Cytology

Not relevant

Diagnostic molecular pathology

This is not clinically relevant for in situ lesions.

Essential and desirable diagnostic criteria

Essential: a proliferation of atypical melanocytes with a lentiginous or pagetoid spread growth pattern; absence of dermal invasion; elastoid degeneration in LMM.

Staging

Not relevant

Prognosis and prediction

Long-term survival approaches 100%. However, LM often recurs: 30–50% of cases will progress to LMM if left untreated, with a latency period varying from 10 to 50 years. The estimated risk of progression to LMM is 3.5% per year {1621,2180,650}.

Surgical excision with evaluation of margins on permanent and delayed reconstruction can lead to excellent local control rates for melanomas of the periocular region {3700}.

Invasive cutaneous melanoma

Mihic-Probst D
Esmaeli B
Moulin A
van Doorn R

Chapter 3

Definition

Invasive cutaneous melanomas of the eyelid are a family of malignant invasive melanocytic neoplasms derived from surface epithelial melanocytes, characterized by a radial or vertical growth phase.

ICD-O coding

8743/3 Low-CSD melanoma (superficial spreading melanoma)
8742/3 Lentigo maligna melanoma
8721/3 Nodular melanoma

ICD-11 coding

2C30.0 Superficial spreading melanoma, primary
2C30.2 Lentigo maligna melanoma, primary
2C30.1 Nodular melanoma, primary

Related terminology

None

Subtype(s)

None

Localization

Lentigo maligna melanoma (LMM) and spindle cell and desmoplastic melanoma, which are strongly related to chronic sun damage, tend to occur commonly on the head and neck, including the eyelid and periocular skin. All other melanoma types (see the *Skin tumours* volume of this series {3597}) may occur at any site of the skin, including the eyelid or periocular region, but are less frequent.

Clinical features

The clinical appearance differs depending upon the type of melanoma. LMM and spindle cell and desmoplastic melanoma occur on chronic actinic damaged skin of elderly patients. In contrast, melanoma in skin with a low degree of cumulative sun damage (low-CSD melanoma) / superficial spreading melanoma (SSM) arises in middle-aged patients, and nearly two thirds of patients are lighter skinned (Fitzpatrick skin types I–III). Dermoscopic examination of lentigo maligna typically reveals perifollicular granular grey dots, with formation of dark rhomboidal structures, in later stages eventuating in obliteration of follicular ostia.

All melanomas range widely in pigmentation, from very dark and heavily melanized to hypomelanotic and amelanotic. Often they are multicoloured. Most tumours are asymmetrical and the borders are poorly defined, with the exception of nodular naevoid, and malignant Spitz tumours (Spitz melanoma). The latter are usually well circumscribed and symmetrical.

Epidemiology

Eyelid melanoma accounts for approximately 1% of all cutaneous melanomas, representing < 1% of all eyelid malignancies.

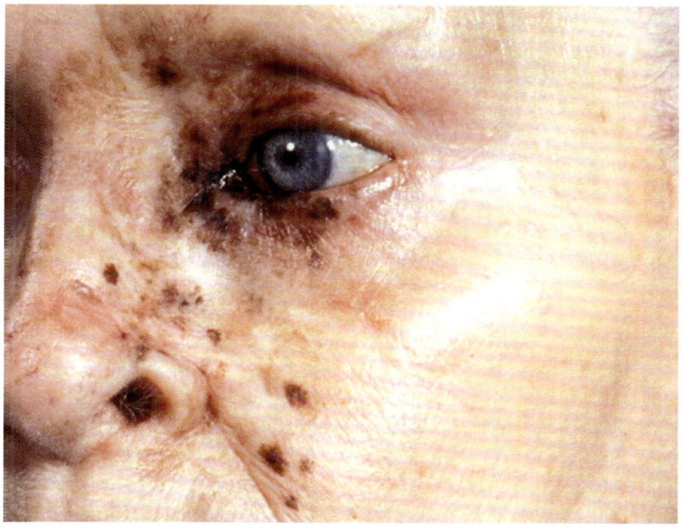

Fig. 3.84 Lentigo maligna and primary acquired melanosis of the conjunctiva. Lentigo maligna / lentigo maligna melanoma involving the face, eyelid, and conjunctiva.

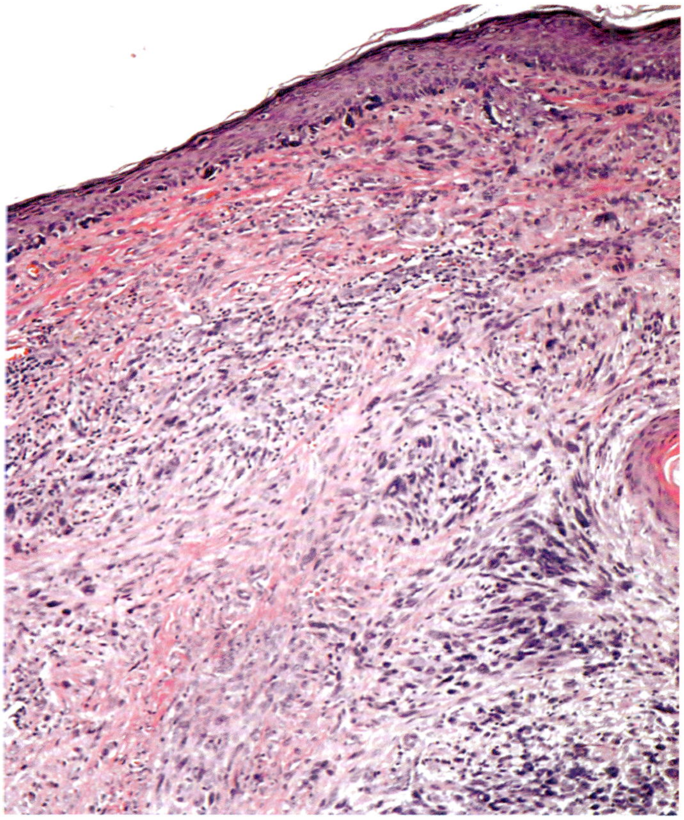

Fig. 3.85 Lentigo maligna with invasive melanoma. An example from eyelid skin showing lentiginous proliferation along the basement membrane of the epidermis with infiltration of the dermis by melanoma cells with a spindled morphology.

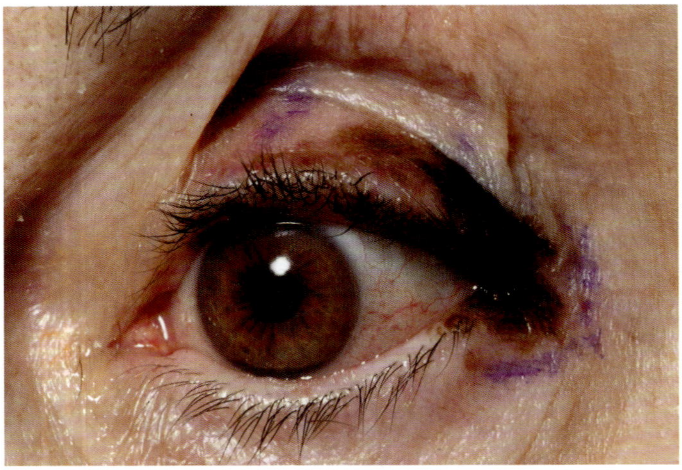

Fig. 3.86 Microinvasive lentigo maligna melanoma. Clinical picture of a 65-year-old woman with microinvasive lentigo maligna melanoma and extensive melanoma in situ.

The incidence rose from 0.2 cases per 1 million person-years in 1978 to 1 case per 1 million person-years in 2016. It affects patients of all ages (range: 4–103 years) but most commonly elderly individuals (median age at diagnosis: 71 years), and it mainly affects White individuals (95.6%). The lower eyelid is more frequently the site of origin than the upper eyelid (66%).

In terms of histological types, LMM is the most commonly diagnosed (24%), followed by low-CSD melanoma / SSM (21.8%), and nodular melanoma (7.7%). The remaining cases (5%) are either rare subtypes or NOS {2054,1182}.

Etiology

Ultraviolet (UV) radiation exposure is the main etiological factor {468}. Other factors include pre-existent naevi with dysplasia, or large congenital naevi {2927}.

Pathogenesis

Most of our understanding of eyelid-skin melanoma is extrapolated from studies of cutaneous melanoma located elsewhere on the body. Melanomas are linked to sun exposure and mostly show a UV radiation mutation signature as recognized by cytosine to thymidine transition at dipyrimidine sites. The use of tanning beds has been linked to an increased rate of melanoma in young women {1874}. Melanomas arise through the accumulation of mutations that activate growth-promoting pathways and ablate tumour suppressor mechanisms. Mutations activating the MAPK pathway and those related to cell-cycle G1/S checkpoint control or chromatin modification are common. *TERT* promoter mutation, which leads to cell immortalization, is the most prevalent in cutaneous melanoma {468,1386}. Although the subtypes share alterations in these pathways, the manner in which the pathways are deregulated shows considerable variation among the subtypes. Melanomas related to high CSD, such as LMM and spindle cell melanoma, have an extremely high mutation burden with approximately 30 mutations/Mb of DNA {1783} and even 62 mutations/Mb in desmoplastic melanoma {2938}. In contrast, low-CSD melanoma / SSM, which is related to sunburn in childhood and intermittent sun exposure throughout life, has about 15 mutations/Mb. Findings from molecular pathology indicate that low-CSD melanoma / SSM mostly derives from a naevus background with or without dysplasia. Therefore, *BRAF* p.V600E or *NRAS* gain-of-function mutations are mostly found. In high-CSD melanomas, inactivation mutations of *NF1* are frequent and *BRAF* mutations rare. If present, these are *BRAF* non-p.V600E {468}. For further details, see the *Skin tumours* volume {3597}.

Macroscopic appearance

Lesions are variably pigmented, flat or nodular, and asymmetrical in shape and structure. They are multicoloured, light brown, dark brown, blue-black, or black, with or without ulceration and mostly with irregular borders.

Histopathology

There is intraepidermal and dermal proliferation of atypical melanocytes or initially dermal atypical proliferation without an epidermal component. Low-CSD melanoma / SSM is characterized by a low degree of sun exposure, in contrast to LMM and spindle cell and desmoplastic melanoma. These melanomas show a high degree of actinic damage with solar elastosis, atrophic epidermis, and often a loss of rete ridges. Low-CSD melanoma / SSM has a prominent intraepidermal pagetoid spread, whereas LMM and spindle cell and desmoplastic melanomas have a

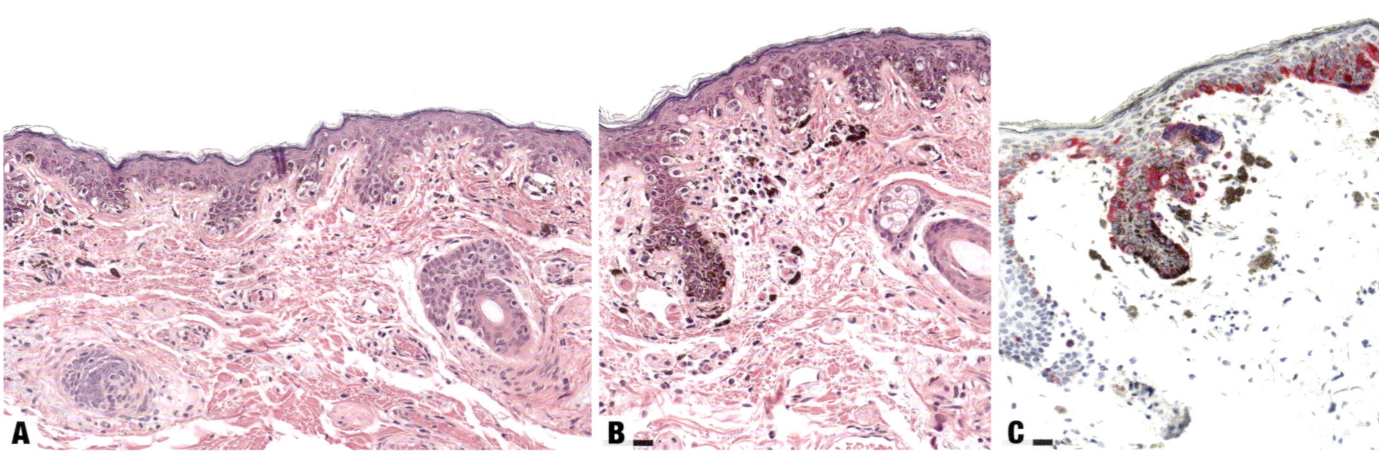

Fig. 3.87 Microinvasive lentigo maligna melanoma. **A** Atrophic epidermis with highly atypical melanocytes occupying the lower third of the epithelium. Single cells are partly confluent, with pleomorphic and hyperchromatic nuclei, perinuclear halo, and pigmentation. **B,C** Higher magnification with H&E (**B**) and melan-A (**C**) showing single dermal atypical melanocytes and melanophages, corresponding to microinvasive lentigo maligna melanoma with immune reaction.

lentiginous intraepidermal pattern with single cell proliferation. Spindle cell melanoma has a spindle-cell morphology, naevoid melanoma is naevus like, and Spitz melanoma shows a Spitz naevus–like morphology. Spindle cell melanoma differs from desmoplastic melanoma only in the cell content, which is much less in desmoplastic melanoma. Malignant blue naevus is dermally located, without an epidermal component, and remnants of blue naevus are often present. In contrast to other melanoma types, nodular melanoma grows vertically without a previous radial growth phase {626,627,628,673,3662,260}.

Further details for each type can be found in the *Skin tumours* volume {3597}. Diagnostic reports should include tumour thickness; Clark level; ulceration; mitoses/mm^2; tumour-infiltrating lymphocytes (brisk/non-brisk); regression (if present, less/more than 50%); vascular invasion; angiotropic, syringotropic, or perineural dissemination; distance to resection margins of invasive and non-invasive melanomas; and associated naevus. Evidence of molecular defects present, particularly *BRAF* mutation, should be included in the integrated report.

Cytology

Not relevant

Diagnostic molecular pathology

In cases difficult to distinguish from naevi, especially Spitz naevi, next-generation sequencing may be helpful to achieve a correct diagnosis. The identification of the driver mutation and a high mutation burden and/or numerous gene amplifications or deletions together with the morphology supports the diagnosis of melanoma {303}. Identification of targetable mutations is important in patients with metastases or at high risk of metastasis.

Essential and desirable diagnostic criteria

Essential: changes supporting a diagnosis of melanoma (a cytologically atypical, nested, and individual cell intraepidermal melanocytic proliferation; an invasive component of similar atypical melanocytes may be seen); low to moderate CSD (solar elastosis) for low-CSD melanoma; pre-existing lentigo maligna for LMM.

Desirable: intraepidermal pagetoid scatter or a confluent lentiginous proliferation; extension of the intraepidermal in situ melanoma three rete ridges beyond any dermal invasive component; mutation status for *BRAF*.

Staging

If metastases are not already present, sentinel node biopsy should be performed for patients at high risk of metastatic disease (> pT2) {2168,2859}.

Prognosis and prediction

Poor prognostic factors include vertical growth phase, increased tumour thickness, ulceration, high mitotic rate, few tumour-infiltrating lymphocytes, lymphovascular invasion, microscopic satellites, and angiotropism.

Surgical excision of eyelid melanoma with 5–10 mm margins, with evaluation of margins on paraffin sections, and delayed reconstruction can lead to excellent local control rates {3700}.

Many melanomas are amenable to tyrosine kinase inhibitor treatment and/or immunotherapy.

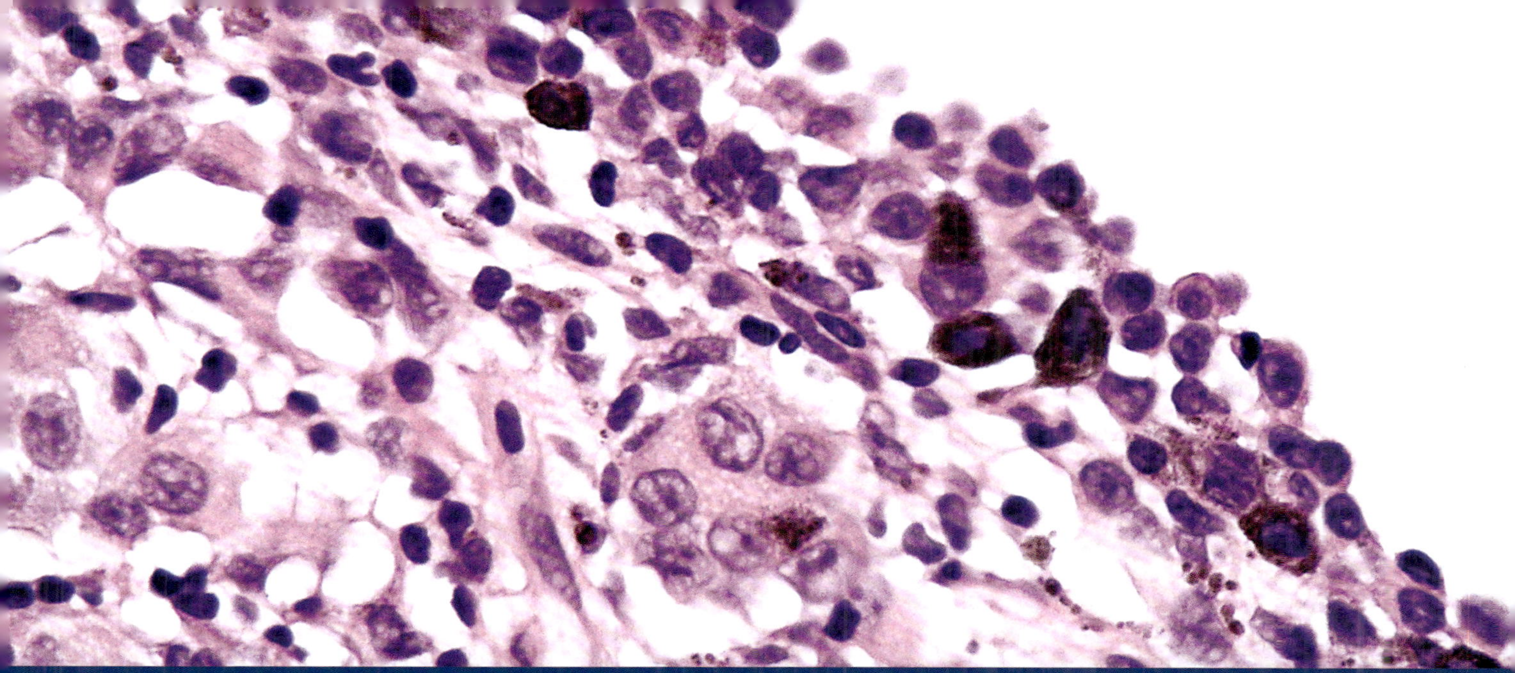

4

Tumours of the uveal tract

Edited by: Cree IA, Jager MJ, Kivelä T, Lazar AJ

Tumours of the uveal tract: Introduction

Kivelä T
Grossniklaus HE
Jager MJ
Lazar AJ
Verdijk RM

The uveal tract – the middle coat of the eye – is divided into the iris, ciliary body, and choroid. As regards the former two, this chapter deals with tumours arising from their stroma. Neuroepithelial tumours and cystic lesions of the iris and ciliary body are described in Chapter 5: *Tumours of the retina and neuroepithelium*.

The main cell types of the uvea are melanocytes, fibroblasts, and smooth muscle of the iris sphincter and ciliary muscles. Additionally, tumours can arise from choroidal blood vessels and nerves (see Chapter 11: *Soft tissue and bone tumours*) (the uvea does not have lymphatics). The uveal tract has resident lymphocytes and macrophages, and it can be infiltrated by neoplastic lymphocytes, plasma cells, leukocytes, and histiocytes (see Chapter 10: *Haematolymphoid tumours*). It is a common site for metastasis (see Chapter 12: *Metastases to the eye and surrounding structures*).

Congenital uveal tumours include ectopic lacrimal and, rarely, thyroid gland tissue. In addition, congenital ocular melanocytosis can predispose to uveal melanoma.

The most frequent benign and malignant uveal tumours are melanocytic. At least in White populations, uveal naevi are estimated to occur in approximately 1 in 20 individuals. A deeply pigmented magnocellular naevus – known as melanocytoma – is a characteristic subtype. Though uncommon for melanomas of the iris, approximately half of melanomas of the ciliary body and choroid result in metastasis. Schwannomas, neurofibromas, and mesectodermal leiomyomas are all rare uveal tumours (see Chapter 11: *Soft tissue and bone tumours*). Lisch nodules in the iris occur in the context of neurofibromatosis.

An intriguing entity is paraneoplastic bilateral diffuse uveal melanocytic proliferation, which is most commonly associated with ovarian or uterine malignancies. We provide an update regarding the pathogenesis of this condition, which may involve autoantibodies to HGF.

Most tumours in the anterior uvea are resected. In case the eye is removed because of a larger tumour, a section should be cut that includes the centre of the pupil, the centre of the tumour, and the optic nerve (PO section). The calottes (caps) from either side can be breadloafed if they contain tumour.

FNAB of uveal tumours is now performed relatively often for prognostic molecular genetic purposes. Such biopsies must be evaluated together with histological or cytological examination to assign correct diagnosis. This chapter now includes descriptions of the cytology of benign and malignant melanocytic tumours of the uveal tract.

Note: Entities that can arise throughout the uveal tract are described in their most common or most prominent site.

Ectopic tissue

Cherepanoff S
Strianese D

Definition
Ectopia represents normal tissue in an abnormal anatomical location, as opposed to a hamartoma, which represents normal but abnormally arranged tissue at its normal anatomical location.

ICD-O coding
None

ICD-11 coding
None

Related terminology
Acceptable: choristoma; heterotopia.

Subtype(s)
Ectopic lacrimal tissue; ectopic thyroid tissue; other ectopic tissues are theoretically possible but have not been reported in the iris

Localization
Ectopic tissue is typically found at fissure lines that form and exist during embryological development. Thus, they are most frequent in the lateral canthus and limbal conjunctiva, in addition to the sclera and orbit. Intraocular ectopic tissue is less common and can involve the uvea, retina, and optic nerve {1682}. The majority reported in the uvea are located anteriorly in the iris and ciliary body, where they tend to be unilateral and nasal, temporal, or inferior {1682}.

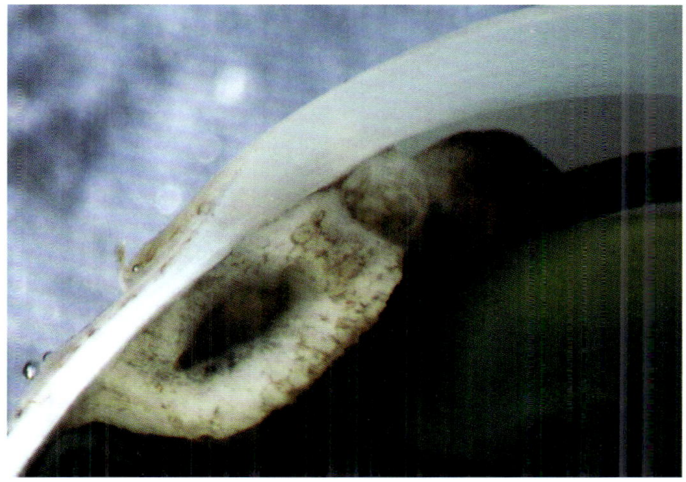

Fig. 4.01 Iris lacrimal ectopia. A macroscopic view shows a pale, solid cut surface with a central cystic area.

Clinical features
Ectopias are typically well-circumscribed, non-pigmented mass lesions, occasionally cystic. Most are asymptomatic until large, when visual disturbance, secondary glaucoma, or uveitis can arise. The majority are diagnosed in infancy and childhood. Lacrimal ectopias are the most frequently reported for anterior uvea, followed by thyroid tissue ectopias {3523,3537}. Lacrimal ectopic tissue is well circumscribed on CT and MRI. Contrast enhancement on CT may correspond to inflammation of adjacent tissues. The solid component appears enhanced compared with the cystic component on MRI {1554}.

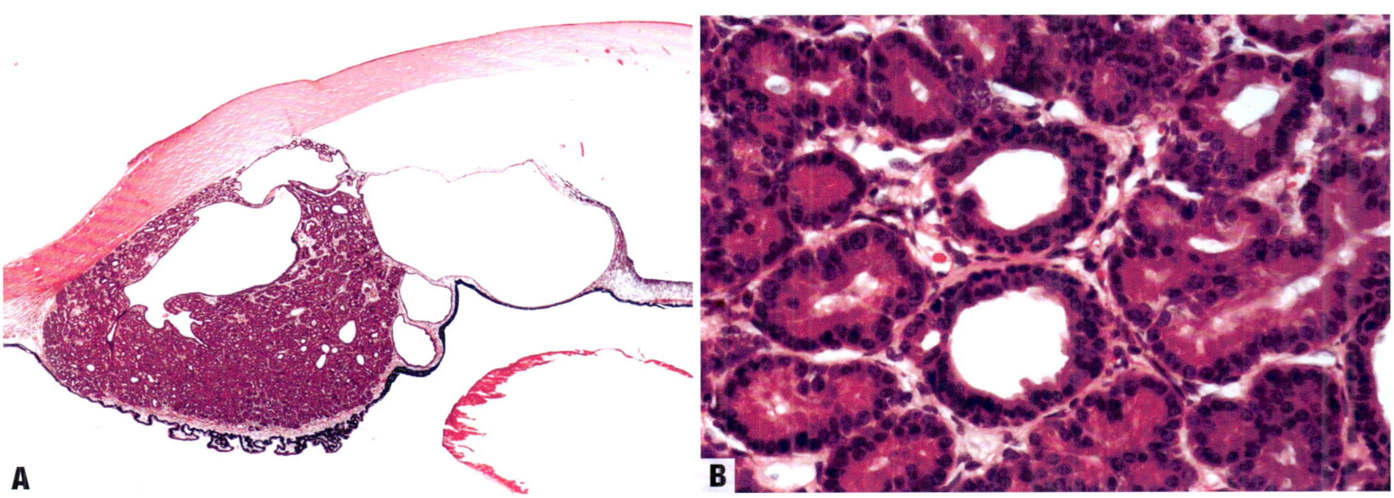

Fig. 4.02 Iris lacrimal ectopia. **A** A low-power view shows ectopic lacrimal tissue that replaces the iris root and involves the par plicata, and obliterates the iridocomeal angle. Well-formed acini and ducts, some of which are cystically dilated, are visible. **B** A high-power view shows lacrimal acini composed of epithelial cells with apical eosinophilic cytoplasmic granules. Intervening lacrimal ducts have an inner epithelial and an outer myoepithelial layer.

Epidemiology

Anterior uveal ectopias are rare. Population-based epidemiological data are not available. However, < 20 cases of ectopic lacrimal tissue {3295} and 3 cases of ectopic thyroid tissue have been reported in peer-reviewed literature.

Etiology

Ectopic tissue is thought to arise from implantations, inclusions, or aberrant differentiation during embryogenesis.

Pathogenesis

An increase in size of ectopic intraocular tissue after embryogenesis may occur during normal developmental growth or secondary to hormonal factors (e.g. during puberty). Release of enzymes, hormones, or other bioactive proteins by ectopic epithelial tissue may cause local tissue damage. Anterior uveal ectopias may raise intraocular pressure if they directly involve the iridocorneal angle or are of a sufficient size to anteriorly displace the iris and obstruct the angle. Reduced visual acuity or visual field defects can be seen if the ectopia is large enough to encroach on the pupillary aperture or cause a peripheral retinal detachment.

Macroscopic appearance

Iris ectopias are typically well circumscribed and may appear lobulated. Lacrimal ectopias have a smooth, pale cut surface {709} and may be cystic. Thyroid ectopias have a red-brown, glistening cut surface similar to that of a thyroid gland.

Histopathology

Microscopically, ectopic tissue resembles its normally sited counterpart. Ectopic lacrimal tissue is composed of acini rich in eosinophilic granules, with or without lacrimal ducts. Thyroid ectopic tissue is composed of thyroid follicles, with or without colloid. Tissue is well differentiated, without cytological atypia or mitoses, and shows low proliferative activity by Ki-67 immunostaining. Histology may raise the differential diagnoses of medulloepithelioma in infants and children {3295} and metastatic well-differentiated carcinoma in adults, so careful clinical correlation is needed.

Cytology

Cytological appearances resemble those of the normal tissue of origin. Given the inherent limitations of cytology, additional care to exclude a benign epithelial or mesenchymal neoplasm, or a metastatic malignancy, should be taken by thorough clinical correlation.

Diagnostic molecular pathology

Not relevant

Essential and desirable diagnostic criteria

Essential: well-differentiated thyroid or lacrimal tissue with formation of acini and ducts (lacrimal) or follicles (thyroid).

Desirable: clinical correlation of well-circumscribed mass with expected findings on imaging; low index of suspicion of metastatic carcinoma.

Staging

Not relevant

Prognosis and prediction

While small asymptomatic lesions can be managed conservatively with close clinical surveillance, excisional biopsy may be required for diagnostic confirmation. For symptomatic ectopias, local excision is typically curative.

Implantation cyst

Auw-Haedrich C
Mudhar HS

Definition
An implantation cyst is a squamous epithelial–lined cyst of the iris that either arises developmentally or is secondary to penetrating ocular injury.

ICD-O coding
None

ICD-11 coding
9A91 Cyst of iris, ciliary body or anterior chamber
9A82 Cyst in the anterior chamber of the eye

Related terminology
None

Subtype(s)
None

Localization
Implantation cysts arise most commonly in the inferior and superonasal sectors in the midperipheral iris.

Clinical features
An implantation cyst appears as a translucent cyst in the iris stroma, containing clear or slightly opaque fluid, which can be associated with secondary glaucoma, corneal oedema, and amblyopia {477,1991,2787}. Secondary posttraumatic implantation cysts are situated adjacent to the former corneal perforation site.

The clinical differential diagnosis includes uveitis-associated cysts that arise from interepithelial fluid accumulation in the iris and ciliary body {1090}, cystic benign naevi, cystic uveal melanoma {3047}, metastases {1092}, intraocular foreign body {1091}, and intraocular parasites {1092}.

Epidemiology
Congenital primary cysts are incidental findings in patients, without sex predilection. Posttraumatic secondary cysts occur months or years after trauma or surgery at any age {1092,1188}.

Etiology
Primary cysts are idiopathic. Secondary cysts follow injury or intraocular surgery.

Pathogenesis
Congenital cysts originate from entrapped epithelium entering the eye during invagination of the surface ectoderm when the lens vesicle forms in the fourth week of embryogenesis {2487, 3520}. Secondary posttraumatic and postsurgical cysts originate from surface epithelium that enters the anterior chamber during injury or surgery.

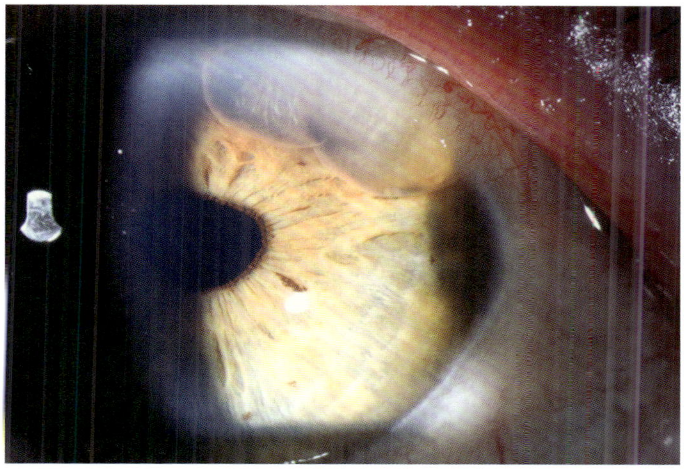

Fig. 4.03 Implantation cyst of the iris. A cyst is located at the upper temporal periphery after a perforating injury 30 years earlier.

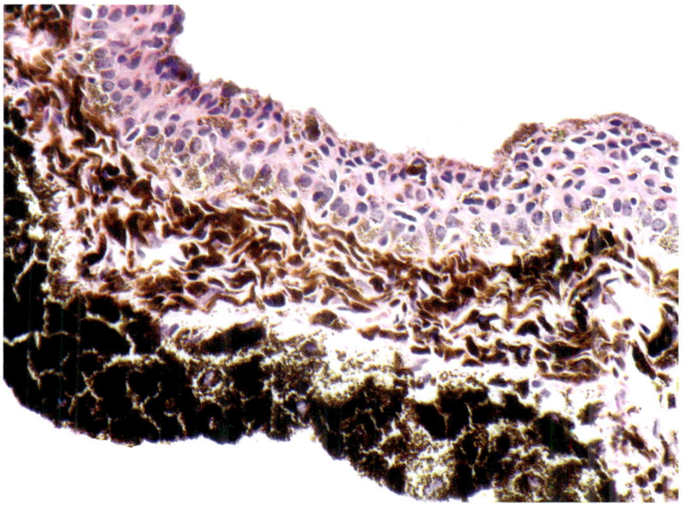

Fig. 4.04 Primary implantation cyst of the iris. The cyst is lined by non-keratinized stratified squamous epithelial cells.

Macroscopic appearance
Cysts are whitish with clear fluid in the lumen.

Histopathology
Primary and secondary cysts are lined by concentric layers of stratified squamous epithelium with or without goblet cells, with or without keratinization {1092}.

Cytology
Not relevant

Diagnostic molecular pathology
Not relevant

Essential and desirable diagnostic criteria
Essential: a cyst lined by surface epithelium consisting of non-atypical non-keratinizing or keratinizing squamous epithelium of varying thickness, with or without goblet cells.

Staging
Not relevant

Prognosis and prediction
An enlarging cyst might cause visual deterioration and precipitate angle-closure glaucoma. Complete excision is curative.

Pigmented epithelial cyst

Auw-Haedrich C
Mudhar HS

Definition
Pigmented epithelial cysts arise from the posterior pigment epithelium of the iris.

ICD-O coding
None

ICD-11 coding
9A91 Cyst of iris, ciliary body or anterior chamber
9A82 Cyst in the anterior chamber of the eye

Related terminology
None

Subtype(s)
None

Localization
The cysts are most common in the peripheral iris but also can be free-floating in the anterior chamber or vitreous cavities {1091}.

Clinical features
Pigmented epithelial cysts are single or multiple dark-brown lesions that bulge the iris stroma anteriorly and can be detected after mydriasis or via ultrasound biomicroscopy or anterior segment optical coherence tomography at the posterior iris. Drug-associated cysts are smaller and located at the pupillary margin {3774}.

The clinical differential diagnosis includes: uveitis-associated cysts that arise from interepithelial fluid accumulation in the iris and ciliary body {1090}, cystic benign naevi, cystic uveal melanoma {3047}, metastases {1092}, intraocular foreign body {1091}, and intraocular parasites {1092}.

Epidemiology
These cysts tend to occur in young adults, with one third of cases diagnosed in the third or fourth decade of life {3048}.

Etiology
Pigmented epithelial cysts are idiopathic, but some cases are secondary to longstanding use of miotic or PGF2α-analogue eye drops {1092,3774}.

Pathogenesis
The pathogenesis of medication-related iris cysts is unclear. In contrast to the other cysts, they resolve after discontinuation of the drug {1092}.

Macroscopic appearance
Dark-brown cysts

Histopathology
Pigmented cysts are lined by a monolayer of iris pigmented epithelial cells, which can be columnar or cuboidal.

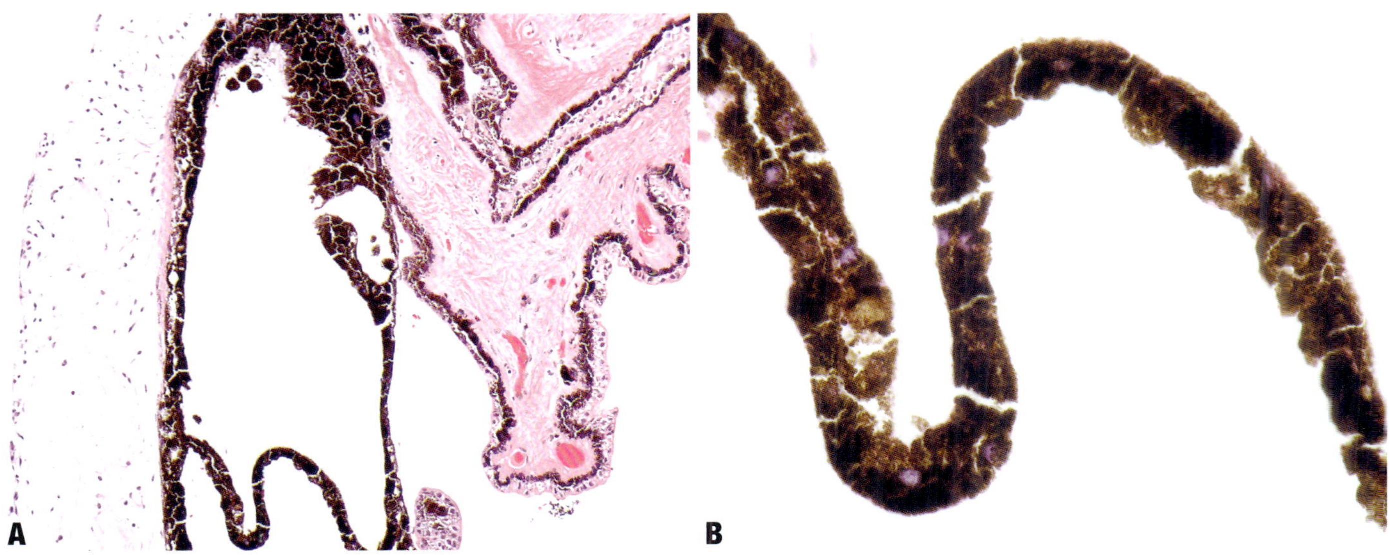

Fig. 4.05 Pigmented epithelial cyst. **A** An iris pigment epithelial cyst located between the posterior iris (to the left) and ciliary body (to the right). **B** A higher magnification showing a monolayer of cuboidal cells containing densely packed melanosomes, obscuring the nuclei.

Cytology
Not relevant

Diagnostic molecular pathology
Not relevant

Essential and desirable diagnostic criteria
Essential: a cyst lined by bland cuboidal or columnar posterior iris pigmented epithelium.

Staging
Not relevant

Prognosis and prediction
An enlarging cyst might cause visual deterioration and precipitate angle-closure glaucoma. Complete excision is curative.

Lisch nodule

Mudhar HS
Rodriguez FJ
Sagoo MS

Definition
A Lisch nodule is a melanocytic hamartoma of the iris consisting of benign, predominantly spindle-shaped melanocytes, in the context of neurofibromatosis type 1 (NF1).

ICD-O coding
None

ICD-11 coding
2F36.1 Benign neoplasm of iris

Related terminology
Acceptable: iris hamartoma; melanocytic hamartoma; Sakurai–Lisch nodule.

Subtype(s)
None

Localization
Lisch nodules are typically multiple and can occur anywhere on the iris, mainly its inferior half {2382}.

Clinical features
The presence of ≥ 2 Lisch nodules constitutes one of the seven clinical diagnostic criteria for NF1 established by the National Institutes of Health (NIH) {2370,1218}. They are bilateral, small, minimally elevated multiple iris nodules, predominantly in the inferior iris {2382}, and usually appear in early childhood, at about 2 years of age. Their colour can vary from tan to cream {12}. They can be mistaken for iris mammillations {2631}.

Epidemiology
In NF1, the prevalence of Lisch nodules rises with age {2002} and skin involvement {3736}. They occur in 63% of patients of all ages, and in > 92% of postpubertal adults with NF1 {2382}. In children with genetically confirmed NF1, the prevalence of Lisch nodules is 34% {986}.

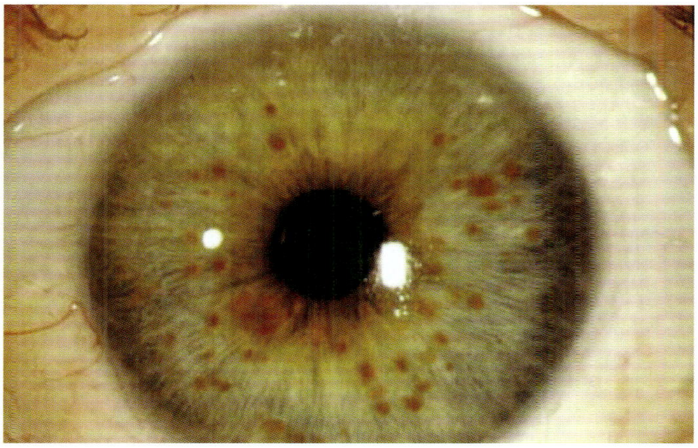

Fig. 4.06 Lisch nodules. Slit-lamp photograph of iris shows multiple small, variably sized, tan-coloured elevations.

Etiology
Haploinsufficiency of the *NF1* gene located on chromosome arm 17q is a necessary event in most cases, according to germline testing {350,367}. A unilateral case without NF1 has been reported, though this may be a forme fruste of NF1 {1840}. Other rare associations described are Cushing disease {394}, familial angiolipomatosis {621}, and neurofibromatosis type 2 {541}.

Pathogenesis
Mutations in *NF1*, leading to dysregulation of RAS signalling, underlie Lisch nodules {256,1518}. DNA damage caused by ultraviolet (UV) radiation may play a role {367}.

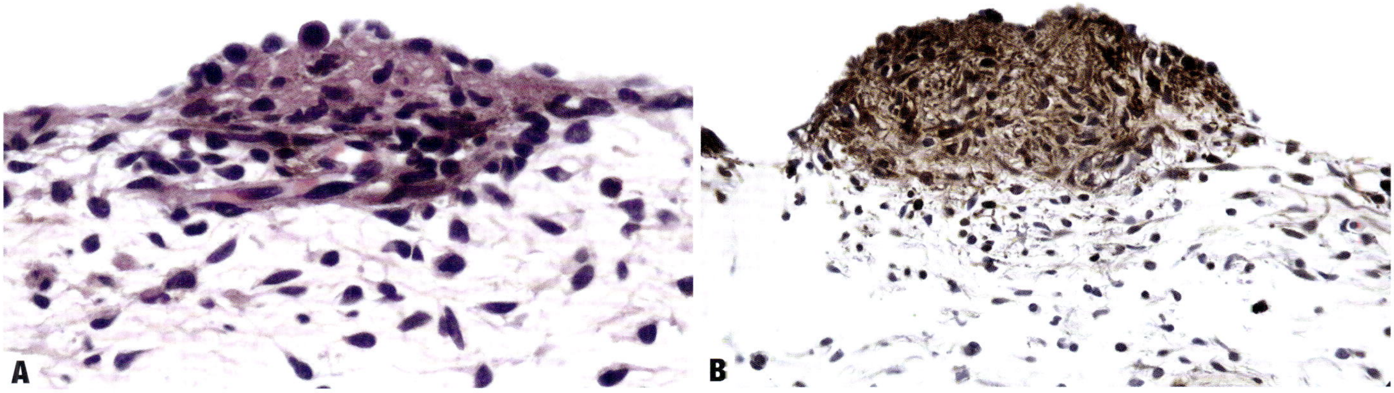

Fig. 4.07 Lisch nodule. **A** The anterior border of the iris shows a nodule composed of bland spindle-shaped melanocytes within the superficial iris stroma. **B** Immunohistochemistry shows S100 positivity of the melanocytic cells.

Macroscopic appearance
See *Clinical features*.

Histopathology
Lisch nodules are usually dome-shaped plaques of mostly spindle-shaped, cytologically bland melanocytes and are arranged haphazardly on the anterior face and anterior stroma of the iris. Nucleoli are not prominent, and mitotic figures are not identified. Ovoid to rounded melanocytes and melanophages can be present. The underlying iris stroma often contains similar melanocytes arranged with a poorly defined margin {2537,3612}. The melanocytes are positive by immunohistochemistry for S100. Transmission electron microscopy shows cells that contain immature and mature melanosomes. No pre-melanosomes are seen {2537}.

Cytology
Not available

Diagnostic molecular pathology
Lisch nodules are not directly tested in clinical practice and detailed molecular genetic studies of the lesions are lacking.

Essential and desirable diagnostic criteria
Essential: bland spindle or ovoid melanocytes, or both, without mitotic activity and with inconspicuous nucleoli, located on the iris surface.
Desirable: immunohistochemical positivity with a melanocytic marker.

Staging
None

Prognosis and prediction
Lisch nodules are not sight threatening and do not undergo malignant transformation.

Ocular melanocytosis

Singh A
Eagle RC Jr
Vishnevskia Dai V

Definition

Congenital ocular melanocytosis is a benign, usually unilateral condition defined as a higher-than-normal population of non-proliferating hyperpigmented melanocytes in the uvea, sclera, and orbit.

ICD-O coding

None

ICD-11 coding

LA1Y Other specified structural developmental anomalies of the eye, eyelid or lacrimal apparatus

Related terminology

Acceptable: ocular melanocytosis; melanosis oculi; congenital melanosis bulbi; congenital oculodermal melanocytosis (naevus of Ota).

Subtype(s)

None

Localization

When associated with adjacent cutaneous melanocytosis, usually at the distributions of the ophthalmic and maxillary divisions of the trigeminal nerves, the condition is known as congenital oculodermal melanocytosis, naevus of Ota, or naevus fuscocaeruleus ophthalmomaxillaris.

In phakomatosis pigmentovascularis, a group of neural-crest disorders found mostly in Asian people, ocular or oculodermal melanocytosis can occur in combination with a cutaneous vascular malformation such as an adjacent port-wine stain {13, 2782}.

Congenital ocular melanocytosis is usually unilateral, but 10% of patients have bilateral involvement (see Fig. 4.08).

The extent of congenital ocular melanocytosis can be classified on the basis of the involved ocular tissue (sclera, iris, ciliary body, choroid) {3501}.

Clinical features

The most typical presenting ocular sign of congenital ocular melanocytosis is iris heterochromia. Iris hyperpigmentation may be associated with iris nodules (iris mammillations), which are dome-shaped small protuberances of the iris surface. The mammillations are composed of aggregates of plump, lightly pigmented naevoid cells interwoven with mature, densely pigmented spindle-shaped uveal melanocytes {3338}. Another clinical feature is loss of iris crypts (see Fig. 4.09).

Patchy hyperpigmentation of the sclera is another very typical and the most common feature. The patches of pigmentation often appear as slate grey or bluish grey areas in the visible anterior sclera. The uvea is involved in a diffuse or sectoral pattern, either anteroposteriorly (subcategories 2–4) or circumferentially (subcategories A–D). The posterior sclera and orbit can also be involved, although this will not be clinically apparent.

In phakomatosis pigmentovascularis, an adjacent port-wine stain is present {13}.

Congenital ocular melanocytosis and phakomatosis pigmentovascularis can be associated with glaucoma {3303,3321, 3302}.

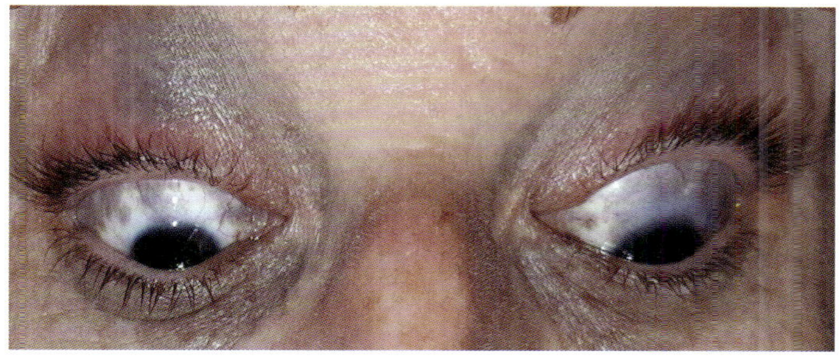

Fig. 4.08 Bilateral naevus of Ota. Bilateral hyperpigmentation. Conjunctival melanosis, scleral melanocytosis, and iris hyperpigmentation. Ocular class 4D–.

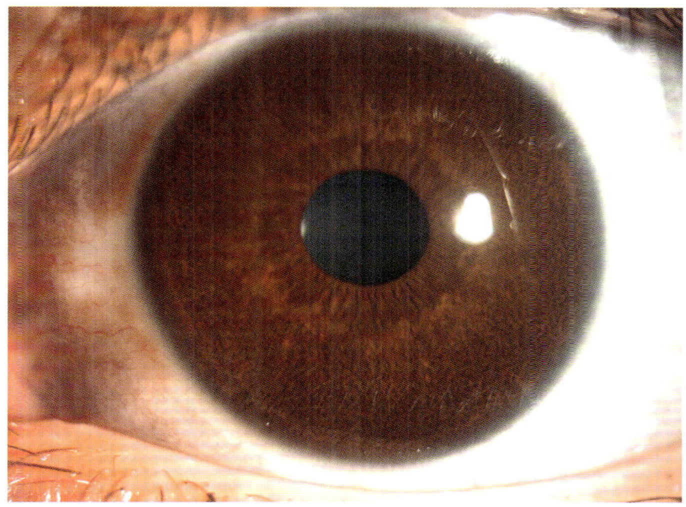

Fig. 4.09 Ocular melanocytosis. Left eye: Class 4D+ naevus of Ota showing loss of iris crypts and the presence of iris mammillations.

Epidemiology

Ocular and oculodermal melanocytosis combined occur in approximately 0.04% of White people, in 1.4–2.7% of patients with uveal melanoma, and in 3.1–4.3% of young patients with uveal melanoma {89,486,1146,2983}. These disorders occur in Asian populations, with a prevalence of 0.014–0.034%, and with an M:F ratio of about 1:5 {584}.

Etiology

Congenital ocular melanocytosis is a hamartoma-like disorder.

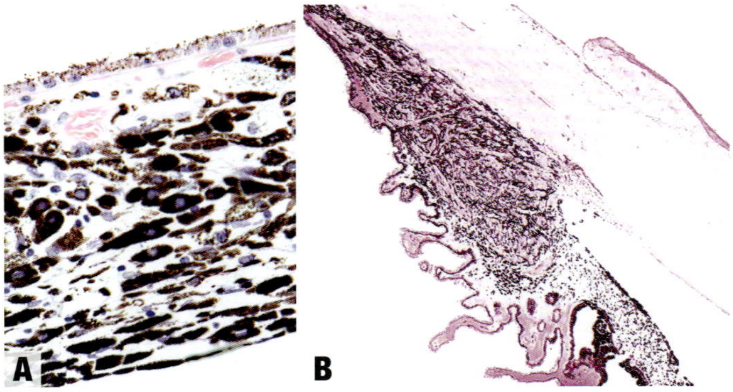

Fig. 4.10 Ocular melanocytosis. **A** Heavily pigmented spindled melanocytic cells of ocular melanocytosis in the choroid, sparing the choriocapillaris. **B** Heavily pigmented spindled melanocytic cells of ocular melanocytosis within the ciliary body.

Pathogenesis

The histogenesis of congenital ocular melanocytosis is similar to that of cellular blue naevus and Mongolian spot. It involves abnormal migration of neural crest–derived melanocytes to the orbit, eye, and dermis, rather than to the dermoepidermal junction {817}. Somatic activating mutations of *GNA11* or *GNAQ* have been found in some patients in association with cutaneous melanocytosis as well as in phakomatosis pigmentovascularis {3328}.

Macroscopic appearance

Striking hyperpigmentation of the periocular skin is seen, along with patchy hyperpigmentation of the conjunctiva, episclera, and sclera, and diffuse or sectoral brown hyperpigmentation of the iris and choroid.

Histopathology

The characteristic histopathology of congenital ocular melanocytosis is overpopulation with spindle-shaped, bipolar, or dendritic melanocytes that may occupy the skin, soft tissues, sclera, uvea, orbit, and even intracranial structures, usually in the distribution of the ophthalmic and maxillary divisions of the trigeminal nerve. The iris and choroid are heavily pigmented and slightly thickened because of increased numbers of heavily pigmented melanocytes; this bears some resemblance to melanocytoma {3683}. Similar melanocytes are abundant, but not clinically visible, in the ciliary body and between scleral lamellae. Mitoses are not seen. Thickened areas should be carefully examined to exclude an embedded early transformation to uveal melanoma.

The differential diagnosis includes diffuse uveal melanoma, bilateral diffuse uveal melanocytic proliferation, and conjunctival melanosis. The differential diagnosis of naevus of Ota includes Hori naevus and naevus of Sun, which are acquired Ota-like facial skin maculae.

Cytology

Not relevant

Diagnostic molecular pathology

Not relevant

Essential and desirable diagnostic criteria

Essential: iris heterochromia and/or scleral pigmentation.

Desirable: abundant spindle-shaped, bipolar, or dendritic melanocytes that may occupy the periocular skin, soft tissues, sclera, uvea, orbit, and intracranial structures, usually in the distribution of the ophthalmic and maxillary divisions of the trigeminal nerve.

Staging

None

Prognosis and prediction

Although this condition is congenital, benign, and non-progressive, it may be associated with two major complications.

Glaucoma is a common ocular complication, caused by angle abnormalities or mechanical occlusion by pigment and melanocytes in an open iridocorneal angle anatomy {3321}.

Uveal melanoma and cutaneous melanoma in oculodermal melanocytosis are important but relatively rare complications with a lifetime risk of 1 in 400 {3102}. Uveal melanoma in a patient with congenital ocular melanocytosis is associated with a higher risk of metastasis {89,2098,2987}.

In atypical cases of uveal melanoma, such as multifocal, bilateral, and paediatric cases, as well as in orbital and leptomeningeal melanomas, underlying congenital melanocytosis should be suspected {1356,1122,2975}. The association with uveal melanoma may be due to a shared predisposing mutation in *GNAQ* or *GNA11* {3447}.

Iris naevus

Laver NM
Damato BE
Singh A
Verdijk RM

Definition
Iris naevus is a benign usually pigmented neoplasm that arises from melanocytes of the iris stroma.

ICD-O coding
8720/0 Iris naevus
8720/0 Circumscribed iris naevus
8720/1 Diffuse iris naevus

ICD-11 coding
2F36.1 & XH4L78 Benign neoplasm of iris & Pigmented naevus, NOS

Related terminology
None

Subtype(s)
Circumscribed iris naevus; diffuse iris naevus

Localization
Most iris naevi are located in the lower half of the iris and tend to be round and small, typically about 3 mm in diameter. Less commonly naevi are located close to the pupillary margin or they are larger, more elongated, or triangular in shape, and in a small number of patients they may be located in the upper half of the iris.

Clinical features
An iris naevus appears as a pigmented or non-pigmented spot or nodule on the iris. The mean age at diagnosis is 51 years {2989}. They can be flat or elevated, may be associated with a cyst, and penetrate deeper into the iris stroma than a freckle would. They fairly often cause uveal ectropion (dragging of the pigmented iris epithelium towards the anterior iris surface) or corectopia. They can be classified into diffuse, sectoral, incomplete sectoral, and solitary in extent {2889}. Circumscribed iris naevi are discrete and often nodular. Diffuse iris naevi involve an entire sector or (rarely) the entire iris. Magnocellular naevus, or melanocytoma, is described in a separate chapter.

Epidemiology
Iris naevi show a predilection for White people and become apparent during puberty or young adulthood {1249,2989} without significant sex predilection.

Etiology
The etiology is unknown but may be multifactorial; sunlight exposure may play a role {3573}.

Pathogenesis
It has been postulated that the formation of iris naevi depends on a time-related embryogenetic alteration of the location, migration, and maturation of normal melanocytes along peripheral nerves, explaining the morphology and extension of benign melanocytic iris lesions {2888,2889,2901}.

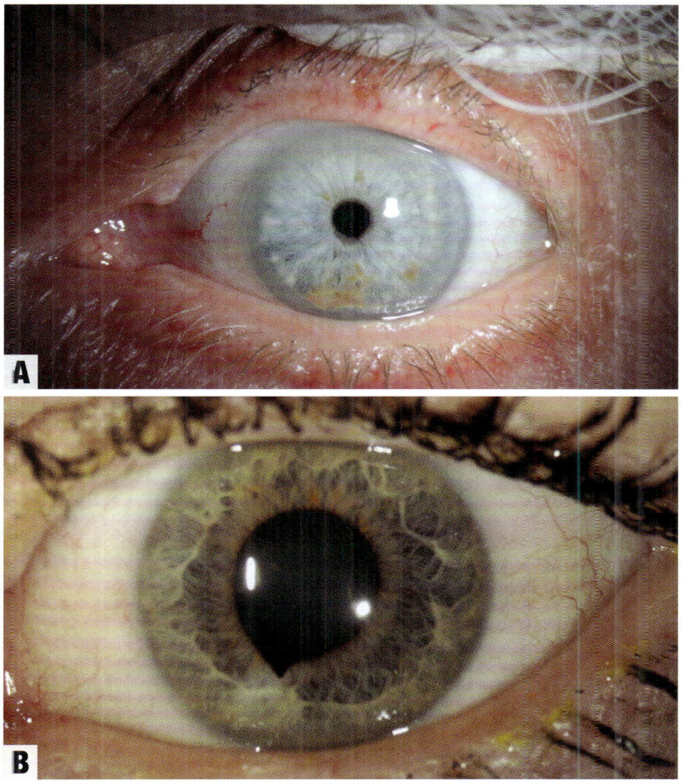

Fig. 4.11 Iris naevus. **A** Pigmented iris naevi. **B** A small non-pigmented iris naevus producing a notch in the iris.

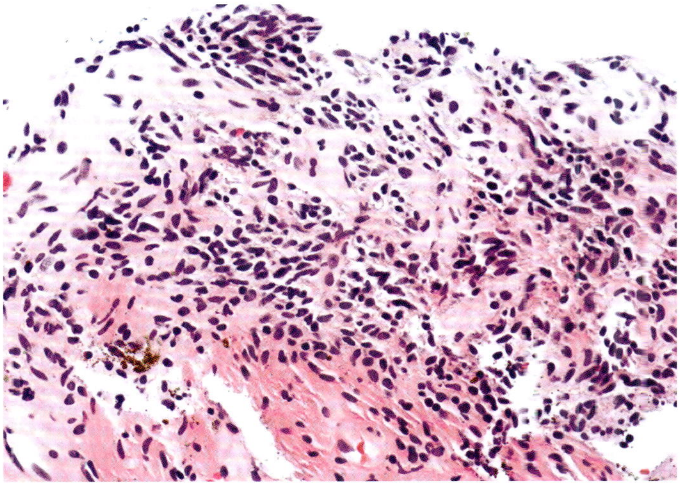

Fig. 4.12 Iris naevus. High-power view of an iris naevus showing mature naevus cells.

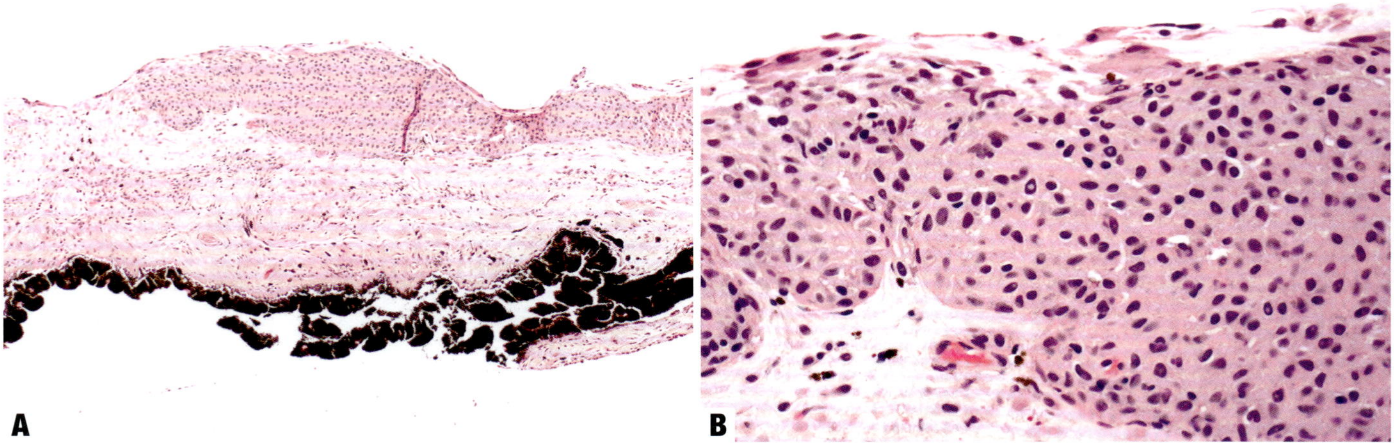

Fig. 4.13 Iris naevus. **A** Neuroid differentiation within a well-circumscribed iris naevus. **B** Neuroid differentiation at high magnification within a well-circumscribed iris naevus, showing a lack of nuclear atypia.

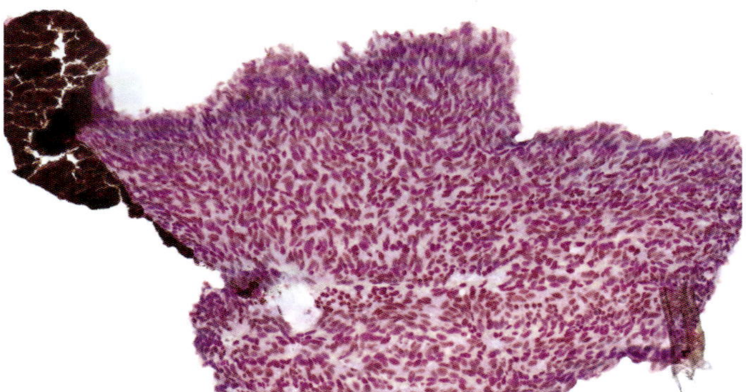

Fig. 4.14 Iris naevus. A cellular lesion composed of spindle cells showing regular elongated nuclei with fine chromatin and inconspicuous nucleoli is seen.

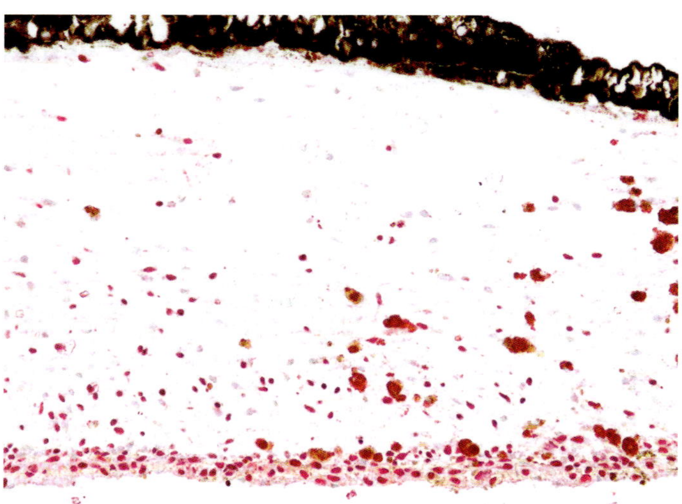

Fig. 4.15 Iris naevus. Immunohistochemistry for SOX10 highlights the unusually numerous melanocytes within the iris stroma and on the anterior iris surface.

Macroscopic appearance

The macroscopic appearance of an iris naevus is generally a brown lesion if pigmented, or a light-beige well-circumscribed lesion if non-pigmented.

Histopathology

Iris naevus cells range from slender spindle to rounded polygonal cells. The nucleolar size of iris naevi is smaller than that of iris melanomas. Differential diagnosis with an iris melanoma can still be challenging {3443}. If epithelioid cells predominate, an iris melanoma should be suspected {3043}.

Immunohistochemistry

A naevus will show rare cycling cells with Ki-67 expression; however, a low-grade iris melanoma may show almost similar findings. Melan-A, S100, and SOX10 immunohistochemistry is positive; HMB45 is usually only focally positive. Nuclear BAP1 is retained; somatic and germline mutations of this gene are frequently found in uveal melanoma, leading to loss of nuclear immunostaining.

Differential diagnosis

This includes metastasis, cysts, and non-melanocytic lesions such as leiomyoma, xanthogranuloma, and neurofibroma {2989}.

Cytology

FNABs of iris naevi are paucicellular and show predominantly small spindle to round cells with or without pigmentation and with small or absent nucleoli. If a melanocytoma, the cells show prominent intracellular pigmentation with centrally located round nuclei and indistinct nucleoli.

Diagnostic molecular pathology

Molecular genetic studies of iris naevi have identified mutations in *GNAQ* and *GNA11* as well as in *NRAS*, *PTEN*, *KIT*, and *TP53* {2882,3445}. Some iris naevi harbour *BAP1* and *EIF1AX* mutations with or without monosomy 3; these tumours are designated iris melanocytic tumours of uncertain malignant potential {3445,2883}. PRAME has been identified as an independent prognostic biomarker in uveal melanoma that identifies gene expression profile class 1 or disomy 3 tumours with increased risk of metastasis. Although PRAME has not been validated for iris melanocytic naevi, it might further increase the accuracy of prognostic testing {969,970}.

Essential and desirable diagnostic criteria

Essential: a cellular, bland melanocytic lesion clinically originating from, or histopathologically mainly located in, the iris.

Desirable: presence of spindle type A melanocytes; immunopositivity for melanocytic markers; retained nuclear BAP1 expression.

Staging

None

Prognosis and prediction

Most naevi show no growth, or very slow growth, over the years. The prognosis for vision and life is excellent. The risk of malignant transformation of an iris naevus to melanoma is < 2%. Diffuse iris naevus is statistically associated with a higher risk of transformation into iris melanoma as compared with a circumscribed naevus {2986}. Periodic examinations with photographic documentation and ultrasound biomicroscopy are recommended to monitor any changes in size or other features that might suggest progression to iris melanoma. This evolution theory is supported by the observation that borderline malignant iris naevi have been reported to harbour mutations that predict clinical and histopathological borderline malignant status {3445,2986,1249}. Clinical factors predictive of iris naevus growth into melanoma are summarized in the mnemonic ABCDEF: A, age < 40 years; B, blood (hyphaema episodes); C, clock-hour inferior; D, diffuse configuration; E, ectropion uveae; and F, feathery margin {2986}.

Iris melanoma

Mudhar HS
Dalvin LA
de Klein A
Sagoo MS
Verdijk RM

Definition

Iris melanoma is a malignant melanocytic neoplasm arising from iris melanocytes.

ICD-O coding

8720/3 Iris melanoma
8720/3 Ring melanoma
8720/3 Diffuse iris melanoma

ICD-11 coding

2D07.2 Melanoma of iris

Related terminology

None

Subtype(s)

Ring melanoma; diffuse iris melanoma

Localization

Iris melanoma is most commonly located in the inferior quadrant {2988}, especially in male patients. In female patients it is more often located in the temporal quadrant {1796}.

Clinical features

Iris melanoma is often asymptomatic but the patient may notice a variably brown enlarging spot or nodule, or diffuse colour change, on the iris. The tumour can be pigmented (82%), non-pigmented (10%), or mixed (8%) in colour. It is associated with corectopia (45%), ectropion uveae (24%), hyphaema (3%), secondary glaucoma (35%), chamber angle seeding (28%), and extraocular extension (3%) {2988}.

Clinical patterns include plateau, dome shaped, or the rare tapioca appearance {2988}.

Epidemiology

The incidence of all uveal melanomas is on average 5.1 per million {3111,3498}, and iris melanomas account for 3–5% of all uveal melanomas {2978}, suggesting an incidence of about 0.2 per million. No sex predilection is known. Most patients are White, and iris melanomas are rare in individuals of Asian or African ancestry.

Etiology

Iris melanoma arises de novo or from a prior iris naevus {1450}. Risk factors for iris melanoma include light-coloured eyes, fair skin, congenital ocular melanocytosis, dysplastic naevus syndrome, and germline *BAP1* pathogenic variants {1781}. Ultraviolet (UV) radiation exposure may play a role in tumorigenesis of iris melanomas given the direct exposure of the iris to sunlight and the more frequent location of iris melanoma on the inferior half of the iris, where sun exposure is most prominent {2986,2173}.

Pathogenesis

Iris melanomas arise from neural crest–derived melanocytes, which are normally scattered within the iris stroma. A tendency for cytological dedifferentiation from normal melanocytes to the spindle-cell morphology, and further to the epithelioid phenotype, is reported during the natural evolution of these lesions {282}. This evolution theory is supported by the observation that borderline malignant iris naevi may harbour driver mutations in *BAP1* and *EIF1AX* that confirm their clinical and histopathological borderline malignant nature {3445}.

Macroscopic appearance

The macroscopic appearance of an iris melanoma specimen is a brown variably pigmented tumour. In the case of a sectoral iridectomy, an effort should be made to document resection margins.

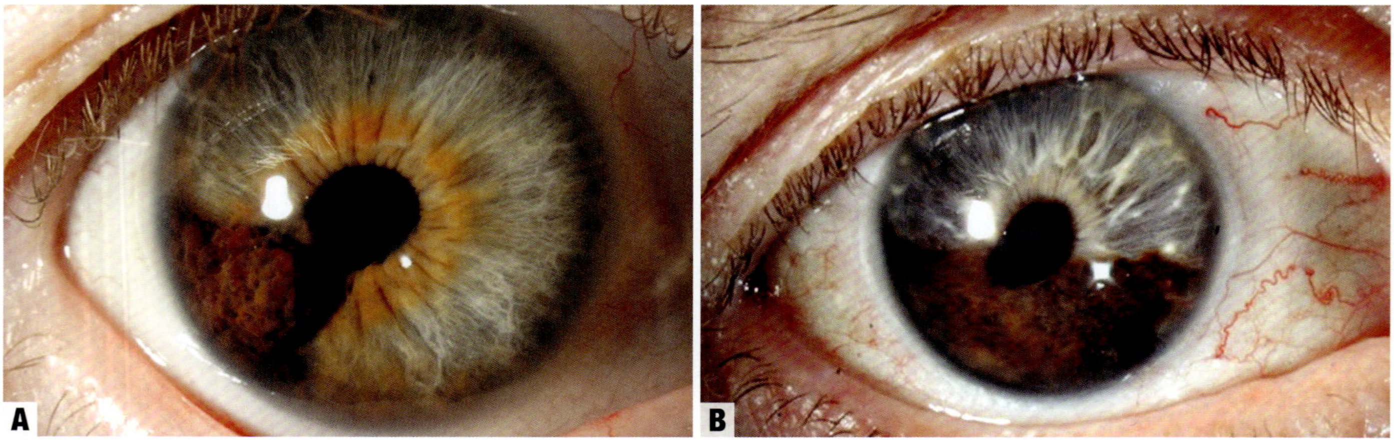

Fig. 4.16 Iris melanoma. **A** Triangular darkly pigmented tumour in the inferolateral quadrant of the right eye. **B** A more diffuse tumour within the inferior half of the right eye.

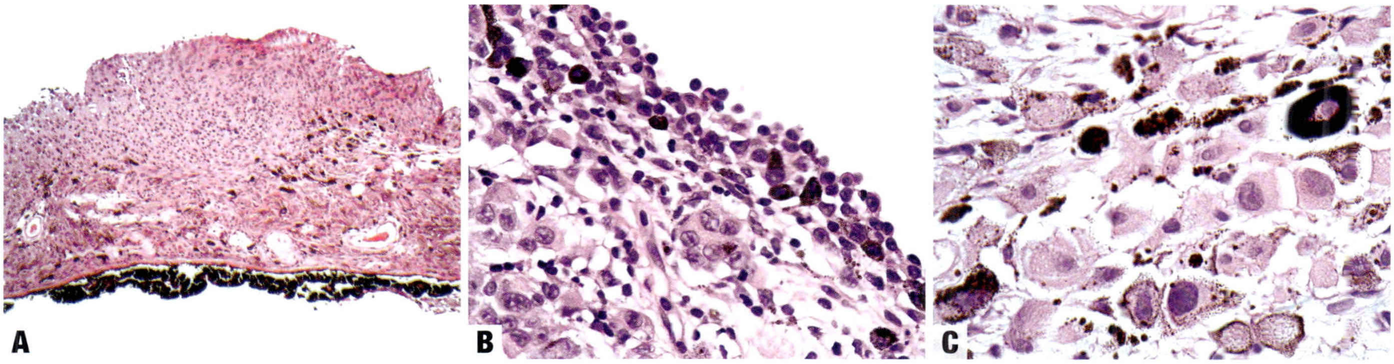

Fig. 4.17 Iris melanoma. **A** A low-power image of an iris melanoma is shown. The posterior iris pigment epithelium is at the bottom of the image. **B** Aqueous modification effect on iris melanoma cells on the anterior tumour surface. Note how the cells become smaller and blander, compared with the cells at the lower left that are deeper in the iris stroma. **C** Abundant epithelioid cells with variable pigmentation.

Histopathology

The Callender system can be applied to iris melanoma cell types. The cells can be spindle shaped and epithelioid. Spindle A cells are fusiform and cohesive, with poorly defined cell borders, eosinophilic tapering cytoplasm, and frequently a longitudinal nuclear groove; nucleoli are inconspicuous. Intranuclear pseudoinclusions are usually absent. Spindle B cells are fusiform and cohesive, and have poorly defined cell borders, eosinophilic tapering cytoplasm, spindle- or cigar-shaped nuclei with aberrant chromatin (clumped and pressed up against the nuclear membrane), and a prominent nucleolus. Epithelioid cells are non-cohesive and possess well-defined eosinophilic cytoplasm, ovoid to circular nuclei, aberrant chromatin, and a prominent nucleolus. Some iris melanomas may show benign naevus cells at the periphery of the tumour {202,1294,2756, 1478,1662,1183,180,3640,1669}. Any of these cell types can be amelanotic or pigmented to varying degrees. Mitotic figures tend to be seen in spindle B and epithelioid cell populations rather than in spindle A cells. Iris melanomas, like their ciliary body and choroidal counterparts as a whole can be of spindle, mixed, and epithelioid type. While most cases are of spindle type {1085,1669}, the diffuse architectural pattern is usually of mixed-cell type {771}.

At low magnification, iris melanoma can be nodular and well defined, multinodular, and diffuse, and a ring melanoma. A particular multinodular pattern is called the tapioca pattern. It is composed of amelanotic tumour cells arranged as multiple nodules over the iris surface. Iris melanoma cells invade the iris stroma as sheets or fascicles, and as individual cells they can efface the normal iris vessels, unlike naevi, and can form a plaque on the surface of the iris. The plaque is cohesive if formed from spindle cells but is rather non-cohesive if formed from epithelioid cells. The cells on the surface tend to be smaller in size compared with the melanoma cells in the deeper stroma {202,1294,2756,1478,1662}. This is thought to be secondary to aqueous humour modification of their cytology {2302,2139}. Melanoma cells can shed into the anterior chamber and lodge in the trabecular meshwork distant from the site of origin; invade the ipsilateral trabecular meshwork; invade the iris pigment epithelium, sclera, cornea, aqueous outflow channels, and ciliary body; and abut the lens inducing a sectoral cataract. Involvement of the circumferential trabecular meshwork with or without the anterior ciliary body produces a ring melanoma {202,1294,2756,1478,1662,180, 3640,1669}.

Ring melanomas that involve circumferentially > 6 clock hours and invade the chamber angle and ciliary body {2433} and the diffuse subtype of iris melanoma {771} are associated with raised intraocular pressure and worse prognosis for vision and life.

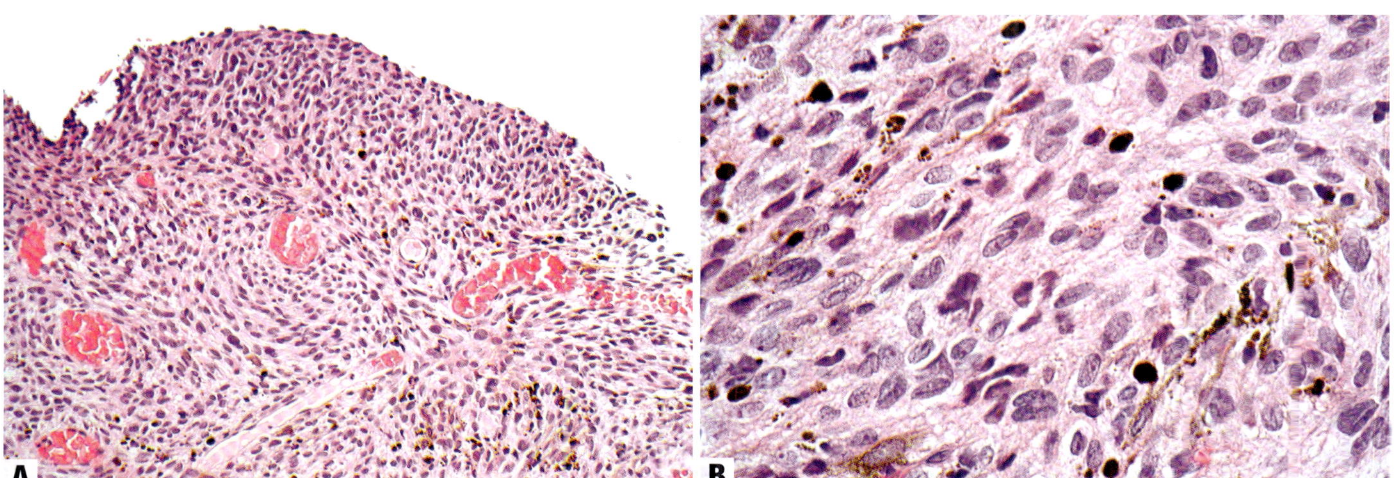

Fig. 4.18 Iris melanoma. **A** A spindle cell–rich iris melanoma with tumour vessels. **B** High-power view of sparsely pigmented spindle-shaped tumour cells.

Table 4.01 Histological differential diagnosis of iris melanoma

Diagnosis	Histological features	Immunohistochemistry	Molecular features	Other features	References
Iris melanoma	See *Histopathology* in *Iris melanoma* (p. 166)	See *Histopathology* in *Iris melanoma* (p. 166)	See *Diagnostic molecular pathology* in *Iris melanoma* (p. 166)	None	See *Iris melanoma* (p. 166)
Iris naevus	Melanocytic cells are commonly spindle shaped with fusiform nuclei, dispersed chromatin, and indistinct regular basophilic nucleoli The nucleus may be grooved and show pseudoinclusions The cytoplasm can be variably pigmented Naevus cells can be ovoid or polyhedral Stroma can be sclerotic The iris vessels are usually not effaced	BAP1 is retained	*GNAQ, GNA11, EIF1AX, NRAS, PTEN, KIT*, and *TP53* mutations	Tumour seeding into iris stroma and anterior chamber angle with secondary glaucoma can occur Malignant transformation to melanoma can occur	{1478,2882,3445, 3162}
Iris melanocytoma	Plump polyhedral melanocytic cells with abundant heavily pigmented cytoplasm that commonly obscures the nucleus After bleaching, small round to oval nuclei, with regular basophilic small nucleoli, and finely dispersed chromatin No mitotic figures Necrosis can be present	n/a	*GNAQ* or *GNA11* mutations	Tumour seeding into iris stroma and anterior chamber angle with secondary glaucoma can occur Malignant transformation to melanoma can occur	{766,619,2810,1424}
Iris melanocytosis	Heavily pigmented spindle, fusiform, or multipolar/dendritic melanocytic cells resembling normal iris stromal melanocytes, dispersed in non-sclerotic stroma or forming cell process tangles Stroma contains melanophages No mitotic figures and no cytological atypia	n/a	*GNA11* or *GNAQ* mutations in association with cutaneous melanocytosis and phakomatosis pigmentovascularis	Iris melanocytosis can be isolated or part of oculodermal melanocytosis Melanocytoma can occur within iris melanocytosis Iris melanoma transformation within melanocytosis can occur	See *Ocular melanocytosis* (p. 161) {3058,1079,697,2615, 3055}
Ciliary body melanoma with anterior extension	Atypical spindle and/or epithelioid melanocytic cells with mitotic activity See *Histopathology* in *Choroidal and ciliary body melanomas* (p. 179)	See *Histopathology* in *Choroidal and ciliary body melanomas* (p. 179)	See *Diagnostic molecular pathology* in *Choroidal and ciliary body melanomas* (p. 179)	Not relevant	See *Choroidal and ciliary body melanomas* (p. 179)

n/a, not applicable.

If a biopsy is rather superficial, it can sample mostly surface melanoma cells that may look bland or naevoid, making it difficult to secure a firm diagnosis of melanoma. Under such circumstances, it is preferable to sample the deeper iris stromal component, which is less modified and will retain a spindle B or epithelioid cytology, or both, facilitating a secure diagnosis {1177,530,973,2520,613,2118}.

Immunohistochemistry

Iris melanomas are positive for S100, melan-A, HMB45, and SOX10. They may show loss of BAP1 nuclear immunoreactivity {1275,1297,3445}.

Differential diagnosis

This is covered in Table 4.01.

Cytology

FNAC shows individually dispersed or small cohesive groups of atypical cells {1798,1177,531} with spindle-shaped or rounded pleomorphic nuclei, with nucleoli, with coarsely hyperchromatic chromatin, within eosinophilic cytoplasm that is spindle shaped in spindle melanoma cells and ovoid in epithelioid melanoma cells. Variable numbers of cytoplasmic finely granular melanosomes are present. Binucleation and mitotic figures can be seen {1177,531}. About 5% of FNAC cases show insufficient cells for a reliable diagnosis {1139}.

Diagnostic molecular pathology

Iris melanomas show chromosomal aberrations similar to those seen in choroidal and ciliary body melanomas. Cytogenetically, most have a low metastatic risk profile, reflecting their relatively indolent clinical course. However, monosomy 3 is well described in some iris melanomas, as well as loss of 9p and gain of 8q {2173,1791,3004}. The prognostic significance of such findings in an iris melanoma is still unclear. Driver mutations in iris melanoma are similar to those in choroidal and ciliary body melanomas, and include mutations of *GNAQ, GNA11, EIF1AX*, and *SF3B1* {2882,3445}, as well as *BAP1* {1211,3445}.

Additionally, in some studies, iris melanomas have occasionally shown mutations similar to those seen in cutaneous melanoma, namely in *NRAS*, *BRAF*, *PTEN*, *KIT*, and *TP53* {3445}. Whole-genome sequencing also suggests genomic features associated with UV radiation damage {1526}.

Essential and desirable diagnostic criteria

Essential: a melanocytic lesion clinically originating from, or histopathologically mainly located in, the iris; highly cellular; composed of cytologically atypical melanocytes.

Desirable: presence of spindle B or epithelioid melanoma cells, or both; loss of nuclear BAP1 protein expression, chromosomal aberrations, or driver mutations may be used in support of the diagnosis of a melanoma or borderline malignancy over a naevus.

Staging

Iris melanomas are staged according to the most recent Union for International Cancer Control (UICC) / American Joint Committee on Cancer (AJCC) edition TNM classification for uveal melanomas that includes a separate system for iris melanomas.

Prognosis and prediction

Prognosis for a melanoma limited to the iris is favourable compared with that for melanomas that involve the choroid or ciliary body, presumably in part because of smaller tumour size at the time of treatment {2797}. Metastases have been reported in 5% of patients by 5 years, 9% by 10 years, and 11% by 20 years {2988}. Risk factors for metastatic disease and tumour-related mortality include initial diagnosis at older age, elevated intraocular pressure, increased tumour thickness, posterior tumour margin at the chamber angle or iris root (vs midzone), and extraocular extension {2797,2988,3019}. Although gene expression profiling may be performed, its prognostic utility in iris melanoma is not well established because of the generally lower risk of metastatic disease compared with in more posterior uveal melanomas, even in the presence of prognostically poor driver mutations {1252}. Treatment modality (i.e. resection, radiotherapy, or enucleation) does not affect metastatic risk {3019}.

Choroidal and ciliary body naevi

Damato BE
Beenakker JWM
Madigan MC

Definition

Choroidal and ciliary body naevi are benign neoplastic proliferations of uveal melanocytes.

ICD-O coding

8720/0 Pigmented naevus
8723/0 Halo naevus
8761/1 Giant pigmented naevus

ICD-11 coding

2F36.0 & XH4L78 Benign neoplasm of choroid & Pigmented naevus, NOS
2F36.2 & XH4L78 Benign neoplasm of ciliary body & Pigmented naevus, NOS

Related terminology

Acceptable: common naevus; melanocytic choroidal tumour of indeterminate malignancy; suspicious naevus.
Not recommended: mole; benign melanoma.

Subtype(s)

Common naevus; pigmented naevus of indeterminate malignancy; giant pigmented naevus; halo naevus

Localization

Most choroidal naevi are postequatorial and evenly distributed throughout both eyes {1793}. Ciliary body naevi are rarely found because this part of the uvea is hidden behind the iris, unless they extend to the iris root or anterior chamber {3255}.

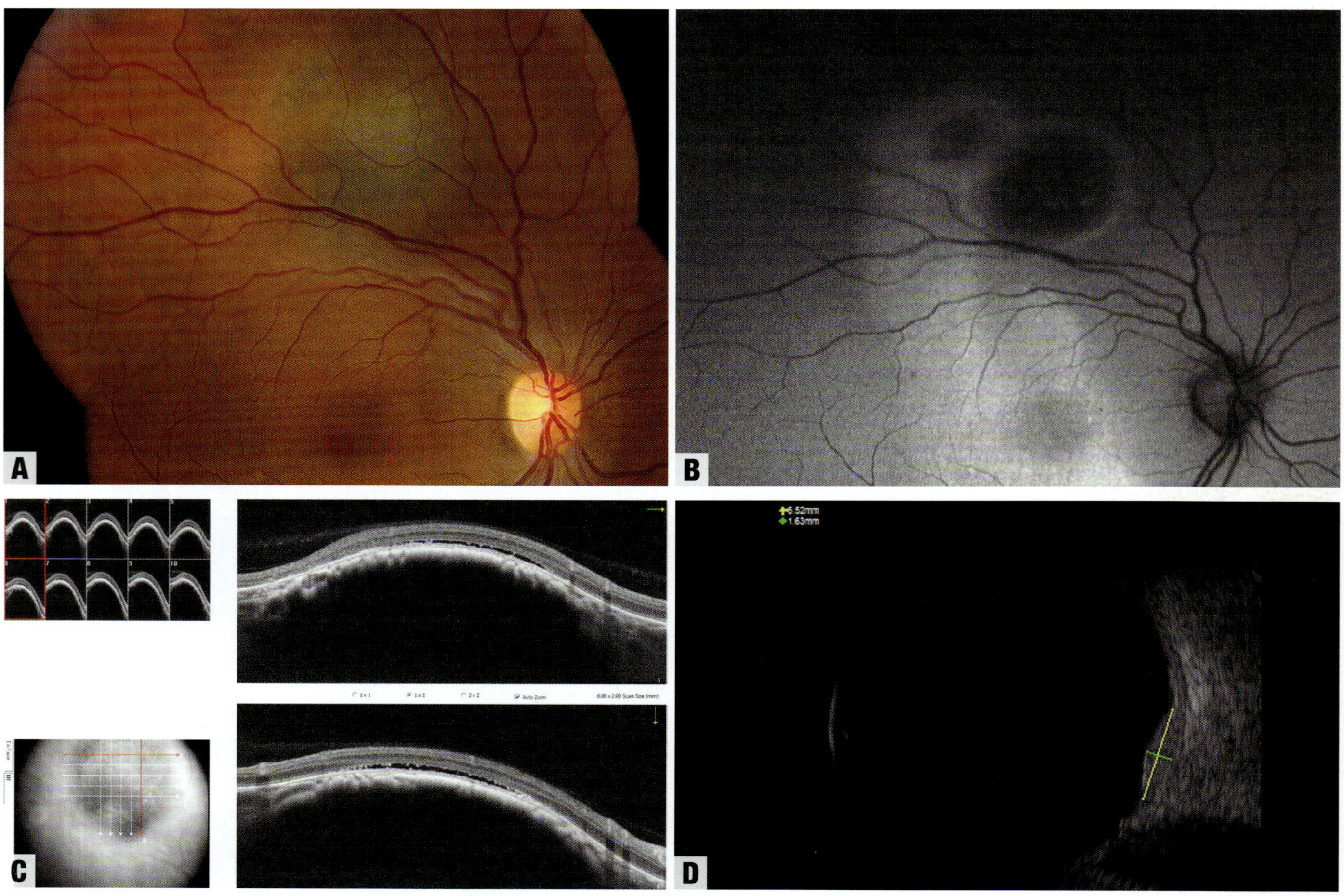

Fig. 4.19 Melanocytic choroidal tumour of indeterminate malignancy. **A** Colour photograph showing a superotemporal melanocytic choroidal tumour of uncertain malignancy. **B** Fundus autofluorescence image showing the tumour to be hypoautofluorescent with adjacent hyperautofluorescence caused by serous retinal detachment. **C** Optical coherence tomography showing disorganization of the retinal pigment epithelium and outer sensory retina with subretinal fluid over the tumour. **D** B-scan ultrasound showing the tumour to be dome shaped, with a basal diameter of 5.5 mm, a thickness of 1.6 mm, and high internal acoustic reflectivity.

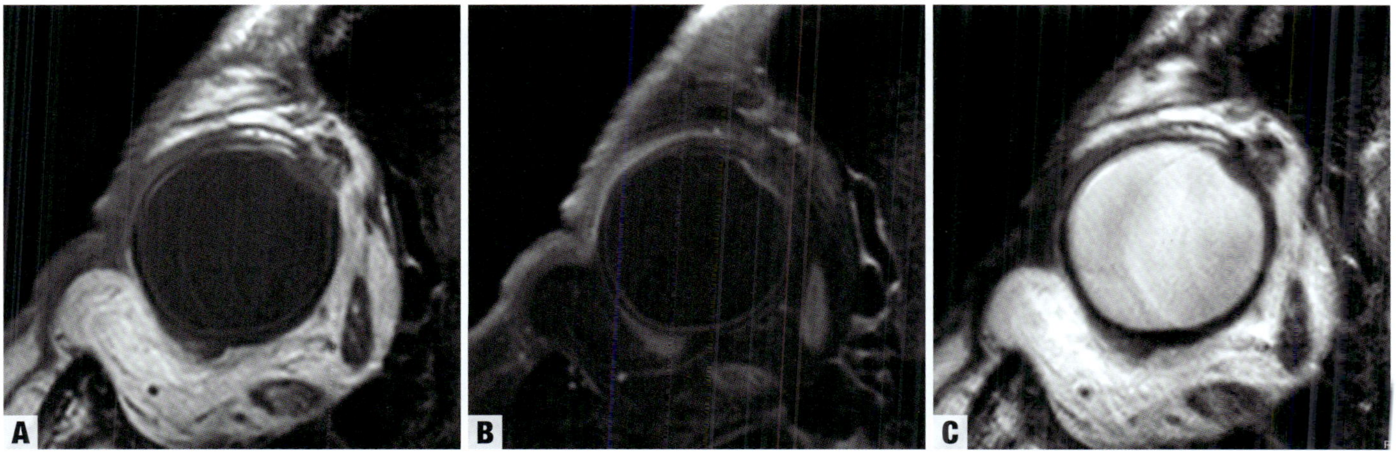

Fig. 4.20 Choroidal naevus. **A** Sagittal oblique 3 Tesla T1-weighted MRI showing a small, choroidal, dome-shaped tumour, which is isointense compared with the choroid. **B** Sagittal oblique 3 Tesla MRI showing enhancement of the naevus after contrast administration. **C** Sagittal oblique 3 Tesla T2-weighted MRI showing the tumour to be isointense compared with the eye muscle.

Clinical features

Choroidal naevi are usually asymptomatic. Most are < 5 mm in diameter and < 1 mm thick {208}. They usually have a greyish surface which is featureless or shows drusen, which indicate chronicity, as does atrophy of the retinal pigment epithelium and intraretinal oedema {1079}. Some are amelanotic and others have amelanotic margins (i.e. halo naevi) {2992}. Melanocytic choroidal tumours of indeterminate malignancy show some features suggestive of uveal melanoma, which include orange lipofuscin (found in 6–10% of choroidal naevi), subretinal fluid (found in 9–15% of choroidal naevi), and large size {2977}. Choroidal naevi usually appear and enlarge in the first two or three decades of life after which time any growth is slow (i.e. ~1% of their diameter or 0.04–0.06 mm per year) {1547,2100}. Retina invasion is rare {3576}. Ciliary body naevi can cause sectoral cataract and can have dilated episcleral feeder blood vessels {3255}.

Imaging

On optical coherence tomography, the naevus may be flat or dome shaped. The tumour obscures the choroidal vasculature and spares the choriocapillaris unless the naevus is thick. The retinal pigment epithelium (RPE) over thick naevi shows irregularity, atrophy or detachment, drusen, and sometimes orange lipofuscin deposits. The neurosensory retina is usually normal over flat naevi, but develops so-called shaggy receptors, outer retinal atrophy, serous detachment, or intraretinal cystoid oedema over larger naevi. These aberrations are more frequently seen in choroidal melanocytic tumours of indeterminate malignancy and choroidal melanomas {1084}. Optical coherence tomography may allow measurement of the diameter and, if the anterior scleral surface is identified, thickness of the naevus. On fundus autofluorescence imaging, any lipofuscin is brightly hyperautofluorescent, whereas RPE atrophy is hypoautofluorescent. On fluorescein angiography, which is rarely necessary, naevi are

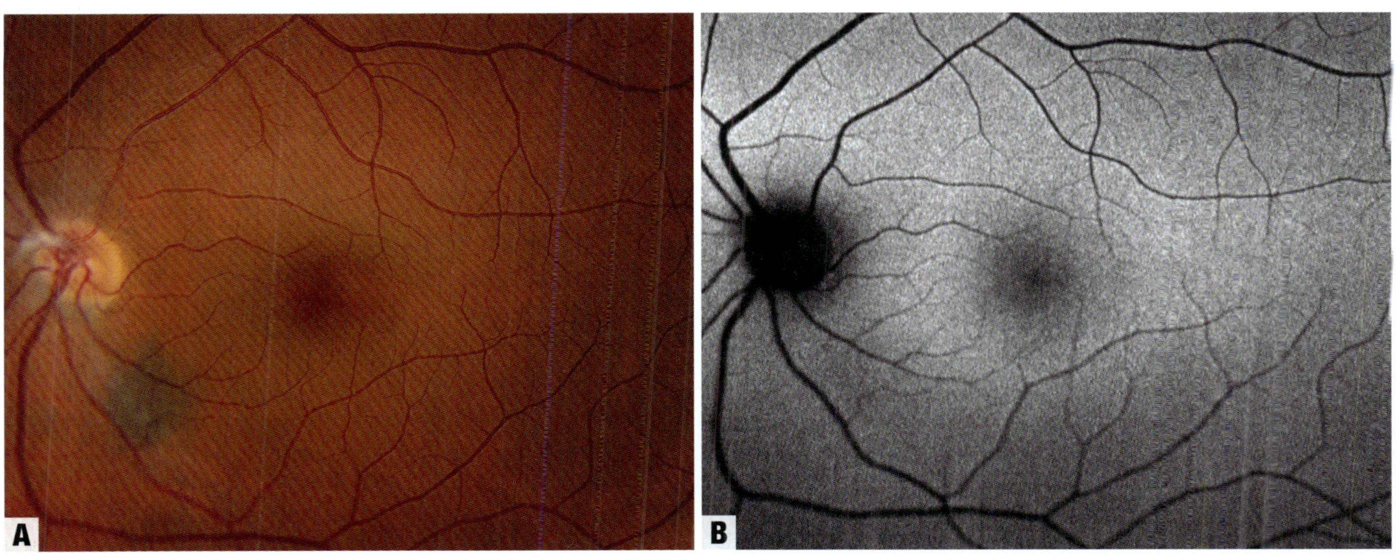

Fig. 4.21 Common choroidal naevus. **A** Small choroidal naevus inferotemporal to the left optic disc. **B** Fundus autofluorescence image showing no retinal pigment epithelial abnormalities over a flat naevus.

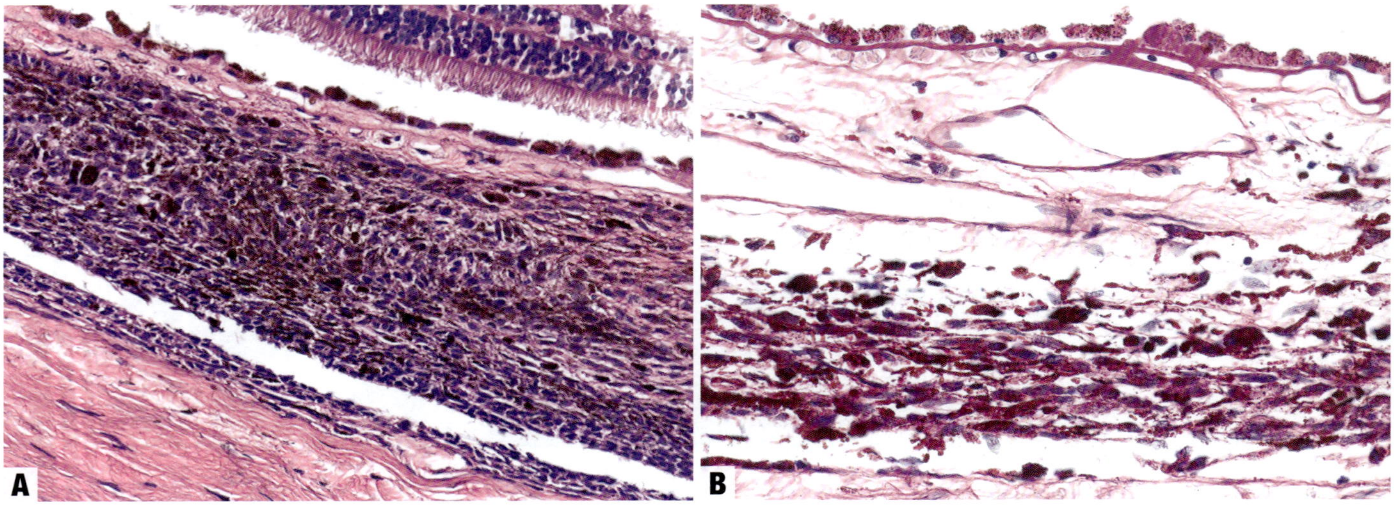

Fig. 4.22 Melanocytic choroidal naevus. **A** Pigmented naevus cells are densely packed and thicken the choroid, with sparing of the choriocapillaris and inconspicuous tumour vasculature. **B** An incidental naevus in a postmortem donor eye is seen; the retina was detached and the retinal pigment epithelium disrupted. There is a pigmented spindle cell naevus in the outer choroid. A PAS-positive drusen is also observed.

relatively hypofluorescent with any hyperfluorescence arising from RPE abnormalities and subretinal fluid. Indocyanine green angiography shows choroidal naevi as hypofluorescent relative to the surrounding choroid, and it may reveal vascular patterns predictive of tumour growth {2305}. If the naevus is large enough, ultrasonography may allow measurement of tumour dimensions and assessment of internal acoustic reflectivity, which tends to be higher than that of choroidal melanomas. On MRI, choroidal naevi show enhancement after contrast administration, but most of them are too small to differentiate them from uveal melanoma using functional imaging {956}.

Differential diagnosis

This includes choroidal or ciliary body melanoma, melanocytoma, metastasis, bilateral diffuse uveal melanocytic proliferation, congenital hypertrophy of the RPE, adenoma and adenocarcinoma of the RPE, and the so-called combined hamartoma of the retina and RPE.

Epidemiology

Choroidal naevi are most common in fair-skinned individuals, with the prevalence ranging from approximately 5.6% in White people to 0.6% in African-American people {2617}. An autopsy study found ciliary body naevi in about 4% of 200 eyes {1231}.

Etiology

The etiology is unknown. Risk factors for choroidal naevi are fair skin and older age.

Pathogenesis

Choroidal and ciliary body naevi arise from uveal melanocytes derived from the neural crest, similarly to blue naevi. In the only known study, almost all choroidal naevi showed low-frequency, almost mutually exclusive *GNAQ* and *GNA11* mutations in 15 of 16 eyes, suggesting a role in their development from normal uveal melanocytes {3421}. Other aberrations included heterogeneous YAP1 expression and, in 1 case, a *CYSLTR2* mutation {2364}.

Macroscopic appearance

See *Clinical features*, above.

Histopathology

Ciliary body and choroidal naevi are typically composed of variably pigmented plump polygonal naevus cells and slender spindle cells, both of which have bland oval nuclei with inconspicuous nucleoli {2359}. About 4% show balloon cells with a foamy cytoplasm {858}. Other possible findings include stromal thickening, obliteration of the overlying choriocapillaris, atrophy of the overlying RPE, intraretinal oedema, and photoreceptor disruption {2359}. Choroidal naevi show intralesional vessels, distended stromal vessels at the naevus border, or both {2784}. Halo naevus histopathology has not been reported.

Cytology

FNAB of melanocytic tumours of indeterminate malignancy may allow differentiation from melanoma by excluding cytological and genetic features of uveal melanoma.

Diagnostic molecular pathology

Choroidal and ciliary body naevi are not usually subject to molecular investigation, although genetic aberrations may be detected when the tumour is sampled for histological or cytological diagnosis to exclude a melanoma. *GNAQ*, *GNA11*, and *CYSTLR2* mutations have been detected in choroidal naevi, but these mutations do not differentiate them from uveal melanoma. A total of 8 naevi showed no loss of nuclear BAP1 immunostaining {3421,2364,3447,3448}. *SF3B1* and *EIF1AX* mutations have not been assessed in choroidal and ciliary body naevi.

Essential and desirable diagnostic criteria

Essential: choroidal naevi (diameter < 5 mm; thickness < 1 mm); flat or shallow dome shape; presence of drusen and/or a halo; minimal or no subretinal fluid; minimal or no orange lipofuscin; minimal or no growth in later life; absence of cytological features of malignancy on histology (if resected).

Staging

No staging exists for choroidal and ciliary body naevi.

The Shields original TFSOM (To Find Small Ocular Melanoma) and the later TFSOM-DIM (Doing IMaging) mnemonics estimate the risk of tumour growth according to Thickness > 2 mm, Fluid under the retina, Symptoms, Orange pigment, Melanoma touching the optic disk or later Melanoma hollow on ultrasonography, and DIaMeter > 5 mm, with the risk increasing with the number of indicators present {2973,2970}.

Damato devised the MOLES acronym to estimate the likelihood of malignancy according to Mushroom shape, Orange pigment, Large size, Enlargement, and Subretinal fluid. Each of these is scored 0, 1, or 2, with tumours categorized as common naevus, low-risk naevus, high-risk naevus, and probable melanoma, according to whether the total score is 0, 1, 2, or > 2, respectively {65,2744,717}.

It has been proposed that the clinician should consider the possibility of a small choroidal melanoma when the observed growth rate of the tumour exceeds the 90th percentile reported for growing benign choroidal naevi, i.e. 0.12 mm per year or 2.6% per year {1547}.

Prognosis and prediction

When a melanocytic choroidal tumour with clinical features of a naevus grows, it is not known how often this is because of normal evolution {2100} or malignant transformation, or because the lesion is a small melanoma that lacks the typical clinical signs of malignancy, which are not yet seen in incipient melanomas {1547}.

Assuming all choroidal melanomas arise from naevi, the risk of malignant transformation is estimated to be 1 per 8845 per year {3104}; however, this average greatly overestimates the risk in younger individuals and underestimates the risk in older individuals. The lifetime risk of malignant transformation is estimated to be approximately 0.2% {1725}.

Uveal melanocytoma

Laver NM
Mudhar HS
Salomao DR

Definition
Uveal melanocytoma is a benign uveal melanocytic neoplasm, consisting of plump polygonal cells with dense intracytoplasmic melanin that obscures the nuclei, which show bland nuclear morphology after bleaching of melanin.

ICD-O coding
8726/0 Uveal melanocytoma

ICD-11 coding
2F36.0 Benign neoplasm of choroid
2F36.1 Benign neoplasm of iris
2F36.2 Benign neoplasm of ciliary body

Related terminology
Acceptable: magnocellular naevus of the uvea.

Subtype(s)
None

Localization
Melanocytomas occur more frequently in the iris {766,1882} and ciliary body {1997} than in the choroid; they are also found adjacent to the optic nerve head {1882,3031}.

Clinical features
Uveal melanocytoma may clinically be similar to an ordinary iris, ciliary body, or choroidal naevus, or a small to medium-sized melanoma {2728,3056}. Most choroidal melanocytomas form a discoid or dome-shaped dark-grey to black mass that elevates the retina. Overlying orange pigment and subretinal fluid can sometimes be seen, which makes the distinction from a choroidal melanoma difficult {914}. Over time, some melanocytomas may spontaneously regress in size. Those in the ciliary body may be associated with cataract, pigment dispersion, or secondary glaucoma.

Epidemiology
Melanocytomas are rare neoplasms and their true incidence in the uvea is not known. The age at diagnosis is variable, ranging from infants to age 90 years {1906,3056}. The frequency in both sexes and in different races is nearly equal {914}. Unlike uveal melanomas, melanocytomas do not show a predilection for White people.

Etiology
Unknown

Pathogenesis
The histogenesis is similar to that of uveal naevi. Uveal melanocytomas originate from neural-crest cells and may harbour *GNAQ* and (possibly) *GNA11* mutations, suggesting a role in their development from normal uveal melanocytes {2293,1027,3162}.

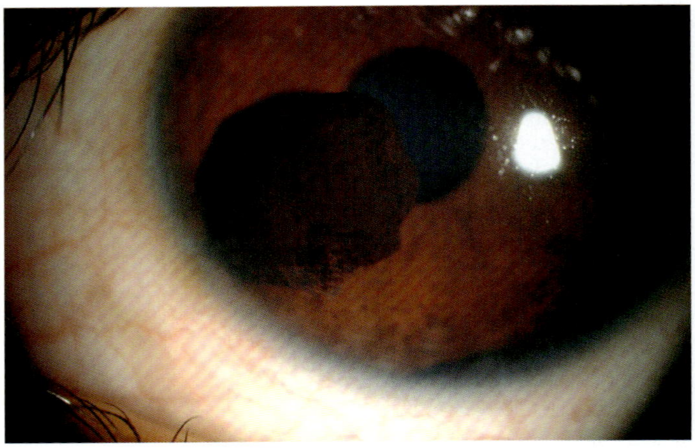

Fig. 4.23 Iris melanocytoma. The image shows a 9-year-old girl with a pigmented iris tumour about 3.4 mm in diameter and located in the lower nasal quadrant (between 7 o'clock and 8 o'clock). Additionally, a smaller inferior crescent-like lesion is seen at 6 o'clock.

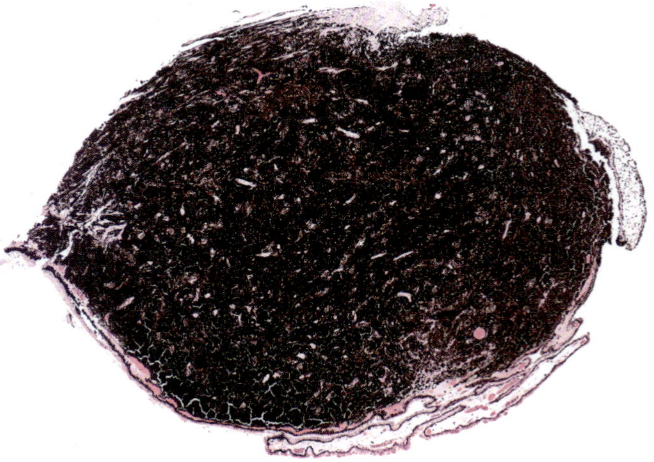

Fig. 4.24 Ciliary body melanocytoma. A resection specimen shows a heavily pigmented dome-shaped mass.

Ciliary body melanocytomas have shown a somatic *GNAQ* p.Q209L missense sequence variant within exon 5 {2293,1027,3162}. The same *GNAQ* variant is typical for uveal naevi and uveal melanoma {2293}. Mutation of *GNA11*, *BAP1*, *SF3B1*, and *BRAF* has so far not been identified {2293,1027,3162}. However, only a few uveal melanocytomas have been evaluated genetically. *GNA11* mutation is reported in melanocytomas in other locations {3760}.

Macroscopic appearance
On gross examination melanocytomas appear dark brown to jet black and generally measure 1–5 mm in thickness. Ciliary body melanocytomas tend to be larger than melanocytomas in other locations before they are detected clinically.

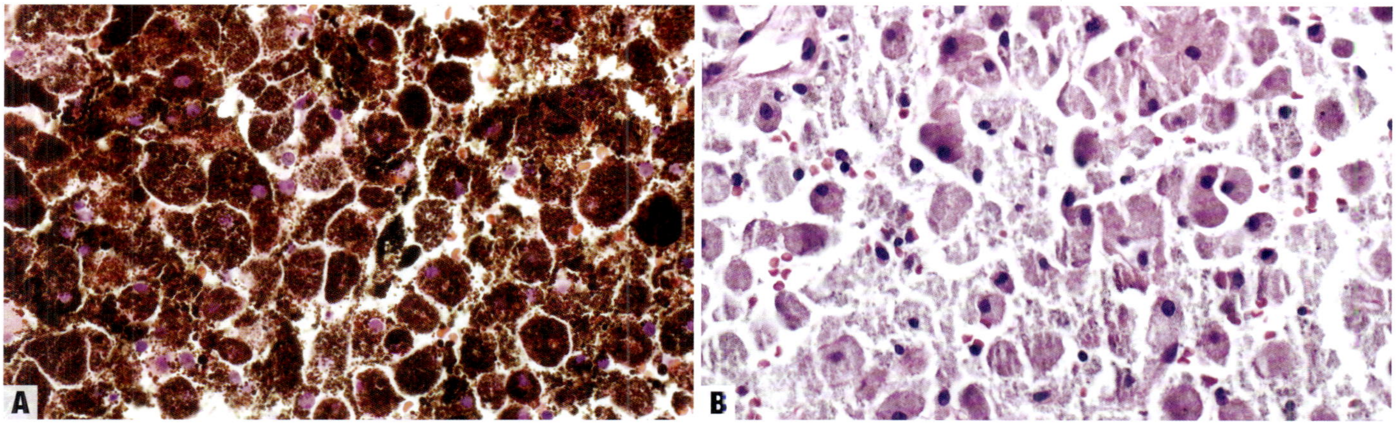

Fig. 4.25 Uveal melanocytoma. **A** Polyhedral tumour cells with abundant cytoplasmic pigmentation that obscures nuclear features are seen. **B** Bleaching allows for removal of cytoplasmic melanin pigment granules, revealing tumour cells with a low N:C ratio and small round nuclei with inconspicuous nucleoli.

Histopathology

Uveal melanocytomas are composed of large, polygonal cells with abundant intracytoplasmic melanin pigment that obscures cellular and nuclear details. Bleaching of melanin is required to adequately evaluate the tumour cells, which show a low N:C ratio, oval to round bland nuclei, and inconspicuous nucleoli. Although partial necrosis may be seen in larger melanocytomas, mitoses are absent and Ki-67 immunohistochemistry does not show cycling cells {1832}, unlike in uveal melanoma and pigmented adenocarcinomas of the ciliary body. BAP1 nuclear expression is retained.

The differential diagnosis includes uveal melanomas and naevi. Adenoma and adenocarcinoma of the ciliary or retinal pigmented epithelium, although rare, should be considered. The melanocytic lineage immunohistochemical markers melan-A, SOX10, and S100 may be useful in challenging cases to rule out pigmented epithelial tumours.

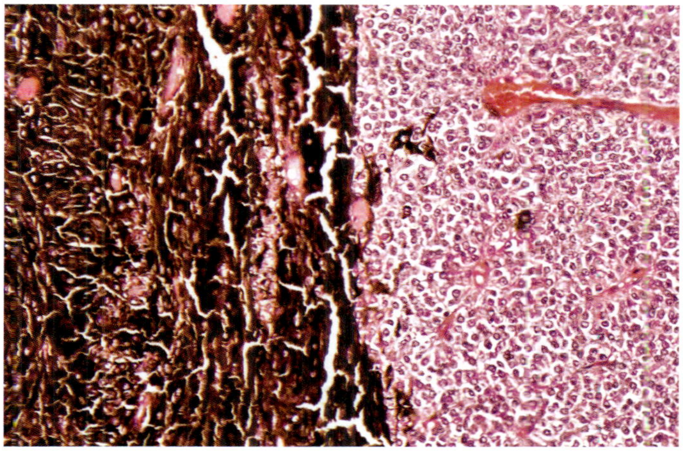

Fig. 4.26 Ciliary body melanocytoma transforming to uveal melanoma. A section showing a ciliary body melanocytoma (on the left) transforming to a uveal melanoma (on the right). Note the loss of pigment and the higher N:C ratio of the uveal melanoma cells.

Cytology

Diagnostic FNAB of melanocytomas shows large, ovoid cells with small centrally located nuclei and heavily pigmented cytoplasm {2853}. The cells are immunoreactive for melanocytic markers and show rare or no cells in cycle with Ki-67 immunostaining.

Diagnostic molecular pathology

Not clinically relevant

Essential and desirable diagnostic criteria

Essential: a deeply pigmented uveal melanocytic tumour with polygonal cells, abundant cytoplasm, small centrally located nuclei, and few indistinct nucleoli.

Desirable: bleaching of melanin and immunohistochemical confirmation of melanocytic lineage with absence of cytokeratin expression.

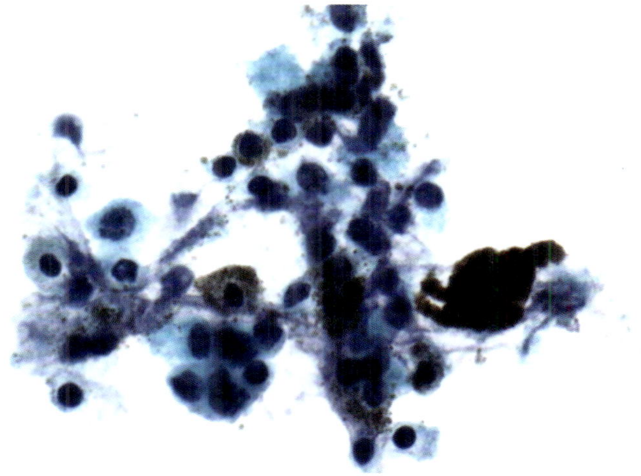

Fig. 4.27 Uveal melanocytoma. FNAB shows a cluster of ovoid cells with centrally located small nuclei and intracytoplasmic pigment (Pap).

Staging

Not relevant

Prognosis and prediction

The prognosis for life is excellent, although in rare instances malignant transformation to uveal melanoma can occur {257, 1911,2293,1813}. *BAP1* mutation was demonstrated in 2 cases of optic nerve melanocytoma with malignant transformation, with 1 of them also harbouring a *GNAQ* mutation. This suggests that mutations in *BAP1* may accompany malignant transformation in ocular melanocytomas {1027}.

Bilateral diffuse uveal melanocytic proliferation

Mudhar HS
Heegaard S

Definition

Bilateral diffuse uveal melanocytic proliferation is a paraneoplastic syndrome characterized by diffuse proliferation of predominantly benign-appearing melanocytes in the uveal tract, usually in both eyes, in patients with an underlying extraocular malignancy, often leading to an exudative retinal detachment and frequently associated with progressive cataracts.

ICD-O coding

None

ICD-11 coding

None

Related terminology

Acceptable: paraneoplastic uveal melanocytic hyperplasia.

Subtype(s)

None

Localization

Paraneoplastic bilateral diffuse uveal melanocytic proliferation may be panuveal (iris, ciliary body, and choroid) or it can affect only a part of the uveal tract, although it usually involves the choroid in all patients.

Clinical features

Patients experience an otherwise inexplicable rapidly progressive bilateral vision loss, which is essentially refractory to treatment. Unilateral ocular involvement is exceptional {3175}. The symptoms can precede the detection of the underlying systemic malignancy. Bilateral diffuse uveal melanocytic proliferation leads to damage to the retinal pigment epithelium, and that destruction is an important part of its fundus (and ancillary histopathological) findings. Important signs include multiple subtle reddish patches at the level of the retinal pigment epithelium corresponding to areas of hypoautofluorescence that are hyperfluorescent upon fluorescein angiography {1744}, multiple pigmented and non-pigmented uveal melanocytic lesions that are hypofluorescent upon indocyanine green angiography, exudative retinal detachment, and rapidly progressive cataracts {1080,2434,1744}. The fundus autofluorescence image with a reticular, often called leopard spot / giraffe, pattern of hyperautofluorescence {1442,1916,1720} is a key diagnostic finding. It corresponds to destruction of the retinal pigment epithelium seen in optical coherence tomography. The ocular findings are associated with an underlying malignancy, most commonly a carcinoma of the ovary or endometrium in women and a carcinoma of the lung in men {505}. Less-common primary sites of the underlying primary neoplasm are the pancreas, lung, colon, and kidney {1744, 2303,2434}. Non-ocular melanocytic proliferation associated with bilateral diffuse uveal melanocytic proliferation affects as many as 25% of patients in the oral and genital mucosa, skin, and conjunctiva {1081,2434,2601,2361,2292}.

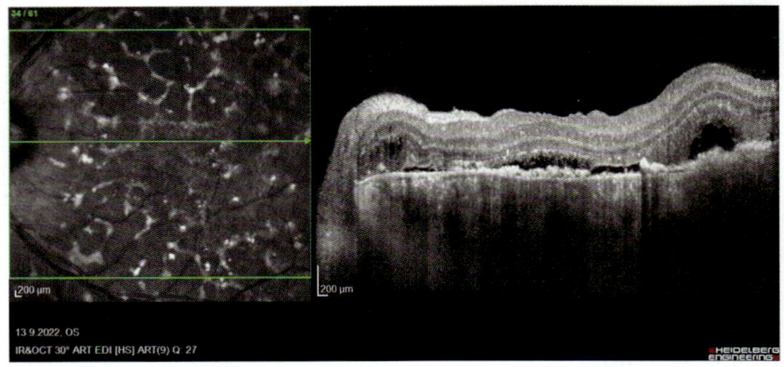

Fig. 4.28 Bilateral diffuse uveal melanocytic proliferation. Optical CT showing destruction of the retinal pigment epithelium.

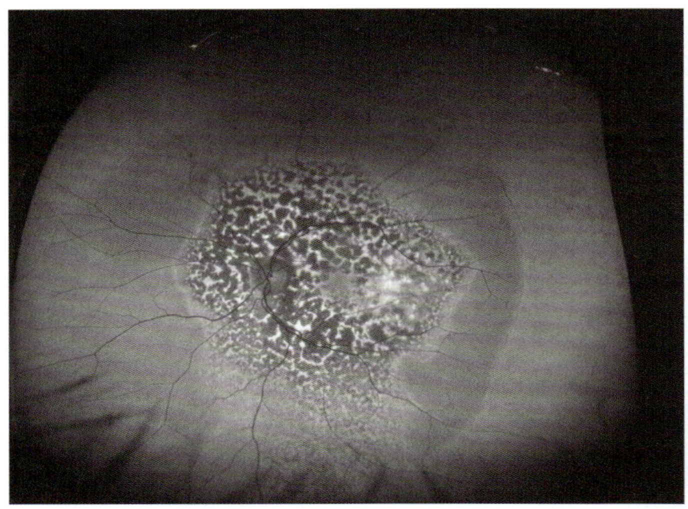

Fig. 4.29 Bilateral diffuse uveal melanocytic proliferation. Fundus autofluorescence image with a reticular pattern (often called a leopard-spot / giraffe pattern) of hyperautofluorescence {1442,1916,1720}, which is a key diagnostic finding.

Epidemiology

The exact incidence is unknown. Median age, depending on the study, ranges from 58 to 65 years, with an average of 64 years; the sex distribution is equal {505,2434,1737}.

Etiology

The precise mechanism has yet to be fully elucidated, but in the IgG fraction of the serum of patients with bilateral diffuse uveal melanocytic proliferation, a cultured melanocyte elongation and proliferation factor (CMEP factor) that stimulates melanocyte proliferation has been detected, which is thought to be released from the underlying extraocular primary malignancy {2203,1499}.

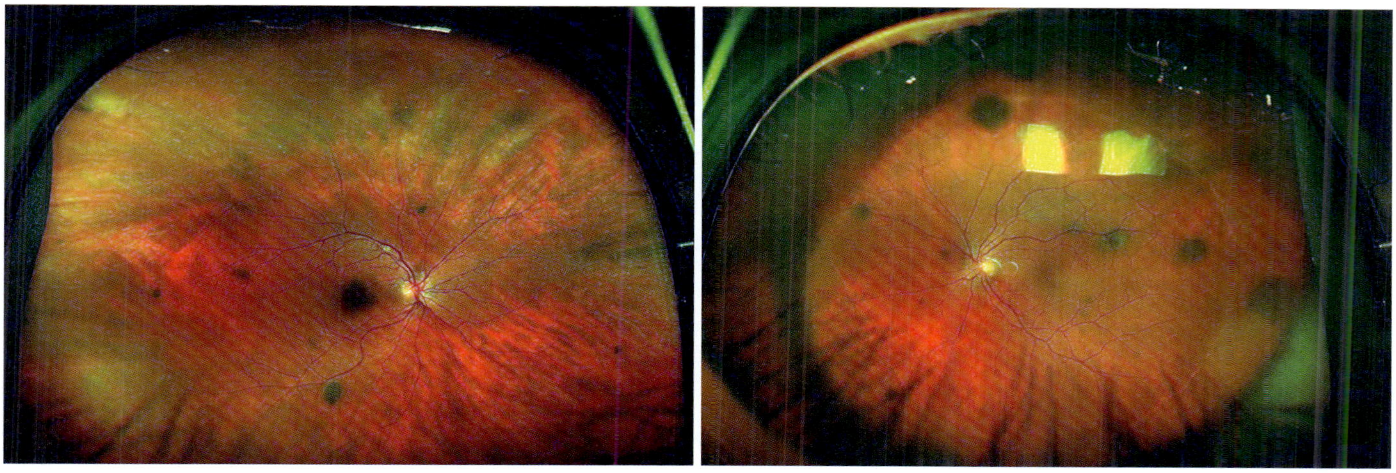

Fig. 4.30 Bilateral diffuse uveal melanocytic proliferation. Optomap false colour clinical images of both fundi that show multiple bilateral red-black spots at the level of the choroid.

Pathogenesis

Circulating CMEP factor, released from the extraocular primary malignancy, induces proliferation and elongation of melanocytes in vitro {2203,1499}. Recently, elevated HGF levels, produced by the extraocular malignancy, and autoantibodies to HGF have been proposed as a novel pathogenesis for bilateral diffuse uveal melanocytic proliferation {2384}. This is supported by the detection by immunohistochemistry of the HGF receptor, c-Met, on melanocytic cells of patients {2292}. Molecular genetics has shown gain of chromosomes 5, 6, and X {2303,2634}, loss of chromosome 19 {2303}, and polysomy 8q {2232}. The lack of consistent chromosomal findings supports a hyperplastic rather than a primary neoplastic process.

Macroscopic appearance

Macroscopic appearance shows diffuse thickening of the uveal tract, usually by a mostly amelanotic lesion coloured cream to tan that may be punctuated with pigmented islands. The thickening, which can be detected by B-scan ultrasonography and ultrasound biomicroscopy, can be panuveal or involve only parts of the uveal tract, but it almost always involves the choroid. An overlying retinal detachment and associated cataract (if the ciliary body is involved) are common, and pigment epithelial cysts of the ciliary body and iris may arise.

Histopathology

The uvea is thickened by a proliferation of melanocytic cells that spare the choriocapillaris. The cells are spindle shaped with elongated oval nuclei, inconspicuous nucleoli, and scant cytoplasmic melanin {262}. In some cases, discrete islands of atypical, pigmented, epithelioid melanocytic cells are observed that can resemble uveal melanoma and can exhibit necrosis {262,2312,2077,2292}. Mitotic activity is rare. In some patients, melanocytic cells can be seen within the scleral emissary channels.

The proliferating melanocytes stain positively for melan-A, HMB45, and SOX10 {2074,329}, do not overexpress p53 {2074}, and show a low proliferation rate with Ki-67 and cyclin D1 {2232, 2434,329}. They are PRAME-negative and retain nuclear BAP1 expression {2292}.

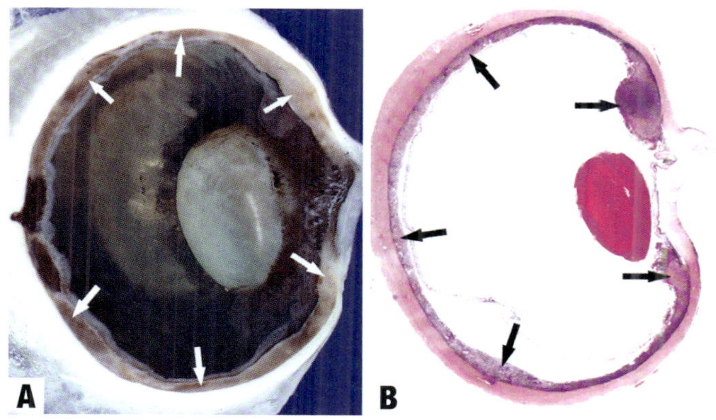

Fig. 4.31 Bilateral diffuse uveal melanocytic proliferation. **A** A macroscopic image shows involvement of the entire uveal tract (arrows) in an enucleated eye. Most of the lesion is lightly pigmented to amelanotic, but some pigmented areas are present posteriorly (left in the image). The other eye was similarly affected. **B** Low-power histology from the same macroscopic specimen shows the thickening of the entire uveal tract (arrows). Note the nodular thickening of the ciliary body anteriorly and the rather flatter thickening of the choroid posteriorly.

Differential diagnosis

This includes diffuse uveal melanoma that will demonstrate widespread cytologically atypical melanocytic cells with spindle, epithelioid, or mixed morphology, demonstrable nucleoli, and choriocapillaris effacement. Islands of tumour divided by extracellular matrix networks and loops, mitotic activity, and necrosis may be associated with the typical genetic findings in uveal melanoma.

Rare cases of histologically confirmed uveal melanoma arising in the setting of bilateral diffuse uveal melanocytic proliferation are reported {1737,2292}.

Cytology

Not relevant

Diagnostic molecular pathology

Molecular analysis can be helpful: *GNAQ*, *GNA11*, and *BRAF* p.V600E mutations and 3p loss have not been reported {2232, 2303}.

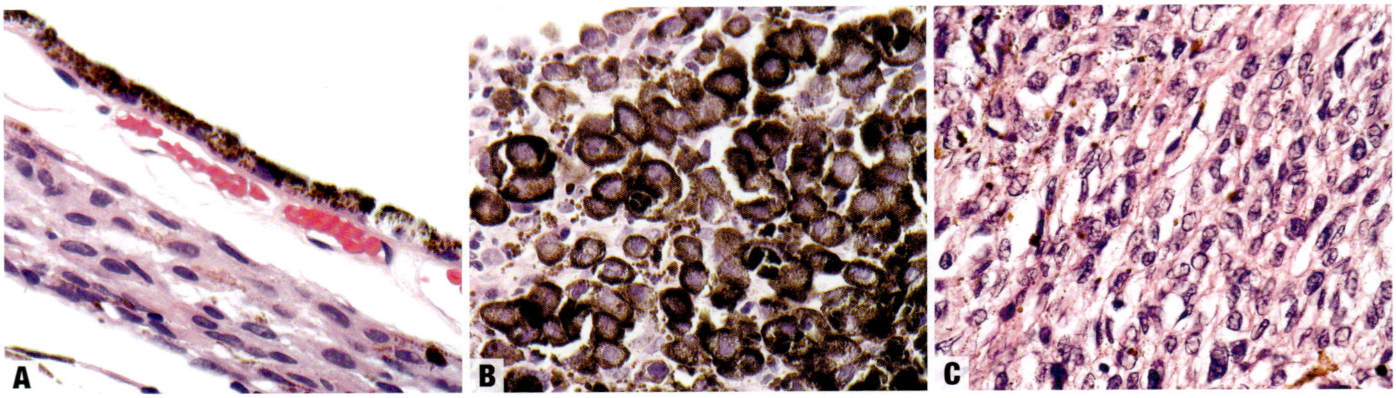

Fig. 4.32 Bilateral diffuse uveal melanocytic proliferation. **A** The choroid shows a syncytial arrangement of bland proliferating amelanotic spindle cells that spare the choriocapillaris. **B** A pigmented epithelioid-cell area of the lesion is seen. **C** The choroid shows abundant, very sparsely pigmented, spindle-shaped proliferating melanocytes.

Essential and desirable diagnostic criteria

Essential: bland, mostly spindle-shaped melanocytic cells diffusely in the uveal tract with sparing of the choriocapillaris with elongated oval nuclei, inconspicuous nucleoli, scant cytoplasmic melanin, and no mitotic activity, in the context of clinical evidence of bilateral uveal involvement and an underlying extraocular primary malignancy.

Desirable: positive immunohistochemistry with one melanocytic marker (melan-A, HMB45, SOX10).

Staging

Staging is not relevant (the initiating tumour should be staged).

Prognosis and prediction

The prognosis for life depends on the response of the extraocular primary tumour to therapy. The mean survival is 16 months, and nearly all patients die from dissemination of the primary malignancy {1737}. Until recently, the loss of vision from bilateral diffuse uveal melanocytic proliferation was considered to be progressive and irreversible, but stabilization of ocular symptoms with plasmapheresis was recently reported {1499}. Some later publications have shown (at least short-term) definite benefit from intravitreal steroids and nonspecific treatment {1089, 1442}.

Choroidal and ciliary body melanomas

Grossniklaus HE
Bastian BC
Beenakker JWM
Cassoux N
de Klein A
Folberg R
Kiilgaard JF
Verdijk RM
Weis E

Definition

Choroidal and ciliary body melanomas are primary malignant melanocytic tumours of the uvea.

ICD-O coding

8772/3 Spindle cell uveal melanoma, NOS
8773/3 Spindle cell uveal melanoma, type A
8774/3 Spindle cell uveal melanoma, type B
8770/3 Mixed epithelioid and spindle cell uveal melanoma
8771/3 Epithelioid cell uveal melanoma
8720/3 Retinoinvasive melanoma
8720/3 Ring melanoma
8720/3 Diffuse melanoma

ICD-11 coding

2D05.0 Melanoma of choroid
2D06.4 Melanoma of ciliary body

Related terminology

Acceptable: uveal melanoma.
Not recommended: intraocular melanoma; ocular melanoma.

Subtype(s)

Spindle cell uveal melanoma NOS; spindle cell uveal melanoma, type A; spindle cell uveal melanoma, type B; mixed epithelioid and spindle cell uveal melanoma; epithelioid cell uveal melanoma; retinoinvasive melanoma; ring melanoma; diffuse melanoma

Localization

Melanoma can arise anywhere in the choroid and ciliary body, and it can extend from one to the other, as well as to the iris, chamber angle, retina, vitreous, and optic nerve, and intrasclerally and extrasclerally {3498,3703}.

Clinical features

Approximately 25% of patients with a ciliary body or choroidal melanoma have no symptoms and are diagnosed during a routine eye examination {2990}. Symptoms include photopsia (perceived flashes of light), floaters, and loss of vision {1784}. Occasionally, large choroidal and ciliary body melanomas result in pain, redness of the eye, and secondary glaucoma {2990}. Multifocal uveal melanomas have been reported {804}. Bilateral primary uveal melanoma occurs rarely {1222,3222}.

Ciliary body melanomas are usually circumscribed and nodular. Diagnosis is often late because the tumour initially is hidden behind the iris and is not apparent on routine examination. They often encroach on and distort the crystalline lens, producing lens dislocation, astigmatism, and ipsilateral cataract. The tumour can also lead to focal shallowing of the anterior chamber. Some ciliary body melanomas grow through the iris root, simulating a primary iris melanoma. Anterior chamber seeding and iris heterochromia can develop in such cases. Mechanisms of secondary glaucoma include anterior displacement of the lens iris diaphragm, invasion of a large segment of the iridocorneal angle, tumour seeding, deposition of melanophages, and iris neovascularization. Ring melanomas usually involve > 180° of the ciliary body and show no or disproportionately less anteroposterior growth to the choroid. The aqueous outflow pathways can be obstructed by a ring melanoma and lead to anterior extraocular extension {1900,3185,3755}. Rare melanomalytic glaucoma develops when melanophages containing necrotic tumour debris obstruct the trabecular meshwork {450}. In contrast, some eyes become hypotonous when the tumour disrupts the ciliary epithelium, causing decreased production of aqueous humour. Hyphaema and vitreous haemorrhage occur rarely when the tumour disrupts blood vessels or undergoes necrosis. Ultrasonography, ultrasound biomicroscopy, anterior segment optical coherence tomography, and transillumination are helpful diagnostic techniques. External ocular signs that can suggest the diagnosis include dilated episcleral (sentinel) blood vessels overlying the tumour, and episcleral nodules from extrascleral extension through emissary canals in the anterior sclera.

Choroidal melanomas appear as a mass that is crescent dome shaped (in 75% of cases), mushroom shaped (in 20%), or diffuse (in 5%). They are pigmented in 55% of cases, non-pigmented in 15%, and of mixed colour in 30% {2935}. Their mean size is 11.3 mm (range: 2–24 mm) in basal diameter by 5.5 mm (0.8–17 mm) in thickness {2978}. The mass is deep to the retina, without feeder vessels, and often associated with an overlying exudative retinal detachment. Necrotic tumours cause painful uveitis, secondary glaucoma, or both. Extraocular extension may occur, anteriorly via aqueous outflow channels, equatorially via vortex veins, and posteriorly along emissary canals in the sclera around the optic disc. The tumour can also invade the optic nerve and its sheath or orbit, or both. Optic nerve invasion occurs in 5–6% of eyes {1957,1956} and especially frequently from retinoinvasive melanomas {1727}.

Imaging

The most common way to localize a choroidal melanoma is by direct visualization with ophthalmoscopy. The tumour should be documented using fundus photography and measured using A-scan and B-scan ultrasonography. The latter is also helpful in excluding extraocular extension {1369}. Optical coherence tomography is generally used to determine the effect of the tumour on the overlying and surrounding retina, and to evaluate subretinal fluid. Fundus autofluorescence imaging can reveal orange lipofuscin pigment overlying the tumour.

Multimodal imaging can be helpful in diagnosing small choroidal melanomas or distinguishing amelanotic melanomas from choroidal metastases. Optical coherence tomography can show subretinal fluid, subretinal lipofuscin pigment, and shaggy

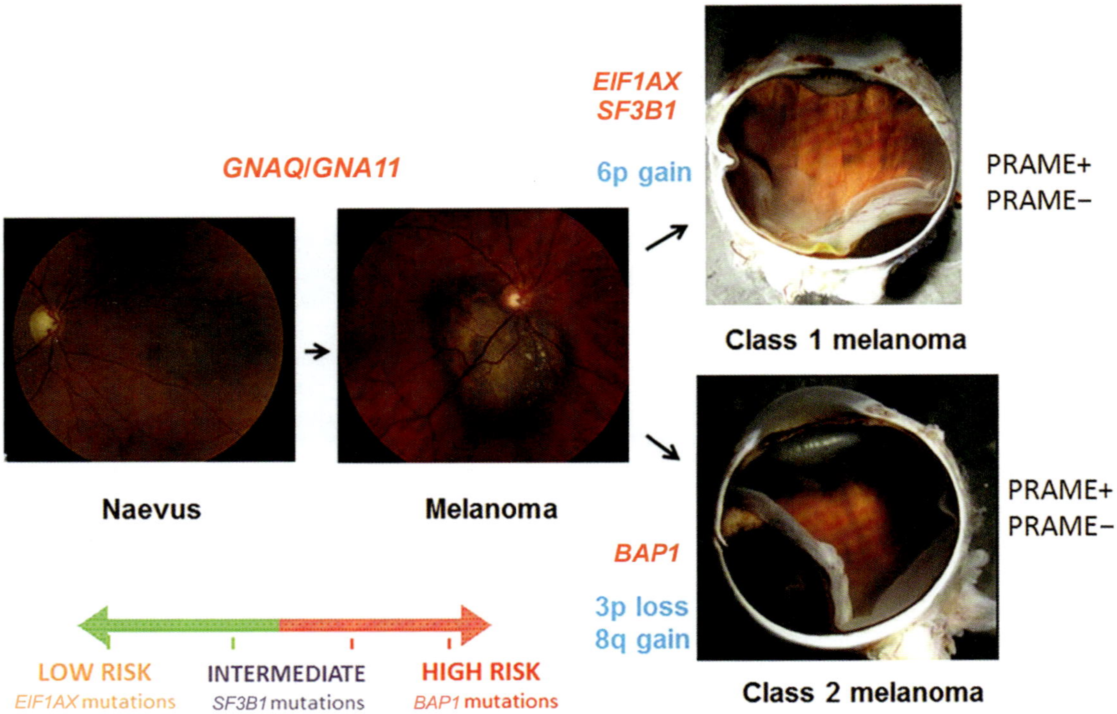

Fig. 4.33 Progression of choroidal naevus to melanoma. A *GNAQ* or *GNA11* mutation appears to occur early in the progression, present also in many uveal naevi. Once the tumour is a melanoma, it may acquire further mutations: mutations in *EIF1AX* or *SF3B1* (typically also 6p gain) result in class 1 melanoma with a low or intermediate risk, respectively, of metastasis, whereas mutations in *BAP1* (typically also 3p loss, 8q gain) result in class 2 melanomas with a high risk of metastasis. PRAME positivity corresponds to worse clinical outcomes for both gene expression profile class 1 and class 2 uveal melanomas {969,970}.

photoreceptors. Fluorescein angiography shows hyperfluorescent lesions with pinpoint leakage and intrinsic vasculature. Indocyanine green angiography may show a dual circulation.

On MRI the signal intensity on T1-weighted imaging correlates with pigmentation, and shows diffuse enhancement after contrast administration {956,1914}. The mean apparent diffusion coefficient is 1.16×10^{-3} mm^2/s and the tumour shows either a washout or plateau perfusion curve {956,3722}. MRI is helpful in diagnosing ciliary body involvement, extrascleral extension, and optic nerve invasion, but it is limited in its ability to identify scleral invasion {956}.

Epidemiology

The worldwide incidence of uveal melanoma is uncertain, but it is estimated to be about 7000 per year {1723}, accounting for 5% of all primary melanomas {865}. Choroidal and ciliary body melanomas are most common in fair-skinned populations (in which 65% of all cases are reported, although only 12% of the world population); they are rare in individuals of Asian and African ancestry {865,1384,3111}. Among Asian people, the risk of developing uveal melanoma is 1.2 times the risk among African-American people; among Hispanic and non-Hispanic White groups, the risk is 5 times and 19 times, respectively, the risk among African-American people {1383}. Worldwide, the incidence rate ranges between 2 and 8 cases per 1 million person-years, being lower at southern latitudes (1.3–2.9 cases per 1 million person-years) and increasing with latitude (to 6.1–8.6 cases per 1 million person-years) {3498,3703}. The age-adjusted incidence has been stable over a 25-year period {3101,3498}. The median age at diagnosis, which has increased

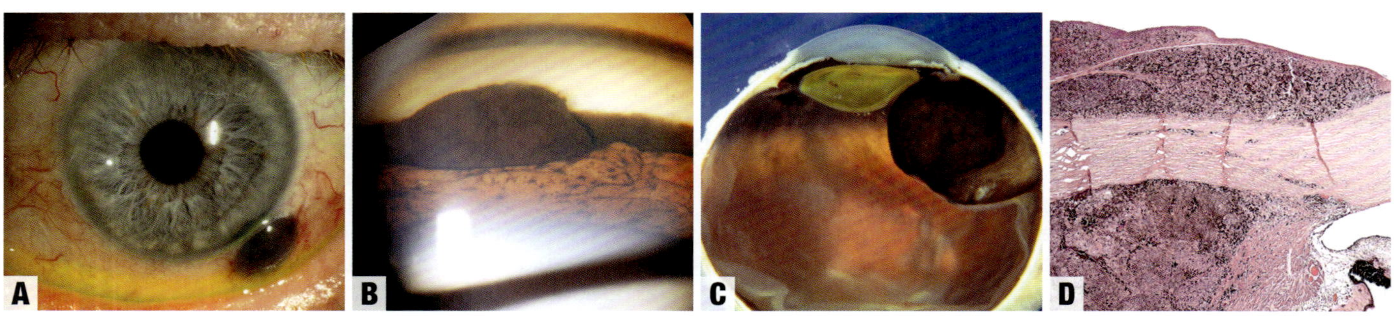

Fig. 4.34 Ciliary body melanoma. **A** Clinical appearance of an epibulbar subconjunctival extension of the underlying melanoma through an emissary channel. **B** A ciliary body melanoma invading the anterior chamber. Gonioscopic examination shows a pigmented melanoma invading the anterior chamber angle: a band of tumour also blankets the adjacent trabecular meshwork. **C** Lens moulding: in this instance, a ciliochoroidal melanoma distorts and dislocates the crystalline lens. **D** The tumour is seen within the trabecular meshwork and intrascleral collector channels, deep to its anterior extrascleral extension.

because of rising life expectancy, is currently 60–64 years in fair-skinned populations and 45 years among Asian people {347,788,1810,3322}. These melanomas are rare before the age of 20 years, accounting for 0.4–0.8% of cases, and are still relatively rare before the age of 45 years {89,3108,1802}. They show no sex predilection {718} and are more common among lightly than darkly pigmented individuals {865,1385,2075,3110}.

Etiology

Most choroidal and ciliary body melanomas appear to develop de novo. Others develop from melanocytes in uveal naevi including melanocytomas {908,1725,3104} or in congenital ocular or oculodermal melanocytosis (naevus of Ota), all with a lifetime risk of about 1 in 400 {3102}. Dysplastic naevus syndrome {3101} and *BAP1* tumour predisposition syndrome {479,3102, 3603} are associated with a higher risk of uveal melanoma. Other risk factors include light skin pigmentation, self-described inability to tan, and light-coloured irises {3573}. In addition, an association with a high number of common cutaneous naevi, atypical cutaneous naevi, cutaneous freckles, and iris naevi has been demonstrated {3574}. The role of ultraviolet (UV) radiation exposure in the development of choroidal and ciliary body melanoma is uncertain. Because of the rarity of the disease, quantitative meta-analytic reviews have provided the majority of information. A statistically significant association with arc welding (odds ratio: 2.05, 95% CI: 1.20–3.51) {2932} and sunlamp use (odds ratio: 2.15, 95% CI: 1.27–3.64) was demonstrated in one series {3571}, but other forms of intermittent and chronic UV radiation exposure were not found to be associated {2932}.

Pathogenesis

Melanoma at this anatomical site is thought to arise from uveal melanocytes through well-defined driver mutations. Most cases develop de novo, but uveal naevi including melanocytomas can also transform into melanoma {908,1725,3104}.

Choroidal and ciliary body melanomas (and many naevi) have mutations in the $G_q\alpha$ signalling pathway, affecting the highly homologous $G\alpha$ subunits $G_q\alpha$ and $G_{11}\alpha$ encoded by the genes *GNAQ* and *GNA11* in > 90% of cases, with the remaining tumours having mutations in the $G_q\alpha$-coupled receptor CYSLTR2 or the downstream effector of $G_q\alpha$ and $G_{11}\alpha$, phospholipase Cβ4 (encoded by *PLCB4*) {751,3448,1525}. Pathogenic *GNAQ* and *GNA11* variants affect codons Q209 and, less commonly, R183, and lead to constitutive activation and relay signals via PKC and the GTP-exchange factor RASGRP3, which is highly overexpressed in uveal melanoma, to the MAPK pathway {567}. The mutations in the $G_q\alpha$ pathway arise early during tumour progression and, in the absence of the additional mutations discussed below, also are found in benign neoplasms such as choroidal naevi, blue naevi, and naevi of Ota.

Transformation to uveal melanoma is caused by additional genetic alterations in one of three genes. Biallelic inactivation of the ubiquitin carboxy-terminal hydrolase *BAP1* at chromosome 3p21, typically by a combination of an inactivating mutation and monosomy 3, is associated with the worst prognosis {3147}. Hotspot mutations in the splice factor *SF3B1*, typically at codon 625 {1251}, result in mis-splicing of genes including *BRD9*, a member of the non-canonical BAF complex involved in epigenetic regulation {1422}. The third gene, *EIF1AX*, located at Xp22.1, encodes a translation initiation factor {2091}, and

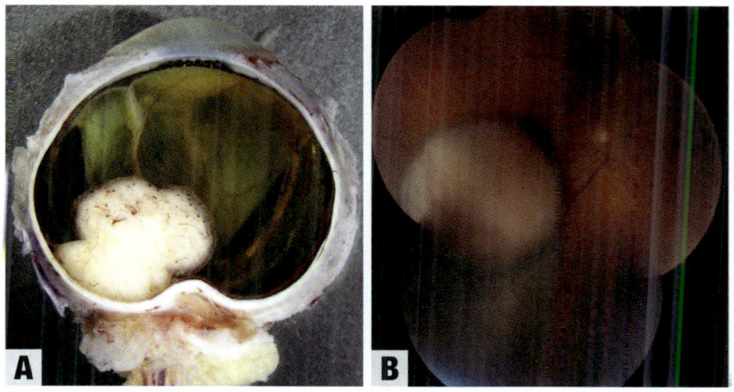

Fig. 4.35 Choroidal melanoma. **A** An amelanotic choroidal melanoma has broken through the Bruch membrane and thus assumed a mushroom (collar-button) shape. Congested vascular channels are visible in the portion of the tumour internal to the Bruch membrane, and a serous retinal detachment is present around the tumour. **B** Fundus photograph showing a mushroom-shaped choroidal tumour.

mutations cluster near the 5′ part of the gene. Less frequently mutated genes of relevance include *TP53* and *RFL5*, encoding an inhibitor of MDM2, which degrades p53 {1526}. Only *BAP1* mutations have been described to occur also in the germ line; the others are always somatic. Metastases often show additional pathogenic mutations involving the PI3K/AKT pathway, inactivation of *CDKN2A*, and activation of PRC2 {2936}.

Loss of chromosome 3 (complete or partial monosomy 3 or isodisomy 3), in particular when associated with polysomy 8q, is associated with metastasis in choroidal melanoma {3447}. *BAP1*, a gene located on chromosome 3 (at 3p21.1), carries inactivating mutations in about 80% of uveal melanomas with metastases {1250}. Somatic or germline *BAP1* loss-of-function mutations are observed in 30–50% of choroidal and ciliary body melanomas. BAP1 appears to be involved with chromatin remodelling {2874} and cell-cycle control {881}. BAP1-deficient cells exhibit stem cell–like qualities {2110}. BAP1 also appears to be involved in transendothelial migration and extravasation of cells to the systemic circulation {2438}. Loss of BAP1 is associated with an increased numbers of tumour-infiltrating macrophages, which are mainly of the proangiogenic M2 type, and

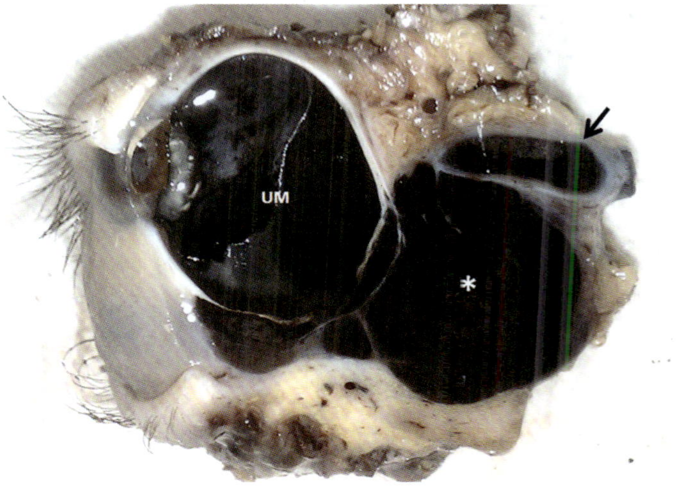

Fig. 4.36 Ciliochoroidal melanoma. An exenteration specimen contains a heavily pigmented choroidal melanoma that fills the eye (UM), invades the optic nerve (arrow), and extends beyond the sclera into the orbit where it forms a large nodule (asterisk)

Chapter 4

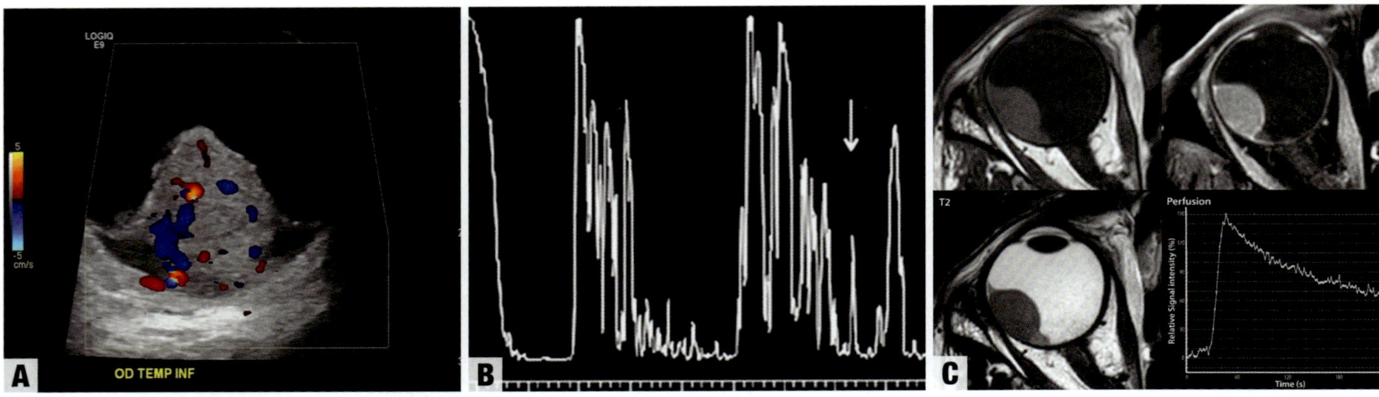

Fig. 4.37 Choroidal melanoma. **A** Ultrasound echography and Doppler showing an intense circulation of blood in intratumoural neovessels suggestive of a uveal melanoma. **B** A-scan ultrasound showing low internal reflectivity in a choroid mass. **C** The typical presentation of a choroidal melanoma on MRI is shown. The mass appears isointense to the choroid on T1-weighted images and enhances after contrast administration. On T2-weighted images it is slightly hyperintense compared with the extraocular muscles. Posterior and anterior to the mass, small retinal detachments can be seen, which do not enhance on T1-weighted images with contrast and are slightly hypointense compared with the melanoma on T2-weighted images. On perfusion-weighted imaging, the choroidal melanoma shows a typical washout curve.

a higher microvascular density {1018,2040,418,423}. Once the neoplastic cells have entered the systemic circulation, a variety of factors, including receptor/ligand gradients (e.g. between c-Met and its ligand HGF) {235,789,790,1313} and the stoichiometric properties of the liver {1179,1185}, appear to be involved in the propensity of uveal melanoma to metastasize to the liver {2661}.

Mutations of codon 625 of *SF3B1* on chromosome 2 are found in 10–23% of uveal melanomas {1251,3147}. SF3B1 is a splice factor involved in intron excision from pre-mRNA, and it may also be associated with chromatin remodelling {1251}. *BAP1*, *SF3B1*, and *EIF1AX* pathogenic sequence variants appear to be mutually exclusive in the vast majority of uveal melanomas {751}.

Gene expression profiling has identified a set of differentially expressed genes in class 1A and 1B (low and intermediate metastatic risk, respectively) versus class 2 (high metastatic risk) uveal melanomas {2439}. Class 1 melanomas retain a differentiated melanocytic phenotype and transcriptome, whereas class 2 melanomas have a dedifferentiated, cancer stem cell–like phenotype and transcriptome {524}. *SF3B1* and *EIF1AX* mutations appear to be associated with a class 1 gene expression profile, while the hemizygous *BAP1* mutation, when combined with monosomy 3, is associated with a class 2 gene expression profile {969}.

A recent study by The Cancer Genome Atlas (TCGA) categorized 80 uveal melanomas into four subsets: two associated with poor prognosis and monosomy 3 and two with better prognosis and disomy 3 {2726}. These four different types (A–D) are characterized by distinct global DNA methylation patterns and distinct genomic, signalling, and immune profiles, which are associated with prognosis {1449,2971}. Types A and B correspond to class 1, and types C and D to class 2 gene expression profile.

In the liver, the melanoma forms relatively dormant micrometastases that have the potential to grow into clinical metastases {1179,1185}. These metastases may form nodules (the nodular pattern), infiltrate the hepatic parenchyma (the infiltrative pattern) {1185}, or both. A variety of factors may contribute to the growth of micrometastases into clinical metastases, including likely abrogation of the host immune response (in particular, NK-cell function) {805,2800} and an increased local VEGF:PEDF ratio {1866}.

Macroscopic appearance

Macroscopically, ciliary body melanomas are either dome-shaped or circumferential ring-shaped tumours of variable colour, ranging from amelanotic to dark brown and variegated. Choroidal melanomas may exhibit a flat to domed shape when confined by the Bruch membrane, or they may exhibit a characteristic collar-button or mushroom-like shape when they break through the Bruch membrane; the portion of the tumour that has broken through is choked off by the membrane, resulting in vascular congestion.

Histopathology

Microscopic examination is necessary to assess for invasion of ocular structures (e.g. the iridocorneal angle, iris, sclera, retina, and optic nerve) as well as for extrascleral extension.

Choroidal and ciliary body melanomas produce variable amounts of melanin pigment and thus appear as amelanotic to mildly, moderately, or heavily pigmented tumours; part of the pigment often resides in tumour-infiltrating melanophages. Their cytological description was traditionally based on the Callender system, which in its abbreviated form includes four morphological subtypes: spindle A (naevus-like) cell, spindle B cell, epithelioid-cell, and mixed-cell (spindle B and epithelioid) melanomas {2145}. Spindle A cells are fusiform and cohesive, and they have poorly defined cell borders. Their spindle-shaped nucleus contains a central nuclear envelope fold (or groove). Spindle B cells are larger, fusiform, and cohesive, and they contain spindle- or cigar-shaped nuclei and prominent nucleoli; this is the most frequent cell type in most tumours. Epithelioid cells are noncohesive and contain large, round nuclei and abundant, prominently eosinophilic cytoplasm; this cell type is associated with a high risk of metastasis. Small epithelioid cells are intermediate between spindle B and epithelioid melanoma cells. The tumour may undergo spontaneous necrosis of variable degree. Those that exhibit 90–100% necrosis are composed of so-called ghost cells; this phenomenon is probably due to a sequence of events that starts with vascular insufficiency within the tumour, followed by cytokine release, tumour necrosis, and secondary glaucoma

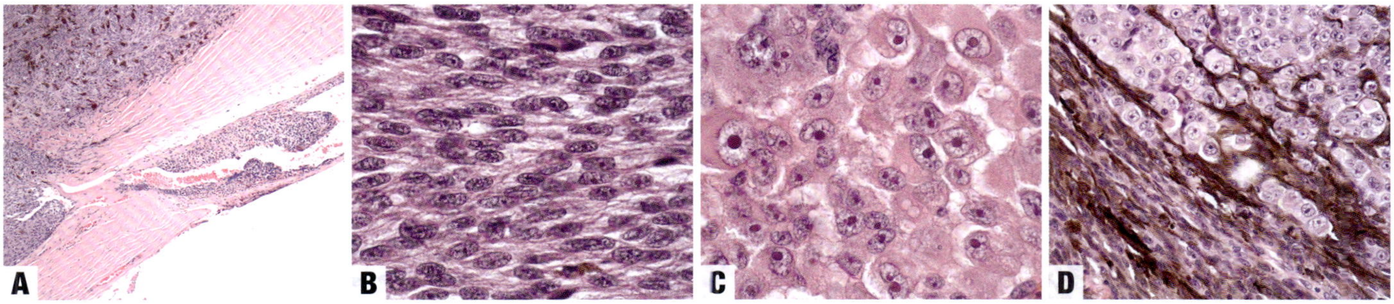

Fig. 4.38 Choroidal melanoma. **A** Tumour extension through an equatorial vortex vein within the sclera. **B** Spindle-cell type. Spindle B cells have prominent nucleoli and form a syncytium. **C** Epithelioid-cell type. Epithelioid cells have distinct cytoplasmic margins and large round or oval nuclei with prominent reddish-purple nucleoli and peripheral margination of chromatin. **D** Mixed cell type. This mixed-cell melanoma comprises clones of pigmented spindle cells (lower left) and amelanotic epithelioid cells (upper right).

{3318}. Balloon cells are sometimes seen {1668}. They have foamy, vacuolated cytoplasm because of faulty production of melanin or degradation of melanosomes, and their cytoplasm contains lipid. Balloon cells are often seen after plaque brachytherapy or proton beam irradiation {2849}. Both dendritic- and scavenger-type tumour-infiltrating macrophages are ubiquitous in uveal melanomas, and they can constitute a substantial portion of the tumour mass {2042}.

Although the cut-off points are arbitrary, spindle cell melanoma is defined as being composed of spindle B cells in ≥ 90% of the tumour, and epithelioid-cell melanoma is defined as being composed of epithelioid cells in ≥ 90% of the tumour; all other tumours are mixed-cell melanomas (the most common type in most series). Epithelioid-cell melanomas are associated with the worst prognosis, and spindle cell melanomas are associated with the best prognosis {2147}.

Other patterns include clear cell melanoma {1180}: the tumour cells have oval, centrally located nuclei and clear cytoplasm because of the dissolution of glycogen granules during fixation. Clear cell melanomas must be distinguished from renal cell carcinoma metastatic to the uvea. Cavitary melanoma is another uncommon pattern which develops cyst-like spaces that may be clinically detected on ultrasonography {281,2895}.

A number of specific subtypes of choroidal and ciliary body melanomas may need to be considered.

Diffuse uveal melanoma is defined as being < 5 mm in thickness and occupying at least one quarter of the uveal tract {535}. This growth pattern may be associated with a high risk of extraocular growth and metastasis, probably related to its large basal dimension {3013}.

Retinoinvasive uveal melanoma tends to evolve from a noncohesive melanoma of the iris or ciliary body, then invades the vitreous, the retina, and through these tissues, sometimes, into the optic nerve {1727,1149}. These tumours express neurotrophin receptors, which may account for the tropism towards the retina {2210}. Other mechanisms of optic nerve invasion include via the adjacent retina after retinal invasion, directly from the peripapillary choroid, and a combination of these mechanisms.

Ring melanoma is another subtype of ciliary body melanoma in which the tumour grows circumferentially up to 360° in the ciliary body typically without significant extension to the choroid {775}. A rare form of ring melanoma, anterior chamber angle melanoma, leads to secondary glaucoma with minimal involvement of the uveal tract {774,3185}.

Immunohistochemistry

Choroidal melanomas are typically positive for immunostaining for HMB45, S100, melan-A, MITF, TYR, and SOX10 {3439,2749,951,2288,2442}. It is advisable to use at least two antibodies, such as those against HMB45 and S100, in case one is negative. Ki-67, a nuclear proliferation marker, may be used to assess proliferative activity. The Ki-67 index has been found to have some prognostic relevance {1613,2262}. Mitotic activity should be reported as the number of mitoses/mm^2 {691}. Mitoses can alternatively be assessed using phosphohistone H3 immunohistochemistry {158}.

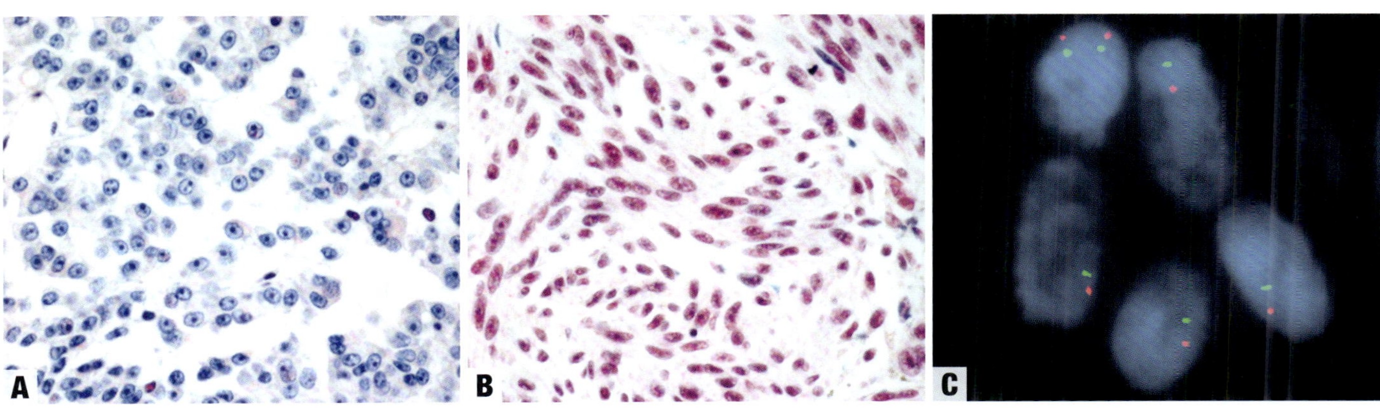

Fig. 4.39 Choroidal melanoma. **A** BAP1 loss. Immunohistochemistry for BAP1 shows no expression in the nuclei. **B** Immunohistochemistry for BAP1 labels the nuclei in this BAP1-preserved case. **C** FISH of an FNAB shows nuclei with monosomy 3, with only single copies of red and green probes (the normal finding is two copies of each); the FISH probe included D3Z1 (centromere CEN3; red) and BCL6 (3q27; green).

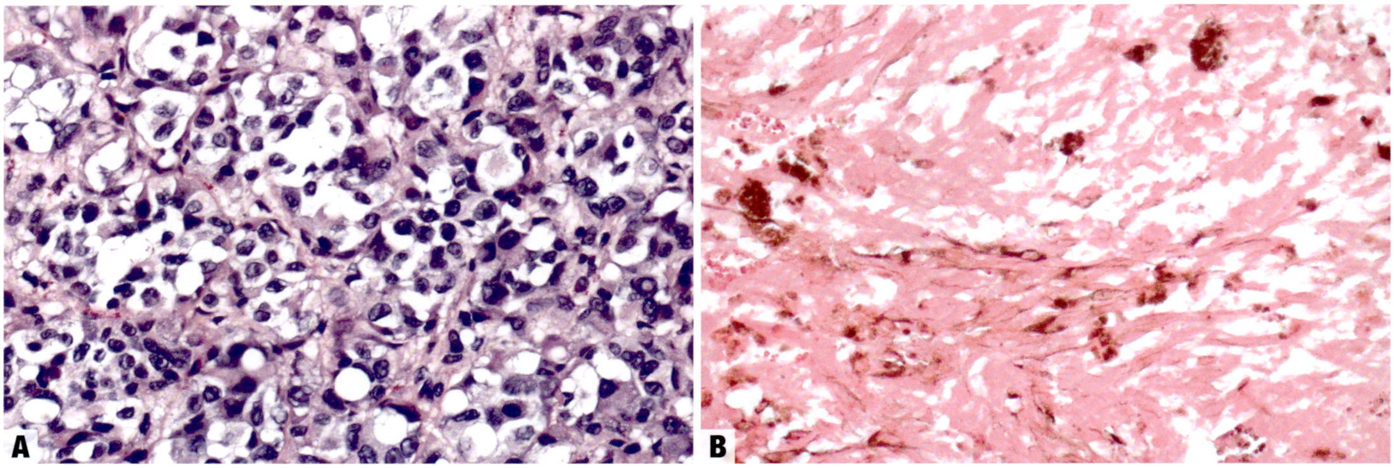

Fig. 4.40 Choroidal melanoma. **A** The image shows the effect of irradiation. This melanoma has undergone treatment-induced changes, with vacuolation of melanoma cells, after plaque radiotherapy. **B** Necrosis of melanoma tissue may occur spontaneously and can be difficult to diagnose (particularly in cases without substantial pigmentation).

A number of additional prognostic features of choroidal and ciliary body melanomas may be considered for reporting to the clinician. Especially, a lack of nuclear immunostaining for the BAP1 protein is strongly associated with a high risk of metastasis {1583,1771,3436}. Several extravascular matrix patterns have been identified, listed from least to most complex: normal, silent, straight, parallel, parallel with crosslinking, arcs, arcs with branching, closed vascular loops, and vascular networks – the last three patterns are associated with a higher risk of metastasis {995,2041}. It has been proposed that the extravascular matrix patterns constitute vasculogenic mimicry {992,1017}. Large tumour cell nucleoli {90,2146} and a high microvascular density also are associated with shorter survival {566,1018, 2040}. Prominent tumour-infiltrating lymphocytes and macrophages are associated with an increased likelihood of metastasis, and they may reflect the presence of high-risk chromosomal abnormalities, in particular monosomy 3 or loss of expression of the BAP1 protein {2017,418,419,1104,2042}.

Cytology

Transvitreal or transscleral FNAB may be performed to detect ciliary body or choroidal melanoma, although it is more commonly undertaken for genetic prognostication purposes {159, 1410,1450,4}. The cytological specimen may contain cells with spindle-shaped cytoplasm or round cells with variable amounts of cytoplasm. Intracytoplasmic melanin pigment granules are often present. Nuclear atypia with margination of chromatin and prominent nucleoli may be present. FNAB can be used to obtain cells for molecular testing {2913,1240}.

Diagnostic molecular pathology

Detection of mutations in the $G_q\alpha$ signalling pathway, affecting *GNAQ* and *GNA11*, can be helpful to distinguish uveal melanoma metastases from other melanomas {2689}. Demonstration of the loss of chromosome 3 or *BAP1*, a gene located on chromosome 3, which has inactivating mutations in about 80% of uveal melanomas with metastases {1250}, can be helpful to assess prognosis.

Gene expression profiling has identified a set of differentially expressed genes in class 1A and 1B (low and intermediate metastatic risk, respectively) versus class 2 (high metastatic risk) uveal melanomas {2439} and can also be used to assess prognosis. The level of PRAME mRNA is an independent prognostic biomarker in uveal melanoma, which identifies increased metastatic risk in patients with class 1 or disomy 3 tumours {969}.

Essential and desirable diagnostic criteria

Essential: melanocytic tumour in the ciliary body or choroid; histological or cytological demonstration of spindle-shaped or epithelioid cells, or both, with round to oval nuclei and prominent nucleoli.

Desirable: if amelanotic, it is desirable to obtain an immunohistochemical confirmation using melanocytic markers; analysis of driver genes may be necessary to distinguish choroidal and ciliary body melanoma from cutaneous and mucous membrane melanoma metastatic to these sites.

Staging

Uveal melanomas are staged according to the Union for International Cancer Control (UICC) / American Joint Committee on Cancer (AJCC) TNM classification, eighth edition, which has a separate staging for ciliary body and choroidal melanomas as distinct from iris melanomas.

According to the UICC/AJCC TNM classification system {1722}, choroidal and ciliary body melanomas are grouped by size as small (T1), medium (T2), large (T3), or very large (T4); and subgrouped by ciliary body involvement and extrascleral growth as choroid only (a), ciliary body involved (b), choroid and extrascleral < 5 mm (c), or ciliary body involved and extrascleral ≤ 5 mm (d), and extrascleral > 5 mm (e). They are staged (stages I–IV) according to size, ciliary body involvement, extraocular extension, and presence of metastasis {1801}.

Staging systems also exist for newly diagnosed metastatic uveal melanoma {1731,3433,2081,2661}.

Prognosis and prediction

Tumour size, ciliary body involvement, and extraocular extension of the melanoma are of independent prognostic significance (see *Staging*, above). The risk of metastasis increases with increasing tumour size, and from invasion of the ciliary body through extraocular invasion to invasion of both compartments {1801,60}.

As many as 50% of patients with a ciliary body or choroidal melanoma ultimately die from haematogenous metastasis, most commonly (in 90% of cases) to the liver {649,1802,2661}. The prognosis for survival is worse for patients with melanomas of the ciliary body and anterior choroid {1936}, and with larger tumours. Other common (often secondary) sites of metastasis are lung (affected in 24% of cases) and bone (in 16%) {649}. The median survival after detection of metastasis is 10–12 months, and the survival rate decreases from 52% at one year to 25% at 2 years, and 13% at 3 years {2660,1675}. In the past, when the liver was not imaged during surveillance, the reported median survival rates for patients with metastases were 15–20% at 6 months and 10% at 1 year {649}; in a recent study in which most patients underwent regular liver imaging, the reported rates were 75% at 6 months and 50% at 1 year {1731}. Liver function tests and imaging, including MRI, CT, PET-CT, and ultrasound, can be used to detect and stage liver metastases {2661}. Older age is a risk factor for shorter survival in patients with uveal melanoma {449}. Patients with metastasis confined to extrahepatic sites may have longer survival times than patients with hepatic metastases {649}.

The reported 5-year survival rates are 88% for the spindle-cell type and 60% for the epithelioid or mixed-cell type overall {649}, but melanomas that have monosomy 3, are of gene expression profile class 2, or show loss of nuclear BAP1 expression are associated with 5-year survival rates of only about 30% {3440}. Some disomy 3 melanomas, in particular *SF3B1*-mutated uveal melanomas, also metastasize, leading to a bimodal metastatic profile with late-onset metastatic disease {3253,3688}. Gain of chromosome 8q is a risk factor for the development of metastases {898}: uveal melanomas with normal copy numbers of 8q are associated with a 5-year survival rate of 83%, while with 8q gain and a normal chromosome 3 status the rate is 67%; addition of more copies of 8q is associated with worse survival {3488}. Additional adverse prognostic factors include larger tumour size {669,809,1801,3536}, extravascular matrix loops and networks {1579,2785}, high microvascular density {566,1018,2040}, high numbers of tumour-infiltrating macrophages {418,419,1104,2042}, and large tumour cell nucleoli {90,2146}. Many of these prognostic factors are associated with the presence of monosomy 3 or loss of BAP1 expression {419,2727}.

Combining genetic information with tumour size results in a more precise prognostication than either parameter alone {3536,227,809,1088}. This is being used in the Liverpool Uveal Melanoma Prognosticator Online (LUMPO) to calculate an individual's risk of metastases {716,1450}. While blue eyes are associated with an increased risk of developing ciliary body or choroidal melanoma, chromosome 3 and 8q aberrations have a greater impact on survival in patients with a light iris versus a dark iris colour {1375,3601}.

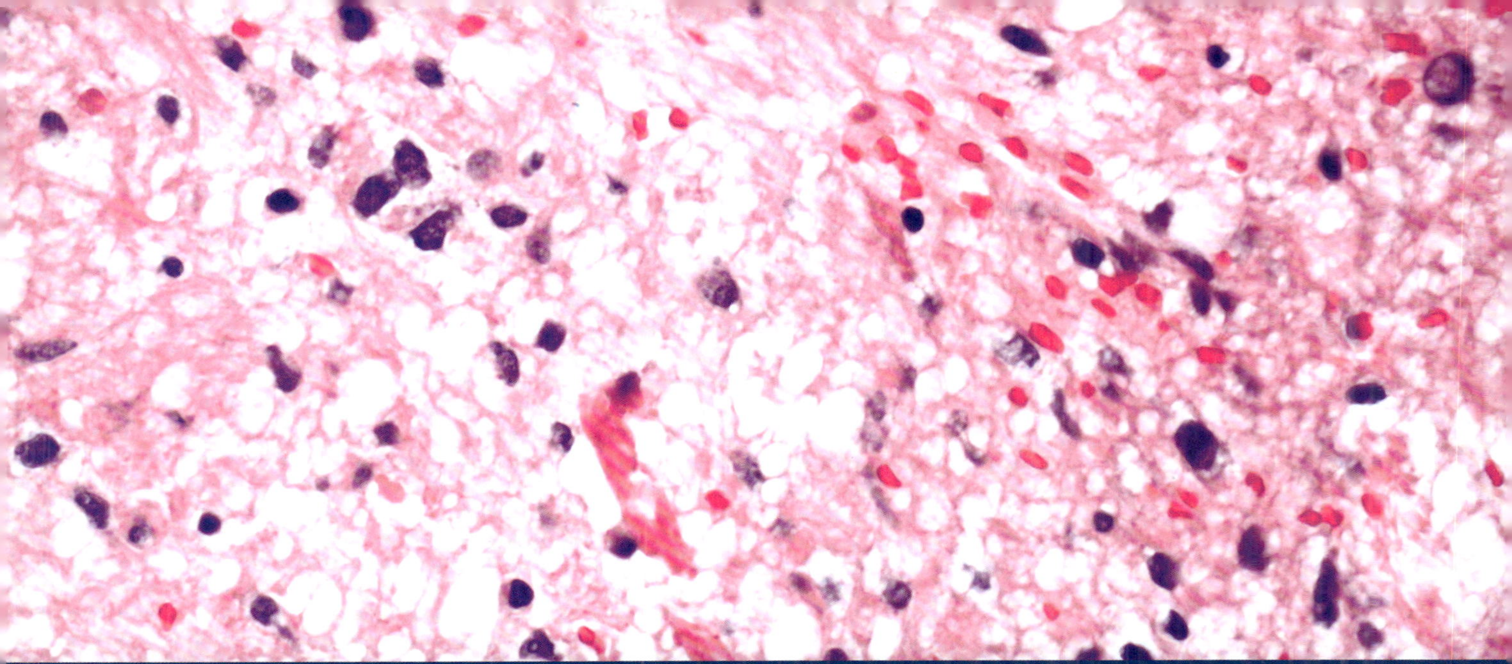

5

Tumours of the retina and neuroepithelium

Edited by: Grossniklaus HE, Heegaard S, Hodge JC, Kivelä T, Vemuganti GK

Tumours of the retina and neuroepithelium: Introduction

Vemuganti GK
Heegaard S
Hodge JC
Kivelä T

The neurosensory retina is a complex neural network consisting of neurons (rod and cone photoreceptors, horizontal cells, bipolar cells, amacrine cells, ganglion cells) and supporting Müller radial glial cells and perivascular astrocytes and their processes organized into nine layers. It is supported by an underlying monolayer of hexagonal retinal pigment epithelial (RPE) cells, and extends to the optic nerve posteriorly and to the non-pigmented inner ciliary epithelium anteriorly. The RPE extends posteriorly around the optic disc and anteriorly to the pigmented outer ciliary epithelium. Embryologically the retina, RPE, and epithelia of the iris and ciliary body derive from the inner (neurosensory retina) and outer layers of the optic cup.

As neuronal, non-proliferating tissues, the neurosensory retina and RPE are not prone to producing tumours, although retinocytoma, retinoblastoma, medulloepithelioma, and adenomas and adenocarcinomas of the RPE and the epithelia of the iris and ciliary body can occur.

In the fourth edition, tumours and tumour-like lesions of the retina and neuroepithelium were categorized together as per anatomical location. In this edition, under the neurosensory retina, RPE, and the iris and ciliary body neuroepithelia, the lesions are further classified to distinguish the clearly identified neoplasms from tumour-like lesions and congenital hamartomas. With emerging evidence of genetics, retinocytoma is classified under premalignant conditions {1064, 2838,801}. A clear distinction is made between reactive and hamartomatous lesions and tumours of the RPE. The tumours of the neuroepithelium are classified as reactive and cystic lesions, or tumours such as adenoma, adenocarcinoma, and medulloepithelioma.

Retinoblastoma is the most common malignant intraocular tumour of childhood with a global incidence of 1 case per 16 000–18 000 live births {1724}, now believed to have increased to 1 case per 13 880 live births because of increasing familial cases {3183}. Rarely, *RB1* sequence variants can result in a stable retinocytoma, although most retinocytomas degenerate into retinoblastoma {801,856}. Exceptional retinoblastomas result from high-level *MYCN* oncogene amplification {2792}. Well-established protocols for genetic testing exist, including prenatal screening and consideration of early delivery {3136,3159}. Newer tools such as liquid biopsies of tumour-derived cell-free DNA from blood and intraocular fluids have emerging utility in prognostication and prenatal testing {1098}.

The retinal glial tumours include astrocytomas, both syndromic (in tuberous sclerosis and, rarely, neurofibromatosis type 1) and non-syndromic forms.

The non-neoplastic RPE lesions include congenital hypertrophy, and simple and combined hamartomas, the latter of which are basically vitreoretinal in nature. Congenital RPE lesions are associated with syndromes like familial adenomatous polyposis {2404,374}, Gardner syndrome, and neurofibromatosis type 2 {206}. The neoplastic tumours of RPE are extremely rare and include RPE adenoma and adenocarcinoma.

This section also covers cysts of the pigmented epithelium of the iris and ciliary body, and medulloepithelioma {1577}, which is a rare congenital tumour of the ciliary body or optic nerve that may be associated with *DICER1* mutations. Initially thought to resemble medulloepithelioma of the brain, later the molecular diversity at the cytogenetic and epigenetic levels enabled the identification of ocular medulloepithelioma as a distinct nosological entity {863}.

Astrocytic tumours

Mendoza P
Chhablani J
Van Ginderdeuren R

Definition

Astrocytic tumours of the retina are low-grade astrocytic neoplasms arising in the inner retina. This category of tumours includes retinal astrocytic hamartoma (RAH) (congenital; typically syndromic and associated most often with tuberous sclerosis and less commonly with neurofibromatosis type 1) and acquired retinal astrocytoma (non-syndromic).

ICD-O coding

9384/1 Giant cell astrocytoma of the retina
9384/1 Retinal astrocytic hamartoma

ICD-11 coding

2F36.Y & XH6PH6 Other specified benign neoplasm of eye or ocular adnexa & Astrocytoma, NOS
2F36.Y & XH1L48 Other specified benign neoplasm of eye or ocular adnexa & Subependymal giant cell astrocytoma

Related terminology

Acceptable: astrocytic hamartoma of the retina; acquired retinal astrocytoma.
Not recommended: intraocular glioma; retinal phakoma.

Subtype(s)

Giant cell astrocytoma of the retina

Localization

Retinal astrocytomas are generally discrete, slightly elevated lesions in the inner retina that expand the nerve fibre layer. They are found most commonly in the posterior pole within the vascular arcades, adjacent to the optic nerve, or (less frequently) in the retinal periphery {196}.

Clinical features

Astrocytic tumours of the retina are usually asymptomatic and are detected incidentally or on screening of patients with suspected phakomatoses. They are discrete, slightly elevated lesions arising in the inner retina. Most tumours grow by direct extension but vitreous seeding has also been reported {645}. Macular tumours or those complicated by haemorrhage {1168}, proliferative retinopathy, or exudation {1114} may cause visual disturbance. RAH is thought to be congenital but may not be clinically apparent until later in life. It has been reported to occur in 36–44% of patients with tuberous sclerosis; the tumours were bilateral in 34–43% of patients and multiple in 40% of patients {196,2777}.

A study of RAH by optical coherence tomography identified a gradual transition between normal retina and the optically hyperreflective mass with associated retinal disorganization (optically empty, so-called moth-eaten spaces) and posterior shadowing as characteristic features {3007}. Presumed retinal pericapillary astrocytic hamartoma has been described as a form of RAH with a glistening granular appearance on fundoscopy and perivascular hyperreflectivity on optical coherence tomography {1880}. Clinically, retinal astrocytomas may mimic retinoblastoma in children, and amelanotic melanoma, haemangioblastoma, and metastatic carcinoma in adults, particularly in patients lacking other syndromic manifestations. The clinical differential diagnosis also includes presumed solitary circumscribed retinal astrocytic proliferation {3027,200}.

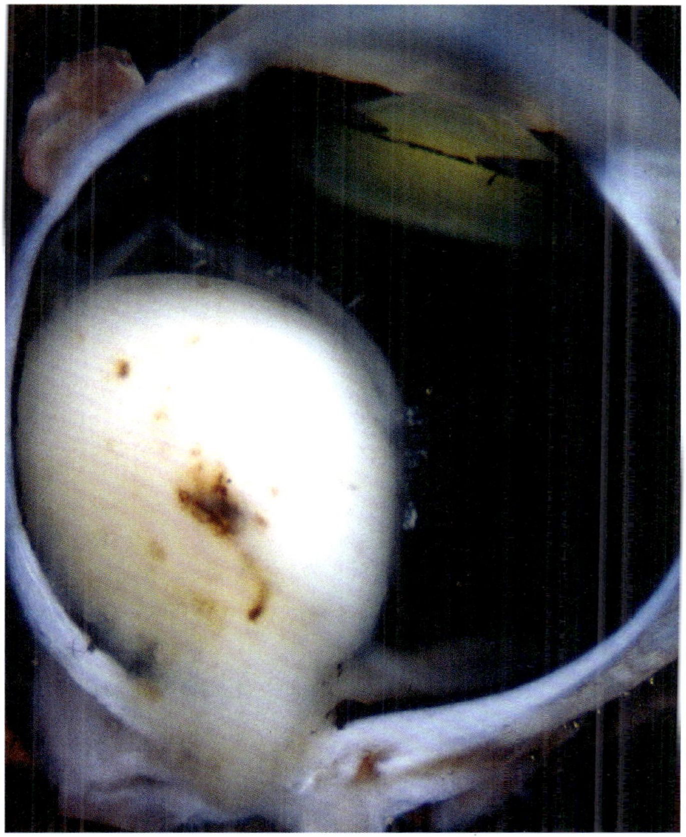

Fig. 5.01 Acquired retinal astrocytoma. This giant cell astrocytoma extends into the subretinal space from the retina.

Epidemiology

Astrocytic hamartomas are often associated with a phakomatosis, most tuberous sclerosis or neurofibromatosis. Tuberous sclerosis has an estimated incidence of 1 case per 6000–10 000 live births {861}. In a review of 42 intraocular astrocytomas confirmed histologically, 57% were associated with tuberous sclerosis, 14% were related to neurofibromatosis, and 29% were sporadic {3411}. A few cases have been reported in patients with retinitis pigmentosa {1428} but most reports lack histopathological confirmation. RAH generally arises in children or young adults although some cases have presented at an older age. Acquired retinal

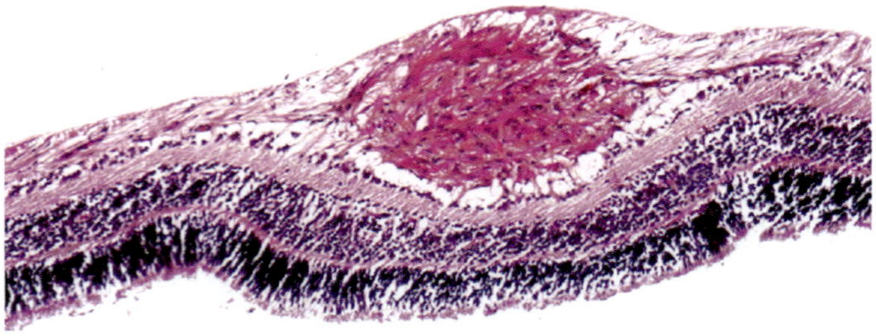

Fig. 5.02 Acquired retinal astrocytoma. A focal astrocytoma arises in the ganglion cell layer of the retina.

astrocytoma generally occurs in older individuals who have no family history or clinical findings of any syndrome.

Etiology

RAH is most commonly associated with tuberous sclerosis, which is caused by a pathogenic variant in either *TSC1* or *TSC2*.

Pathogenesis

The protein product of *TSC1* is hamartin while that of *TSC2* is tuberin, both part of a heteromeric protein complex known as TSC that inactivates the mTOR protein kinase pathway {3301}. Disruption of TSC results in upregulation of the mTOR pathway and increases proliferation and cell growth. Elucidation of the pathobiology has led to the use of mTOR inhibitors in the treatment of tuberous sclerosis–associated tumours {1028,3512}. Many are centred in the inner retina, suggestive of the tumours originating from astrocytes of the nerve fibre layer. One case of giant cell astrocytoma of the retina displayed ultrastructural features of a Müller glial cell origin {1462}.

Macroscopic appearance

Retinal astrocytic tumours are well-circumscribed, slightly elevated, yellow to grey-white lesions arising in the inner retina. RAHs are more poorly defined and translucent than acquired retinal astrocytomas, and they have associated calcifications {3049,12}.

Histopathology

Two main histopathological patterns have been described {3049,2609}. The first is characterized by fascicles of spindle-shaped cells with cytologically bland nuclei. The second, seen in giant cell astrocytomas of the retina subtype, shows larger tumour cells, abundant glassy eosinophilic cytoplasm (gemistocytic), round nuclei, and prominent nucleoli {1551}, morphologically similar to subependymal giant cell astrocytoma in the brain, and demonstrates a greater propensity for invasive growth. As is the case with subependymal giant cell astrocytoma, both glial and neuronal immunohistochemical markers can be expressed. Calcifications and necrosis are common in this second subtype of tumour. Although mitotic figures are rare or absent, these

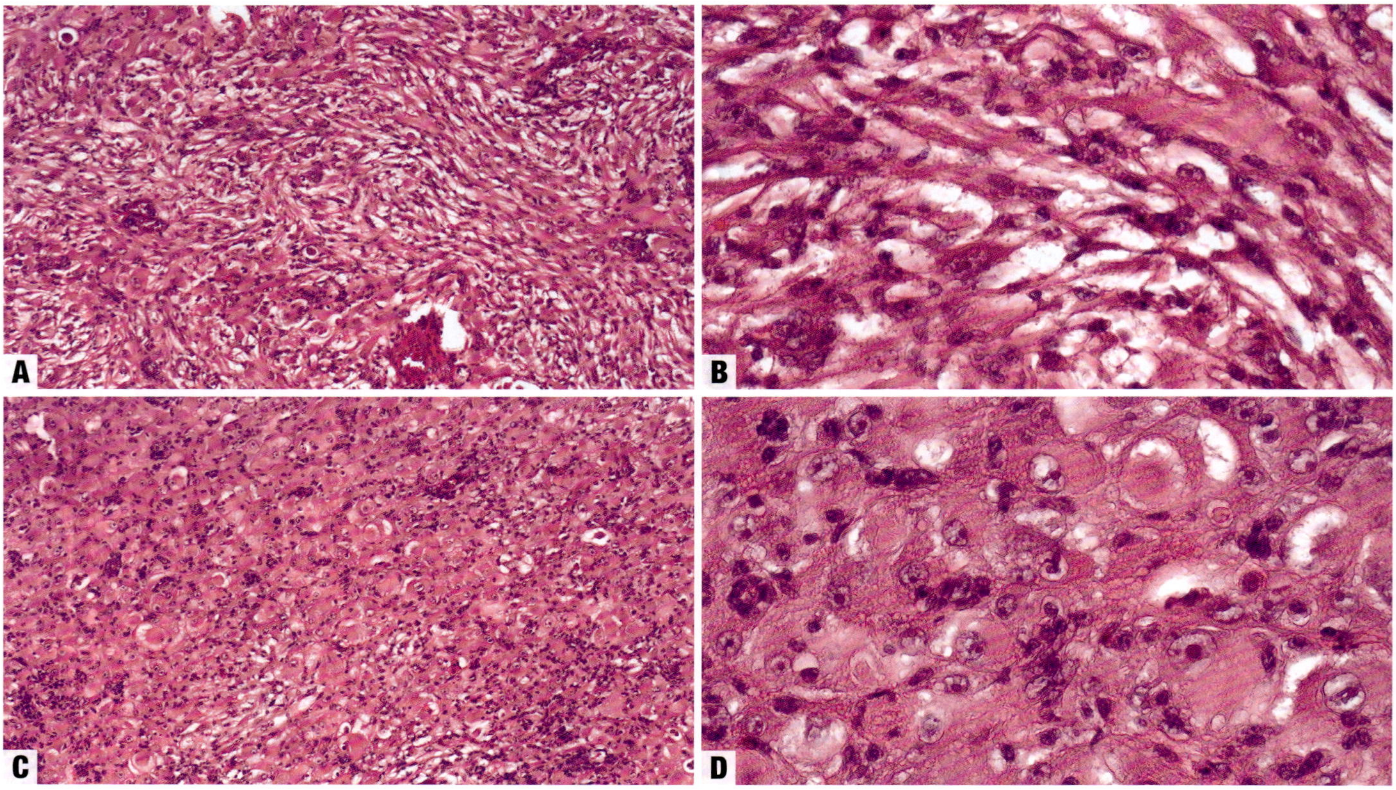

Fig. 5.03 Acquired retinal astrocytoma. **A** Giant cell astrocytoma of the retina may also contain spindle-shaped cells with fibrillary cytoplasm and fusiform nuclei. **B** Giant cell astrocytoma of the retina may also contain spindle-shaped cells with fibrillary cytoplasm and fusiform nuclei, with prominent nuclei. **C,D** Giant cell astrocytoma of the retina containing gemistocytic cells with billowing, eosinophilic cytoplasm and eccentric nuclei.

tumours can grow and eventually fill the posterior globe and are then termed aggressive retinal astrocytomas {3036,3358}. Rosenthal fibres, eosinophilic granular bodies, and other features of pilocytic astrocytoma are generally absent.

Immunohistochemistry

Retinal astrocytomas are usually diffusely positive for GFAP and S100. Most tumours are negative for neuronal markers; however, the larger gemistocytic cells may coexpress NSE and have variable staining for GFAP and S100 {2609}.

Differential diagnosis

The histological differential diagnosis would include nodular and massive retinal gliosis, which lack abundant eosinophilic cytoplasm, do not have features similar to subependymal giant cell astrocytoma, and have a very low (usually < 1%) Ki-67 proliferation index {2579}. RAH is also distinguished from a combined hamartoma of the retina and retinal pigment epithelium, which is associated with neurofibromatosis type 2.

Cytology

FNAB reveals bland spindle cells with fibrillar cytoplasm {645, 3015}.

Diagnostic molecular pathology

Not clinically relevant

Essential and desirable diagnostic criteria

Essential: a tumour arising in the inner retina; spindle-shaped and/or gemistocytic astrocytes; low mitotic activity.

Staging

Not clinically relevant

Prognosis and prediction

RAH generally remains stable and is not clinically aggressive {3768}, but progressive growth and severe local complications have been reported in exceptional cases. The cases with large gemistocytic cells and necrosis sometimes develop iris neovascularization and glaucoma {3036}. In contrast to RAH, acquired retinal astrocytoma exhibits a more aggressive clinical course with slow enlargement and progressive exudation {3015}. Current treatment modalities include photodynamic therapy {2126, 2171} in combination with verteporfin {909}, laser photocoagulation, and plaque brachytherapy {829}. Aggressive retinal astrocytomas may require enucleation of the globe.

Nodular and massive retinal gliosis

Mendoza P
Chan ASY
Eberhart CG
Edward DP

Definition

Nodular and massive retinal gliosis encompasses a spectrum of retinal glial proliferations with a vascular component, hence the clinical term "vasoproliferative tumour of the retina", ranging from focal nodules to massive lesions that can fill the eye.

ICD-O coding

None

ICD-11 coding

2F36.Y Other specified benign neoplasm of eye or ocular adnexa

Related terminology

Not recommended: vasoproliferative tumour; peripheral retinal angioma; angioma-like mass; retinal angiomatous mass; neovascular fundus abnormalities; peripheral nodular retinal telangiectasis; presumed acquired retinal haemangioma; reactive retinal glioangiosis; focal nodular gliosis; reactive retinal astrocytic tumour.

Subtype(s)

None

Localization

The lesions are most commonly located in the inferotemporal pre-equatorial retina.

Clinical features

Lesions may be asymptomatic or may present with blurring of vision, primarily from macular exudation or exudative retinal detachment. Clinically, they are yellow-orange to pink-red masses with a vascular appearance (hence the name "vasoproliferative tumour"). Although commonly unilateral and solitary, they can be bilateral {1374}, multiple, or diffuse {2982}. Retinal pigment epithelial hyperplasia is often seen at the base of the

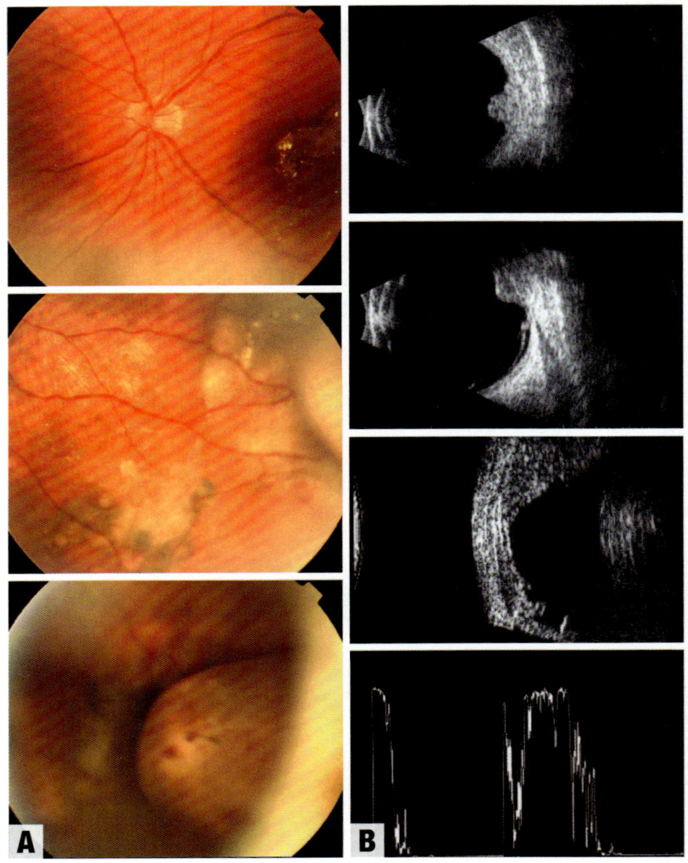

Fig. 5.04 Nodular gliosis. **A** Fundus photos show an elevated inferotemporal white-yellow mass anterior to the equator with an associated shallow exudative retinal detachment. **B** Ultrasound shows a solid dome-shaped lesion.

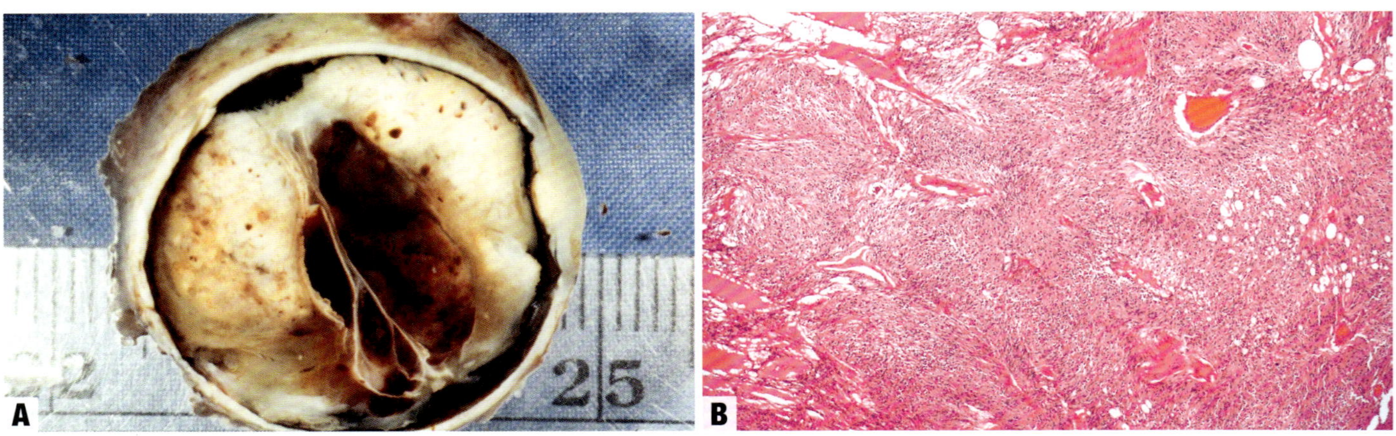

Fig. 5.05 Massive retinal gliosis. **A** Macroscopic view of a mass filling the vitreous cavity. **B** Microscopic examination shows a proliferation of glial cells.

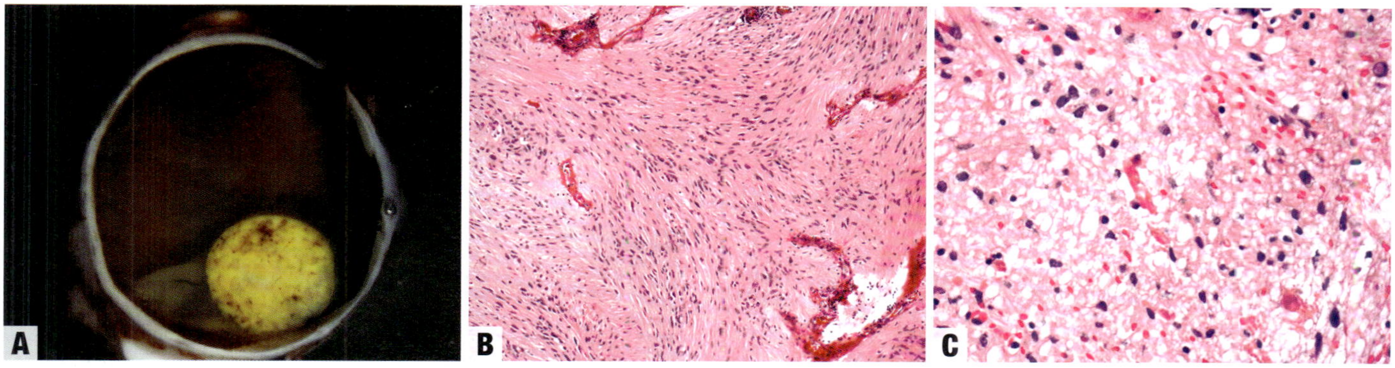

Fig. 5.06 Nodular retinal gliosis. **A** Macroscopic view of a discrete yellow-white retinal mass with scattered vessels. **B** The lesion is composed of spindle-shaped fibrous astrocytes with filamentous cytoplasm and hyalinized vessels. **C** Occasional Rosenthal fibres may be present.

lesions. Sight-threatening complications include cystoid macular oedema, epimacular membrane, and vitreous haemorrhage. On fluorescein angiography, these lesions are hyperfluorescent and leak. Ultrasonographically, nodular gliosis appears solid and dome shaped {2982,3011}.

Based on size, these lesions can be categorized as {1484} nodular retinal gliosis, which occupies < 25% of the vitreous cavity; submassive retinal gliosis, which occupies 25–50%; and massive retinal gliosis, which occupies > 50%.

Epidemiology

These lesions are non-familial with no sex predilection, and they occur in adults about 40 years of age.

Etiology

In one series, 80% of cases were primary/idiopathic and 20% were secondary {2982}. Secondary lesions can occur in relation to neurofibromatosis {1475}, retinitis pigmentosa, uveitis {2548}, retinopathy of prematurity {1374}, Coats disease, retinal detachment surgery, cryotherapy, trauma, infections (toxoplasmosis and toxocariasis), and idiopathic inflammatory retinal disease {2982}. Massive retinal gliosis is commonly associated with phthisis bulbs and congenital diseases or malformations {1484}.

Pathogenesis

These lesions are thought to be reactive in nature, arising from retinal astrocytes or Müller glial cells {2396}. Findings that support this include clinical progression of nodular gliosis to the advanced stage of massive retinal gliosis {1396}, polyclonality of massive retinal gliosis in 1 case {1420}, the lack of *KIAA1549::BRAF* fusions and *IDH1* p.R132H mutation {2579}, and expression of genes associated with reactive astrocytes {2958}. The production of angiogenic cytokines and angiogenesis are likely to be secondary events driven by glial proliferation {2958}.

Macroscopic appearance

Lesions appear as discrete white-yellow retinal masses. An outer rim of calcification may be present.

Histopathology

Lesions are composed of elongated spindle-shaped fibrous astrocytes with filamentous eosinophilic cytoplasm. The astrocytic cells are positive for GFAP and S100. The nuclei are mostly bland and oval or fusiform in shape. Rosenthal fibres and cells with hair-like (piloid) processes can sometimes be observed. Within the lesion, there are often scattered PAS-positive hyalinized/sclerotic vascular channels. Glial cells may have a perivascular orientation {3298}. Subretinal proteinaceous exudates may extend beyond its borders and contain cholesterol clefts or even a granulomatous response. Fibrous or osseous metaplasia and pseudoadenomatous hyperplasia of the retinal pigment epithelium are often present. Mitotic figures are absent or rare, and the Ki-67 proliferation index is generally < 5% {1484,2579}. Ultrastructural features include interweaving cells with intermediate cytoplasmic filaments corresponding to GFAP and small cellular processes that contain lysosomes.

Differential diagnosis includes pilocytic astrocytoma {3451}, infiltrating astrocytoma, astrocytic hamartoma, and haemangioblastoma.

Cytology

Fine-needle biopsy shows cells with uniform nuclei, abundant fibrillary cytoplasm, and GFAP-positive elongated processes {3109}.

Diagnostic molecular pathology

Not clinically relevant

Essential and desirable diagnostic criteria

Essential: a proliferation of spindle-shaped astrocytes with scattered hyalinized vessels.

Staging

Not relevant

Prognosis and prediction

Although lesions are benign, patients can have poor visual outcomes and a long, protracted clinical course. Treatment may include laser photocoagulation, cryotherapy, plaque brachytherapy, vitreoretinal surgery, and possible enucleation. While massive retinal gliosis generally remains confined to the eye, extrascleral extension with reactive microscopic features has been reported {663}.

Retinocytoma

Eagle RC Jr
Al Hussaini M

Definition

Retinocytoma is a benign primary tumour of the neurosensory retina with biallelic *RB1* sequence alterations in photoreceptor precursor cells showing differentiation and a lack of proliferation. Dedifferentiation and acquisition of additional mutation may lead to malignant transformation into retinoblastoma.

ICD-O coding

9510/0 Retinocytoma
9514/1 Retinoblastoma, spontaneously regressed

ICD-11 coding

2F36.Y & XH5AV1 Other specified benign neoplasm of eye or ocular adnexa & Retinocytoma

Related terminology

Not recommended: retinoma; spontaneously regressed retinoblastoma; spontaneously arrested retinoblastoma; retinoblastoma group 0; benign variant of retinoblastoma; spontaneous cure of retinoblastoma.

Subtype(s)

None

Localization

Retinocytomas are primary tumours of the neurosensory retina with no preferential localization {3106}.

Clinical features

While retinocytomas are often asymptomatic {3106}, blurred vision and strabismus occasionally develop {3106}. These tumours can occur in the same or contralateral eye with retinoblastoma, and have been found in phthisical eyes {244}. Leukocoria, a frequent presentation in retinoblastoma, is rarely seen in retinocytoma and usually occurs in younger patients {3022}. While 13% of cases can be bilateral {244,3106,3716}, the tumour can be unifocal or multifocal. Unifocal tumours prevail in asymptomatic patients with no family history and tend to be larger with more calcification, alteration in the retinal pigment epithelium, and chorioretinal atrophy {3022}. Second malignancies have developed in some patients with germline *RB1* sequence alterations {244,1774,18}. Retinocytomas can also be revealed after overlying retinoblastoma treatment {802,801}. Enhanced depth optical coherence tomography and high-resolution (20 MHz) ultrasonography can help to narrow the differential diagnosis {2462,1076}, but optical coherence tomography alone cannot differentiate between retinoblastoma and retinocytoma {2331}.

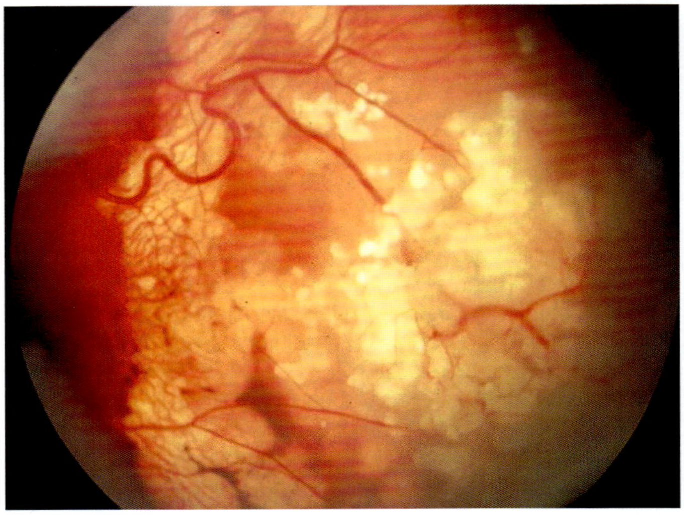

Fig. 5.07 Retinocytoma. Retinal tumour is composed of translucent cytoplasm. It contains cartilage and is bordered by a zone of atrophic retinal pigment epithelium.

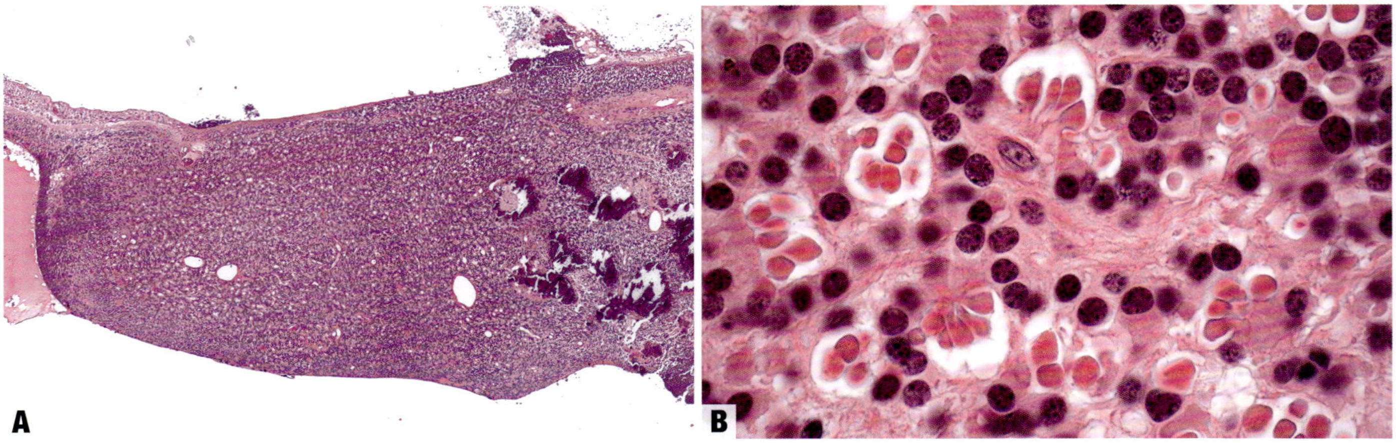

Fig. 5.08 Retinocytoma. **A** The retinal tumour is composed largely of cells showing photoreceptor differentiation. Foci of calcification are present within viable parts of the tumour. **B** Inner segments of neoplastic photoreceptors form bouquet-like aggregates called fleurettes. Cells have bland round nuclei, and mitoses and apoptosis are not present.

Clinically, the differential diagnosis includes mainly retinoblastoma, and astrocytic hamartoma.

Epidemiology

Retinocytoma is usually diagnosed at an older age than retinoblastoma, affecting only 14% of patients under 5 years of age. In two large series, the mean age at diagnosis of retinocytoma was 9 years and 28.7 years {3022,18}. The reported incidence of retinocytomas is variable and they can be found incidentally or through familial testing {2818}. It has been estimated that 2% of patients with mutated *RB1* have retinocytoma. In a large series of patients with retinoblastoma, 3% had retinocytomas {3022}. Based on histopathological examination, a 15.6–20.4% incidence was found of well-differentiated tumour areas consistent with retinocytoma within eyes enucleated for retinoblastoma {801,856}. One fourth of retinocytomatous foci are located in the base of endophytic retinoblastomas consistent with precursor lesions {856}. There appears to be no race or sex predilection, but the total number of reported cases is low.

Etiology

Like retinoblastoma, retinocytoma results from biallelic mutation of the *RB1* tumour suppressor gene located at chromosome 13q14.2. However, compared with retinoblastoma, it has low levels of genomic instability and high expression of senescence-associated proteins {801}.

Pathogenesis

Retinoblastoma and retinocytoma share the same genetic changes {19}. However, retinocytoma may develop if the second mutant allele occurs at a later stage of cell maturation, when the precursor cell has limited mitotic capability {2108}. Other possible explanations include low-penetrance *RB1* variants {1402} or epigenetic modification through *RB1* promoter hypermethylation {3326}. Upregulation of senescence-associated proteins p16 (p16INK4A) and p130 may account for the non-proliferative nature of retinocytoma {801}. Retinocytoma displays greater genomic stability than retinoblastoma {801}, although both entities have copy-number changes in *MDM4*, *MYCN*, and *E2F3*. *MDM4* gain may affect the early transition from normally developing retina to retinocytoma, while *MYCN* and *E2F3* progressive gain may help drive tumour progression {2838}.

Macroscopic appearance

Retinocytomas appear as small semitranslucent tumours at the level of the retinal pigment epithelium that contain foci of calcification and are surrounded by mild to moderate pigmentary changes.

Histopathology

Retinocytoma replaces the neurosensory retina and expands into the vitreous, but does not invade the choroid. Within eyes enucleated for retinoblastoma, foci of viable retinocytoma appear relatively eosinophilic and paucicellular compared with adjacent undifferentiated tumour on low-magnification microscopy of H&E-stained sections. Retinocytoma is composed of a uniform population of bland cells that have round or oval nuclei that are relatively uniform in size and have evenly dispersed chromatin. Necrosis, apoptotic cells, and mitotic activity are

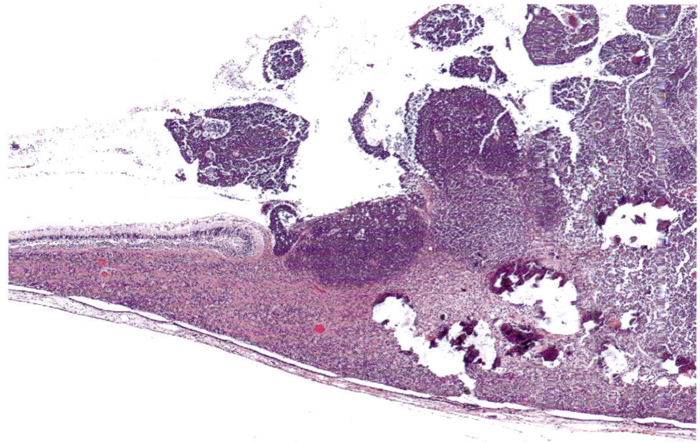

Fig. 5.09 Malignant transformation of retinocytoma. The base of the lesion is relatively eosinophilic and paucicellular compared with overlying retinoblastoma, which is seeding into the vitreous. A portion of the retinocytoma contains fractured foci of calcification. Malignant transformation was observed clinically.

absent {2067}. In some cases, the cytoplasm appears clear rather than eosinophilic. Photoreceptor differentiation is a characteristic feature, but it is not present in all cases. Advanced photoreceptor differentiation is characterized by linear arrays and bouquet-like aggregates of bulbous eosinophilic neoplastic photoreceptor inner segments called fleurettes that are joined by zonulae adherentes forming short segments of neoplastic external limiting membrane {3391}. The cellular processes of the neoplastic photoreceptors are often surrounded by Alcian blue–positive, hyaluronidase-resistant acid mucopolysaccharide. Flexner–Wintersteiner rosettes generally are not present in retinocytoma. Foci of calcification are common, tend to be denser, lack cellular profiles, appear fractured, and occur in viable parts of the tumour, unlike the dystrophic calcification in retinoblastoma that occurs within necrosis.

Retinocytomas do not express Ki-67, consistent with a lack of proliferation, or p53 {802} and lack nuclear staining for RB1 protein. As noted above, about one fifth of retinoblastomas that are enucleated contain foci of retinocytoma thought to represent tumour precursors. Foci of well-differentiated tumour consistent with retinocytoma also can be encountered as a residual mass after eye-conserving therapy for retinoblastoma. The benign tumour probably persists because it is relatively unresponsive to treatment that destroys the contiguous retinoblastoma. It is believed that retinocytoma is relatively rare clinically because the vast majority of cases progress to retinoblastoma after they acquire additional mutations in critical cancer pathways {801, 2169}.

Cytology

FNAB of eyes containing retinocytoma generally is not performed, owing to concerns about extraocular extension.

Diagnostic molecular pathology

Retinocytoma is initiated by germline and/or somatic loss-of-function mutation in both alleles of *RB1* {671,801}. Sequencing to detect *RB1* germline mutation in blood or buccal swabs {3649} and somatic mutation in tumour tissue {3649} can help establish the diagnosis.

Essential and desirable diagnostic criteria

Essential: retinal tumour composed of small bland cells with round or oval nuclei; no evidence of pleomorphism, mitosis, or necrosis.

Desirable: photoreceptor differentiation (fleurettes); low Ki-67 proliferative index.

Staging

The same staging system is used as for retinoblastoma.

Prognosis and prediction

Retinocytoma typically remains stable with no evidence of progression over an extended period of time {3324}; malignant transformation to retinoblastoma occurs in 4–12% {3106,18} of cases, reaching 15.3% by 10–20 years {3022}. Histopathologically confirmed cases of malignant transformation of retinocytoma have been reported {857}. Late malignant change of retinocytomas is a plausible explanation for the development of retinoblastoma in adults {2109}. Increasing thickness is the only factor predictive of malignant transformation {3022}.

Patients diagnosed with retinocytoma should receive close lifelong observation and they and their offspring should be offered genetic counselling {3022}. Evaluation of first-degree relatives of patients with retinoblastoma is recommended to exclude retinocytoma {2818}.

Retinocytoma has been associated with two patterns of reactivation: benign cystic growth or malignant transformation {18}, which can be rapid with vitreous seeding {857,3106}. Occasional cases of retinocytoma may regress spontaneously {1843}. However, aggressive endophytic and exophytic growth before spontaneous regression can occur {18}. Occasional cases may result in vitreous haemorrhage necessitating vitrectomy {1162}. Cases progressing to retinoblastoma have been treated successfully with intra-arterial chemotherapy {1712}. Malignant transformation of retinocytoma in an adult with a fatal outcome has been reported {2109}.

Retinoblastoma

Chevez-Barrios P
Al Hussaini M
de Graaf P
Dorsman JC
Eagle RC Jr
Gallie BL
Kaliki S
Mendoza P
Moll AC
Radvanyi F

Definition

Retinoblastoma is a malignant neoplasm derived from the developing retina that usually develops in early childhood.

ICD-O coding

9510/3 Retinoblastoma
9510/3 Unilateral retinoblastoma
9510/3 Bilateral retinoblastoma
9510/3 Trilateral retinoblastoma

ICD-11 coding

2D02.2 Retinoblastoma

Related terminology

Not recommended: glioma retinae.

Subtype(s)

Clinical subtypes: unilateral retinoblastoma (non-heritable or heritable); bilateral retinoblastoma (heritable); trilateral retinoblastoma (heritable; associated with primary intracranial tumour [pineoblastoma or suprasellar tumour])

For histological and genetic subtyping, see Table 5.01.

Localization

Retinoblastoma is a tumour of the neurosensory retina which can also involve the vitreous cavity. Tumour progression leads to involvement of the anterior segment, ocular coats, optic nerve, and periocular tissues.

Clinical features

Leukocoria, a white pupillary reflex, secondary to the retinal tumour, is the hallmark clinical feature of retinoblastoma identified in 63% of cases {1128}. Leukocoria is often detected by parents, who bring it to the attention of their health care provider {23}. Identification of leukocoria is dependent upon ambient lighting and the direction of the child's gaze. Larger pupils in dimmer lighting may facilitate detection of leukocoria while tumours arising outside the centre of vision may only be apparent in extreme positions of gaze {2324}. Differential diagnosis of childhood disease that cause leukocoria include congenital and acquired lesions. Strabismus is the second most common presenting sign (10% of cases) {1128}, while the combination of leukocoria and strabismus is seen less frequently (4% of cases) {1679}. Clinical features associated with advanced disease at presentation include iris heterochromia (neovascularization of iris), glaucoma with buphthalmos, pseudohypopyon, uveitis, hyphaema, and aseptic orbital cellulitis {2446}. In advanced cases, extraocular disease extension may produce proptosis or a cauliflower-like mass arising from the front of the eye. Proptosis, a symptom of advanced disease, is reported in 7% of cases worldwide and is more common in low-income countries than in high-income countries, owing to delayed diagnosis {1128}.

In most cases, the diagnosis of retinoblastoma can be confirmed in the clinic by dilated eye examination. Ocular ultrasound is a non-invasive diagnostic imaging modality to detect the mass and the characteristic dystrophic calcifications within the tumour. However, an examination under anaesthesia is needed for a detailed evaluation of the tumour and the affected eye, to evaluate the contralateral eye, and to stage the tumour. After examination of eyelids and adnexa, the diameter and clarity of the cornea and the intraocular pressure are recorded. The anterior segment is evaluated for the presence of tumour cells, iris neovascularization, and lens opacification. The number and location of the tumours in each eye and associated serous fluid along with vitreous and subretinal seeding are detailed in a fundus drawing and/or documented by fundus photography.

Table 5.01 Retinoblastoma subtypes (genetic and histological features)

General type	Subtype	Definition
Genetic	Sporadic (H0)	No history of hereditary retinoblastoma; patient without a germline *RB1* mutation (normal *RB1* alleles in blood, high-sensitivity assays) Normal *RB1* in blood, < 1% risk of mosaicism {1989}
	Hereditary (H1)	Bilateral retinoblastoma with or without intracranial CNS midline embryonic tumour (i.e. trilateral retinoblastoma); family history of retinoblastoma or molecular definition of germline *RB1* gene mutation
	Unknown (HX)	Unknown *RB1* mutation
	MYCN amplified	High-level amplification of the *MYCN* gene (approximately > 28 copies) with no detectable mutation in *RB1*
Histopathology	Growth patterns	Exophytic, endophytic, combined exophytic and endophytic, diffuse, diffuse anterior, indeterminate extensively necrotic (> 90%)
	Degree of differentiation (grade) {2209A}	1. Areas of retinocytoma (fleurettes / neuronal differentiation) 2. Many rosettes (Flexner–Wintersteiner or Homer Wright) 3. Occasional rosettes 4. Poorly differentiated cells without rosettes and/or > 50% anaplasia
	RB1 mutated / conventional	Neuroendocrine type, irregular nuclei, without nucleoli, with rosettes
	MYCN amplified	Unilateral retinoblastoma with round nuclei and prominent nucleoli without rosettes

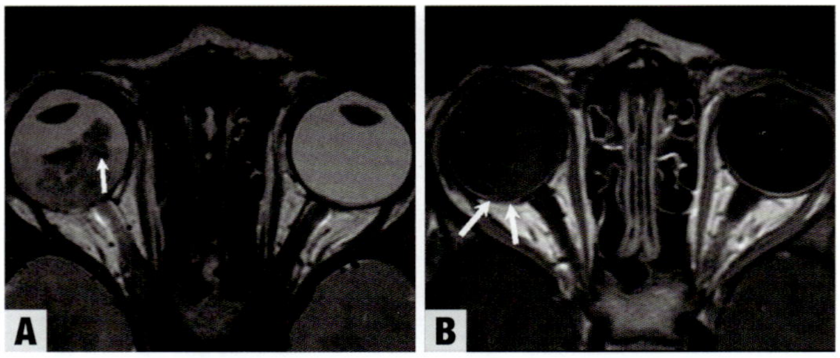

Fig. 5.10 Retinoblastoma. **A** T2-weighted MRI with an exophytic retinoblastoma of the right eye with focal calcifications (arrow). A total retinal detachment is present. **B** On contrast-enhanced T1-weighted MRI the tumour shows marked enhancement combined with massive choroidal invasion (arrows).

On clinical examination, retinoblastoma appears as a white mass. Exophytic tumours arise from the outer layers of the retina. As the tumour increases in size, serous fluid accumulates detaching the retina. Total serous retinal detachments that can touch the crystalline lens may occur. Exophytic tumours often seed the subretinal space, resulting in new tumour loci that may invade below the retinal pigment epithelium and eventually the choroid. Endophytic tumours grow into the vitreous cavity producing small pieces of tumour that detach from the main mass (seeds) that can appear as dust, spheres, or clouds {1026}. The type of seed is associated with diverse treatment response {2979,3717,147}. Vitreous seeding has the worst prognosis for eye preservation. Diffuse infiltrative retinoblastoma, the rarest growth pattern (2% of cases) is found typically in older children (mean age: 4 years), can masquerade as uveitis or hyphaema or keratic precipitates, and is associated with extensive vitreous seeding. However, a well-circumscribed mass and calcification can be absent {2979,147}.

Imaging

MRI of the orbits and brain is performed {736} to confirm the clinical diagnosis, to exclude differential diagnoses {1500}, and to evaluate extraocular extension into the orbital soft tissues and/or overt tumour invasion into the optic nerve. Brain images are reviewed to exclude trilateral retinoblastoma (pineoblastoma or suprasellar mass), which is associated with germline (constitutional) *RB1* gene pathogenic variants {741}. Although MRI continues to improve as a diagnostic modality, histopathology remains the gold standard for assessing high-risk features associated with metastasis.

Epidemiology

Retinoblastoma is the most common primary intraocular malignant tumour in infants and young children and is thought to be the most common primary malignant intraocular neoplasm {1724}. It accounts for approximately 3% of all cancers occurring in young children. There is no race or sex predilection; however, some report a preponderance of boys over girls, which may reflect culture-based medical care bias {2316}.

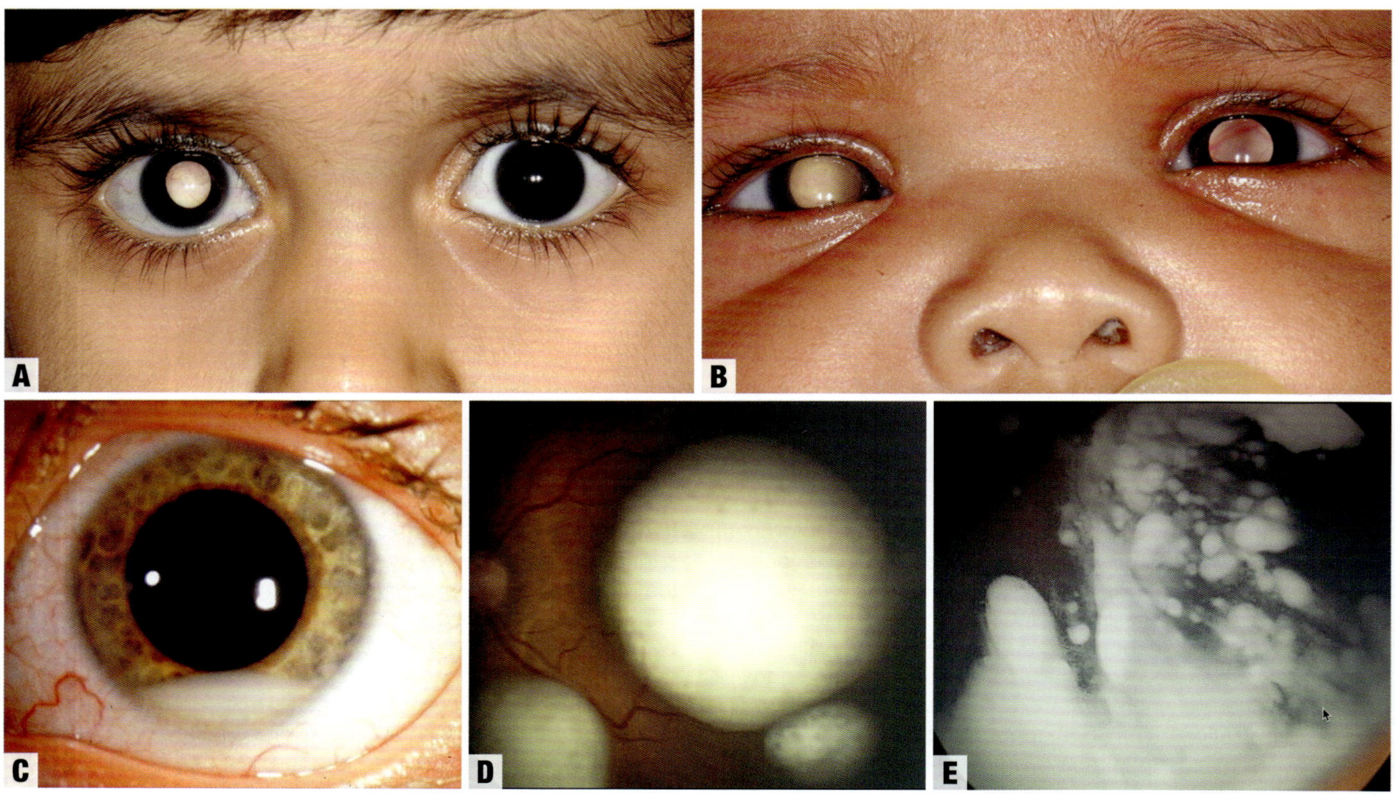

Fig. 5.11 Retinoblastoma. **A** The hallmark of retinoblastoma is leukocoria (white pupillary reflex), evident here in the right eye. **B** Bilateral leukocoria indicates bilateral retinoblastoma in this infant with germline *RB1* mutation. **C** The image shows a diffuse infiltrative retinoblastoma in which a pseudohypopyon of tumour cells in the inferior anterior chamber was the presenting manifestation; the eye shows no inflammatory signs. **D** Endophytic growth pattern. A fundus photograph shows multiple encephaloid tumours projecting into the vitreous from attached retina; the patient had bilateral tumours and germline *RB1* mutation. **E** A fundus photograph shows numerous tumour seeds in the vitreous, dispersed from endophytic retinoblastoma.

The incidence of retinoblastoma is reported as 1 case in 16 000–18 000 live births {3495,416,1724}. About 80% to 95% of cases are diagnosed before the age of 3 and 5 years, respectively {416,2019}. About 7980 retinoblastomas were predicted to have been diagnosed in 2015 worldwide {2316}. Predictions for Africa, representing 16% of the world population, are 2293, or 29% of the total. Almost double the number (4258 or 53%) is predicted for Asia, with 60% of the world population. Latin America, North America, and Europe, with 8%, 3%, and 6% of retinoblastomas, also have fewer incident cases relative to their percentage of the world population of 9%, 5%, and 10%, respectively. These discrepancies can be explained by differences in birth rates that range from 33.6 per 1000 population in Africa to 10.5 per 1000 population in Europe {2316}. Incidence of retinoblastoma must always consider birth rate and infant mortality {800}, since median age at diagnosis is 24 months for unilateral disease, and 12 months for bilateral disease. Retinoblastoma cases rarely occur in older children and adults. The Global Retinoblastoma Outcome Study, a cross-sectional international study, showed in the analysis of retinoblastoma at the time of diagnosis important differences in presentation among patients from different countries, depending on their national income level. Patients with retinoblastoma from high-income countries present with early disease and are, therefore, likely to survive {800,1128,927,1127}. In contrast, patients from lower-income settings present with late disease, many with extraocular extension and some already with metastasis, and their prognosis is poorer, with a 3-year survival rate of 57% (52–63%), while those in high-income countries have a 3-year survival rate of 99.5% (98.8–100%) {1127}. The incidence of trilateral retinoblastoma, which is retinoblastoma combined with an intracranial midline tumour in the pineal gland or around the sella turca, is 3.8% in patients with bilateral disease and 3.5% among all patients with hereditary retinoblastoma {740}.

Etiology

Retinoblastoma originates from developing retinal cells, most probably from cone progenitors {3661,3114}. In most cases (> ~98%; *RB1*$^{-/-}$ tumours), carcinogenesis is initiated by the inactivation of the *RB1* tumour suppressor gene {2792}. Inactivation of the *RB1* gene may also be caused by promoter methylation or chromothripsis, the latter being a mutational phenomenon characterized by massive, clustered genomic rearrangements {2138,725}.

Pathogenesis

Heritable retinoblastoma is caused by a germline mutation (first hit) followed by a somatic alteration (second hit), while non-heritable retinoblastoma can be initiated when two alterations arise in the same vulnerable cell. Although this event is required for initiation, it is probably not sufficient, because benign retinal lesions (retinocytoma) also have biallelic *RB1* mutations {801}. Several chromosomal regions have been found to be recurrently altered in retinoblastoma tumours; these include large gains of regions at 1q, 2p, and 6p, and losses of regions at 16q {671,1768}. The most likely candidate oncogene for 2p is *MYCN* (2p24.3), while the other candidate oncogenes are the *MDM4* gene (1q32), coding for a p53 regulator, and the *E2F3* and *DEK* genes (6p22), coding for proteins involved in transcription. Candidate tumour suppressor genes at 16q are the *RB1*-related

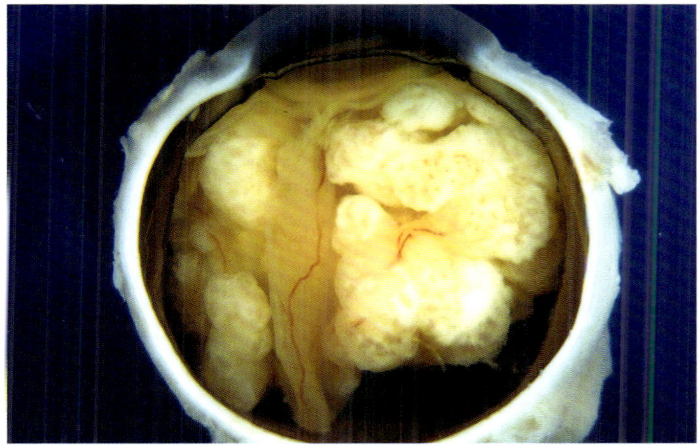

Fig. 5.12 Retinoblastoma. In this example with an exophytic growth pattern, encephaloid lobules of tumour fill most of the subretinal space beneath the totally detached retina.

gene *RBL2* (16q12) and the *CDH11* gene (16q22) belonging to the cadherin superfamily. In line with other paediatric tumours, the frequency of gene mutations is low. Besides *RB1*, the only gene found to be recurrently mutated is the *BCOR* gene, a chromatin remodelling–related gene {3743,1769,1967}.

Two retinoblastoma subtypes have recently been proposed and characterized at the clinical, histopathological, and molecular levels {1967}. Subtype 1 corresponds to a later cone differentiation, presents significantly fewer genomic alterations, and has an early onset. Subtype 2 contains all *MYCN*-amplified and *BCOR*-mutated tumours, presents a less-differentiated cone state, expresses ganglion/neuronal genes, and has been suggested to be more aggressive {1967}. Subtype 2 has more intratumoural and intertumoural heterogeneity and the *MYCN*-amplified tumours display fewer genomic changes than other tumours belonging to this subtype {1967}. Another study suggested that the small group (< 2% of unilateral tumours) of *RB1*-wildtype and *MYCN*-amplified tumours (28–121 *MYCN* copies) might be initiated by overexpression of MYCN. These primary tumours seem to have fewer overall genomic copy-number changes in genes characteristic of retinoblastoma than the *RB1*$^{-/-}$ tumours, although the number of tumours analysed of this type is still limited {2792}.

Macroscopic appearance

Retinoblastoma arises from and destroys the neurosensory retina. Macroscopically, the tumour has a white encephaloid appearance that typically contains more intensely white flecks of calcification. Several growth patterns are recognized. Endophytic retinoblastomas arise from the retina, which remains attached, and invade the vitreous. Endophytic tumours may be confused with inflammation. Exophytic retinoblastomas arise from the outer layers of the retina and cause retinal detachment, which often is high and bullous and may cause anterior displacement of the lens iris diaphragm and secondary angle closure. In more-advanced cases, the growth pattern may be indeterminate or a combined endophytic/exophytic pattern. Diffuse infiltrating retinoblastoma diffusely thickens the retina and typically does not form a discrete tumour. Calcification typically is absent in such cases and the tumour often blankets the ciliary body and infiltrates the zonule. Many cases present with tumour clumps or a pseudohypopyon of tumour cells in the anterior chamber. Diffuse infiltrating retinoblastomas typically arise in older children (mean age: 6 years) and may be misdiagnosed clinically. Extensively necrotic tumours found in patients who present with aseptic orbital cellulitis are often bloodstained or orange in colour and may have additional signs of necrosis such as pigment dispersion and lens dislocation. Posterior uveal invasion manifests as thickening by white tumour tissue. Seeds of tumour may be found in the vitreous or subretinal space. They include diffuse vitreous infiltrates called dust or clouds and larger clumps or spherules of tumour cells. The latter may have a targetoid appearance reflecting a central core of necrotic tumour cells. Dust comprises scattered tumour cells alternating with macrophages, while clouds are composed largely of necrotic cells. Multiple tumours may occur in the same eye of patients who harbour germline mutations in *RB1*. However, it often is difficult to distinguish multiple primary retinoblastomas from tumour dispersion if the eye is full of tumour.

To assess high-risk features, adequate handling of the enucleated eye is key. A block of the optic nerve margin should be obtained before opening the eye, to avoid contamination by tumour. After fixation, the eye should be oriented and cut into three pieces in a posterior to anterior manner. The goal is to obtain a central pupil–optic nerve section including the centre of the eye, lens, pupillary region, and entire thickness of the optic nerve (avoiding cuts through the nerve). The resulting two pieces, the caps (calottes), are further sectioned (anterior to posterior with a bread-slicing approach) to increase the choroidal surface examined. As a result, the entire eye is processed in four cassettes: (1) the central pupil–optic nerve section, (2) and (3) the calottes, and (4) the optic nerve margin (blocked so that the surgical margin is cut first). Histological sectioning of the central pupil–optic nerve should include early sections of the surface cut grossly and then sections that show the centre of the optic nerve (optic nerve head in contact with retina/tumour) to evaluate invasion. Incomplete sections may hinder interpretation, possibly impacting adequate adjuvant treatment of the patients {2856}.

Histopathology

Retinoblastoma is composed of poorly differentiated neuroblastic cells (retinoblasts) that have hyperchromatic nuclei and scant cytoplasm. Apoptosis and mitotic figures are common. Viable

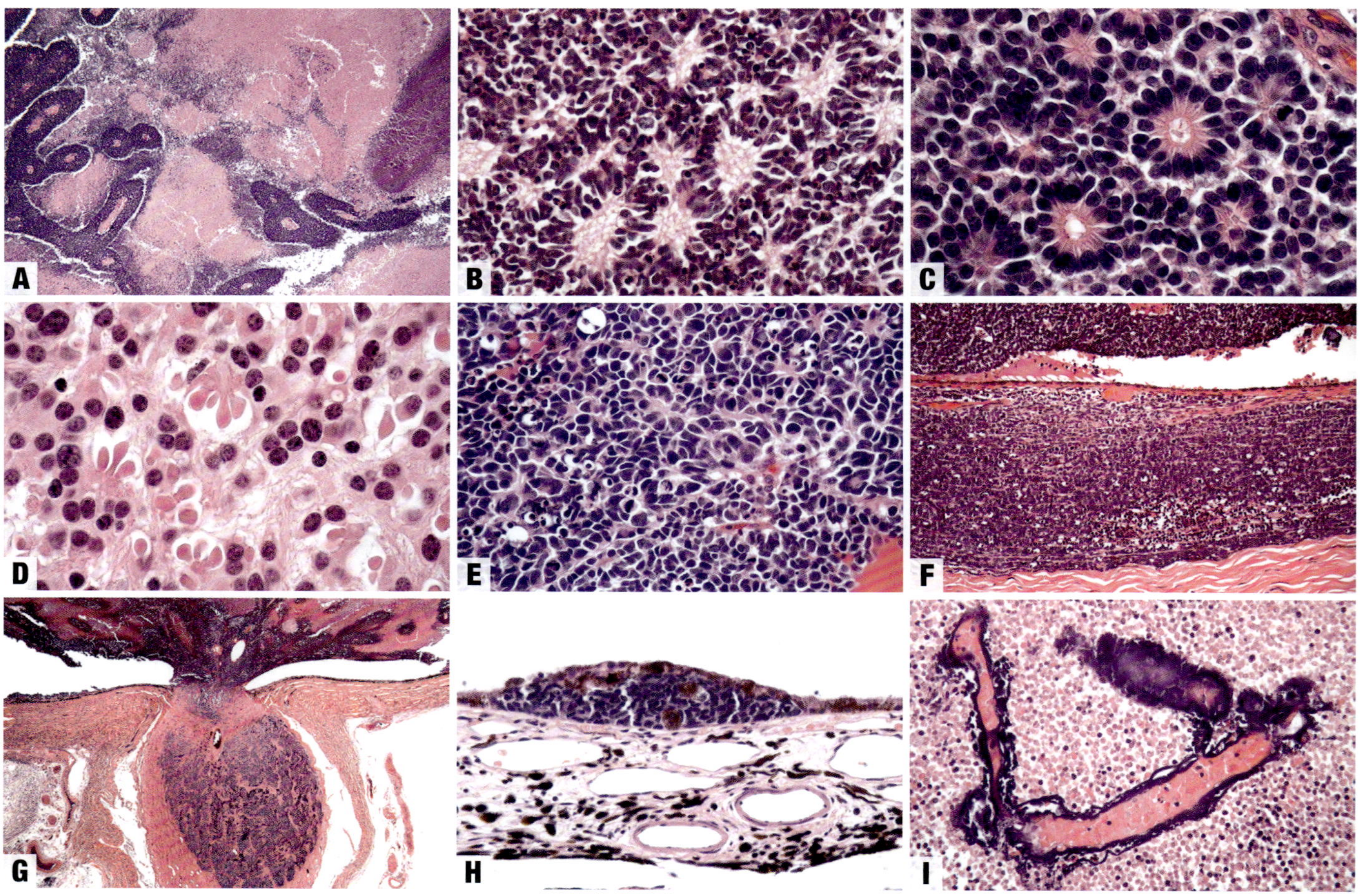

Fig. 5.13 Retinoblastoma. **A** Necrotic tumour containing foci of dystrophic calcification surrounds perivascular cuffs and sleeves of viable retinoblastoma cells. **B** Primitive Homer Wright rosettes lack a central lumen. **C** Consistent with early retinal differentiation, Flexner–Wintersteiner rosettes have a central lumen that corresponds to the subretinal space. **D** Fleurettes comprise eosinophilic bouquet-like aggregates of neoplastic photoreceptor inner segments; the nuclei are bland and mitotic activity and apoptosis are absent. **E** A severely anaplastic focus contains large, extremely pleomorphic nuclei, cellular wrapping, and mitotic figures. **F** A sheet of tumour cells infiltrates the full thickness of the posterior choroid. Massive posterior choroidal invasion is defined as > 3 mm. **G** Tumour invading the optic nerve extends posterior to the lamina cribrosa; postlaminar invasion is a high-risk feature. **H** A segment of retinal pigment epithelium has been detached by retinoblastoma; the tumour is located on the inner surface of the Bruch membrane and does not represent choroidal invasion. **I** Basophilic deposits of DNA surround vessels within necrotic tumour.

retinoblastoma appears intensely basophilic. The tumour has a propensity to outgrow its blood supply and undergo necrosis. This typically occurs approximately 90–110 µm away from a vessel and is responsible for the characteristic appearance of basophilic perivascular cuffs and sleeves of viable cells that are surrounded by sheets of necrotic cells that have lost their nuclear DNA and appear eosinophilic. Foci of dystrophic calcification, which are a helpful clinical diagnostic feature, often occur within the necrotic tumour. Endophytic retinoblastoma may have vitreous seeding (dust, sphere, or cloud types) {142}.

Varying degrees of retinal differentiation may be evident as rosettes or photoreceptor differentiation. Homer Wright rosettes contain a central tangle of neurofilamentary neuropil ringed by nuclei. They represent neuroblastic differentiation and are a typical finding in neuroblastoma, and are also seen in other neuroendocrine tumours. Flexner–Wintersteiner rosettes represent early retinal differentiation. They have a central lumen filled with mucopolysaccharide that corresponds to the subretinal space. The apices of the surrounding cells are joined by intercellular connections analogous to the external limiting membrane. Flexner–Wintersteiner rosettes are a characteristic finding in retinoblastoma but also occur in ocular medulloepithelioma. Rosettes are more common in retinoblastomas that are enucleated from very young patients {856}. Retinoblastoma tends to become less well differentiated with increasing age. Foci of retinal differentiation are found in areas of viable tumour and appear relatively eosinophilic compared with retinoblastoma. These areas of well-differentiated retinal tumour are consistent with foci of precursor retinocytoma and often contain photoreceptor differentiation evident as fleurettes. The latter comprise bouquet-like aggregates of photoreceptor inner segments with a fleur de lis–like aspect aligned along a segment of neoplastic external limiting membrane. The nuclei are bland and apoptosis and mitotic figures are absent. Some areas of well-differentiated tumour lack fleurettes and are composed of cells with bland round or oval nuclei in a glial matrix (neuroglial differentiation). Rarely, retinoblastomas may undergo true spontaneous regression. Such cases typically are phthisical eyes with evidence of widespread necrosis that contain characteristic aggregates of calcified retinoblastoma cells. It is thought that these findings are the result of vascular occlusion secondary probably to severe neovascular glaucoma. This may be an end point in patients that originally had an orbital cellulitis presentation and went unrecognized. In some cases, viable tumour may persist in the orbital optic nerve. High-risk histopathological features for metastasis include extraocular extension, massive posterior uveal invasion defined as > 3 mm in diameter and/or full-thickness choroidal involvement, and retrolaminar optic nerve invasion. In a recent large prospective study, patients who had a combination of massive (> 3 mm) peripapillary choroidal invasion and 1.5 mm of retrolaminar optic nerve invasion had the poorest prognosis for CNS recurrence and death from the disease {582}. Focal detachments of the retinal pigment epithelium by invasion of retinoblastoma cells are observed frequently but do not represent uveal invasion, because the tumour cells are situated internal to the Bruch membrane.

Anaplasia has been reported to be an additional risk factor for metastasis and death in the absence of other high-risk features {1395}. Anaplastic features include the presence of cells with large, extremely pleomorphic hyperchromatic nuclei that are

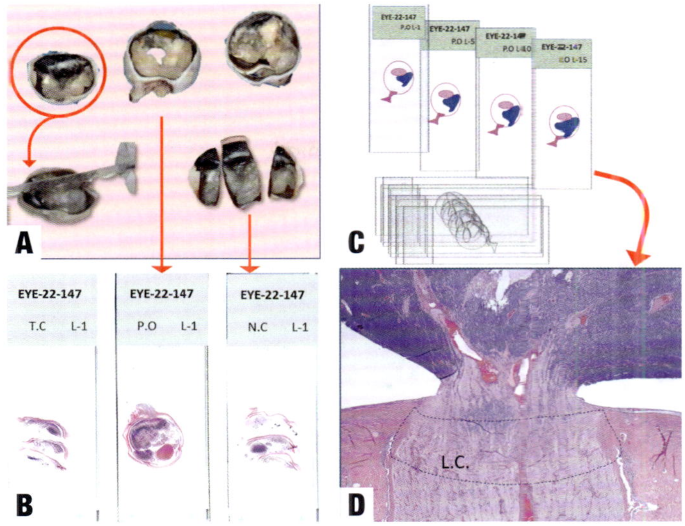

Fig. 5.14 Handling and processing of enucleated eyes with retinoblastoma. **A** After adequate fixation the eye is sectioned to obtain a central pupil–optic nerve section that contains the intact optic nerve (upper centre). The caps (calottes) (upper right and left) resulting from the sectioning are further serially sectioned anteriorly to posteriorly (lower left) to obtain segments of the calottes (lower right), maximizing the surface of choroid to be studied. **B** The entire eye is then submitted in three cassettes for histological sectioning. The resulting slides show the segments of the calottes on the cut edge to evaluate the choroid and sclera and the central pupil–optic nerve to evaluate the optic nerve in relation to the intraocular tumour. **C** Histopathological examination of several sections and levels of the central pupil–optic nerve segment is recommended to evaluate possible invasion and if present the depth of invasion into the optic nerve. Sections may be cut serially and stained every five levels keeping the unstained slides (bottom) for possible staining with immunohistochemistry or H&E if necessary. **D** Sectioning should continue until the complete centre of the optic nerve is seen on the slides as represented in this microphotograph of the optic nerve. Notice the central vessels in the optic nerve and in the retina/tumour, and the presence of the lamina cribrosa (LC). The tumour is barely touching the inner layers of the lamina cribrosa in this example.

angular, rhomboid, or fusiform in shape, as well as cell wrapping and numerous mitotic figures.

About 1.5% of unilateral retinoblastomas lack mutations in the *RB1* gene and are thought to be caused by *MYCN* amplification. These $RB1^{+/+}$ tumours have an early onset, behave aggressively, and lack Flexner–Wintersteiner rosettes. Characteristically the tumours are poorly differentiated and certain cells with large oval nuclei with nucleoli. They also exhibit nuclear immunoreactivity for RB1 protein, which is absent in retinoblastomas with *RB1* mutation {2792}.

Tumours are graded by the growth pattern of the tumour in relationship with intraocular tissues and by specific characteristics of the tumour. These patterns translate to clinical presentations and associate with high-risk features (see *Histopathology* and Table 5.01, p. 197). Histological grades are defined by the degree of differentiation (College of American Pathologists [CAP] protocol {2209A}). Grades 1–4 represent very well differentiated to poorly differentiated tumours. Histological features suggesting *MYCN* amplification include unilateral retinoblastoma with a loose cellular pattern, round nuclei, and prominent nucleoli.

The pathology report in enucleated eyes with retinoblastoma must include confirmation of diagnosis, with the presence of small blue round cell tumour, composed of primitive embryonal cells with a high N:C ratio, basophilic nuclei, and scant

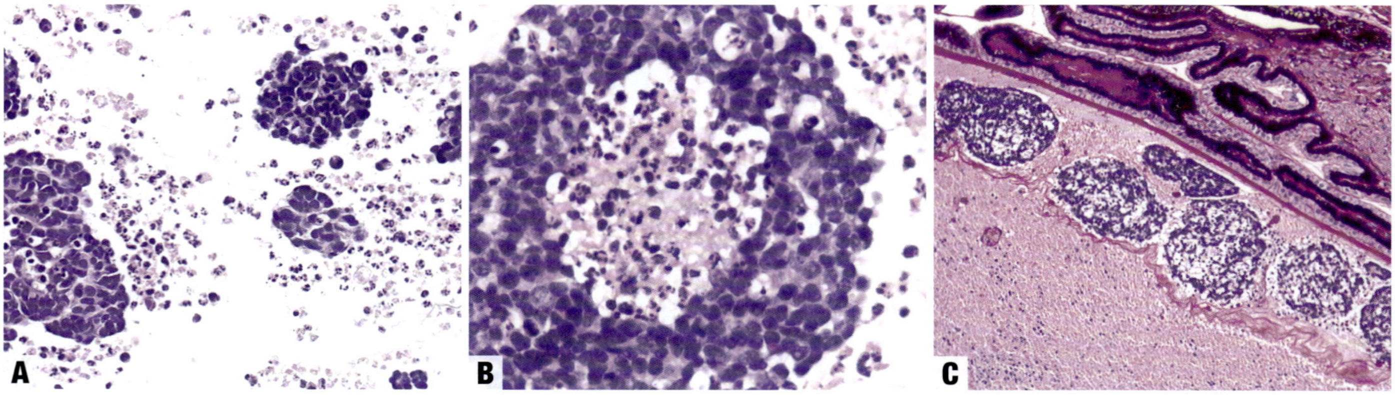

Fig. 5.15 Vitreous retinoblastoma tumour seeding. **A** The background shows dust-type vitreous seeding, where there is a combination of necrotic cells, macrophages, and scattered single tumour cells. The nests of floating tumour cells are sphere type 1, which are those that have solid centres and clinically appear as translucent spheres. Notice the small budding tumour cells that detach from the main sphere and create new tumour seeds. **B** Sphere type 2 tumour seeding shows a central area of necrosis and clinically these appear as spheres with a white or yellow centre. **C** A close-up shows an area of cloud-type seeding in which most of the cloud corresponds to large areas of tumour necrosis (lower left), rimmed by viable spheres. In this example the cloud is behind and adjacent to the lens and the ciliary body (upper right). Notice the PAS-positive basement membranes of these structures.

cytoplasm, with increased mitosis and apoptosis. Tumour invasion status is given, in the choroid (and if present the amount in millimetres and if it reaches the sclera) and in the optic nerve (location and depth of invasion in millimetres measured either from the inner limiting membrane of the optic nerve or from the Bruch membrane to the deepest point of invasion at the centre of the optic nerve), along with status of the optic nerve margin, whether the tumour in the optic nerve encroaches on the meninges, and whether there is an extraocular extension (including the site). Also to be mentioned are the degree of differentiation (Homer Wright rosettes, Flexner–Wintersteiner rosettes, and fleurettes), presence or absence of calcification, percentage of tumour necrosis, and other findings such as neovascularization of the iris, extensive necrosis of intraocular structures, or treatment effect {2856}.

Cytology

Retinoblastoma should not be biopsied routinely as it may induce extraocular recurrence and metastasis. Cytological samples often have pitfalls (sampling of retinal neurons, scant material, and others) that may mislead. Diagnostic features of malignancy such as necrosis, mitosis, and nuclear atypia should be present when diagnosing retinoblastoma by cytology. Consultation with a trained ophthalmic cytopathologist is recommended if a biopsy is considered.

Diagnostic molecular pathology

Genetic risk subtypes are divided by absence of a pathogenic germline *RB1* mutation based on blood evaluation using a high-sensitivity assay (sporadic = H0), and presence of a mutation, family history of retinoblastoma, or bilateral or trilateral retinoblastoma (hereditary = H1). Heritable retinoblastoma syndrome is further detailed in *Retinoblastoma syndrome* (p. 494). About 1.5% of sporadic unilateral retinoblastoma tumours have high-level *MYCN* amplification with no detectable pathogenic mutation in *RB1* (see Table 5.01, p. 197).

Patients with the hereditable form of retinoblastoma due to germline *RB1* mutation may present with bilateral tumours, and a delay in the occurrence of tumour in the second eye, or with a unilateral tumour {800}. Knowledge of *RB1* mutation status is very important for patient care, case management, and counselling of family members. In high-income countries, the assessment of *RB1* mutation detection is therefore common clinical practice. To perform DNA diagnostics of the *RB1* gene, blood of the retinoblastoma proband and if available retinoblastoma tumour is collected, ideally fresh (kept frozen until used), but formalin-fixed paraffin-embedded tissue may be used. Inactivation of *RB1* can result from small or large DNA alterations, complex rearrangements such as chromothripsis, loss of heterozygosity, and promoter methylation {2707,1989,2138,725}. The methodology for *RB1* DNA diagnostics may differ; however, it is important to use suitably accredited laboratories (e.g. ISO15189) that have the high sensitivity and range of testing necessary for a reliable result. Increasingly, sensitive next-generation sequencing is used to analyse the exons of the *RB1* gene and is instrumental in determining complex rearrangements {1937,725}. *RB1* RNA analysis may identify pathogenic splice variants caused by deep intronic mutations {811}. Specific protocols, including next-generation sequencing, are used to detect mosaic *RB1* mutations or *RB1* promoter methylation {2791,1937,2591}. *MYCN* amplification testing should also be considered in very young children with unilateral retinoblastomas that have wildtype *RB1* to detect *RB1*$^{+/+}$ *MYCN*^{A} (*MYCN*-amplified) tumours. Immunohistochemistry to detect RB1 protein is not reliable as about 20% of *RB1* biallelic mutation tumours are positive owing to the presence of a non-functional protein {2792}. Double immunostaining using RB1 and MYCN antibodies is also available {1937}.

The use of cell-free DNA analysis is increasing as biopsies of intraocular retinoblastoma are contraindicated owing to the risk of metastatic spread. Sources of cell-free DNA include aqueous and blood samples for detection of both *RB1* variants and *MYCN* amplification {1099,3659}. Aqueous enriched cell-free DNA, and to a lesser extent plasma analysis, may be useful to identify copy-number alterations for tumour prognosis based on relative chromosomal instability level {1691}. It has also been proposed that blood cell-free DNA may aid in detection of second primary malignancies {20}. Single nucleotide variation or relative haplotype dosage may be determined in maternal plasma to test the *RB1* status of the fetus. In a small study, the prenatal diagnosis was 100% concordant with the postdiagnostic result {1097}. Capture-based targeted sequencing and relative haplotype dosage analysis of maternal plasma can evaluate fetal *RB1* status for paternal or de novo variants; in a small study, the prenatal diagnosis was 100% concordant with the postdiagnostic result {1097}.

Genetic counselling of the family is warranted by an expert clinical geneticist / genetic counsellor. For the H1 proband, counselling includes the increased risk for developing secondary primary malignancies. In addition, risk stratification based on proband testing directs screening of children at elevated risk of development of retinoblastoma {3136}. Wildtype *RB1* with amplified *MYCN* (*RB1*$^{+/+}$ *MYCN*^{A}) is not a heritable form of retinoblastoma; thus, no extensive genetic counselling is required.

Essential and desirable diagnostic criteria

Essential: patient age < 5 years; intraocular tumour, unilateral or bilateral; histology – small blue round cell tumour with frequent mitoses, rosettes, and necrosis.

Desirable: germline alteration of *RB1*; assessment of *MYCN* mutation in *RB1*-wildtype tumours.

Staging

Classification schemes for staging stratify prognosis for ocular salvage and guide treatment. The current tumour grouping is based on tumour response to primary systemic chemotherapy. The two systems initially proposed were the International Intraocular Retinoblastoma Classification (IIRC) {1959} and the International Classification of Retinoblastoma (ICRB) {2996}. Both group eyes based on tumour size, location, the extent of serous fluid, and the presence of vitreous or subretinal seeding, with tumour size the most significant difference. More recently, the American Joint Commission on Cancer (AJCC) developed a clinical Tumour Node Metastasis classification system (cTNM) for retinoblastoma with broad international input and data {2049}. This incorporates additional prognostic features such as cellulitis, extraocular extension (clinical or radiographic evidence), and proptosis.

Staging is according to the AJCC and the Union for International Cancer Control (UICC) eighth-edition TNMH classification {2049}. This comprehensive system includes both clinical and pathological findings, and incorporates intraocular, extraocular, and systemic disease aspects within the same system. The AJCC staging system serves to standardize data reporting, prognostication (predicting globe salvage, metastatic risk, and patient survival), and selection of the most suitable treatments. Retinoblastoma staging is also the first to acknowledge the role of genetic predisposition by including heritable trait (H) in the staging system {3353,3354}. Primary retinoblastoma (T) is divided into four groups, with several subgroups and additional descriptors. The stages from cT1a to cT3b closely reflect the five stages of the IIRC and ICRB. Stage cT3 (IIRC/ICRB Group E) indicates a high risk for tumour extension outside the eye and the need for urgent removal of the eye. Stages pT2 and pT3 confirm local invasion of tumour. Stages cT4, pT4, N, and M involve disease dissemination beyond the eye. When both eyes are affected, each eye is staged independently. The stage for a bilaterally affected child is based on the worse-affected eye, as an indicator of risk to the child's life.

Prognosis and prediction

Priorities for treatment of retinoblastoma are first the life of the child, second vision, and third globe salvage. The natural history of retinoblastoma without therapy is 100% mortality {3754}. Currently, therapies to salvage an eye have been greatly optimized to achieve 98% survival. Patients presenting with clinical high-risk features, including any suggestion of optic nerve enlargement or enhancement on MRI, are offered enucleation {1192}. For advanced unilateral retinoblastoma in eyes with limited visual potential, primary enucleation provides the hope of complete curative resection with no need for additional therapy {3754}. The extent of intraocular disease predicts the likelihood to successfully treat an eye with retinoblastoma. Eye salvage treatments historically relied on external beam radiation (EBRT), an option that is now replaced by chemotherapy, sometimes with focal treatment, to minimize radiation-induced secondary malignancies {1690}, radiation retinopathy, and dry eyes. Proton beam therapy delivers an adequate radiation dose to the tumour, with minimal dose to the adjacent tissue and bone, but still carries increased risk of a second primary malignancy in H1 patients.

Chemotherapy is the basis of saving an eye with retinoblastoma. It is delivered by different routes including systemic {2997,1578}, intra-arterial {21,2870,3006}, intravitreal {2317, 2974,2315}, periocular (for locally advanced or recurrent retinoblastoma) {2991}, and more recently intracameral {2318, 146}. In cases of tumour seeding, it is important to adequately

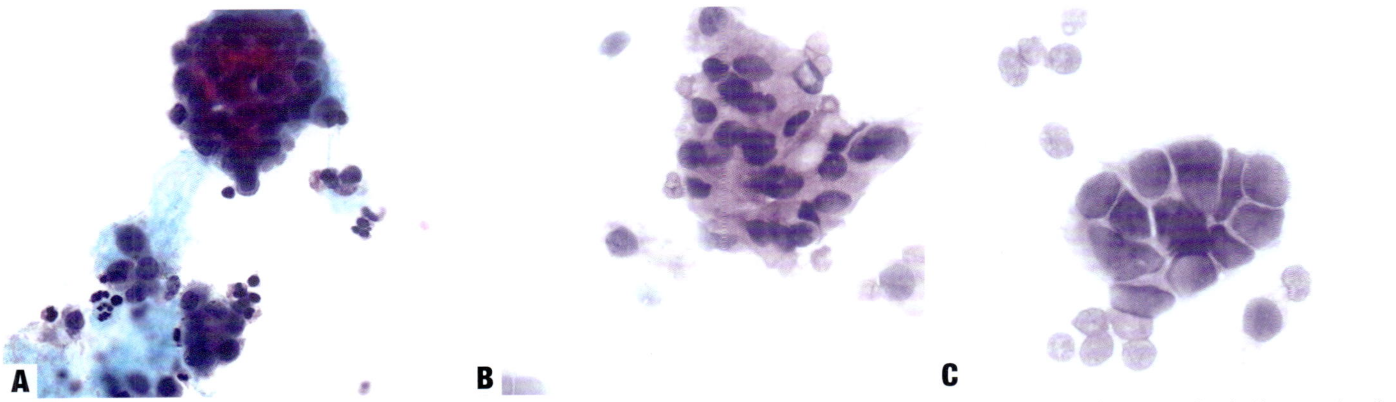

Fig. 5.16 Cytology of retinoblastoma. **A** FNAB of tumour in the anterior chamber shows groups and rosettes of atypical cells with a high N:C ratio associated with apoptotic cells as seen in this Pap-stained liquid-based cytology. **B** An H&E-stained touch imprint of a newly sectioned optic nerve near the true margin shows groups of meningothelial cells (top right), blood, and two atypical retinoblastoma cells with a high N:C ratio (lower left). **C** Nearby the area of meningothelial cells there is a large group of retinoblastoma cells that have a rosette configuration.

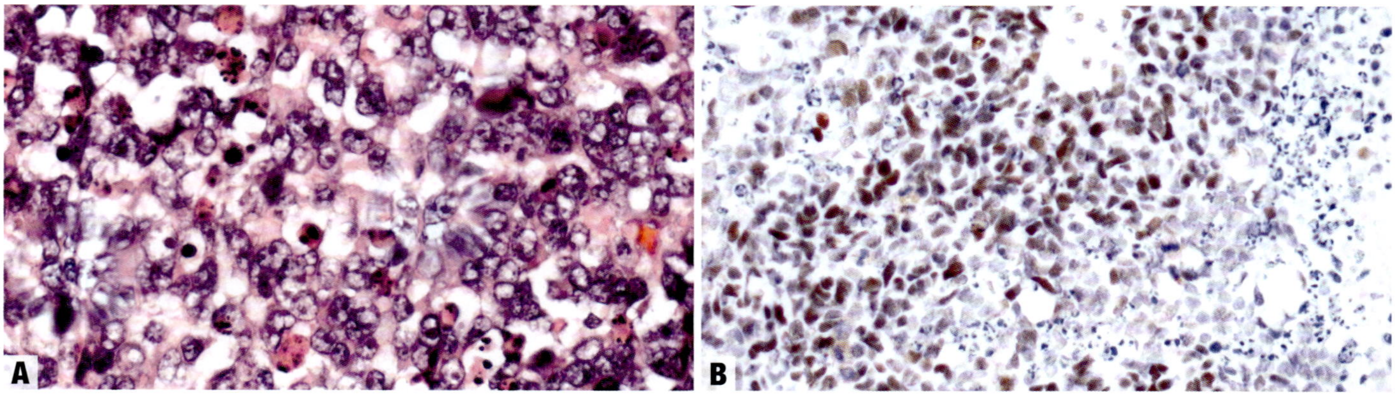

Fig. 5.17 Retinoblastoma with *MYCN* amplification. **A** Histology shows oval-shaped nuclei with large, prominent nucleoli. There are also scattered apoptotic retinoblastoma cells with nuclear debris present. **B** There is positive nuclear staining for RB1 protein, indicating that there is no mutation in *RB1*.

treat the tumour source of the seeding. The presence and type of vitreous seeds {142} can impact the response to chemotherapy {2315,317}. Systemic chemotherapy is paired with focal consolidating treatments to the eye that include cryotherapy, laser photocoagulation, and episcleral plaque brachytherapy {3014}. Among some new therapies being assessed within clinical trials are tylectomy ("tulos", Greek for "lump", surgical resection of retinoblastoma) after standard chemotherapy using chemotherapy infusion during the procedure, and chemoplaque for local chemotherapy control {1954}. Treatment choices depend on the size, number, and location of the tumour deposits within the eye. Regimens vary but most achieve similar efficacies.

The treatment of extraocular retinoblastoma requires the use of systemic chemotherapy, and radiation to the involved orbit and regional lymph nodes. Metastatic retinoblastoma is best treated with bone morrow transplantation {2742,2468}. However, the prognosis for CNS metastases remains poor.

The prognosis for retinoblastoma is excellent, with survival rates reaching 98% in high-income countries {3355,1128}. This can be attributed to radical improvements in understanding of the molecular biology, diagnostics, and therapeutic interventions of the disease. The life salvage rates worldwide vary between 90% and 99%, owing to the differences in age at presentation {1574}, health care facilities within the reach of an affected child {1573}, national income level and health care facilities in the country {3355,1128}, stage of disease at presentation {3628}, and socioeconomic factors {474} across different geographical regions.

Globe salvage rates parallel life salvage trends with failure to salvage the globe in eyes which do not undergo primary enucleation ranging from 25% to 30% {3355}. A paradigm shift from EBRT to combination therapy with focal treatment, chemotherapy (intravenous, intra-arterial, intravitreal, periocular), and plaque brachytherapy has improved the scope of globe salvage, especially in group D retinoblastoma {140}. After resolution of the tumour, periodic surveillance is warranted for early detection of tumour recurrence, metastasis, and development of second primary malignancies {1581,1206,3466,1575,3756}. Multifocal tumours and the presence of retinal detachment are risk factors for tumour recurrence with most occurring within 5 years of completion of primary treatment {1581}. Extraocular extension is an important risk factor for metastatic retinoblastoma {1206}. However, metastasis from intraocular retinoblastoma can also occur. Sites of metastatic deposits include the CNS, lymph nodes, viscera, skull, and long bones {3466}. Children with metastatic disease sparing the CNS fare better than those with CNS involvement {1206}. Retinoblastoma survivors also run a lifetime risk of development of various second primary cancers such as sarcoma, leukaemia, and carcinomas of the breast and genitourinary system. The risk is greater for those with bilateral tumours, germline mutations, and a history of radiotherapy {1575,3756}. Lifelong surveillance is thus warranted for retinoblastoma survivors.

Hamartoma of the retinal pigment epithelium

Eagle RC Jr

Definition

Simple and combined hamartomas of the retinal pigment epithelium (RPE) are hamartomas that are composed of normal retinal elements but lack the distribution and organization of the normal retina and RPE. Congenital simple hamartoma of the RPE involves only the RPE, whereas combined hamartoma of the retina and RPE (CHR-RPE) involve cellular elements of both the retina and the RPE.

ICD-O coding

None

ICD-11 coding

2F36.Y Other specified benign neoplasm of eye or ocular adnexa

Related terminology

Not recommended: retinal hamartoma; hyperplasia of the retinal pigment epithelium; juxtapapillary hamartoma of the retina.

Subtype(s)

None

Localization

Simple RPE hamartoma usually is located in the macula. Combined hamartoma occurs most commonly on, or adjacent to, the optic disc, but also may occur in extrapapillary areas of the fundus.

Clinical features

Combined hamartoma of the retina and RPE typically appears as a poorly defined grey retinal mass with blood vessels that are tortuous or straightened by secondary retinal traction caused by excessive glial tissue on the lesion's surface {1007,2863, 3023}. Variable amounts of pigment, telangiectatic vessels, and white glial tissue occur. CHR-RPE can vary markedly in size, ranging from 1 mm to > 10 mm in diameter with a mean diameter of 7.6 mm {3023}. The lesions may be slightly elevated, and their thickness can gradually increase over time. Visual acuity is variable and depends on the size and location of the lesion and the amount of retinal traction. Affected children often present with visual loss when they fail preschool screening. Macular tumours can cause profound visual loss {3023}. Most combined hamartomas are stable lesions. but retinal traction secondary to glial proliferation can cause progressive visual loss. Vitreous haemorrhage, exudation, and choroidal neovascularization occur rarely.

Fluorescein angiography shows early hypofluorescence due to blockage in hyperpigmented areas. Abnormal dilated capillaries, tortuous vessels, and leakage may be observed in the later phases {2863}.

Ocular coherence tomography of CHR-RPE discloses a thickened mass of focally disorganized retina with a sawtooth or folded pattern of retinal folds caused by vitreoretinal traction secondary to prominent epiretinal membranes {183}.

Simple hamartomas of the RPE are very rare small, dark, elevated lesions that usually are located within the macula {3018}.

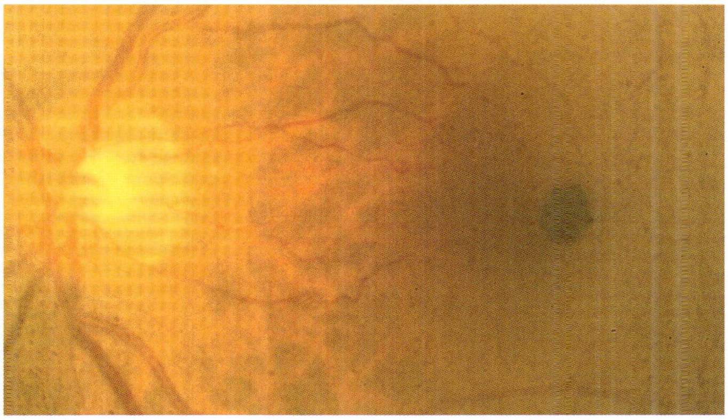

Fig. 5.18 Congenital simple hamartoma of the retinal pigment epithelium. This discrete heavily pigmented simple retinal pigment epithelium hamartoma is located near the fovea.

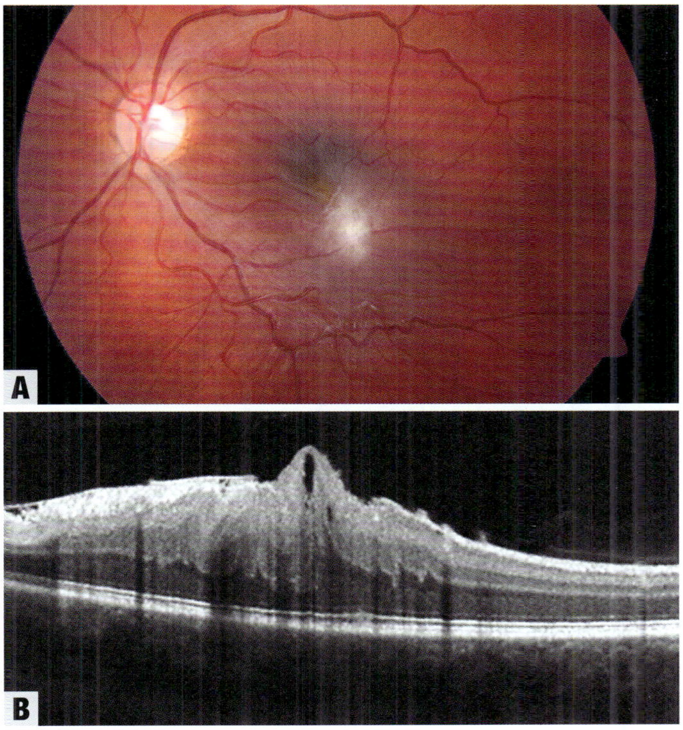

Fig. 5.19 Combined hamartoma of the retina and retinal pigment epithelium. **A** The epiretinal glial component of this grey subfoveal combined hamartoma exerts vitreoretinal traction on retinal vessels. **B** Optical coherence tomography of this combined hamartoma discloses a focal area of thickened disorganized retina with an epiretinal membrane and retinal folds.

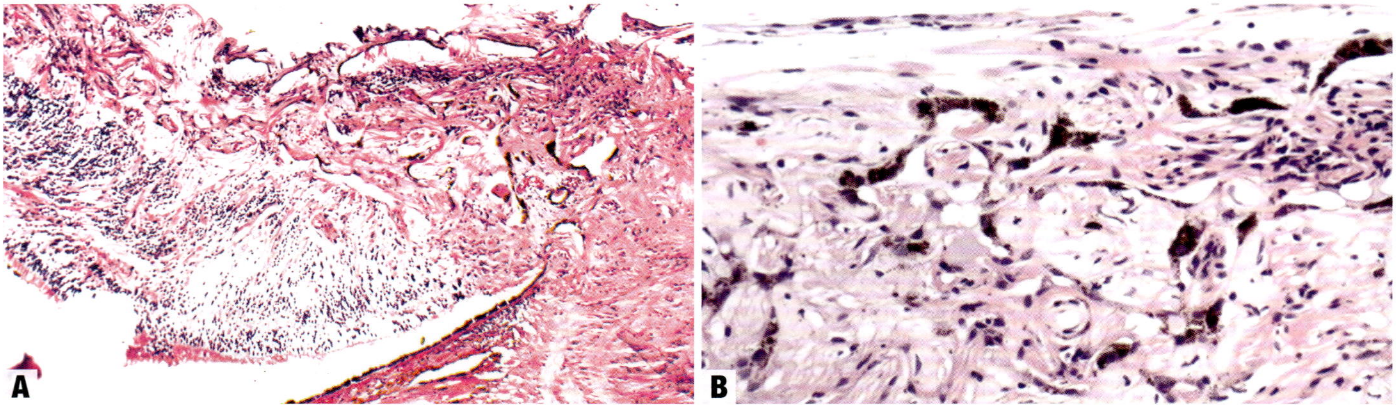

Fig. 5.20 Combined hamartoma of the retina and retinal pigment epithelium. **A** There is abnormal organization of the retinal layers of the juxtapapillary retina; pigmented cells are evident in the retinal layers. **B** There is a thin epiretinal membrane on the surface of the retina; the organization of the retinal layers is abnormal and pigmented cells are evident within the superficial retinal layers.

They are asymptomatic and most are found incidentally in eyes with good vision. Optical coherence tomography discloses a full-thickness retinal lesion with abrupt margins, high-surface reflectivity, and deep optical shadowing.

Epidemiology

Combined hamartomas of the retina and RPE are rare lesions. There is a slight male predominance of affected patients {1007,2863,3023}. The mean and median patient age at initial diagnosis in one large series was 11.9 months and 7.5 months, respectively, with a range of 0.4–60 months {3023}. The lesions are almost always unilateral and sporadic. However, CHR-RPE is associated with neurofibromatosis type 1 {3384,3492} and type 2 {1161,2717,974,3129}, and also has been reported in association with naevoid basal cell carcinoma syndrome (Gorlin syndrome) {2842,746}, branchio-oculo-facial syndrome {3053,770}, branchio-otic syndrome {1560}, benign branchial cleft cysts {226}, juvenile nasopharyngeal angiofibroma {1002}, and Poland anomaly {3221}. Bilateral combined hamartomas have been reported as the presenting feature of a severe phenotype of neurofibromatosis type 2 {974}.

Etiology

Simple and combined hamartomas of the RPE are probably congenital lesions; the median age at diagnosis is quite young, and the lesions have been observed in infants. A number of systemic associations have been reported including neurofibromatosis type 1 and neurofibromatosis type 2.

Pathogenesis

Unknown

Macroscopic appearance

See *Clinical features*, above.

Histopathology

CHR-RPEs are composed of disorganized glial tissue intermixed with numerous blood vessels and with cords and tubules of proliferated RPE. A glial epiretinal membrane is present on the surface of the retina. Pigmented cells may be present in the membrane {1007}.

Histopathology of a single case of congenital simple hamartoma of the RPE revealed a nodular proliferation of hyperplastic RPE that had undergone fibrous metaplasia {259}.

Differential diagnosis

The differential diagnosis may be influenced by the patient's age at presentation. In younger patients presenting with leukocoria, retinoblastoma is an important differential diagnostic consideration. In older patients, the differential diagnosis of pigmented CHR-RPE includes uveal melanoma and melanocytoma. Most cases of CHR-RPE can be readily distinguished from retinoblastoma and uveal melanoma. Less-common conditions that should also be considered are adenoma of the RPE, persistent fetal vasculature, and morning glory disc malformations.

Cytology

Insufficient information

Diagnostic molecular pathology

Not relevant

Essential and desirable diagnostic criteria

Essential: well-circumscribed, mostly flat, pigmented lesion in the posterior pole.

Desirable: glial tissue intermixed with numerous blood vessels and with cords and tubules of proliferated RPE; linear dragging of vessels by vitreoretinal traction; normal retinal elements with abnormal distribution and organization.

Staging

Not relevant

Prognosis and prediction

RPE hamartomas are benign. Patients with CHR-RPE can experience progressive visual loss due to tumour growth or complications associated with the tumour. In one series, 60% of patients with macular tumours lost three or more lines of Snellen visual acuity at 4 years, compared with 13% of those with extramacular tumours {3023}. Some patients have visual loss due to amblyopia, which can be improved with treatment. Vitreoretinal surgery can improve vision in some patients' progressive vitreoretinal traction {647}.

Congenital hypertrophy of the retinal pigment epithelium

Materin MA

Definition

Congenital hypertrophy of the retinal pigment epithelium (CHRPE) is a congenital patch of hypertrophic, benign retinal pigment epithelial (RPE) cells containing macromelanosomes.

ICD-O coding

None

ICD-11 coding

2F36.Y Other specified benign neoplasm of eye or ocular adnexa

Related terminology

Acceptable: solitary congenital hypertrophy of the retinal pigment epithelium.

Subtype(s)

None

Localization

These lesions usually affect the peripheral or midperipheral fundus, but 2% of cases occur in the macular or peripapillary region {209,1794}.

Clinical features

CHRPE presents as a unilateral, sharply demarcated, flat or minimally elevated plaque of abnormally tall RPE cells {2607, 2998}. The lesions are typically asymptomatic and are found incidentally during ophthalmoscopy. Most lesions are round or oval, 13% are geographical with smooth margins marked by focal convexities, and 85% are jet black or dark brown. Rare non-pigmented cases in adults probably result from the confluence of characteristic depigmented intralesional lacunae, which develop in 43% of CHRPE lesions and have been documented to enlarge gradually in 32% of cases. The reported mean and median largest diameters are 4.7 mm and 4.5 mm, respectively (range: 1–13 mm). Most lesions are surrounded by a narrow pigmented or depigmented ring or halo. Of lesions followed up for > 3 years, 83% have shown subtle enlargement {182,366,2998,3617}. Nodules develop in about 1% of cases and have been confirmed to be RPE adenocarcinomas in several instances {3039,3057,3071,3373}. Optical coherence tomography reveals thinning and photoreceptor loss in the overlying retina {780,1050,1734,2441,2999}. Careful perimetry may disclose a focal scotoma corresponding to the lesion {2607}. CHRPE appears dark on fundus autofluorescence imaging {3002,3258}.

CHRPE must be distinguished from choroidal naevus, small choroidal melanoma, congenital grouped pigmentation (so-called bear tracks), adenoma and adenocarcinoma of the RPE, solitary hamartoma of the RPE, torpedo maculopathy, and pigmented ocular fundus lesion (POFL) or hamartoma

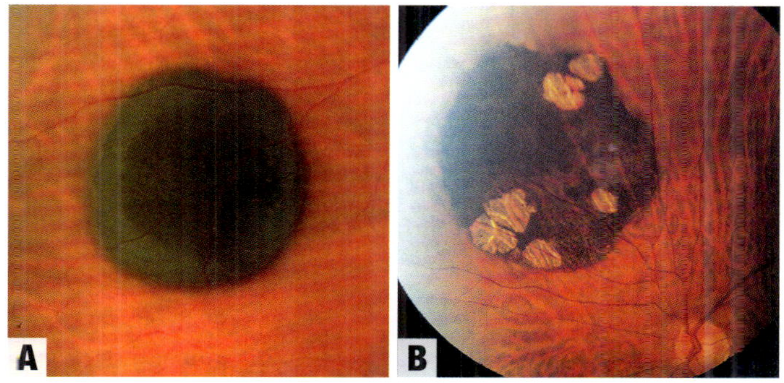

Fig. 5.21 Congenital hypertrophy of the retinal pigment epithelium. **A** Ophthalmoscopy discloses a round, deeply pigmented lesion with no lacunae. **B** A larger lesion has smooth, scalloped margins and multiple depigmented lacunae.

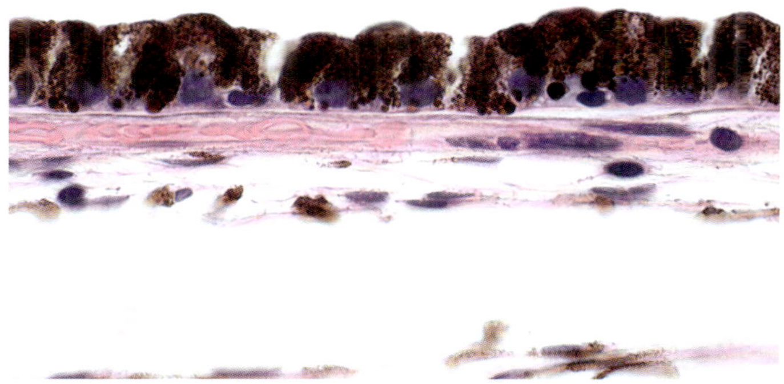

Fig. 5.22 Congenital hypertrophy of the retinal pigment epithelium. The cytoplasm of tall retinal pigment epithelial cells is packed with large round melanosomes (including macromelanosomes).

of the RPE in familial adenomatous polyposis (FAP). Unfortunately, the term "congenital hypertrophy of the retinal pigment epithelium" is often used erroneously in the non-ophthalmic literature to designate POFLs or hamartomas of the RPE that occur in some kindreds with FAP. Unlike CHRPE, hamartoma of the RPE tends to be multiple and bilateral, and it has less well defined margins {3367,3368}. In a clinicopathological study, three types of POFLs were identified: one type similar to CHRPE and two types consistent with hamartomatous RPE malformations in a patient with FAP {3369}. In 1 patient with a POFL and FAP, optical coherence tomography disclosed retinal invasion {3405}. CHRPE should not be used to determine the presence of hereditary FAP, though ophthalmoscopy may be helpful in addition to other investigations {2688}.

Epidemiology

These lesions are believed to be congenital, but the mean patient age at diagnosis is 43 years (range: < 1 year to 83 years). There is no race predilection. A mild female predominance has been reported, with 64% of cases occurring in female patients {514,2998,3082}.

Etiology

CHRPE is believed to be a developmental lesion {1982} and is associated with FAP, where it may be present in as many as 80% of patients {2688}.

Pathogenesis

The lesion originates from the RPE. There is no genetic profile and no germline mutations have been found in the *APC* gene within the lesions.

Macroscopic appearance

See *Clinical features*.

Histopathology

Light microscopy reveals a monolayer of thickened RPE cells. The cytoplasm is packed with large round melanosomes, which often obscure the nucleus {437,514,1982,2501}. Lacunae show segmental loss of the RPE and focal chorioretinal adhesions. Fluorescence microscopy confirms the absence of lipofuscin in dysfunctional RPE cells. The sharply circumscribed patches of abnormal RPE cells are readily apparent on scanning electron microscopy {514,1982}.

An increased amount of melanin pigment is also found focally in RPE cells in congenital grouped pigmentation (so-called bear tracks), but the granules retain their normal ellipsoidal configuration and do not fill the entire cytoplasm {2687,3074}.

Cytology

Not relevant

Diagnostic molecular pathology

Not clinically relevant

Essential and desirable diagnostic criteria

Essential: unilateral, sharply demarcated, flat or minimally elevated plaque of abnormally tall RPE cells.

Staging

None

Prognosis and prediction

Most cases are benign and asymptomatic and require no treatment. Rarely, RPE adenoma or low-grade RPE adenocarcinoma may develop from CHRPE {3039,3057,3071,3373}. Typical CHRPE does not appear to be associated with FAP or colorectal adenocarcinoma {1315,2192,3070}.

Reactive hyperplasia of the retinal pigment epithelium

Materin MA

Definition

Reactive hyperplasia of the retinal pigment epithelium (RPE) is a non-neoplastic proliferation of RPE cells.

ICD-O coding

None

ICD-11 coding

9B7Y Other specified disorders of the retina

Related terminology

Acceptable: nodular hyperplasia of the retinal pigment epithelium.
Not recommended: pseudoepitheliomatous hyperplasia; pseudoadenomatous hyperplasia; reactive hyperplastic lesion of the retinal pigment epithelium; ringschwiele.

Subtype(s)

None

Localization

Reactive hyperplasia of the RPE can occur anywhere in the retina {1298}.

Clinical features

RPE hyperplasia is classified as localized, multifocal, or diffuse. It presents as darkly pigmented deposits. The pigment may be associated with retinal blood vessels, resulting in a spiculated appearance.

Nodular reactive RPE hyperplasia can be confused with adenomatous RPE tumours or choroidal melanoma. On fluorescein angiography, reactive RPE hyperplasia shows early hypofluorescence, with areas of hyperfluorescence in the late phase. It shows high reflectivity on ultrasound {1298}.

Epidemiology

The incidence is unknown. Reactive hyperplasia of the RPE can occur in patients of any age and either sex. Multifocal hyperplasia may be seen in older people.

Etiology

The etiology of primary hyperplasia is unknown. Secondary hyperplasia can occur secondary to congenital abnormalities, inflammation, degenerative diseases, intoxications, radiation-induced choroiditis, chronic retinal detachment, subretinal haemorrhage, sequelae of traumatic retinopathy, or retinitis pigmentosa {1030, 1298}. There may be a chronic vitreous base and zonular traction.

Pathogenesis

The proliferation of RPE cells is induced by growth factors.

Macroscopic appearance

See *Clinical features*.

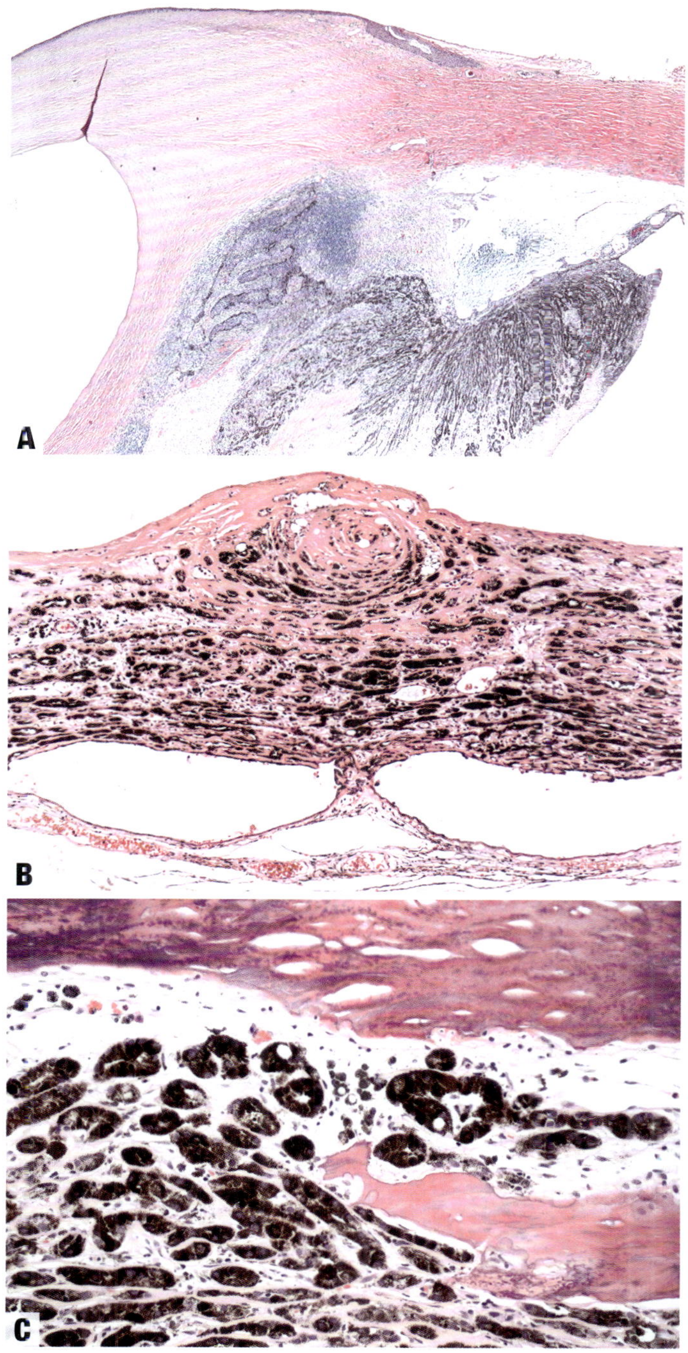

Fig. 5.23 Reactive hyperplasia of the retinal pigment epithelium. **A** The ringschwiele shows lymphocytic infiltration close by, a possible source of growth factors. **B** Layers of proliferating pigmented retinal pigment epithelial cells over the choroid (lower field) alternate with extracellular basement membrane material. **C** Cords and tubules of proliferating retinal pigment epithelial cells are seen adjacent to metaplastic bony tissue in a phthisical eye.

Histopathology

Reactive RPE hyperplasia can range from simple duplication of cells to massive proliferations with intervening basement membrane material; in advanced, late-stage cases, the hyperplasia may be accompanied by collections of connective and osteoid tissue {1030}.

In nodular reactive proliferation of the RPE, the cells are arranged in a tubular pseudoadenomatous pattern, with a large amount of basement membrane–like material. Areas of extracellular material alternate with areas of cellular proliferation. Neoplastic features, mitotic figures, and necrosis are absent {3390}.

Differential diagnosis

Reactive hyperplasia of the RPE must be distinguished from choroidal melanoma, RPE adenoma, RPE adenocarcinoma, congenital hypertrophy of the RPE, combined hamartoma of the retina and RPE, and simple hamartoma of the RPE.

Cytology

Not relevant

Diagnostic molecular pathology

Not relevant

Essential and desirable diagnostic criteria

Essential: darkly pigmented deposits in the retina, which may be associated with retinal blood vessels and/or nodular; proliferation of the RPE, often with intervening basement membrane material.

Staging

Not relevant

Prognosis and prediction

These lesions are benign; the survival prognosis is excellent. The visual prognosis depends on the underlying process. Longstanding RPE hyperplasia in disorganized, blind eyes may rarely give rise to RPE adenocarcinoma {862,1307,1985,2803}.

Adenoma and adenocarcinoma of the retinal pigment epithelium

Eagle RC Jr
Mori T

Definition

Adenomas and adenocarcinomas of the retinal pigment epithelium (RPE) are benign and malignant neoplasms derived from the RPE.

ICD-O coding

8140/0 Retinal pigment epithelial adenoma
8140/3 Retinal pigment epithelial adenocarcinoma

ICD-11 coding

2F36.Y & XH3DV3 Other specified benign neoplasm of eye or ocular adnexa & Adenoma, NOS
2D02.0 Adenocarcinoma of retinal pigment epithelium

Related terminology

Acceptable: epithelioma of the retinal pigment epithelium; retinal pigment epithelial carcinoma; malignant epithelioma of the retinal pigment epithelium.

Subtype(s)

None

Localization

RPE adenomas typically affect the peripheral retina but may occur adjacent to the optic disc {361,3040}. RPE adenocarcinomas have no predilection for laterality or retinal location.

Clinical features

Patients typically present with blurred vision, but can be asymptomatic. Choroidal melanoma is a common referring diagnosis. RPE neoplasms are solitary, unilateral tumours located on the inner surface of the choroid. They typically are oval and dome shaped with an abrupt vertical elevation at the edge of the tumour and a derby-hat configuration. They are 6 mm in mean basal diameter and 3.5 mm in thickness. Although adenomas and adenocarcinomas of the RPE typically are dark grey or jet black in colour, about 8% are amelanotic or yellow. Perforation of the overlying retina occurs frequently, and many cases develop a retinal blood supply with dilated and tortuous retinal feeder arteries and draining veins. In contrast to uveal melanoma, more than half of RPE neoplasms often have prominent yellow intraretinal and subretinal exudates, and 22% have exudative retinal detachments {3611,3053}. B-scan ultrasonography discloses mostly dome-shaped or derby hat–shaped lesions that are acoustically solid and lack extraocular extension or choroidal excavation. They often are hypofluorescent in the early stages of intravenous fluorescein angiography, are isofluorescent or hyperfluorescent in the mid/late phases with leakage or staining, and also lack the double circulation pattern of internal vascularity found in many melanomas. Optical coherence tomography of RPE adenocarcinomas typically shows retinal invasion and posterior shadowing, high anterior reflectivity with an irregular or rugged surface and occasional vitreous seeds. Some tumours appear to contain optically empty cavities {3611,3181}.

Epidemiology

These tumours occur in adults. The mean patient age at diagnosis is 51 years (range: 18–83 years) {3611}. There is no race predilection {3066,3053}. Two thirds of cases occur in women {3611}.

Etiology

These are acquired neuroepithelial neoplasms that arise from the RPE. About one fifth are associated with congenital hypertrophy of the RPE. Several RPE adenocarcinomas that have arisen from CHRPE have been confirmed histopathologically {3611,3039,3057,3373}.

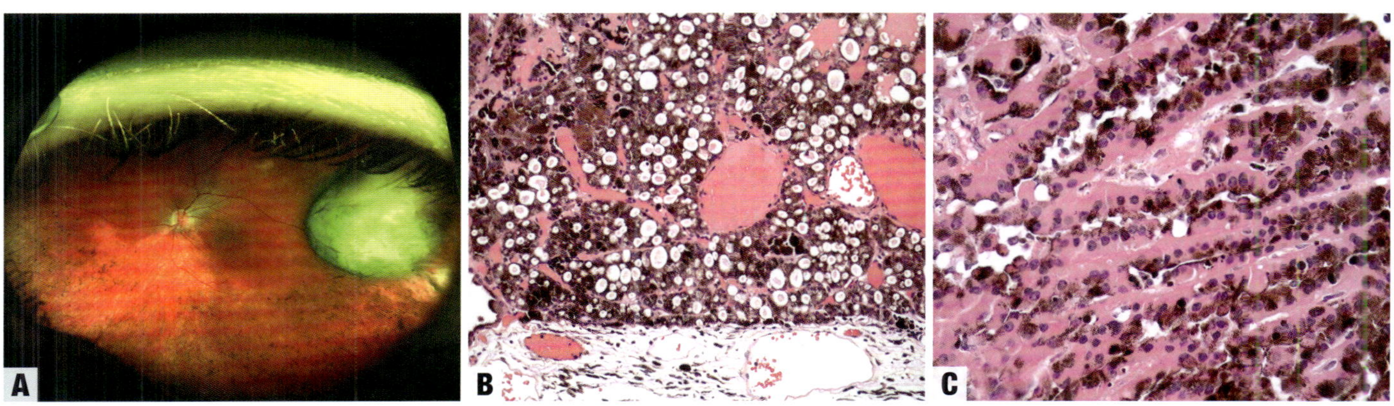

Fig. 5.24 Adenoma of the retinal pigment epithelium. **A** A mass lies below the retina in this clinical image. **B** Cystic adenoma. This heavily pigmented tumour is located on the inner surface of the choroid as a cytologically bland neoplasm containing cyst-like spaces. **C** The cells form characteristic linear bands and have bland nuclei.

Pathogenesis

Some cases may develop from reactive RPE hyperplasia in blind disorganized eyes after trauma or inflammation {3053}. About 12% of patients have a history of ocular trauma, a potential nidus for RPE hyperplasia {3611}.

Macroscopic appearance

Most RPE tumours appear as heavily pigmented oval and dome-shaped lesions with abruptly elevated margins situated on the inner surface of the choroid. Exudative retinal detachment, lipid exudation, retinal invasion with perforation, and vitreous seeding often are present.

Histopathology

Contiguous with the adjacent RPE, RPE tumours are situated on the inner surface of the Bruch membrane. The location on the inner surface of the choroid is one of the most important features that serve to differentiate RPE tumours from choroidal melanoma on routine histopathological examination. Invasion, and often perforation, of the overlying retina occurs in all cases and vitreous seeding may be present. Much of the tumour is often situated anterior to the plane of the surrounding retina. Choroidal invasion occurs in some cases and is evidence of aggressive behaviour. It is one of the histological criteria for malignancy, which also include nuclear atypia and mitotic activity, which is minimal or absent in most cases.

RPE tumours may be solid, vacuolated, or combined {1010,1298}. Tumours arising from the peripheral RPE often have vacuolated cells similar to those in pigmented ciliary epithelial tumours {2274}. The cells of posterior RPE tumours typically are arranged in linear arrays or strands on prominent PAS-positive connective tissue septa. The tumour cells also can form tubules, lobules, or pseudoglandular structures. The cells of RPE adenocarcinoma often are quite atypical with nuclear pleomorphism and prominent nucleoli and are easily confused with epithelioid melanoma cells, especially on FNAB. Mitotic activity typically is low. Foci of heavily pigmented RPE cells consistent with residual CHRPE are observed at the base of some tumours {3039}. Transmission electron microscopy discloses intercellular junctions in RPE tumours {2274,1010}.

Immunohistochemistry

Immunoreactivity is variable and somewhat nonspecific. RPE tumours typically show variable immunoreactivity for the epithelial markers CK7, AE1/AE3, CAM 5.2, and EMA as well as vimentin, but also may stain for melanocytic markers that are expressed by uveal melanoma. In one large series of RPE neoplasms, 100% stained with S100, 44% with melan-A (MART1), and 22% with HMB45 {3611}.

The commonly used melanocytic marker SOX10 stains both melanocytes and RPE cells. Although staining for epithelial markers is suggestive, uveal melanomas occasionally are immunoreactive for cytokeratin {1312}.

Considering this significant immunohistochemical overlap between RPE tumours and uveal melanoma, care should be taken in interpreting immunohistochemical reaction of pigmented intraocular tumours. Routine histopathological features

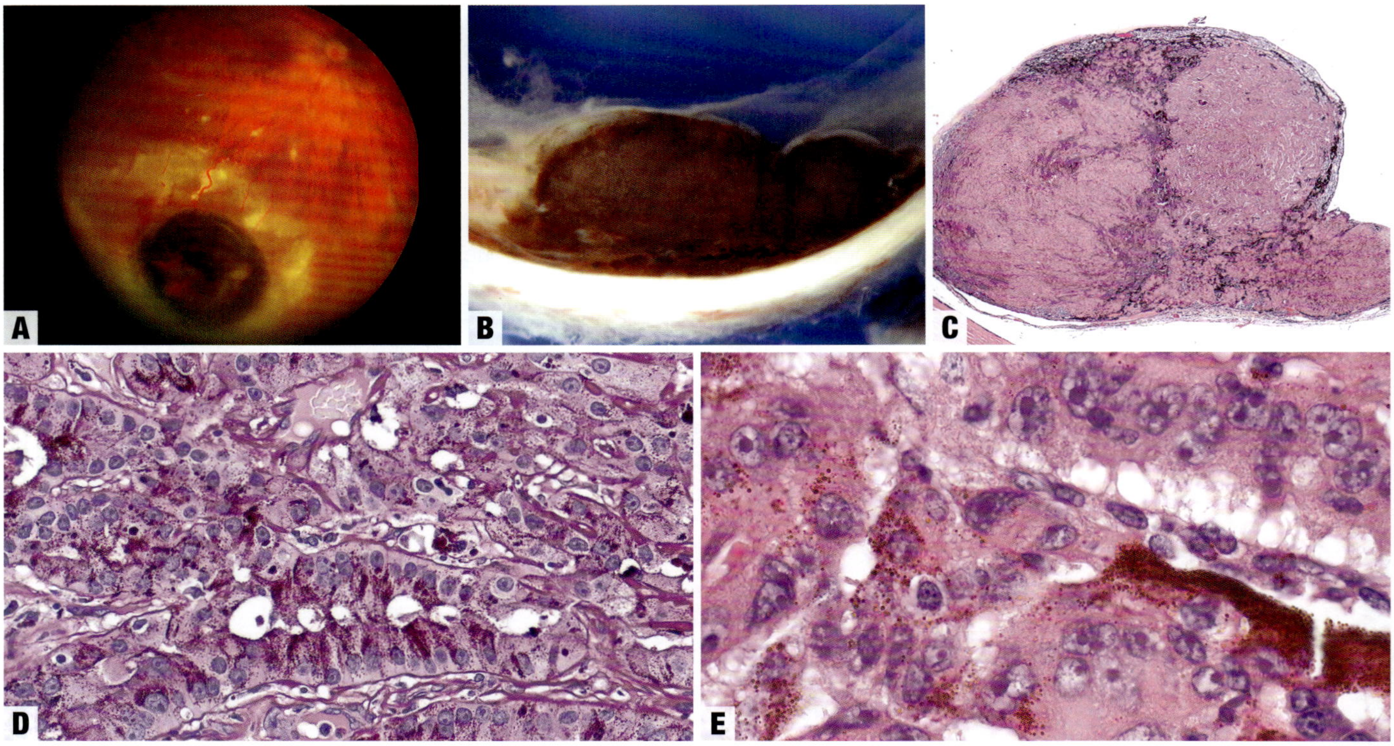

Fig. 5.25 Adenocarcinoma of the retinal pigment epithelium (RPE). **A** A clinical ophthalmoscopy image shows a darkly pigmented tumour with abrupt margins. The tumour has perforated the retina and is surrounded by exudates. **B** A heavily pigmented tumour rests on the inner surface of the choroid and invades the overlying retina. **C** A largely non-pigmented RPE adenocarcinoma with abrupt margins is seen. The tumour rests on the inner surface of the choroid and invades the overlying retina. This tumour was observed clinically to arise from a congenital hypertrophy of the RPE. **D** Linear bands of tumour cells rest on PAS-positive septa. The tumour cells have prominent nucleoli (PAS stain). **E** The nuclei of pleomorphic RPE tumours have prominent nucleoli and peripheral chromatin margination.

including tumour location on the inner surface of the choroid, a characteristic linear arrangement of cells on PAS-positive septa, and scant mitotic activity should be the major diagnostic criteria for diagnosis of RPE tumours, not immunohistochemistry.

Differential diagnosis

Differentiating RPE adenomas from adenocarcinomas generally is impossible clinically and is often challenging histopathologically. Histopathological features that favour adenocarcinoma include cellular pleomorphism and nuclear atypia, mitotic activity, choroidal invasion and other evidence of aggressive behaviour.

Cytology

Cytological assessment can be difficult. Adenocarcinoma cells and epithelioid melanoma cells can appear similar and there is significant immunohistochemical overlap between RPE tumours and uveal melanoma {3032}. It is very important to correlate the cytological findings with clinical and imaging findings.

Diagnostic molecular pathology

Not relevant

Essential and desirable diagnostic criteria

Essential: tumour location on the inner surface of the choroid; characteristic linear arrangement of cells on septa; scant mitotic activity.

Staging

Not relevant

Prognosis and prediction

Prognosis for life is excellent if the tumour has not spread extraocularly. There are very few documented cases of metastatic RPE carcinoma {3181,1307,1913}. Poor vision and enucleation are associated with larger thicker tumours and exudative retinal detachment {3611}.

Reactive epithelial hyperplasia of the ciliary epithelium

Roberts F
Loeffler KU

Definition
Reactive epithelial hyperplasia of the ciliary epithelium is an increase in the number and volume of the ciliary epithelial cells, usually in response to injury or inflammation.

ICD-O coding
None

ICD-11 coding
9A90.Y Other specified degeneration of iris or ciliary body

Related terminology
Not recommended: pseudoadenomatous hyperplasia.

Subtype(s)
None

Localization
Reactive epithelial hyperplasia occurs over the pars plana or pars plicata of the ciliary body, often with extension into the adjacent posterior chamber or vitreous base.

Clinical features
Reactive epithelial hyperplasia is typically an incidental finding in eyes enucleated because of other substantial pathology. It is almost always clinically obscured by opaque media of the diseased eye.

Epidemiology
The incidence is unknown. Reactive epithelial hyperplasia is seen mostly in eyes that have been subject to significant injury.

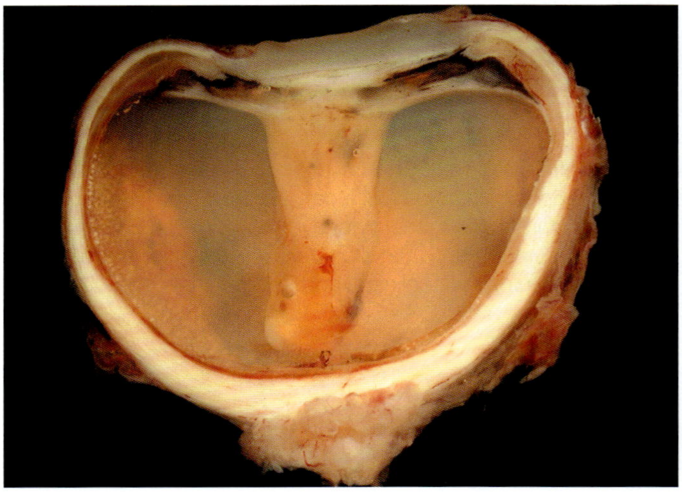

Fig. 5.26 Cyclitic membrane showing reactive epithelial hyperplasia. A macroscopic photo of an aphakic eye with longstanding retinal detachment and formation of a cyclitic membrane forming a fibrous sheet extending from the ciliary body.

Etiology
Reactive epithelial hyperplasia of the ciliary body occurs in reaction to physical injury, surgery including cryotherapy, inflammation including pars planitis {660}, and longstanding retinal detachment. It occurs fairly often in end-stage, blind, phthisical eyes {3376}.

Pathogenesis
Reactive hyperplasia may be induced by growth factors released during and after the inciting insult.

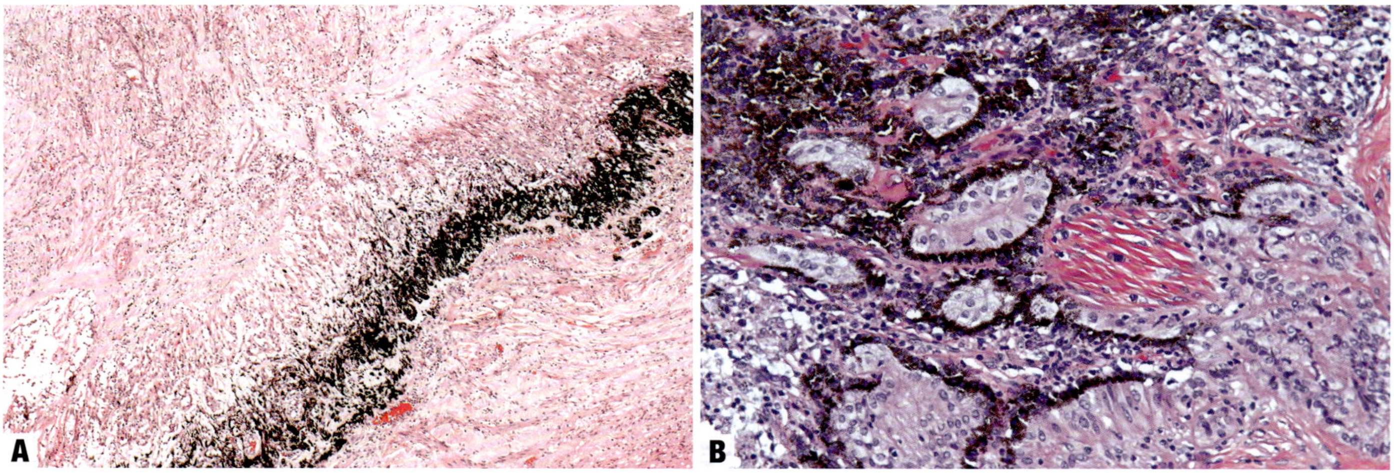

Fig. 5.27 Reactive epithelial hyperplasia. **A** A reactive proliferation of the non-pigmented ciliary epithelium forming cords and glandular structures within the fibrous tissue of a cyclitic membrane in an enucleation specimen after failed treatment of retinal detachment. **B** A multilayered proliferation of cells of the non-pigmented inner layer of the ciliary epithelium flanked by its non-proliferating pigmented outer layer, in an enucleated eye from a 3-year-old child with persistent fetal vasculature (previously called persistent hyperplastic primary vitreous).

Macroscopic appearance

Although generally obscured by opaque refractive media of the diseased eye, reactive epithelial hyperplasia, typically with accompanying fibrous metaplasia, may form a cyclitic membrane: a variably pigmented fibrous sheet that extends from the ciliary body behind and around the lens.

Histopathology

The hyperplastic ciliary epithelium either proliferates as cords and strands or forms pseudoacinar structures. The proliferating cells derive predominantly from the inner, non-pigmented layer of the ciliary epithelium, but cells from the outer, pigmented epithelial layer may also contribute. The cells are entrapped within a variable amount of fibrous stroma, induced by the underlying insult, and they may appear stretched within this fibrous tissue. Together, the reactively proliferating epithelial cells and fibrous stroma may form a tumour-like mass or, more commonly, a diffuse cyclitic membrane over the ciliary body, extending towards the lens {2864}.

Cytology

The proliferating cells vary in shape but show bland cytological features, minimal mitotic activity, and no invasive features.

Diagnostic molecular pathology

Not available

Essential and desirable diagnostic criteria

Essential: predominantly non-pigmented ciliary epithelial cells with bland cytological features that proliferate as cords and strands or form pseudoacinar structures, forming a membrane together with associated fibrous metaplasia.

Desired: a phthisical eye after past injury or inflammation.

Staging

Not relevant

Prognosis and prediction

The prognosis for vision depends on the inciting pathology and its effect on the eye. These proliferations generally become increasingly fibrous with time after the inciting pathology has subsided. It is suspected that a longstanding reactive proliferation of the ciliary epithelium in a phthisical eye may occasionally give rise to an adenocarcinoma of the ciliary body {3034,3234, 831,1264,1870,1772}.

Nodular hyperplasia of the ciliary epithelium

Roberts F
Loeffler KU

Definition
Nodular hyperplasia of the ciliary epithelium is a well-circumscribed proliferation of the inner non-pigmented epithelium of the pars plicata of the ciliary body not associated with injury.

ICD-O coding
None

ICD-11 coding
9A90.Y Other specified degeneration of iris or ciliary body

Related terminology
Acceptable: adenomatous hyperplasia of the ciliary body; Fuchs adenoma.
Not recommended: coronal adenoma; age-related hyperplasia of the non-pigmented ciliary body epithelium; pseudoadenomatous hyperplasia of the ciliary body epithelium.

Subtype(s)
None

Localization
Hyperplasia of the ciliary epithelium is located in the pars plicata of the ciliary body and is usually confined to a single ciliary process.

Clinical features
Hyperplasia of the ciliary epithelium is typically an incidental finding in an enucleated eye, because it is generally small and asymptomatic. It can be imaged by ultrasound biomicroscopy {2166}. It can occasionally cause a sectoral cataract or grow to sufficient size to involve the iris root. Rarely, a larger hyperplasia may mimic a malignant tumour of the ciliary body {3522}. These lesions can be solitary or multiple and unilateral or bilateral.

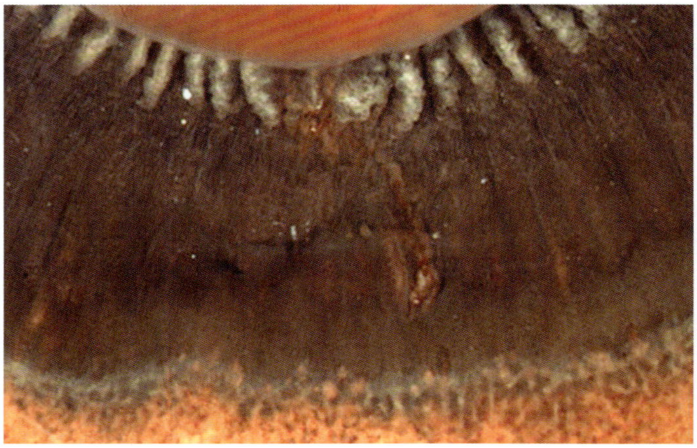

Fig. 5.28 Nodular hyperplasia of the ciliary body. A macroscopic image of an example presenting as a small nodular expansion of a single ciliary process.

Epidemiology
Hyperplasia of the ciliary epithelium is associated with age. At autopsy, these lesions are found in only about 5% of eyes from individuals < 50 years of age, but in about 60% of eyes from individuals > 80 years {3034}.

Etiology
Hyperplasia of the ciliary epithelium is an age-related degenerative lesion.

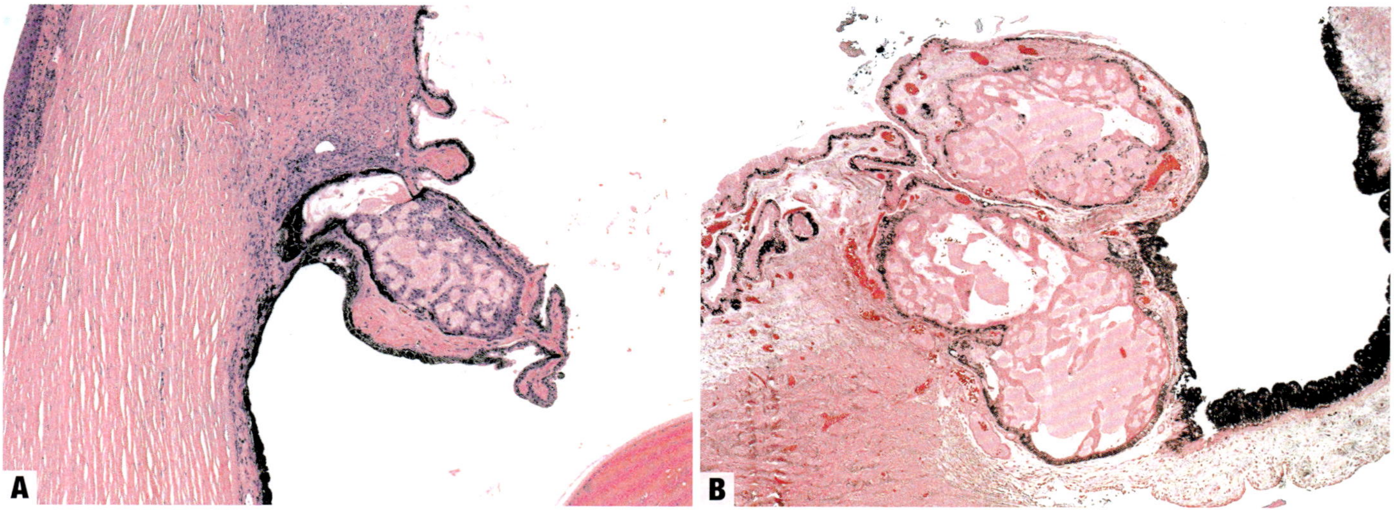

Fig. 5.29 Nodular hyperplasia of ciliary body. **A** A single ciliary process is expanded by non-pigmented cells (derived from the ciliary epithelium) in interlacing cords, separated by hyaline extracellular material. **B** Rarely, larger nodules composed of non-pigmented ciliary epithelium with variable amounts of extracellular matrix can extend behind the iris.

Pathogenesis
This type of hyperplasia of the ciliary epithelium results in a nodular growth pattern. It appears to be associated with ageing. No genetic profile has been published.

Macroscopic appearance
Hyperplasias of the ciliary epithelium appear as small, yellowish-white or slightly pigmented nodules in a single ciliary process in the pars plicata of the ciliary body.

Histopathology
Hyperplasia of the ciliary epithelium forms a small nodule that is composed of interlacing cords of uniform non-pigmented ciliary epithelial cells, surrounded by amorphous extracellular hyaline material that stains with PAS. The nodules may be pedunculated, countersunk, or embedded in the stroma of the ciliary body. In some cases, the extracellular material may be the predominant feature, with only occasional strands of epithelial cells. The extracellular material is immunoreactive for collagen IV and laminin {3034}. Immunoreactivity for vimentin is reported {2416}.

Cytology
Not relevant

Diagnostic molecular pathology
Not relevant

Essential and desirable diagnostic criteria
Essential: a nodule of interlacing cords of uniform non-pigmented ciliary epithelial cells surrounded by PAS-positive amorphous extracellular hyaline material.

Staging
Not relevant

Prognosis and prediction
Hyperplasia of the ciliary epithelium is a benign reactive proliferation and usually an incidental finding in an enucleated eye. The prognosis for vision is excellent. Occasionally, it can cause sectoral cataract or grow to sufficient size to involve the iris root and simulate a malignant neoplasm of the ciliary body necessitating removal {3522}.

Glioneuronal hamartoma of the ciliary body

Kivelä T
Rodriguez FJ

Definition
Glioneuronal hamartoma of the ciliary body is a tumour-like neuroglial lesion occurring at the margin of the optic cup, often with an adjacent chorioretinal coloboma.

ICD-O coding
None

ICD-11 coding
LA11.Y Other specified structural developmental anomalies of the anterior segment of eye

Related terminology
Acceptable: glioneuroma of the ciliary body.

Subtype(s)
None

Localization
Localization is in the ciliary body, typically in the temporal quadrant, with frequent extension to the iris and retina {27,1726,2062, 3177}.

Clinical features
Lesions appear as a tan, slowly growing mass, usually detected before the first year of life, often at birth. Extraocular extension may be present {3177,1726}. A chorioretinal coloboma may coexist but not be clinically detectable {1726, 3177}. The eye may secondarily be smaller or larger than the contralateral eye, the cornea and lens may be cloudy {3177, 27}, a persistent pupillary membrane or hyaloid artery may be present {2062,3177}, and the intraocular pressure may be elevated {1726,3177}. The tumour enhances with contrast medium on CT {1726}.

Epidemiology
Lesions are very rare. Fewer than 10 cases have been published {27,1726,2062,3177}.

Etiology
Lesions arise as a congenital developmental mass {1726,3177}. There is no association with neurofibromatosis type 1 or 2.

Pathogenesis
One possibility is that the developing choristoma interferes with the normal development of the adjacent iris, ciliary body, choroid, and retina, and causes a secondary coloboma. Alternatively, faulty differentiation of the optic cup could result in formation of both heterotopic brain tissue and a coloboma {1726}.

Macroscopic appearance
Lesions appear as a pink, greyish, or yellowish mass in the ciliary body.

Histopathology
The tumour consists of fibrillary astrocytes, an eosinophilic matrix of glial and neuronal processes, clusters of neuronal cells with small round nuclei, and scattered large ganglion cells. Calcospherites, dysplastic rosettes, and tubules composed of several rows of cells that resemble Homer Wright and Flexner–Wintersteiner rosettes may be present. Mitotic figures are very rare or absent. The glial component is immunopositive for GFAP and the neuronal component for synaptophysin and neurofilament proteins {1726}. The ciliary epithelium over the mass shows reactive proliferation. The adjacent retina may be dysplastic and may extend to the chorioretinal coloboma when one is present {1726,3177}. Glioneuroma of the ciliary body must be distinguished from teratoid medulloepithelioma containing mature brain tissue {421,1726,2062}.

Cytology
Not reported

Diagnostic molecular pathology
Not reported

Essential and desirable diagnostic criteria
Essential: histologically mature neuroglial tissue unassociated with neoplastic neuroepithelium; an adjacent coloboma, when present, is a helpful sign.

Staging
Not available

Prognosis and prediction
Lesions are curable early on by surgical excision, with negligible risk of recurrence.

Adenoma and adenocarcinoma of the ciliary body

Mudhar HS
Laver NM
Mori T
Moulin A

Definition

Ciliary body adenoma and adenocarcinoma are benign and malignant neoplasms, respectively, that arise from the pigmented or non-pigmented ciliary epithelium.

ICD-O coding

8140/0 Ciliary body adenoma
8140/3 Ciliary body adenocarcinoma

ICD-11 coding

2F36.2 & XH3DV3 Benign neoplasm of ciliary body & Adenoma, NOS
2D06.0 Adenocarcinoma of ciliary epithelium

Related terminology

None

Subtype(s)

None

Localization

Adenoma and adenocarcinoma both arise from the ciliary body epithelium, which has a non-pigmented inner and a pigmented outer layer. The adenocarcinomas can infiltrate the iris and anterior chamber angle and, eventually, the sclera anteriorly to form an extrascleral epibulbar mass {102,1186,1264,1870,2736}, or posteriorly through scleral channels.

Clinical features

Adenomas and adenocarcinomas of the ciliary body are often asymptomatic, but they may be associated with visual disturbances because of local inflammation, secondary glaucoma from angle invasion, or lens subluxation and sectoral cataract from lens touch. They can protrude into the posterior chamber and anteriorly to involve the iris and anterior chamber {3035,3037}.

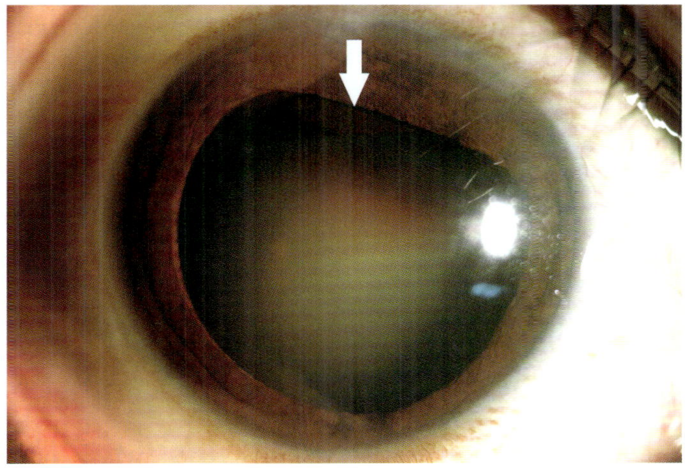

Fig. 5.30 Adenoma of the ciliary body. A dark-brown, well-defined, solid mass (arrow) located behind the iris.

Non-pigmented adenomas and adenocarcinomas are greyish-white, yellowish, or pinkish, vascularized, multilobular masses that transmit light on transillumination. Pigmented adenomas and adenocarcinomas appear dark grey to black-brown, and they block light on transillumination.

Ultrasound biomicroscopy of both non-pigmented and pigmented adenomas and adenocarcinomas reveals a solid mass with medium to high internal reflectivity and abrupt borders. The median diameter of adenomas is about 5 mm. On MRI, non-pigmented adenoma and adenocarcinoma is T1 isointense and T2 isointense to hyperintense relative to the lacrimal gland tissue, whereas pigmented adenomas and adenocarcinomas

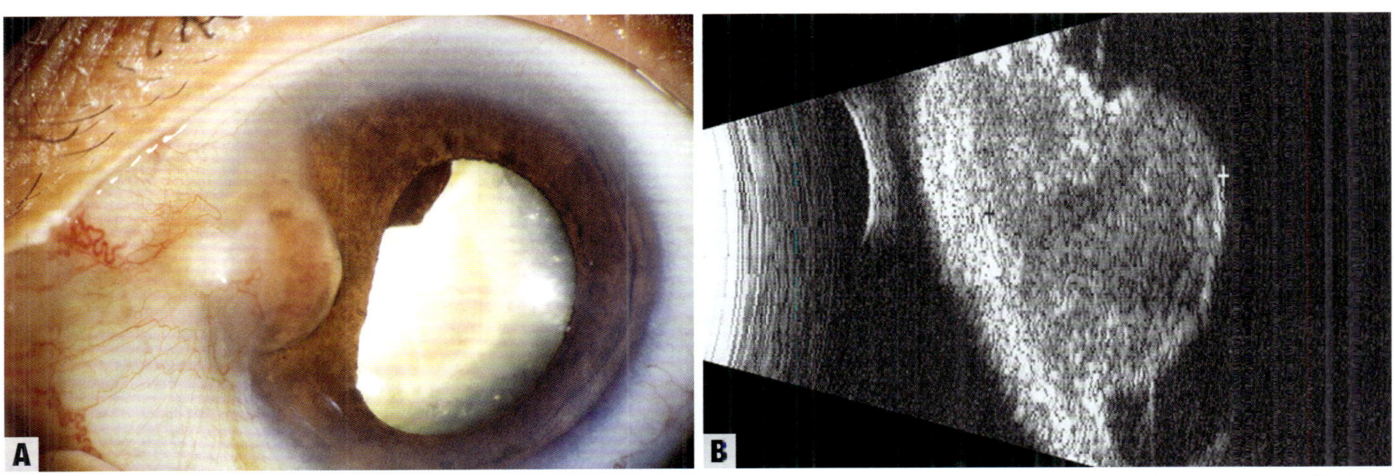

Fig. 5.31 Adenocarcinoma of the ciliary body. **A** A partially pigmented ciliary body mass extends to the iris surface. **B** B-scan ultrasonography shows a mass with abrupt borders.

are T1 hyperintense and T2 hypointense relative to brain tissue {525,3653}.

Epidemiology

Adenoma and adenocarcinoma are rare tumours of the ciliary body. Adenomas generally occur in middle-aged individuals, with no sex predilection {525}. The incidence of adenocarcinomas is highest in the fifth decade of life, with no sex predilection. The age at diagnosis tends to be slightly younger than that of choroidal melanoma. Pleomorphic adenocarcinoma usually affects patients in their eighth decade of life. Most patients are White. Few adenomas and adenocarcinomas have been reported in African-American {1186,2069} or Asian {1898,3234, 1154} patients or in children {2482}.

Etiology

The etiology is unknown. Several cases are reported in phthisical eyes several years after blindness from injury or chronic inflammation {3234,831,1264,1870,1772}.

Pathogenesis

Adenomas of the ciliary body derive from the ciliary epithelium that is a SOX10-negative region of the optic cup {3234,2275}. Adenocarcinomas are presumed to arise de novo, from long-standing reactive hyperplasia, or from a prior adenoma {3034}.

Macroscopic appearance

Lesions appear as a pigmented, greyish-white, or yellowish mass behind the lens in the ciliary body.

Histopathology

Non-pigmented and pigmented adenomas: These are composed of nests, cords, and tubules of polygonal epithelial cells that have round to oval nuclei and small nucleoli, with minimal cytological atypia and very rare mitotic figures {3674,3035, 525,3065}. Some adenomas can show spindle-cell morphology {3035}. These tumours can exhibit solid and papillary patterns, with delicate fibrous septa and basement membrane. Non-pigmented adenomas show variable acid mucopolysaccharide matrix {3674,3035}. Pigmented adenomas contain large spherical melanin granules, and the neoplastic cells are often vacuolated, the latter containing a hyaluronidase-resistant acid mucopolysaccharide {525,3065}. Pigmented adenomas can show pigment dispersion into the anterior chamber and infiltration of the trabecular meshwork {803}. This is not an indication of malignancy as long as the cytology remains bland.

Both non-pigmented and pigmented adenomas show consistent strong nuclear expression of PAX8 {2297}, vimentin, and S100, and variable expression of cytokeratins, most consistently CK8 and CK18 {2515,3674,3035,525,3065,1941}. In pigmented adenomas, variable immunoreactivity for the melanocytic marker melan-A has been documented {2515}.

Non-pigmented and pigmented adenocarcinomas: These are composed of strands, cords, and duct-like structures of cuboidal to epithelioid cells that are cytologically atypical with enlarged and irregular nuclei containing prominent nucleoli. The cells are frequently surrounded by a meshwork of basement membrane material that is PAS-positive. Papillary, solid,

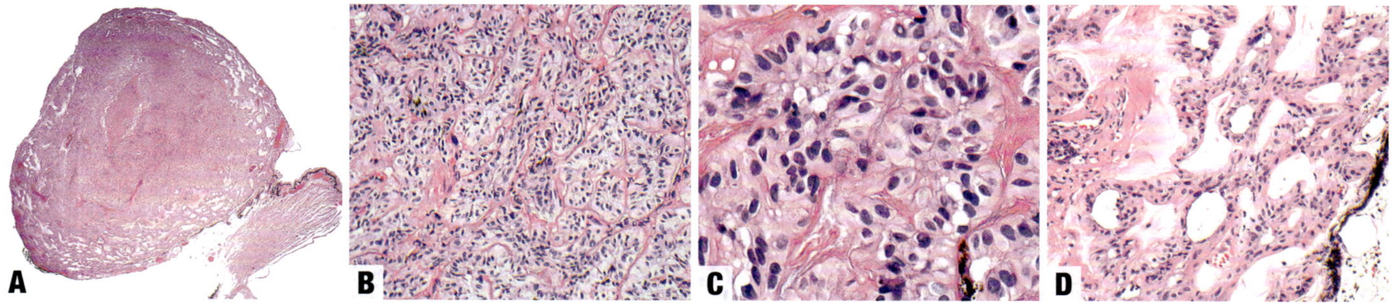

Fig. 5.32 Non-pigmented adenoma of the ciliary body. **A** Low-power view of a non-pigmented ciliary body adenoma. **B** Trabecular pattern with hyalinized stroma. **C** High-power view showing the bland cytological features. **D** Tubuloglandular pattern with extracellular mucopolysaccharide elaboration.

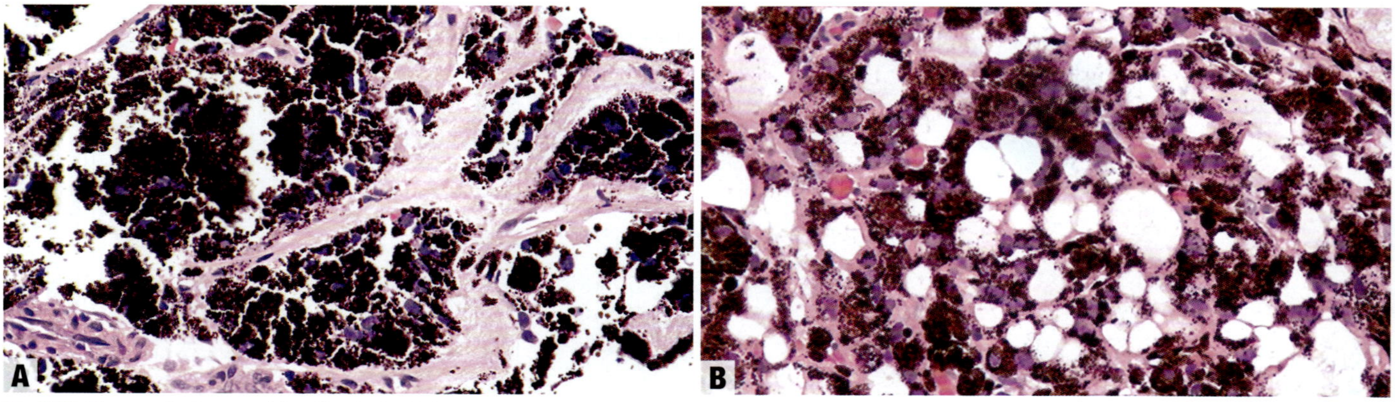

Fig. 5.33 Pigmented adenoma of the ciliary body. **A** Cords and nests of pigmented epithelial cells separated by fibrous septa. **B** Vacuolated tumour cells containing numerous intracellular melanin granules.

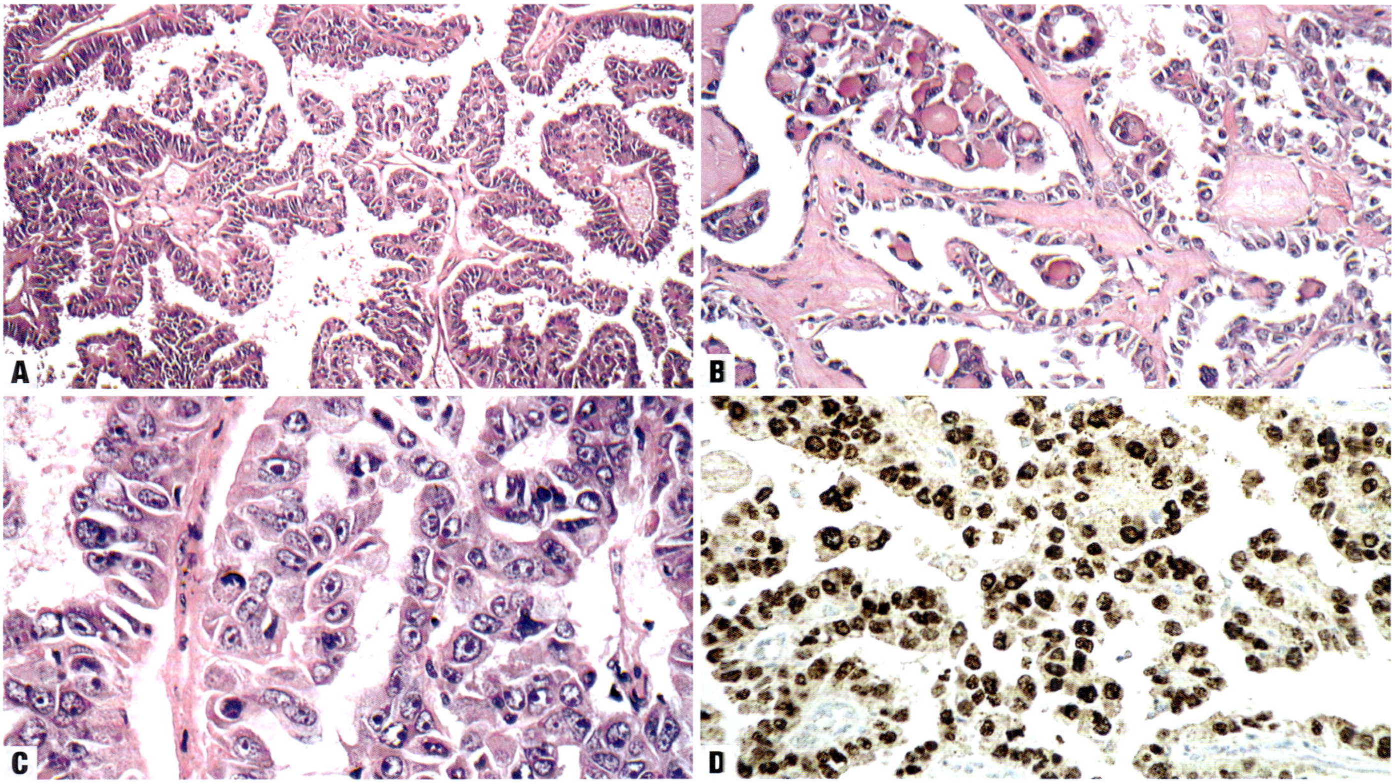

Fig. 5.34 Non-pigmented adenocarcinoma of the ciliary body. **A** A tubulopapillary pattern. **B** Prominent basement membrane elaboration. **C** High-power view showing malignant, atypical cells. **D** PAX8 nuclear immunopositivity; a pigmented adenocarcinoma would show an identical pattern.

and pleomorphic growth patterns have been described {3772, 1870}. The term "pleomorphic" has been used to describe the variation in differentiation across the tumour, with extraocular extension often showing poorly differentiated tumour compared with a better differentiated intraocular tumour component {1870}. Extracellular mucopolysaccharide deposits can be present in their stroma {1490}. Pigmented adenocarcinomas contain heavily pigmented cells, commonly associated with vacuoles that are thought to be extracellular {3216}. Features of malignancy include widespread cytological atypia, conspicuous mitotic figures that may include abnormal forms, destructive local invasion, and necrosis.

Adenocarcinomas are immunoreactive with uniform nuclear staining for PAX8 {2297}, vimentin, S100 {1870}, and pancytokeratin (AE1/AE3), and often CK8, CK18, and CK5/6 {3234, 1870}. In pigmented adenocarcinomas, variable immunoreactivity for the melanocytic markers melan-A, MITF, and HMB45 has been documented {2868,3234}.

Differential diagnosis

Adenomas: The differential diagnosis for non-pigmented adenomas includes adenomatous hyperplasia of the ciliary epithelium, amelanotic melanoma and adenocarcinoma of the ciliary body, and medulloepithelioma of the ciliary body. For pigmented adenomas, it includes melanocytoma, pigmented melanoma, and pigmented adenocarcinoma of the ciliary body.

Adenocarcinoma: Non-pigmented ciliary adenocarcinoma includes amelanotic melanoma and metastatic adenocarcinoma in the ciliary body. For pigmented adenocarcinoma, the main differential diagnosis is pigmented ciliary body melanoma. In small biopsy specimens, the differential diagnosis with a ciliary body adenoma can be difficult if the atypia is not striking.

Cytology

Adenoma of the ciliary body: FNAB shows polygonal epithelial cells with bland round to oval nuclei and small nucleoli, with

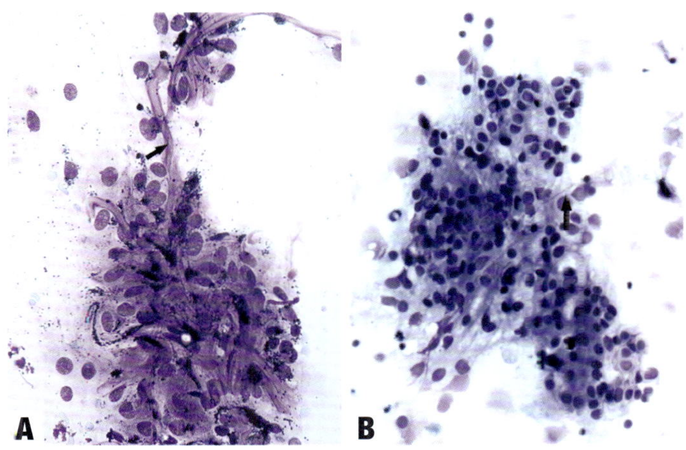

Fig. 5.35 Ciliary body tumours. **A** Adenoma. FNAB shows nests of polygonal epithelial cells with round to oval nuclei, small nucleoli, and focal pigmentation. Note the prominent basement membrane material (arrow) (Giemsa). **B** Adenocarcinoma. FNAB shows a cohesive cluster of atypical cuboidal epithelial cells with large hyperchromatic nuclei, vacuolated cytoplasm, and associated basement membrane material (arrow). Pigment is absent (Giemsa).

or without melanin granules. The presence of basement membrane material is helpful in differentiating this tumour from melanocytic and mesenchymal tumours {534,533,2297,3065}. The melanosomes of an adenoma are larger and more spherical than those of uveal melanoma. PAX8 immunohistochemistry is useful in distinguishing adenomas from melanocytic lesions of the ciliary body {2297}.

Adenocarcinoma of the ciliary body: FNAB shows cohesive clusters of atypical cuboidal to large epithelioid epithelial cells with hyperchromatic, enlarged nuclei, prominent nucleoli, vacuolation, and basement membrane material. Similarly to adenomas, the cells may be pigmented or non-pigmented. The presence of basement membrane material differentiates these tumours from melanoma and metastatic adenocarcinoma in the ciliary body. PAX8 immunohistochemistry is useful in distinguishing an adenocarcinoma from melanocytic lesions {2297}.

Diagnostic molecular pathology

BRAF p.V600E mutations are commonly found in pigmented ciliary body adenomas and adenocarcinomas, whereas mutations in *GNAQ* or *GNA11* are absent from them, in contrast to uveal melanoma {2275}.

Essential and desirable diagnostic criteria

Adenoma

Essential: bland polygonal epithelial cells arranged as nests, cords, and tubules with delicate fibrous septa and basement membrane; pigmented adenomas additionally show large cytoplasmic spherical melanin granules.

Desirable: hyaluronidase-resistant acid mucopolysaccharide matrix; immunohistochemical positivity for cytokeratins and PAX8; pigmented adenomas additionally show vacuolation and frequent immunohistochemical positivity for BRAF p.V600E.

Adenocarcinoma

Essential: cytologically atypical, mitotically active, cuboidal to epithelioid cells with enlarged and irregular nuclei containing prominent nucleoli, arranged in strands, cords, sheets, or duct-like structures; pigmented adenocarcinomas additionally contain large spherical melanin granules and are commonly associated with vacuoles.

Desirable: a meshwork of basement membrane around tumour that is PAS-positive indicates a primary ciliary body malignancy because metastases do not elaborate prominent basement membrane; hyaluronidase-resistant acid mucopolysaccharide matrix; immunohistochemical positivity for cytokeratins and PAX8; pigmented adenocarcinomas show frequent immunohistochemical positivity for BRAF p.V600E.

Note: Adenomas of the ciliary body with bland cytological features can be locally invasive with iris infiltration, angle closure, ciliary body invasion, and even extraocular extension, which do not necessarily indicate a malignant nature. Cytological atypia, mitotic activity, necrosis, and destructive local tissue invasion are the most reliable criteria to distinguish an adenoma from an adenocarcinoma of the ciliary body.

Staging

None

Prognosis and prediction

Adenoma of the ciliary body: Local resection is usually curative. Enucleation may be necessary when an adenoma is large and associated with loss of vision from tumour-related complications {3035}.

Adenocarcinoma of the ciliary body: The prognosis is usually favourable, although a few patients have died after extraocular extension associated with orbital recurrence {1772}, intracranial invasion {831,1870,1243}, or metastasis {1870,1772}.

Medulloepithelioma of the ciliary body

Eagle RC Jr
Stagner AM

Definition

Medulloepithelioma of the ciliary body is a primary intraocular embryonal neuroectodermal tumour characterized by cords of multilayered neuroepithelial cells resembling the medullary epithelium of the optic cup.

ICD-O coding

9501/0 Medulloepithelioma, benign
9501/3 Medulloepithelioma, malignant
9502/0 Teratoid medulloepithelioma, benign
9502/3 Teratoid medulloepithelioma, malignant

ICD-11 coding

2F36.2 & XH28W9 Benign neoplasm of ciliary body & Medulloepithelioma, benign
2F36.2 & XH5NR7 Benign neoplasm of ciliary body & Teratoid medulloepithelioma, benign
2D06.1 Malignant medulloepithelioma of ciliary body
2D06.1 & XH0AM8 Malignant medulloepithelioma of ciliary body & Teratoid medulloepithelioma

Related terminology

Not recommended: diktyoma.

Subtype(s)

Medulloepithelioma, benign; medulloepithelioma, malignant; teratoid medulloepithelioma, benign; teratoid medulloepithelioma, malignant

Localization

Most medulloepitheliomas are ciliary body tumours located on the surface of the ciliary body {2858}. Rarely they can develop in the optic nerve {2611,1165,346,550} and, exceptionally, in the retina {3422}.

Clinical features

Medulloepithelioma presents typically with poor vision or blindness (27%), leukocoria (20%), strabismus (12%), or a red, painful eye (20%) {1577}. Clinical diagnosis is challenging: diagnoses on referral include medulloepithelioma (12%), an undetermined mass (22%), cataract (20%), glaucoma (17%), and retinoblastoma (7%) {1577,3256}. Unusual clinical presentations include translucent neoplastic cysts in the posterior or anterior chamber {3762}. More than half of patients have intratumoural cysts, which are a helpful diagnostic clue on imaging studies. One fifth show notching or coloboma of the lens caused by segmental loss of lens zonules {1577,2538,3256}. A neoplastic membrane of tumour tissue is present behind the lens in half of patients and may cause leukocoria {1577, 2955,2538}. One half lead to neovascularization of the iris, and about 45% to secondary glaucoma {1577}. Treatment and diagnosis often are delayed. In one series, the average age at

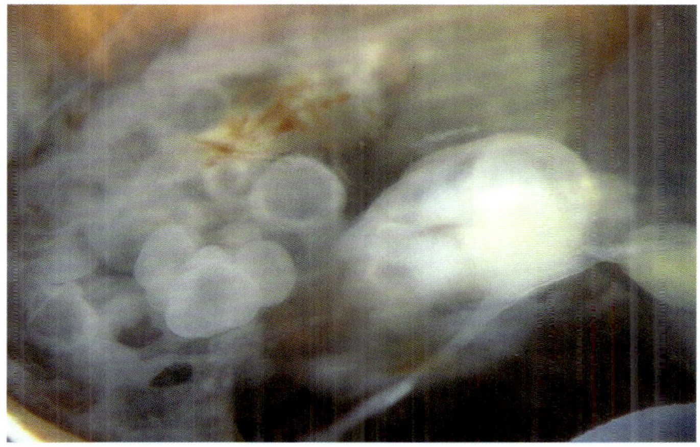

Fig. 5.36 Medulloepithelioma of the ciliary body. A whitish tumour on the inner surface of the ciliary body with numerous intratumoural cysts.

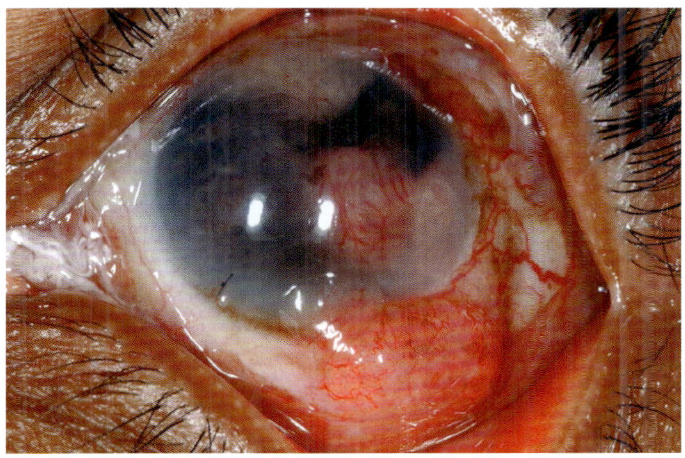

Fig. 5.37 Malignant medulloepithelioma of the ciliary body. Because of a delayed diagnosis in an adult, the tumour has extended extraocularly to form an epibulbar mass. The patient developed metastases.

presentation was about 4 years, but the tumour was diagnosed at the age of 5 years {421}. Before diagnosis, some patients are treated for cataract or glaucoma. An epibulbar mass may be present from extraocular extension, which has been observed after local resection {1729} or misguided tube shunt surgery for neovascular glaucoma {1572}. Some medulloepitheliomas are found incidentally in blind, painful eyes after enucleation or evisceration.

Epidemiology

Most medulloepitheliomas occur in children who are typically 2–5 years of age, but exceptional ones are reported in adults (range: 0–66 years) {3477,82}. Sixty-three per cent occur in females and there is no race predilection {1577}.

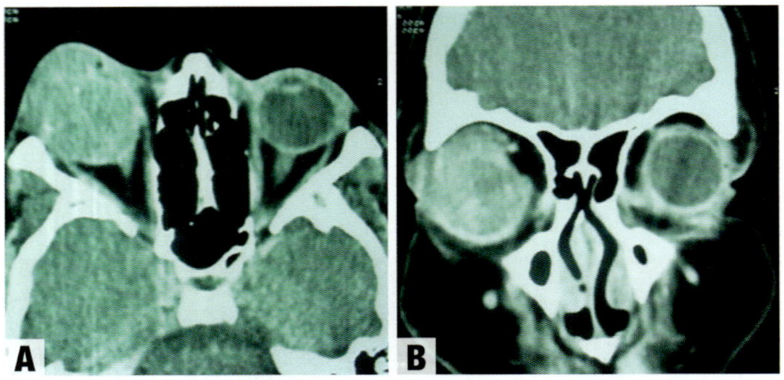

Fig. 5.38 Teratoid medulloepithelioma. **A** CT of a malignant teratoid medulloepithelioma of the ciliary body in an 11-year-old girl. **B** Coronal CT of a malignant teratoid medulloepithelioma of the ciliary body in an 11-year-old girl.

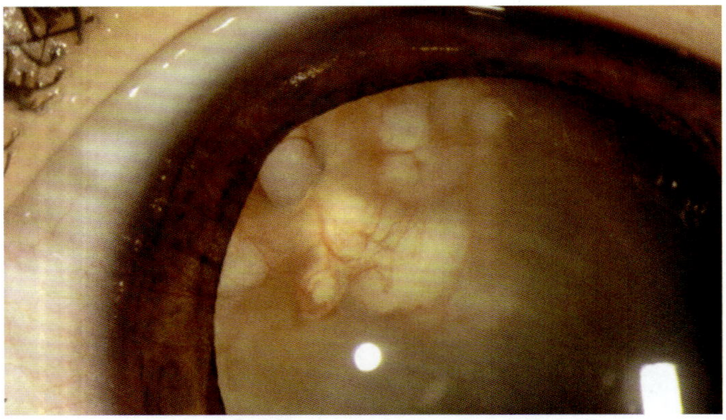

Fig. 5.39 Teratoid medulloepithelioma of the ciliary body. A tumour is seen behind the iris. Intratumoural cysts and whitish foci of heteroplastic cartilage are evident.

Etiology

Intraocular medulloepitheliomas are congenital tumours thought to arise from anlagen of medullary epithelium that lines the forebrain and optic vesicle {421,3038,3034}. No risk factors for intraocular medulloepithelioma are known. Most are sporadic and unassociated with any congenital malformation or cytogenic abnormality. However, a minority (5%) arise in patients with pleuropulmonary blastoma familial tumour and dysplasia predisposition syndrome (MIM number 601200) caused by germline mutations in *DICER1* {2594,1779,1837}. Conversely, in this syndrome, only < 1% of patients have developed an intraocular medulloepithelioma.

Pathogenesis

The neoplastic multilayered medullary epithelium appears to arise from a simple premedullary epithelial monolayer of cells that are S100-positive {1485}. Immunostaining for CRX and the neuronal marker NeuN suggests that the anteriormost layers of the optic cup retain the potential for retinal and neuroglial differentiation. Although intraocular medulloepitheliomas share histomorphological features with CNS medulloepitheliomas, the evidence suggests that they do not share a common origin and biological behaviour. The latter is a rare entity grouped with several other primitive neuroectodermal tumours as embryonal tumours with multilayered rosettes. Although both intraocular and CNS medulloepitheliomas express LIN28A, the former show numerous copy-number aberrations that involve entire chromosomes or chromosome arms. In addition, they show no amplification of the C19MC cluster of microRNA typical of CNS medulloepitheliomas, and they have strikingly different DNA methylation patterns {1773,1470,3188}. Conversely, RNA expression profiling of genes in the sonic hedgehog and WNT signalling pathways displays common upregulated target genes in both intraocular and CNS tumours, suggesting these pathways as critical drivers of both medulloepithelioma types {819}.

Cytogenetic analysis of intraocular medulloepitheliomas shows recurrent aberrations in chromosomes 1p, 4, 8, and 16p {1773}. Mutation of *DICER1* in some sporadic intraocular medulloepitheliomas is not associated with pleuropulmonary blastoma syndrome {850,2815,863}. Expression profiling shows significantly upregulated and downregulated microRNAs in a fashion different from that in CNS medulloepitheliomas. Instead, the microRNA dysregulation profiles are similar to those seen in glioblastoma and retinoblastoma {863}. Mutation of *KMT2D* has been reported {2815}. Unsupervised hierarchical clustering of DNA methylation showed that intraocular medulloepitheliomas have signatures distinct from CNS medulloepitheliomas {1773}. The targetable epigenetic tumour protein EZH2 is enriched in intraocular medulloepithelioma {216}.

Macroscopic appearance

Medulloepithelioma appears as a greyish-white mass typically with intralesional cysts behind the lens on the surface of the ciliary body, sometimes with freely floating cysts.

Histopathology

Medulloepitheliomas reside on the inner surface of the ciliary body and extend into the vitreous cavity and posterior chamber. Involvement of the iris and anterior chamber occurs occasionally. Aggressive lesions can invade the stroma of the ciliary body and the sclera to extend extraocularly. Sheets of tumour can grow posteriorly on the inner surface of the retina and reach the posterior pole of the eye. These tumours range in size from 2 to 30 mm (mean: 11 mm) {1577}. They are composed of anastomosing cords, bands, and ribbons of polarized neuroepithelial cells that resemble embryonic medullary epithelium. A meshwork of thin interweaving strands of neuroepithelium characterizes a diktyomatous pattern. The polarized neuroepithelial elements secrete a relatively acellular myxoid stroma rich in hyaluronidase-sensitive mucopolysaccharide (neoplastic vitreous).

The side of the neuroepithelium abutting the myxoid stroma is lined by a thin basement membrane, whereas the lumina of the neuroepithelial clefts and rosettes contains zonulae adherentes analogous to the external limiting membrane of the retina. Approximately half of medulloepitheliomas contain intralesional cystoid spaces, and one third contain areas of intrinsic pigmentation {1577,3041}. Sheets of poorly differentiated neuroblastic cells resembling retinoblastoma is a histopathological criterion of malignancy. Such areas may contain Homer Wright or Flexner–Wintersteiner rosettes. Additional criteria for malignancy include invasion of adjacent tissues including the uvea, sclera, cornea, and optic nerve, extraocular extension, sarcomatous dedifferentiation in areas of heterologous tissue, cellular pleomorphism, atypia, and mitotic activity. Altogether, 66–80% of medulloepitheliomas are classified as malignant {421,1577}.

Because the histopathological criteria for malignancy do not correlate with clinical behaviour, and molecular genetic studies have disclosed no differences between histologically benign and malignant medulloepitheliomas, a simple grading scheme has been proposed to replace the prevailing dichotomous classification {3477}. The proposed scheme divides intraocular medulloepitheliomas into grade 1, corresponding to the current WHO designation "benign"; grade 2 with progression evidenced by pleomorphism, mitotic activity, and local invasion; and grade 3 with metastatic potential evidenced by extrascleral extension or existing metastasis. Metastatic disease occurs only after extraocular extension.

Non-teratoid medulloepitheliomas consist exclusively of neuroepithelial elements. Teratoid medulloepitheliomas additionally contain heterotopic elements, such as cartilage and striated muscle. Medulloepitheliomas are therefore designated as teratoid if they contain heteroplastic elements including hyaline cartilage, muscle, myoblasts, and brain-like tissue. About one third of all intraocular medulloepitheliomas are teratoid {1577}: about one fifth of benign and one half of malignant ones {421,1577}. The presence of heteroplastic elements does not alter prognosis. Hyaline cartilage is the most common heteroplastic element. Cartilage has even developed in non-teratoid tumours that recurred after local resection.

Pigmented tumours occasionally occur {2954,507}.

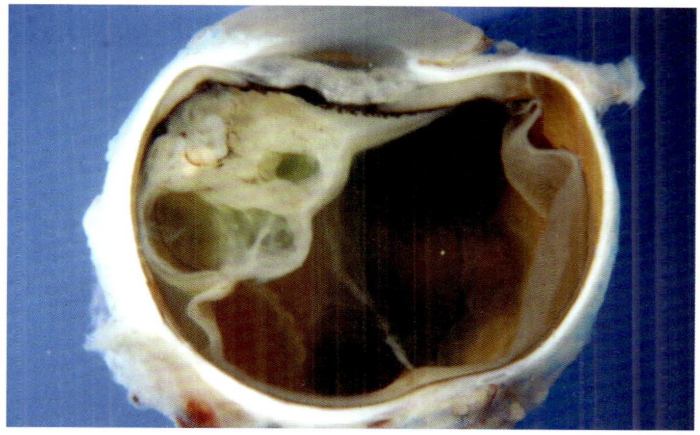

Fig. 5.40 Malignant teratoid medulloepithelioma of the ciliary body. A tumour on the inner surface of the ciliary body is seen. Intralesional cysts, a neoplastic retrolental membrane, and an incidental persistent hyaloid artery are present.

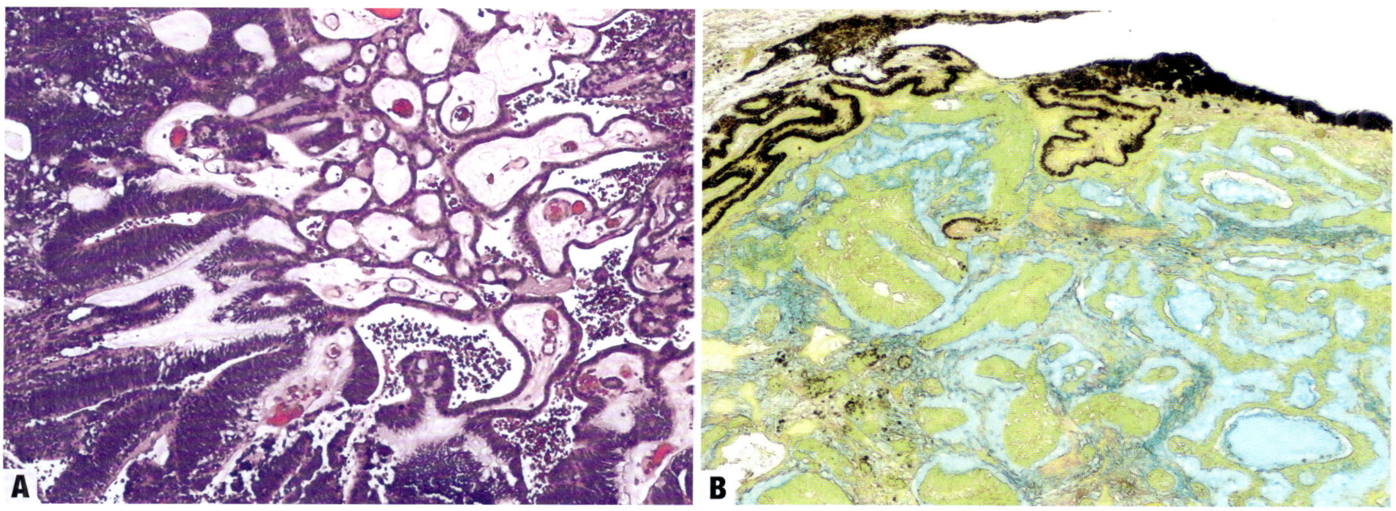

Fig. 5.41 Medulloepithelioma of the ciliary body. **A** Thick bands of polarized neuroepithelium, which resembles medullary epithelium, and a diktyomatous meshwork pattern consisting of thinner strands are present. Pools of hyaluronic acid surround the neuroepithelial elements. PAS stain. **B** Myxoid stroma of hyaluronidase-sensitive mucopolysaccharide surrounds the neuroepithelioid elements. Colloidal iron stain.

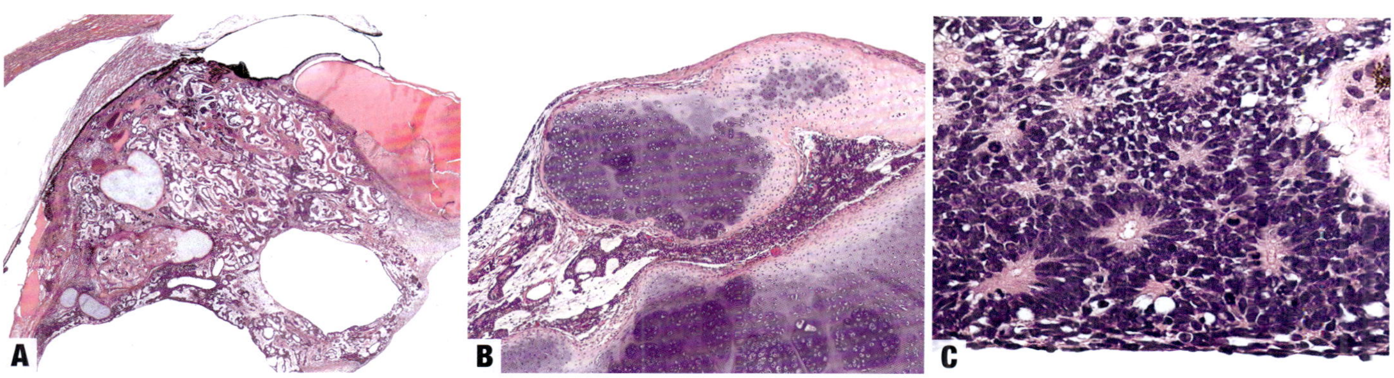

Fig. 5.42 Malignant teratoid medulloepithelioma of the ciliary body. **A** A tumour on the inner surface of the ciliary body with cystoid spaces and foci of heteroplastic hyaline cartilage abuts the posterior surface of the lens. **B** A teratoid tumour with a prominent island of heteroplastic hyaline cartilage is seen. Retinoblastoma-like tissue also is present between foci of cartilage. **C** A poorly differentiated area that resembles retinoblastoma is seen. Several Flexner–Wintersteiner rosettes are present.

Immunohistochemistry

The non-teratoid component of medulloepitheliomas typically is immunoreactive for vimentin and NSE {1729}. Limited and sometimes conflicting results are reported for chromogranin, synaptophysin, GFAP, S100, and HMB45. Immunoreactivity for pancytokeratin and CK18 with no reactivity for CK7, CK20, and EMA has been described {1476,2858}. Almost all medulloepitheliomas stain positively for LIN28A as CNS medulloepitheliomas do, and the intensity of staining may correlate with aggressive behaviour {1470}. As regards intraocular tumours, LIN28A might be specific for medulloepithelioma, because 19 of 20 were found to stain positive, while 0 of 10 retinoblastomas were immunopositive. PAX8 also showed diffuse immunoreactivity in ciliary body medulloepitheliomas, and this may be another useful immunostain for distinguishing poorly differentiated ones from retinoblastoma {2297}.

Cytology

The polymorphous nature of medulloepithelioma can reduce the sensitivity and specificity of aspiration cytology {3112,2032, 2858,223}. In many reports, diagnosis is limited to a malignant round cell tumour, although more-specific rosettes and focal epithelial-like fragments with cellular polarity and multilayering occasionally are observed {3112}.

Diagnostic molecular pathology

Not clinically relevant

Essential and desirable diagnostic criteria

Essential: a tumour composed of non-pigmented or pigmented cords and bands of polarized neuroepithelial cells with a myxoid matrix located on the surface of the ciliary body.

Desirable: teratoid subtypes contain heteroplastic elements, most often cartilage.

Staging

None

Prognosis and prediction

Most eyes with a medulloepithelioma are still enucleated. Prognosis for vision is thus poor. Recurrence often follows local resection because of clinically inapparent tumour cells {1729}. Plaque brachytherapy is sometimes used, but its role is not clearly defined. Prognosis for life is excellent if the tumour remains intraocular. Metastases are infrequent but can develop after extraocular extension: in one series, 4 of 41 medulloepitheliomas developed metastases, all of which had extraocular extension because of a delayed diagnosis {1577}.

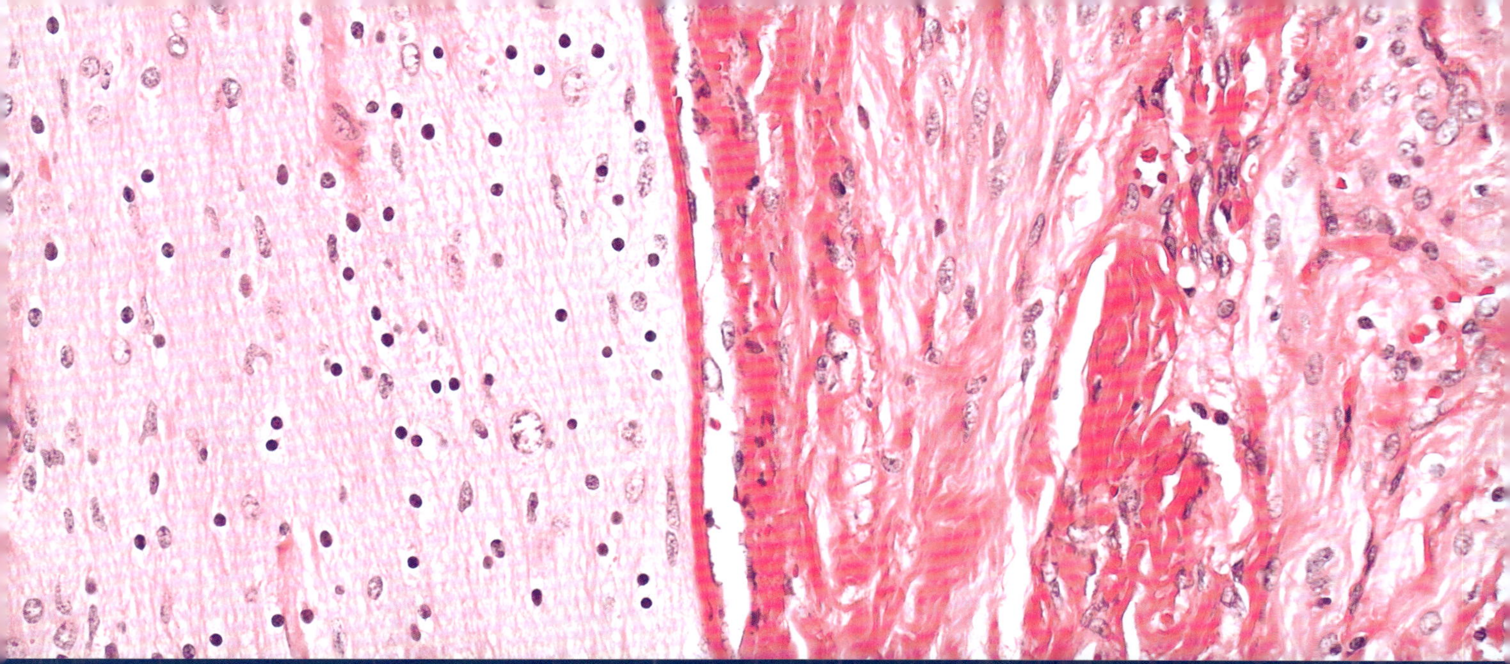

6

Tumours of the optic disc and optic nerve

Edited by: Verdijk RM

Tumours of the optic disc and optic nerve: Introduction

Eberhart CG

The optic nerve arises from the embryonal optic stalk and contains axons extending from the retinal ganglion cells to the brain. These axons exit the globe through the lamina cribrosa, a connective tissue meshwork continuous with the sclera. Within the globe, the axons are unmyelinated; posterior to the lamina cribrosa, the axons are myelinated by oligodendrocytes, with additional support provided by astrocytes and microglia. The optic nerve is surrounded by the same layers as the rest of the CNS (the dura mater, arachnoid mater, and pia mater), with invaginations of the pia dividing bundles of axons into individual fascicles. This section focuses on prechiasmal lesions.

Consistent with the derivation of the optic nerve from diencephalic extensions, tumours in the optic nerve make up a subset of those seen in the CNS and its coverings. Choristomas containing heterotopic smooth muscle and adipose tissue can also be found around the optic nerve and optic disc {1266}. Astrocytomas most commonly arise in children, are of low-grade, and have the microscopic features of pilocytic astrocytoma {1035,2693}. They are often associated with neurofibromatosis type 1, and they can be bilateral in such cases {2740}. High-grade astrocytomas and gangliogliomas can also be encountered in the optic nerve, but only rarely {1972, 2752}. High-grade B-cell lymphoma and medulloepithelioma can also involve the optic nerve. Interestingly, IDH-mutant gliomas, including diffuse infiltrating astrocytoma and oligodendrogliomas of various grades, are almost never found in the optic nerve. Meningioma, solitary fibrous tumour / haemangiopericytoma, melanocytoma, melanoma, and other neoplasms of the CNS coverings can also arise in the optic nerve.

In this, the fifth edition, tumours metastatic to the optic nerve are covered in a separate chapter on metastases to the eye and surrounding structures.

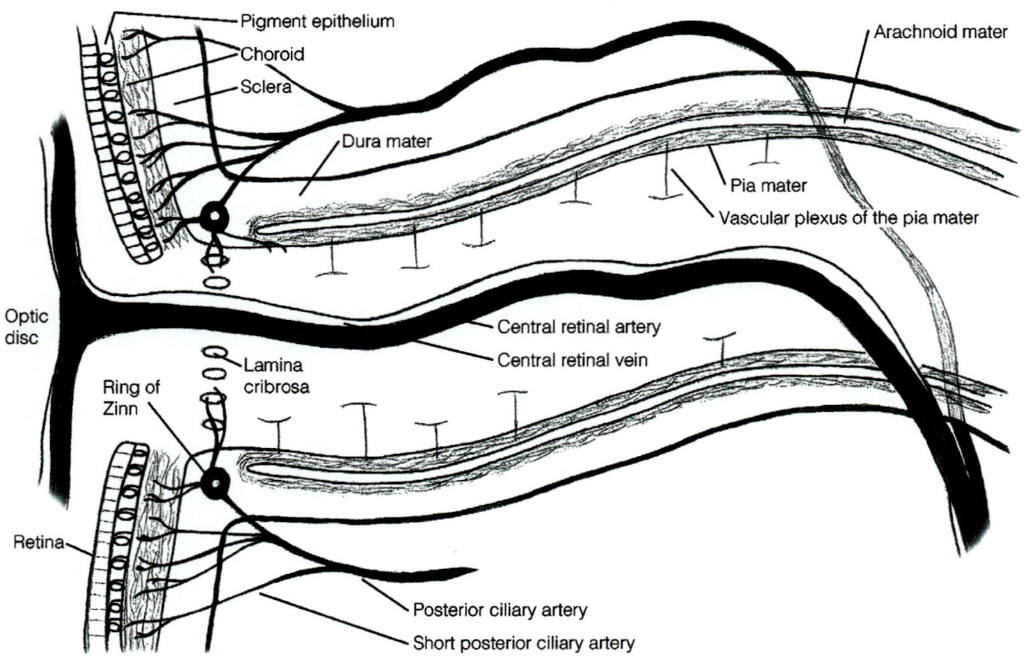

Fig. 6.01 Normal anatomy. The normal anatomy of the optic disc and optic nerve.

Optic nerve choristoma

Cummings TJ

Definition
Optic nerve choristoma is a rare, benign, and probably developmental/malformative choristomatous lesion composed of smooth muscle and adipose tissue within and around the optic nerve.

ICD-O coding
None

ICD-11 coding
LA13.7Y Other specified congenital malformation of optic disc

Related terminology
None

Subtype(s)
None

Localization
There is equal left:right optic nerve involvement. The location within the nerve may be intracanalicular, intraorbital, and intracranial involving the optic chiasm {1107}.

Clinical features
There is a painless, slow, progressive decrease in visual acuity, associated with optic atrophy. In rare cases, the visual loss may be rapid and progressive. MRI shows enlargement of the nerve and hyperintense signal that disappears with fat suppression, suggestive of a fat-containing lesion. Differential diagnostic considerations may include optic nerve glioma, optic nerve meningioma, lipoma, an inflammatory process, and a secondary process involving the optic nerve {2225}.

Epidemiology
Rare single case reports in the literature show an approximately equal sex distribution and an age range from 9 to 63 years.

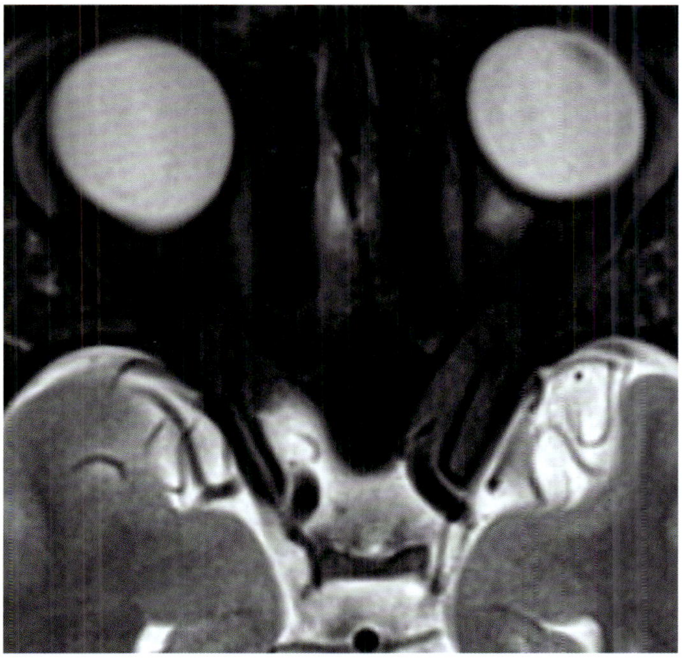

Fig. 6.02 Optic nerve choristoma. Axial MRI, T2-weighted, bright signal in right optic nerve proximal to optic chiasm.

Etiology
Unknown

Pathogenesis
This is believed to be a developmental malformation with heterotopic smooth muscle and adipose tissue within and around the optic nerve. Optic disc colobomas may be associated with heterotopic adipose tissue and/or smooth muscle {3773}. A rare case showed mixed features of both optic nerve coloboma and morning glory anomaly.

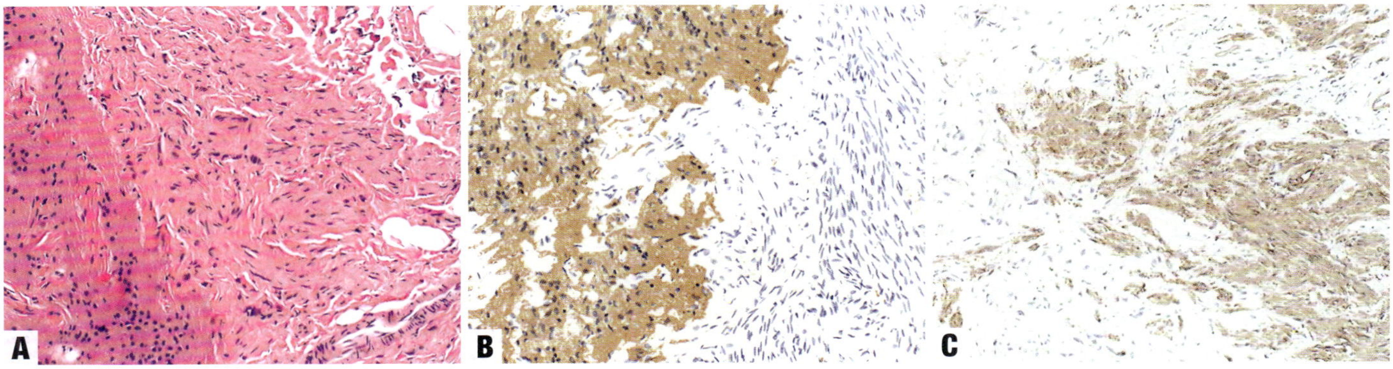

Fig. 6.03 Optic nerve choristoma. **A** The biopsy exhibits optic nerve glial tissue (left), smooth muscle (centre), and adipose tissue (right). **B** Immunohistochemistry for GFAP highlights glial tissue. **C** The smooth muscle component is highlighted by SMA.

Macroscopic appearance

Optic nerve choristoma may appear as a yellow/tan mass.

Histopathology

Histology shows adipose tissue and bundles of smooth muscle in variable amounts within or adjacent to atrophic optic nerve tissue. Immunohistochemistry for SMA highlights the smooth muscle component, and GFAP staining highlights optic nerve tissue {1107,3176,2225,1266}.

Cytology

Limited experience

Diagnostic molecular pathology

Not relevant

Essential and desirable diagnostic criteria

Essential: variable amounts of adipose tissue and smooth muscle.

Staging

Not relevant

Prognosis and prediction

There is slow growth, with benign, progressive visual loss.

Gliomas of the optic nerve

Rodriguez FJ
Eberhart CG
Rushing EJ

Definition

Gliomas of the optic nerve are a family of defined tumour types. Astrocytomas of the optic disc and optic nerve are tumours with an astrocytic phenotype developing from glial precursor cells and located within the optic nerve and chiasm. Optic nerve gliomas are most frequently pilocytic astrocytomas. However, other diffuse gliomas (including glioblastoma) may rarely involve the nerve, usually by secondary extension from the CNS.

ICD-O coding

9421/1 Pilocytic astrocytoma
9425/3 Pilomyxoid astrocytoma
9400/3 Astrocytoma, IDH-mutant, grade 2
9440/3 Glioblastoma, IDH-wildtype

ICD-11 coding

2A02.12 & XH29Q5 Malignant neoplasm of the optic nerve & Pilomyxoid astrocytoma
2A02.12 & XH2HK4 Malignant neoplasm of the optic nerve & Diffuse astrocytoma, IDH-mutant
2A02.12 & XH5571 Malignant neoplasm of the optic nerve & Glioblastoma, IDH-wildtype

Related terminology

Acceptable: optic pathway glioma (not a pathological category).
Not recommended (obsolete): juvenile pilocytic astrocytoma.

Subtype(s)

Pilocytic astrocytoma; pilomyxoid astrocytoma; glioblastoma and other diffuse gliomas: malignant optic nerve glioma; primary and secondary glioblastoma

Localization

The most common location is the optic nerve or chiasm. Bilateral involvement can be seen in patients with neurofibromatosis type 1 (NF1). Intraocular tumour extension and vitreous spread are rare {3366}. Local recurrence of high-grade gliomas is inevitable, with frequent extension into the adjacent brain tissue. The tumour may spread via the optic radiations to the occipital pole. There have been documented cases of malignant optic nerve glioma occurring in the context of multifocal glioblastomas {503, 3366}. Transtentorial spread to the cerebellum has been documented {2107}.

Clinical features

Individuals with optic nerve gliomas present clinically with a wide spectrum of ophthalmic abnormalities, including visual impairment, optic atrophy, and proptosis {866,1667,2338,2392}. Patients with high-grade glioma present with rapidly progressive unilateral vision loss, often eventually developing bilateral blindness. Pain may be an accompanying symptom {3366}, along with headaches, motor deficits, and behavioural changes {2107}.

Epidemiology

Optic nerve gliomas account for approximately 5% of all intracranial gliomas and 66% of primary optic nerve tumours {851, 1963,2013,3083}. About 90% are diagnosed within the first two decades of life. The median patient age at diagnosis is 7 years (range: from birth to the eighth decade of life). The M:F ratio is approximately 2:3. Both sexes appear to be equally affected when the neoplasm involves the optic chiasm. About 15% of patients with NF1 develop optic pathway gliomas. Diffuse gliomas of the optic nerve are rare, with < 100 cases reported in adults. There is a male predominance, with a mean patient age at diagnosis of 62 years (range: 26–83 years) {254,1953,2107}. Rare cases have been reported in children {3776}. The novel molecular class of high-grade astrocytoma with piloid features is typically cerebellar tumours in adults, and does not tend to affect the optic pathways {2692,2738}.

Etiology

Optic nerve gliomas probably derive from glial progenitors and have an astrocytic phenotype. Light stimulation during specified developmental periods is important for the formation of optic nerve gliomas in NF1 mouse models, which explains in

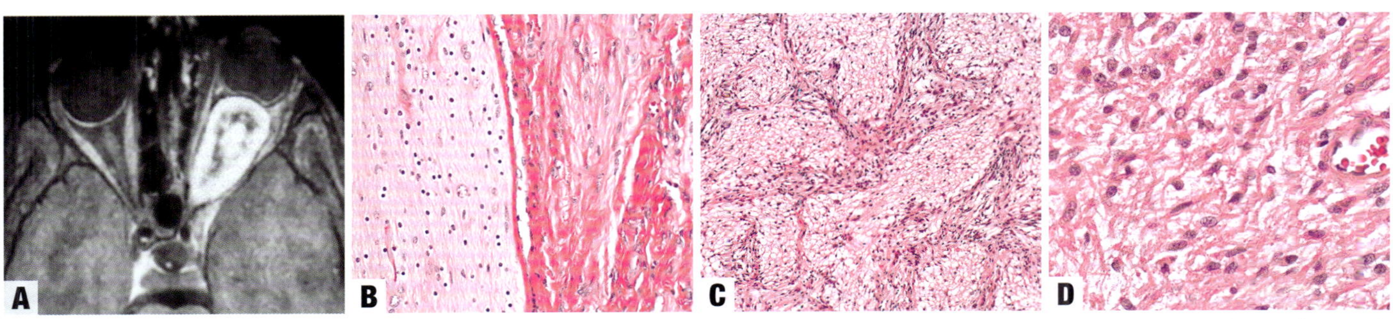

Fig. 6.04 Pilocytic astrocytoma of the optic nerve. **A** T1-weighted axial MRI shows a left optic nerve tumour with strong enhancement in an individual with neurofibromatosis type 1. **B** Pilocytic astrocytomas involving the optic nerve may extend into the adjacent subarachnoid space. **C** This pilocytic astrocytoma arising in the optic nerve demonstrates piloid morphology and expansion of the optic nerve septa. **D** Bright eosinophilic processes characterize these neoplastic astrocytes in a pilocytic astrocytoma of the optic nerve.

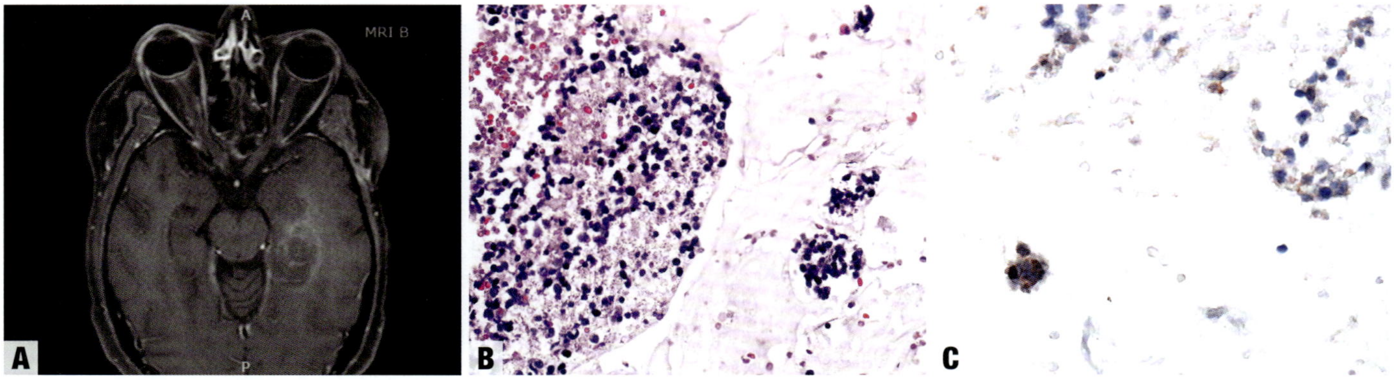

Fig. 6.05 Astrocytoma, IDH mutant. **A** T1-weighted postcontrast axial MRI demonstrates mild enhancement of the right optic nerve and flattening of the globe posteriorly resulting from optic nerve and intraocular extension from a hemispheric astrocytoma, IDH mutant. **B** A cell block from a vitreous cytology preparation demonstrates a cellular astrocytic neoplasm with necrosis resulting from optic nerve and intraocular extension of a hemispheric astrocytoma, IDH mutant. **C** Immunohistochemistry detected IDH1 p.R132H mutant–positive cells in a vitrectomy specimen.

part a predilection for the optic pathways in this patient population {2472}. Radiation therapy has been implicated in the formation of some high-grade gliomas {2808}.

Genetic susceptibility

NF1 has a recognized association with gliomas of the optic pathways {760,1962}. About 70% of optic pathway gliomas are associated with the syndrome {1961}, and these tumours generally have a more favourable outcome than sporadic gliomas. Approximately 20% of optic nerve tumours in patients with NF1 affect both nerves {906}. Tumour enlargement and progressive visual impairment occasionally occur in children with NF1 {1960, 1962}, and malignant change at this site is exceptional {384}.

Pathogenesis

Pilocytic astrocytomas of the optic pathway may show deletions and allelic losses involving the *NF1* gene at chromosome 17q11.2, with homozygous inactivation of the gene a uniform feature in the NF1 population. It appears that various mechanisms involving the *NF1* tumour suppressor gene may play an important primary genetic role in the promotion or initiation of NF1-associated pilocytic astrocytomas {1217,3615}. Pilocytic astrocytomas associated with NF1 typically lack the genetic changes associated with diffuse gliomas {1932}. Mutations of the *TP53* gene are rare {1853}. Sporadic optic nerve pilocytic astrocytomas harbour *KIAA1549*::*BRAF* fusions typical of pilocytic astrocytomas in other locations. Unlike in diffuse or infiltrating astrocytomas, IDH mutations are absent in pilocytic astrocytomas {652,2739}.

Very few optic pathway glioblastoma cases have been subject to molecular genetic profiling. In a single case report, FISH / microsatellite analyses showed 1p36 and 19q13 loss in a high proportion of cells, deletion of *PTEN* at chromosome 10q23 in 28% of cells, monosomy 7 in 40% of cells, and polysomy 7 in 15%. No *EGFR* or *EGFRvIII* amplification or *MGMT* methylation was observed {203}. *MGMT* promoter methylation was found in a case with transtentorial spread to the cerebellum {2107}.

Macroscopic appearance

Most pilocytic astrocytomas are soft, grey, and relatively discrete. Intratumoural or paratumoural cyst formation, including mural tumour nodules, is common. Optic nerve tumours often circumferentially infiltrate the optic sheath {384}.

Histopathology

Pilocytic astrocytomas expand the septa of the optic nerve and frequently exhibit a biphasic growth pattern. They can also extensively involve the leptomeninges. The tumour cells are characterized by delicate bipolar hair-like processes. Rosenthal fibres (eosinophilic corkscrew or beaded structures) are frequently found in pilocytic astrocytomas in addition to eosinophilic granular bodies and protein droplets {2780}. Verhoeff described three histological patterns of optic nerve pilocytic astrocytoma: coarsely reticulated, coarsely fibrillated, and finely reticulated {2531}. Oligodendrocyte-like cells may be present as in other sites. The pilomyxoid subtype of pilocytic astrocytoma has a distinct predilection for the chiasm / hypothalamic region, affecting infants. Immunohistochemical staining for GFAP highlights the tumour cells and their processes.

Pilomyxoid astrocytoma

Pilomyxoid astrocytoma {3341} shares many features with classic pilocytic astrocytoma but differs in some important clinicopathological respects {1762,952}. It is a tumour of infancy occurring in the hypothalamic/chiasmatic region, has a higher rate of recurrence and a poorer outcome than classic pilocytic astrocytoma, and shows a propensity for cerebrospinal dissemination {1762,1515}. It is characterized by monomorphic cytology and a diffuse myxoid background {3341}. It also has a prominent angiocentric arrangement of tumour cells and typically lacks Rosenthal fibres and eosinophilic granular bodies. Some pilomyxoid astrocytomas develop into a classic pilocytic astrocytoma on recurrence {1528}.

Diffuse gliomas

Diffuse gliomas are characterized by single cell parenchymal infiltration, with higher grades demonstrating brisk mitotic activity, microvascular proliferation, necrosis, or a molecular profile typical of high-grade tumours as described in the current *Central nervous system tumours* volume of this series {1998}. Molecularly confirmed primary diffuse gliomas of the optic nerve and pathways are scant and usually represent secondary extension of supratentorial primaries. An IDH-mutant high-grade astrocytoma with secondary infiltration of the optic nerve and vitreous seeding has been reported {1972}.

Differential diagnosis

Piloid gliosis can mimic and be difficult to distinguish from pilocytic astrocytoma. Optic nerve gliosis may include arachnoid gliomatosis {3207} and diffuse hyperplastic gliosis, and may be seen in patients with or without NF1 {2790}. Diffuse leptomeningeal glioma can involve the optic nerve sheath {310}. Arachnoid enhancement of the optic nerve sheath on MRI may mimic optic nerve meningioma in some cases. Optic nerve gliomas can be associated with meningothelial hyperplasia, and a superficial biopsy of the meninges may result in an erroneous diagnosis of meningioma {662}. On a tiny biopsy specimen, it might not be possible to histologically distinguish pilocytic astrocytoma from a diffuse or fibrillary (WHO grade 2) astrocytoma {2740}.

Rare examples of glioneuronal tumours (predominantly ganglioglioma) involving the optic nerve and chiasm have been reported, and they are histologically identical to similar tumours elsewhere in the CNS {2752,2802,1344}. They contain the same combination of neoplastic mature ganglion cells admixed with neoplastic glial cells that typically constitutes a pilocytic astrocytoma. Because the optic nerve is normally a pure white matter fibre tract that lacks ganglion cells, explanations for the presence of ganglion cells in optic nerve gangliogliomas include ectopic neurons {588} and undifferentiated neuroepithelium of the optic stalk lumen, which could conceivably differentiate concurrently into both glial and ganglionic derivatives with neoplastic potential {2000}. When a ganglioglioma involves the region of the optic chiasm and hypothalamus, the pathologist must determine whether the neuronal component constitutes entrapped non-neoplastic hypothalamic neurons. Chiasmal–optic nerve rosette-forming glioneuronal tumours associated with NF1 have been reported {2871}.

For diffuse gliomas, the most important aspect of the differential diagnosis is distinguishing malignant optic nerve gliomas from metastases, lymphoma, meningioma, ganglioglioma, and pilocytic astrocytoma. Not surprisingly, biopsy specimens consisting largely of necrosis may pose a particular challenge {239}, as can the vascular proliferation commonly seen in pilocytic lesions.

Cytology

Intraoperative smears of pilocytic astrocytoma are characterized by cells with long, fine, hair-like processes. The cells usually show uniform, round to spindled nuclei with minimal atypia. Rosenthal fibres, eosinophilic granular bodies, and glomeruloid vessels can be present. In some cases, there may be degenerative atypia, with multinucleated cells. Vitreous sampling may detect glioma cells in the rare tumours extending to the retina {1972}.

Diagnostic molecular pathology

The most frequent genetic alteration in pilocytic astrocytoma is a chromosome 7q34 rearrangement resulting in a *KIAA1549::BRAF* tandem duplication and fusion {1538,2543,1016}. In small numbers of cases, alternative *BRAF* fusions have also been identified, occurring by various genetic rearrangements (including deletions and translocations) but all resulting in loss of the N-terminal regulatory region of the BRAF protein, with retention of the kinase domain {1537,3745,1308,3357}. Other MAPK pathway gene alterations also occur (see Table 6.01) {1537,3745}. *BRAF* duplications and MAPK pathway activation are detected in almost all sporadic optic nerve gliomas {2739,2693}.

Essential and desirable diagnostic criteria

Pilocytic astrocytoma

Essential: classic histological features of pilocytic astrocytoma, such as biphasic compact and loose growth patterns, piloid cytology, and low proliferative activity, with or without Rosenthal fibres and/or eosinophilic granular bodies; OR a low-grade piloid astrocytic neoplasm with a solitary MAPK pathway alteration, such as *KIAA1549::BRAF* fusion.

Table 6.01 Molecular alterations and their prevalence in pilocytic astrocytomas

Genetic alteration	% of tumours	Prevalence	References
***KIAA1549::BRAF* fusion**	> 60%	Common, particularly cerebellar; rare in other tumour forms except diffuse leptomeningeal glioneuronal tumour	{1538,3094B}
Other *BRAF* fusions	< 5%	Occasional; very rare in other entities	{1308}
***BRAF* mutations (especially p.V600E)**	~5–10%	Occasional, mainly supratentorial; also in many other glial and glioneuronal tumours	{2875A,1537A}
***NF1* mutation**	~10–15%	Typically germline; common with optic pathway tumours	{1217,1218A}
***FGFR1* mutation**	< 5%	Found mainly in midline tumours; also observed in other low-grade gliomas	{1537,3376A,3094A}
***FGFR1* fusions (especially *FGFR1::TACC1*)**	< 5%	*FGFR1::TACC1* fusion more common; also observed in other low-grade gliomas	{1537,3094A}
NTRK family fusions	~2%	Rare; also observed in other glial/glioneuronal tumours	{1537,2509A}
***KRAS* mutation**	Single cases	Very rare in pilocytic astrocytoma; extremely rare in other entities	{2954A,1501A}
***RAF1* fusion**	Single cases	Very rare in pilocytic astrocytoma; extremely rare in other entities (with the possible exception of pleomorphic xanthoastrocytoma)	{1537A,1016,3690A}
***ROS1* fusions**	Single cases	Very rare in pilocytic astrocytoma; more common in infantile hemispheric glioma; extremely rare in other entities	{2706A,2794A}
Other alterations (of *MET*, *RET*, etc.)	Single cases	Very rare in pilocytic astrocytoma; frequency in other entities not determined (probably extremely rare)	{2794A}

Chapter 6

Pilomyxoid astrocytoma

Essential: a monomorphic, loose, myxoid neoplasm with piloid cytology and a prominent angiocentric pattern, often without Rosenthal fibres and eosinophilic granular bodies; OR an astrocytic neoplasm with pilomyxoid features and a solitary MAPK pathway alteration, such as *KIAA1549*::*BRAF* fusion.

Diffuse glioma

Essential: a diffusely infiltrating glioma; molecular alterations typical of a specific diffuse glioma subtype (see the *Central nervous system tumours* volume).

Staging

For supratentorial pilocytic astrocytomas, including those involving the optic pathways, spinal MRI is performed if there is evidence of intracranial dissemination. Cerebrospinal fluid cytology is only done if radiological findings indicate disseminated disease {1131}.

Prognosis and prediction

Pilocytic astrocytomas are typically slow growing and have a favourable prognosis. Some remain stable for extended periods of time, and some may regress. Others, despite years of relative quiescence, retain the ability to grow and invade the optic chiasm and hypothalamus, resulting in considerable morbidity and mortality and a worse prognosis {3630}. Malignant transformation is rare.

Like analogous tumours of the brain and spinal cord, high-grade astrocytomas in the optic pathways have a dismal prognosis, with most patients dying of the disease in < 2 years despite radiation and/or chemotherapy {2107,3366}.

Medulloepithelioma of the optic disc and optic nerve

Eagle RC Jr
Rushing EJ

Definition

Medulloepithelioma of the optic disc and optic nerve is a rare primary intraocular embryonal tumour characterized by cords of multilayered neuroepithelial cells resembling the medullary epithelium of the optic cup.

ICD-O coding

9501/0 Medulloepithelioma, benign
9501/3 Medulloepithelioma, malignant
9502/0 Teratoid medulloepithelioma, benign
9502/3 Teratoid medulloepithelioma, malignant

ICD-11 coding

2A02.3 & XH28W9 Benign neoplasm of cranial nerves & Medulloepithelioma, benign
2A02.12 & XH2WK5 Malignant neoplasm of the optic nerve & Medulloepithelioma, NOS
2A02.3 & XH5NR7 Benign neoplasm of cranial nerves & Teratoid medulloepithelioma, benign
2A02.12 & XH0AM8 Malignant neoplasm of the optic nerve & Teratoid medulloepithelioma

Related terminology

Not recommended: diktyoma, teratoneuroma.

Subtype(s)

Benign non-teratoid medulloepithelioma; malignant non-teratoid medulloepithelioma; benign teratoid medulloepithelioma; malignant teratoid medulloepithelioma

Localization

Rare medulloepitheliomas involve the orbital optic nerve and optic disc. Most ocular medulloepitheliomas are located on the inner surface of the ciliary body.

Clinical features

Of reported cases, 86% involve the orbital optic nerve. Most are large orbital tumours that often extend to the orbital apex and can invade the CNS and cavernous sinus {1955,670,585,2505}. Optic nerve tumours typically present with symptoms of an orbital mass {1955,2611}. Misdiagnosis as optic nerve glioma is common. Fewer tumours form optic disc masses without significant optic nerve involvement {670,2420}. These can cause leukocoria and often are misdiagnosed as retinoblastoma {2420}. Ophthalmoscopically, the optic disc lesions appear as round or multilobular, well-circumscribed white tumours with a smooth convex surface that cover and obscure the optic nerve head {670,1237}.

Epidemiology

About three quarters of optic nerve cases occur in boys. The mean age at presentation is 3.5 years (median: 3.5 years, range: 1–12 years) {1955,2505}.

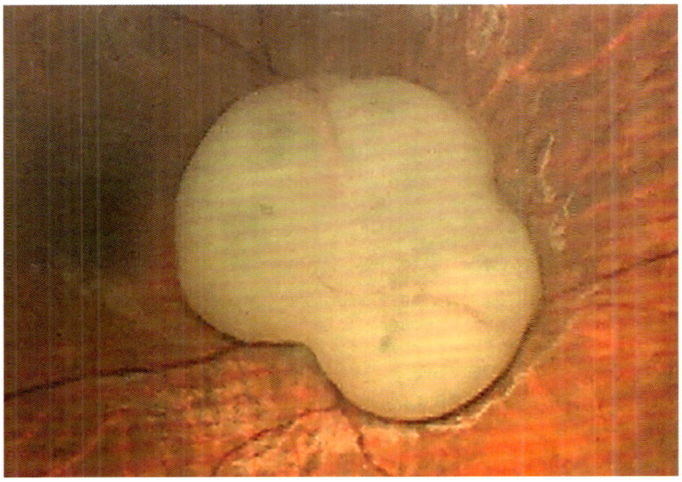

Fig. 6.06 Medulloepithelioma of the optic disc. Clinically the tumour obscures the optic disc and has smooth curved margins.

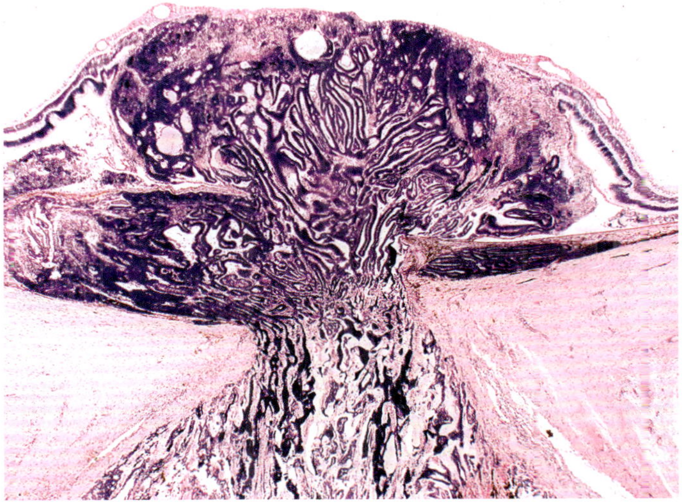

Fig. 6.07 Medulloepithelioma of the optic nerve. The tumour involves the optic nerve, optic nerve head, and peripapillary choroid.

Etiology

Most intraocular medulloepitheliomas occur sporadically and are not associated with known risk factors. Medulloepithelioma of the ciliary body (but not the optic nerve) has been reported in patients with the pleuropulmonary blastoma familial tumour predisposition syndrome caused by germline mutation of *DICER1* {1577}.

Pathogenesis

Unknown

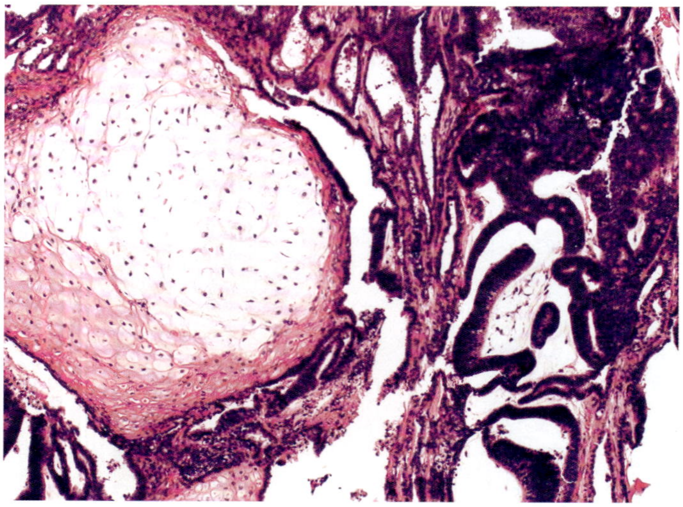

Fig. 6.08 Malignant teratoid medulloepithelioma. The tumour contains polarized bands of neuroepithelium and heteroplastic cartilage.

Macroscopic appearance

Optic nerve medulloepithelioma appears as marked thickening of the optic nerve or a lobulated perineural mass {1165,2611}. Intraocular extension may be present.

Histopathology

Medulloepitheliomas are composed of bands or cords of polarized neuroepithelial cells, resembling embryonic medullary epithelium, that are surrounded by myxoid stroma rich in hyaluronidase-sensitive mucopolysaccharide. A net-like diktyomatous pattern of thinner interweaving neuroepithelium strands, sheets of poorly differentiated neuroblastic cells resembling retinoblastoma, multilayered rosettes, and cystoid spaces are additional features. Medulloepitheliomas are subclassified as benign and malignant, and teratoid and non-teratoid. Teratoid tumours contain heteroplastic elements including cartilage (most common), muscle, rhabdomyoblasts, and brain-like tissue. Criteria for malignancy include the sheets of poorly differentiated neuroblastic cells that can contain Flexner–Wintersteiner and Homer Wright rosettes, evidence of aggressive behaviour including invasion of ocular tissues and extraocular extension, sarcomatous change, atypia, and mitotic activity {421,2858}. Immunoreactivity for LIN28A, PAX8, and RB1 can help to distinguish poorly differentiated tumours from retinoblastoma {1470,2297}.

Cytology

Cytological diagnosis is limited to malignant round cell tumour in most reported cases of ciliary body medulloepithelioma {3263,3112,2032,2858,223}. Rosettes and focal epithelial-like fragments with cellular polarity and multilayering occasionally are observed {3112}.

Diagnostic molecular pathology

Not relevant

Essential and desirable diagnostic criteria

Essential: a tumour composed of bands of polarized neuroepithelial cells within a myxoid matrix located in the orbital portion of the optic nerve or on the optic disc.

Desirable: teratoid tumours contain heteroplastic elements, most often cartilage.

Staging

Not relevant

Prognosis and prediction

The prognosis for optic nerve medulloepithelioma appears to be worse than for ciliary body tumours owing to direct access to the CNS {1955}. Patients in several reported cases of optic nerve medulloepithelioma with direct intracranial extension invasion died within 18 months of tumour resection {585}, and another developed brain metastases {346}. The relationship between malignant histopathological features and clinical outcome has been questioned {3477}.

Meningioma of the optic nerve

Pekmezci M
Rodriguez FJ
Rushing EJ

Definition
Meningioma of the optic nerve is a neoplasm arising from precursors in the optic nerve sheath.

ICD-O coding
9530/0 Meningioma of the optic nerve

ICD-11 coding
2A01.0Z Meningiomas, unspecified

Related terminology
Acceptable: optic nerve sheath meningioma.

Subtype(s)
Morphological subtypes are similar to intracranial meningiomas.

Localization
Primary optic nerve sheath meningioma (ONSM) arises from the intraorbital (92%) or intracanalicular (8%) portion of the optic nerve sheath. Secondary involvement of the optic nerve and orbit by intraorbital extension of intracranial sphenoid wing tumours is more common {2206}. Rarely, meningiomas develop ectopically in the orbit, unassociated with the optic nerve sheath {934}.

Clinical features
The classic triad at presentation consists of visual loss, optic atrophy, and optociliary shunts, with visual loss being the most common {852}. Although considered infrequent initial symptoms, proptosis and strabismus affect approximately half of patients. Orbital compartment syndrome is only rarely encountered {1451,2495}. Tumour growth may accelerate during pregnancy {560,2948}. Nearly all optic nerve meningiomas are unilateral. Bilateral cases are more likely to be secondary tumours extending from the skull base and/or tuberculum sella. Bilateral primary ONSMs typically affect children and may be associated with neurofibromatosis type 2 (NF2) {1260,2948,2495}. Diagnosis often is made based on clinical presentation and imaging findings, and a tissue diagnosis is not always pursued owing to the surgical risk to sight. ONSMs are often hypointense on T1- and hyperintense on T2-weighted MRI and show contrast enhancement in a tubular pattern, which looks like rings on coronal and tram tracks on axial sections {2034}. Given the elevated SSTR2 density in meningiomas, 68Ga-DOTATOC PET-CT can be useful in challenging cases {2034}.

Epidemiology
Primary optic nerve (sheath) meningiomas account for 2–10% of all orbital tumours and 1–2% of all meningiomas {2034}. There is a female predilection with the majority presenting in the fourth decade of life (range: from childhood to the eighth decade of life). The age at presentation is earlier in men {1453,2495}.

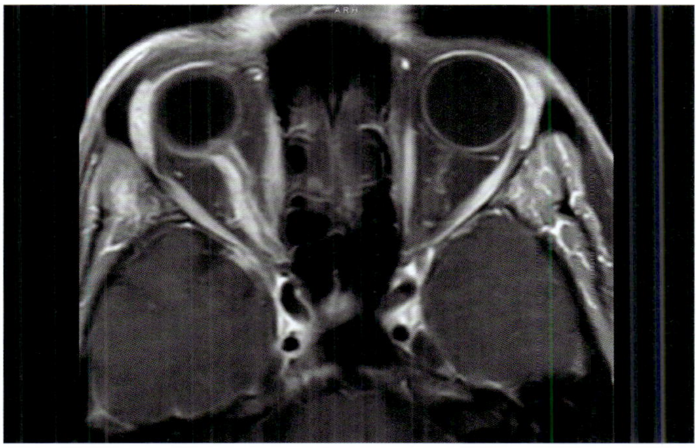

Fig. 6.09 Meningioma of the optic nerve sheath. T1-weighted postcontrast axial MRI demonstrates a tubular pattern enhancement along the right intraconal optic nerve (tram-track appearance).

Paediatric cases are even less common, comprising < 5% of ONSMs {1921}.

Etiology
Most ONSMs are sporadic and their etiology is unknown. A subset arises in the setting of NF2 syndrome or after radiation. Incidence of NF2 in the setting of paediatric ONSM is higher than in the adult population and has been reported as 29% {2349}. The incidence of ONSMs in the setting of NF2 is 2–8%, much higher than in the general population {387,919}.

Pathogenesis
Genetic alterations of ONSMs, especially sporadic cases, are not well studied given they are uncommon and only a small subset of cases undergoes surgical intervention. Based on a small series of mostly sporadic intraorbital tumours, primary ONSM and secondary meningioma extending from intracranial locations appear to be genetically distinct {1345}.

Macroscopic appearance
Optic nerve meningiomas are well circumscribed and surround the nerve, imparting a tubular appearance. Orbital apex tumours tend to cause bulbous expansion of the optic nerve with distal tubular enlargement. Occasionally, tumours invade the nerve itself {2206}.

Histopathology
Morphological classification and grading conform to the same criteria used for CNS meningiomas with most cases assigned to WHO grade 1. Meningothelial and transitional subtypes predominate at this location {1260,1453}. However, the true distribution of morphological subtypes is not clearly defined, since surgical intervention is less frequent. Meningothelial

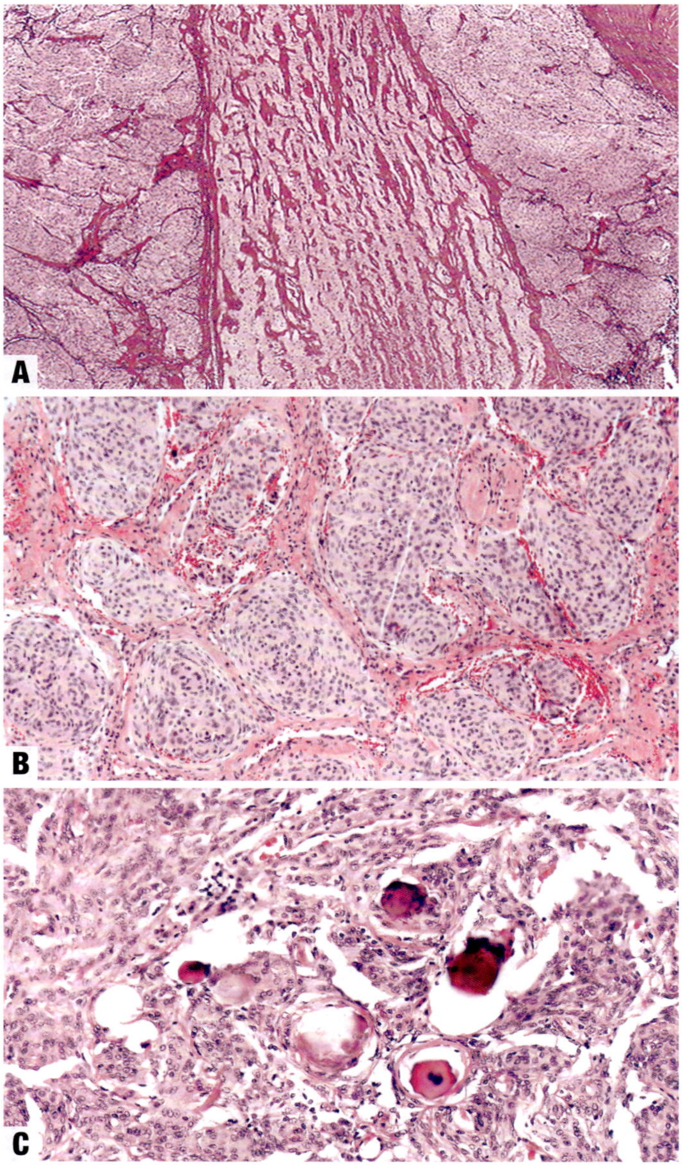

Fig. 6.10 Meningothelial meningioma of the optic nerve sheath. **A** Optic nerve surrounded by tumour within the optic nerve sheath. **B** Sphenoid meningioma extending along the optic nerve showing a meningiothelial growth pattern. **C** Tumour characterized by syncytial growth, whorls, and psammoma bodies.

meningiomas are composed of lobules of epithelioid cells with eosinophilic cytoplasm and indistinct cell borders separated by delicate collagenous septa. Nuclear holes and pseudoinclusions are common. Transitional meningiomas contain a mixture of meningothelial and fibrous features, often accompanied by psammoma bodies. Fibrous meningiomas are characterized by spindle cells arranged in fascicles, with variable amounts of intercellular collagen. In a series that included 21 ONSMs, only 1 case with angiomatous features (abundant, often hyalinized, small blood vessels) fulfilled WHO grade 2 criteria on the basis of increased mitotic activity {1453}. Other grade 2 cases have been reported, including 2 cases in children with local recurrences {1174,2328}. However, studies critically evaluating the value of histological grading in ONSMs are lacking. CNS WHO criteria do not explicitly address whether invasion of the optic nerve proper is equivalent to brain invasion, owing to the rarity of such cases. Optic nerve invasion has been reported in 5 of 47 cases in two relatively large series, but follow-up was available for only 1 patient, who was alive and well after 28 years {2804,1453}.

Immunohistochemistry

Meningiomas stain positive for EMA and SSTR2A, with fibrous meningiomas exhibiting less extensive EMA staining. Fibrous meningiomas are also more likely to stain positive for S100.

Cytology

Intraoperative smear preparations reveal cohesive clusters of epithelioid cells with eosinophilic cytoplasm and short, wispy cytoplasmic processes. Whorls, psammoma bodies, and intranuclear holes or pseudoinclusions may be present.

Diagnostic molecular pathology

Diagnostic molecular pathology is not relevant in most cases. While most secondary meningiomas harbour monosomy 22 or 22q loss, along with deletions of chromosomes 1p, 6q, and 19p, primary ONSMs seem to harbour alterations in chromosomes 2, 10, 17, and 20 {1345}. The presence of *CDKN2A* homozygous deletion or *TERT* promoter mutation would be sufficient for designation of CNS WHO grade 3 in intracranial tumours {2536, 2816,2817}. ONSM has not been studied regarding the presence or prognostic role of these alterations. But they are predicted to be associated with a worse prognosis, similar to in intracranial tumours.

Essential and desirable diagnostic criteria

Essential: classic histopathological features matching with at least one of the meningioma subtypes, or suggestive histopathological features combined with molecular changes supportive of meningioma.

Desirable: EMA immunopositivity.

Staging

Staging might be relevant only for grade 3 meningiomas with the potential for metastasis.

Prognosis and prediction

Patients with primary optic nerve meningioma have an excellent prognosis for survival, but the visual prognosis is poor, with most patients experiencing permanent vision loss in the affected eye {385,2948}. Of note, patients with tumours that demonstrate radiographic evidence of stabilization in size may even show vision improvement {2495}.

Melanocytoma of the optic disc and optic nerve

Rushing EJ
Cummings TJ
Eberhart CG

Definition
Melanocytoma is a benign, densely pigmented melanocytic tumour that is classically located in the optic disc and anterior portion of the optic nerve but can be found anywhere in the uveal tract.

ICD-O coding
8726/0 Melanocytoma of the optic disc and optic nerve

ICD-11 coding
2A02.3 & XH2RY7 Benign neoplasm of cranial nerves & Meningeal melanocytoma

Related terminology
Acceptable: magnocellular naevus; hyperpigmented magnocellular naevus.

Subtype(s)
None

Localization
Melanocytoma is usually unilateral and found on or adjacent to the optic disc. Bilateral involvement is more common in children {769,3031}. Multiple tumours in the same eye are recognized {3030}. Lesions average 1–2 disc diameters {878,3031,3029}. Rare giant examples may extend as far as the ora serrata {1003, 3091}.

Clinical features
Melanocytoma is classically asymptomatic, with visual symptoms occurring in 24% of patients and pupillary defects in < 10%. The visual field is abnormal in 90% of patients, with enlargement of the blind spot ranging from minimal to marked. Vision loss can result from central retinal vein obstruction and/or spontaneous tumour necrosis and is not necessarily related to malignant transformation {1057,3031,3029,3030}. Fluorescein angiography shows blocked fluorescence rather than alternating hyperfluorescence and hypofluorescence as seen in melanoma {3031}. Optical coherence tomography is characterized by a gradual transition from normal retina into nodular tumour. Optically empty internal details and a bright anterior border facilitate the distinction from melanoma {3001,2677}.

Epidemiology
The incidence is unknown and there is no race predilection. Optic nerve melanocytoma is proportionally more common than uveal melanoma in dark-skinned individuals. There is a slight female predilection, with an M:F ratio of approximately 1:1.5. The mean age at diagnosis is 50 years, with a range from infancy to 91 years {3029,3056}.

Etiology
Melanocytoma is considered to be of congenital origin.

Pathogenesis
Melanocytomas of the optic nerve may be related to other melanocytic lesions of the uveal tract and CNS. They are hypothesized to originate from extraepithelial melanocytes derived from the cranial neural crest {274}. It should be noted that in the *Skin tumours* volume, the term "melanocytoma" is used to delineate a completely different type of lesions at that site.

Few intraocular melanocytomas have been subject to genetic analysis. In a targeted sequencing study that included 5 melanocytomas of the optic nerve, a mutation of *GNAQ* was present in 1 case {1027}. *GNAQ* and *GNA11* encode alpha subunits of the Gq class and are frequently mutated in uveal melanoma and melanocytomas of the CNS. Interestingly, 2 cases that had a *BAP1* sequence variant plus monosomy 3 (one of which was a case with *GNAQ* mutation) progressed to melanoma. In another study, gene expression profiling of three optic nerve

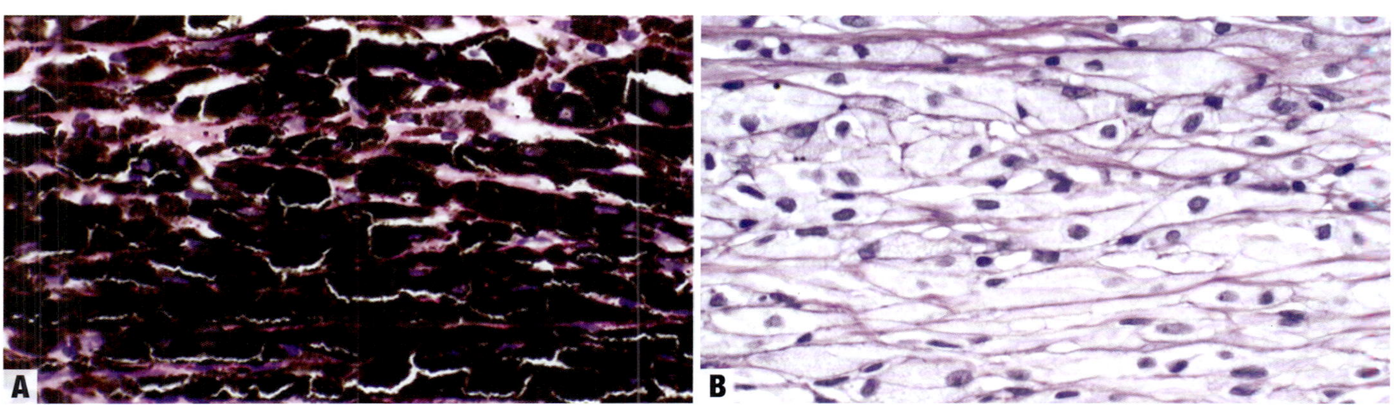

Fig. 6.11 Melanocytoma. **A** A heavily pigmented melanocytoma. **B** Bland cytological features revealed after potassium permanganate bleaching.

melanocytomas revealed that all 3 cases showed a class 1A genetic signature, which is associated with a low risk of metastatic disease in uveal melanoma {731}.

Macroscopic appearance

Typical features include a well-demarcated, flat or elevated, dark-brown to black lesion.

Histopathology

Since the tumours are densely pigmented, bleaching is required in order to identify the round to oval or polyhedral cells with small nuclei, abundant cytoplasm, and generally inconspicuous nucleoli {1997,3031,3056,3769}. Mitoses are exceptional; however, necrosis is frequent, often accompanied by pigment-laden macrophages and lymphocytic inflammation. Extensive spontaneous tumour necrosis may occur in some cases. Melanocytic markers such as HMB45, melan-A (MART1), and S100 are variably positive {1003,3031,3029,3769}.

Cytology

Smear preparations reveal cohesive nests of elongated to polygonal, intensely pigmented cells with small, uniform nuclei and inconspicuous nucleoli. Macrophages containing melanin may be present {2853}. FNAB can assist with documentation of malignant transformation to melanoma.

Diagnostic molecular pathology

Not clinically relevant

Essential and desirable diagnostic criteria

Essential: circumscribed, highly pigmented melanocytic tumour of the optic disc/nerve; limited cytological atypia and (almost) no mitoses; dense pigmentation.

Staging

Not relevant

Prognosis and prediction

Progressive growth with local invasion is common, with minor enlargement seen in as many as one third of all patients by 10 years after diagnosis. Malignant transformation is reported in 1–2% of cases, usually within 5 years of the initial diagnosis {3031,3029}; however, malignant transformation has been documented as late as 33 years after diagnosis {174,3089}.

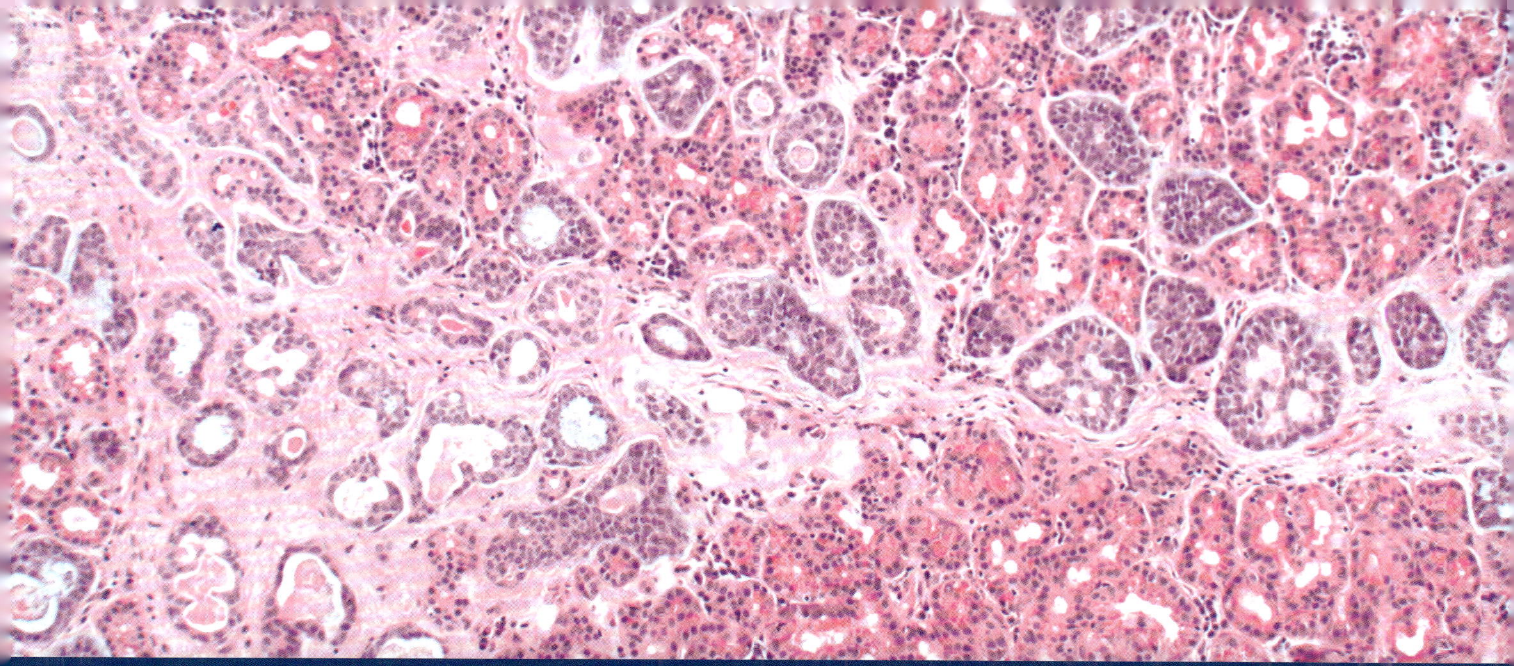

7

Tumours of the lacrimal gland

Edited by: Esmaeli B, Heegaard S, Rodríguez-Reyes AA, White VA

Tumours of the lacrimal gland: Introduction

Heegaard S
Chan ASY
Iacob CE
Milman T
Salomao DR
White VA

The lacrimal gland is composed of lobules of glands with acini that drain via interlobular ducts into excretory ducts. The acini are lined internally by acinar epithelium and externally by myoepithelium. The ducts are lined internally by low-cuboidal epithelium and externally by myoepithelium. The most common causes of lacrimal gland enlargement are inflammatory processes, but neoplasms can also arise within the gland. There are few changes in this edition, though some new molecular and other advances in knowledge are included in relevant entries.

Lacrimal gland tumours are rare and constitute a wide spectrum of different entities ranging from benign epithelial and lymphoid lesions to high-grade carcinomas, lymphomas, and sarcomas with large differences in prognosis and clinical management {150,3634}. Epithelial neoplasms of the lacrimal gland are classified along a continuum on the basis of their origin in the gland. At one end of the continuum are acinic cell tumours, which arise in the inner epithelial layer of the acinus; at the other end are monomorphic adenomas, which arise from the inner layer of the duct. Pleomorphic adenomas contain two components: an epithelial component (probably arising from the inner layer of the duct) and a myoepithelial (stromal) component. Carcinomas, such as squamous cell carcinoma, adenocarcinoma, and poorly differentiated carcinoma, can arise from the inner epithelial lining of the duct in pleomorphic adenoma (carcinoma ex pleomorphic adenoma). Lymphoid aggregates in the gland may give rise to lymphomas; these are most commonly extranodal marginal zone lymphoma of mucosa-associated lymphoid tissue (MALT lymphoma), although other forms of lymphoma may also arise in the gland.

There are many similarities between the neoplasms that occur in the salivary gland and in the lacrimal gland, but there are also some differences in terms of the frequency of the different subtypes and treatment considerations between lacrimal gland and salivary gland tumours. Salivary gland carcinomas comprise several morphologically and clinically heterogeneous subtypes, of which adenoid cystic carcinoma, mucoepidermoid carcinoma, and salivary duct carcinoma are the most commonly encountered, representing 70% of cases (see the *Head and neck tumours* volume of this series {3595}). In the lacrimal gland, adenoid cystic carcinoma is the most common carcinoma accounting for about 70% of cases, with carcinoma ex pleomorphic adenoma being the next most frequently encountered carcinoma. Mucoepidermoid carcinomas occur very rarely in the lacrimal gland.

For disease coding, and also in the published literature, there is some lumping of lacrimal drainage apparatus (lacrimal sac/duct) tumours with lacrimal gland tumours. We believe this to be inappropriate, and potentially confusing, as the most common tumour types, the anatomical structures involved, and thus the functional outcomes and treatments required differ substantially between lacrimal gland tumours and lacrimal drainage (sac/duct) tumours. For classification of tumours of the lacrimal drainage pathway, see the separate chapter in this volume.

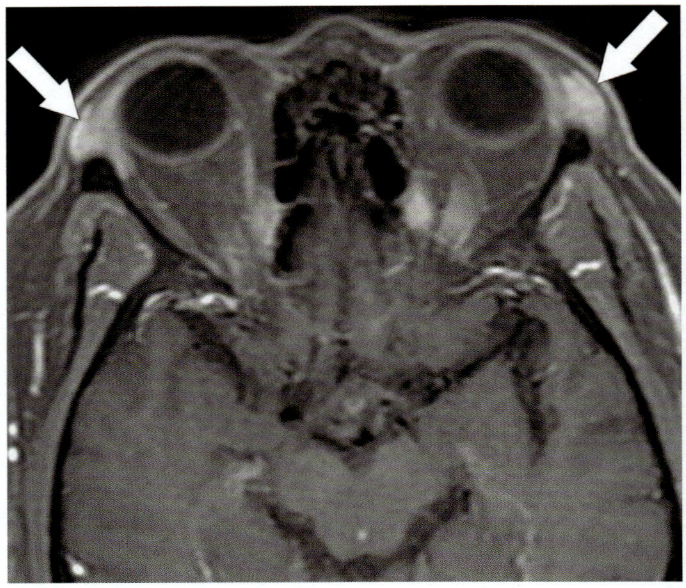

Fig. 7.01 Prolapsed lacrimal glands. Axial T1-weighted postcontrast MRI shows prolapse of bilateral lacrimal glands outside of the lacrimal fossa to a location anterior to the zygoma (arrows).

Several lacrimal gland neoplasms harbour specific genetic alterations that have been implicated in tumour pathogenesis. Gene fusions in *MYB* or *MYBL1* with *NFIB* have been reported in lacrimal gland adenoid cystic carcinoma. Recent studies of whole exome and genome performed in salivary gland carcinomas suggest that adenoid cystic carcinomas of salivary gland tend to generally fall into two molecular categories: the ones that have the canonical fusion genes and those that harbour the *NOTCH* mutation, the latter being of more aggressive biological behaviour and having a more solid histological (basaloid) appearance {1615}.

Requirements for resection

In general, when pleomorphic adenoma is the clinical diagnosis, it is advisable to excise the tumour in toto, including with an intact capsule. Rupture of the capsule can spread the tumour, and it may then recur and give rise to carcinoma ex pleomorphic adenoma, or to benign multifocal recurrence that is difficult to treat. Tumours that appear nodular on imaging (CT or MRI) and do not mould to the adjacent bone are probably epithelial (pleomorphic adenoma), whereas tumours that mould to the adjacent bone are probably lymphoid (e.g. lymphoma). Adenoid cystic carcinoma, the most common carcinoma of the lacrimal gland, usually presents as a more rapidly growing mass compared with pleomorphic adenoma, and on imaging studies such as MRI it extends posteriorly and laterally along the lateral wall of the orbit towards the superior orbital fissure. In locally advanced cases of adenoid cystic carcinoma, bony erosion and dural and CNS extension as well as extension into the temporal fossa are seen. The second most common carcinoma of the lacrimal gland is carcinoma ex pleomorphic adenoma, which as mentioned above may be an adenocarcinoma (of varying grade) or squamous carcinoma. Carcinoma ex pleomorphic adenoma of the lacrimal gland has varying clinical and radiological presentation and can have a slow growth pattern if low-grade, and be more rapid in presentation and degree of tissue expansion and bony destruction when it is of high grade {3351,3138}.

It is important for the surgeon to recognize the possibility of a pleomorphic adenoma as the diagnosis when evaluating a patient with a lacrimal gland mass based on imaging. Incisional biopsies of lacrimal gland pleomorphic adenoma should be avoided for fear of seeding and increased risk of local recurrence and potential malignant transformation. In contrast, an incisional biopsy is the most appropriate first step for lacrimal gland lesions suspected to be carcinoma based on imaging findings and clinical presentation. Definitive surgical treatment for lacrimal gland carcinoma can then be carried out after diagnosis is established and is usually followed by adjuvant radiotherapy and/or chemotherapy {1015,3351}. FNAB is commonly used to assess salivary gland tumours, but it has not been widely used in clinical practice for lacrimal gland tumours.

Lymphomas

See Chapter 10: *Haematolymphoid tumours.*

For lacrimal gland lesions suspected to be lymphoid, a biopsy to establish the diagnosis and the exact histological type of lymphoma is the appropriate first step; FNAB has been successful for lymphoid lesions of the lacrimal gland, but again with limited application in clinical practice since open biopsies of most lymphoid lesions are easy to do, have limited morbidity, and provide larger amounts of tissue for ancillary studies. Ultra-low-dose radiation therapy (only 4 Gy total dose) {2558} has been successfully used for low-grade lymphomas of the orbit and lacrimal gland, whereas chemotherapy and monoclonal antibody therapy (rituximab) are appropriate for higher-grade lymphomas such as diffuse large B-cell lymphoma or mantle cell lymphoma of the lacrimal gland {3490}.

Dacryops cyst

Mittal R
Cherepanoff S

Definition
Dacryops cyst results from dilatation of the lacrimal gland duct/ductules.

ICD-O coding
None

ICD-11 coding
9A10.Y Other specified disorders of lacrimal gland

Related terminology
Not recommended: ranula of the lacrimal gland.

Subtype(s)
None

Localization
Dacryops cysts are most common in the palpebral lobe (simple dacryops); less common in the deeper orbital lobe, accessory lacrimal glands of Krause and Wolfring, ectopic (choristomatous) lacrimal glands; and least common in the glands of Popoff in the caruncle {3208,1489,3274,125}.

Clinical features
Dacryops cyst commonly presents as an asymptomatic swelling, eyelid fullness, or mild irritation. Symptoms differ based on location.

On CT, these are usually well-defined, commonly uniloculated fluid-dense lesions anterior to the orbital rim, with absence of nodular enhancement, and bony changes. T2-weighted MRI helps in the delineation of the cystic lesion, which is isointense with the vitreous.

Epidemiology
Lesions are rare, with reported incidence varying from 1% to 17% among lacrimal gland lesions and from 0.5% to 2% among orbital lesions. They commonly arise in the fourth to fifth decade of life but can occur at any age (reported range: 18 months to 78 years), with a variable sex preponderance {2587,1489,3069}. They are commonly unilateral but may be bilateral {946,3389, 3382}.

Etiology
Most cysts are thought to be caused by persistent chronic inflammation, trauma, chemical injury, or infection {2273,1489}.

Pathogenesis
Proposed mechanisms for duct dilatation resulting in cyst formation include lacrimal gland hypersecretion or outflow obstruction by chronic periductal inflammation or fibrosis of the parenchyma, and dysfunction of the periductal/ductular neural plexus {3563,3274,1489,1846}.

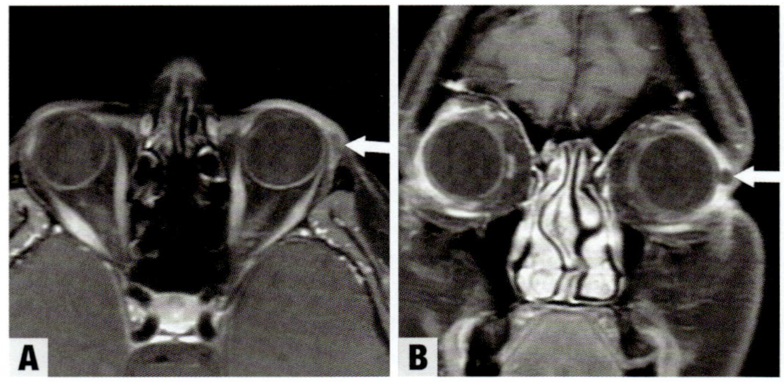

Fig. 7.02 Dacryops cyst. **A,B** Axial and coronal T1-weighted postcontrast MRI shows a non-enhancing cyst in the left lacrimal gland (arrows).

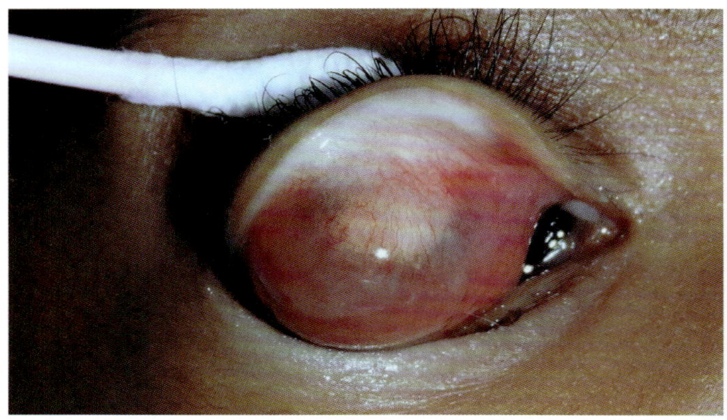

Fig. 7.03 Dacryops cyst. Eyelid eversion shows a large cystic lesion in the subconjunctival region.

Macroscopic appearance
Cysts appear as a uniloculated to (rarely) multiloculated smooth-walled cystic mass.

Histopathology
The cyst is lined by non-keratinized, double-layered columnar to cuboidal epithelium with dispersed goblet cells. The luminal cells may show focal apical projections and microvilli. Lumina may show globular eosinophilic to mucoid secretions. The wall of the cyst shows remnants of lacrimal gland acinar and variably dilated ductal structures. There may be patchy chronic inflammation and fibrosis.

Immunohistochemistry
CK7 and CK18 highlight the lining epithelium; the latter is more intense superficially. Epithelial cells are negative for CK17, SMA,

S100, and GCDFP-15. The luminal surfaces of luminal cells have been reported to strongly express IgA {1489,2587,1846}.

Differential diagnosis

Dacryoadenitis, prolapsed orbital fat, prolapsed lacrimal gland, dermolipoma, epithelial tumours of the lacrimal gland, foreign body granuloma, respiratory cyst, conjunctival inclusion cyst, dermoid or epidermoid cyst, mucocoele, sarcoidosis, and lymphoma can all mimic dacryops cysts {1489,3274}.

Cytology

Not clinically relevant

Diagnostic molecular pathology

Not relevant

Essential and desirable diagnostic criteria

Essential: cystic lesion lined by non-keratinized double-layered epithelium, with dispersed goblet cells; presence of lacrimal gland acini and variably dilated ducts in the wall of the cyst.

Staging

Not relevant

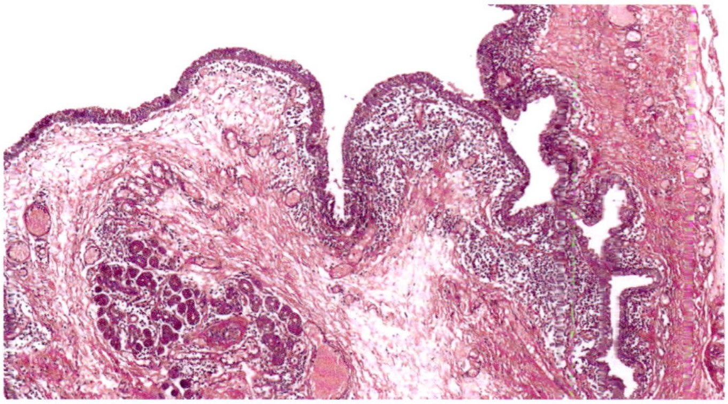

Fig. 7.04 Dacryops cyst. A cyst lined by non-keratinized pseudostratified columnar epithelium with dispersed goblet cells is seen. The wall of the cyst shows lacrimal gland acini, variable fibrosis, oedema, and patchy mild chronic lymphomononuclear cell infiltration (PAS staining).

Prognosis and prediction

The outcome is good after complete surgical removal and marsupialization. However, recurrences, fistula formation after marsupialization, and secondary tear deficiency have been reported {2823,1489,3274}.

Chapter 7

Pleomorphic adenoma of the lacrimal gland

Salomao DR
Chan ASY
Paridaens D

Definition
Pleomorphic adenoma (PA) is a benign primary lacrimal gland neoplasm consisting of a mixture of epithelial, myoepithelial, and mesenchymal-appearing components.

ICD-O coding
8940/0 Pleomorphic adenoma

ICD-11 coding
2F36.Y & XH2KC1 Other specified benign neoplasm of eye or ocular adnexa & Pleomorphic adenoma

Related terminology
Not recommended: benign mixed tumour.

Subtype(s)
None

Localization
PA arises in the lacrimal gland, most commonly from the orbital lobe (90%), occasionally from the palpebral lobe {3452,2085, 2656,2583,2497}, and rarely from accessory lacrimal gland tissue {129,2310}. It may also arise from sweat glands in the eyelid skin {2467,2443,3538}.

Clinical features
PA usually presents as a slow-growing mass causing painless enlargement of the lateral upper eyelid, progressing to proptosis and globe displacement. Some patients experience diplopia and visual impairment {3714,1267}.

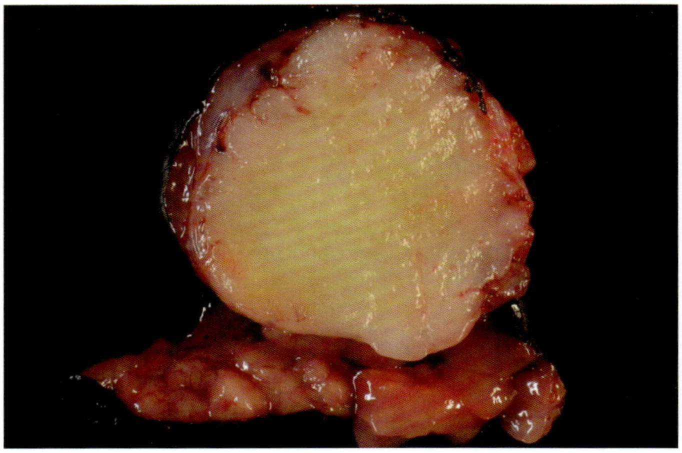

Fig. 7.05 Pleomorphic adenoma. A well-demarcated, encapsulated nodule with a yellowish glistening cut surface.

Imaging
CT and MRI are important to visualize surrounding bone and possible extension to adjacent structures, assisting with the differential diagnosis with malignant lacrimal neoplasms. On MRI, PAs are usually well-circumscribed, round to oval isointense lesions with regular margins, located in the lacrimal fossa {1267}. Cystic areas, foci of calcification, and bony excavation may be seen {3559}. There is often bony expansion (remodelling) of the lacrimal fossa without destruction owing to the slowly enlarging mass. Significant differences are observed between primary and recurrent PA in imaging studies. Recurrent PA tends to present with uneven density, unclear boundaries, adjacent

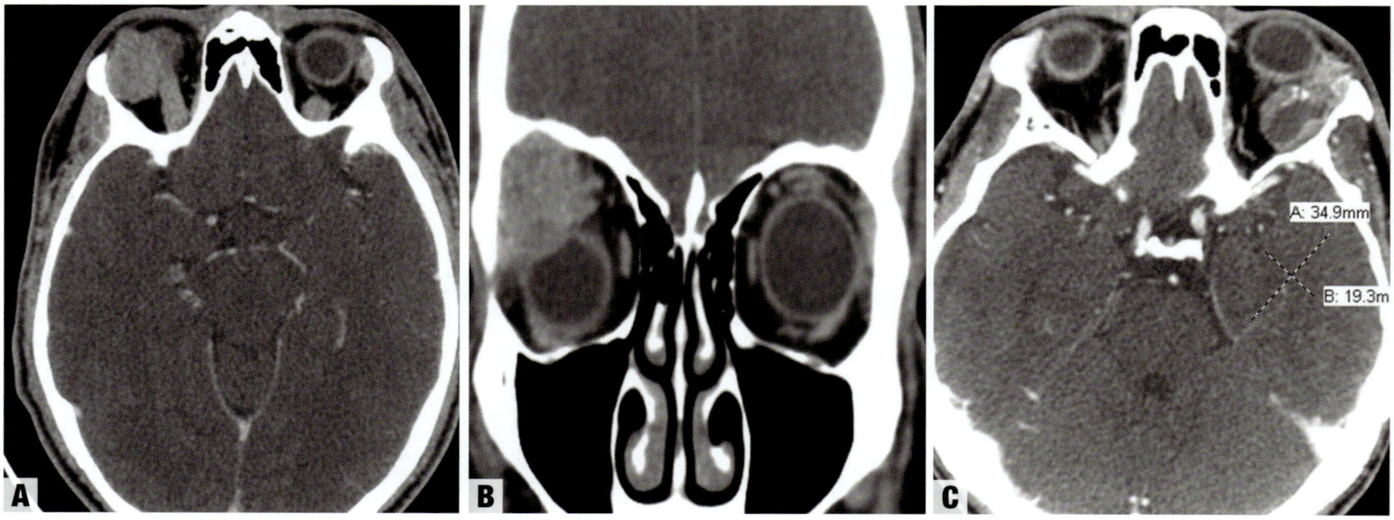

Fig. 7.06 Pleomorphic adenoma. **A** Axial CT image of a pleomorphic adenoma; note the well-circumscribed round lacrimal gland mass. **B** Coronal CT image of a pleomorphic adenoma; note the bony expansion of the lacrimal gland fossa and lack of frank bony erosion. **C** Axial CT image of a cellular pleomorphic adenoma of the left lacrimal gland; this lesion was benign but with a higher proliferation rate than the typical pleomorphic adenoma.

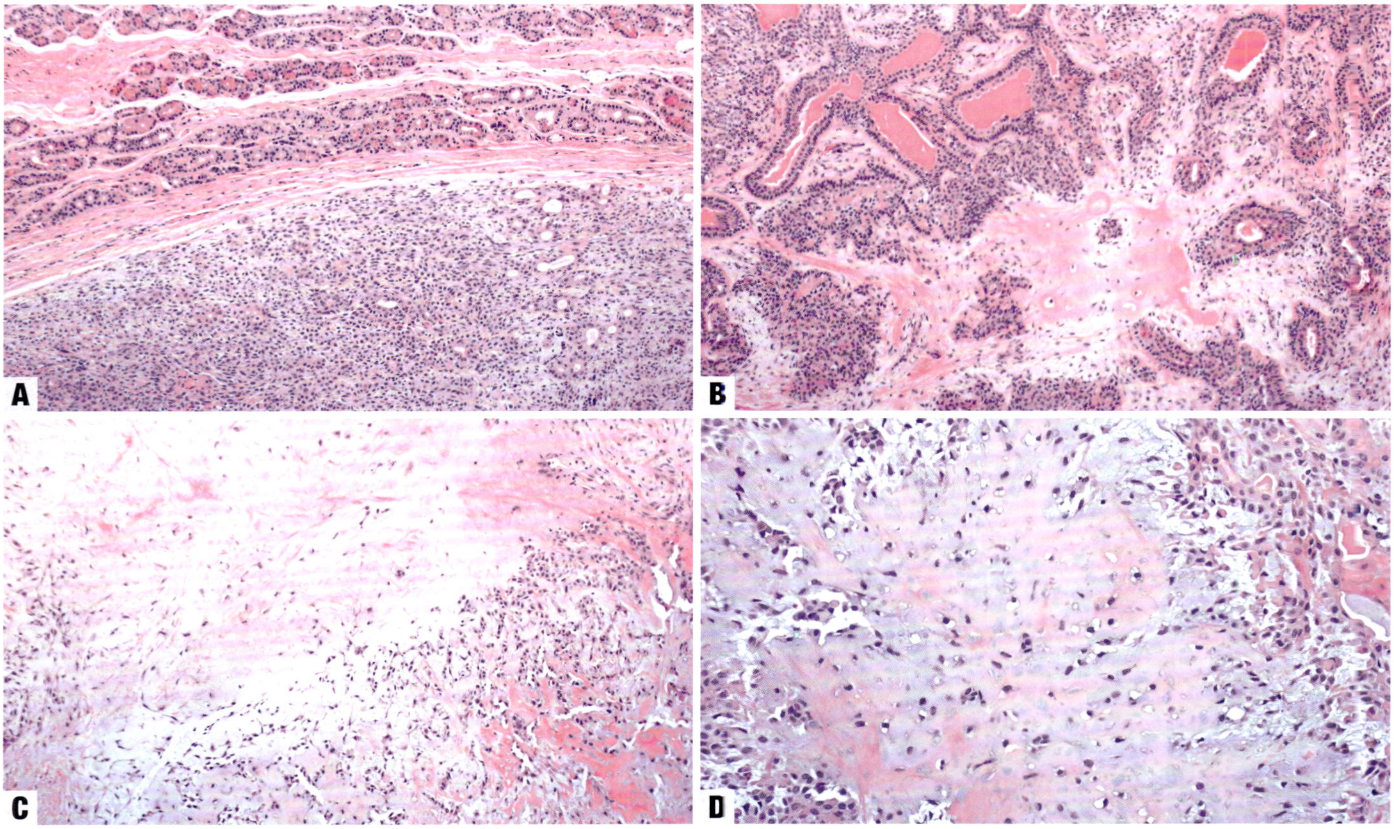

Fig. 7.07 Pleomorphic adenoma. **A** A low-power microscopic view shows a sharp demarcation between the benign lacrimal gland tissue and the pleomorphic adenoma due to the presence of a pseudocapsule. **B** The classic pattern shows a balanced representation of epithelial, myoepithelial, and stromal components. **C** The stromal component, derived from myoepithelial cells, is often represented by fibrous and myxoid areas. **D** Chondroid areas are often seen in the stroma.

bone destruction, and adherence to surrounding tissues {2152, 3714,1971}.

Epidemiology

Although PA accounts for only 0.6–2% of all orbital lesions, it is the most common epithelial neoplasm of the lacrimal gland and represents approximately 50–70% of lacrimal gland tumours in most series {3152,3572,552,96}. The mean patient age at presentation is 40 years, with a broad range from childhood {1213} to the ninth decade of life {592,127,1971}. No race, sex, or geographical location predilection has been identified {127,1971,592}.

Etiology

Unknown

Pathogenesis

Recurrent translocations of *PLAG1*, an adenoma-associated gene located at chromosome 8q12, result in the overexpression of the PLAG1 oncoprotein in PAs {153,1267}. *PLAG1* gene translocation t(5;8)(p13;q12) is highly specific for PA {1267}. Translocations of *HMGA2*, located at chromosome 12q14, have also been reported in PAs although to a lesser extent {1267}.

Macroscopic appearance

PAs are usually well-circumscribed, pseudoencapsulated, round to bosselated masses with a firm, whitish surface with occasional cysts, calcification, or cartilaginous areas {2918}. Protrusions outside the pseudocapsule and satellite nodules may be observed infrequently. Recurrent PAs tend to be multinodular and multifocal.

Histopathology

The histological hallmark of PA is its morphological diversity because of the relative proportions of each component in each tumour {3507,2012,3572}. The epithelial component is characterized by bilayered ductal structures, and the epithelial cells may show a squamous, clear, round, oncocytic, and/or plasmacytoid appearance. The stromal component, derived from myoepithelial cells, may be fibrous, myxoid, hyaline, chondroid, or osseous or occasionally show adipose differentiation. The epithelial component predominates in the so-called cellular pattern, and the stromal component predominates in the stroma-rich pattern. The classic pattern has a balanced representation of epithelial and stromal components. Cyst formation and crystals may be present. Extensive squamous and focal mucinous metaplasia may be observed in some tumours. Although a few mitoses are usually present, overt cytological atypia and areas of carcinoma should raise the possibility of malignant transformation (carcinoma ex pleomorphic adenoma). There is a pseudocapsule, with protrusions of the tumour within it, explaining the tendency of these tumours to recur if not completely excised with surrounding tissue.

Immunohistochemistry

The luminal epithelial cells stain with cytokeratins (CK7 and CAM5.2), while the myoepithelial cells are positive for p40, p63,

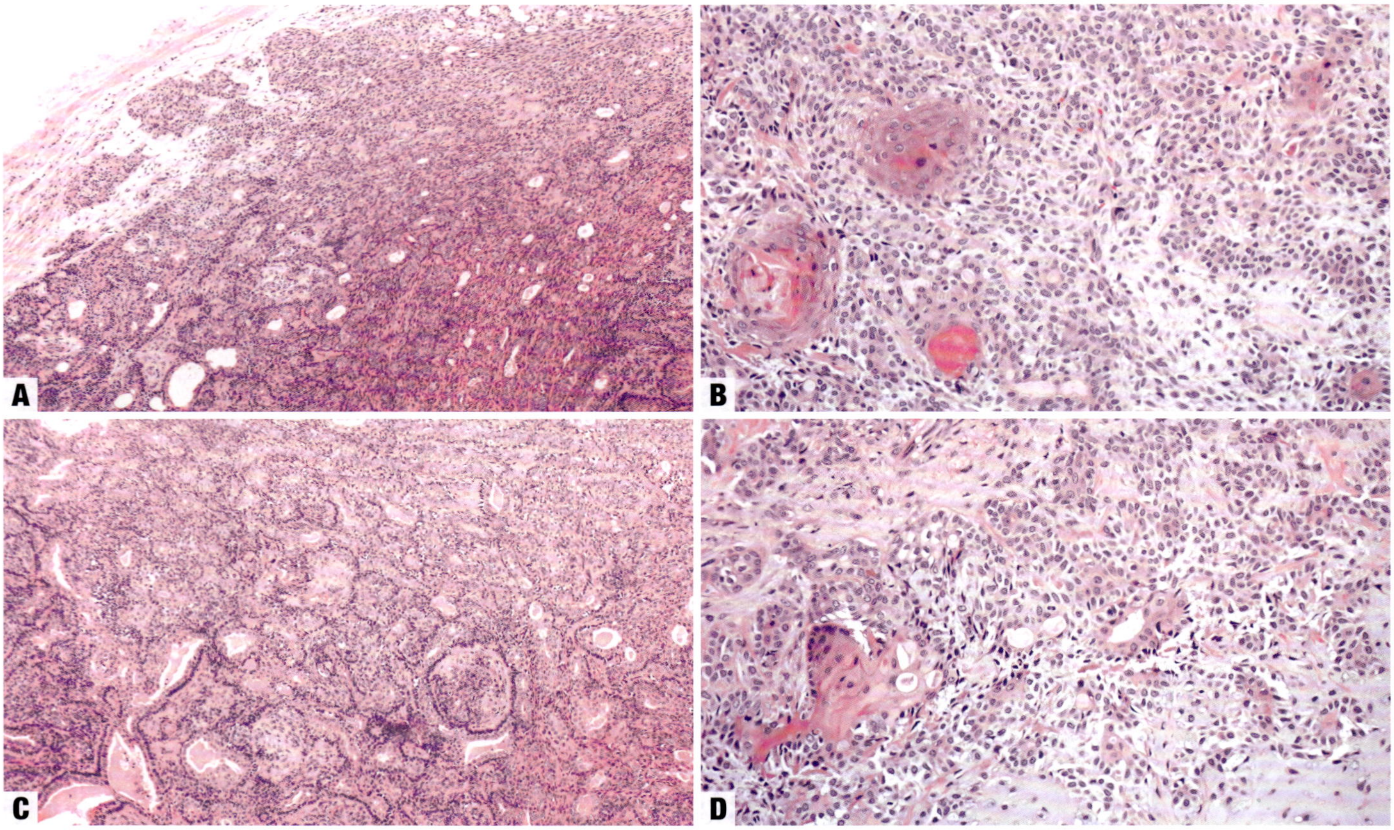

Fig. 7.08 Pleomorphic adenoma. **A** In a few cases, protrusions into and through the pseudocapsule can be seen. These might cause recurrences if the tumour is incompletely excised. **B** Areas of squamous metaplasia may be observed. **C** In more cellular-pattern tumours, the epithelial component predominates, raising the differential with other epithelial neoplasms. **D** Note the clearing of the myoepithelial cells and a focus of squamous metaplasia in this field.

SMA, and calponin. KIT (CD117) is negative and the proliferative index with Ki-67 immunostain should be very low. Positive staining for PLAG1 (nuclear) is consider specific {2170,1481} along with HMGA2 {153}, and the tumours may also stain with GFAP {2934,696}.

Differential diagnosis

Differential diagnoses include basal cell and canalicular adenoma, carcinoma ex pleomorphic adenoma, adenoid cystic carcinoma, myoepithelioma, and epithelial-myoepithelial carcinoma. Tumours with extensive squamous or mucous metaplasia should be differentiated from squamous cell carcinoma and mucoepidermoid carcinoma.

Cytology

Cytological preparations are characterized by a mixture of small cuboidal epithelial cells in clusters or small sheets, and myoepithelial cells (usually numerous, discohesive, bland, elongated, or plasmacytoid in appearance). Variable amounts of fibrillary and chondromyxoid stroma, metachromatic on Giemsa staining or greyish blue on Pap staining, are observed in the background {1839,1213}.

Diagnostic molecular pathology

Not relevant in most cases

Essential and desirable diagnostic criteria

Essential: lacrimal fossa mass; round or bosselated tumour with an admixture of bilayered ducts, myoepithelial cells, and chondromyxoid/fibrous stroma in the absence of invasion and malignant cytomorphological features.

Desirable: PLAG1 or *HMGA2* alteration in select cases.

Staging

Not relevant

Prognosis and prediction

Two major factors determining prognosis in lacrimal gland PA are the probability of recurrence as a result of incomplete resection, and evidence of malignant transformation {3572,1971}. Biological behaviour is not affected by histological pattern. Multifocal benign recurrences as well as malignant transformation can be observed in lacrimal gland PA after previous incomplete excision and can be challenging to treat surgically. Spontaneous malignant transformation has also been reported {3351}. Multiple recurrences and longstanding tumours seem to be associated with increased risk of malignant transformation {2152,1267, 3434}. Although cases of histologically benign-appearing PA demonstrating metastatic behaviour (benign metastasizing PA) have been described in salivary glands {1745,3558}, to date, such cases have not been reported in the lacrimal gland.

Lacrimal gland oncocytoma

Iacob CE
Chan ASY
Paridaens D

Definition
Oncocytoma of the lacrimal gland is a neoplasm composed of epithelial cells with a large amount of granular eosinophilic cytoplasm, rich in mitochondria.

ICD-O coding
8290/0 Oncocytoma
8290/3 Oncocytic carcinoma

ICD-11 coding
2F36.Y & XH9Z86 Other specified benign neoplasm of eye or ocular adnexa & Oxyphilic adenoma

Related terminology
Acceptable: oncocytic adenoma; oxyphilic adenoma.

Subtype(s)
None

Localization
Periocular oncocytoma arises in the ducts of the main and the accessory lacrimal glands. Oncocytomas of accessory lacrimal glands can involve the caruncle and, less frequently, the palpebral and forniceal conjunctiva as well as the plica semilunaris {2517}. In the lacrimal drainage apparatus, oncocytoma can involve the lacrimal sac, nasolacrimal duct, and lacrimal canaliculus (peripunctal) {1418}.

Clinical features
Oncocytoma of the main lacrimal gland can cause fullness of the temporal aspect of the orbit, proptosis, nasal deviation of the eye, and eyelid ptosis. Oncocytomas are well-delineated masses causing compressive phenomena according to their location: enlargement of the caruncle, swelling of the conjunctiva or eyelid, and obstruction of the lacrimal drainage system.

Epidemiology
Oncocytomas are uncommon, accounting for < 1% of lacrimal gland neoplasms. They are tumours of adulthood with incidence peaking in the sixth to eighth decades of life. They tend to have slight female predominance {2450}. Periocular oncocytic carcinomas are extremely rare; 1 case arising in the setting of neurofibromatosis has been described {313}, another 1 in plica semilunaris {1147}.

Etiology
Unknown

Pathogenesis
While the precise mechanism of mitochondrial multiplication and its link to the proliferation of oncocytes remains unclear, a variety of deletions, SNPs, and gene rearrangements have been described in oncocytomas of the thyroid, kidney, salivary gland, and adrenal cortex. It appears that mutations in the mitochondrial rather than nuclear genes encoding for enzymes involved in oxidative phosphorylation are involved in the genesis of oncocytomas {2125}. In a single lacrimal gland oncocytoma investigated, trisomy 8 and monosomy 22 were identified, together with an additional 33 sequence variants in mitochondrial DNA {2201}. The large diversity of genetic changes found in oncocytomas in general precludes a unifying understanding of their pathogenesis.

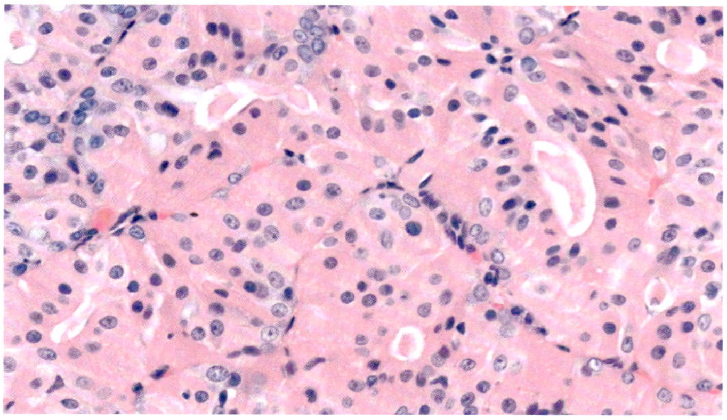

Fig. 7.09 Lacrimal gland oncocytoma. Eccentric smoothly bordered nuclei with vesicular chromatin and a single conspicuous nucleolus, accompanied by abundant granular cytoplasm.

Macroscopic appearance
Oncocytomas are well-circumscribed lobulated red-brown masses that are solid and/or cystic on the cut surface.

Histopathology
Oncocytomas are well-delineated neoplasms that display solid, papillary, or cystic architecture. They are composed of proliferating polygonal epithelial cells with a low N:C ratio, smoothly bordered nuclei, and large amounts of eosinophilic granular cytoplasm (highlighted by phosphotungstic acid–haematoxylin stain). The oncocytes are arranged in sheets, nests, or trabeculae, separated by thin fibrovascular bands. Their nuclei display vesicular chromatin, typically with a single conspicuous nucleolus. Ultrastructural analysis reveals a plethora of cytoplasmic mitochondria {461}.

Oncocytic carcinomas display nuclear atypia, mitoses, and invasion of neighbouring structures (soft tissue and bone) {1553,3343}.

Immunohistochemistry
Positivity with an antimitochondrial antibody (e.g. MU213-UC) may be helpful. Oncocytomas stain similarly to the lacrimal ducts: they are positive for CK4, CK5/6, CK7, CK8, CK17, CK18, S100, and EMA, but negative for CK20, CEA, and for markers of

keratinizing epithelium {2450}. Ki-67 shows a low nuclear labelling index (< 1%) and mitoses are exceptional {2201}.

Cytology

Oncocytes are readily identified by their specific morphology in salivary gland FNA cytology preparations, but such a method has limited application in lacrimal neoplasms.

Diagnostic molecular pathology

Not relevant

Essential and desirable diagnostic criteria

Essential: a mass composed of oncocytic epithelial cells; eosinophilic granular cytoplasm.

Desirable: a well-delineated mass; variably solid or cystic growth; arising in lacrimal gland parenchyma.

Staging

Oncocytic carcinomas are staged according to Union for International Cancer Control (UICC) TNM or the American Joint Committee on Cancer (AJCC) *Cancer staging manual*, eighth edition, 2017.

Prognosis and prediction

No specific prognostic features have been delineated. Complete surgical excision is the treatment of choice for oncocytomas and oncocytic carcinomas of the lacrimal glands.

Myoepithelioma

Iacob CE
Chan ASY
Paridaens D

Definition

Myoepithelioma is a benign epithelial neoplasm of the lacrimal gland with myoepithelial differentiation. Its malignant counterpart is myoepithelial carcinoma.

ICD-O coding

8982/0 Myoepithelioma
8982/3 Myoepithelial carcinoma

ICD-11 coding

2F36.Y & XH3CQ8 Other specified benign neoplasm of eye or ocular adnexa & Myoepithelioma
2D0Y & XH43E6 Other specified malignant neoplasms of eye or ocular adnexa & Myoepithelial carcinoma

Related terminology

Not recommended: myoepithelial cell tumour; myoepithelial adenoma.

Subtype(s)

None

Localization

Myoepitheliomas of the main lacrimal gland have been reported in > 10 published papers {29,368,2503}. Myoepitheliomas have also been reported in the orbital apex without a connection to the lacrimal gland; such lesions are thought to arise from glandular embryonic remnants along the Rathke pouch {1287}.

Clinical features

Myoepitheliomas of the main lacrimal gland are usually nontender, slow-growing, well-circumscribed superotemporal orbital masses causing proptosis, internal deviation of the eye, or eyelid ptosis. Myoepithelial carcinomas can arise de novo or as clonal expansions in other tumours, such as pleomorphic adenomas {321}.

Epidemiology

Myoepithelial tumours account for < 1% of lacrimal gland neoplasms {29}. Patients' age at presentation varies widely and both sexes are equally affected.

Etiology

Unknown

Pathogenesis

Salivary gland myoepitheliomas show chromosomal alterations (12q), a feature shared with pleomorphic adenomas {2029}. In addition, myoepithelial carcinomas of the salivary gland, especially the clear cell pattern, show *EWSR1* gene rearrangement {3144}. Other studies on salivary gland tumours found that malignant transformation in myoepithelial cells requires, in addition to p16 pathway deregulation, inactivation of p53 {3464}. These findings have not yet been validated in lacrimal gland myoepithelial neoplasms.

Macroscopic appearance

Myoepitheliomas are solid well-delineated masses with a tan to yellow appearance and glistening cut surfaces.

Histopathology

Myoepitheliomas are usually well circumscribed and sometimes surrounded by a variably thick fibrous capsule. They are densely cellular and display spindle, plasmacytoid, epithelioid, or clear cells proliferating in trabeculae or sheets. Occasional rudiments of ducts or microcysts as well as mucinous foci can be encountered. Interlacing fibrous fascicles with hyalinized areas can be present. The nuclei are normochromatic, smoothly bordered, and round to oval, and lack mitoses. Light-pink to clear cytoplasm is seen in variable amounts and is more abundant in the plasmacytoid pattern. The neoplastic cells are consistently positive for cytokeratins (CK7 and CK14) and variably

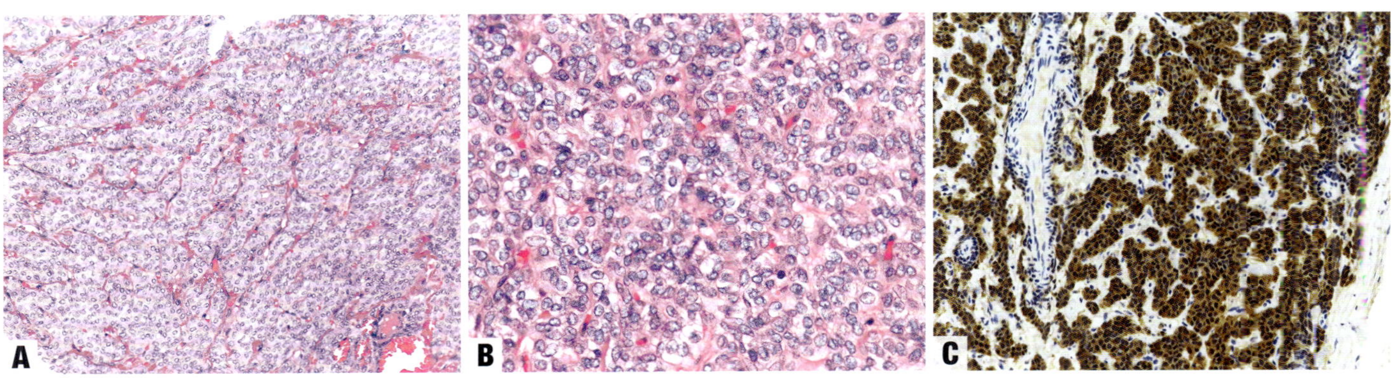

Fig. 7.10 Myoepithelioma of the lacrimal gland. **A** Trabecular growth pattern. **B** Sheets of cells with monotonous oval nuclei and variable pink cytoplasm. **C** A well-delineated neoplasm with consistently S100-positive myoepithelial cells.

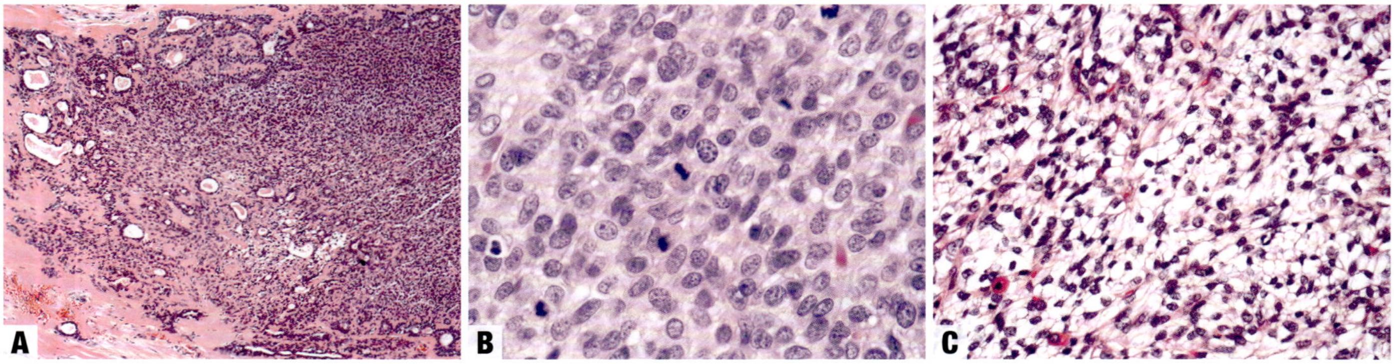

Fig. 7.11 Myoepithelial carcinoma of the lacrimal gland. **A** A lacrimal gland pleomorphic adenoma on the left gives rise to a myoepithelial carcinoma on the right; the carcinoma is cellular. **B** The image shows pleomorphic nuclei with mitoses (oil immersion). **C** Cells in this example have clear cytoplasm.

immunoreactive for myoepithelial markers (S100, SMA, MSA, p63, calponin, and less for GFAP) {1184}.

Myoepithelial carcinomas show invasion into neighbouring structures (lacrimal gland, orbital soft tissue, bone, or perineural spaces). They can have cytologically bland nuclei or display nuclear pleomorphism and mitotic activity.

Cytology

Myoepithelial cells can be recognized based on their spindle morphology with limited cytoplasm on cytology from FNAB of salivary glands {56,1558}, but this method is of limited use for lacrimal gland neoplasms.

Diagnostic molecular pathology

Not relevant

Essential and desirable diagnostic criteria

Essential: monotonous epithelial cells coexpressing myoepithelial markers.

Desirable: tumours are encapsulated.

Staging

Myoepithelial carcinomas are staged according to the Union for International Cancer Control (UICC) TNM or American Joint Committee on Cancer (AJCC) *Cancer staging manual*, eighth edition, 2017.

Prognosis and prediction

Myoepitheliomas are benign and treated by complete local excision. There are no specific prognostic criteria for myoepithelial carcinomas, which have a recurrence rate of > 20% after surgical resection and late metastases {2271}.

Intraductal carcinoma

Hyrcza MD
Dubovy SR
Paridaens D

Definition

Intraductal carcinoma (IDC) is a biphasic carcinoma characterized by round tumour lobules with variable architecture and low-grade cytology that are surrounded by a single continuous layer of myoepithelial cells

ICD-O coding

8500/2 Intraductal carcinoma

ICD-11 coding

2E6A.Y & XH1H31 Carcinoma in situ of other and unspecified part of the eye and adnexa & Intraductal carcinoma, noninfiltrating, NOS

Related terminology

Acceptable: intercalated duct carcinoma; low-grade intraductal carcinoma.

Not recommended: low-grade cribriform cystadenocarcinoma; low-grade salivary duct carcinoma.

Subtype(s)

None

Localization

One case has been described in the lacrimal gland {451}. Most cases occur in the major salivary glands {400,3569} and oral cavity {561,575}.

Clinical features

The lacrimal tumour caused proptosis with inferomedial globe displacement {451}.

Epidemiology

This is a rare type of lacrimal carcinoma with only a single case described so far {451}.

Etiology

Unknown

Pathogenesis

The single lacrimal case was not analysed for molecular changes. Intraductal carcinoma of the salivary glands tends to harbour *NCOA4::RET* and *TRIM33::RET* fusions {2342,3143, 3139}. *RET* gene rearrangement was shown to be present in both luminal and myoepithelial cells, suggesting both components are neoplastic {343}.

Chapter 7

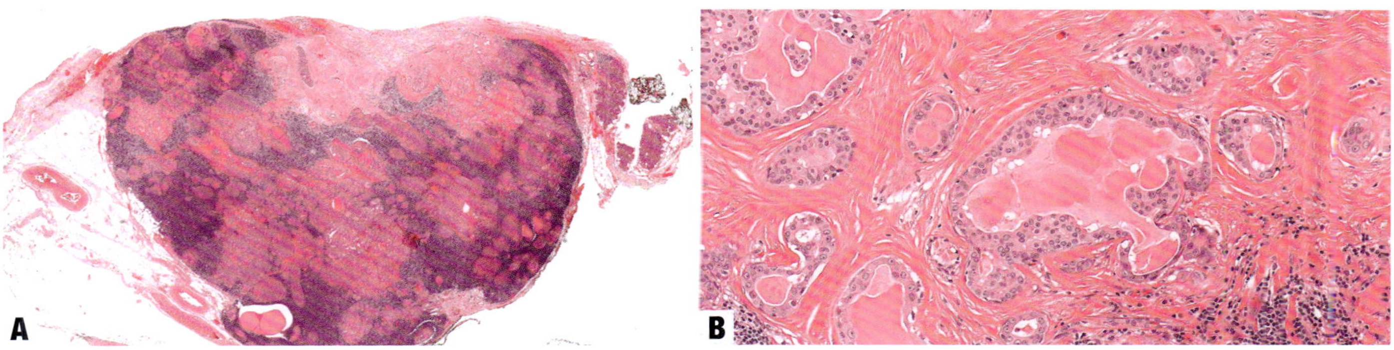

Fig. 7.12 Lacrimal intraductal carcinoma. **A** The well-circumscribed tumour consists of islands surrounded by lymphoid tissue and focally dense collagenous stroma. **B** Tumour cells show low-grade cytology with central nuclei, small single nucleoli, and ample eosinophilic cytoplasm.

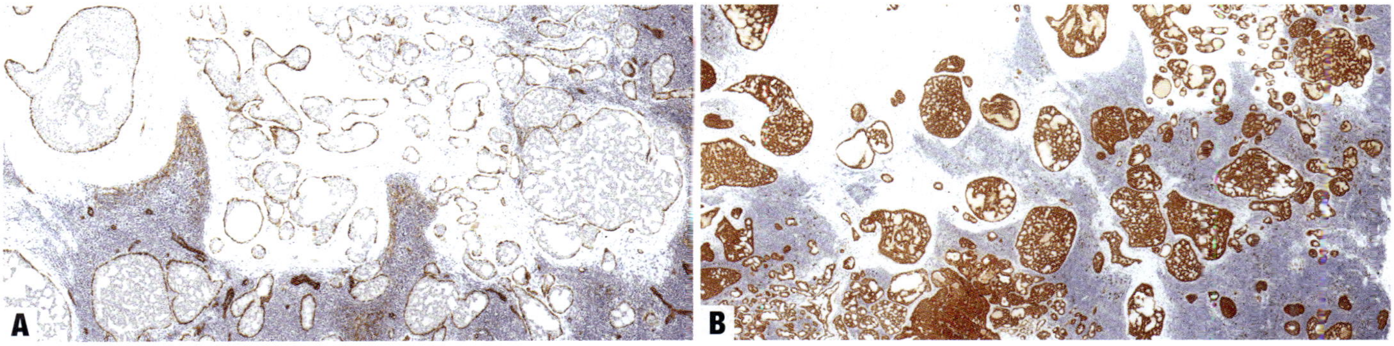

Fig. 7.13 Lacrimal intraductal carcinoma. **A** SMMHC immunohistochemistry highlights a thin layer of myoepithelial cells surrounding each tumour island. **B** The tumour shows diffuse positivity for S100 by immunohistochemistry.

Macroscopic appearance

Not reported

Histopathology

Unencapsulated, well-circumscribed carcinoma consists of round lobules with variable solid, papillary-cystic, cribriform, and micropapillary architecture, surrounded by a single, continuous, flat layer of myoepithelial cells. The ductal cells are large and polygonal with abundant amphiphilic or oncocytic cytoplasm and mild nuclear atypia. Small nucleoli and intranuclear inclusions may be seen. Eosinophilic secretions fill the cystic spaces. The surrounding stroma may be densely fibrotic and contain lymphocytic infiltrate. Intercalated duct, oncocytic, and apocrine subtypes have been described in the salivary IDCs. The 1 lacrimal case had intercalated morphology {451}.

Immunohistochemistry

Intraductal cells of the intercalated and oncocytic types are positive for CK19, S100, SOX10, and mammaglobin, and negative for AR and GCDFP-15. The opposite staining pattern is seen in apocrine IDCs. Myoepithelial cells are positive for p63, p40, CK5, CK14, calponin, SMA, and SMMHC.

Cytology

Not reported

Diagnostic molecular pathology

Demonstration of *RET* gene rearrangement may help with diagnosis; however, break-apart FISH is often falsely negative in IDC with *NCOA4*::*RET* fusion owing to a tight inversion {3569,3143, 343}.

Essential and desirable diagnostic criteria

Essential: round lobules of ductal cells surrounded entirely by a single layer of myoepithelial cells.
Desirable: presence of *RET* gene rearrangement.

Staging

IDC is currently regarded as in situ disease by Union for International Cancer Control (UICC) staging of invasive carcinoma ex IDC, according to the UICC TNM classification.

Prognosis and prediction

The single lacrimal IDC did not recur in the 6 years after complete excision {451}.

Carcinoma ex pleomorphic adenoma

Salomao DR
Chan ASY
Mittal R

Definition
Carcinoma ex pleomorphic adenoma is a malignant lacrimal gland epithelial neoplasm that shows the presence of an epithelial and/or myoepithelial malignancy arising in association with primary or recurrent pleomorphic adenoma (PA).

ICD-O coding
8941/3 Carcinoma ex pleomorphic adenoma

ICD-11 coding
2D0Y & XH42V2 Other specified malignant neoplasms of eye or ocular adnexa & Carcinoma ex pleomorphic adenoma

Related terminology
Not recommended: carcinoma ex benign mixed tumour; malignant mixed tumour; carcinoma arising in mixed tumour; carcinoma arising in pleomorphic adenoma.

Subtype(s)
None

Localization
Lesions arise in the orbital and palpebral lobes of the main lacrimal gland {3351,3427,3429} and accessory and ectopic lacrimal gland tissue.

Clinical features
Patients may present with a previously slow-growing mass in the lacrimal fossa, causing proptosis or inferior globe displacement, or with recurrent PA that abruptly shows rapid growth and/or becomes symptomatic with pain, skin ulceration, and/or fixation {3050,3427}.

Imaging
Although simple X-rays can show an orbital wall lytic lesion, CT and MRI are able to demonstrate the infiltrative pattern of an aggressive malignancy {1267,3351}.

Epidemiology
Carcinoma ex pleomorphic adenoma (CEPA) is the second most common lacrimal gland malignancy, although rare. Review of the literature of 40 cases showed no sex predilection and a median age at diagnosis of 56 years (range: 17–76 years) {312,3572,1971,3351,153,3748}.

Etiology
CEPA may arise de novo {3351} or secondary to malignant change after incomplete excision of PA {1267}.

Pathogenesis
Recurrent translocations of *PLAG1* (chromosome 8q) and *HMGA2* (chromosome 12q), involved in PA pathogenesis, are also seen in CEPA {1267,153,3351,2363}. CEPA development follows progressive sequential loss of heterozygosity of 8q, 12q, and finally 17p {1267,3351,2363}. Malignant transformation has been associated with alterations in 12q genes (*HMGA2* and *MDM2*), 17p loss leading to loss of p53 {153,1267,3351,2363}, and copy-number alterations involving 9p and 22q, resulting in activation of *NFIB* and *PDGFB* {1267}. Overexpression of the IL-6/JAK/STAT3 pathway may also play a role in the malignant transformation {152}.

Macroscopic appearance
Lesions appear as a heterogeneous mass, often with areas resembling residual PA, or possible invasion of surrounding tissue.

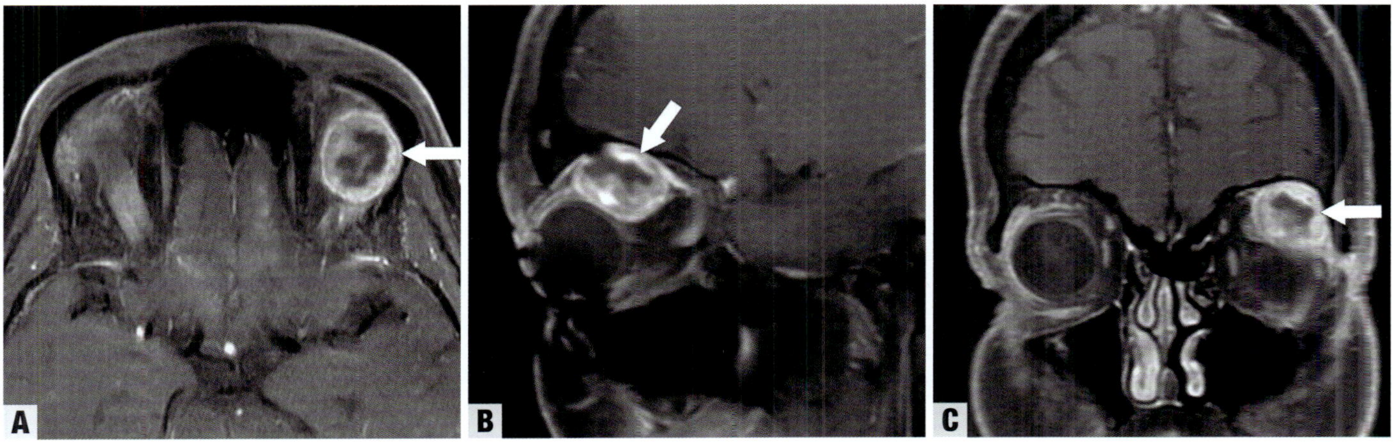

Fig. 7.14 Carcinoma ex pleomorphic adenoma. Axial (**A**), sagittal (**B**), and coronal (**C**) T1-weighted postcontrast MRI shows a peripherally enhancing mass involving the superotemporal left orbit (arrows) with mass effect upon an inferiorly displaced globe.

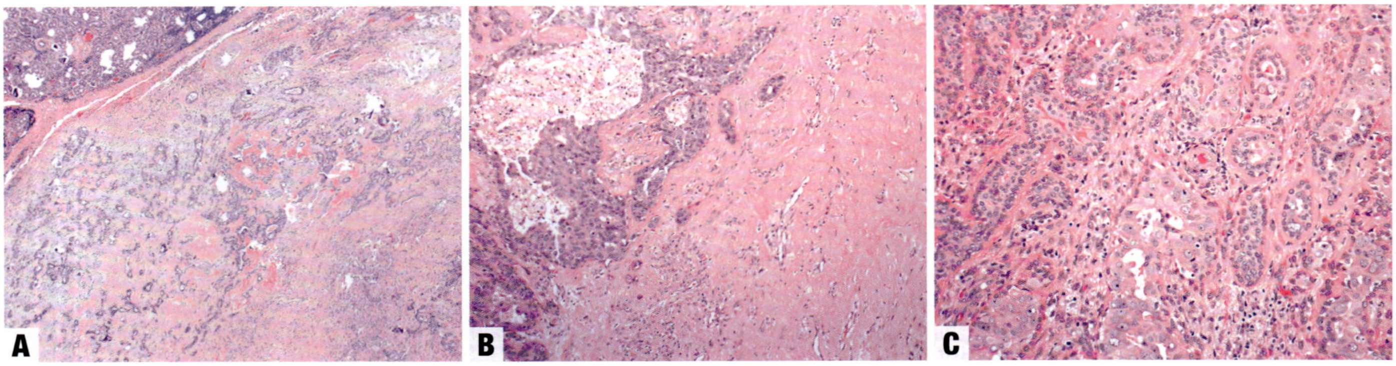

Fig. 7.15 Carcinoma ex pleomorphic adenoma. **A** Intracapsular carcinoma ex pleomorphic adenoma characterized by the presence of glands lined by atypical cells, and still confined within the pseudocapsule of a pre-existing pleomorphic adenoma. **B** Hyalinized nodule adjacent to an area of adenocarcinoma indicating a pre-existing pleomorphic adenoma. **C** Higher magnification showing malignant glands intermixed with benign ducts from the pre-existing pleomorphic adenoma.

Histopathology

Microscopically, transition between the malignant component and residual PA is observed. The carcinoma component may be of any type: adenocarcinoma of salivary duct appearance (most common) {201}, mucoepidermoid carcinoma {721,3361}, myoepithelial carcinoma, squamous cell carcinoma {2047}, or adenoid cystic carcinoma {3507}. Extensive sampling may be required for identification of a prior PA component, which may be represented by densely hyalinized, sclerotic, or hypocellular stroma. Intravascular, perineural, and/or bone invasion may be present.

Based on cases arising in the salivary glands, by convention, CEPA is considered intracapsular (non-invasive) when confined within the capsule, minimally invasive if there is minimal breach of the capsule (< 4–6 mm), and widely invasive if extension beyond the capsule is > 6 mm {2719}. The terms "intracapsular" and "minimally invasive" should only be applied to uninodular tumours with a well-delineated interface after the entire lesion border has been microscopically evaluated. These terms should not be used for carcinomas arising in multinodular recurrent PA.

Immunohistochemistry

Immunohistochemistry is usually not necessary for diagnosis. Carcinoma areas may show increased expression of p53, MYC, and Ki-67. PLAG1 and HMGA2 expression may assist identification of the PA component {1481,1622,3748}, and can be useful in separating CEPA from de novo lacrimal gland carcinomas {153}. AR positivity may indicate lacrimal gland ductal adenocarcinoma differentiation.

Differential diagnosis

This includes pleomorphic adenoma, mucoepidermoid carcinoma, adenocarcinoma, carcinosarcoma, myoepithelial and epithelial-myoepithelial carcinoma, and adenoid cystic carcinoma.

Cytology

Smears can show variable morphology depending on sampling. Features of poorly differentiated adenocarcinoma, mucoepidermoid or adenosquamous carcinoma, carcinosarcoma, or another lacrimal gland malignancy, in addition to classic PA features, may be seen {1738,1739,2419,2066}.

Diagnostic molecular pathology

PLAG1 or *HMGA2* rearrangements, detected by FISH, serve as markers of pre-existing PA. These rearrangements in CEPA can assist in differentiating CEPA from de novo lacrimal gland carcinomas {153}.

Essential and desirable diagnostic criteria

Essential: mass arising from the lacrimal gland; presence of an epithelial and/or myoepithelial malignant component; histological areas compatible with PA or history of previous PA in the same site.

Staging

Lesions are staged according to the Union for International Cancer Control (UICC) / American Joint Committee on Cancer (AJCC) *Cancer staging manual*, eighth edition.

Prognosis and prediction

Based on a small series, distant metastases were seen in 11% of cases. Treatment included complete excision, orbital bone resection, radiotherapy, and chemotherapy {3351}. No current biomarkers are available to predict the risk of malignant transformation in PA.

Adenoid cystic carcinoma of the lacrimal gland

Chan ASY
Alkatan H
Dubovy SR
Wolkow N

Definition

Adenoid cystic carcinoma (AdCC) is a malignant epithelial neoplasm composed of epithelial and myoepithelial cells that are arranged in tubular, cribriform, and solid patterns associated with a basophilic matrix and reduplicated basement membrane material, frequently accompanied by *MYB::NFIB* gene rearrangements.

ICD-O coding

8200/3 Adenoid cystic carcinoma

ICD-11 coding

2D0Y & XH4302 Other specified malignant neoplasms of eye or ocular adnexa & Adenoid cystic carcinoma

Related terminology

None

Subtype(s)

None

Localization

AdCCs arise most commonly from the orbital lobe of the lacrimal gland {3064}, occasionally from the palpebral lobe {835}, and rarely from accessory lacrimal gland tissue in the conjunctiva and orbit {1004,2360,3535}.

Clinical features

Clinically, AdCC may present initially with lacrimal gland enlargement causing ptosis, but the most common presentation is inferomedial globe displacement followed by non-axial proptosis {592,3507,1202,96}. The duration of symptoms is short, with a median of 7 months {96}. Pain and paraesthesia, secondary to perineural, muscle, or bone invasion, are cardinal signs distinguishing AdCC from benign lacrimal gland lesions {3507,592,1202}. Decreased motility, diplopia, and loss of vision have also been reported in more-advanced disease {592}. AdCCs most frequently metastasize to distant sites including lung, liver, and bone. Metastases to regional lymph nodes including preauricular, submandibular, and cervical lymph nodes occur less often {1202}.

On CT or MRI, AdCCs may present initially as circumscribed masses but more often will appear as nodular lesions with irregular margins, infiltration of adjacent tissue, bony destruction, and calcification {3507,1202}. MRI may be useful for detecting small tumours, infiltration, and perineural invasion {298,3507}.

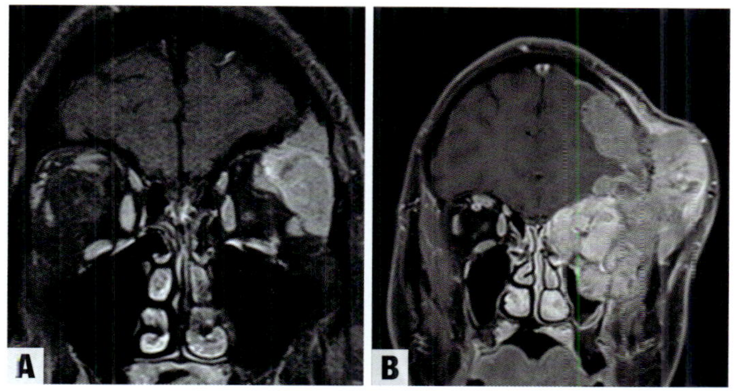

Fig. 7.16 Adenoid cystic carcinoma. Coronal MRI demonstrates a left lacrimal gland adenoid cystic carcinoma with extradural extension superiorly (**A**) and a recurrent lacrimal gland adenoid cystic carcinoma after failed treatment with intra-arterial chemotherapy and radiation, extending intracranially (**B**).

Epidemiology

Although they are rare, accounting for approximately 1.6–4.8% of all orbital lesions {592,2360,298}, AdCCs are the most common primary malignant epithelial tumour of the lacrimal gland, accounting for as many as 60% of cases {3064,298}. AdCC has a bimodal age distribution, with the first peak in middle age

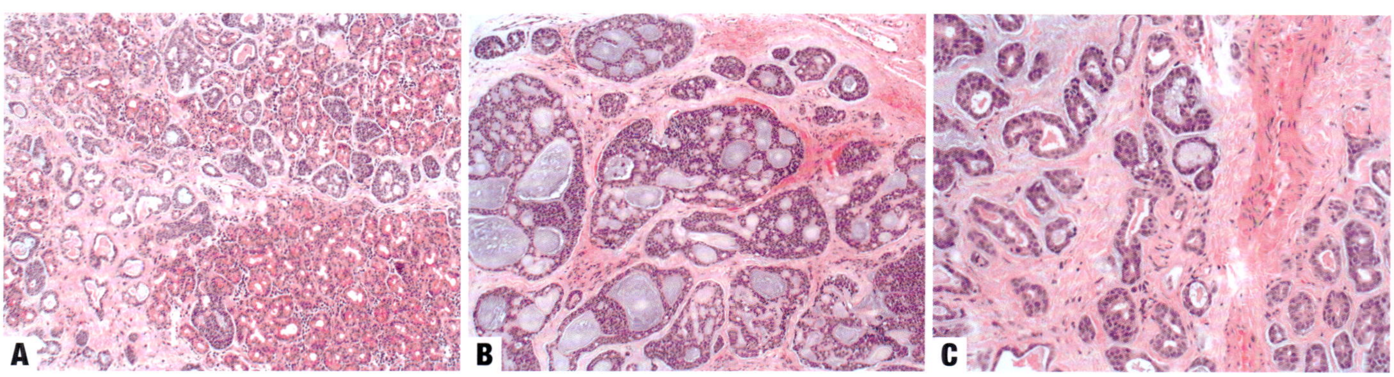

Fig. 7.17 Adenoid cystic carcinoma. **A** The carcinoma infiltrates the normal lacrimal gland. **B** Cribriform pattern with a Swiss-cheese appearance, composed of cystic structures containing basophilic amorphous glycosaminoglycans and eosinophilic hyalinized basal lamina. **C** The tubular pattern is composed predominantly of small glandular structures.

Chapter 7

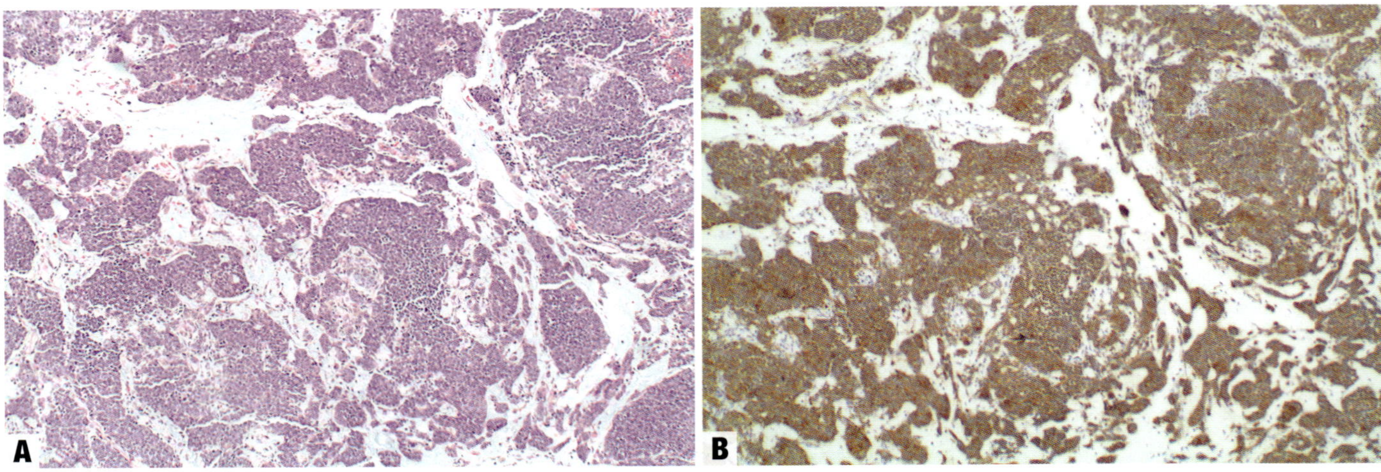

Fig. 7.18 Adenoid cystic carcinoma. **A** The solid/basaloid pattern is composed of compact, sheet-like, proliferating basaloid myoepithelial cells that lack the cribriform or tubular architecture. **B** Diffuse KIT staining is seen in this tumour with a solid/basaloid pattern.

(majority in their forties) and a smaller peak in the first decade of life {835,3507}. There is a slight female predominance with a reported M:F ratio of 4:7 {96,3069}.

Etiology

Unknown

Pathogenesis

Similarly to salivary gland AdCCs, lacrimal gland AdCCs frequently (as many as 50%) carry a t(6;9)(q22-23;p24-23) chromosomal translocation that results in *MYB*::*NFIB* gene fusion, and activation of the *MYB* oncogene and associated target proteins such as KIT and BCL2, which are involved in cell growth, apoptosis, transcription, and cell-cycle regulation {3509,563}. Other than losses in chromosome 6q, AdCCs in the lacrimal gland also show losses in chromosome 12q and 17p, and gains in chromosomes 19q, 8q, and 11q {3509}. Whole-exome sequencing has implicated aberrant NOTCH pathway signalling in lacrimal gland AdCCs {2848}. Other oncogenic mutations that may occur include those of *KRAS*, *NRAS*, and *MET* {294}.

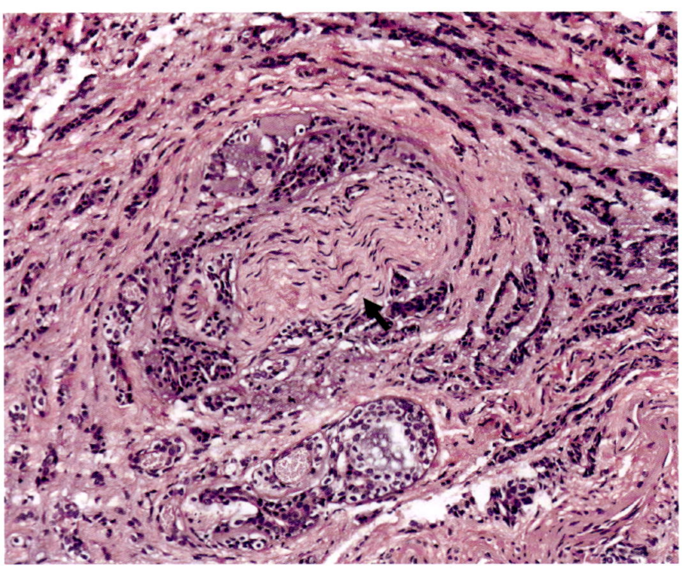

Fig. 7.19 Adenoid cystic carcinoma. Perineural invasion is commonly seen.

Macroscopic appearance

AdCCs present as unencapsulated firm, white nodular lesions with irregular borders.

Histopathology

AdCCs are biphasic tumours composed of proliferating modified myoepithelial cells and luminal ductal cells {191,3507}. There are three histological growth patterns that may be present in variable combinations: cribriform, tubular, and solid/basaloid {3507,2667,2170}. The most common histological pattern is the cribriform followed by the solid then the tubular {96}. The cribriform pattern, classically described as a Swiss-cheese pattern, is most commonly seen and is composed of cystic structures where the connective tissue stroma is filled with basophilic amorphous glycosaminoglycans and/or eosinophilic hyalinized basal lamina. The tubular pattern is composed predominantly of small glandular structures {3507,2170}. The solid/basaloid pattern carries the worst prognosis. It is composed predominantly of compact sheet-like proliferating basaloid myoepithelial cells that lack the cribriform or tubular architecture {2667,3507}. Mitotic figures are infrequent but more commonly seen in the solid/basaloid pattern. Perineural invasion is commonly seen {3507}.

High-grade transformation/dedifferentiation can occur with comedonecrosis, increased nuclear atypia, mitoses {3310}, and rarely sarcomatoid or myoepithelial components {191,2476}. Differential diagnosis includes adenocarcinoma, myoepithelial carcinoma, epithelial-myoepithelial carcinoma, polymorphous adenocarcinoma, and basal cell adenocarcinoma {3507,2667}.

Immunohistochemistry is not usually required for diagnosis. However, immunostaining for MYB and its downstream target KIT, although less sensitive and specific, may be used as a surrogate for *MYB* rearrangement molecular studies {2170}. The mean Ki-67 index is 30% and p53 may be expressed in 39% of cases {2170}.

Cytology

Tumour cells are basaloid with small, angulated hyperchromatic nuclei and scant cytoplasm. These basaloid cells may encircle large well-demarcated spherules of acellular hyaline globules {610}.

Diagnostic molecular pathology

FISH for *MYB* rearrangement is not usually required, but may be helpful in difficult cases {563,835}.

Essential and desirable diagnostic criteria

Essential: a malignant biphasic tumour composed of proliferating myoepithelial cells and luminal ductal cells.

Desirable: perineural invasion; positive MYB and/or KIT immunohistochemistry; FISH for *MYB* rearrangement may be useful in challenging cases.

Staging

Staging is according to the Union for International Cancer Control (UICC) / American Joint Committee on Cancer (AJCC) TNM, eighth edition, for lacrimal gland carcinoma.

Prognosis and prediction

The mainstay of treatment is surgical excision such as orbital exenteration or eye-sparing surgery together with adjuvant radiotherapy or chemoradiation, both having similar recurrence outcomes {1015}. The prognosis for AdCC has improved owing to earlier diagnosis and improved treatment. Poor outcomes such as higher rates of local/regional recurrence, distant metastasis, and death are associated with basaloid patterns of growth, perineural invasion, and larger tumours (> 25 mm) {49, 1202}. Several immunohistochemistry markers, i.e. NOTCH1 and activated NICD1 overexpression, and nuclear expression of BIRC5 (survivin), have been shown to be associated with a worse prognosis {162,2309}. NOTCH1-directed targeted clinical trials are in progress and have yet to be reported.

Primary ductal adenocarcinoma of the lacrimal gland

Grossniklaus HE
Mittal R
Pekmezci M

Definition

Primary ductal adenocarcinoma (PDA) of the lacrimal gland is a rare high-grade adenocarcinoma and a counterpart of salivary duct carcinoma, resembling invasive ductal carcinoma of the breast.

ICD-O coding

8500/3 Primary ductal adenocarcinoma of the lacrimal gland

ICD-11 coding

2D03.0 & XH7KH3 Adenocarcinoma of the lacrimal apparatus & Infiltrating duct carcinoma, NOS

Related terminology

Acceptable: unclassified adenocarcinoma; ductal carcinoma/ adenocarcinoma; lacrimal duct carcinoma.

Not recommended: cystadenocarcinoma; mucinous cystadenocarcinoma; intestinal-type adenocarcinoma.

Subtype(s)

None

Localization

PDA arises throughout the main lacrimal gland and (rarely) in accessory lacrimal glands.

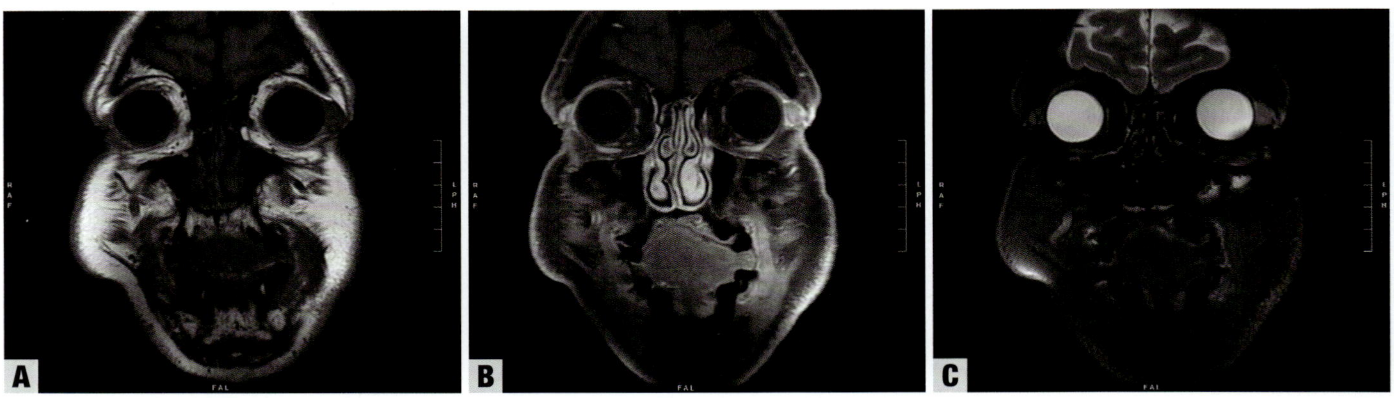

Fig. 7.20 Primary ductal adenocarcinoma of the lacrimal gland. **A** Coronal T1-weighted MRI shows a well-circumscribed isointense mass in the left lateral orbit. **B** Coronal MRI shows a well-circumscribed mass in the left lateral orbit, with diffuse enhancement on T1-weighted postcontrast imaging. **C** Coronal T2-weighted MRI shows a well-circumscribed mass in the left lateral orbit, hyperintense on T2-weighted fat-suppression imaging.

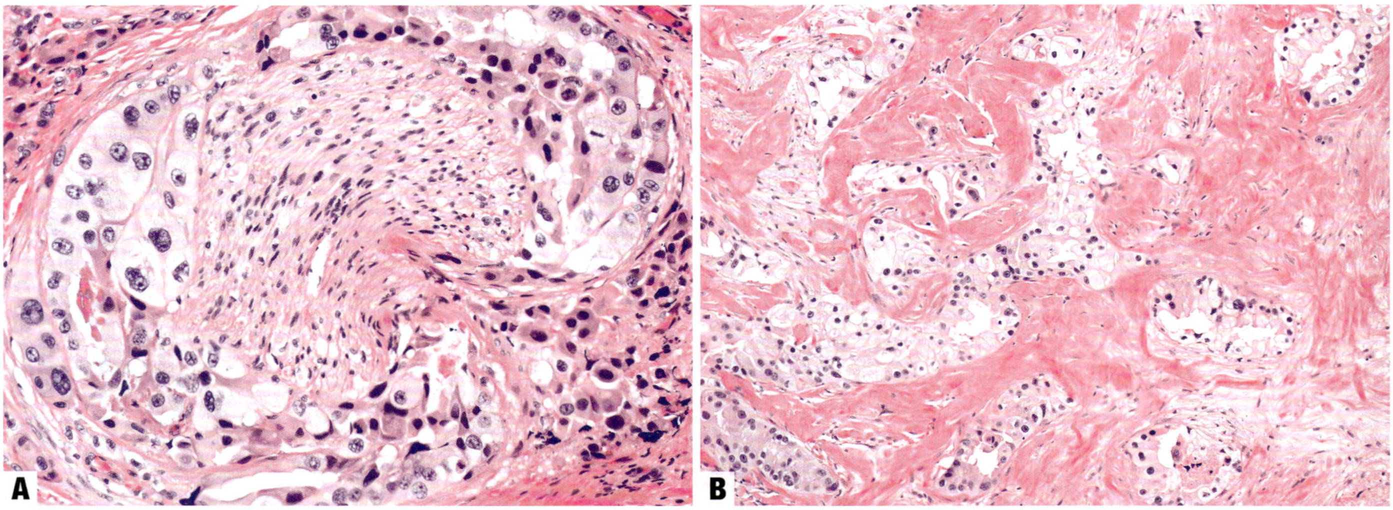

Fig. 7.21 Primary ductal adenocarcinoma of the lacrimal gland. **A** High-grade carcinoma composed of large epithelial cells with abundant eosinophilic cytoplasm, prominent nucleoli, mitotic activity, and perineural invasion. **B** High-grade carcinoma composed of large epithelial cells with abundant eosinophilic cytoplasm in the background of significant hyalinization.

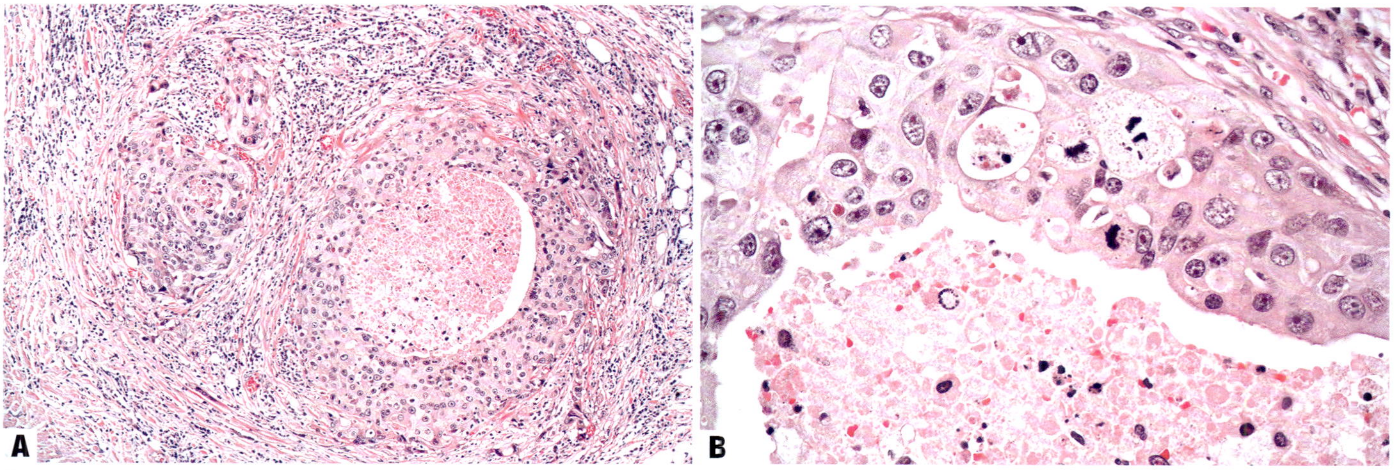

Fig. 7.22 Primary ductal adenocarcinoma. **A** A low-power photomicrograph shows infiltrating adenocarcinoma with a desmoplastic background and inflammatory cells. **B** A high-power photomicrograph shows large cells with abundant eosinophilic granular cytoplasm, numerous mitotic figures, and central comedonecrosis.

Clinical features

PDA of the lacrimal gland presents with painless proptosis (31%), palpable mass (25%), swelling (22%), diplopia (16%), mechanical ptosis (15%), pain (13%), and decreased vision (12%) {2902}. The average duration of symptoms is 25 months. Left and right lacrimal glands are involved equally, without any bilateral cases reported to date. The average size of the tumours ranges from 11 to 50 mm, with a mean diameter of 30 mm.

Orbital imaging (CT, MRI) features include an irregularly shaped, heterogeneous, enhancing mass in contrast T1-weighted MRI. Bony erosions, muscle involvement, and calcifications may be present.

Epidemiology

PDA is rare, accounting for only 2% of all epithelial lacrimal gland tumours {3572}. The exact incidence is not known, with < 40 cases reported to date {2902,3374,1689}. It appears to occur more commonly in men than women (M:F ratio: 3:1), with an average age at diagnosis of 58 years (range: 34–78 years) {1800,1867,2902}. Interestingly, this predominance in men is greater than that seen in the salivary counterpart. It remains unclear whether this is a true trend, or whether women are underrepresented owing to misdiagnosis of these tumours as metastatic ductal adenocarcinoma of the breast.

Etiology

Unknown

Pathogenesis

The pathogenesis of this tumour is currently unknown, although at least a subset of cases show ERBB2 (HER2) overexpression by immunohistochemistry and/or *ERBB2* gene amplification similar to that seen in salivary duct carcinoma {151,1800,3766, 2902}.

Macroscopic appearance

The tumour appears as a poorly defined mass surrounding the lacrimal gland and within the soft tissue.

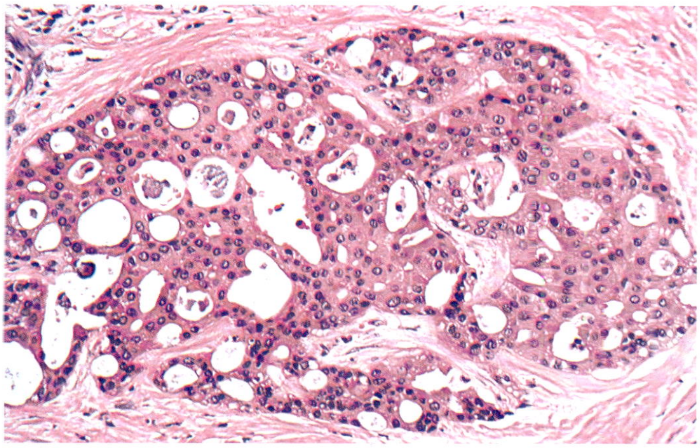

Fig. 7.23 Primary ductal adenocarcinoma. Adenocarcinoma with apocrine features.

Histopathology

Tumour cells are polygonal with granular eosinophilic cytoplasm, pleomorphic and vesicular nuclei, prominent nucleoli, and mitoses. The cells are arranged in ductal structures of varying patterns (glandular, cribriform, and solid) with frequent central comedonecrosis resembling intraductal adenocarcinoma of the breast and salivary gland {2902}; extracellular mucin may also be present {2219}. Perineural, vascular, lymphatic, and bony invasion have been reported, all in approximately 25% of cases {2902}. Dense hyalinization and sclerosis with interspersed myoepithelial cells favour an adenocarcinoma ex pleomorphic adenoma over a PDA.

Positive immunohistochemical markers include markers for epithelia (AE1/AE3, CK7, CK19, EMA), apocrine differentiation (AR, GCDFP-15), and cell growth (ERBB2). ER, PR, and PSA are usually negative, and the Ki-67 proliferation index may reach 70% {151,1800,3766}. Expression of p53 and cyclin D1 is also reported {3766,1800,3374}. Myoepithelial markers including SMA, p63, and calponin are negative in most of the cases.

Differential diagnoses are adenocarcinoma NOS, adenocarcinoma ex pleomorphic adenoma, and mucoepidermoid carcinoma

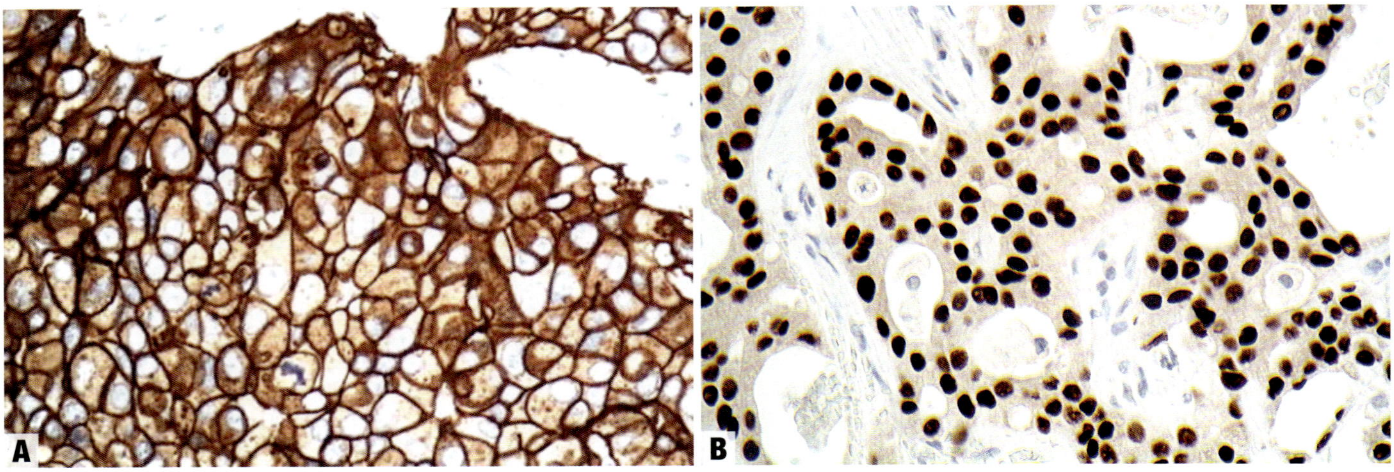

Fig. 7.24 Primary ductal adenocarcinoma. **A** There is strong membranous immunostaining for ERBB2, similar to that seen in ductal carcinoma of the breast. **B** Positive nuclear staining for AR is seen.

Cytology
Individual tumour cells display moderate to marked pleomorphism, contain round nuclei with prominent nucleoli and abundant eosinophilic/granular cytoplasm, and form gland-like structures in a necrotic background.

Diagnostic molecular pathology
Amplification of *ERBB2*, which is present in approximately 25% of salivary duct carcinomas, has also been reported in lacrimal duct carcinoma {151}.

Essential and desirable diagnostic criteria
Essential: an invasive adenocarcinoma with ductal differentiation, arising de novo (not arising from a benign tumour such as pleomorphic adenoma) in the lacrimal gland.
Desirable: tumour comedonecrosis.

Staging
PDA of the lacrimal gland is staged according to the eighth edition of the Union for International Cancer Control (UICC) / American Joint Committee on Cancer (AJCC) TNM classification for carcinoma of the lacrimal gland.

Prognosis and prediction
The reported 5-year survival rate of patients with PDA is 44% (indicating a more aggressive course than that of adenoid cystic carcinoma of the lacrimal gland, but a less-aggressive course than that of salivary duct carcinoma with a 5-year mortality rate of 60–80%) {1800,1867,2902}. Based on a large case series with literature review, lymph node and distant metastases are seen in 24% and 50% of patients, respectively. Treatments include complete excision, lymph node dissection, orbital bone resection, and radiotherapy {1811,1867}. Poor prognosis for PDA may be associated with overexpression of ERBB2 and p53 {1800}. GCDFP-15, AR, and ERBB2 have been proposed as biomarkers for treatment guidance and prognosis in PDA {3766}.

Secretory carcinoma

Hyrcza MD
Milman T

Definition
Secretory carcinoma (SC) is a monophasic carcinoma characterized by a rearrangement of the *ETV6* gene resulting in *ETV6::NTRK3* fusion in most cases.

ICD-O coding
8502/3 Secretory carcinoma

ICD-11 coding
2D0Y & XH44J4 Other specified malignant neoplasms of eye or ocular adnexa & Secretory carcinoma

Related terminology
Acceptable: mammary analogue secretory carcinoma.

Subtype(s)
None

Localization
Two cases of SC have been described in the main lacrimal gland {1412,386}, and cases have been described in the eyelid, arising in the accessory lacrimal gland and in the sweat gland {251,193}.

Clinical features
SC presents with painless diplopia and proptosis, and as a circumscribed subcutaneous nodule {1412,386,193}. CT and MRI show a heterogeneous circumscribed mass in the lacrimal fossa causing inferomedial displacement of the globe {1412}.

Epidemiology
Reported lacrimal SC occurred in a 28-year-old man and a 52-year-old man. One tumour was identified in a retrospective review of 350 lacrimal tumours, suggesting low incidence in lacrimal glands {1412}. Eyelid-skin SC occurred in a 55-year-old woman.

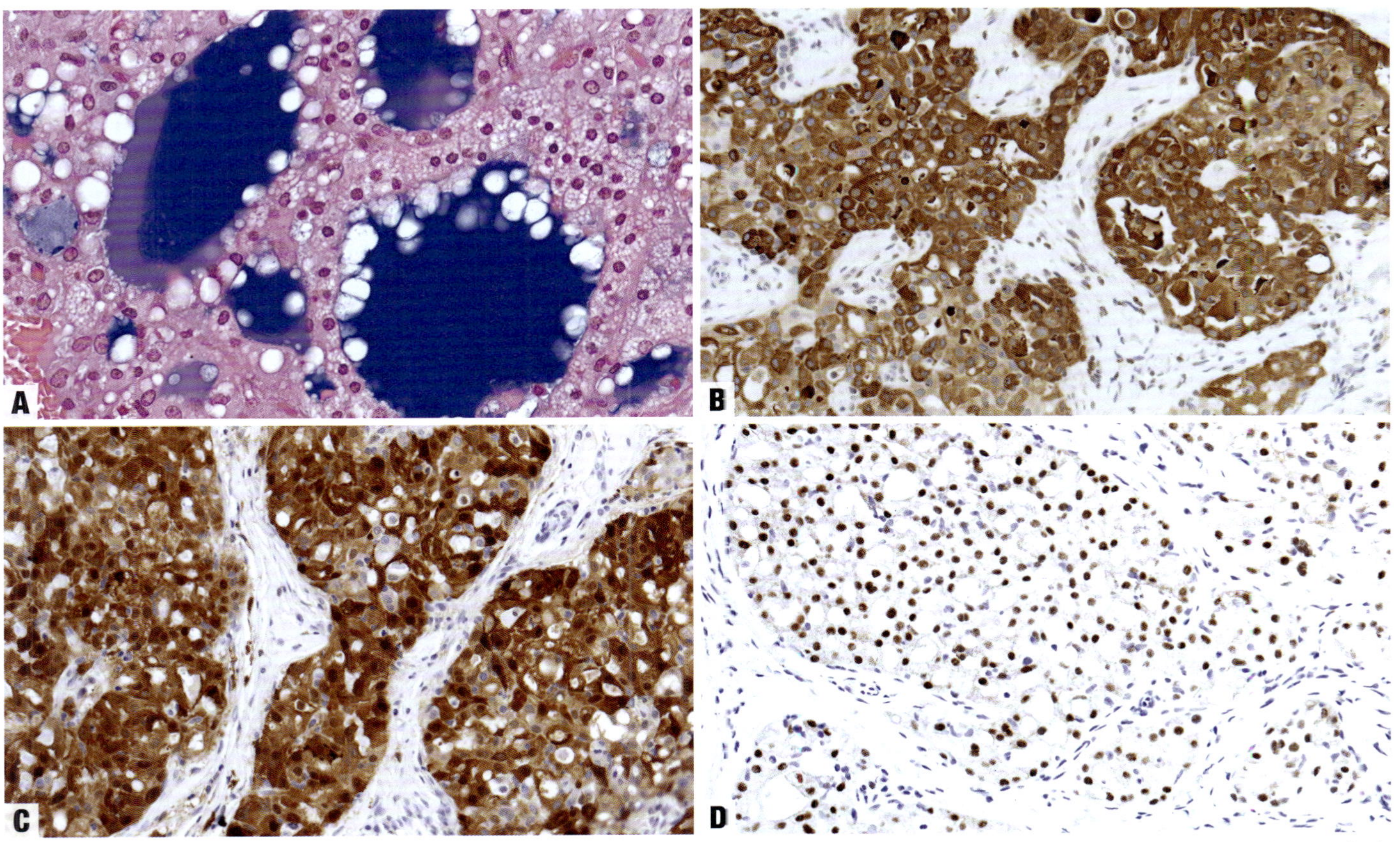

Fig. 7.25 Lacrimal secretory carcinoma. **A** Mucin stains such as Alcian blue highlight the extracellular secretions within the microcystic lumina. **B** Mammaglobin expression is a hallmark of secretory carcinoma. **C** S100 shows strong cytoplasmic expression in secretory carcinoma. **D** Most cases of secretory carcinoma harbour *NTRK3* fusion resulting in NTRK protein expression, which can be shown with pan-TRK immunohistochemistry.

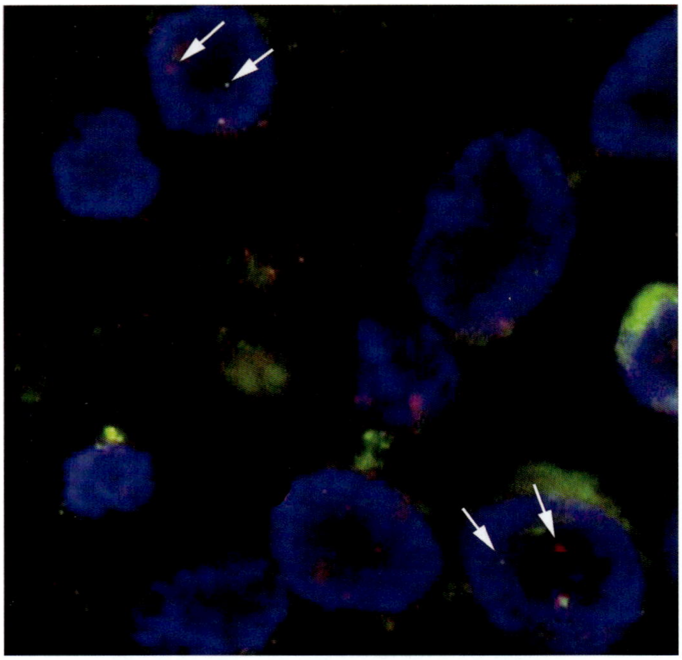

Fig. 7.26 Lacrimal secretory carcinoma. *ETV6* gene rearrangement can be demonstrated by *ETV6* break-apart FISH, showing one intact (yellow) probe and a pair of separated red and green probes (arrows).

Etiology

Unknown

Pathogenesis

ETV6 gene rearrangement was present in reported cases {1412,386}. RNA sequencing demonstrated a fusion transcript of exon 5 of the *ETV6* gene and exon 14 of the *NTRK3* gene in 1 case {1412}. In salivary glands, alternative fusions include *ETV6::RET* {1438,3142,3141}, *ETV6::MET* {2758}, *ETV6::MAML3* {1196}, and *VIM::RET* {3137}.

Macroscopic appearance

Lacrimal gland tumours are encapsulated and partially cystic {1412,386}.

Histopathology

SC demonstrates papillary-cystic, solid, and microfollicular patterns {1412,386,251}. A dense collagenous capsule with capsular invasion was present in both cases of main lacrimal gland SC. Tumour cells are round to ovoid, with mildly pleomorphic nuclei and abundant pale, eosinophilic, focally vacuolated cytoplasm. Clear cytoplasm can be present focally {1412}. Goblet cells and intracytoplasmic zymogen granules are absent. Haemosiderin deposition can be focally prominent. No necrosis or perineural or lymphovascular invasion is identified. PAS staining highlights only luminal secretions.

Immunohistochemistry

Tumour cells are positive for S100, mammaglobin, CK18, CAM5.2, and NTRK proteins. They lack expression of p63, CK5, DOG1, and AR. The Ki-67 proliferation index is below 5% {1412, 386,251,193}. SOX10, GCDFP-15, and vimentin positivity has been demonstrated in salivary cases.

Cytology

There are no reports of lacrimal SC cytology to date. Salivary SC shows loosely cohesive sheets, papillary or cribriform tissue fragments composed of cells with abundant finely granular or vacuolated cytoplasm, and uniform round to oval nuclei with fine chromatin, single nucleoli, and mild atypia {345,1171,1336,1566,2197}.

Diagnostic molecular pathology

ETV6 gene rearrangement can be demonstrated by break-apart FISH. Detection of *NTRK3* fusion by RT-PCR or RNA sequencing may be predictive of response to NTRK inhibitors for unresectable or metastatic cases {826,825}.

Essential and desirable diagnostic criteria

Essential: a monophasic tumour with vacuolated secretory material, lacking cytoplasmic granules; immunohistochemical positivity for S100, mammaglobin, and NTRK, and negativity for p40/p63 and CK5.

Desirable: ETV6 and/or *NTRK3* gene rearrangement.

Staging

The eighth-edition Union for International Cancer Control (UICC) / American Joint Committee on Cancer (AJCC) TNM staging system for lacrimal gland tumours applies.

Prognosis and prediction

SC is an indolent carcinoma which may be cured with a complete surgical resection. One reported lacrimal case showed no recurrence 12 years after resection {826}.

Mucoepidermoid carcinoma of the lacrimal gland

Roberts F
Alkatan H
Iacob CE
von Holstein SL

Definition

Mucoepidermoid carcinoma (MEC) of the lacrimal gland is a malignant epithelial tumour characterized by squamous (epidermoid) cells, mucous cells, columnar cells, and intermediate cells.

ICD-O coding

8430/3 Mucoepidermoid carcinoma

ICD-11 coding

2D0Y & XH1J36 Other specified malignant neoplasms of eye or ocular adnexa & Mucoepidermoid carcinoma
2D03.1 Mucoepidermoid carcinoma of lacrimal apparatus

Related terminology

Not recommended: mixed epidermoid and mucus-secreting carcinoma; mucoepidermoid tumour.

Subtype(s)

None

Localization

MEC can arise throughout the main lacrimal gland and in accessory lacrimal glands.

Clinical features

MEC usually presents as a slow-growing mass in the lacrimal gland region, clinically indistinguishable from more-common tumours such as pleomorphic adenoma {96,552}. Occasionally it may cause painful proptosis. On CT, MEC is usually a well-circumscribed enhancing mass in the lacrimal gland region {96}.

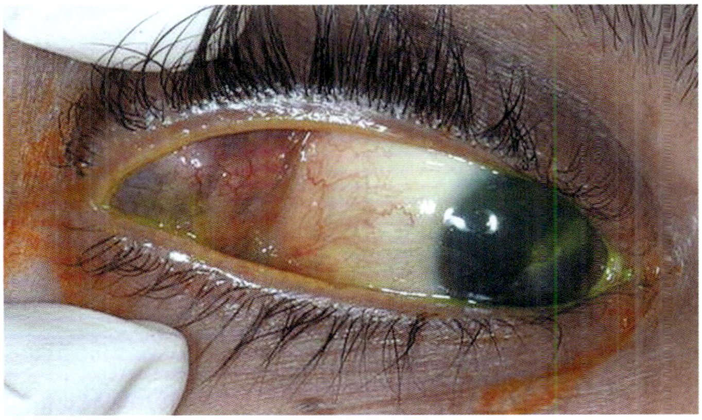

Fig. 7.27 Mucoepidermoid carcinoma. Tumour bulging from the superotemporal orbit.

Epidemiology

MEC is relatively rare, accounting for 1.5–4% of all epithelial tumours and about 7% of all malignant tumours in the lacrimal gland {552,96}. The mean age at presentation is 50–52 years, although it may occur at younger ages {3511}.

Etiology

Etiological factors have not been described for lacrimal gland carcinoma. MEC of the salivary gland is associated with radiation exposure {2753}.

Pathogenesis

Lacrimal gland and salivary gland MECs share a common histogenesis: they are composed of varying proportions of luminal and myoepithelial cells. This is supported by reports describing MEC arising in pleomorphic adenoma {721,3361,3426}.

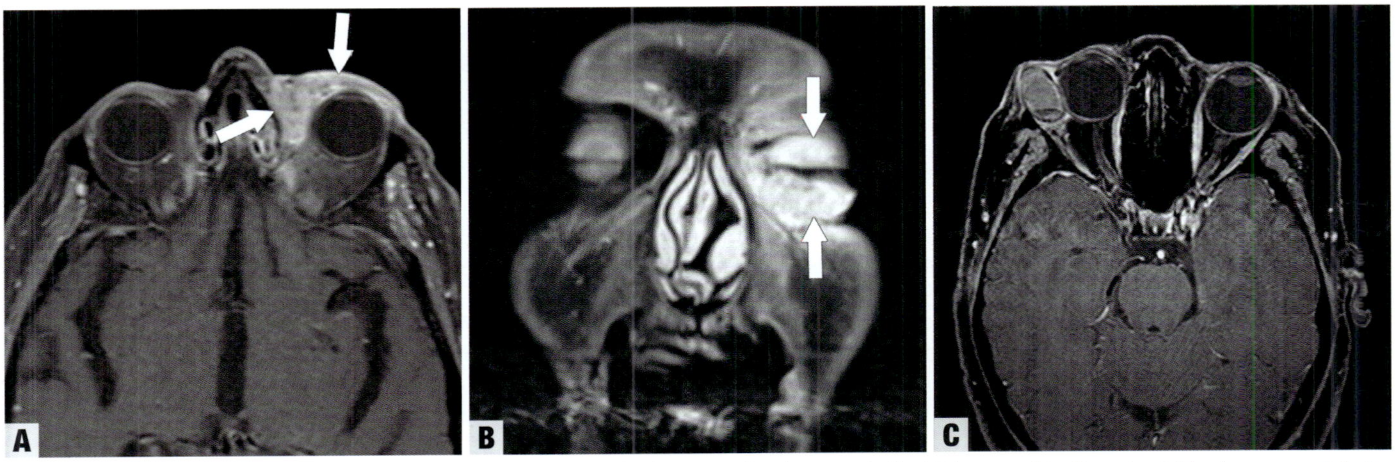

Fig. 7.28 Mucoepidermoid carcinoma. **A** Axial T1-weighted postcontrast MRI shows an enhancing mass in the left lower eyelid with postseptal involvement medially (arrows). **B** Coronal T1-weighted postcontrast MRI shows an enhancing mass involving the left upper and lower eyelids (arrows). **C** Axial T1-weighted postcontrast MRI shows an enhancing mass in the right lacrimal gland.

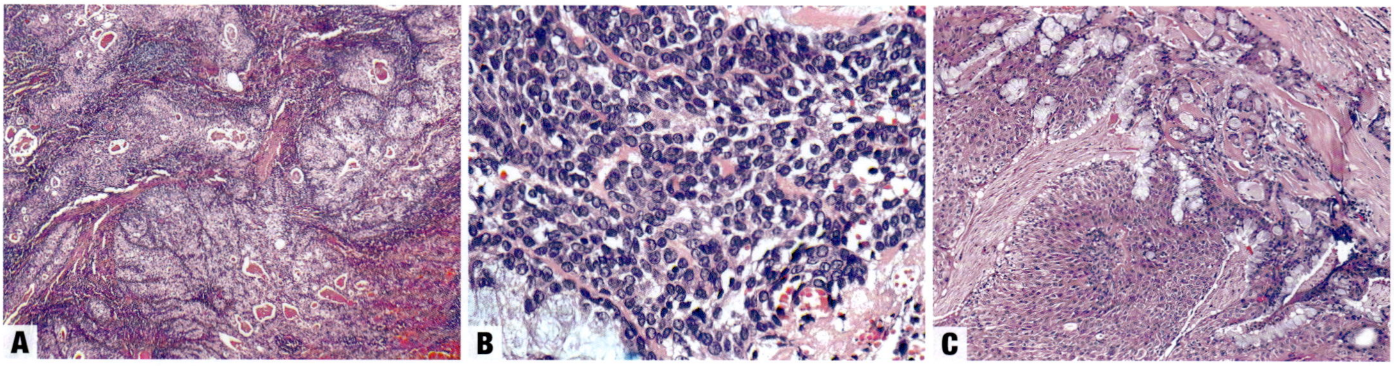

Fig. 7.29 Mucoepidermoid carcinoma of the lacrimal gland. **A** A low-power view showing the mixture of solid and mucinous components. **B** An intermediate cell area. **C** Solid sheets of intermediate cells juxtaposed with mucous cells.

A *CRTC1::MAML2* gene fusion is present in the majority of tumours and is considered a key oncogenic driver {3140,571}. This fusion transactivates expression of the EGFR (HER1) ligand {571}. RAS and PIK3 family mutations also involved in the EGFR pathway have been detected in poorly differentiated tumours {2276}. In the salivary gland, *ERBB2* and *EGFR* are upregulated in high-grade MEC {2345}.

Macroscopic appearance

These tumours usually appear circumscribed, with a greyish-white lobulated cut surface. Cystic areas may be evident depending on tumour grade. Calcification has been described {552}.

Histopathology

MEC of the lacrimal gland is composed of variable proportions of three cells types: squamous, mucin-secreting, and intermediate. The squamous cells have medium to large nuclei with eosinophilic cytoplasm and intercellular bridges between cells, but keratinization is rare. Mucous cells form small glands, tubules, and cysts; the cysts contain inspissated mucin (which may calcify) and are lined by mucous cells, looking deceptively bland. The intermediate (or transitional) cells are oval, with a round nucleus and faintly eosinophilic cytoplasm. In addition, columnar, clear, and oncocytic cells may be admixed. PAS or Alcian blue may be required to visualize mucin. The stroma may be hyalinized with calcification and ossification. A granulomatous reaction to extravasated mucus may be seen.

There are several systems for grading salivary gland MEC {2613,623,944}. Most divide tumours into three levels (low-grade, intermediate-grade, and high-grade). The systems are based on the proportions of cystic areas, proportion of necrosis, perineural invasion, mitoses, nuclear pleomorphism, invasion front, and lymphovascular invasion. More recently a binary grading system separating low- and intermediate-grade tumours from high-grade tumours using the Brandwein system has been shown to best stratify patients into groups based on risk of recurrence {623}.

The differential diagnosis includes squamous cell carcinoma, sebaceous carcinoma, adenosquamous carcinoma, and pleomorphic adenoma.

Cytology

In the salivary gland, the cytology of low-grade lesions consists predominantly of mucus and macrophages with occasional bland epithelial cells {1740}. Higher-grade lesions show an admixture of cell types, and pleomorphism, mitoses, and necrosis can be present. There are few reports of the cytology of lacrimal gland MEC although associated inflammation can cause diagnostic error {529}.

Diagnostic molecular pathology

A *CRTC1::MAML2* fusion protein has been identified in lacrimal gland MECs {3508}; this fusion, resulting from a t(11;19)(q21;p13.1) translocation, is present in 80% of salivary gland MECs {944} and may be used as diagnostic maker.

Essential and desirable diagnostic criteria

Essential: squamous cells, intermediate cells, and mucous cells in varying proportions; for lower-grade tumours: cystic, mucous cell–rich, and well circumscribed; for higher-grade tumours: solid, higher proportion of squamous and intermediate cells.

Desirable: CRTC1::MAML2 fusion on genetic analysis.

Staging

Mucoepidermoid carcinoma is staged according to the eighth-edition Union for International Cancer Control (UICC) TNM classification for carcinoma of the lacrimal gland.

Prognosis and prediction

Prognostic factors have not been formally reported for MEC of the lacrimal gland. In the salivary glands, the prognosis for MEC varies with tumour grade. Low/intermediate-grade tumours have a survival rate of 97% whereas high-grade tumours have poorer survival at 67% {636}.

The *CTRC1::MAML2* fusion is associated with better prognosis {2039,571}. *RAS* and *PIK3* mutations may be associated with higher-grade tumours {2276}.

Epithelial-myoepithelial carcinoma

Mittal R
Chan ASY
Salomao DR

Definition

Epithelial-myoepithelial carcinoma (EMC) is a low-grade malignant biphasic tumour of the lacrimal gland characterized by tubular structures, usually composed of tightly coupled inner ductal and prominent outer myoepithelial cells.

ICD-O coding

8562/3 Epithelial-myoepithelial carcinoma

ICD-11 coding

2D0Y & XH9JP2 Other specified malignant neoplasms of eye or ocular adnexa & Epithelial-myoepithelial carcinoma

Related terminology

None

Subtype(s)

None

Localization

Lacrimal gland

Clinical features

EMC usually presents as a slow-growing painless orbital mass with proptosis. It may present with a history of a rapid increase in size, diplopia, pain, and restriction of ocular movements {1928, 521,3620,2952,3113}. Associated lymphadenopathy is rare.

Imaging

EMC is frequently well defined and multilobulated on CT and MRI, with intermediate signals in T1- and T2-weighted images. It enhances heterogeneously.

Epidemiology

EMC is extremely rare in the lacrimal gland {161,2952}, with an M:F ratio of 3:2. The median age at diagnosis is approximately 59.6 years (range: 29–86 years).

Etiology

EMC arises from intercalated ducts {3570}. It may arise as a de novo lesion or in a pre-existing pleomorphic adenoma {161, 3469,2952}.

Pathogenesis

A significant number of EMCs harbour *HRAS* mutations, most commonly at codon 61 {3417,727}.

Macroscopic appearance

The cut surface shows a greyish-white, lobulated, firm mass {161}. Cystic changes may be noted {1928}.

Histopathology

EMC generally exhibits a multinodular invasive growth pattern. The histological hallmark is the biphasic arrangement of inner, smaller, eosinophilic ductal epithelial cells and outer, relatively larger, often clear myoepithelial cells {665,2904}. The myoepithelial component varies from single layered to multilayered or even with solid areas. Nuclear atypia tends to be mild to moderate. Cribriform, basaloid, sebaceous, oncocytic and double-clear histological variations have been described {2904,2905, 1411,344}. High-grade transformation rarely occurs {2778}.

Immunohistochemistry

The inner cells are positive for pancytokeratin and CK7, whereas the outer myoepithelial cells are usually positive for p63, SMA, calponin, and S100 {2904,2340}. Diffuse and membranous/cytoplasmic RAS p.Q61R expression, almost always restricted to myoepithelial cells, has been observed in 65% of

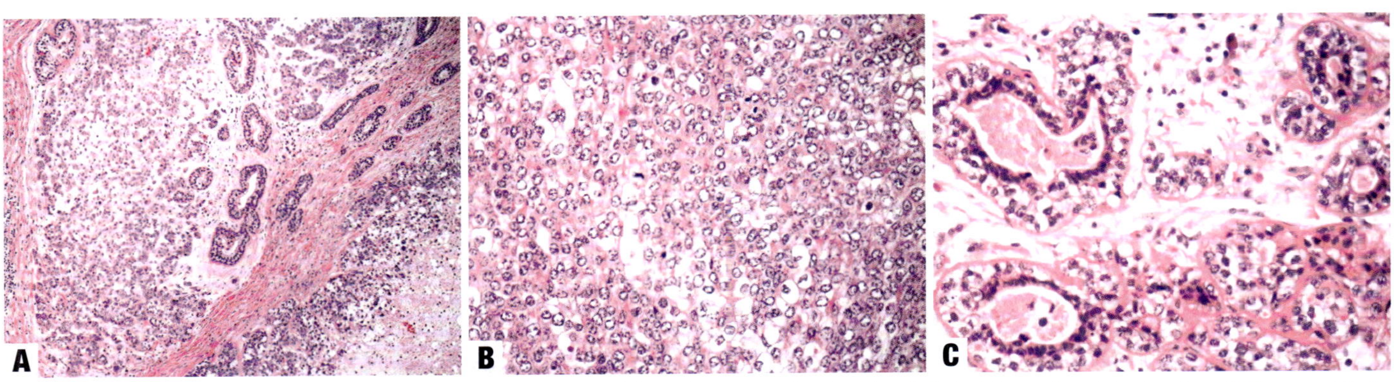

Fig. 7.30 Epithelial-myoepithelial carcinoma. **A** This tumour shows areas of high-grade transformation (dedifferentiation) with loss of the biphasic pattern. **B** The areas of high-grade transformation (dedifferentiation) show solid areas with loss of the biphasic pattern, increased pleomorphism, and mitoses. **C** The typical biphasic pattern with an inner cuboidal layer and an outer layer of myoepithelial cells, which are often clear, is seen.

Chapter 7

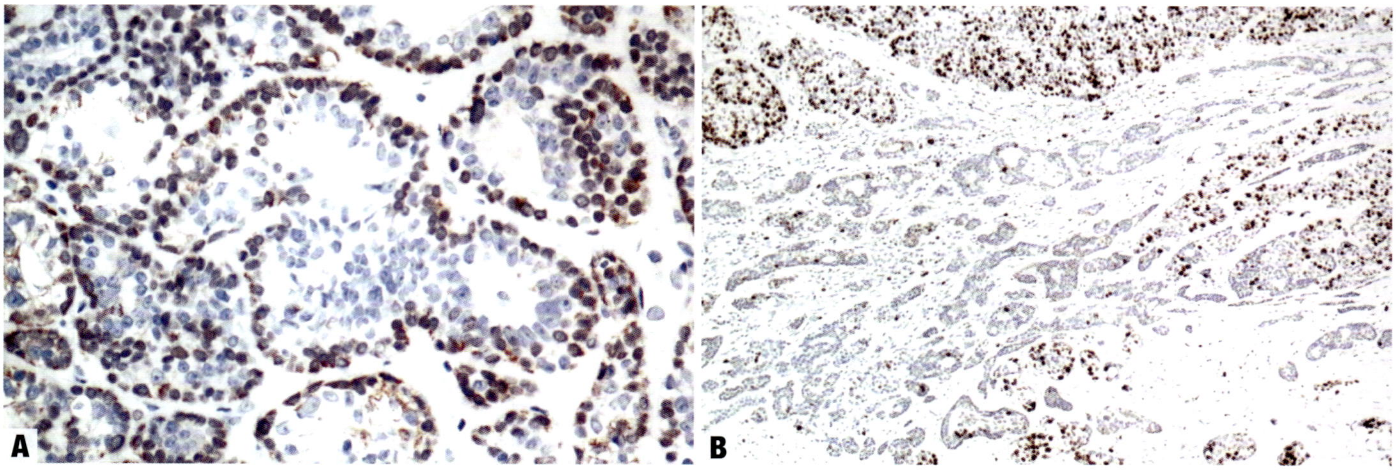

Fig. 7.31 Epithelial-myoepithelial carcinoma. **A** p63 immunohistochemistry highlights the outer layer of myoepithelial cells, demonstrating the biphasic pattern. **B** Ki-67 immunohistochemistry shows the difference in proliferative activity between the typical epithelial-myoepithelial carcinoma pattern (centre) and the high-grade area (top and bottom).

EMCs {2341,3417} and helps in their differentiation from EMC ex pleomorphic adenoma and also from its histological mimics {3417}.

Differential diagnosis

The entities include other lacrimal gland tumours with biphasic or/and clear cell morphology, such as adenoid cystic carcinoma, basal cell adenoma/adenocarcinoma, pleomorphic adenoma, myoepithelial carcinoma, and clear cell carcinoma {2340,727,3417}.

Cytology

Aspirates classically show tubular structures with a dual epithelial and myoepithelial cell population with mild to moderate atypia {1741,2204,161}.

Diagnostic molecular pathology

Assessment of *HRAS* mutations is useful for diagnosing EMC and excluding its mimics {3417,2340}. Identification of *MYB* fusion by FISH or immunohistochemistry may help in differentiation of these tumours from adenoid cystic carcinoma and hybrid tumours {344}.

Essential and desirable diagnostic criteria

Essential: usually multinodular invasive growth; at least partly with a dual arrangement of inner ductal cells and outer prominent, and usually clear, myoepithelial cells.

Staging

EMC is staged according to the eighth-edition Union for International Cancer Control (UICC) TNM staging system for lacrimal gland tumours.

Prognosis and prediction

EMC has a favourable prognosis but occasionally recurs locally; lymph node and distant metastases are rare. High-grade transformation, myoepithelial differentiation, solid growth pattern, increased mitotic activity, Ki-67 > 10%, perineural invasion, and necrosis are indicators of aggressive biology and might indicate poor prognosis {161,74,2778}.

Acinic cell carcinoma

Salomao DR
Chan ASY
Iacob CE

Definition

Acinic cell carcinoma is a rare malignant lacrimal gland neoplasm displaying predominantly serous acinar differentiation.

ICD-O coding

8550/3 Acinic cell carcinoma

ICD-11 coding

2D0Y & XH3PG9 Other specified malignant neoplasms of eye or ocular adnexa & Acinar cell carcinoma

Related terminology

Acceptable: acinic cell adenocarcinoma; acinar cell carcinoma.

Subtype(s)

None

Localization

The rare cases occurring in the lacrimal gland have involved the palpebral {249} and orbital lobes {945,748}, and a few cases extended to adjacent soft tissues {2770} or intracranially {1497}.

Clinical features

Patients may be asymptomatic {157} or present with a slow-growing painless mass causing inferior globe displacement {1497} or proptosis {748}.

Imaging

CT shows a circumscribed mass located in the lacrimal fossa {157}. MRI provides better detail of the involvement of adjacent structures.

Epidemiology

This is an extremely rare lacrimal gland neoplasm with slight female predominance. The majority of the patients are in their fifties; however, a case was reported in an 18-year-old patient {2770}.

Etiology

Unknown

Pathogenesis

Studies performed in salivary gland cases revealed the recurrent genomic rearrangement t(4;9)(q13;q31) as a characteristic genetic driver event in acinic cell carcinomas, enabling upregulation of the transcription factor *NR4A3* through enhancer hijacking {1233,1234}.

Macroscopic appearance

Tumours are often well-circumscribed, tan-greyish, firm to soft solid masses with occasional cystic areas. Infiltrative borders and multinodularity are mostly seen in recurrences {3450}.

Histopathology

Microscopically, the tumour may show solid (trabecular or acinar arrangements), microcystic, papillary-cystic (lattice-like), and follicular growth patterns. A prominent lymphoid infiltrate may be seen in the background. The typical tumour cell is characterized by a polygonal shape, abundant basophilic granular cytoplasm with poorly defined borders, central/eccentric small nuclei, and distinct nucleoli {748,1497}; oncocytic and clear cells might be present. Cytoplasmic granules are PAS-positive and diastase-resistant. Tumours with high-grade transformation exhibit areas of nuclear enlargement and pleomorphism increased mitoses, necrosis, and perineural and vascular invasion {3138,2333}.

Immunohistochemistry

DOG1 and SOX10 positivity is found in tumours with acinar and intercalated duct cell features, but it is not necessary

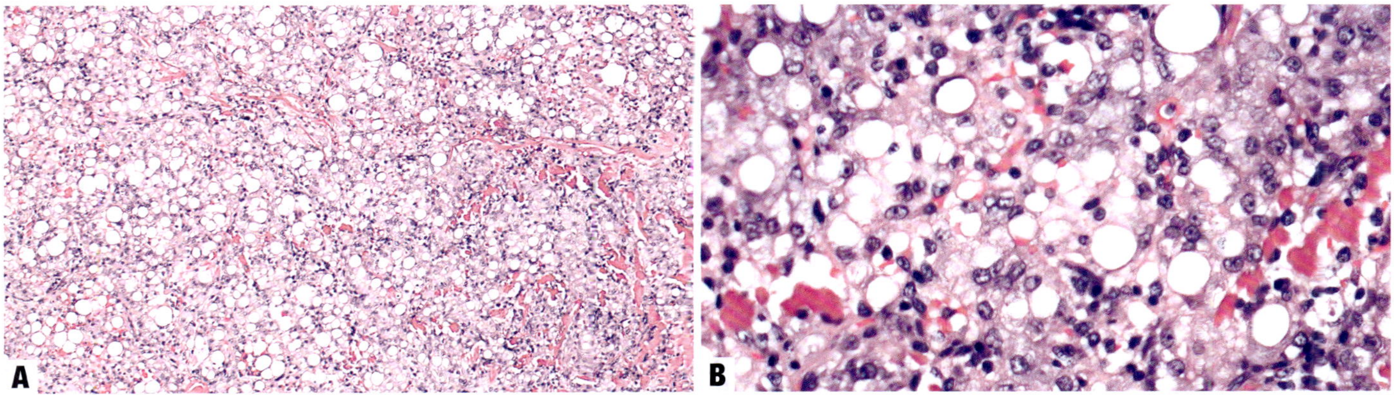

Fig. 7.32 Acinic cell carcinoma. **A** The carcinoma is composed of sheets of cells similar to glandular acini. **B** There are scattered lumina of glandular acini present within sheets of tumour cells with round vesicular nuclei, prominent nucleoli, and numerous microcystic vacuoles.

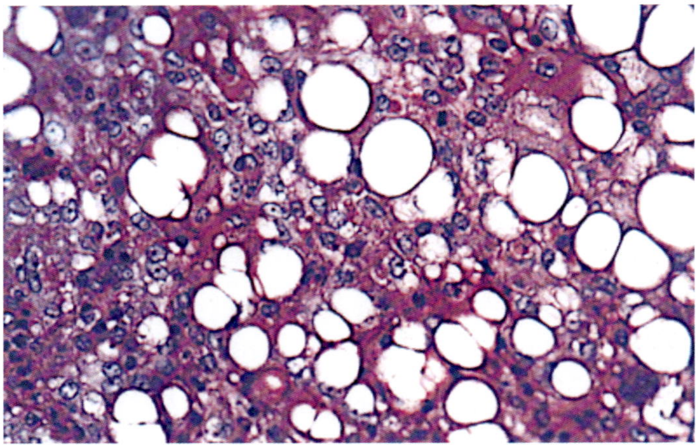

Fig. 7.33 Acinic cell carcinoma. PAS staining showing the cytoplasmic granularity as PAS-positive secretions {2770}.

for diagnosis. Recently described immunohistochemistry for NR4A3 or NR4A2 has been reported to be more specific and sensitive for diagnosis {1234,3631}.

Acinic cell carcinomas are usually negative for p63, S100, and mammaglobin, which assists differentiation from secretory carcinoma, a tumour that has a characteristic *ETV6::NTRK3* translocation.

Differential diagnosis

This includes normal lacrimal gland tissue, secretory carcinoma, mucoepidermoid carcinoma, and papillary cystadenocarcinoma, especially cases with papillary-cystic areas and stromal lymphoid aggregates. The most important differential is with secretory carcinoma, as on further testing most lacrimal gland acinic carcinomas turn out to be secretory carcinomas.

Cytology

Cellular smears composed of large, polygonal, serous cells with round, uniform nuclei and delicate, vacuolated, or finely granular basophilic cytoplasm. Stripped nuclei and small lymphocytes can be seen in the background. Uncommonly, mitoses, necrosis, and marked nuclear atypia may indicate high-grade transformation.

Diagnostic molecular pathology

Diagnostic molecular pathology is not needed in most cases. However, challenging cases may require demonstrating NR4A subfamily rearrangements via immunohistochemistry {3631, 1234}.

Essential and desirable diagnostic criteria

Essential: tumour cells with acinar differentiation; zymogen granules in focal areas.

Desirable: nuclear staining for NR4A3 (NOR1) or NR4A2 (NUUR1); molecular demonstration of *NR4A3* rearrangement.

Staging

Stage according to the eighth-edition Union for International Cancer Control (UICC) / American Joint Committee on Cancer (AJCC) TNM staging system.

Prognosis and prediction

Acinic cell carcinomas are low-grade malignancies, with a total any-year disease-specific survival rate of nearly 90%. Histological features associated with poor prognosis include extracapsular extension, increased mitoses, a desmoplastic and lymphoid stromal reaction, perineural and vascular invasion, and high-grade features {1974,3450}.

Adenocarcinoma NOS of the lacrimal gland

Chan ASY
Alkatan H
Roberts F

Definition
Adenocarcinoma NOS of the lacrimal gland is a malignant epithelial neoplasm with a solid and glandular growth pattern that lacks the histopathological features characteristic of other specific carcinoma types.

ICD-O coding
8140/3 Adenocarcinoma, NOS

ICD-11 coding
2D0Y & XH74S1 Other specified malignant neoplasms of eye or ocular adnexa & Adenocarcinoma, NOS

Related terminology
Not recommended: unclassified adenocarcinoma; primary ductal adenocarcinoma.

Subtype(s)
None

Localization
Adenocarcinoma NOS arises from the orbital lobe of the lacrimal gland and rarely in accessory lacrimal glands {2211, 352}.

Clinical features
Patients present with similar clinical features to those of other lacrimal gland tumours. These include upper eyelid swelling, ptosis, non-axial proptosis, restriction of ocular movement, diplopia, and loss of vision secondary to the mass effects of the enlarged lacrimal gland {3507,2211}. Symptoms are usually present for < 1 year before presentation {3507}. Pain is often a feature although is not as common as in adenoid cystic carcinoma of the lacrimal gland {3507}. Imaging is non-diagnostic and shows typical features of a malignant lacrimal mass with irregular margins, bony erosion or invasion, and calcification {3507,150}. Adenocarcinoma NOS has a propensity to spread by lymphatic and haematogenous routes, and may metastasize to regional lymph nodes as well as distant sites including the lung, brain, and mediastinum {1721,1202}.

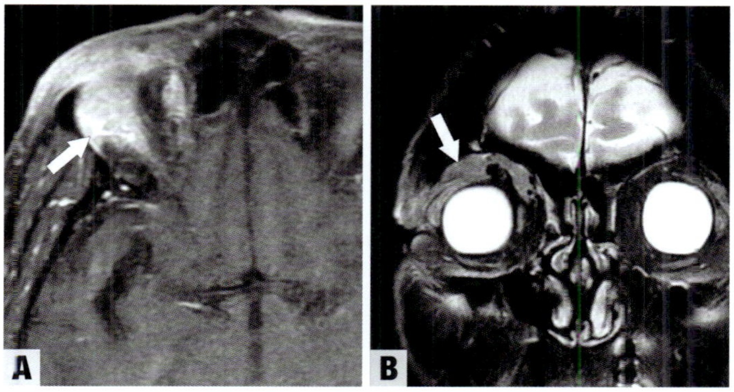

Fig. 7.34 Adenocarcinoma NOS. **A** Axial T1-weighted postcontrast MRI shows an enhancing mass in the superior right orbit and periorbital soft tissues (arrow). **B** Axial T2-weighted MRI shows an isointense mass in the superior right orbit (arrow).

Epidemiology
Adenocarcinoma NOS is the third most frequent malignant epithelial tumour of the lacrimal gland occurring in 5–10% of cases {312,150,1721}. It is reported to be more common in men {3507} and occurs in the older population with a mean age at presentation of 50–52 years {3507,1202}.

Etiology
These tumours may occur de novo or within a pleomorphic adenoma {1721}.

Pathogenesis
Unknown

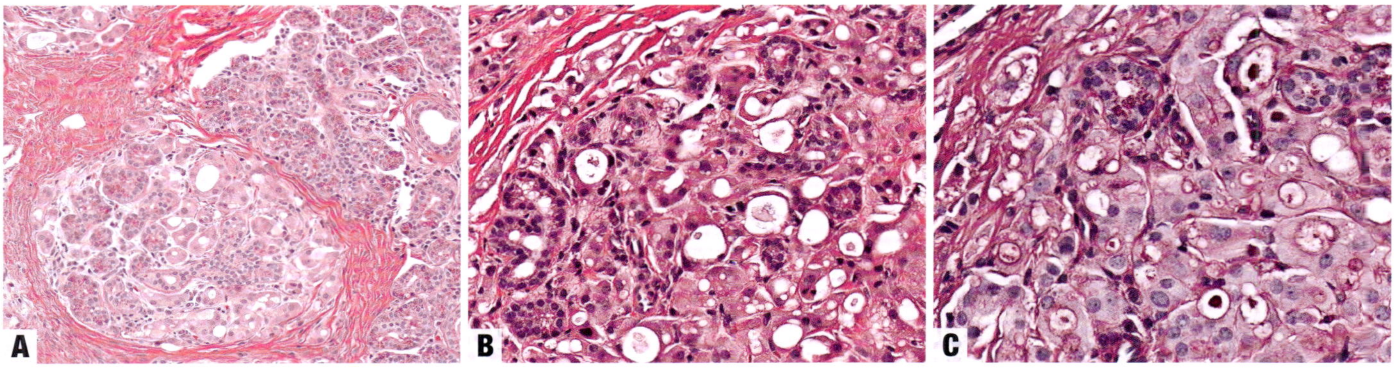

Fig. 7.35 Adenocarcinoma NOS. **A** At scanning magnification, the neoplasm arises in the lacrimal gland lobules. **B** Higher magnification demonstrates neoplastic cells with abundant eosinophilic cytoplasm with focal intracytoplasmic vacuoles arranged in ductules with eosinophilic secretory material. **C** Focal mucin is seen in the neoplastic cells adjacent to the non-neoplastic lacrimal gland acinar cells with PAS-positive zymogen granules.

Macroscopic appearance

Tumours may present as unencapsulated irregular masses {2211}.

Histopathology

Adenocarcinoma NOS lacks the distinctive histological features that characterize other specific carcinoma types. It shows variable gland formation with duct-like configurations, and nests of clear cells {3507,3572}. Mitoses reported in these tumours vary from less than occasional to many {3572}. These tumours can also show a higher grade of anaplastic cell proliferation with prominent glandular formation and extensive necrosis {3572}.

Immunohistochemistry

Although nonspecific for diagnosis, the tumour cells have been reported to stain for cytokeratins {3370}, CK7 {3370,2211}, GATA3 {3370}, p63 {3370}, E-cadherin {3370}, GCDFP-15 {2211}, and AR {2211,440}, and focally for CEA {2211}.

Differential diagnosis

As this is a diagnosis of exclusion, differential diagnoses of all other specific primary lacrimal gland carcinomas must be considered and excluded {3507}. Unlike primary ductal carcinoma, the majority of adenocarcinoma NOS reported show absence of ERBB2 expression {2211,3370,440}.

Cytology

Cytological diagnosis has not been described.

Diagnostic molecular pathology

Diagnostic molecular pathology is nonspecific without alterations that would categorize these tumours elsewhere.

Essential and desirable diagnostic criteria

The diagnosis of adenocarcinoma NOS is made strictly by exclusion of other known primary lacrimal gland carcinomas {3507}.

Staging

Staging is according to the eighth-edition Union for International Cancer Control (UICC) / American Joint Committee on Cancer (AJCC) TNM staging system.

Prognosis and prediction

Prognosis is poor with an average survival of 1.5 years and mortality ranging from 50% to 80%. Earlier treatment intervention has been reported to decrease metastases and increase long-term survival {1293}. A 10-year overall survival rate of 27.7% and 10-year disease-specific survival rate of 51.4% has been reported with early treatment intervention {154}. Tumour histology has been suggested to correlate with disease-specific survival {154}. Treatment consists of complete surgical excision by exenteration with lymph node dissection accompanied by adjuvant radiotherapy and rarely chemotherapy. Immunotherapy with checkpoint inhibitors such as pembrolizumab {2211} and nivolumab {440} has also been used.

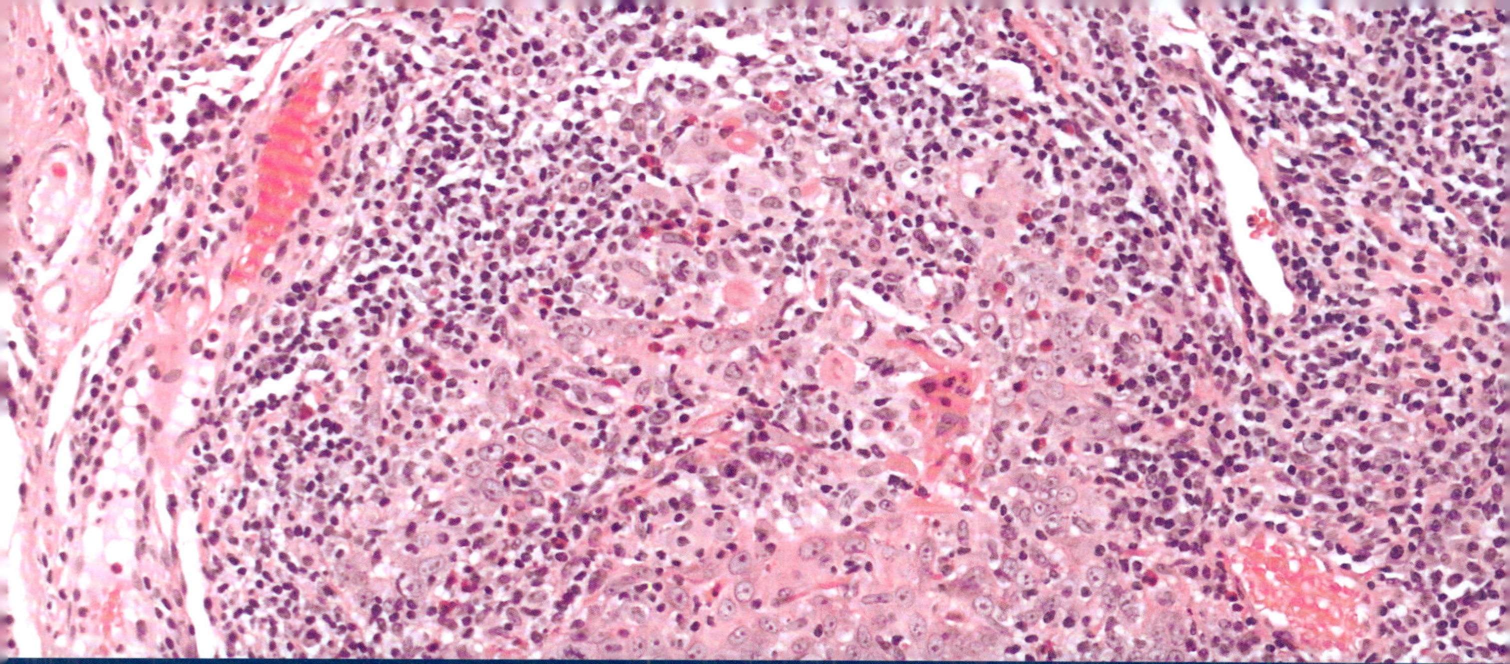

8

Tumours of the lacrimal drainage system

Edited by: Esmaeli B, Heegaard S, Rodríguez-Reyes AA

Tumours of the lacrimal drainage system: Introduction

Heegaard S
Farmer J
Irion LCD
Rodríguez-Reyes AA

The lacrimal drainage system (LDS) serves as a conduit for the exit of tears from the eye into the nasal cavity. Tears on the ocular surface enter the canaliculi through puncta on the medial aspects of the upper and lower eyelids. Both the puncta and canaliculi are lined by stratified, non-keratinized epithelium, which is generally 5–10 cells thick. The tears then drain into the lacrimal sac, which is lined by stratified columnar epithelium containing mucus-secreting goblet cells, and exit via the similarly lined nasolacrimal duct into the nasal cavity.

Disorders of the LDS are relatively common, accounting for approximately 3% of clinical visits in some series {1743}. Most cases are associated with chronic inflammation and fibrosis of the lacrimal sac wall. Infectious organisms are identified in some cases of chronic dacryocystitis, but many cases represent nonspecific processes. A discrete dacryolith composed of variably mineralized inflammatory and shed epithelial cells, often containing bacteria or other infectious organisms, is sometimes removed and sent for microscopic evaluation.

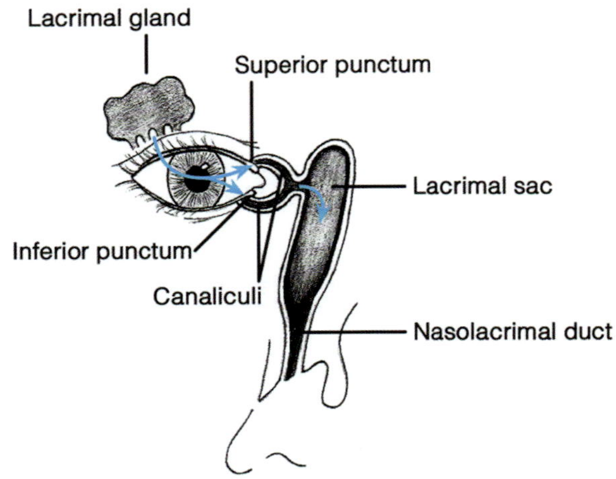

Fig. 8.01 Lacrimal drainage system. The normal anatomy of the lacrimal drainage system.

Epithelial tumours

Although neoplasms of the LDS are relatively rare, they must be considered whenever patients present with obstructive lesions {2652}. Epithelial neoplasms are the most common tumours of the LDS {1306}. Papillomas can be covered with squamous or so-called transitional epithelium, and they display exophytic or inverted/endophytic growth patterns. Inverted papillomas are more likely to recur and progress to carcinoma {3542}. Early clinical symptoms are nonspecific and may include epiphora, bloody tears, or symptoms of dacryocystitis. A progressive mass in the area of the lacrimal sac / nasolacrimal duct makes the diagnosis more obvious {1805}, particularly if it is a firm mass. Extension above the medial canthal tendon or with extension into the paranasal sinuses and nasal cavity makes the diagnosis of a malignant tumour of the lacrimal sac more likely. In some instances the diagnosis is made intraoperatively during routine dacryocystorhinostomy when the surgeon notes a mass or other abnormal findings.

Squamous cell carcinoma is by far the most common epithelial malignant tumour of the lacrimal drainage apparatus. It can be divided into keratinizing and non-keratinizing squamous cell carcinoma. HPV infection has been identified in both benign/papillomatous and malignant (keratinizing or non-keratinizing squamous) lesions {33,3135}. Less-common primary epithelial neoplasms at this anatomical site include adenocarcinoma, mucoepidermoid carcinoma, adenoid cystic carcinoma, and lymphoepithelial carcinoma.

The treatment of primary lacrimal sac / nasolacrimal duct carcinomas is multidisciplinary and typically involves surgery followed by radiation therapy and/or chemotherapy {889,2422}. In the majority of cases, eye-sparing treatments can be achieved and orbital exenteration is rarely needed.

Non-epithelial tumours

Those neoplasms originating in the LDS include malignant lymphoma and soft tissue tumours. Most arise from the lacrimal sac.

Haematolymphoid malignancies, including diffuse large B-cell lymphoma (DLBCL), extranodal marginal zone lymphoma, and chronic lymphocytic leukaemia / small lymphocytic lymphoma, occur at this site and must be differentiated from reactive lymphoid hyperplasia {1306} (see Chapter 10: *Haematolymphoid tumours*). LDS lymphomas represent 2–11% of LDS tumours, with a patient age > 50 years and a female predilection, and are usually found incidentally during a dacryocystorhinostomy procedure {1790,3120,2088}. Malignant lymphoma arises from LDS-associated lymphoid tissue, although DLBCL is known to arise de novo {3120}. EBV has been associated with DLBCL and NK/T-cell lymphoma of the LDS {3120}. DLBCL makes up one third of LDS lymphomas, followed by extranodal marginal zone lymphoma (20%), chronic lymphocytic leukaemia / small lymphocytic lymphoma (15%), and other low-grade B-cell lymphomas {3120,3132}. The morphological features of periocular lymphomas are described in Chapter 10: *Haematolymphoid tumours*. Periocular lymphoma–related deaths range from 2% to 12% for extranodal marginal zone lymphoma and from 38% to 48% for DLBCL {3120,3132}.

Soft tissue tumours have been reported {3120} and represent 12–14% of LDS tumours, the most common being fibrous histiocytoma (FH) and solitary fibrous tumour (SFT) {2523,1790, 2268,3560} (see Chapter 11: *Soft tissue and bone tumours*). The average age at diagnosis of FH is 34 years, and there is no sex predilection; for SFT, the average age is 58 years, with a female predominance {3120,2268,2523,3560}. Gene fusions involving *PRKCB* and *PRKCD* (encoding protein kinase isoforms) are described in a subset of cases of in FH {3537}. SFT involves a *NAB2::STAT6* fusion {590,762} (see *Solitary fibrous tumour*, p. 395, for further details). FHs are composed of spindle to polymorphous cells in a storiform collagenous background and express vimentin, CD68, and factor XIIIa, and are negative for CD34 {1474}. Wide and complete surgical excision is the management for FH and SFT. The prognosis is excellent for FH and SFT without histological features of aggressiveness {2523, 1306,2268}.

Metastatic tumours are only rarely seen in the LDS, and generally also involve orbital soft tissue or other surrounding structures {1306}.

Melanocytic tumours of the LDS are very rare, and the lacrimal sac is the most common location.

Chapter 8

Papillomas (squamous and inverted)

Krishna Y
Farmer J
Mittal R

Definition
Papillomas of the lacrimal drainage system are benign neoplasms characterized by an exophytic or an inverted growth of acanthotic, maturing multilayered epithelium.

ICD-O coding
8052/0 Squamous papilloma, exophytic
8053/0 Squamous papilloma, inverted
8052/0 Squamous papilloma, mixed

ICD-11 coding
2F36.Y & XH0TP8 Other specified benign neoplasm of eye or ocular adnexa & Sinonasal papilloma, exophytic
2F36.Y & XH8FH7 Other specified benign neoplasm of eye or ocular adnexa & Sinonasal papilloma, inverted

Related terminology
Not recommended: Schneiderian papilloma; everted papilloma; fungiform papilloma; endophytic papilloma; transitional papilloma.

Subtype(s)
Exophytic papilloma; inverted papilloma; mixed papilloma

Localization
Papillomas usually arise from the epithelium in the lacrimal sac and may secondarily involve the lower canaliculus, nasolacrimal duct, and nasal cavity as they grow. Inverted papillomas (IPs) may also originate from the nasolacrimal duct {3198,1306, 3527}.

Clinical features
Most are unilateral and present with persistent/chronic epiphora, recurrent dacryocystitis, and/or a non-tender mass above the medial tendon. Serosanguineous punctal discharge, epistaxis, and pain are rare. About 40% of cases have been discovered incidentally during dacryocystorhinostomy or dacryocystectomy {724,923,1364,2498,2794,3432,1295,1790}.

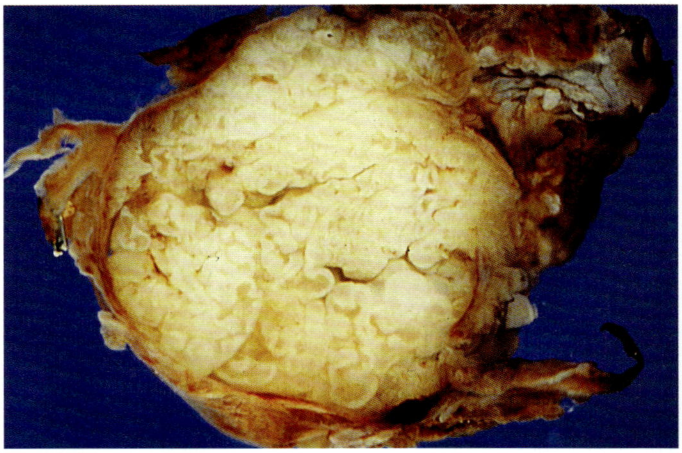

Fig. 8.02 Inverted papilloma. A dacryocystectomy specimen with an inverted papilloma filling the lumen of the lacrimal sac is seen; ribbons of thickened epithelium can be identified within the mass.

Epidemiology
Papillomas usually arise in the fourth to fifth decades of life but can occur at any age, with no sex predilection; IP is the most common {2379,2794,3198,1306}.

Etiology
Low-risk HPV6 and HPV11 genotypes have been reported {3198,2344,1125,2648}. Statistically associated increased risk with cigarette smoking and dust and aerosol exposure has also been shown {3542,1253}.

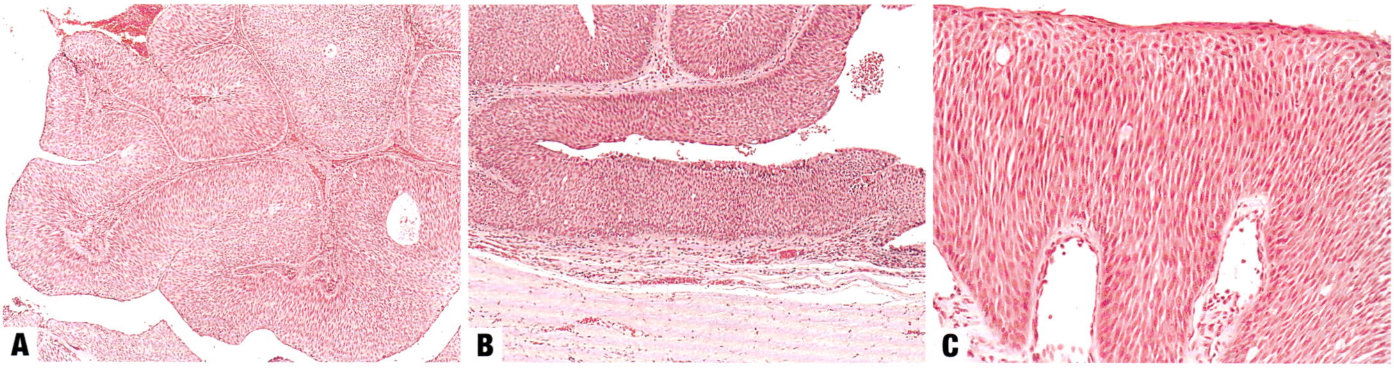

Fig. 8.03 Inverted papilloma. **A** An example with thickened surface epithelium in which there are two microcysts is shown. **B** Adjacent to the papilloma, the junction between normal lacrimal sac epithelium and transitional epithelium is seen. **C** An example with thickened surface epithelium composed of closely packed, vertically aligned, spindle-shaped cells with scattered goblet cells is shown; intercellular bridges cannot be identified, although there is slight surface keratinization.

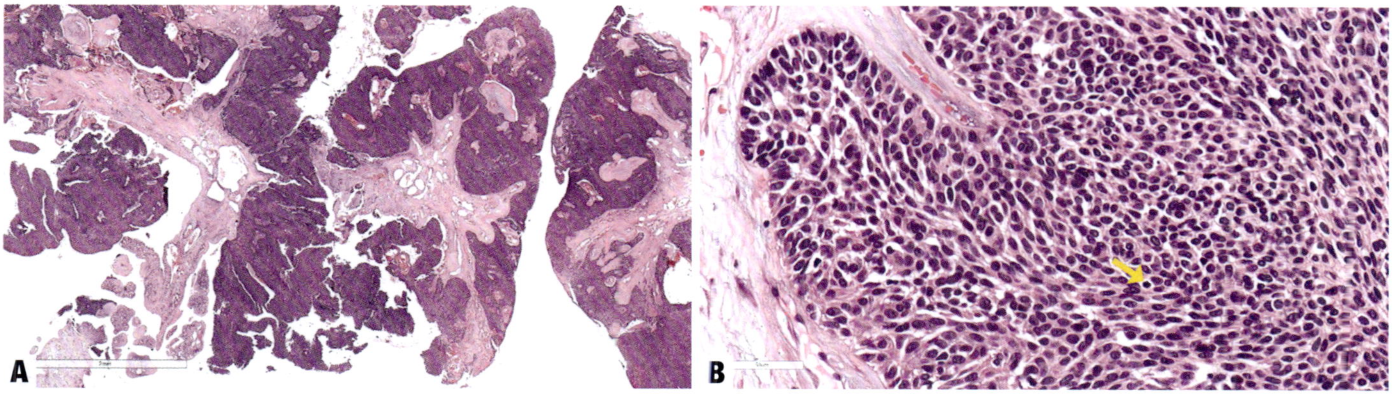

Fig. 8.04 Exophytic papilloma. **A** Outward growth of papillary fronds with branching fibrovascular cores is seen. **B** Higher magnification shows the hyperplastic epithelium, predominantly lined by transitional cells; a typical mitotic figure is present (yellow arrow).

Pathogenesis

IPs are histopathologically identical to inverted sinonasal papillomas and their pathogenesis is similarly related {1295}. Over 70% have activating *EGFR* mutations in the tyrosine kinase domains {2155}.

Macroscopic appearance

Squamous papillomas (SPs) appear as single polypoidal or confluent, firm, fleshy greyish-pink/tan masses. IPs are firm, tan/reddish polyps often with a convoluted cerebriform surface {341}.

Histopathology

SPs are composed of outward/exophytic proliferations of finger-like projections of multilayered epithelium 5–20 cells thick, variably squamous, squamotransitional, or columnar, but most often squamous, with a central fibrovascular core {341}.

IPs show an inward/endophytic growth of epithelial nests from the surface epithelium, surrounded by an intact basement membrane; mixed endophytic/exophytic tumours are not uncommon {923,1790}. The epithelium is the same as in SPs but is more frequently transitional {1295,341}. Pools of mucin with neutrophils are common {1295}. Stromal changes include submucosal oedema and chronic inflammation {341}. Condylomatous changes (marked acanthosis with scattered koilocyte-like cells) are features of HPV infection {2155}. Mitoses are rare and not atypical; although varying grades of dysplasia have been observed in papillomas {724,1498}, malignant change in SPs is extremely rare {612}. IPs can erode bone, but this alone does not indicate malignant transformation; there are no histopathological features predictive of subsequent malignant transformation {341}.

Immunohistochemistry

Papillomas are positive for pancytokeratin {265}.

Differential diagnosis

Exclude squamous cell carcinoma and mucoepidermoid carcinoma.

Cytology

Not relevant

Diagnostic molecular pathology

Not relevant

Essential and desirable diagnostic criteria

Squamous papilloma

Essential: proliferative, exophytic, papillary growth; lined by an acanthotic multilayered epithelium; no evidence of high-grade squamous dysplasia; absence of inverted, destructive, or infiltrative growth.

Inverted papilloma

Essential: prominent endophytic growth of hyperplastic epithelium into the stroma with an intact basement membrane; absence of malignant cellular features and necrosis.

Staging

Not relevant

Prognosis and prediction

Complete en bloc surgical excision is the treatment of choice for both SPs and IPs of the lacrimal drainage system. Recurrence and progression to malignancy is distinctly uncommon in SP, if completely excised {3542}. IP recurrence rate is 11–14%; smoking increases the risk to 50% {3542,1253}. Invasion into the orbit, paranasal sinuses, and intracranial cavity can occur with risk increasing in recurrent cases {3542}. The rate of malignancy of IP confined to the lacrimal drainage system is 22%, increasing to 27% when orbitally invasive cases are included {3542}. The types of carcinomas identified include squamous cell carcinoma, mucin-producing carcinoma, and Schneiderian/transitional carcinoma {1790,3542}.

There are currently no histopathological, immunohistochemical, or molecular features predictive of aggressive behaviour.

Squamous cell carcinoma of the lacrimal drainage system

Krishna Y
Mittal R

Definition

Squamous cell carcinoma (SCC) of the lacrimal drainage system is a malignant epithelial neoplasm originating from surface epithelium. Keratinizing squamous cell carcinoma (KSCC) shows squamous differentiation and keratin production, whereas non-keratinizing SCC (NKSCC) shows histological and/or immunohistochemical evidence of squamous differentiation, but with no or minimal keratinization.

ICD-O coding

8070/3 Squamous cell carcinoma
8071/3 Squamous cell carcinoma, keratinizing, NOS
8072/3 Squamous cell carcinoma, non-keratinizing, NOS

ICD-11 coding

2D03.2 Squamous cell carcinoma of the lacrimal apparatus
2D03.2 & XH4CR9 Squamous cell carcinoma of the lacrimal apparatus & Squamous cell carcinoma, keratinizing, NOS
2D03.2 & XH6705 Squamous cell carcinoma of the lacrimal apparatus & Squamous cell carcinoma, large cell, non-keratinizing, NOS

Related terminology

Not recommended: squamous cell carcinoma NOS; epidermoid carcinoma; Schneiderian carcinoma; transitional cell carcinoma.

Subtype(s)

Keratinizing squamous cell carcinoma (KSCC); non-keratinizing squamous cell carcinoma (NKSCC)

Localization

SCC arises predominantly in the lacrimal sac but may involve the canaliculi and rarely the nasolacrimal duct {3198,3204, 2820,1306,79,1790,902,1295,3527}.

Clinical features

The majority of SCCs arising from the lacrimal drainage system are unilateral and present with persistent/chronic epiphora, recurrent dacryocystitis, and/or a non-tender, incompressible mass above the medial tendon. Serosanguineous punctal discharge, epistaxis, pain, nasal obstruction, and medial canthal skin ulceration/telangiectasia may occur. Some cases have been discovered incidentally during dacryocystorhinostomy or dacryocystectomy {2498,2794,3432,1295,1790,79,889,1306, 1743,3204}.

Direct extension into the orbit, paranasal sinuses with bony destruction, and cranium, and rarely regional lymphadenopathy or metastases have been described {370,889,1623,3204}. CT and MRI are helpful to delineate tumour extension through bone and soft tissues.

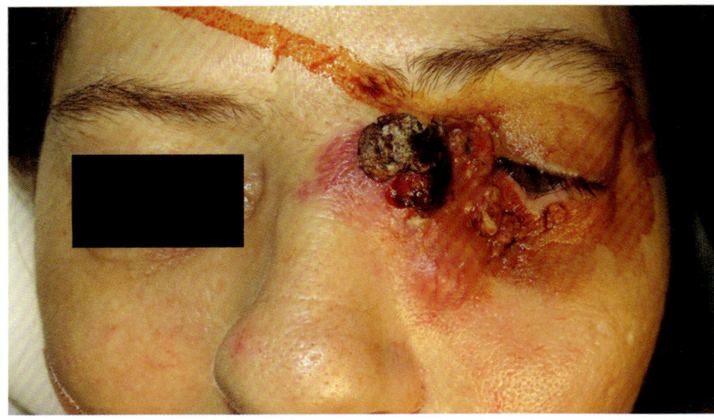

Fig. 8.05 Squamous cell carcinoma of the lacrimal drainage system. An example presenting as a large ulcerating mass over and below the left medial canthal ligament in a middle-aged woman.

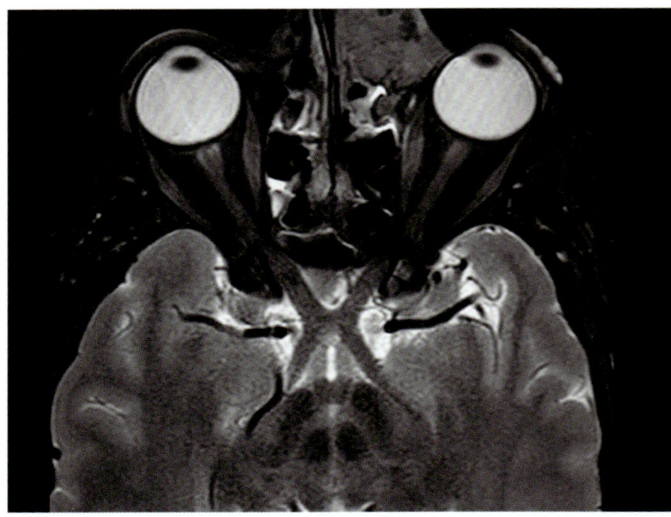

Fig. 8.06 Squamous cell carcinoma of the lacrimal drainage system. T2-weighted fat-suppressed axial MRI shows a tumour in the left lacrimal sac area, with ethmoid sinus and nasal cavity involvement.

Epidemiology

SCC of the lacrimal sac is rare and accounts for about 14% of all lacrimal sac neoplasms {2379,2633,2794}. They typically present in the fifth to eighth decades of life, with no sex predilection {33,370,2633,3204,1295,2379}.

Etiology

High-risk HPV genotypes (HPV16, HPV18, or HPV33) have been reported in about 60% of lacrimal sac SCCs with predominantly non-keratinizing histomorphology {2024,2344,3135,33, 1790,2648}.

SCC in the lacrimal sac may arise as a de novo lesion or in a pre-existing inverted papilloma as an invasive carcinoma or carcinoma in situ ex inverted papilloma in about 10–15% of cases {2826}.

Increased risk with cigarette smoking has also been shown in small studies {3542,1253}. Lesions may originate from pre-existing squamous metaplasia and chronic inflammation has been implicated in inducing malignant transformation {2826}.

Pathogenesis

The genomic landscape in lacrimal sac SCCs is poorly defined. Gene mutations in *EGFR*, *PTEN*, *CDKN2A*, and *KMT2D*, and p53 expression dysregulation have been reported in sinonasal SCCs. SCCs arising from inverted papillomas have been shown to harbour the *EGFR* mutation {3408,1359}.

HPV16-associated SCC exhibits mutations of *PIK3CA*, *FGFR3*, *AKT1*, and/or *PIK3R1*; wildtype *TP53*; p16 overexpression; and deregulated high-risk E6/E7 transcription {2654}. HPV testing by in situ hybridization or PCR identifies those tumours with associated HPV infection. In sinonasal SCC, HPV-associated p16 overexpression reflects oncogenic HPV in SCC pathogenesis {342,1857}.

Macroscopic appearance

Lesions appear as an endophytic or exophytic mass with a friable white-tan surface with or without haemorrhage and/or necrosis.

Histopathology

KSCC comprises infiltrating nests and strands of polygonal squamous cells with eosinophilic cytoplasm, large hyperchromatic nuclei, and a moderately high mitotic count; extracellular or intracellular keratinization with intercellular bridging and squamous eddies; comedonecrosis; desmoplastic stromal reaction; and a dense inflammatory background. There may also be koilocytosis {33,370,1759}.

NKSCC demonstrates large expansile nests, lobules, and ribbons of malignant epithelial cells with variable eosinophilia of their cytoplasm. Squamous differentiation may not always be obvious, especially in poorly differentiated carcinomas, and keratinization is usually minimal or absent. The carcinoma comprises atypical transitional-like epithelium with a lack of maturation and cell polarity, and an invasive acanthotic inverted/endophytic growth pattern or a mixed papillary and inverted growth

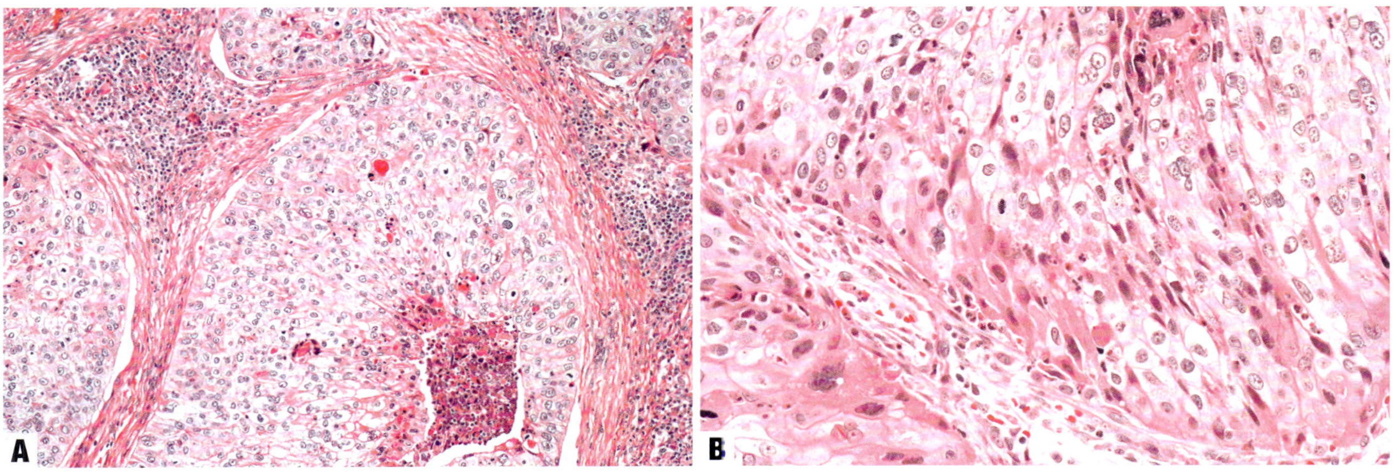

Fig. 8.07 Non-keratinizing squamous cell carcinoma of the lacrimal drainage system. **A** Invasive tumour islands showing acanthosis, increased cellularity, nuclear pleomorphism, and prominent nucleoli. **B** Atypical transitional epithelium with spindled and elongated tumour cells with prominent nucleoli.

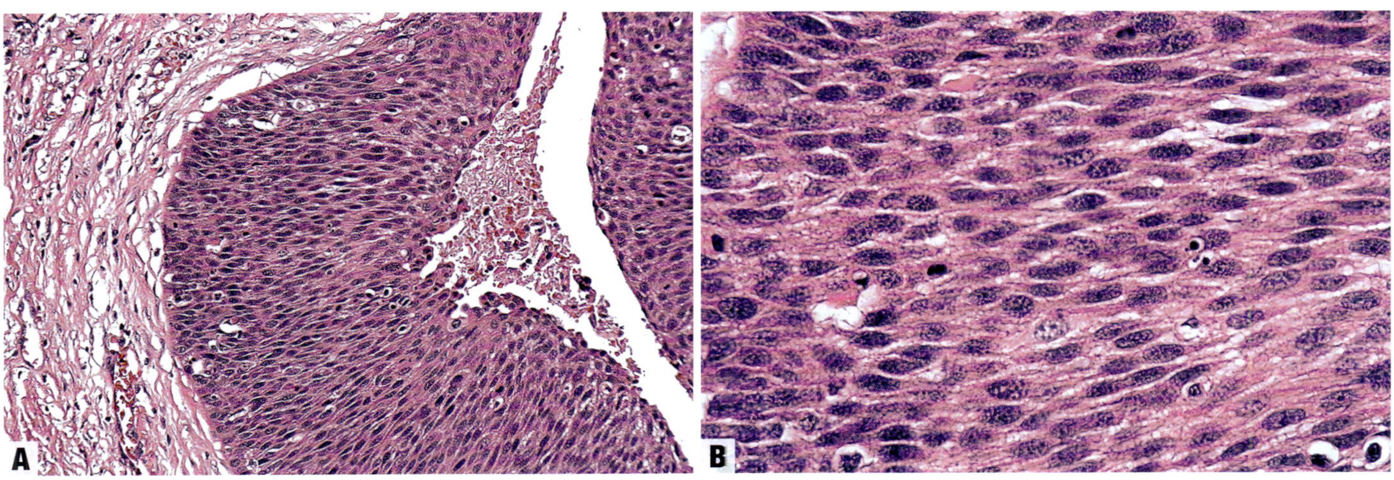

Fig. 8.08 Non-keratinizing squamous cell carcinoma. **A** Invasive non-keratinizing squamous cell carcinoma (also called transitional cell carcinoma) of the lacrimal sac. **B** Higher magnification showing cell morphology.

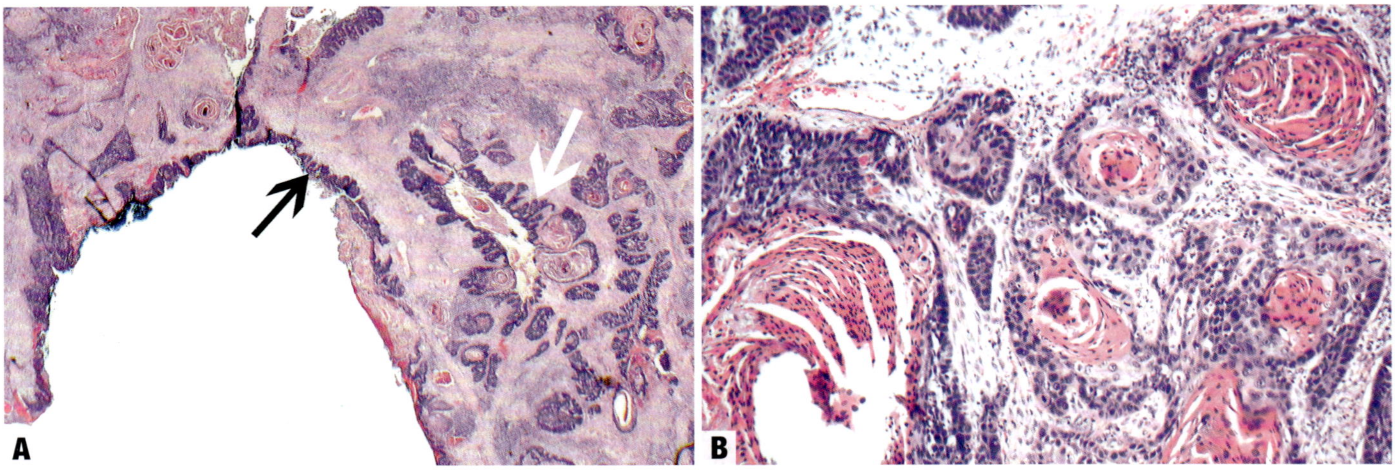

Fig. 8.09 Lacrimal sac keratinizing squamous cell carcinoma. **A** A low-power view shows the inner lining of the lacrimal sac (black arrow) and invasive lobules of keratinizing squamous cell carcinoma (white arrow). **B** At higher magnification, keratin can be seen among the invasive squamous cell carcinoma islands.

pattern with fibrovascular cores. Occasional goblet cells may be present {79,148,2794}.

Numerous abnormal mitoses and lymphovascular and perineural invasion can be seen in both subtypes. The SCC can be well, moderately, or poorly differentiated.

Immunohistochemistry

Immunohistochemistry is usually not required for KSCC, but it may be helpful in cases without keratinization or small biopsies. The carcinoma cells are positive for pancytokeratin, CK5/6, CK7, p40, p63, and EMA. They are negative for CK20, adipophilin, and other soft tissue, neuroendocrine, or melanoma markers, and with BerEP4.

Differential diagnosis

Poorly differentiated KSCCs and NKSCCs need differentiation from basaloid SCC, sinonasal malignancies, sebaceous cell carcinoma, amelanotic melanoma, and neuroendocrine carcinomas.

Cytology

Not relevant

Diagnostic molecular pathology

HPV detection is not currently used in this setting.

Essential and desirable diagnostic criteria

Essential: for KSCC: malignant epithelial cells with morphological evidence of squamous differentiation and keratinization; for NKSCC: malignant epithelial cells with morphological and/or immunohistochemical evidence of squamous differentiation, and with no or minimal keratinization.

Staging

While there is currently no separate TNM classification for carcinomas of the lacrimal drainage system, the eighth-edition Union for International Cancer Control (UICC) / American Joint Committee on Cancer (AJCC) TNM staging system for lacrimal gland tumours can be applied.

Prognosis and prediction

In a recent large series of lacrimal sac SCCs, the reported 5-year overall survival and progression-free survival were 88% and 76%, respectively {3167}. Long-term follow-up is recommended owing to high rates of recurrence and metastases. NKSCCs, poorly differentiated KSCCs, and those with orbital/and or sinonasal invasion are associated with a higher recurrence rate and poor prognosis {2588,3198,889,1790,2256,3167}. There are as yet no data on PDL1 expression and response to immunotherapy in this setting.

Lymphoepithelial carcinoma

Roberts F
Stagner AM

Definition

Lymphoepithelial carcinoma of the lacrimal drainage system is a poorly differentiated / undifferentiated squamous cell carcinoma accompanied by reactive lymphoplasmacytic infiltration strongly associated with EBV.

ICD-O coding

8082/3 Lymphoepithelial carcinoma

ICD-11 coding

2D03.2 & XH1E40 Squamous cell carcinoma of the lacrimal apparatus & Lymphoepithelial carcinoma

Related terminology

Not recommended: lymphoepithelioma-like carcinoma; non-keratinizing undifferentiated nasopharyngeal-type carcinoma; undifferentiated carcinoma with lymphocytic stroma; lymphoepithelioma

Subtype(s)

None

Localization

At this anatomical site, lymphoepithelial carcinomas present in the lacrimal sac and nasolacrimal duct.

Clinical features

The duration of symptoms is 1–24 months. Epiphora and swelling over the lacrimal sac are common, and a hard, non-tender, immobile mass above the medial tendon is characteristic {1483, 1999}.

Epidemiology

Lymphoepithelial carcinoma is rare in the lacrimal drainage system, with only 12 reported cases {786}, in women (10 cases) and men (2 cases) aged 20–82 years; 10 of these patients were Asian, 1 was African-American, and 1 was White {786}

Etiology

Nearly all lymphoepithelial carcinoma cases are strongly associated with EBV infection; 78% of cases in the lacrimal sac were found to be EBV-positive {1640,786}.

Pathogenesis

It is presumed that EBV plays an oncogenic role in these tumours.

Macroscopic appearance

Macroscopically, the tumour is polypoid, whitish, and firm.

Histopathology

Microscopically, the tumour is characterized by polygonal, undifferentiated malignant epithelial cells occurring in sheets, in clusters, and as isolated cells, mixed with an intense lymphoid infiltrate. The malignant cells have round vesicular nuclei and a single large central nucleolus. The background lymphoid infiltrate is composed of a mixture of B lymphocytes, T lymphocytes, plasma cells, and macrophages. Immunohistochemically, the epithelial tumour cells are positive for CK5/6, CK14 CK19, EMA, and p63 {1483,786}. Cytokeratin staining can be focal {1640}. The lymphoid infiltrate is polyclonal.

Cytology

There are no reports in lacrimal sac lymphoepithelial carcinoma, but the cytological findings of polygonal and spindled cells with prominent nucleoli and a heterogeneous background

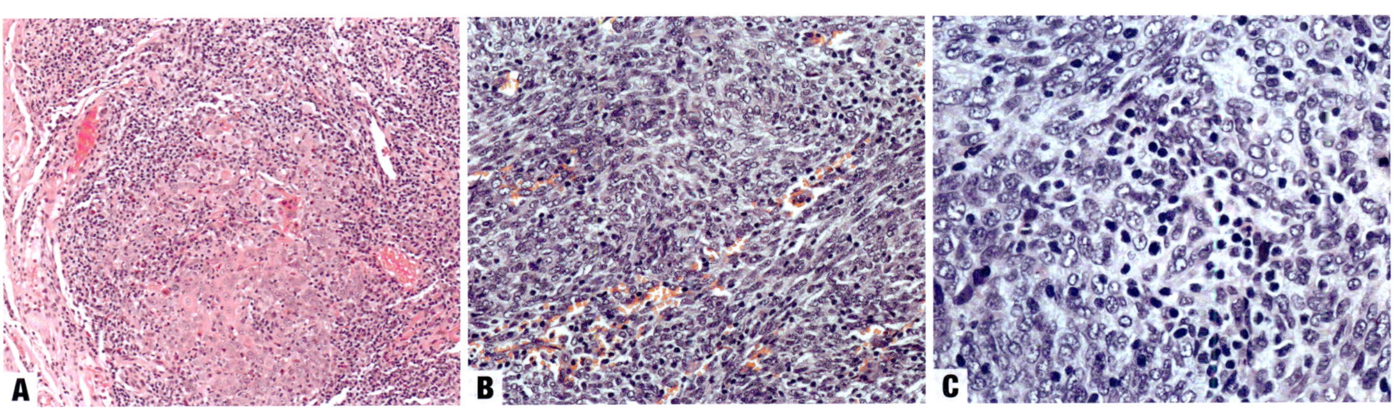

Fig. 8.10 Lymphoepithelial carcinoma. **A** The image shows the histological appearance with islands of poorly differentiated squamous cell carcinoma infiltrated and surrounded by large numbers of lymphocytes. **B** Clusters of undifferentiated malignant epithelial cells associated with a lymphoid infiltrate are seen. **C** The malignant epithelial cells have round vesicular nuclei and a single large central nucleolus; lymphocytes and plasma cells are scattered between the tumour cells.

population of lymphoid cells are described in salivary gland tumours {607}. These findings are identical to those in metastatic nasopharyngeal carcinoma {607}.

Diagnostic molecular pathology

EBV-encoded small RNA (EBER) may be helpful in establishing the presence of EBV infection.

Essential and desirable diagnostic criteria

Essential: pleomorphic epithelial cells with a heterogeneous background population of lymphocytes and plasma cells.
Desirable: EBV positivity.

Staging

While there is currently no separate TNM classification for carcinomas of the lacrimal drainage system, the eighth-edition Union for International Cancer Control (UICC) / American Joint Committee on Cancer (AJCC) TNM staging system for lacrimal gland tumours can be applied.

Prognosis and prediction

The reported disease-free survival is 15–33 months. Three patients developed locoregional relapses or metastases despite treatment. Lymphoepithelial carcinoma can be life-threatening if diagnosed late, with a mortality rate of about 50% {786}.

Mucoepidermoid carcinoma of the lacrimal drainage system

Roberts F
Alkatan H
Iacob CE

Definition
Mucoepidermoid carcinoma (MEC) of the lacrimal drainage system is a malignant glandular epithelial neoplasm characterized by squamous (epidermoid) cells, mucous cells, columnar cells, and intermediate cells.

ICD-O coding
8430/3 Mucoepidermoid carcinoma

ICD-11 coding
2D03.1 Mucoepidermoid carcinoma of lacrimal apparatus

Related terminology
Not recommended: mixed epidermoid and mucus-secreting carcinoma; mucoepidermoid tumour.

Subtype(s)
None

Localization
At this anatomical site, MEC arises in the lacrimal sac.

Clinical features
MEC presents with unilateral epiphora which can occasionally be sanguineous, usually followed by the development of a palpable mass in the medial canthal area {3121,1101,1495}. This mass is usually firm, solid, and non-inflamed. Other clinical features include eye pain and irritation, recurrent dacryocystitis, and nasal congestion {3121,1101,1495}. The average duration of symptoms is 18 months (range: 3–36 months) {3121,1101,1495}.

Epidemiology
MEC of the lacrimal sac occurs in adults with a median age of 50 years (range: 30–78 years) {3121}. There is a slight male predominance {3121,1495}.

Etiology
In the salivary gland, MEC is associated with radiation exposure {2753}. This has not been reported in the lacrimal sac.

Pathogenesis
Unlike in the analogous tumour at other body sites including salivary and lacrimal gland, a *CRTC1*::*MAML2* or *CRTC3*::*MAML2* fusion has not been identified {1101,1413}. Two cases have arisen in HPV-associated papillomas but HPV is not considered to be involved in malignant transformation {1413,1427}.

Macroscopic appearance
Lacrimal sac mass

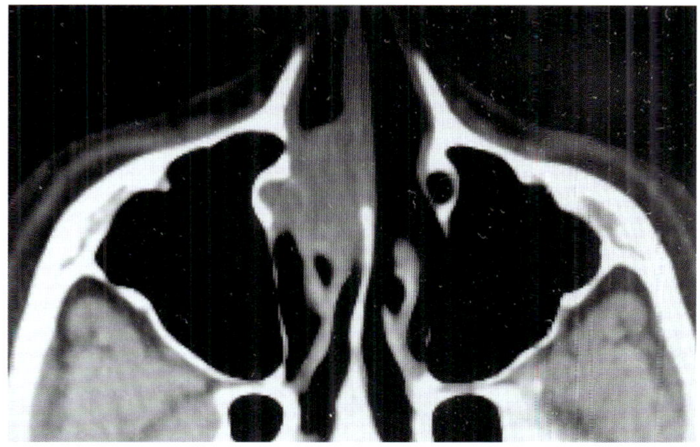

Fig. 8.11 Mucoepidermoid carcinoma. CT shows a tumour in the right lacrimal sac, as well as signs of bone invasion.

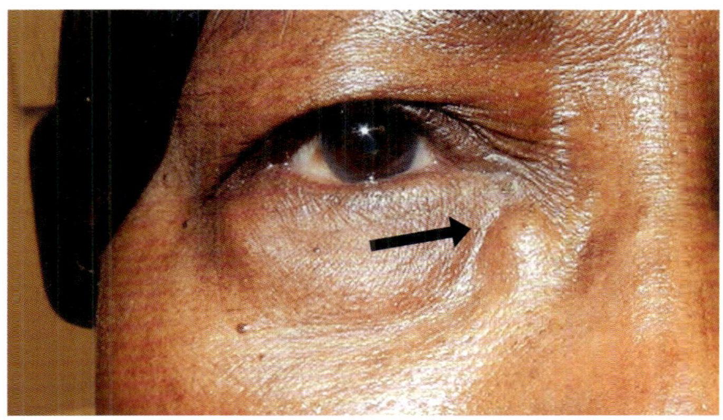

Fig. 8.12 Mucoepidermoid carcinoma. An example presenting as a mass in the medial canthal area; the tumour (arrow) is firm, solid, non-inflamed, and painless.

Histopathology
MEC of the lacrimal sac is composed of variable proportions of three cells types: squamous, mucous secreting, and intermediate. The squamous cells have medium to large nuclei with eosinophilic cytoplasm and intercellular bridges between cells, but keratinization is usually absent. Mucous cells form small glands, tubules, and cysts; the cysts contain inspissated mucin (which may calcify) and are lined by mucous cells, looking deceptively bland. The intermediate (or transitional) cells are oval, with a round nucleus and faintly eosinophilic cytoplasm. In addition, columnar, clear, and oncocytic cells may be admixed. PAS or Alcian blue staining may be required to visualize mucin. The stroma may be hyalinized with calcification and ossification. A granulomatous reaction to extravasated mucus may be seen.

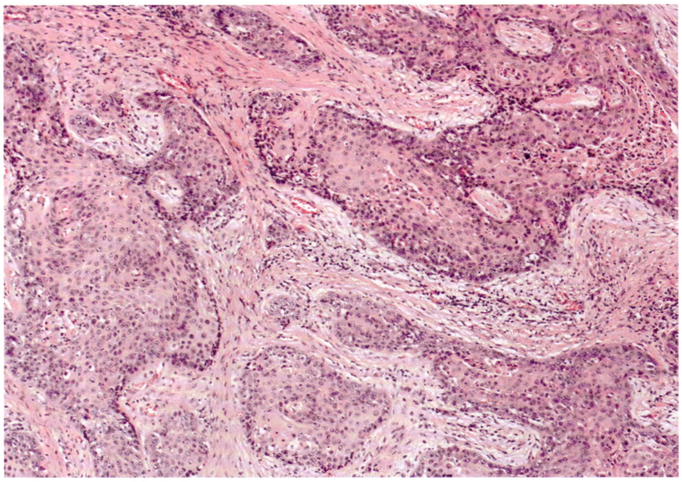

Fig. 8.13 Mucoepidermoid carcinoma. A high-grade example composed of a mixture of intermediate cells, with scant cytoplasm and large polygonal hyperchromatic pleomorphic nuclei, and squamous (epidermoid) cells, with abundant eosinophilic cytoplasm; very few mucous cells are seen.

There are several systems for grading salivary gland MEC {2613,623,944}. Most divide tumours into three levels (low-grade, intermediate-grade, and high-grade). The systems are based on the proportions of cystic areas, proportion of necrosis, perineural invasion, mitoses, nuclear pleomorphism, invasion front, and lymphovascular invasion. More recently a binary grading system separating low- and intermediate-grade tumours from high-grade tumours using the Brandwein system has been shown to best stratify patients into groups based on risk of recurrence {623}.

Immunohistochemistry

Lesions are positive for EMA (common in high-grade tumours), MUC2, MUC4 (common in low-grade tumours), MUC5AC, and MUC5B. MECs are usually positive for CK5/6, CK7, and CK14, and with BerEP4, and negative for CK20. The tumour cells can be focally positive for vimentin, CEA, and p63 {1427}. Myoepithelial markers are negative.

Differential diagnosis

Exclusion of squamous cell carcinoma, sebaceous carcinoma, adenosquamous carcinoma, and metastatic carcinomas is important. There should be no in situ component.

Cytology

Not relevant

Diagnostic molecular pathology

Unlike in MEC at other body sites, a *CRTC1::MAML2* or *CRTC3::MAML2* fusion has not been identified in lacrimal sac tumours {1101}.

Essential and desirable diagnostic criteria

Essential: squamous cells, intermediate cells, and mucous cells in varying proportions; for lower-grade tumours: cystic, mucous-cell rich, and well circumscribed; for higher-grade tumours: solid with a higher proportion of squamous and intermediate cells.

Staging

While there is currently no separate TNM classification for carcinomas of the lacrimal drainage system, the eighth-edition Union for International Cancer Control (UICC) TNM staging system for lacrimal gland tumours can be applied.

Prognosis and prediction

These tumours are locally aggressive but rarely metastasize. Of the 26 cases in the literature the majority were treated successfully with combined surgery and radiotherapy with a few patients requiring more extensive surgery. Local recurrence has been reported in 4 patients but there have been no tumour-related deaths (mean follow-up: 39 months, range: 6–98 months) {3121}.

Other salivary gland–type carcinomas of the lacrimal drainage system

Farmer J
Irion LCD

Definition

Salivary gland–type carcinomas of the lacrimal drainage system are a family of primary epithelial adenocarcinomas that morphologically resemble their salivary gland counterparts. They include adenoid cystic carcinoma (AdCC), duct adenocarcinoma (DA), oncocytic carcinoma, epithelial-myoepithelial carcinoma (EMC), carcinoma ex pleomorphic adenoma (CEPA), and sebaceous carcinoma.

ICD-O coding

8290/3 Oncocytic carcinoma
8200/3 Adenoid cystic carcinoma
8562/3 Epithelial-myoepithelial carcinoma
8941/3 Carcinoma ex pleomorphic adenoma
8410/3 Sebaceous carcinoma

ICD-11 coding

2D03.0 Adenocarcinoma of the lacrimal apparatus
2D03.Y & XH09D6 Other specified malignant neoplasm of lacrimal apparatus & Oxyphilic adenocarcinoma
2D03.Y & XH4302 Other specified malignant neoplasm of lacrimal apparatus & Adenoid cystic carcinoma
2D03.Y & XH9JP2 Other specified malignant neoplasm of lacrimal apparatus & Epithelial-myoepithelial carcinoma
2D03.Y & XH42V2 Other specified malignant neoplasm of lacrimal apparatus & Carcinoma ex pleomorphic adenoma
2D03.Y & XH4VR2 Other specified malignant neoplasm of lacrimal apparatus & Sebaceous carcinoma

Related terminology

Not recommended: for ductal adenocarcinoma: salivary duct carcinoma; for epithelial-myoepithelial carcinoma: adenomyoepithelioma.

Subtype(s)

None

Localization

These tumours arise from stromal seromucinous glands predominantly in the lacrimal sac {1433}.

Clinical features

Most tumours present with unilateral tearing (74–100%) and a mass in the lacrimal fossa or swelling in the medial canthus {2652,3121,1790}.

Features of concern for malignancy are a palpable, firm, non-compressible, immobile mass above the medial canthal tendon chronic dacryocystitis which irrigates or partially irrigates and sanguineous reflux on irrigation {1790}.

Imaging modalities of the orbit and paranasal sinuses include contrast-enhanced thin-sectioned CT for tumour extent, MRI with contrast to differentiate between a solid mass and cystic o

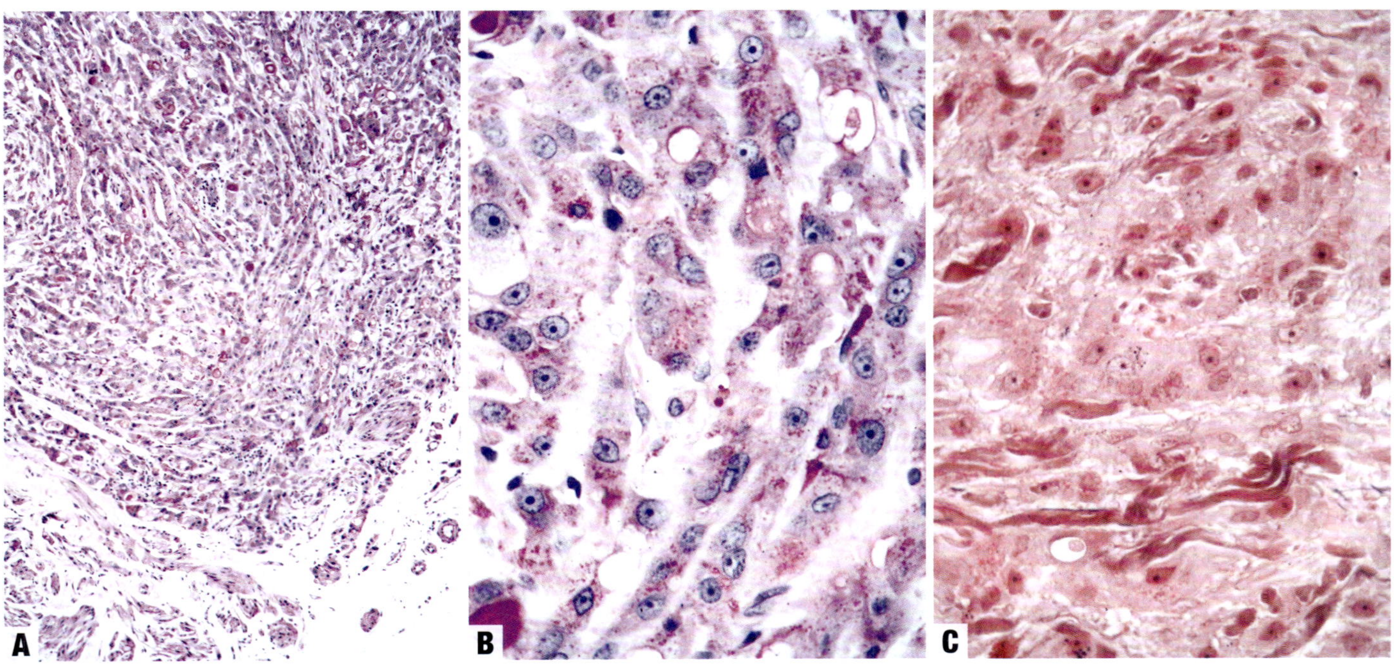

Fig. 8.14 Oncocytic adenocarcinoma. **A** The tumour has an infiltrative pseudoglandular pattern. **B** Large polyhedral cells with granular cytoplasm (PAS staining). **C** Phosphotungstic acid–haematoxylin demonstrates positive staining for mitochondria (purple point staining).

inflammatory disease, and dacryocystography to demonstrate a filling defect and delayed draining of contrast medium {2652}.

Epidemiology
Salivary gland–type carcinomas affect middle-aged and elderly individuals, with a median age at diagnosis of 57.5 years {2652}. There is a slight male predominance in all tumour types except for AdCC which is largely (80%) seen in women {2652}.

Etiology
Chronic inflammation (as many patients present with or have been treated for presumed dacryocystitis) and previous probing or surgery of the lacrimal drainage system are thought to be risk factors for tumour development {2652}. The occurrence of sebaceous carcinoma in the lacrimal sac is thought to arise from ectopic sebaceous glands within the stroma or sebaceous gland metaplasia of the lacrimal sac epithelium {3425}.

Pathogenesis
Adenocarcinoma may arise from a pleomorphic adenoma and recurrent oncocytoma may undergo malignant transformation {2652}. Activation of mTOR pathway proteins has been reported in DA {2490,3424}.

Macroscopic appearance
DA has been described as a polypoidal mass {250}, AdCC as a gelatinous mass {2657}, and EMC as a grey-tan homogeneous mass {2952}.

Histopathology
DA consists of polygonal tumour cells with granular eosinophilic cytoplasm, pleomorphic and vesicular nuclei arranged in ductular structures of varying patterns (glandular, cribriform, and solid), and frequent central comedonecrosis. Extracellular mucin may be present {2902}. Tumour cells express cytokeratins, AR, GCDFP, and ERBB2 {2902}.

AdCC, EMC, CEPA, and sebaceous carcinoma show the same morphological features as their salivary gland counterparts, which have been detailed elsewhere (see Chapter 7: *Tumours of the lacrimal gland*).

Oncocytic carcinoma displays large polyhedral cells with nuclear atypia and granular eosinophilic cytoplasm arranged in an infiltrative pseudoglandular pattern. Evidence of the increased mitochondrial content of the tumour cells is achieved with positive phosphotungstic acid–haematoxylin cytoplasmic staining and/or immunohistochemical expression of antimitochondrial antibodies {2652,1553,3723}.

Differential diagnosis
The differential diagnosis of AdCC, EMC, CEPA, and sebaceous carcinoma is the same as for their salivary gland counterparts (see Chapter 7: *Tumours of the lacrimal gland*).

DA is distinguished from oncocytic carcinoma by the absence of excessive and abnormal mitochondria in the cytoplasm of the tumour cells, demonstrated by immunohistochemistry or electron microscopy.

Sebaceous carcinoma must be distinguished from direct extension from the conjunctiva or caruncle.

Cytology
Not reported

Diagnostic molecular pathology
Demonstration of *MYB* or *MYBL1* rearrangements or gene fusions may be helpful for the diagnosis of AdCC.

Essential and desirable diagnostic criteria
See individual tumour types in Chapter 7: *Tumours of the lacrimal gland*.

Staging
While there is currently no separate TNM classification for carcinomas of the lacrimal drainage system, the eighth-edition Union for International Cancer Control (UICC) TNM staging system for lacrimal gland tumours can be applied.

Prognosis and prediction
Wide surgical excision (including exenteration) and/or radiotherapy are the preferred courses of management for these carcinomas {2652,3121}. AR and ERBB2 are potential therapeutic targets for salivary-type ductal adenocarcinomas {2652,2490}. Large tumour size and positive lymph node status correlate with a decreased overall and disease-free survival {2652}. The 5-year overall survival is reported to range from 61% to 88% {2652}.

Adenocarcinoma NOS of the lacrimal drainage system

Stagner AM
Irion LCD

Definition

Adenocarcinoma NOS of the lacrimal sac/duct is a rare primary malignant epithelial tumour with glandular differentiation, not otherwise classifiable.

ICD-O coding

8140/3 Adenocarcinoma, NOS, of the lacrimal drainage system
8147/3 Basaloid / basal cell adenocarcinoma

ICD-11 coding

2D03.0 Adenocarcinoma of the lacrimal apparatus

Related terminology

None

Subtype(s)

Basaloid/basal cell adenocarcinoma

Note: Oncocytic and ductal adenocarcinomas are covered in *Other salivary gland–type carcinomas of the lacrimal drainage system* (p. 285).

Localization

Adenocarcinoma of the lacrimal drainage system usually originates in the lacrimal sac and/or nasolacrimal duct, but it can extend into the canaliculi {255,1306,1790}. Involvement of the adjacent sinonasal cavities or orbit, particularly if poorly differentiated {2269}, is relatively common {3121}.

Clinical features

Nearly all patients with adenocarcinoma present with epiphora and/or a firm, slow-growing, immobile lacrimal fossa mass lesion in the region of the medial canthus. Pain and bloodstained epiphora are uncommonly noticed but are concerning features for malignancy {3121,1433,2256,3424,3744}. Some tumours are incidentally found at dacryocystorhinostomy or present as recurrent dacryocystitis {250,402 1306,1790}. Non-axial proptosis, blepharoptosis, periorbital oedema, and regional lymphadenopathy may be found in more-advanced cases {255,402,1306,3506}.

Epidemiology

Adenocarcinoma is rare (< 30 reported cases), accounts for < 5% of cases of malignant epithelial tumours, and is a tumour of middle-aged and older patients {332,402,1790,3506}. It is typically diagnosed in the sixth to seventh decades of life (mean age: 67 years) and shows a slight male predilection {1790,2521,3121}.

Etiology

Although HPV infection is increasingly reported as an etiological agent in the development of nasolacrimal drainage carcinomas

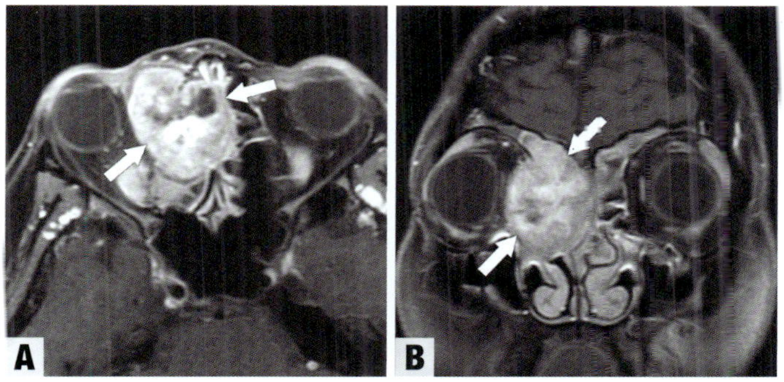

Fig. 8.15 Nasolacrimal duct carcinoma. **A,B** Axial and coronal T1-weighted post-contrast MRI shows a large, heterogeneously enhancing mass in the region of the right lacrimal sac with involvement of the medial right orbit and the sinonasal cavity (arrows).

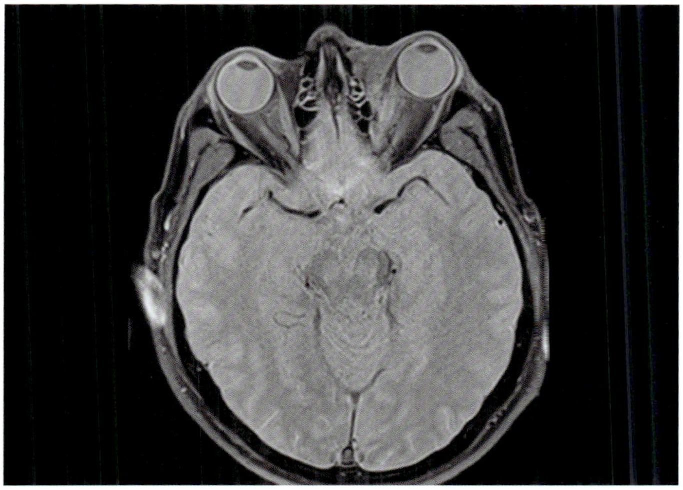

Fig. 8.16 Adenocarcinoma NOS of the lacrimal drainage system. T2-weighted fat-suppressed axial MRI shows a tumour in the left lacrimal sac area, with medial rectus muscle invasion.

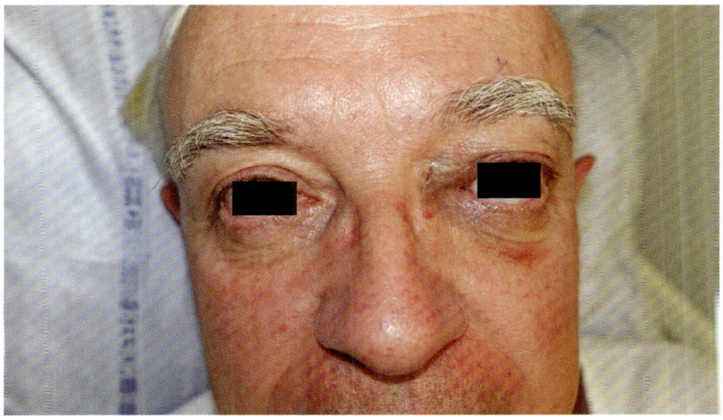

Fig. 8.17 Adenocarcinoma NOS of the lacrimal drainage system. A tumour mass over the left medial canthus area, with overlying skin ulceration and telangiectasia

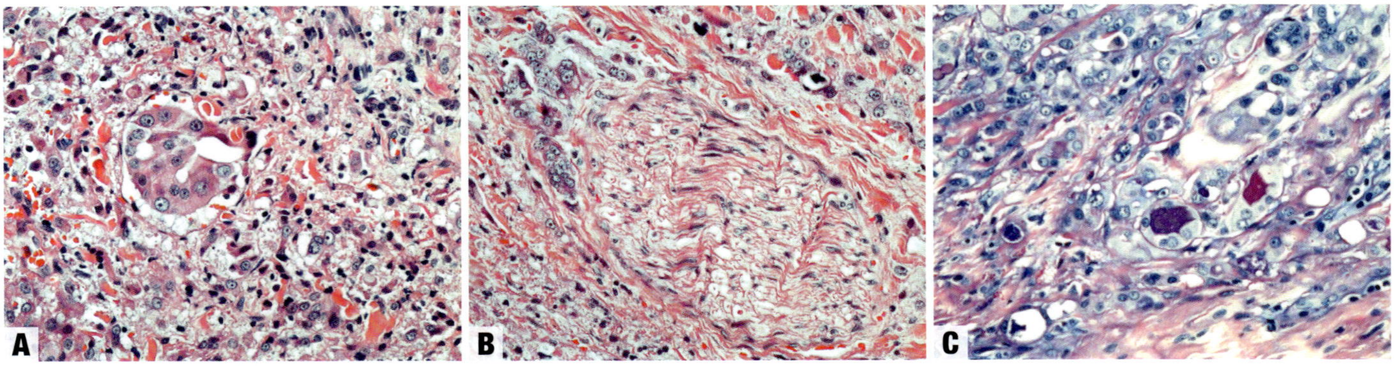

Fig. 8.18 Adenocarcinoma NOS of the lacrimal drainage system. **A** Cuboidal epithelial cells with eosinophilic granular cytoplasm and uniform nuclei. **B** Perineural invasion of adenocarcinoma cells. **C** Malignant cells with marked nuclear pleomorphism, a single central prominent nucleolus, mitotic figures, and mucin production, highlighted by PAS staining.

{3135}, HPV infection has not been specifically demonstrated in adenocarcinoma.

Pathogenesis

Adenocarcinoma is believed to arise from the seromucinous accessory salivary-type glands within the lacrimal sac and/or nasolacrimal duct {323,2521}.

Macroscopic appearance

These are lacrimal fossa mass lesions, often with invasion of surrounding tissue.

Histopathology

Adenocarcinoma of the lacrimal drainage system may show sheets, cords, nests, or single cell infiltration of pleomorphic cells forming lumina (glandular differentiation) with variable mucin production {402,1433,2521,3198}. Cribriform and tubular structures may be seen. Cytomorphologically, cells are often cuboidal with eosinophilic granular cytoplasm and prominent nucleoli; nuclei may be highly pleomorphic to more uniform {1433,1790,67}. Mitotic figures, an inflammatory cell infiltrate, invasion into the fibrous lacrimal sac wall, and lymphovascular and perineural invasion are often present {402,1433,2521,2794}.

Immunohistochemistry

Tumours are typically immunoreactive for pancytokeratin (AE1/AE3), CK7, AR, EMA, and GCDFP-15. CK20, ER, PR, chromogranin A, and synaptophysin do not often stain in these tumours, while ERBB2 expression is variable {250,1433,3424,2490,22}.

Differential diagnosis

Nasolacrimal adenocarcinoma may be encountered as part of a biphasic tumour {2393} or occur in the setting of malignant transformation of a benign precursor tumour (carcinoma ex pleomorphic adenoma or oncocytoma) {255}. Adenocarcinomas in the NOS category may be low-grade or high-grade, well differentiated or poorly differentiated, and show variable oncocytic/apocrine {67} and mucinous features. Ductal adenocarcinoma resembles salivary duct carcinoma {1433,2490}. Metastases should also be excluded.

Cytology

Not reported

Diagnostic molecular pathology

Fusion assays based on next-generation sequencing or FISH may be useful to exclude other diagnoses defined by specific translocations (e.g. mucoepidermoid or adenoid cystic carcinoma).

Essential and desirable diagnostic criteria

Essential: pleomorphic, gland-forming neoplasm, often with abundant eosinophilic cytoplasm, and not categorized as another specific salivary-type adenocarcinoma.

Desirable: AR immunoreactivity; proof of absence of other translocation-defined salivary-type neoplasia.

Staging

While there is currently no separate TNM classification for carcinomas of the lacrimal drainage system, the eighth-edition Union for International Cancer Control (UICC) TNM staging system for lacrimal gland tumours can be applied.

Prognosis and prediction

Given the paucity and heterogenicity of cases, significant prognostic data is not available {1306,1790,2256,3506}. Current practices are based on information from a few case series {2379,2794,3198} and individual case reports. However, recurrence with local destruction seems to be relatively common {1306,1790,2256,2498,2393,402}, and metastases can occur, usually to lung or bone {3121}. Certain low-grade subtypes such as basaloid adenocarcinoma may fare better {1399}. AR-expressing tumours have been treated with androgen deprivation {22,3424}.

Melanoma involving the lacrimal drainage system

Vemuganti GK
Eberhart CG

Definition
Melanoma of the lacrimal drainage system is a rare invasive melanocytic neoplasm.

ICD-O coding
8720/3 Melanoma involving the lacrimal drainage system

ICD-11 coding
2D03.Y & XH4846 Other specified malignant neoplasm of lacrimal apparatus & Malignant melanoma, NOS

Related terminology
Acceptable: lacrimal drainage system melanoma.

Subtype(s)
None

Localization
The lacrimal sac is the most common location, but tumours can invade other parts of the lacrimal drainage system or adjacent soft tissue and bone (e.g. the lacrimal crest) {2599}. Rare cases arising in the nasolacrimal duct have also been reported {916}.

Clinical features
The most common presentations include unilateral epiphora, mass lesions in the medial canthal area, bloody discharge, epistaxis, and (rarely) pain {3496}. Lesions are often misdiagnosed as dacryocystitis and repeated biopsies are sometimes necessary {2026,2697}. CT and MRI generally show a partially defined soft tissue mass in the lacrimal sac fossa, with possible extension into the nasolacrimal duct or anterior ethmoid sinus {2947}.

Epidemiology
Melanomas of the lacrimal drainage system are extremely rare, accounting for 1–4% of tumours at this site {2947,1306,3198}. The mean age of patients is 59 years.

Etiology
The etiology is unknown, but it is probably similar to that of melanomas occurring at other mucosal sites not exposed to the sun.

Pathogenesis
These melanomas probably originate from melanocytes associated with the epithelial mucosa lining the lacrimal drainage apparatus.

Macroscopic appearance
The tumour may be seen as an irregular dark-brown mass adherent to the lacrimal sac wall {2697}.

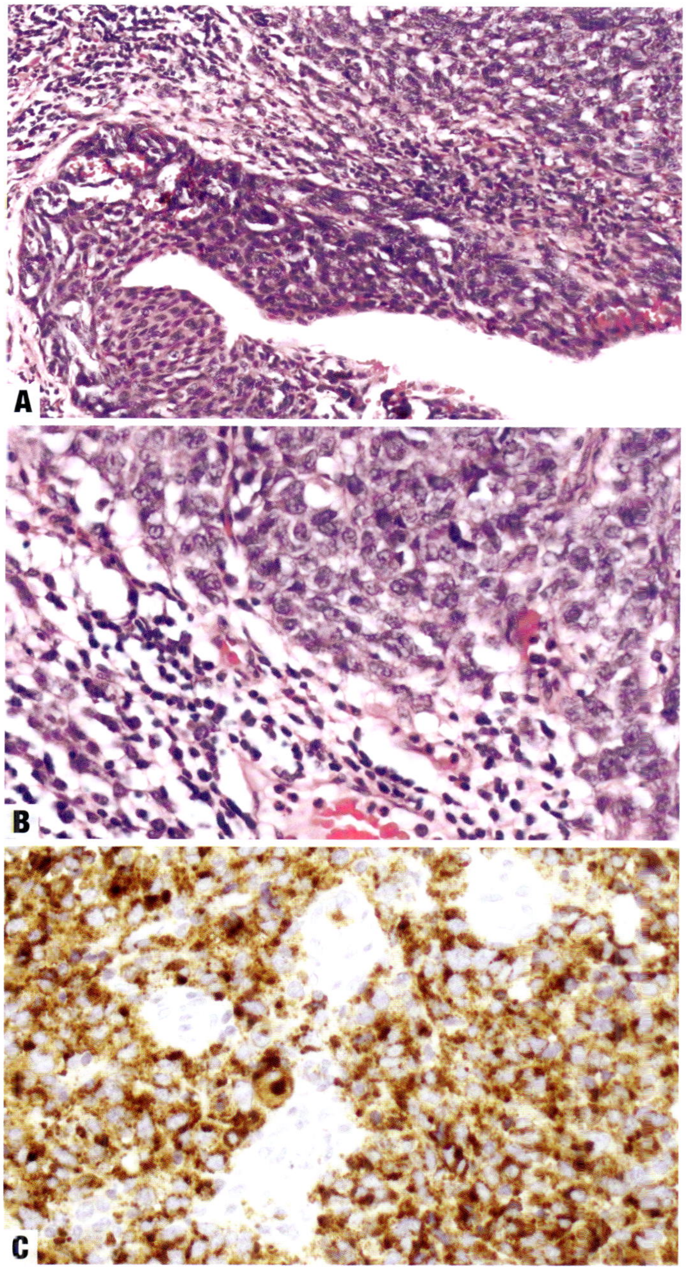

Fig. 8.19 Melanoma of the lacrimal sac. **A,B** The image shows an invasive melanoma arising in the lacrimal sac of a 52-year-old White man who presented with increased tearing but no pain or bleeding. **C** The melanoma was centred in the lacrimal sac but diffusely invaded the orbit and the extraocular muscles (HMB45 expression).

Histopathology
The mucosal lining of the lacrimal sac and surrounding soft tissues is infiltrated by variably pigmented spindled or epithelioid

melanocytes with moderate to abundant pigmented granular cytoplasm, often showing large vesicular nuclei with prominent nucleoli. Nuclear pleomorphism and variable numbers of mitotic figures are present. Tumour cells are immunoreactive for HMB45, melan-A, and S100 {1760}.

Cytology

Not reported

Diagnostic molecular pathology

One lacrimal sac melanoma has been reported to have *BRAF* p.V600E mutations {2116}.

Essential and desirable diagnostic criteria

Essential: demonstrated malignancy with melanocytic differentiation; relation to the mucosa of the lacrimal tract; no evidence of previous or synchronous melanoma outside the lacrimal tract.

Staging

Stage according to the eighth-edition Union for International Cancer Control (UICC) / American Joint Committee on Cancer (AJCC) TNM staging system for sinonasal tumours.

Prognosis and prediction

The primary treatment modality is surgery (i.e. dacryocystectomy). Poor prognostic factors include positive surgical margins, large tumour size, and dissemination of the tumour {3224}. Local recurrence is common. For advanced cases, treatment may range from wide en bloc resection to radiotherapy, chemotherapy, and immunotherapy in a variety of combinations {2839, 573}.

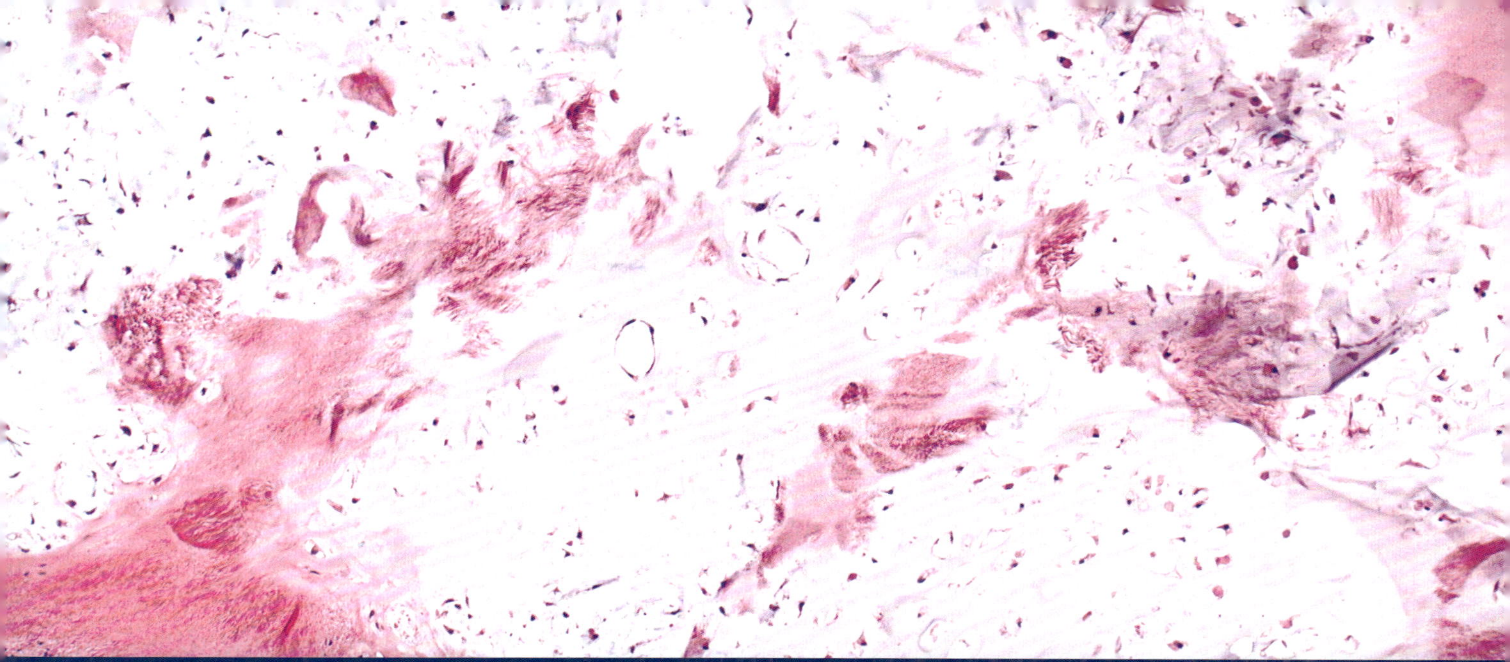

9

Tumours of the orbit

Edited by: Esmaeli B, Kivelä T, Milman T, White VA

Tumours of the orbit: Introduction

White VA
Alkatan H
Kivelä T
Mudhar HS

The orbit is the space behind and around the eye that nestles the latter within the bony orbital cavity of the skull and allows for its movement. The volume of the adult orbit is approximately 30 cm^3 and its shape is a square-based pyramid with four bony walls and the apex pointing posteriorly {3293}. It contains the main lacrimal gland, the optic nerve, and the extraocular muscles, with the remainder of the space occupied by adipose tissue, fascia, blood vessels, and peripheral nerves. The space inside the cone formed by the extraocular muscles is designated the intraconal space, while that outside the muscles is extraconal.

The orbit can be the location for a diverse array of tumours, similar to those in many other parts of the body (see Table 9.01). Thus, the possibility of a primary tumour, metastatic tumour, or direct extension from adjacent structures must be considered. The latter includes tumours of the eye, eyelids, conjunctiva, nasolacrimal drainage system, brain, and paranasal sinuses.

As the orbit is a confined space, larger tumours produce effects on the eye, such as proptosis, displacement, and compression, as well as restriction of extraocular motility. Rapid

Table 9.01 Types and frequency of orbital tumours, with an emphasis on soft tissue tumours (continued on next page)

	All ages combined				Adults				Children					
Author	Shields {3069}		Ohtsuka {2418}		Demirci {773}		Alsamalah {120}		Shields {3026}		Alkatan {99}		Bajaj {233}	
Data collection time frame	1971–2002		1981–2002		1974–2000		2000–2017		1962–1983		2000–2013		1991–2000	
Lesion category[a]	***N***	**%[b]**	***N***	**%**	***N***	**%**	***N***	**%**	***N***	**%**	***N***	**%**	***N***	**%**
Soft tissue tumours total	**243**	**30%**	**40**	**19%**	**23**	**14%**	**45**	**43%**	**30**	**15%**	**44**	**42%**	**54**	**51%**
Fibrous, fibroblastic total	15	2%	5	2%	3	2%	4	4%	0	0%	4	4%	1	1%
Solitary fibrous tumour	2	< 1%	2	1%	3	2%	4	4%	0	0%	1	1%	0	0%
Fibrous histiocytoma	6	1%	0	0%	0	0%	0	0%	0	0%	0	0%	1	1%
Myofibroma	2	< 1%	0	0%	0	0%	0	0%	0	0%	0	0%	0	0%
Angiofibroma	2	< 1%	0	0%	0	0%	0	0%	0	0%	0	0%	0	0%
Nodular fasciitis	2	< 1%	0	0%	0	0%	0	0%	0	0%	0	0%	0	0%
Juvenile fibromatosis	0	0%	0	0%	0	0%	0	0%	0	0%	3	3%	0	0%
Fibrosarcoma	1	< 1%	1	< 1%	0	0%	0	0%	0	0%	0	0%	0	0%
Adipocytic total	3	0%	0	0%	0	0%	2	2%	0	0%	0	0%	0	0%
Lipoma	2	< 1%	0	0%	0	0%	0	0%	0	0%	0	0%	0	0%
Liposarcoma	1	< 1%	0	0%	0	0%	2	2%	0	0%	0	0%	0	0%
Skeletal muscle	35	4%	2	1%	0	0%	0	0%	10	5%	11	11%	29	28%
Rhabdomyosarcoma family	35	4%	2	1%	N/A	N/A	N/A	N/A	10	5%	11	11%	29	28%
Smooth muscle	0	0%	0	0%	0	0%	2	2%	0	0%	0	0%	0	0%
Leiomyosarcoma	0	0%	0	0%	0	0%	2	2%	0	0%	0	0%	0	0%
Peripheral nerve sheath total	21	3%	11	5%	0	0%	13	12%	3	1%	7	7%	4	4%
Schwannoma	14	2%	7	3%	0	0%	9	9%	1	< 1%	N/A	N/A	2	2%
Neurofibroma	6	1%	2	1%	0	0%	4	4%	2	1%	N/A	N/A	2	2%
MPNST	1	< 1%	0	0%	0	0%	0	0%	0	0%	N/A	N/A	0	0%
Granular cell tumour	0	0%	2	1%	0	0%	0	0%	0	0%	N/A	N/A	0	0%

AVM, arteriovenous malformation; MPNST, malignant peripheral nerve sheath tumour; N/A, not available.
[a]Excluded for consistency: histiocytic-dendritic neoplasms, inflammatory, infectious, traumatic (haematoma), structural (varix, fistula, deformity, high myopia, herniated fat), lacrimal gland, amyloid deposits. [b]All per cent values are rounded to the nearest whole number. [c]Both malformations and neoplastic lesions are included because of the inconsistent use of terminology before the 2018 International Society for the Study of Vascular Anomalies (ISSVA) classification {3557}.

enlargement of a tumour within the orbit, such as owing to haemorrhage into a lymphangioma, may produce a visual emergency, similar to those in the intracranial cavity, because of lack of space for expansion. Malignant orbital tumours may invade the surrounding bony walls of the orbit or extend through the cavernous sinus into the brain.

Table 9.01 Types and frequency of orbital tumours, with an emphasis on soft tissue tumours (continued)

	All ages combined				Adults				Children					
Author	Shields {3069}		Ohtsuka {2418}		Demirci {773}		Alsamalah {120}		Shields {3026}		Alkatan {99}		Raja {233}	
Data collection time frame	1971–2002		1981–2002		1974–2000		2000–2017		1962–1983		2000–2013		1991–2000	
Lesion category[a]	*N*	%[b]	*N*	%	*N*	%	*N*	%	*N*	%	*N*	%	*N*	%
Vascular total[c]	168	21%	24	12%	20	12%	23	22%	16	8%	17	16%	18	17%
Cavernous haemangioma / cavernous venous malformation	77	9%	18	9%	15	9%	20	19%	2	1%	N/A	N/A	5	5%
Haemangioma NOS	0	0%	0	0%	0	0%	0	0%	0	0%	N/A	N/A	0	0%
Lymphangioma / lymphatic-venous malformation	54	7%	3	1%	4	2%	1	1%	4	2%	N/A	N/A	7	7%
Capillary haemangioma / infantile haemangioma	36	4%	3	1%	0	0%	0	0%	10	5%	N/A	N/A	1	1%
Masson tumour	1	< 1%	0	0%	1	1%	0	0%	0	0%	N/A	N/A	0	0%
Vascular malformation / AVM	0	0%	0	0%	0	0%	2	2%	0	0%	N/A	N/A	5	5%
Tumours of uncertain derivation	1	< 1%	0	0%	0	0%	1	1%	1	< 1%	1	1%	2	2%
Epithelioid sarcoma	0	0%	0	0%	0	0%	0	0%	0	0%	1	1%	0	0%
Alveolar soft part sarcoma	1	< 1%	0	0%	0	0%	0	0%	1	< 1%	0	0%	2	2%
Undifferentiated/unclassified sarcoma	0	0%	0	0%	0	0%	1	1%	0	0%	0	0%	0	0%
Tumours of orbital bone total	**22**	**3%**	**6**	**3%**	**0**	**0%**	**1**	**1%**	**3**	**1%**	**3**	**3%**	**4**	**4%**
Osteogenic total	9	1%	2	1%	0	0%	0	0%	0	0%	0	0%	0	0%
Osteosarcoma	5	1%	0	0%	0	0%	0	0%	0	0%	0	0%	0	0%
Osteoma	4	0%	2	1%	0	0%	0	0%	0	0%	0	0%	0	0%
Chondrogenic	0	0%	0	0%	0	0%	0	0%	1	< 1%	2	2%	0	0%
Fibrous, fibroblastic total	10	1%	2	1%	0	0%	0	0%	2	1%	1	1%	0	0%
Fibrous dysplasia	7	1%	2	1%	0	0%	0	0%	0	0%	N/A	N/A	0	0%
Ossifying fibroma	3	< 1%	0	0%	0	0%	0	0%	2	1%	N/A	N/A	0	0%
Vascular tumours of bone	0	0%	0	< 1%	0	0%	1	1%	0	0%	0	0%	0	0%
Osteoclast-rich giant cell tumours	1	< 1%	1	< 1%	0	0%	0	0%	0	0%	0	0%	0	0%
Ewing sarcoma family	2	< 1%	1	< 1%	< 1%	0%	0	0%	0	0%	0	0%	4	4%
Other lesions total	**549**	**67%**	**161**	**78%**	**140**	**86%**	**59**	**56%**	**168**	**84%**	**57**	**55%**	**47**	**45%**
Haematolymphoid	132	16%	104	50%	56	34%	29	28%	6	3%	5	5%	4	4%
Cysts	70	9%	16	8%	3	4%	6	6%	130	65%	47	45%	12	11%
Optic nerve sheath / meningeal	101	12%	10	5%	10	6%	2	2%	6	3%	1	1%	9	9%
Melanocytic	11	1%	0	0%	0	0%	0	0%	0	0%	0	0%	0	0%
Miscellaneous	3	< 1%	0	0%	0	0%	3	3%	17	8%	2	2%	0	0%
Secondary	141	17%	23	11%	48	29%	16	15%	9	4%	0	0%	21	20%
Metastatic	91	11%	8	4%	20	12%	3	3%	0	0%	2	2%	1	1%
Total orbital tumours	**814**	**100%**	**207**	**100%**	**163**	**100%**	**105**	**100%**	**201**	**100%**	**104**	**100%**	**105**	**100%**

AVM, arteriovenous malformation; MPNST, malignant peripheral nerve sheath tumour; N/A, not available.
[a]Excluded for consistency: histiocytic-dendritic neoplasms, inflammatory, infectious, traumatic (haematoma), structural (varix, fistula, deformity, high myopia, herniated fat), lacrimal gland, amyloid deposits. [b]All per cent values are rounded to the nearest whole number. [c]Both malformations and neoplastic lesions are included because of the inconsistent use of terminology before the 2018 International Society for the Study of Vascular Anomalies (ISSVA) classification {3557}.

After clinical examination, patients presenting with a presumed orbital tumour are usually assessed by CT, MRI, or both. Most patients will require a core needle or open biopsy for definitive diagnosis before a decision on treatment, which may be complex and multidisciplinary. As the orbit is also host to a variety of inflammatory processes that can masquerade as neoplasms, it may be difficult to distinguish between these without an adequate tissue sample. The orbit is accessible for cytological examination which may be particularly helpful in assessing recurrent or metastatic tumours {2252,104}.

This chapter, new in the fifth edition, covers tumours not seen elsewhere in the ophthalmic structures. Tumours of the optic nerve, lacrimal gland, and lacrimal drainage system are discussed separately in Chapter 6: *Tumours of the optic disc and optic nerve*, Chapter 7: *Tumours of the lacrimal gland*, and Chapter 8: *Tumours of the lacrimal drainage system*, respectively. Haematolymphoid and soft tissue and bone tumours of all of the ocular structures, including the orbit, are discussed in Chapter 10: *Haematolymphoid tumours* and Chapter 11: *Soft tissue and bone tumours*.

In this volume, vascular anomalies are divided into malformations and tumours, according to the recommendation of the International Society for the Study of Vascular Anomalies (ISSVA) {1436,2801,2254,1809}, though this may not apply well to some orbital tumours. Vascular malformations are covered in Chapter 9: *Tumours of the orbit* and vascular tumours in Chapter 11: *Soft tissue and bone tumours*.

Finally, there are many tumours which have been described in the orbit in only a few instances and did not warrant a full section. These are briefly described in Table 11.02 (p. 383) in Chapter 11: *Soft tissue and bone tumours*.

Orbital dermoid cyst and other orbital cysts

Alkatan H

Definition

Dermoid cyst is a developmental lesion that is considered a choristoma with ectodermal and mesodermal components that are not normally present at the involved site but are histopathologically normal.

ICD-O coding

None

ICD-11 coding

9A23.0 Congenital orbital cyst
9A23.1 Acquired orbital cyst
9A23.Z Orbital cyst, unspecified

Related terminology

None

Subtype(s)

See Table 9.02.

Localization

The incidence of periocular dermoid cysts is approximately 1 in 650 live births {234}. About one third of the epidermoid and dermoid cysts in the head and neck region occur in the orbit {2606}. Orbital dermoid cysts have been classified as superficial (simple) or deep (complicated) based on their location with respect to the orbital septum {1187}. Deep cysts can be medial,

Table 9.02 Cysts in the differential diagnosis of orbital dermoid cysts

Cyst type	Lining	Other characteristics
Conjunctival cyst {1461,3586,2879}	Non-keratinizing stratified squamous epithelium and goblet cells but without appendages	Tumour tends to present later in life, is usually soft, results in minor symptoms (eyelid fullness with no proptosis), and is mostly anterior and superomedial in location without bony defect
Conjunctival dermoid cyst {1461}	Non-keratinizing stratified squamous epithelium with goblet cells and adnexal structures in the wall	Symptoms usually develop over years; usually involves the superomedial quadrant of the orbit, lacks osseous defect, and may cause proptosis {655}
Epidermoid cyst {53}	Keratinizing stratified squamous epithelium with absent adnexal structures	Can be either primary (congenital) or secondary (implantation);[a] the primary cysts are usually slowly growing and deep in the orbit, and present at a relatively older age
Respiratory epithelial choristomatous cyst[a] {2372,2279,1645,3565}	Pseudostratified ciliated columnar epithelium with goblet cells, filled with mucoid material; believed to arise from sequestered respiratory epithelium from paranasal sinuses during development	Located in orbital sites that are atypical for dermoids but may be associated with bony defect {2154}; has been reported also in the eyelid {3692}; usually follow a benign course but may result in strabismus and amblyopia in young children {1645}; can be intraconal in location causing difficulty in the management {3565}
Choristomatous lacrimal gland cyst {3586,2789}	Thin ductal epithelial lining with or without fibrous capsule and adjacent nest of ectopic lacrimal gland tissue	Develops in relation to ectopic lacrimal gland tissue with ductal-like cyst formation
Ossifying cystic odontogenic and Schneiderian choristoma {2299}	Lined by Schneiderian cystic epithelium with adjacent mucinous oral glands, tooth, and lamellar bone	A single reported case of a 12-year-old girl with infraorbital-located recurrent mass {2299}
Phakomatous choristoma {2923,2630}	Islands of lenticular-like material surrounded by thick basement membrane	Rare, benign congenital tumour of lenticular anlage that can be partially cystic; almost always located in the medial lower eyelid and anterior orbit
Others		
Cystic teratoma {3673}	Teratomatous cyst showing tissue from two to three germ cell layers	Teratomas can be either mature or immature and their clinical diagnosis might be challenging {107,101}
Congenital cystic eye {1212,3673}	A thin-walled cyst with no identifiable ocular structures	Rare; diagnosed at birth; may attain large size and be associated with facial dermal appendages
Microphthalmos with cyst {106}	Cystic portion lined by retinal and neuroglial tissue	Cyst is found in relation to microphthalmic globes with coloboma
Haematic cyst {93}	Cyst with reactive fibrosis and pseudocapsule formation but no epithelial lining; haemorrhage and haemosiderin deposits are common with possible formation of cholesterol granuloma	Etiology is unclear but might be related to a pre-existing vascular lesion; mean age of 44 years at presentation; diagnosis can be aided by radiological findings

[a]Secondary implantation cysts in the orbit may arise from conjunctival or respiratory epithelium after trauma, surgery, or chronic sinus disease {1492,3316}, or from ectopic lacrimal gland tissue {1598}.

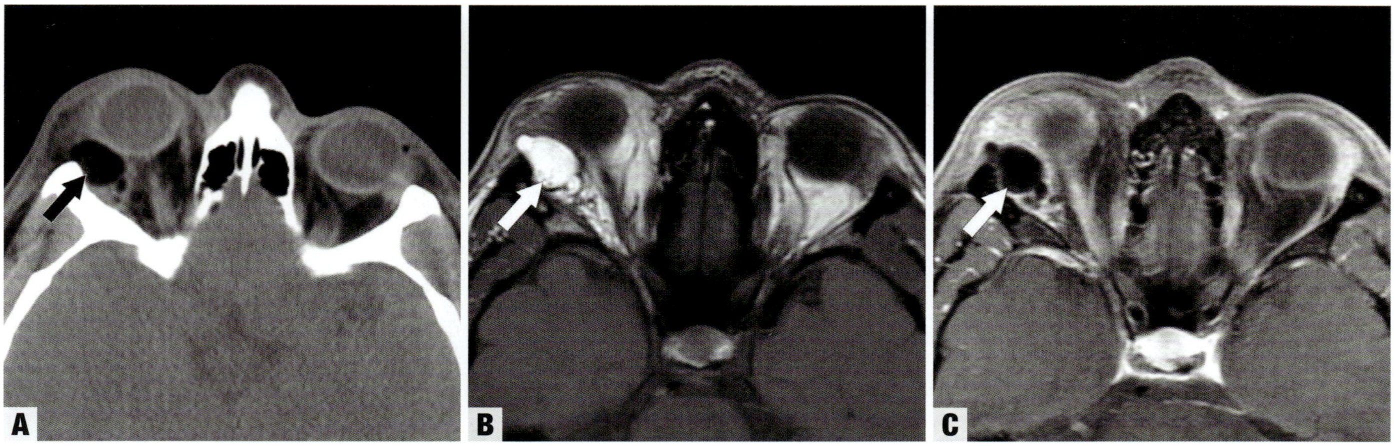

Fig. 9.01 Dermoid cyst. **A** Axial CT without contrast shows a fat-density mass in the lateral right orbit (arrow), causing exophthalmos. **B** Axial T1-weighted non-contrast MRI without fat saturation shows a hyperintense appearance of the mass (arrow). **C** Axial T1-weighted postcontrast MRI with fat saturation shows a hypointense, non-enhancing appearance of the mass due to the fat saturation (arrow).

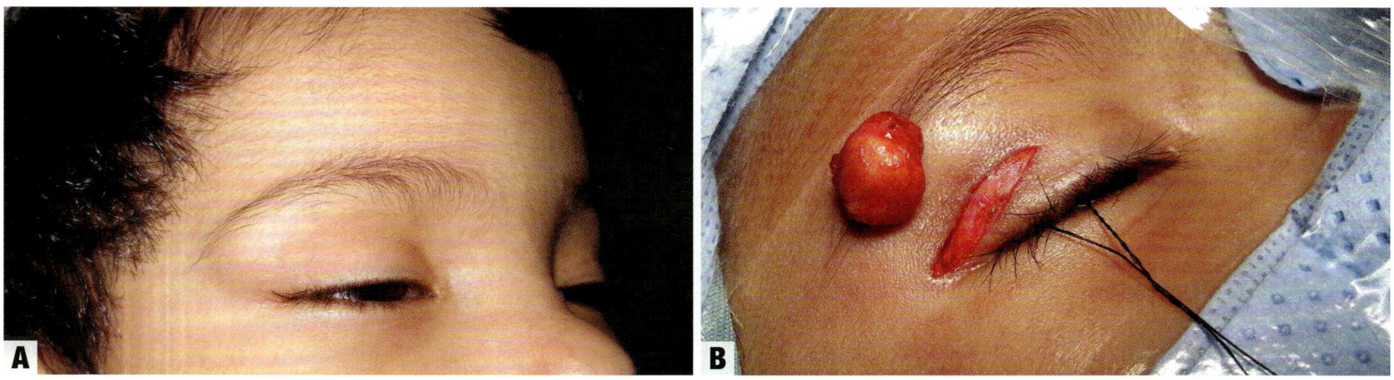

Fig. 9.02 Dermoid cyst. **A** The clinical appearance of a superficial dermoid cyst in a child. **B** Intraoperative appearance of the fully excised cyst in the same patient.

lateral, superolateral, retrobulbar, or inferior, with the commonest (60–80%) being superotemporal in relation to the frontozygomatic suture {369,3042,551,496,879}. In a large series, superficial dermoid cysts accounted for 71%, while 29% were deep in location {2610}. Dumbbell dermoid cysts with connection to the temporalis fossa may cause visual disturbance and were observed in 5.7% in one series {894,1950,2610}.

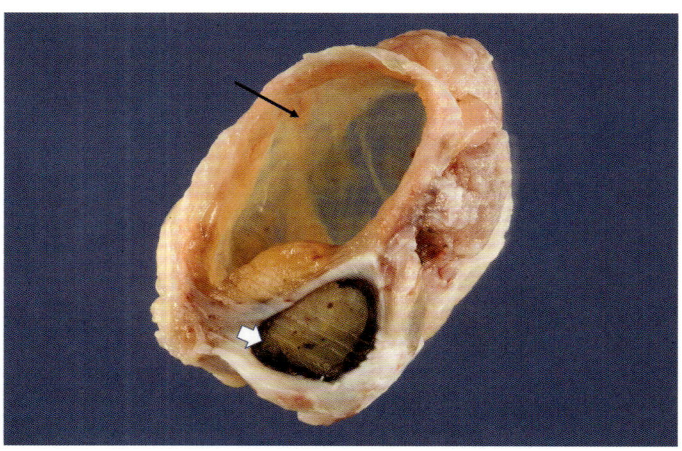

Fig. 9.03 Microphthalmos with cyst. The image shows a gross cross-section of a large developmental cyst (black arrow) in association with a microphthalmic globe (white arrow). The cyst develops in a coloboma and is lined by neuroglial tissue.

Clinical features

The clinical features of dermoid cysts depend on their location. Superficial dermoid cysts present earlier, before the age of 1 year, as asymptomatic, slowly progressive, painless, palpable subcutaneous masses, and are usually fixed to the underlying bone {879,2610}. Ocular sequelae such as amblyopia in these cases are rare {234}. Deep cysts are usually detected later in life, are clinically partially palpable or non-palpable, and may present with globe dystopia {369,879, 2610}. These deep dermoid cysts are associated with possible bone destruction and invasion especially if they have a subperiosteal component or undergo spontaneous rupture of the wall. Thus, they are better evaluated by radiological imaging {551,1915,1062,595}.

Dermoid cysts may have a characteristic dumbbell appearance with two cystic components: one involving either the superficial or deep orbit and the other involving the temporalis fossa or nearby spaces such as the frontal sinus, or the cranial fossa, with a narrow intraosseous communication through the bone resulting in a bony defect or even destruction of the lateral orbital wall depending on the location of the two interconnected cystic components {2229,3173}.

Epidemiology

Dermoid cysts account for 46% of orbital lesions in children {3051} and are the commonest cystic lesion of the orbit in the

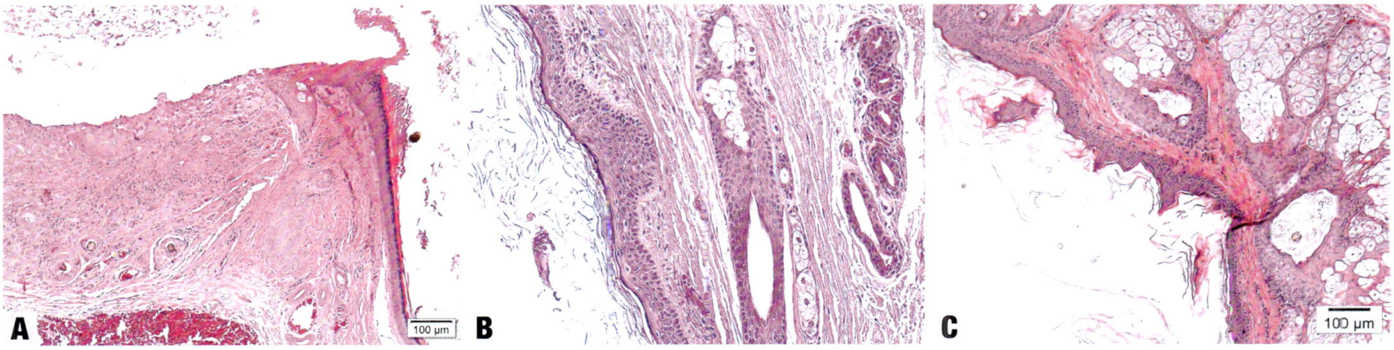

Fig. 9.04 Dermoid cyst. **A** High-power view of an area of ruptured dermoid cyst wall with numerous foreign body–type giant cells on the left and intact epithelium on the right. **B** The wall of a dermoid cyst with pilosebaceous units and sweat glands. **C** Histopathological appearance of a dermoid cyst wall consisting of keratinizing stratified squamous epithelium with skin appendages.

paediatric age group accounting for 62% of all cysts, followed by developmental cysts in association with microphthalmos in 25.5% {442,99,120}. The incidence of dermoid cysts is 1 in 638 live births {234}. Age at presentation ranges from one month to 27 years for superficial dermoid cysts, while deep cysts tend to present later at 3–45 years {2610}. A male predominance has been found {2610}, but not consistently reported in the literature {234}.

Etiology

Dermoid cysts result from entrapment of surface ectoderm near sites of embryological bony suture lines {496,2610}.

Pathogenesis

The entrapped surface ectoderm continues to slowly grow producing a cystic mass.

Macroscopic appearance

A dermoid cyst is usually oval or round in shape. The cystic mass is firm in consistency with a thin wall often showing protruding hair. Upon sectioning of the cyst, keratin-like cheesy material fills the cavity of the cyst with possible protruding hairs inside the cyst.

Histopathology

The wall of a dermoid cyst is typically keratinizing stratified squamous epithelium with skin appendages {3042}. In a large clinicopathological study, hair shafts were observed in the wall and/or the cavity of the cyst in 99% of specimens, sebaceous glands in 75%, and (eccrine) sweat glands in 20% {3042}. Chronic inflammation with collections of foreign body–type giant cells has been variably reported in nearly two thirds of cases in relation to the spontaneous rupture of the cyst wall and leakage of the contents {3042,654,2610,1062}. The inflammatory response may completely replace the epidermal wall without collapse of the cyst (in 16%) {654}. This rupture of the dermoid cyst wall with granulomatous reaction has been reported to be significantly associated with a higher median age of patients {654,1062}.

The differential diagnosis includes a wide array of other cystic lesions which may occur in the orbit. These may be lined by various types of epithelia or may be non-epithelial. The latter include both developmental abnormalities of the eye, such as microphthalmos with cyst, and infectious entities, such as those due to *Echinococcus*. The features of some other orbital cysts are described in Table 9.02 (p. 295).

Chapter 9

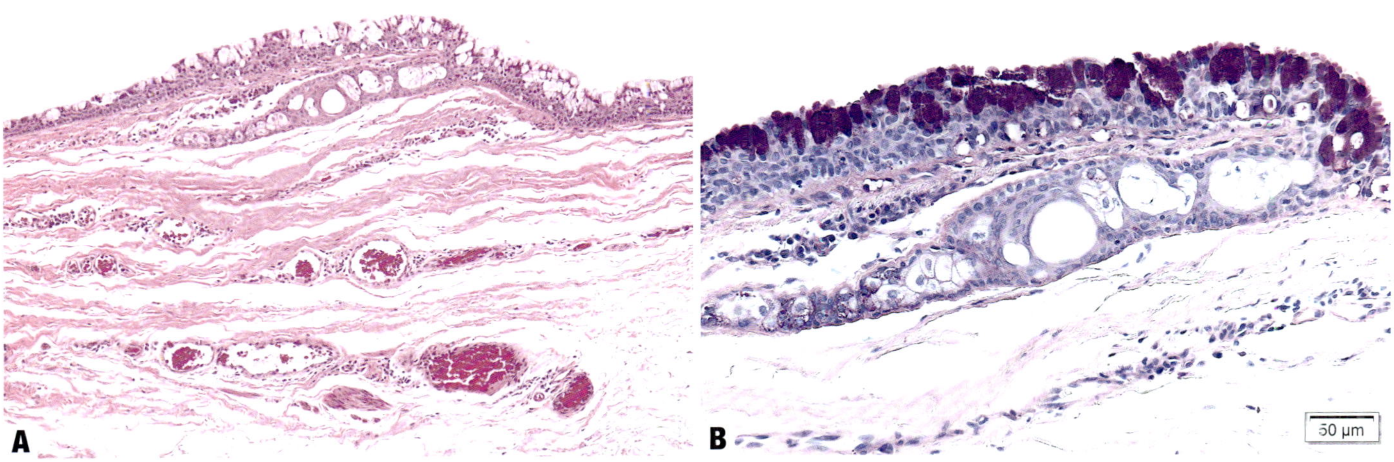

Fig. 9.05 Dermoid cyst. **A** The wall of a conjunctival dermoid cyst with pilosebaceous units. **B** Histopathological appearance of the conjunctival component of an orbital dermoid cyst with goblet cells stained by PAS and skin appendages.

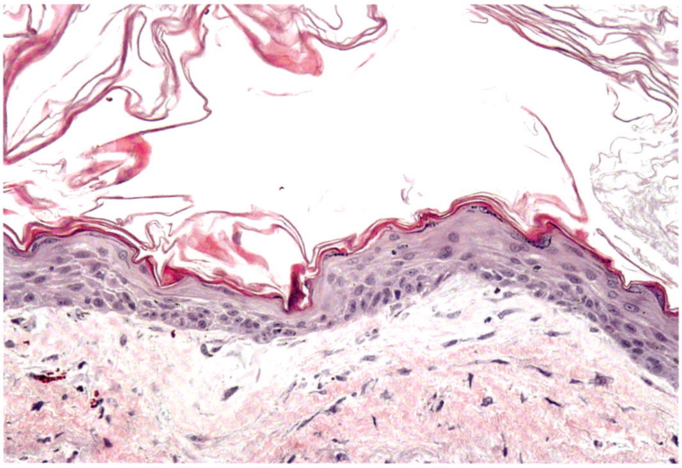

Fig. 9.06 Epidermoid cyst. Histopathological appearance of the keratinizing squamous epithelial wall of an epidermoid cyst. Note the absence of skin appendages in contrast to the typical dermoid cyst.

Cytology
Not clinically relevant

Diagnostic molecular pathology
Not relevant

Essential and desirable diagnostic criteria
Essential: cystic structure lined by keratinizing stratified squamous epithelium with epidermal appendages within the wall of the cyst.

Desirable: eccrine sweat glands and possible granulomatous reaction in the case of spontaneous rupture of the cyst wall.

Staging
Not relevant

Prognosis and prediction
Dermoid cysts require complete surgical excision. There is a risk of intraoperative rupture of the cyst in about 10% of the cases as a whole reaching 56.3% in exophytic cysts that are removed via skin crease incision {879,234}. Cysts may require decompression before surgical excision {2610}. Location of the cyst (superotemporal versus superomedial) does not seem to affect the morbidity or risk of cyst rupture {1915}. Intraoperative cyst rupture or incomplete surgical excision increases the chance of recurrence, postoperative inflammation, and fistula formation {2573,3552}. Recurrence is reported to range from 4.2% to 6.3% {1917,879,234}.

Cavernous vascular malformation

Flucke U
Kaliki S
Rootman DB
Singh A

Definition
Cavernous vascular malformation (CVM) is an encapsulated mass composed of numerous dilated vein-like structures.

ICD-O coding
9121/0 Cavernous vascular malformation

ICD-11 coding
2F36.Y & XH1GU2 Other specified benign neoplasm of eye or ocular adnexa & Cavernous haemangioma

Related terminology
Acceptable: cavernous haemangioma; cavernous venous malformation.

Subtype(s)
None

Localization
CVMs are typically (75%) located at least partially in the intraconal space, mostly in the mid and posterior orbit {2761,460}.

Clinical features
The presence of an orbital mass with development of progressive axial proptosis is the most common sign. Pain can be noted in as many as a third of patients {2761}. Visual impairment is typically due to optic neuropathy or hyperopic shift. Diplopia is uncommon {460}. With imaging (ultrasound, CT, or MRI), CVMs tend to present as well-circumscribed T2-hyperintense ovoid or lobular lesions and demonstrate progressive enhancement with contrast {2761}.

Epidemiology
CVM is the most common benign orbital lesion of adults and the third most common diagnosis after lymphoid tumours and orbital inflammatory syndromes. Lesions typically become symptomatic in the fourth and fifth decades of life. About 60% occur in women {460}.

Etiology
Vascular malformations arise during embryogenesis owing to mosaic mutations or, more rarely, germline mutations leading to developmental errors in the vascular system {987,2401,2620}.

CVM may be associated with blue rubber bleb naevus syndrome (predominantly sporadic and rarely hereditary [autosomal dominant]) (MIM number 112200).

CVM associated with Maffucci syndrome (sporadic) has a relationship with spindle cell haemangioma, another vascular malformation {460} (MIM number 614569).

Pathogenesis
CVMs have been postulated to undergo growth owing to repeated cycles of thrombosis and recanalization leading to slow enlargement of the mass {2761}. In other venous malformations, *TEK* is commonly affected by somatic or germline mutations, but this has not been studied in CVM. CVMs in Maffucci syndrome usually harbour *IDH1* or *IDH2* hotspot mutations {460}.

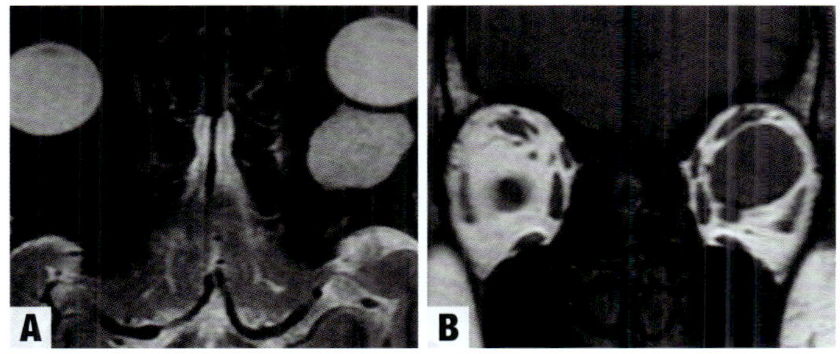

Fig. 9.07 Cavernous vascular malformation. **A** MRI of the orbit reveals a well-defined hyperintense lesion in the mid-orbit. **B** The lesion is superolateral to the optic nerve

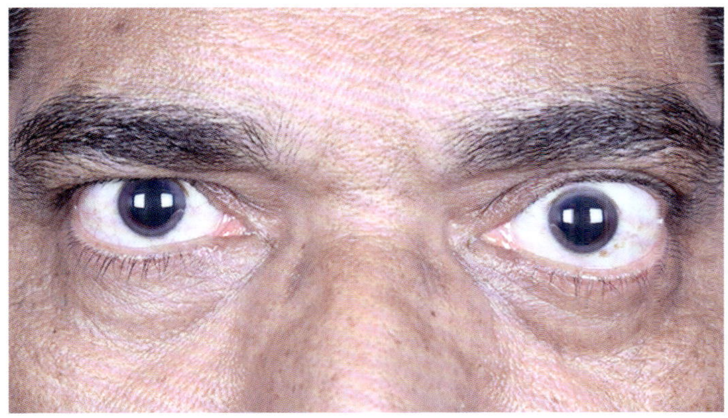

Fig. 9.08 Cavernous vascular malformation. A 53-year-old male patient presented with a history of proptosis in the left eye for 2 years.

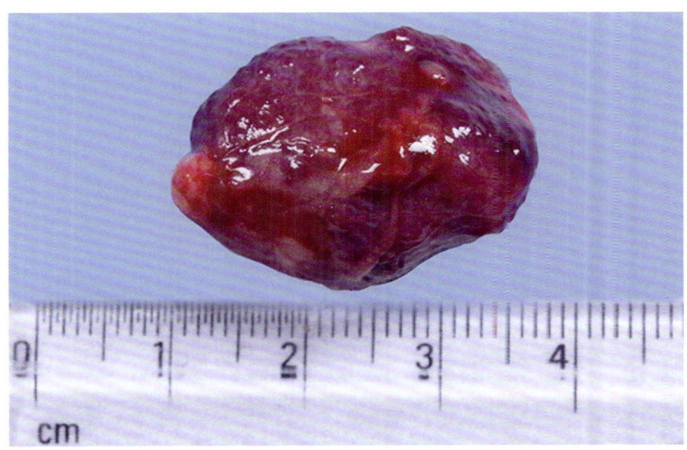

Fig. 9.09 Cavernous vascular malformation. Complete excisional biopsy was performed by transcutaneous orbitotomy. Gross examination revealed a well-defined reddish-purple lesion.

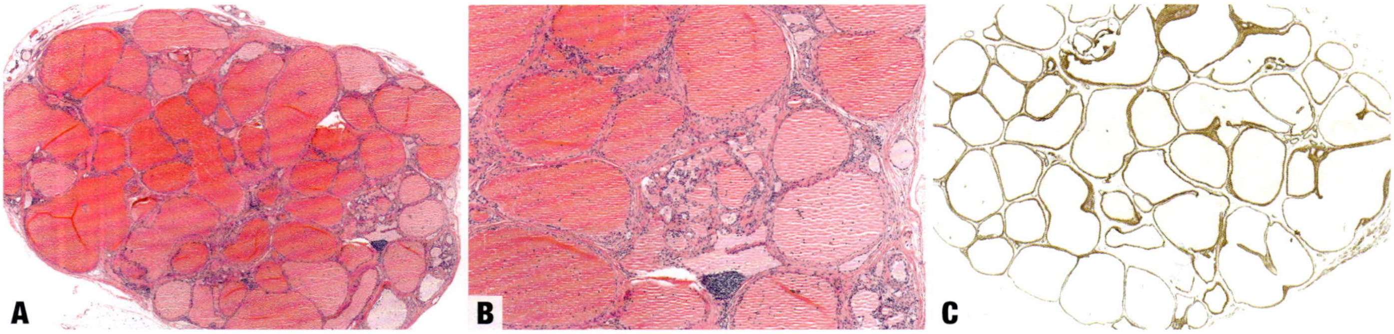

Fig. 9.10 Cavernous vascular malformation. **A** A circumscribed lesion consists of dilated/cavernous veins. **B** Higher magnification shows the flattened vessel walls with normal endothelial cells and a focus of vascular proliferation. **C** SMA highlights the walls of the veins.

Recently, two studies have shown mutation of *GJA4* in a high proportion of these tumours {1358}. *GJA4* encodes a transmembrane protein involved in gap junctions and hemichannels in vessels, and the mutation is found within the endothelial cell component of these tumours. *GJA4* mutation is also seen within cutaneous cavernous malformations and hepatic haemangiomas {3409}.

Macroscopic appearance
CVMs form nodular encapsulated spongy lesions filled with blood. The size distribution is not documented, but most are 10–25 mm in diameter.

Histopathology
CVM is usually a circumscribed encapsulated lesion characterized by clustered cavernous dilated veins. The veins are lined by normal-appearing endothelial cells {460}. Focal areas of microvascular proliferation adjacent to the larger vascular spaces and organizing thrombi may be present {2761}.

Cytology
Not clinically relevant

Diagnostic molecular pathology
Not clinically relevant

Essential and desirable diagnostic criteria
Essential: typical clinical and imaging features; circumscribed mass composed of dilated, cavernous venous channels.

Staging
Not clinically relevant

Prognosis and prediction
CVMs generally progress slowly. Treatment is determined by progression and symptomatology. Surgery, typically direct orbital approaches, is the mainstay of treatment; however, some have described endoscopic-assisted and purely radiological approaches {2762}. Recurrences are rare after complete excision. Sclerotherapy can be used in challenging lesions {460}.

Combined lymphatic-venous malformation of the orbit

Flucke U
Alkatan H
Colmenero I
Kaliki S
Mudhar HS
Roctmar DB
Thway K

Definition
Combined lymphatic-venous malformation (LVM) is a congenital low-flow vascular malformation consisting of both malformed veins and lymphatic channels often interspersed with lymphoid follicles, areas of fibrosis, and old haemorrhage.

ICD-O coding
9170/0 Combined lymphatic-venous malformation of the orbit

ICD-11 coding
LA90.2Y Other specified peripheral venous malformations
LA90.12 Lymphatic malformations of certain specified sites

Related terminology
Acceptable: lymphatic malformation.
Not recommended: lymphangioma; venous anomaly.

Subtype(s)
None

Localization
Orbital LVM can be superficial in location or deep within the orbit, or have combined superficial and deep components {2764}. Complex lesions involve other head and neck structures including the infratemporal, intracranial, and temporalis fossae {2812}. Most cases of conjunctival involvement constitute the superficial component of an orbital lymphatic malformation {1503,2899,3046}.

Superficially these lesions tend to be more microcystic whereas orbital lesions tend towards being macrocystic. Deeper components tend to be more predominantly venous {3088}.

Clinical features
LVMs can present in childhood or later in life, depending on the size and activity of the lesion. Superficial components tend to present as a subcutaneous or subconjunctival mass, whereas orbital components may present with unilateral proptosis, with or without extraocular motility disturbance, ptosis, and visual loss {2764,1061,3398,1584,3635}. They can expand in times of viral illness and/or present with intralesional haemorrhage and/or thrombosis, the latter being characterized by the subacute onset of pain, proptosis, and/or ecchymosis. They can lead to vision impairment / optic neuropathy and amblyopia {1973, 3088}.

Orbital LVMs can be misdiagnosed as rhabdomyosarcoma, haemangioma, or lymphoma on imaging studies {1066}.

Epidemiology
There is a female preponderance with most lesions presenting in infancy and childhood {1978,3088}. Orbital LVM accounts for 0.3–4% of orbital lesions {2764,1197,3088}.

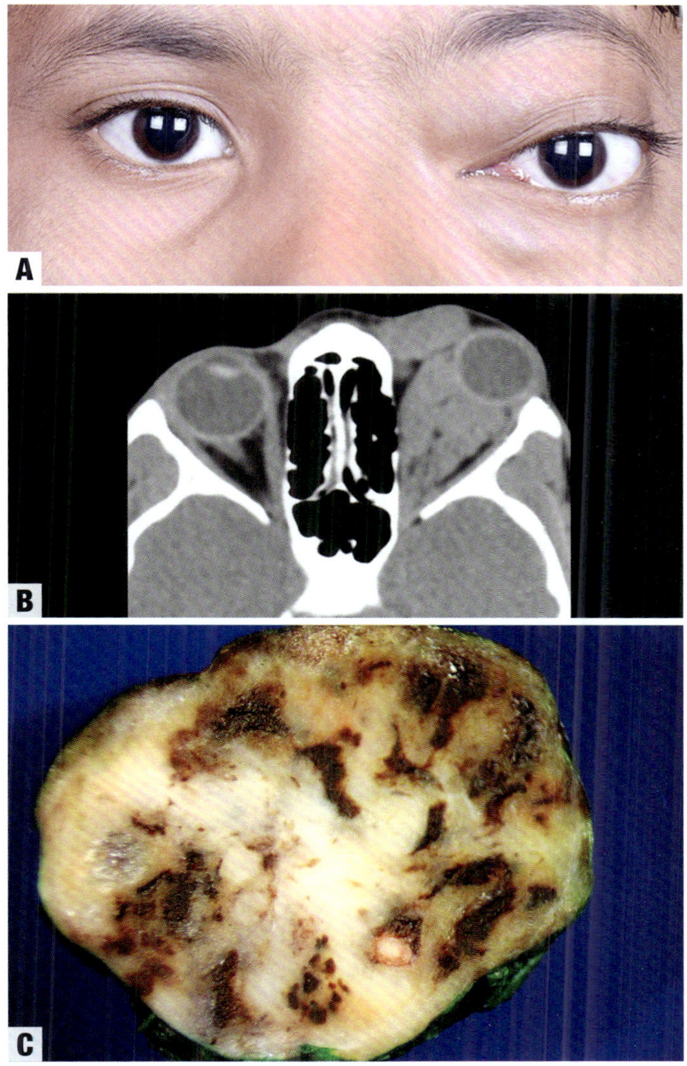

Fig. 9.11 Combined lymphatic-venous malformation of the orbit. **A** A 10-year-old girl presented with sudden proptosis of the left eye. **B** CT of the orbit reveals a poorly defined heterogeneous lesion in the preseptal tissues and intraconal space of the left orbit. **C** A tan lesion with multiple compartments and cysts filled with blood, and irregular margins.

Etiology
Systemic vascular malformations arise during embryogenesis and can be due to mosaic mutations or, more rarely, germline mutations leading to developmental errors in the vascular system {2401, 987,2620}. Orbital LVMs have not been studied in this regard

Pathogenesis
Some systemic LVMs have been found to be due to somatic mosaic mutations in *PIK3CA* which lead to activation of the

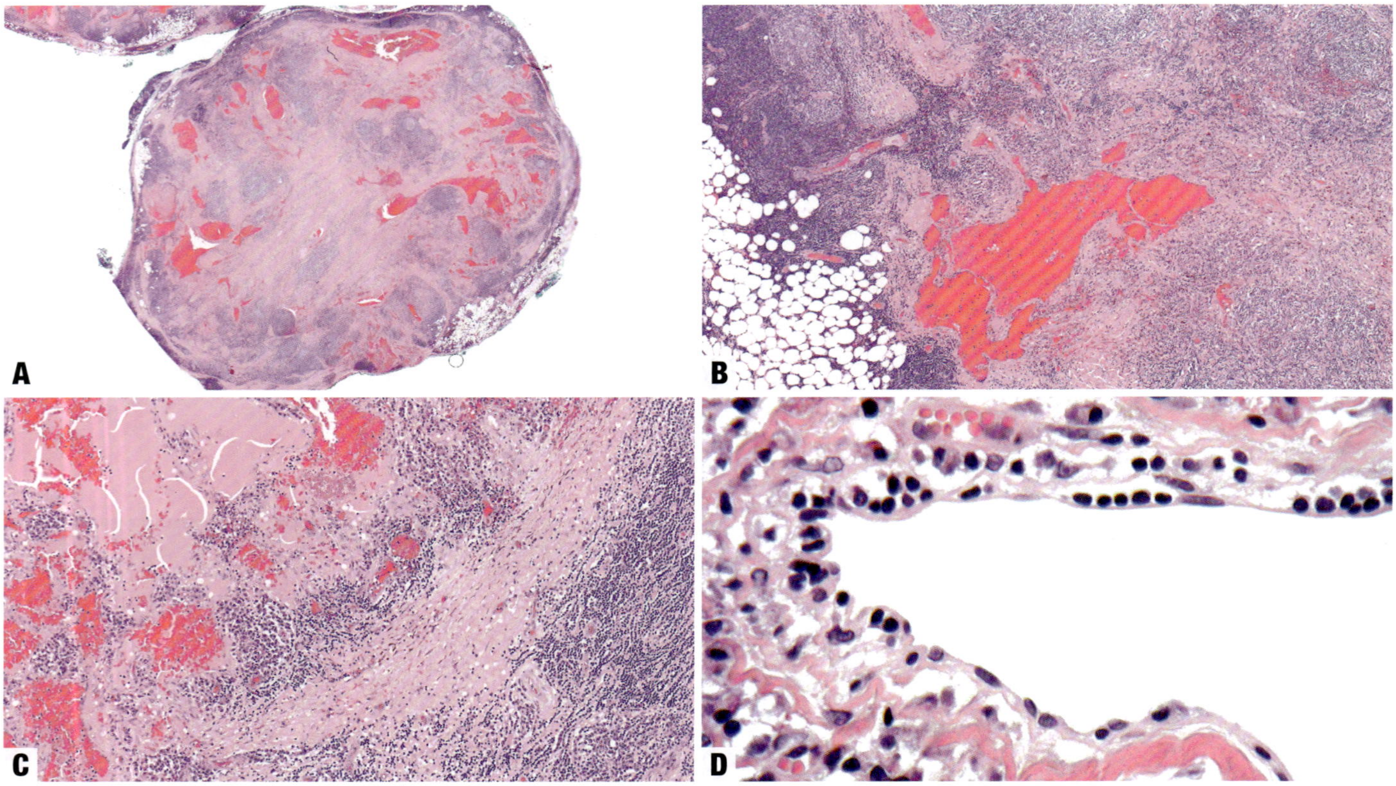

Fig. 9.12 Combined lymphatic-venous malformation of the orbit. **A** An irregular mass of malformed vascular channels of various sizes. **B** The lesion is unencapsulated. **C** Intervening fibroconnective tissue septa contain numerous lymphocytes forming aggregates, and lymphoid follicles separate the malformed vascular channels. **D** Endothelial cells line the dilated channels of an orbital lymphatic-venous malformation. Note lymphocytes at a subendothelial location.

AKT/mTOR signalling pathway with consequent increased cell growth, proliferation, and migration {356,949,2449,388,2378}.

Macroscopic appearance

LVM is tan to reddish or brownish in colour and unencapsulated, with multiple compartments and cysts filled with blood, and irregular margins due to its infiltrative nature {617}.

Histopathology

LVM forms an unencapsulated irregular mass of malformed endothelial-lined channels of various sizes separated by fibroconnective tissue septa that lack smooth muscle. The connective tissue may show aggregates of small mature lymphocytes, which may form lymphoid follicles. Haemosiderin-laden macrophages may be present, reflecting prior haemorrhage. The lymphatic channels often contain proteinaceous fluid, blood, or both. Lymphatic endothelial cells express CD31 and stain with D2-40 {330,2461,3117,1486,504,1978}.

Cytology

Not clinically relevant

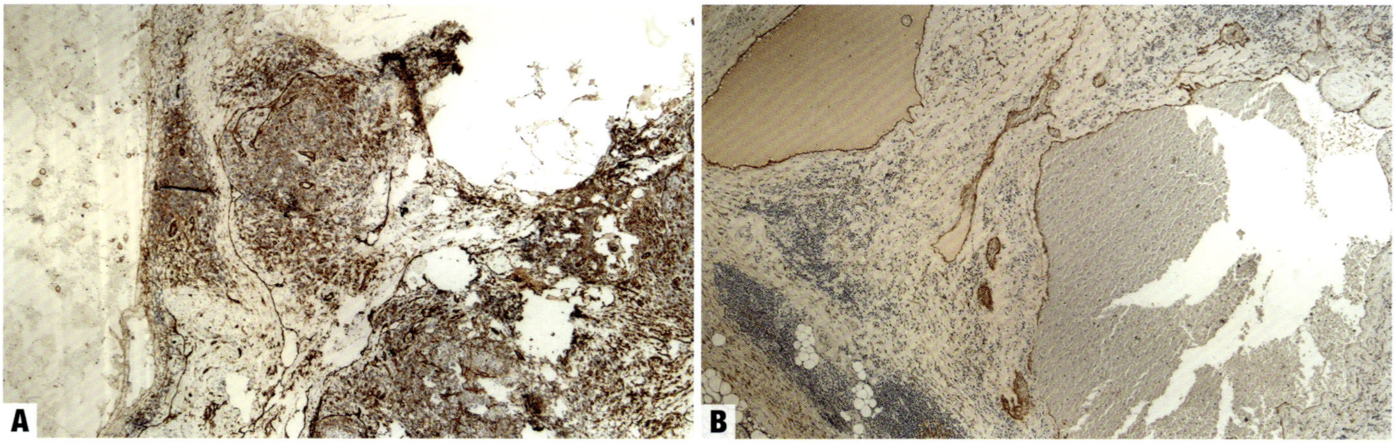

Fig. 9.13 Combined lymphatic-venous malformation of the orbit. **A** CD31 demonstrates vascular endothelium lining mostly clumps of smaller vessels in the stroma. **B** D2-40 demonstrates lymphatic endothelium lining larger and medium-sized serous channels.

Diagnostic molecular pathology

Detection of somatic mutations can support the use of specific treatments in select cases (mTOR or PI3K inhibitors).

Essential and desirable diagnostic criteria

Essential: characteristic clinical, radiological (MRI: vascular mass) findings; proliferation of dilated, variably sized lymphatic and venous channels

Desirable: immunohistochemical expression of CD31 and CD34, and staining with D2-40 in the endothelial cells.

Staging

Not clinically relevant

Prognosis and prediction

LVMs typically progress slowly. The clinical course is variable, ranging from spontaneous regression to gradual progression. Treatment is reserved for vision-threatening lesions or those causing severe disfigurement, while less severe lesions can be observed. Treatment options include sclerotherapy, medical treatment with sildenafil (PDE5 inhibitor) or sirolimus (mTOR inhibitor), anti-VEGF medications, and surgical debulking {2355, 1848,3247,3635}. Lymphatic and venous components can be treated separately {2655}.

Chapter 9

Orbital venous malformation

Flucke U
Kaliki S
Rootman DB

Definition

Orbital venous malformations (VMs) are defined as a vein-to-vein diversion of blood in the absence of an interceding arterial bed.

ICD-O coding

9122/0 Orbital venous malformation

ICD-11 coding

LA90.2Z Peripheral venous malformations, unspecified

Related terminology

Not recommended: orbital varix; venous haemangioma.

Subtype(s)

None

Localization

Owing to developmental defects, VMs can affect any tissue and organ. Involvement of the skin and subcutis is frequently seen as well as deeper tissues within the orbit. They can be complex, crossing into associated anatomical regions including the intracranial space, the infratemporal fossa, and the temporalis fossa. Intraosseous components are not uncommon {2620, 3557}. They are usually unifocal and infrequently multifocal.

Clinical features

VMs can present as bluish subdermal lesions when superficial and, though they can be noted at birth, typically present later in life. Subcutaneous lesions are typically soft and can be emptied by digital pressure. If found deeper in the orbit, Valsalva manoeuvre may lead to expansion of the lesion, manifesting as proptosis, strabismus, and globe dystopia. As they are venous in nature, there is typically no thrill, bruit, or pulsation. Symptomatology relates to repeated cycles of filling and emptying, leading to Valsalva-induced pain and globe dystopia during filling and enophthalmos when emptying owing to chronic tissue atrophy. Acute intralesional thrombosis may occur and this can be painful, with associated signs of orbital compression including optic neuropathy and strabismus {1387,1173,2355,2760,2763,642,813}.

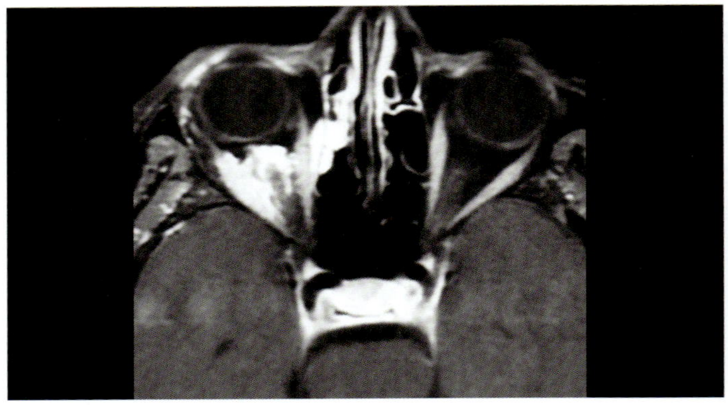

Fig. 9.14 Orbital venous malformation. MRI of the orbits reveals a poorly defined lesion on the ocular surface with a diffuse lesion in the right orbit and ipsilateral ethmoidal sinus mucosa, with intense contrast enhancement suggestive of right-sided orbito-conjunctivosinus venous malformation.

Epidemiology

VMs affect as much as 1.5% of the population. They are the most common slow-flow vascular malformations and a common orbital disease {813,3680}.

Etiology

Venous malformations arise during embryogenesis owing to mosaic mutations or, more rarely, germline mutations leading to

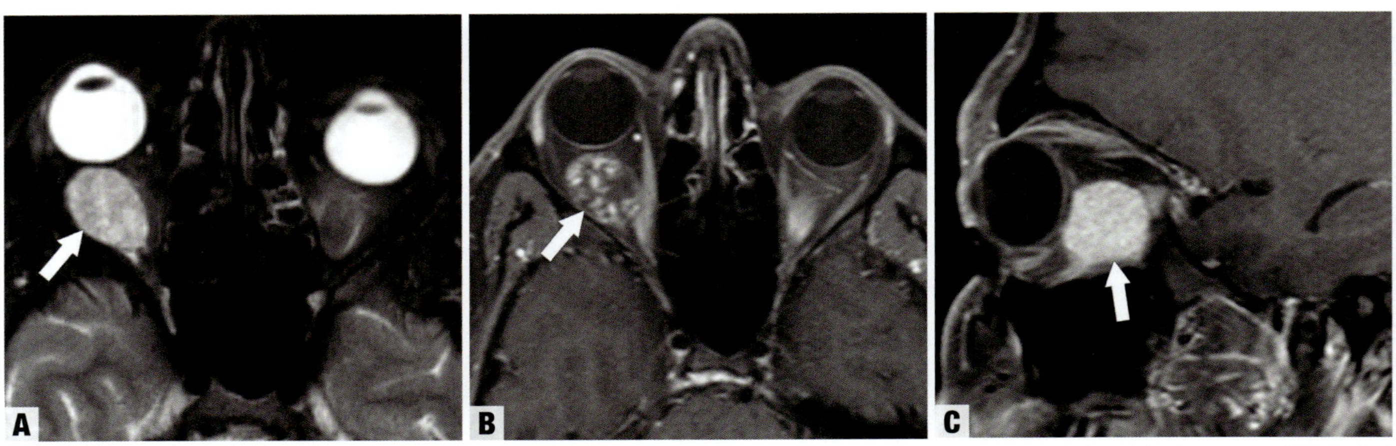

Fig. 9.15 Orbital venous malformation. **A** Axial T2-weighted MRI shows an isointense to hyperintense right orbital mass (arrow). **B** Axial T1-weighted postcontrast MRI obtained immediately after contrast administration shows heterogeneous enhancement of the mass (arrow). **C** Sagittal T1-weighted postcontrast MRI (delayed image) shows complete filling-in of the mass with contrast (arrow) over time.

developmental errors in the vascular system {2620,987,2401}. VMs are mainly sporadic and rarely inherited, and can be associated with lymphatic or other tissue in complex malformations (lymphatic-venous malformation, capillary lymphatic-venous malformations, etc.) {813}.

VMs are associated with cutaneomucosal venous malformation (distensible and non-distensible; autosomal dominant inheritance), blue rubber bleb naevus (Bean syndrome; sporadic), and glomuvenous malformation (sporadic or autosomal dominant inheritance) {813,381}.

Pathogenesis

Sporadic systemic cases show activating somatic mosaic mutations predominantly in *TEK*. Inherited malformations harbour a combination of a germline mutation with a postzygotic somatic second hit leading also to overexpression and autophosphorylation of the corresponding endothelial receptor tyrosine kinase TIE2. TIE2 activates the PI3K/AKT/mTOR signalling pathway. In a few sporadic cases *PIK3CA* is an alternatively affected gene. Glomuvenous malformations harbour inactivating mutations in *GLMN* {2620,3557,2378}. Orbital lesions have not been studied molecularly.

Macroscopic appearance

These lesions show a vascular/haemorrhagic circumscribed or diffuse spongy lesion with variable fibrous tissue, although they often collapse after removal. The cavities are communicating, separated by septa. Thrombi (often calcified) may be observed.

Histopathology

The lesions comprise an abnormal collection of enlarged veins that are superficial or deep, diffuse or localized, and solitary or multiple. Veins show a variable diameter and a variably thick smooth muscle layer, absence of an internal elastic lamina, and inconspicuous endothelium. Small venules and capillaries may also be present. Thrombi and phleboliths with signs of recanalization are relatively common. The presence of Masson lesions (intravascular papillary endothelial hyperplasia) can be confused with malignancy {987,3557,2401}.

In glomuvenous malformations the media of the veins contain cuboidal glomus cells with relatively monomorphic round nuclei. The glomus cells can also be seen in the wall of arteries and capillaries. They are highlighted by SMA immunohistochemistry {3557}.

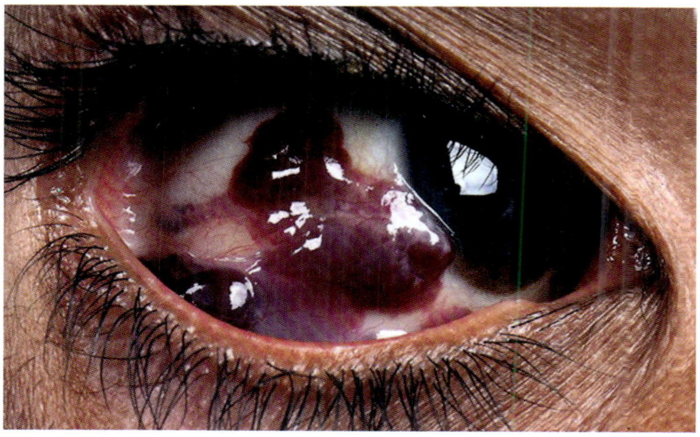

Fig. 9.16 Orbital venous malformation. A 48-year-old woman presented with a progressively increasing violet-red lesion in her right eye extending anteriorly from the orbit.

Cytology

Not clinically relevant

Diagnostic molecular pathology

Not clinically relevant

Essential and desirable diagnostic criteria

Essential: slow-flow vascular lesion with characteristics described in *Clinical features*; histological features of a dilated venous channel.

Desirable: Valsalva-augmented CT can be useful in diagnosis and characterization; phleboliths common by imaging; MRI may be additionally helpful in cases of combined lymphatic-venous malformation.

Staging

Not relevant

Prognosis and prediction

Treatment is indicated for improvement of quality of life and to prevent or treat complications. Embolization, sclerotherapy and targeted treatment (e.g. rapamycin) with or without surgery can be performed {1825,1317}. Recanalization and recurrence is common with intravascular therapy alone {813,2620, 642,2760}.

Chapter 9

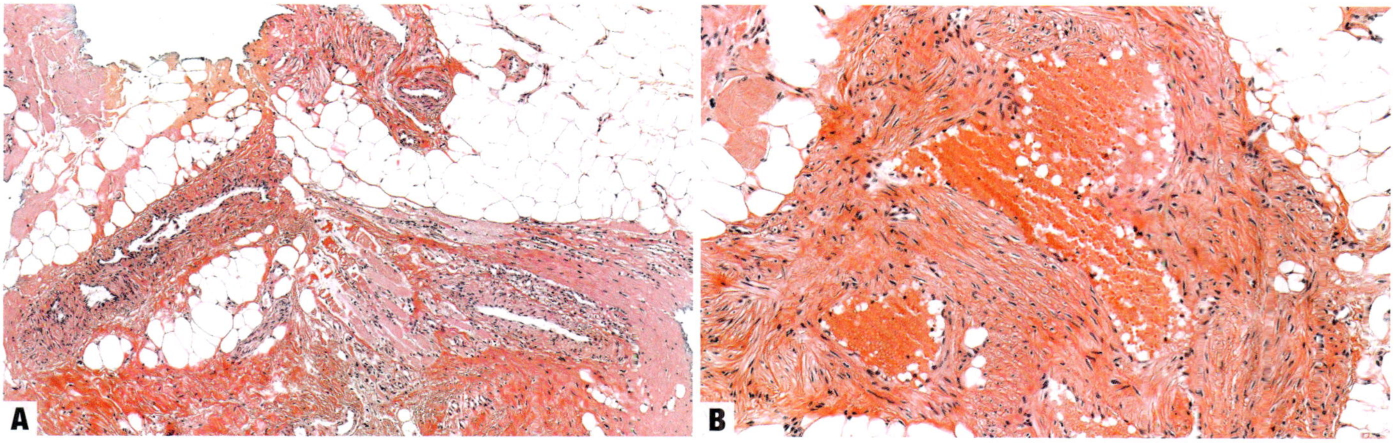

Fig. 9.17 Venous malformation. **A** Abnormal veins are arranged in clusters. **B** Higher magnification shows the abnormal texture of the malformed vessel wall.

Arteriovenous malformation

Flucke U
Kaliki S
Rootman DB

Definition
Arteriovenous malformations (AVMs) are rare fast-flow vascular lesions composed of anomalous arterial and venous vessels connected directly without an intervening capillary bed.

ICD-O coding
9123/0 Arteriovenous malformation

ICD-11 coding
LA90.3Y Other specified peripheral arteriovenous malformations

Related terminology
Not recommended: arteriovenous haemangioma.

Subtype(s)
None

Localization
Lesions arise within the orbit and may extend into the surrounding tissues (e.g. nasal cavity, paranasal sinuses, deep facial tissues, intracranial space) {1612}. Different structures of the eye can be affected {1254,3294}.

Clinical features
AVMs are usually present at birth showing a significant arteriovenous shunting with raised skin temperature and pulsation if superficial. Haemorrhage and ischaemia due to arterial steal are relatively uncommon in the periorbital region. Deep-seated lesions may become apparent at a later age when shunting is low-grade {3557,2401,987}. Orbital AVMs can cause significant morbidity including chronic pain, decreased vision, and cosmetic disfigurement with exophthalmos {752}. When the compromised vessels rupture, the consequences can be devastating {2378}. Doppler ultrasonography and MRI are the techniques most often used for their investigation {1387}.

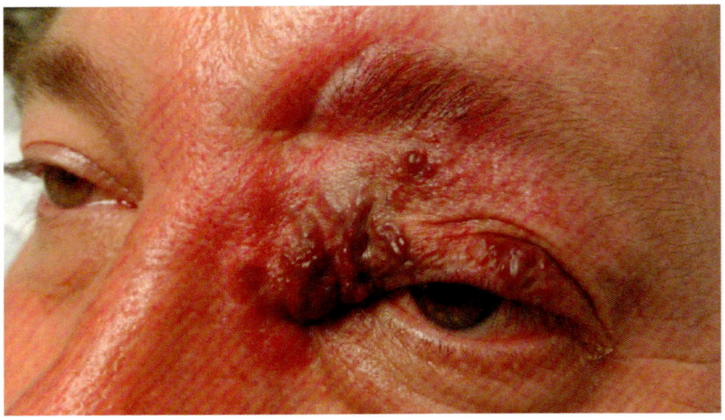

Fig. 9.18 Orbital arteriovenous malformation. Clinical image demonstrating arteriovenous malformation of the left upper eyelid, medial brow, glabella, and medial orbit.

Epidemiology
AVMs in the orbit and eye are rare {752}. There is no sex predilection {1387}.

Etiology
Vascular malformations arise during embryogenesis owing to mosaic mutations or, more rarely, germline mutations leading to developmental errors in the vascular system {987,2401,2620}. Most AVMs are sporadic with a few cases occurring within familial disorders {2378}.

Pathogenesis
Several members of the MAPK signalling pathway have been implicated in sporadic AVMs. They include hyperactivating changes in the RAS genes and *MAP2K1* {2378}. AVMs in familial disorders are driven by changes in *RASA1* and *EPHB4* {2378}.

Macroscopic appearance
AVMs are composed of a tangle of large thick-walled vessels and cystic cavities.

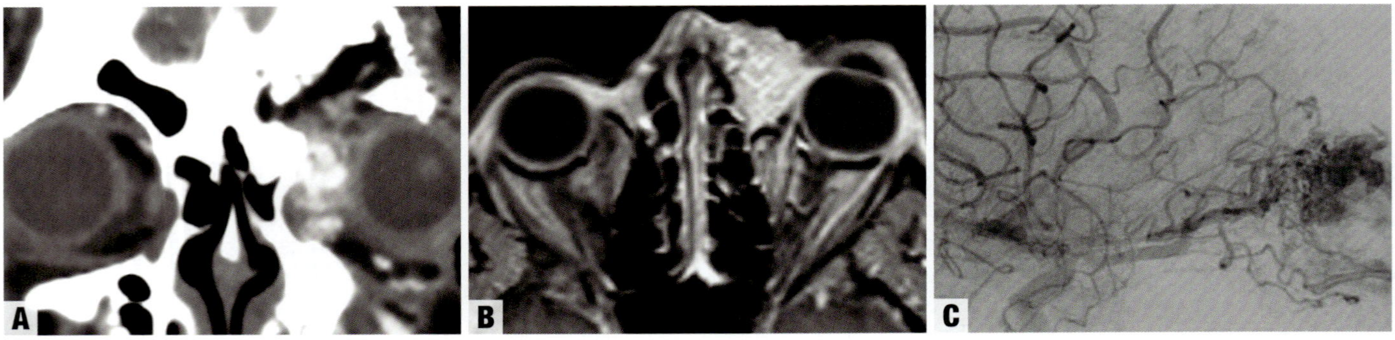

Fig. 9.19 Orbital arteriovenous malformation. **A** CT with contrast demonstrating a tangle of arterialized vessels in the medial orbit, with frontal sinus floor defect from previous surgery. **B** MRI with contrast demonstrating arterialized mass in the medial orbit, glabella, and lateral radix. **C** Subtraction angiogram demonstrating arterialized veins in the orbit, with feeders from the supraorbital, infraorbital, and superficial temporal arteries.

Histopathology

The histological appearance of AVMs is variable. There are numerous large-calibre arteries and thick-walled veins. The arteries are often tortuous and the veins show intimal and adventitial fibrosis. Arterioles, venules, capillaries, dilated lymphatics, and undefined vessels may be present. The background is often fibrous or fibromyxoid. The overlying skin may show a proliferation of small vessels probably due to arteriovenous shunt–related tissue ischaemia {2401,987}.

Cytology

Not clinically relevant

Diagnostic molecular pathology

Not clinically relevant

Essential and desirable diagnostic criteria

Essential: specific clinical findings (pain, warmth, and bleeding episodes) and radiological features (see *Clinical features*).

Desirable: histology showing vessels of different sizes, including both arteries and veins; fibrointimal thickening in veins.

Staging

The Schobinger staging system describes four stages of progression {1387,3557}:

Stage I: asymptomatic pink patches or maculae that often mimic capillary malformation; increased warmth or thrill to palpation

Stage II: vessels becoming dilated and prominent; increased warmth and thrill; prominent draining veins; skin may thicken and become more purple

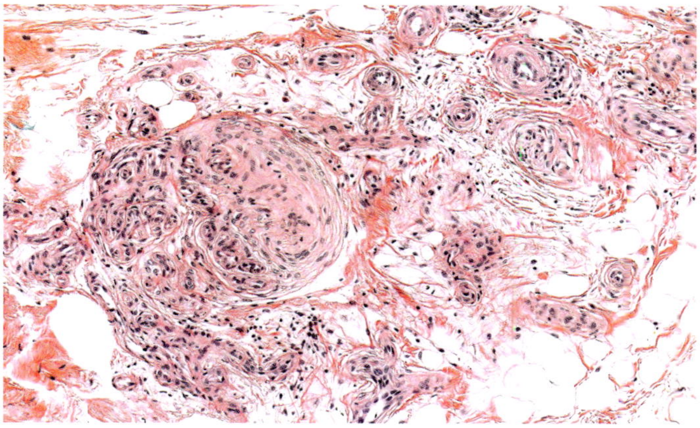

Fig. 9.20 Arteriovenous malformation. Clusters of arterioles and small veins are directly connected without a capillary bed.

Stage III: destruction of deeper tissues, including bone; pain and haemorrhage

Stage IV: cardiac compromise from increased blood flow.

Prognosis and prediction

AVMs are the most problematic vascular lesions to manage. They never regress spontaneously {2378}. When treatment is indicated (pain, bleeding, enlargement, ulceration), a multidisciplinary approach, including embolization and resection is often necessary {752,1387}. Recurrence is common, particularly when the nidus is fed from small vessels {1387,1612}. Newer strategies including mTOR and VEGF inhibitors show promise for future medical management {2378,2620,1612}.

Chapter 9

Orbital glial heterotopia

Herwig-Carl MC
Cummings TJ

Definition

Orbital glial heterotopia is an isolated orbital focus of non-teratomatous CNS tissue occurring entirely outside the intracranial and intraspinal cavities in the absence of a skull defect and microphthalmia with cyst.

ICD-O coding

None

ICD-11 coding

LA14.2 Structural developmental anomalies of orbit

Related terminology

Acceptable: ectopic glial-meningeal tissue; neuroglial heterotopia.

Not recommended: heterotopic brain choristoma; ectopic brain tissue.

Subtype(s)

None

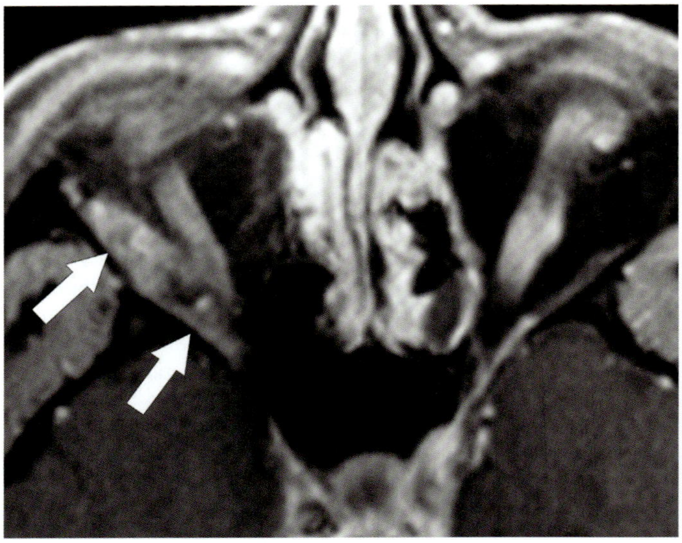

Fig. 9.21 Orbital glial heterotopia. Contrast-enhanced T1-weighted MRI with extraconal enhancing lesion (arrows) in the right orbit extending posteriorly to the orbital apex.

Localization

Glial heterotopia can rarely be found in the orbit (without any dural connection) {2157} and only single reports of extraorbital lesions (lower eyelid, retina) exist {83,2513}.

Clinical features

Based on the approximately 30 reported cases, the most common signs are swelling, strabismus, and proptosis. One case of blindness due to orbital glial heterotopia has been reported {3127}. Microphthalmia and anophthalmia can also be present {2704}; however, the symptoms depend on the location and the size of the orbital lesion. The lesion is usually unilateral, but a patient with bilateral orbital lesions has been described {2421}. Leukocoria has been clinically noted in a case of intraocular glial heterotopia mimicking a retinoblastoma {2513}. CT or MRI is recommended for localization of the lesion.

The differential diagnosis may include encephalocoele and microphthalmia with cyst. In order to suggest the diagnosis of orbital glial heterotopia, it must be shown clinically that there is no skull defect to suggest an encephalocoele and that the eye is otherwise without evidence of microphthalmia with cyst.

Epidemiology

For orbital lesions the age at presentation is typically before 5 years {2157}. Some of the reported cases were described in neonates. Glial heterotopia is rarely found in adults {3243,2593}.

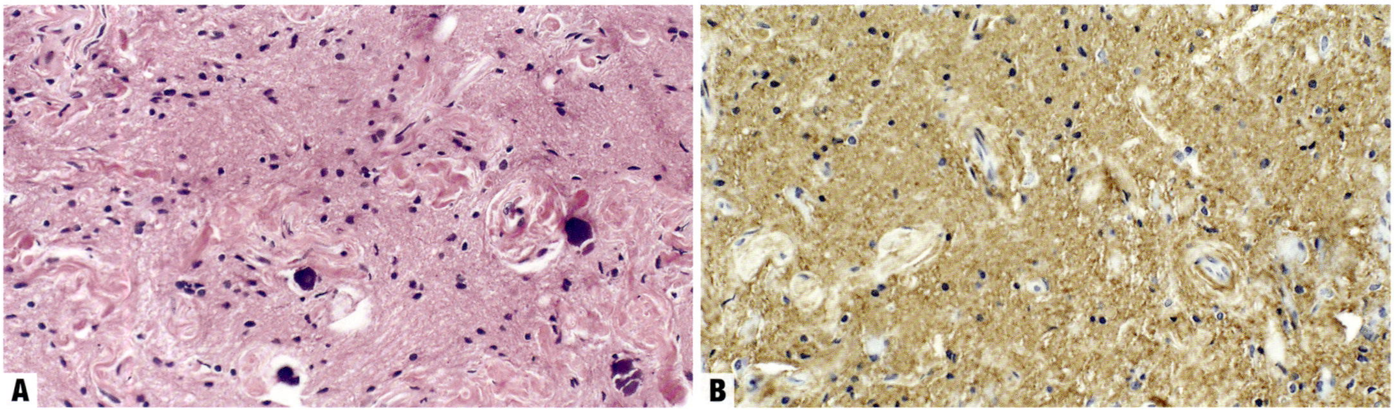

Fig. 9.22 Orbital glial heterotopia. **A** Benign neuroglial tissue with microcalcifications is seen. **B** The glial tissue is immunoreactive for GFAP.

Etiology
Unknown

Pathogenesis
The pathogenesis is unclear. Embryological hypotheses include abnormal migration of neural tissue and abnormal maturation of neural crests.

Macroscopic appearance
The reported size of lesions has varied between a few and 80 mm.

Histopathology
The lesions are composed of benign and mature brain tissue including glial and neural components. Microcalcifications and psammoma bodies may be present {2448}. The tissue is typically positive for S100 and GFAP {78}. Neurofilament protein may identify axons within the tissue. Ependyma, choroid plexus, and cerebellar tissue are rarely present. One report described an orbital lesion composed of glial tissue intermixed with muscle fibres {1714}.

Cytology
Not reported

Diagnostic molecular pathology
Not relevant

Essential and desirable diagnostic criteria
Essential: mature brain tissue in the orbit without connection to the dura/meninges; absence of a skull defect and absence of microphthalmia with cyst.

Staging
Not relevant

Prognosis and prediction
No malignant transformation has been reported. The lesions can exhibit slow growth. A diagnostic and therapeutic approach is necessary to rule out other tumours and to prevent further ocular sequelae {3127}. Complete excision should be achieved but is often not possible. Subtotally excised lesions often remain stable {237} but can recur {1714}.

Mesenchymal hamartoma of the orbit

Proia AD
McKelvie PA

Definition
Orbital mesenchymal hamartomas are a family of benign malformations of mesenchymal cells found in the orbit including rhabdomyomatous mesenchymal hamartoma (RMH), chondromesenchymal hamartoma (CMH), and fibrous hamartoma of infancy (FHI).

ICD-O coding
None

ICD-11 coding
LA14.2 & XH2P15 Structural developmental anomalies of orbit & Mesenchymal hamartoma

Related terminology
Rhabdomyomatous mesenchymal hamartoma
Acceptable: striated muscle hamartoma.
Not recommended: hamartoma of cutaneous adnexa and mesenchyme; congenital midline hamartoma.

Chondromesenchymal hamartoma
Acceptable: chondroid hamartoma.
Not recommended: mesenchymoma; nasal hamartoma.

Fibrous hamartoma of infancy
Not recommended: subdermal fibromatous tumour of infancy.

Subtype(s)
None

Localization
RMH presents most often in the subcutis of the head and neck {867}. Three primary orbital RMHs have been reported {2124, 2544}. CMH typically occurs in the sinonasal tract in children (nasal CMH), with possible orbital and skull involvement {1140}. There are two reports of primary orbital CMH {395,1205}, and several reports of nasal cases extending into the orbit {3096, 2852,1140}. FHI presents in the axilla, back, or upper arm in about one half of cases and is distributed widely over the body in the other half {86}. Two FHIs have arisen in the orbit {86,599}.

Clinical features
All three subtypes can present as a painless orbital mass resulting variably in proptosis, ptosis, and altered ocular motility. Although nasal CMH is benign, it can be locally invasive with potential intracranial or paranasal sinus invasion {1140}. MRI distinguishes primary orbital CMH from nasal CMH {1205}.

Epidemiology
RMH is rare, and 80% of tumours have a clinical onset before 18 years of age {867}. Both reported orbital RMHs were in children {2124,2544}. Nasal CMHs are rare {1140,3460} with the majority presenting in newborn infants and young children and more rarely in adolescents {1140}. The two reported orbital CMHs were in young children {395,3096}. FHI is also rare, with 91% of cases in children < 2 years of age and an M:F ratio of 2.7 {1140}.

Etiology
Unknown

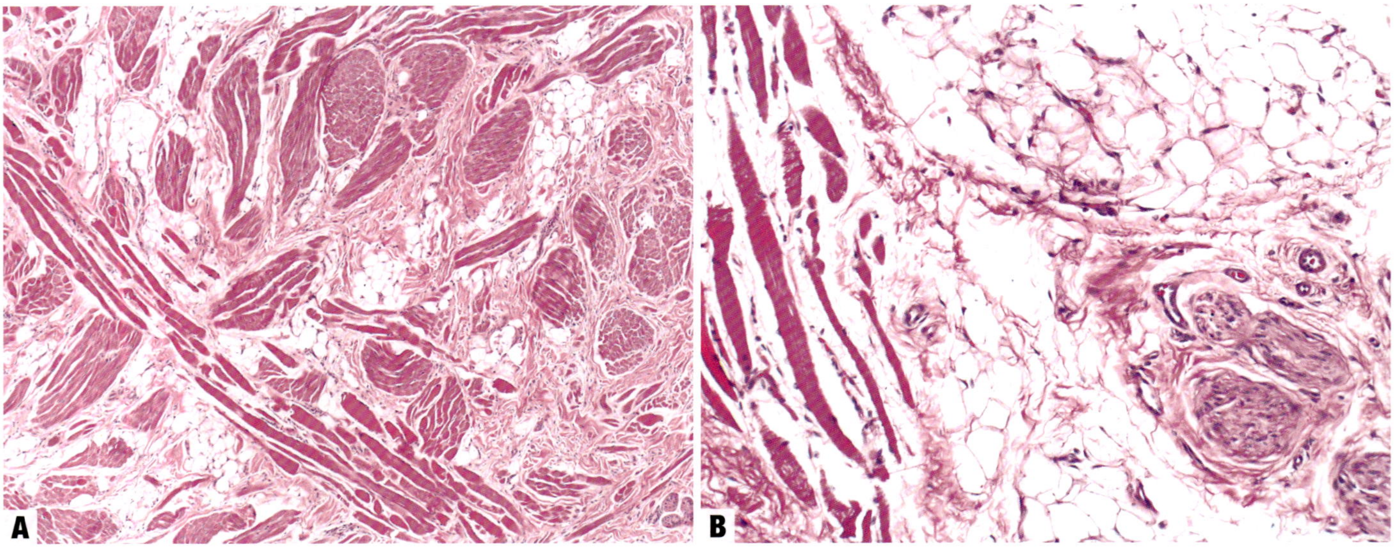

Fig. 9.23 Rhabdomyomatous mesenchymal hamartoma. **A** Low-power view showing randomly arranged bundles of mature striated muscle fibres and benign admixed adipose tissue, collagen, and blood vessels. **B** Medium-power view showing mature striated muscle, adipose tissue, collagen, blood vessels, and peripheral nerves.

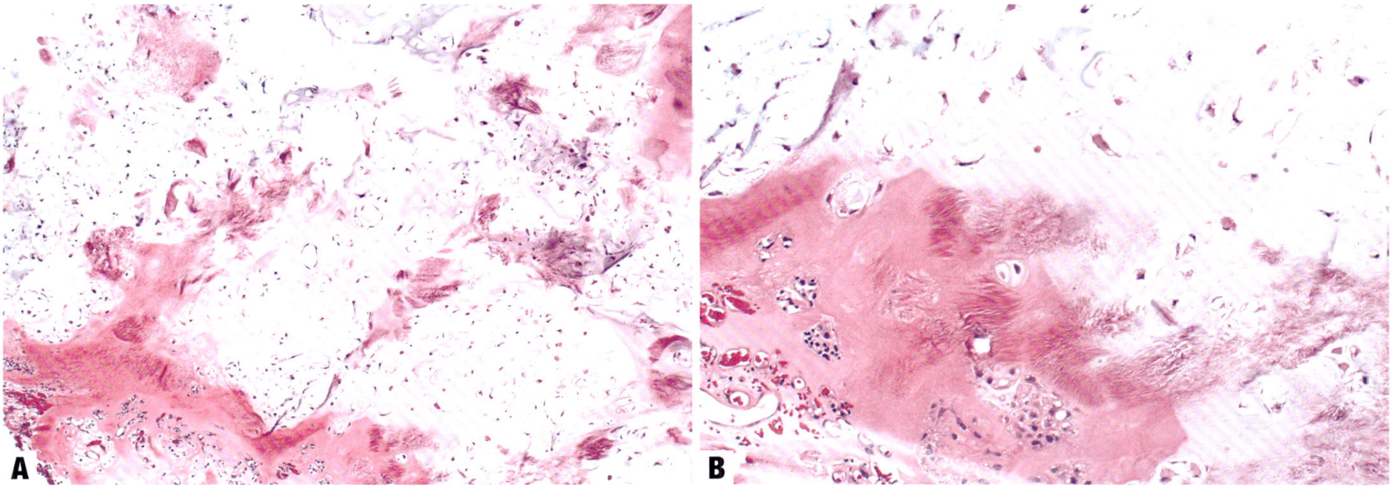

Fig. 9.24 Chondromesenchymal hamartoma. **A** Low-power view showing irregular islands of mature hyaline cartilage separated by collagenous septa. **B** Medium-power view showing vascularized fibrocollagenous tissue merging with mature hyaline cartilage.

Pathogenesis

RMH is considered a congenital hamartoma in 80% of cases and an acquired tumour in 20% {867}. Nasal CMH is regarded as a congenital hamartoma analogous to mesenchymal hamartoma of the chest wall {2136}. Nasal CMH is associated with pathogenic germline *DICER1* variants that give rise to *DICER1*-related tumour predisposition syndrome {3460}. A review of 58 reported cases of nasal CMH showed that 38% had at least one additional *DICER1*-associated tumour {3460}. A recent study of 12 FHI tumours, none from the orbit, identified *EGFR* exon insertion/deletion mutations in all cases {2492}.

Macroscopic appearance

Nasal CMHs are usually removed in fragments that vary from firm and white, typical of cartilage, to soft, fleshy, and tan {2136}. The primary orbital CMH reported by Bowen et al. was "pearly white, firm, well-circumscribed, and composed of several lobules" {395}. Dermal and subcutaneous FHIs are mostly rounded or bosselated with firm, glistening, greyish-white tissue intermixed with islands of yellow fat {900}.

Histopathology

RMH shows randomly arranged mature striated muscle fibres with an admixture of adipose tissue, collagen, blood vessels, and peripheral nerves {2681,2124}. Orbital RMH may be composed predominantly of bland spindle-shaped cells with scattered skeletal muscle fibres and intermixed collagen {2544}. Nasal CMH shows irregular islands of hyaline cartilage with variable components of mesenchyme and fibro-osseous tissue {3418,1382}. Both of the reported primary orbital CMHs had mature hyaline cartilage {395,1205}. FHI has varying proportions of mature adipose tissue, intersecting fascicles of fibroblastic/myofibroblastic cells, and myxoid nodules of primitive-appearing spindled to stellate mesenchymal cells {900,86} with 30% of cases having hyalinized zones {86}

Cytology

FNAB of FHI shows fibroblastic-appearing cells, fatty tissue, and collagenous material without significant nuclear atypia or mitoses {1447}.

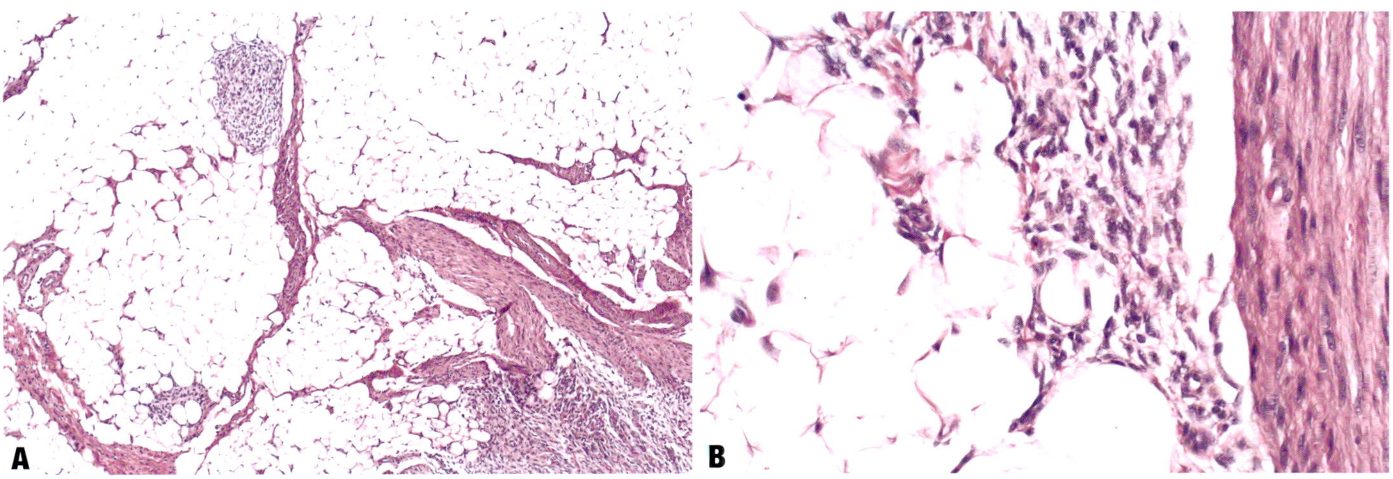

Fig. 9.25 Fibrous hamartoma of infancy. **A** Low-power view showing the triphasic morphology with mature adipose tissue, bundles of bland fibroblastic/myofibroblastic cells, and areas of primitive mesenchyme. **B** Medium-power view of mature adipose tissue, primitive mesenchyme, and bland fibroblastic/myofibroblastic cells.

Diagnostic molecular pathology

A diagnosis of CMH should prompt referral for *DICER1* genetic testing and lifelong surveillance if positive {3460}.

Essential and desirable diagnostic criteria

Rhabdomyomatous mesenchymal hamartoma

Essential: randomly arranged mature striated muscle fibres and benign admixed adipose tissue, collagen, and blood vessels.
Desirable: peripheral nerves.

Chondromesenchymal hamartoma

Essential: irregular islands of benign hyaline cartilage with variable components of mesenchyme.
Desirable: DICER1 testing.

Fibrous hamartoma of infancy

Essential: triphasic morphology with varying proportions of mature adipose tissue, bundles of cytologically bland fibroblastic/myofibroblastic cells, and nodules of primitive mesenchyme.

Staging

Not clinically relevant

Prognosis and prediction

Nasal CMH may recur if not completely excised {1140}, and there are rare reports of malignant transformation of adult tumours {1939,651}. FHIs may recur in about 1% of cases, but there were no metastases in a series of 145 cases {86}.

Teratoma

Mulay K
Mishra DK

Definition
Teratomas are a family of embryonic tumours comprising tissues derived from all three germ cell layers: ectoderm, mesoderm, and endoderm.

ICD-O coding
9080/0 Mature teratoma
9080/3 Immature teratoma
9080/3 Malignant teratoma

ICD-11 coding
2F36.3 & XH3GV5 Teratoma of orbit & Teratoma, benign
2F36.3 & XH7YZ9 Teratoma of orbit & Teratoma, malignant, NOS

Related terminology
None

Subtype(s)
Mature teratoma; immature teratoma; adult teratoma; infantile (congenital) teratoma

Localization
Lesions are found in the orbit and occasionally within the eye.

Clinical features
Congenital (infantile) orbital teratomas present in healthy newborns as rapidly growing, tense, and fluctuating masses causing massive, unilateral proptosis with chemosis, exposure keratopathy, and eyelid distension with elongation of the palpebral fissure {3392,2528,2857}. Intracranial extension, although rare, has been documented and may be seen at presentation or occur later {2857,1130,2926}.

Adult orbital teratomas are mostly unilateral and present as mobile, non-tender, slow-growing masses that are easily dissectible from the surrounding tissue {2665}.

At imaging, teratomas are well circumscribed and cystic, revealing hyperintense T1- and T2-weighted sequences due to the sebaceous content on MRI {2665}. Fat attenuation in a cyst is diagnostic of mature cystic teratoma. Cartilage, calcification, and fibrosis result in echogenic foci.

Epidemiology
True congenital (infantile) orbital teratomas represent 0.3–1.3% of childhood orbital tumours {3392}. Adult orbital teratomas are extremely rare compared with those in infants; they mostly involve the lacrimal gland {2665,3116}. No definitive sex bias has been observed.

Etiology
Unknown

Pathogenesis
Origin from a primordial germ cell is the most likely possibility. The exact stimuli for differentiation and mechanisms of development are not yet elucidated.

Macroscopic appearance
The tumours are soft to firm, and frequently nodular. The cut sections show heterogeneity due to the presence of several tissue types and usually appear solid and cystic. Solid areas are firm to soft and grey-white to tan. Cysts are filled with serous, mucoid, or keratinous material. Rokitansky tubercles from which hair typically arises, may be seen in the wall. Cartilage, bone, and tooth may be identified grossly

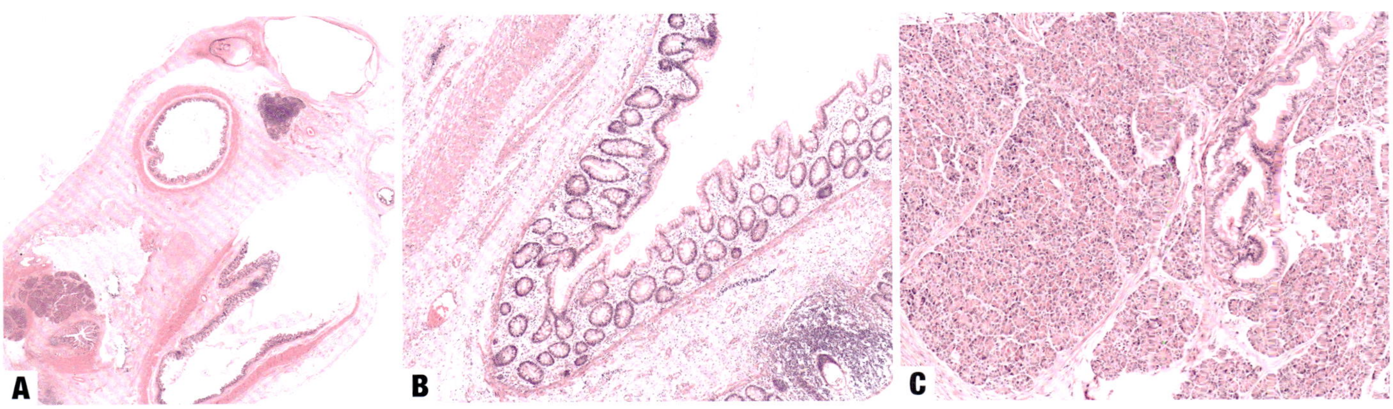

Fig. 9.26 Orbital teratoma. **A** A tumour with solid and cystic areas is seen. **B** Intestinal-type epithelium and glands are frequently observed endodermal derivatives in these tumours. **C** Pancreatic tissue of endodermal origin may be seen in these tumours.

Histopathology

Ectodermal derivatives include squamous epithelium, cutaneous adnexal structures, hair, and tooth enamel; neuroectodermal tissues are glia, ependyma, and cerebellum. Mesodermal derivatives include adipose, bone, cartilage, and smooth muscle. Endodermal derivatives include gastrointestinal and respiratory/bronchial epithelium, thyroid, pancreas, and salivary glands. Stroma may show fibroblastic, myofibroblastic, smooth muscle, and even skeletal muscle differentiation. Fat necrosis and foreign body reaction to keratin may be present.

Immature teratomas contain variable amounts of immature tissues, mostly neuroectodermal tubules and rosettes. Immature orbital teratomas have not been described in adults.

Cytology

Not reported

Diagnostic molecular pathology

Not relevant

Essential and desirable diagnostic criteria

Essential: tissue derived from at least two of the three germ layers (ectoderm, mesoderm, or endoderm); the tissue types may range from mature and completely differentiated to immature and undifferentiated.

Staging

Pure extragonadal teratomas are benign and are not staged.

Prognosis and prediction

Since most orbital teratomas are benign, complete surgical excision is the treatment of choice. Given that infantile teratomas may extend intracranially or recur or undergo malignant transformation, close follow-up is recommended {2411,2528,59, 3051,2033,2857,1130,2926}.

Yolk sac tumour

Proia AD
Mishra DK

Definition
Yolk sac tumour (YST) is a malignant germ cell neoplasm with variable histological patterns reflecting stages in the phylogenetic development of extraembryonic membranes such as the allantois and the yolk sac.

ICD-O coding
9071/3 Yolk sac tumour

ICD-11 coding
2D04 & XH09W7 Malignant neoplasm of orbit & Yolk sac tumour

Related terminology
Not recommended: endodermal sinus tumour.

Subtype(s)
None

Localization
YST occurs in the orbit, most often in the extraconal space, with possible extension into the nasopharynx, paranasal sinuses, or cranium {1586}.

Clinical features
Orbital YST usually presents in early childhood with an average presentation age of 27 months {1586,98,2570,1806}. One orbital YST arose at age 14 years {50}, but all others arose at ≤ 4 years of age. The M:F ratio is 1:1.6 (7 male patients vs 11 female patients). Common clinical features include progressive proptosis, ptosis, ophthalmoplegia, vision loss, relative afferent pupillary defect, exposure keratopathy, and inflammatory symptoms and signs {1586}. Orbital YST may be well delineated or infiltrative on CT or MRI {1586}. Serum AFP was elevated in the cases where it was measured {411,2242,1806,2570}.

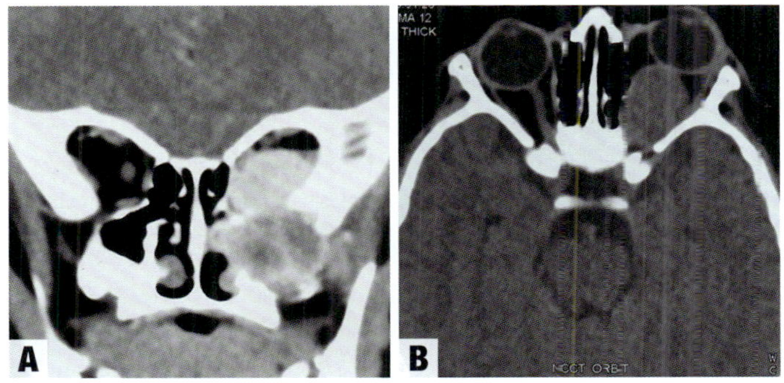

Fig. 9.27 Yolk sac tumour. **A** Contrast-enhanced CT shows a well-defined mass with multiple cysts extending from the left pterygopalatine fossa through the inferior orbital fissure. **B** Contrast-enhanced CT shows the well-defined mass extending to the left globe inferior to the optic nerve.

Epidemiology
Orbital YST is rare, with only 19 reported cases {1586,98,2570,1806}.

Etiology
Unknown

Pathogenesis
Orbital YST is postulated to arise from ectopic extraembryonic germ cells or defective embryogenesis {1586,1728}.

Macroscopic appearance
Not available

Histopathology
Orbital YSTs feature a meshwork of spaces lined by flat to cuboidal epithelium with marked cellular anaplasia and conspicuous mitoses {2070}. There may be a microcystic, macrocystic,

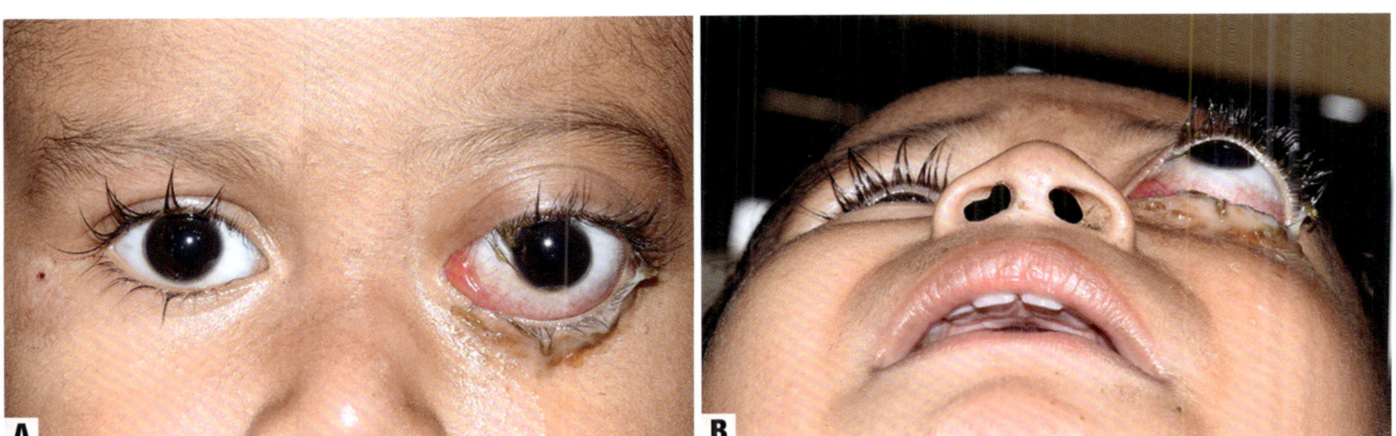

Fig. 9.28 Yolk sac tumour. **A,B** Clinical image of a yolk sac tumour in a 3-year-old boy who presented with an acute-onset painless progressive protrusion of the left eye

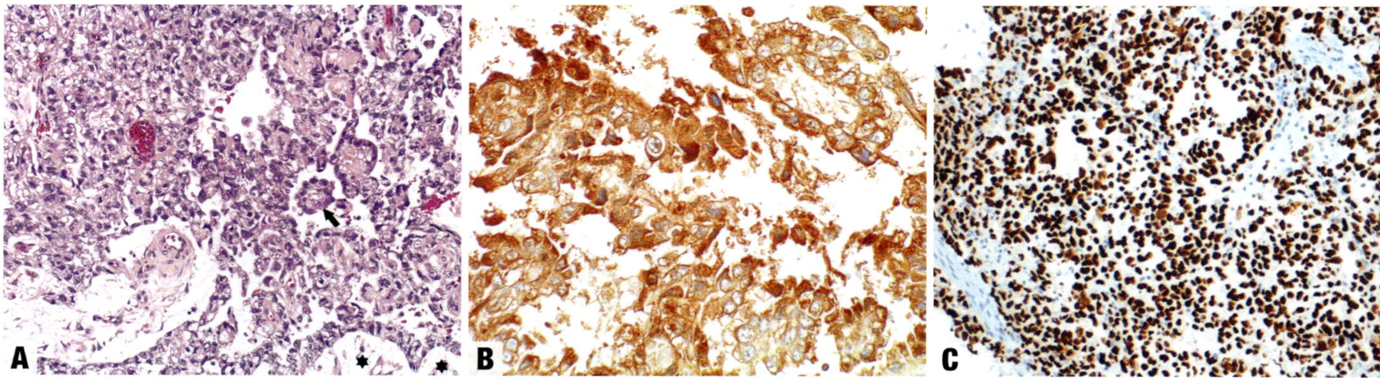

Fig. 9.29 Yolk sac tumour. **A** Irregular anastomosing channels are lined by cuboidal tumour cells with formation of cystic spaces (asterisks). A Schiller–Duval body is near the centre (arrow). **B** The tumour cells have strong cytoplasmic staining for AFP. **C** The tumour cells exhibit strong nuclear expression of SALL4.

reticular, alveolar-glandular, or myxomatous pattern {1586}. Schiller–Duval bodies (fibrovascular cores covered by a layer of embryonic epithelium) may be present or absent {1586}. The stroma and tumour cells contain hyaline globules that are PAS-positive and diastase resistant {2070,1586}. There is strong cytoplasmic staining for AFP, CAM5.2 {1586}, and glypican-3 (GPC3) {2570}, and nuclear expression of SALL4 {2570}, similarly to other extragonadal YSTs {3540}.

Cytology

Not clinically relevant / not described for orbital YSTs

Diagnostic molecular pathology

Not clinically relevant

Essential and desirable diagnostic criteria

Essential: primitive germ cell tumour exhibiting stages in the phylogenetic development of extraembryonic membranes.

Desirable: positive immunohistochemical staining for AFP, GPC3, or SALL4.

Staging

Not clinically relevant / not described for orbital YSTs

Prognosis and prediction

Prognostic and management guidelines are not available for primary orbital YST. Proptosis allowing early tumour detection may result in a better prognosis for orbital YST than other extragonadal YSTs {2070}. Chemotherapy and radiotherapy may provide long-term disease-free survival {2070,1710}.

Primary orbital melanoma

Mudhar HS
Coupland SE

Definition
Primary orbital melanoma is a primary malignant melanocytic neoplasm of the orbital soft tissue, without a prior history of conjunctival, uveal, or non-ocular melanoma.

ICD-O coding
8720/3 Primary orbital melanoma

ICD-11 coding
2D04 & XH1G74 Malignant neoplasm of orbit & Blue naevus, malignant

Related terminology
None

Subtype(s)
None

Localization
The tumour is located in the orbital soft tissues, can affect any quadrant, and can be extraconal or intraconal {3305,2769,971, 3069,2294,30}. It has been reported in the left orbit in 58% of cases, and the right in 42%.

Clinical features
The commonest presentations are unilateral proptosis, decreased visual acuity, periorbital pain, and diplopia. Other signs include ptosis, eyelid swelling, visual disturbances, and relative afferent pupillary defect. Imaging shows a well-circumscribed enhancing lesion, resembling a benign vascular lesion. The duration of symptoms varies between 3 and 156 months. There may be signs of ocular or oculodermal melanocytosis {3305,2769,971,3069,2294,30}.

Epidemiology
The age range of presentation is 5–91 years, with a median of 45 years. There is a male predilection (58% male and 42% female patients). Most patients are White European (95%), with very occasional cases recorded in South Asian and African Black patients {3305,2769,971,3069,2294,30}.

Etiology
Unknown

Pathogenesis
Primary orbital melanomas are thought to arise from melanocytic cells of the leptomeninges or ciliary nerves, or from ectopic intraorbital nests of melanocytes. They can occur de novo but are usually in association with pigmentary changes of the periocular tissues – such as naevus of Ota, cellular blue naevus, or oculodermal melanocytosis. The underlying genomic alterations vary and include some that are similar but not identical to those occurring in ocular melanomas. These include mutations in *GNAQ*, *GNA11*, *EIF1AX*, and *SF3B1*, with copy-number variations including chromosomal gains in 6p, 8q, 17q, 6q, and 20p, and losses in 1p, 9p, 16q, and 17p {2768,2294}.

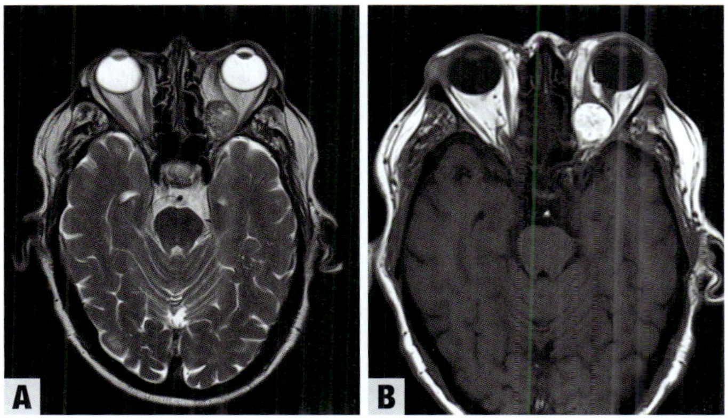

Fig. 9.30 Primary orbital melanoma. **A** T1-weighted axial MRI shows a hyperintense well-defined lesion of primary orbital melanoma, located in the left medial rectus muscle close to the orbital apex. **B** On T2-weighted axial MRI the primary orbital melanoma is hypointense when compared with the vitreous.

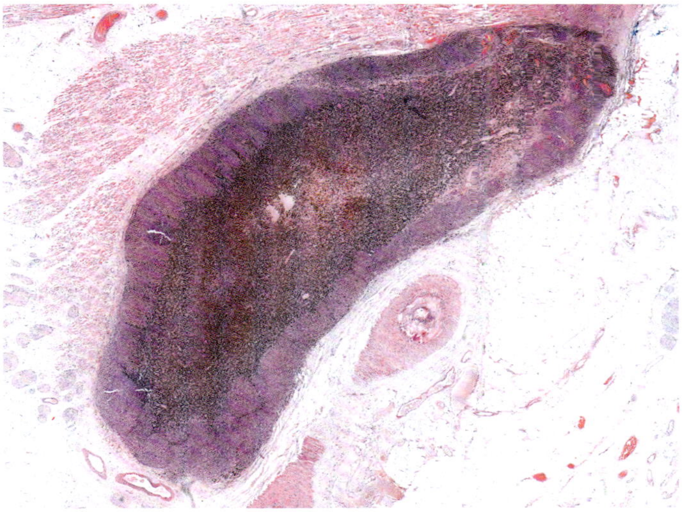

Fig. 9.31 Primary orbital melanoma. Scanning power showing a well-defined deposit of primary orbital melanoma, situated between the optic nerve and a dilated orbital blood vessel on the left and extraocular muscle to the right.

Macroscopic appearance
The cut surface shows a well-defined tumour that can be amelanotic or variably pigmented. The tumour can be extraconal or intraconal. There may be involvement of orbital fat, fascial planes, extraocular muscle, and moulding against the sclera.

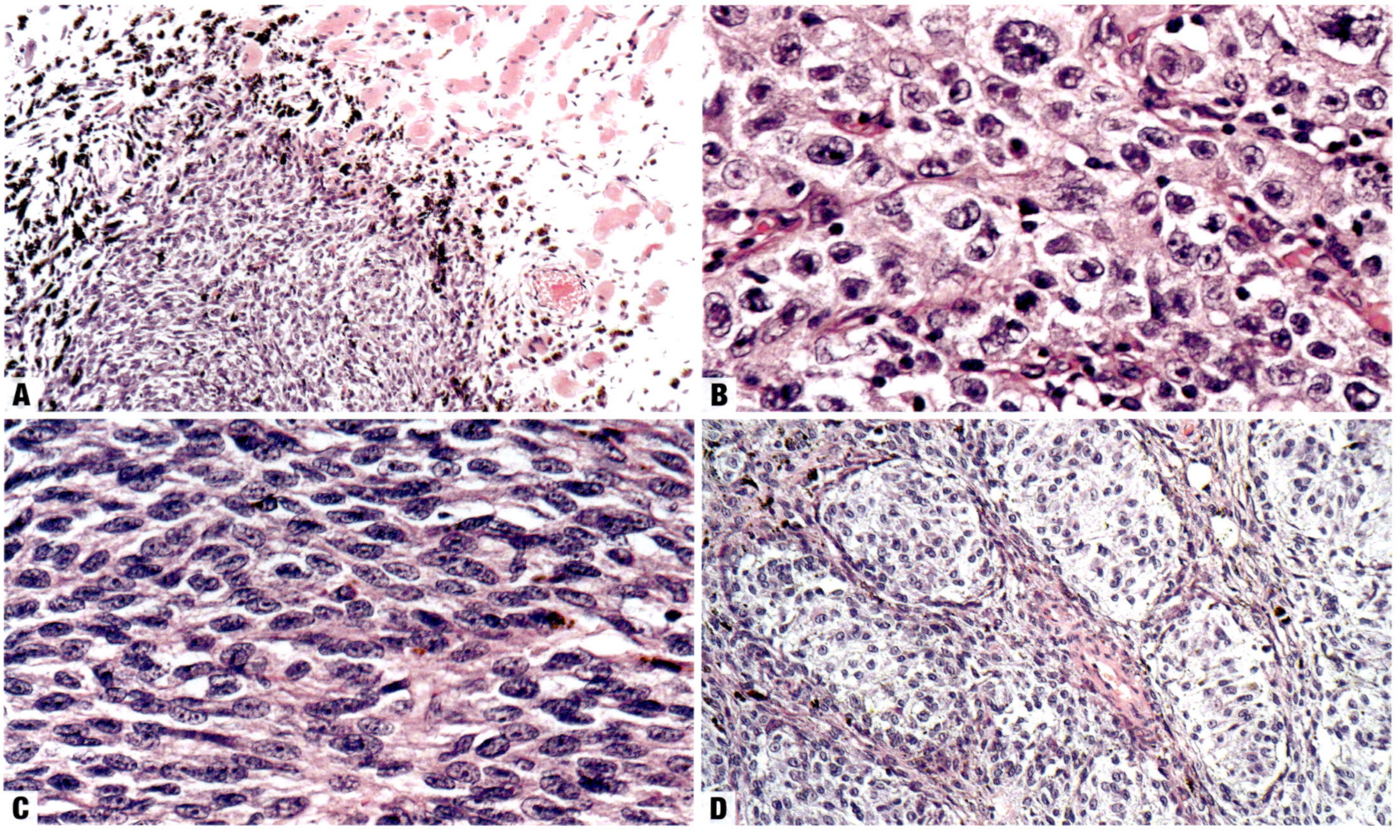

Fig. 9.32 Primary orbital melanoma. **A** The melanoma is surrounded by melanophages and interfaces with orbital fat and extraocular muscle tissue. **B** Epithelioid cells within a primary orbital melanoma. **C** Spindle melanoma cells in a primary orbital melanoma. **D** Clones in a primary orbital melanoma arranged as back-to-back ovoid nodules.

Histopathology

Two types of melanoma cells can be identified – spindle and epithelioid – identical to uveal melanoma (see *Choroidal and ciliary body melanomas*, p. 179) {3305,2294}, giving rise to spindle, mixed, or epithelioid melanomas. Mitotic figures are present, and necrosis is seen in some cases. The melanoma cells can exhibit a packeted arrangement of clones separated by extracellular matrix {3305,2294}. Some cases show balloon cell change {2294}. Melanophages are commonly seen throughout the tumour. The background orbital soft tissue may show orbital melanocytosis, oculodermal melanocytosis, or orbital blue naevi (conventional and cellular) {3305,2294, 797}. These are characterized by benign pigmented or non-pigmented melanocytic cells that can be spindle or multipolar,

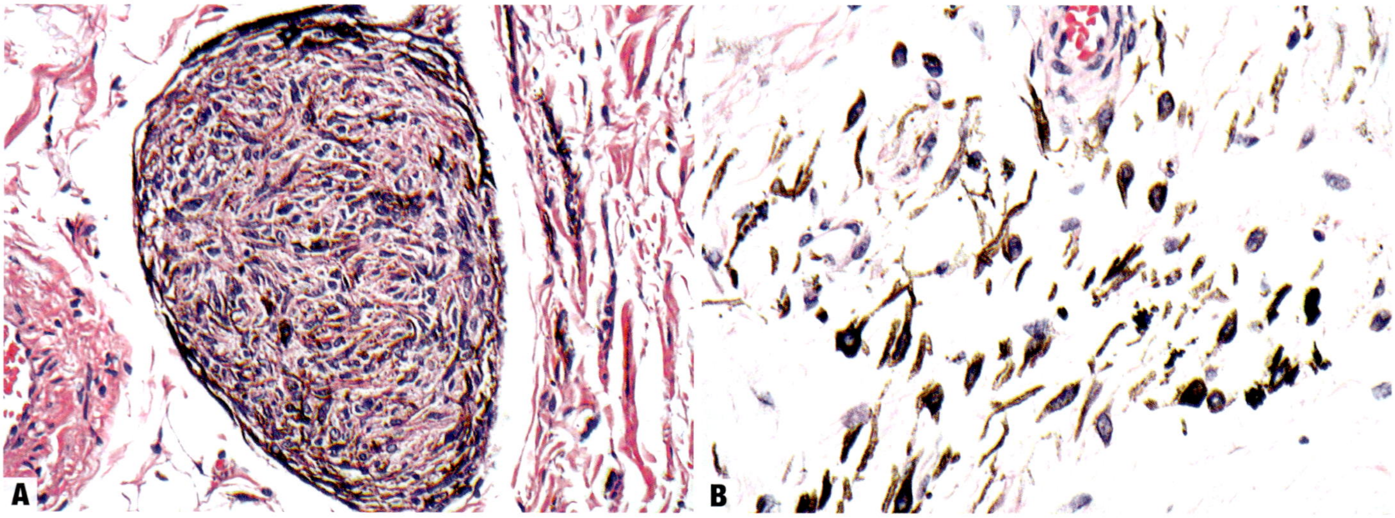

Fig. 9.33 Primary orbital melanoma precursor lesions. **A** Cellular blue naevus in the orbital soft tissue from which primary orbital melanoma can arise. **B** Benign, pigmented spindle cells of oculodermal melanocytosis, present in the orbital adipose tissue, from which primary orbital melanoma can arise.

scattered individually or as groups or larger cohesive swathes, associated with sclerotic stroma and melanophages.

Immunohistochemistry

The melanoma cells are positive for S100, melan-A, HMB45, and SOX10. Some cases are nuclear BAP1-negative {2768, 2294}.

Differential diagnosis

Differential diagnosis includes spread or metastasis of conjunctival, uveal, or non-ocular melanoma to the orbit (secondary orbital melanoma) {2766} and orbital clear cell sarcoma {2294}. The latter can be tested for the presence or absence of the *EWSR1::ATF1* fusion gene.

Cytology

No cases reported

Diagnostic molecular pathology

A mutation panel comprising the following aids in the diagnosis of primary orbital melanoma in the context of the clinical history and findings: *GNAQ*, *GNA11*, *BRAF*, *NRAS*, *TERT* promoter, *SF3B1*, and *EIF1AX* {2768,2294}.

Essential and desirable diagnostic criteria

Essential: cytologically malignant melanocytic cells arising in the orbital soft tissue; no previous history of conjunctival, uveal, or non-ocular melanoma.

Desirable: immunohistochemical positivity with melanocytic markers; presence of blue naevus (conventional or cellular), or oculodermal melanocytosis in background orbital soft tissue.

Staging

American Joint Committee on Cancer (AJCC) TNM staging for orbital tumours can be applied after detailed imaging investigations are undertaken to confirm the primary site of origin of the tumour and the extent of its spread.

Prognosis and prediction

Most cases are treated by exenteration, followed by adjuvant radiotherapy and chemotherapy in a smaller number of cases {30}. Adjuvant radiotherapy confers a better survival advantage. Proton beam therapy can control local orbital recurrences {30}. Metastases develop in 36% of patients, 15% develop local recurrence, and 32% die of metastatic disease {30}.

Some genetic evidence suggests that mutations in *SF3B1* and *EIF1AX* confer a more favourable prognosis {2768}.

Chapter 9

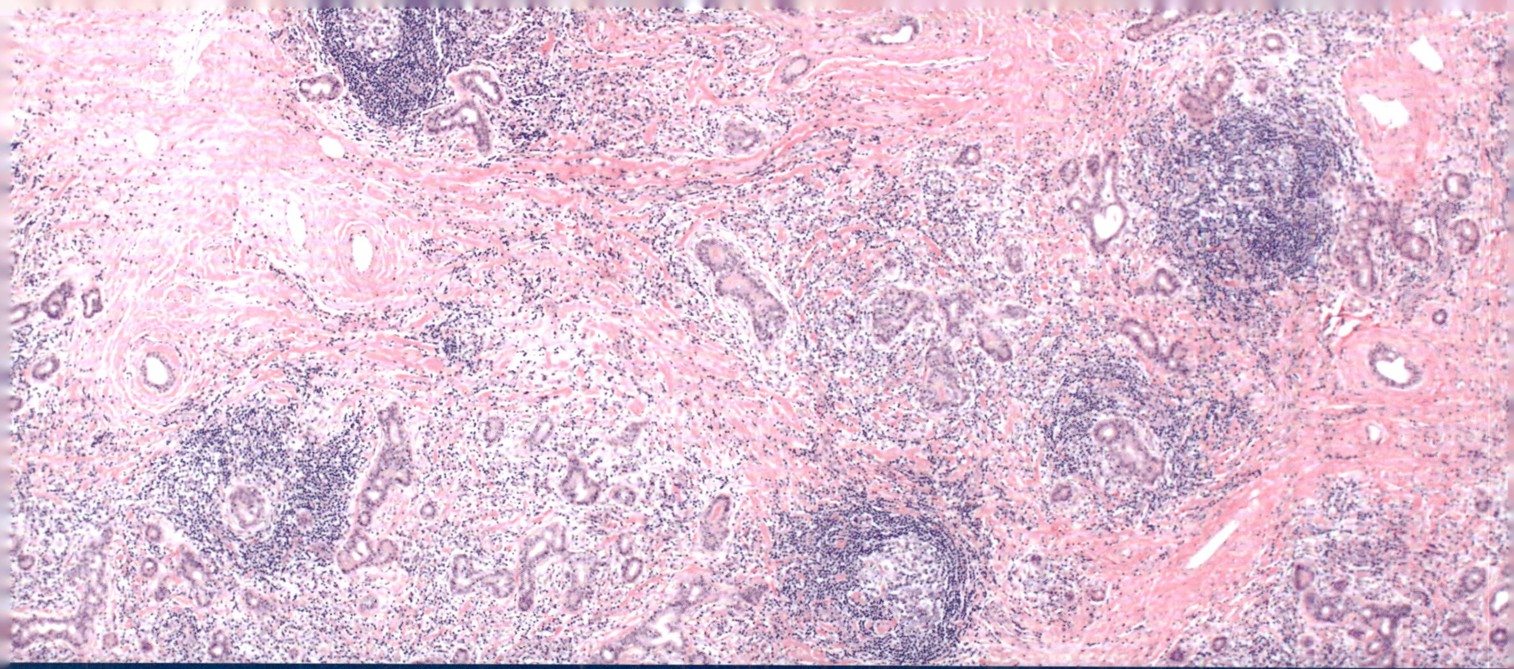

10

Haematolymphoid tumours

Edited by: Coupland SE, Heegaard S, Khoury JD

Haematolymphoid tumours: Introduction

Heegaard S
Khoury JD

This chapter on tumours of haematolymphoid origin of the ocular region describes reactive lesions of the conjunctiva and orbit, intraocular lymphomas (i.e. vitreoretinal lymphoma and primary choroidal lymphoma), ocular adnexal lymphoma of B-cell type and T/NK-cell type, myeloid tumours, and histiocytic and dendritic neoplasms.

All of these tumours are extranodal neoplasms, as there are no lymph nodes in the ocular region. Each of the haematolymphoid and histiocytic/dendritic neoplasms are described in more detail in the *Haematolymphoid tumours* volume {3594}.

The ocular adnexa are affected by many reactive conditions and are part of the eye-associated lymphoid tissue and mucosa-associated lymphoid tissue system {1746}. A table is provided in this chapter (see Table 10.01, p. 324, in *Reactive lymphoid hyperplasia*) to help enable the differentiation between reactive lymphoid hyperplasia and some common B-cell non-Hodgkin lymphomas (NHL) that affect the ocular adnexa. An entity that is commonly asked to be excluded is IgG4 disease, which is dealt with in *IgG4-related disease* (p. 326), clearly outlining the required features to make this diagnosis {1677}, and with an emphasis on clinicopathological correlation.

The B-cell NHLs are the most common lymphoma type affecting this region. T-cell lymphomas are rare; however, they may occur in the eyelids as primary or secondary tumours. The chapter commences with the intraocular lymphomas – vitreoretinal lymphoma and primary choroidal lymphoma – each differing from the other significantly with respect to NHL subtype and clinical course.

Vitreoretinal lymphoma – a high-grade B-cell lymphoma, arising in an immune-privileged environment {2153} – is notoriously difficult to diagnose and is a masquerader in chronic uveitis cases. It should always be considered in the differential diagnosis, in both immunocompetent and immunodeficient patients, to decrease diagnostic delays. Repeated vitrectomies and/or chorioretinal biopsies may be required before a definitive diagnosis is achieved. Molecular testing for either clonality or *MYD88* and/or *CD79B* mutations is of value {379}. In contrast, primary choroidal lymphoma is a low-grade B-cell lymphoma, mimicking uveal effusion syndrome and typically diagnosed on FNAB. It responds well to low-dose radiotherapy {677}.

A major advantage when diagnosing ocular adnexal lymphomas is that they are usually visible, and more accessible for biopsy. This provides the unique opportunity to correlate clinical appearance and clinical behaviour with the histological, immunophenotypic, and genetic features of these conditions. The most common orbital tumours are NHLs, with the extranodal marginal zone B-cell lymphoma being the most frequent type {1341}.

In recent years, genome-wide studies have contributed to a better understanding of molecular pathways involved in the pathogenesis of the various types of NHL. This has resulted in the identification of additional diagnostic and prognostic criteria, and of new potential therapeutic targets. Thus, the integration of histological, immunophenotypic, and genetic markers, together with clinicopathological correlation, is essential for an accurate diagnosis of ocular lymphoma.

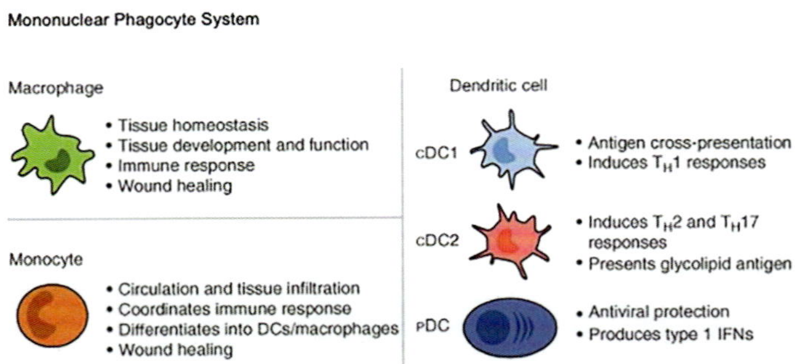

Fig. 10.01 Mononuclear phagocyte populations. The self-maintaining haematopoietic stem cells in the bone marrow give rise to common monocyte progenitors and common dendritic cell (DC) precursors. The latter differentiate into either conventional (cDC) or plasmacytoid (pDC) dendritic cells. Monocytes can further differentiate into monocyte-derived cells, macrophages, and DCs under certain conditions. Macrophages originally present in tissues have an embryonic origin and maintain themselves. TH, T helper; IFN, interferon.

Finally, this chapter briefly addresses the histiocytic and dendritic cell disorders seen in the ocular region, predominantly in the ocular adnexa. They are supposed to originate from and/or show differentiation towards cells of the mononuclear phagocyte system, which includes monocytes, macrophages, and dendritic cells. The term "histiocyte" has been variably defined and used, equating with macrophages or also including dendritic cells. In contrast, the adjective "histiocytic" has been used for a broad spectrum of disorders, which morphologically show large "epithelioid" cells with poorly defined, mostly moderately stained cytoplasm (e.g. histiocytic haemangioma, histiocytic breast carcinoma metastases). In general, clinicopathological correlation is the gold standard of diagnosis for histiocytic and dendritic cell disorders. Amendments since the last edition relate to genetic alterations which are shown to be linked to biological behaviour such as in Langerhans cell histiocytosis, in which *BRAF* p.V600E is highly associated with increased risk of relapse {1321}. In those cases, *BRAF* p.V600E can serve as a therapeutic target {111}. In addition, other genetic alterations such as rearrangements in *RET* and *ALK* that may be targeted by selective inhibition have recently been identified in patients with histiocytosis {848}.

Reactive lymphoid hyperplasia

Salomao DR
Eberhart CG

Definition
Reactive lymphoid hyperplasia (RLH) is a benign, reactive, polyclonal lymphoid proliferation without cytological or architectural atypia, which may resemble B-cell lymphoma.

ICD-O coding
None

ICD-11 coding
9A22.Z Orbital inflammation, unspecified

Related terminology
Acceptable: lymphoid hyperplasia; (florid) follicular hyperplasia.
Not recommended: benign lymphoid proliferation; pseudotumour.

Subtype(s)
None

Localization
RLH may involve the ocular adnexa including eyelids, conjunctiva, orbital soft tissues, lacrimal gland, and drainage ducts {1426,589,1747,126}, as well as intraocular structures, such as the choroid {2959}.

Clinical features
Signs vary according to the tissues involved; however, RLH typically results in a unilateral, red or orange, painless swelling or tumour mass, leading to corresponding symptoms, such as proptosis, eyelid or conjunctival mass, decreased ocular motility and visual acuity, and diplopia, among others {3619}. Manifestations may be more severe in immunodeficient patients {2496,1799}. Because RLH is clinically and radiologically indistinguishable from low-grade lymphoma, a tissue biopsy is recommended in all cases {675}.

Epidemiology
RLH accounts for approximately 8–19% of cases categorized as ocular adnexal lymphoproliferative disease {155,3476}. It affects patients in their fifth to seventh decades of life, with no sex or race predilection {155}. RLH is uncommon in children {116,326,66}.

Etiology
The etiology is unknown, but RLH is probably caused by chronic antigen stimulation (either exogenous or endogenous antigens) leading to chronic inflammation and ultimately RLH. Implicated exogenous antigens include antigens associated with *Chlamydia psittaci*, *Chlamydophila pneumoniae*, *Chlamydia trachomatis*, *Helicobacter pylori*, EBV, and HTLV-1 {155}. Implicated endogenous antigens include those occurring in autoimmune diseases {1458}.

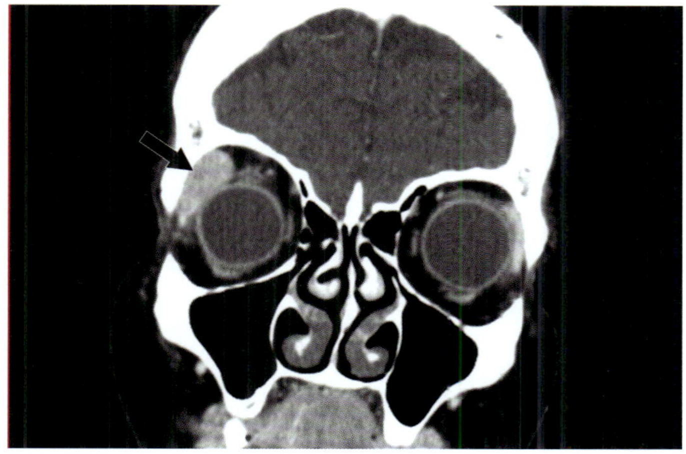

Fig. 10.02 Reactive lymphoid hyperplasia. Coronal CT with contrast shows an enlarged right lacrimal gland (arrow) with inferomedial displacement of the globe.

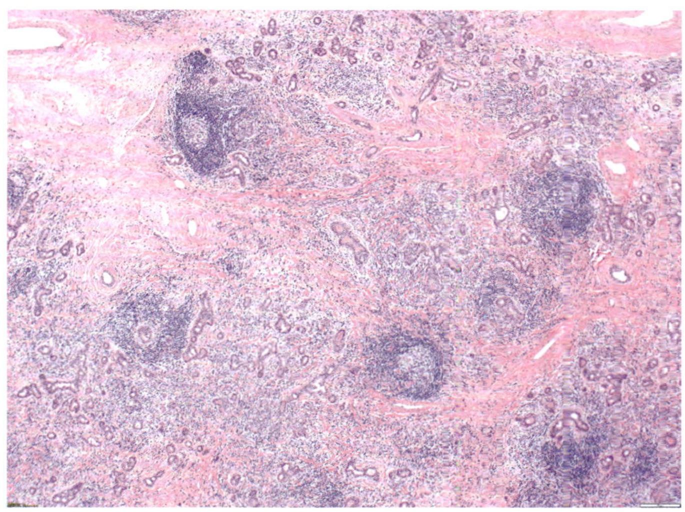

Fig. 10.03 Reactive lymphoid hyperplasia. Lacrimal gland biopsy shows acinar atrophy and lymphoid hyperplasia with numerous reactive follicles

Pathogenesis
It is proposed that either endogenous or exogenous chronic antigen stimulation leads to polyclonal expansion of B cells and T cells {1431}.

Macroscopic appearance
Macroscopic appearance is variable according to the site of involvement.

Histopathology
RLH shows a polymorphous infiltrate of mature lymphocytes within the stroma, as well as scattered irregular secondary

Table 10.01 Reactive follicular hyperplasia and differential diagnosis

Reactive follicular hyperplasia	Follicular lymphoma	Extranodal marginal zone B-cell lymphoma
Morphology		
Low density of follicles	High density of follicles	Low density of follicles
Follicles of uneven size and shape	Follicles usually of similar size and shape	Moth-eaten follicles of uneven size and shape
Mixture of cell types in GC	Monomorphic or polymorphic GC population	Mixture of cell types in GC
Tingible-body macrophages present	Tingible-body macrophages usually rare	Tingible-body macrophages present
Usually moderate to high mitotic rate	Usually low to moderate mitotic rate	Usually moderate to high mitotic rate
Cell polarization in GC often seen	Cell polarization in GC usually absent	Cell polarization in GC often seen
Mantle zone usually distinct	Mantle zone usually indistinct	Mantle zone compressed by enlarged marginal zone
Large interfollicular areas with admixed cells	Compressed interfollicular areas	Interfollicular areas filled by expanded marginal zones with centrocyte-like cells, monocytoid cells, and/or plasmacellular differentiated cells and extrafollicular blasts
		Lymphoepithelial lesions
Immunoprofile		
Normal distribution of B cells and T cells within and outside the GCs	Dominance of B cells on CD20, CD79a, or PAX5 staining, particularly in GC, with loss of follicular T cells and macrophages	Dominance of B cells on CD20, CD79a, or PAX5 staining in marginal zone
GC cells negative for BCL2; regular follicular dendritic cell network on CD23 immunohistochemistry	GC cells positive for BCL2, CD10, and BCL6; expanded follicular dendritic cell network on CD23 immunohistochemistry	GC cells negative for BCL2; residual follicular dendritic cell network on CD23 immunohistochemistry
Cell polarization in GC highlighted by Ki-67	Irregular scattered staining for Ki-67 without polarization	Cell polarization in GC highlighted by Ki-67
Mantle zone usually present in IgD stain	Mantle zone thinned or lost in IgD stain	Mantle zone thinned in IgD stain
Dominant T-cell population within interfollicular zone	Compressed T-cell interfollicular zone	Interfollicular zone replaced by neoplastic marginal zone B cells (CD20, CD79a, and/or PAX5)
Molecular pathology		
Polyclonal IgH PCR and TR PCR	Usually monoclonal on IgH PCR but can be polyclonal owing to a large number of somatic mutations	Usually monoclonal on IgH PCR
No demonstrable translocations, deletions, or mutations	Most common: t(14;18)(q32;q21) translocation associated with IGH::*BCL2* fusion	Trisomy of chromosomes 3 and 18 common; gain of 6p and loss of 6q as well as *TNFAIP3* mutation/deletion seen often in ocular adnexa

GC, germinal centre.

lymphoid follicles with regular germinal centres and narrow marginal and mantle zones {155,684}.

Immunohistochemistry

The infiltrate comprises a mixture of B and T cells arranged physiologically. The germinal centres are immunoreactive for CD10 and BCL6 but negative for BCL2 {155}.

Differential diagnosis

Differential diagnosis includes reactive lesions such as sarcoidosis, idiopathic orbital inflammation, IgG4-related disease {156}, Sjögren disease involving the lacrimal gland {2496}, and small cell B-cell lymphomas (extranodal marginal zone lymphoma, mantle cell lymphoma, follicular lymphoma).

Cytology

The distinction between reactive B-cell–rich lymphoid proliferations and small cell B-cell lymphoma is challenging on FNA specimens and is not advised as a primary diagnostic modality. However, flow cytometry immunophenotyping on aspiration material may be a helpful adjunct to confirm polytypic light chain expression by reactive B cells.

Diagnostic molecular pathology

Occasional cases may show distortion of normal architecture or cytological atypia, raising the question of lymphoma. Molecular studies may be helpful in such cases to demonstrate polyclonal or oligoclonal immunoglobulin gene rearrangement {2057, 2950,938}.

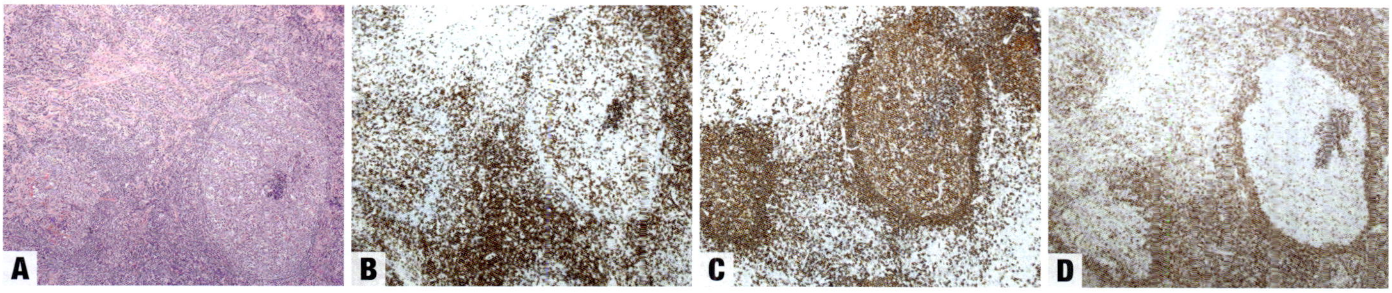

Fig. 10.04 Reactive lymphoid hyperplasia. **A** A right lateral orbital biopsy demonstrates reactive lymphoid hyperplasia. **B** CD3 immunostaining shows physiological distribution of T cells in the perifollicular region. **C** CD20 immunostaining demonstrates physiological distribution of B cells. **D** Centrocytes and centroblasts in the germinal centres are negative with BCL2 immunostaining.

Essential and desirable diagnostic criteria

Essential: identification of appropriate histological features and supporting ancillary studies (immunohistochemistry, flow cytometry, and clonal analyses); no diagnostic evidence of lymphoma or other neoplasm (see Table 10.01).

Desirable: identification of an infectious agent or evidence of underlying autoimmune disease, immunodeficiency, or other inflammatory condition on clinical and/or laboratory data.

Staging

Not applicable

Prognosis and prediction

RLH has a favourable outcome, which is dependent on the size of the lesion and available therapy. Most cases resolve spontaneously or respond to antibiotics or low-dose radiotherapy. Some larger lesions have been treated with intralesional steroids and/or rituximab {3619,3084}.

IgG4-related disease

Salomao DR
Eberhart CG
Verdijk RM

Definition

IgG4-related disease (IgG4-RD) is a chronic, fibroinflammatory process that can affect multiple organs, histologically characterized by storiform fibrosis and lymphoplasmacytic infiltration, with numerous IgG4-positive plasma cells and an increased ratio of IgG4:IgG positive cells (> 40%) and often with an elevated serum IgG4 titre.

ICD-O coding

9760/1 IgG4-related disease

ICD-11 coding

4A43.0 IgG4-related disease

Related terminology

Acceptable: IgG4-related orbital disease.

Not recommended: IgG4-related autoimmune disease; IgG4-related sclerosing disease; Küttner tumour; pseudotumour.

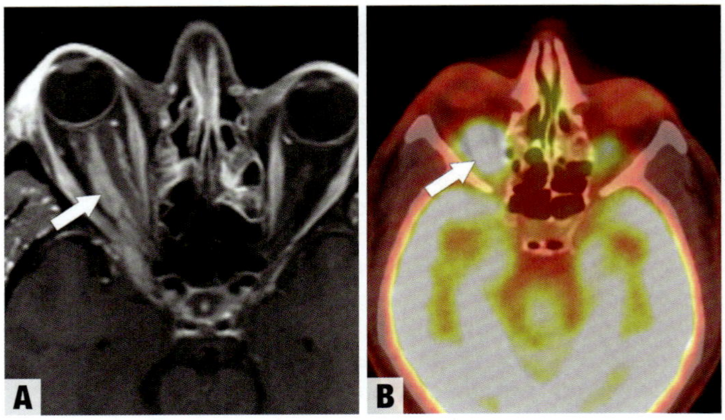

Fig. 10.05 IgG4-related disease. **A** Axial T1-weighted postcontrast MRI shows homogeneously enhancing soft tissue in the intraconal space of the right orbit (arrow) with proptosis. Enhancing soft tissue is also present in the right periorbital region. **B** Axial PET-CT shows FDG-avid disease in the right orbit (arrow).

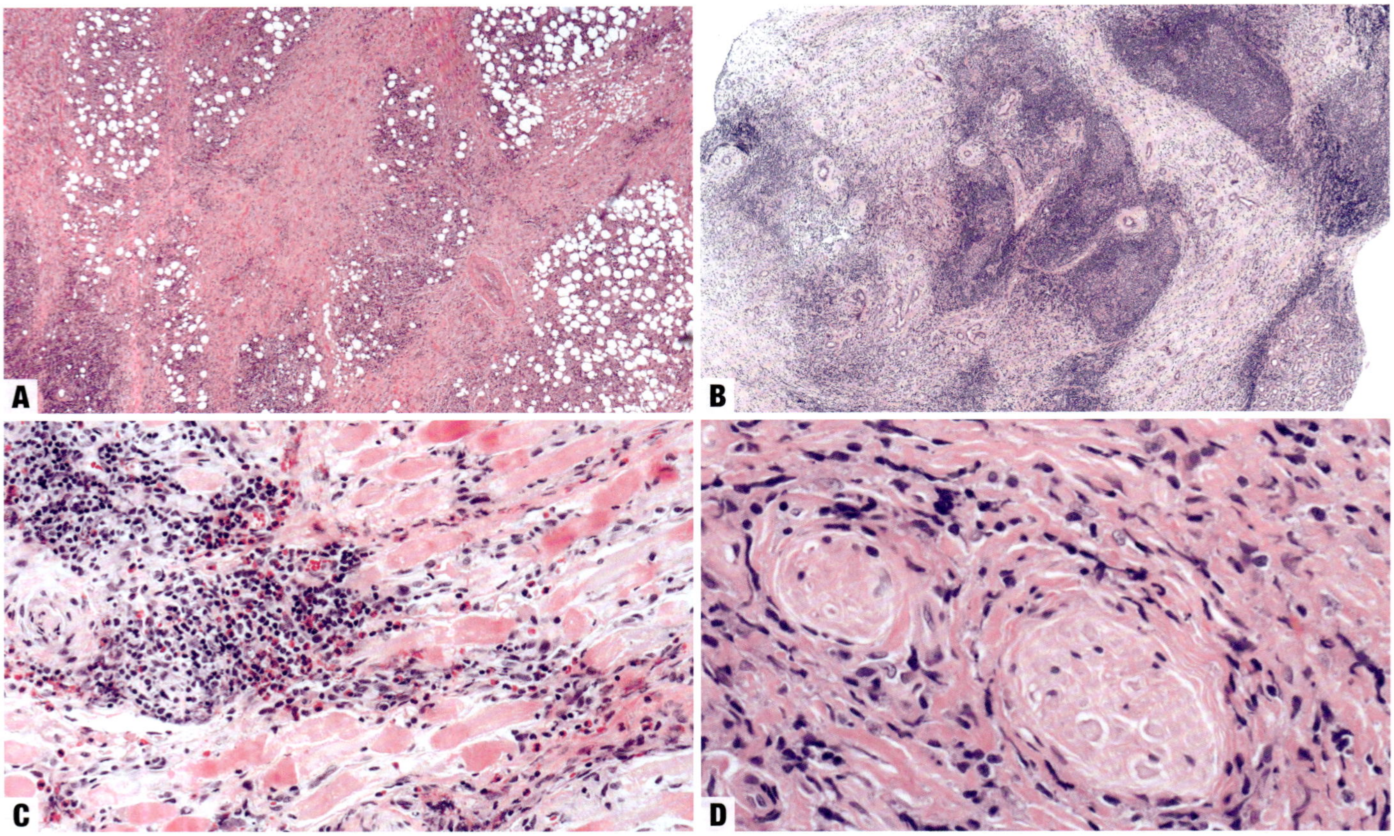

Fig. 10.06 IgG4 related disease. **A** Orbital biopsy shows background fibrosis and chronic inflammation. **B** Isolated unilateral IgG4-positive dacryoadenitis. Serum status unknown. Fibrotic phase with a dense lymphoplasmacellular inflammation with sparse eosinophils. **C** Isolated unilateral IgG4-positive orbital myositis. Serum IgG4 not elevated. Very good response on corticosteroids. Lymphoplasmacellular inflammation with eosinophils and fibrosis. **D** IgG4-related disease in the orbit characteristically shows involvement of trigeminal nerve branches.

Subtype(s)

None

Localization

IgG4-RD can affect almost any organ, and may affect single or multiple organs simultaneously or metachronously. The most common sites of ophthalmic involvement are the lacrimal glands {781,1389,779} and orbital soft tissues, mainly involving infraorbital nerves {1507,3156,885} and extraocular muscles {2149,860,1693}. More recently, tarsal, scleral, choroidal, and orbital bone involvement has been reported {3483,1610,3531,1068,1671,784}.

Table 10.02 Common sites involved by IgG4-related disease (IgG4-RD) and the salient clinical features (continued on next page)

Affected sites	Nomenclature (related/obsolete terminology)	IgG4+ cell count[a]	Salient clinical features
Pancreas	IgG4-related pancreatitis (autoimmune pancreatitis type 1; lymphoplasmacytic pancreatitis)	> 40/mm² (biopsy) > 200/mm² (excision)	• Parenchymal mass lesion mimicking pancreatic carcinoma (painless obstructive jaundice, pancreatic mass, abdominal pain) and/or pancreatic insufficiency (new-onset diabetes mellitus, steatorrhoea) • Sausage-shaped pancreas with delayed enhancement, capsule-like low-density rim, main pancreatic duct narrowing without upstream dilatation on contrast CT/MRI {3259}
Hepatobiliary system	IgG4-related sclerosing cholangitis	> 40/mm² (biopsy) > 200/mm² (excision)	• Biliary obstruction mimicking cholangiocarcinoma (obstructive jaundice, abnormal liver function tests) or primary sclerosing cholangitis but exhibiting dramatic response to steroids; frequently associated with IgG4-related pancreatitis • Diffuse or segmental narrowing of bile ducts and wall thickening on cholangiogram {1589}
	IgG4-related cholecystitis	> 40/mm² (biopsy) > 200/mm² (excision)	• Mass lesion mimicking cancer (right upper quadrant pain, jaundice) {943}
	IgG4-related hepatic inflammatory pseudotumour	> 40/mm² (biopsy) > 200/mm² (excision)	• Probably represents intrahepatic involvement of IgG4-related sclerosing cholangitis • Hepatic mass and abnormal liver function tests; contrast-enhancing mass lesion with dilatation of intrahepatic and peripheral bile ducts {1889}
Orbit, including lacrimal glands	IgG4-related ophthalmic disease, IgG4-related orbital inflammation, IgG4-related orbital myositis (orbital pseudotumour, idiopathic fibroinflammatory disease, idiopathic orbital inflammation)	> 400/mm²	• Unilateral or bilateral painless orbital swelling, proptosis and diplopia; rarely eye pain and visual impairment • Contrast-enhancing soft tissue mass; preferentially affecting lateral rectus muscle in contrast to Graves ophthalmopathy; bilateral infraorbital nerve involvement on imaging is pathognomonic of IgG4-related ophthalmic disease {1403,1696,578}
Salivary glands	IgG4-related sialadenitis (Küttner tumour, chronic sclerosing sialadenitis)	> 400/mm²	• Unilateral or bilateral painless swelling most commonly involving submandibular gland; occasionally simultaneous bilateral lacrimal, parotid, and submandibular gland involvement (Mikulicz disease); xerostomia is usually mild and responds well to steroids in contrast to Sjögren syndrome; sialography normal {1935}
Retroperitoneum, mediastinum, and aorta	IgG4-related retroperitoneal fibrosis (Ormond disease)	> 120/mm²	• Asymptomatic or nonspecific constitutional symptoms (fatigue, anorexia, fever, weight loss), low back or flank pain, leg oedema, abnormal renal function test • Imaging shows soft tissue mass over paravertebral area and pelvis, frequently involving abdominal aorta and iliac arteries (IgG4-related periaortitis), and entrapping the ureter causing hydronephrosis {2239,600}
	IgG4-related mediastinal fibrosis	> 120/mm²	• Thoracic counterpart of retroperitoneal fibrosis and often manifest simultaneously; frequently involves thoracic aorta (IgG4-related aortitis/periaortitis); asymptomatic or dyspnoea, haemoptysis, dysphagia, and chest pain {3260}
	IgG4-related aortitis / periaortitis / periarteritis	> 200/mm²	• Most commonly involves infrarenal abdominal aorta and iliac arteries in the context of retroperitoneal fibrosis or thoracic aorta, less commonly other medium-sized arteries (coronary and mesenteric arteries); asymptomatic or low back pain; some may present with aortic aneurysm or dissection • Imaging shows vessel wall thickening (media and adventitia), mass-like lesion with contrast enhancement with or without luminal dilatation (aneurysm) or reduction; PET-CT useful to assess disease activity and detect asymptomatic lesions {2386,2239}

[a]IgG4-RD cannot be diagnosed solely on the basis of IgG4-positive plasma cell count.

Table 10.02 Common sites involved by IgG4-related disease (IgG4-RD) and the salient clinical features (continued)

Affected sites	Nomenclature (related/obsolete terminology)	IgG4+ cell count[a]	Salient clinical features
Lymph node	IgG4-related lymphadenopathy	> 400/mm²	• Incidental lymphadenopathy on imaging, painless non-tender lymph nodes, often adjacent to organs affected by IgG4-RD, local mass effects (hydronephrosis, lower limb swelling for pelvic lymph nodes) • Lymph nodes usually mildly enlarged (mean: 20 mm) with homogeneous enhancement and no calcification or necrosis {579,3346}
Kidney	IgG4-related kidney disease	> 40/mm² (biopsy) > 120/mm² (excision)	• Incidental finding on imaging or abnormal renal function tests/urinalysis, hypocomplementaemia or elevated serum IgE is common • Contrast CT shows multiple low-density lesions, diffuse kidney enlargement, and hypovascular solitary masses {2806}
Dura and pituitary	IgG4-related pachymeningitis (idiopathic hypertrophic pachymeningitis)	> 40/mm²	• Headache, cranial nerve palsies, visual impairment, motor weakness, numbness, seizures, cognitive decline, and gait instability {11,2158}
	IgG4-related hypophysitis (lymphocytic hypophysitis)	> 40/mm²	• Headache, visual field defect, hyperprolactinaemia (galactorrhoea), hypopituitarism (diabetes insipidus, fatigue, amenorrhoea) {1938,1918}
Skin and soft tissue	IgG4-related skin disease (cutaneous pseudolymphoma) IgG4-related soft tissue disease (Idiopathic cervical fibrosis; cutaneous pseudolymphoma)	> 800/mm²	• Plaques or indurated nodules frequently in the head and neck region; local neurological symptoms (numbness and shoulder drop) due to associated nerve involvement are common {576}
Lung and pleura	IgG4-related lung disease, IgG4-related pleuritis	> 80/mm² (biopsy) > 200/mm² (excision)	• Incidental finding of abnormal chest imaging or cough, chest pain, dyspnoea, and haemoptysis • Nodules, ground glass opacities, bronchial wall / bronchovascular bundle thickening, interlobular septal wall thickening, infiltrative shadow, pleural thickening or effusion {2114,2264}
Thyroid	IgG4-related thyroiditis (Reidel thyroiditis; fibrosing Hashimoto thyroiditis)	> 80/mm²	• At least some Reidel thyroiditis and the fibrosing variant of Hashimoto thyroiditis represent IgG4-RD; presents with goitre and/or hypothyroidism {3265}

[a]IgG4-RD cannot be diagnosed solely on the basis of IgG4-positive plasma cell count.

Clinical features

Patients may present with periocular swelling, painless proptosis, decreased vision, or other symptoms depending on the ocular tissue involved {2567,779,3531,2151}. Bilateral involvement is common but may not be symmetrical {2567,2084}. IgG4 serum levels may be elevated (> 135 mg/dL), although 30–40% of patients have normal levels {781,2811,489}.

Orbital CT and MRI may show enlargement of the lacrimal gland, trigeminal nerve branches, and/or extraocular muscle, and whole-body 18F-FDG PET imaging is useful for evaluating systemic involvement {3365,1115,3340,2151}.

Epidemiology

Patients with IgG4-RD have a median age range of 58–67 years, with slight male predominance {3530,1152,1065}. The disease is rare in children {1568,2233,1611,3146}. IgG4-RD disease may occur in all ethnic groups. A potential prevalence in Asian populations might be the result of numerous reports in the literature {3214,1952,467}. Overall frequency of ophthalmic involvement in systemic IgG4-RD ranges from 4% to 34% {3531,860}.

Etiology

IgG4-RD appears to be immune-mediated, and may be linked to genetic predisposition, autoimmunity, and perhaps environmental factors {3741,383,1379,1965}.

Pathogenesis

Recent studies have proposed that T-helper 2 and regulatory T lymphocytes lead to activation of B cells including IgG4-expressing B cells in a modified Th2 response {3741,1301,568}. Increased cytokine secretion of IL-4, IL-5, IL-10, IL-13 (Th2 cells), IL-1, TGF-β, and interferon-γ by CD4+ cytotoxic T cells and TGF-β by T regulatory cells is implicated in the pathogenesis of this disease {2417,1588,3663,1379}.

Macroscopic appearance

IgG4-RD varies according to the proportion of inflammation and fibrosis, resulting in soft tan-coloured to firm grey tissue fragments.

Histopathology

Characteristic histological findings include dense, polyclonal lymphoplasmacytic infiltrate, with increased IgG4+ cells, and fibrosis of collagenous and focally storiform type with a radiating pattern of closely packed fibroblasts. Obliterative phlebitis is rarely present in ocular IgG4-RD. It is characterized by transmural inflammatory infiltrate and fibrous occlusion of venous lumen, which can be demonstrated by elastic stain. However, it is seldom observed in ocular tissue biopsies. Eosinophilia and non-obliterative phlebitis can be found {781}. The histopathology is a spectrum evolving from an early lymphoid-predominant tissue infiltration to paucicellular fibrosis {1304}. The presence of necrosis, vasculitis, granulomas, and acute inflammation generally excludes IgG4-RD {781}. The diagnostic IgG4+ plasma cell count is different according to sites. Elevation of both the absolute IgG4+ cell count and the IgG4:IgG ratio (> 40%), nevertheless, is required for the diagnosis (see Table 10.02, p. 327) {781}.

Immunohistochemistry

Immunohistochemical staining is essential to demonstrate increased IgG4+ plasma cells, a hallmark of this disease. While the count of IgG4+ cells may vary from 40/mm^2 (in orbital myositis) to > 400/mm^2 (as required for the lacrimal gland lesions), the IgG4:IgG ratio should be > 40% {3413,781}. These numbers are determined as the mean of three separate hotspot counts (often less than a square millimetre in total).

Differential diagnosis

See Table 10.02 (p. 327). Differential diagnoses include follicular hyperplasia, lymphoma, sarcoidosis, antineutrophil cytoplasmic antibody (ANCA) positive granulomatosis with polyangiitis (Wegener granulomatosis), thyroid-related orbitopathy, idiopathic orbital inflammation, Sjögren syndrome, and infectious processes {3504,1608,3360}. In cases of sclerouveitis, collagen-vascular disorders should also be considered. IgG4+ cells can be seen in several inflammatory conditions that do not meet diagnostic criteria for IgG4-RD {3217,3479} and xanthogranulomas.

Immunostaining or in situ hybridization for κ and λ light chains is recommended in select cases of IgG4-RD to demonstrate polyclonality and exclude an IgG4-expressing lymphoma with plasmacytic differentiation or plasma cell neoplasm {354,1103,3468}. Rarely, oligoclonal expansions of IgG4+ plasma cells may be encountered in nodal or extranodal sites, which may raise the possibility of lymphoma or a plasma cell neoplasm {353}.

Cytology

Not applicable

Diagnostic molecular pathology

In select cases immunoglobulin gene rearrangement studies may be performed in order to exclude IgG4-expressing lymphoma.

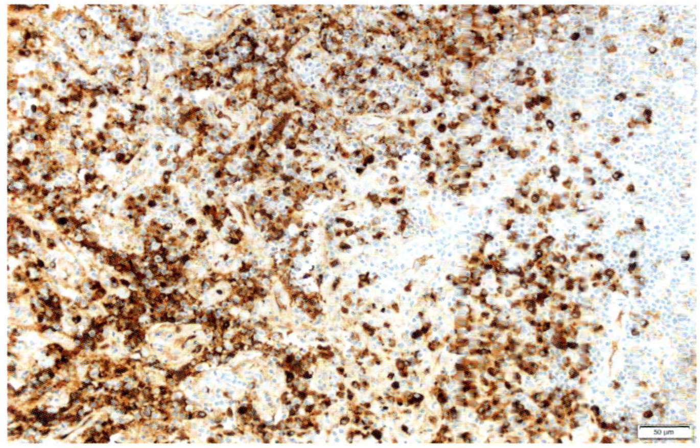

Fig. 10.07 IgG4 related disease. IgG4 immunostain demonstrates numerous (> 100) IgG4-positive cells in a single field.

Essential and desirable diagnostic criteria

Essential: dense lymphoplasmacytic infiltrate; fibrosis, at least focally storiform; increased IgG4+ plasma cells with an IgG4:IgG ratio > 40%; clinicopathological correlation required; exclusion of well-defined entities that mimic IgG4-RD.

Desirable: phlebitis (that may rarely be obliterative); 40–400 IgG4+ cells per mm^2 (mean within three high-power field hotspots per mm^2); elevated serum IgG4 levels; response to steroids/rituximab.

Staging

Not applicable

Prognosis and prediction

Overall prognosis is favourable with a good response to steroid treatment. Some patients experience relapse and others might require long-term steroids and/or immunosuppressive therapy. Rituximab has been shown to be very effective as a steroid-sparing drug in recurrent disease {2151,783}. An association between amyloidosis, carcinoma, and lymphoma has been suggested in patients with IgG4-RD {1397,1309,671,577,2457,1132,2097,199,3283,57}, but a causal relationship is still unsettled {1342,1423,1990}.

Primary choroidal lymphoma

Damato BE
Krishna Y
Mittal R

Definition
Primary choroidal lymphoma (PCL) is a low-grade, B-cell lymphoma of the choroid without evidence of systemic lymphoma at diagnosis.

ICD-O coding
9699/3 Primary choroidal lymphoma

ICD-11 coding
2D05 & XH6JB5 Malignant neoplasm of choroid & Primary choroidal lymphoma

Related terminology
Not recommended: uveal (benign) lymphoid neoplasia; choroidal benign lymphoid hyperplasia; choroidal pseudotumour; choroidal lymphosarcoma.

Subtype(s)
None

Localization
PCL is usually unilateral and localized but can be diffuse, sometimes extending into the adjacent ciliary body and iris. Extraocular extension may occur, in advanced stages.

Clinical features
PCL usually presents in later life, with a male preponderance. Symptoms and signs include gradual visual loss, painful angle-closure glaucoma (where there is involvement of the ciliary body and iris), and/or a visible extraocular episcleral salmon-pink tumour nodule {677}. Posterior extension of the tumour into the orbit may cause symptoms due to the mass lesion.

Ophthalmological examinations usually reveal choroidal thickening caused by a tumour of low internal reflectivity on ultrasound, with obscuration of the normal choroidal vasculature {2526}. The overlying retina may be detached with changes in the retinal pigment epithelium; however, its vasculature is usually intact and the vitreous clear.

Epidemiology
PCL is relatively rare, with about 100 reported cases, and its prevalence is unknown {683,2099,679,677}.

Etiology
Unknown

Pathogenesis
The morphological, immunohistochemical, and genetic alterations of PCLs are similar to those of extranodal marginal zone lymphoma {679}. As such, PCL represents a clonal expansion of post–germinal-centre B lymphocytes. Although extranodal marginal zone lymphomas can be associated with various microorganisms (e.g. *Helicobacter pylori*, *Borrelia burgdorferi*) and autoimmune diseases {3641,959,2629}, no such association has been identified for PCL.

MYD88 gene mutations and dysregulation of the NF-κB, BCR, and PI3K signalling pathways have also been implicated {2094,2006}.

Chromosome translocation t(11;18)(q21;q21) has been reported {677}.

Macroscopic appearance
Enucleation specimens demonstrate a diffuse white thickening of the choroid, with a detached overlying retina.

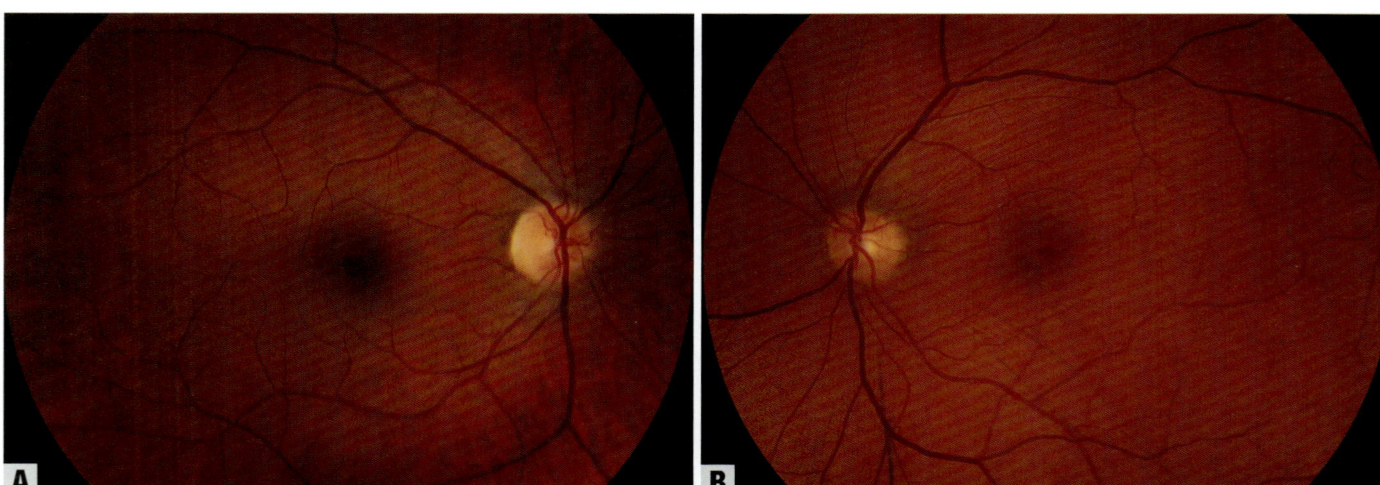

Fig. 10.08 Choroidal lymphoma of left eye. **A** Colour photograph showing a normal right fundus in a 39-year-old man with choroidal lymphoma of the left eye. **B** Left fundus showing obscuration of choroidal vasculature by lymphoma.

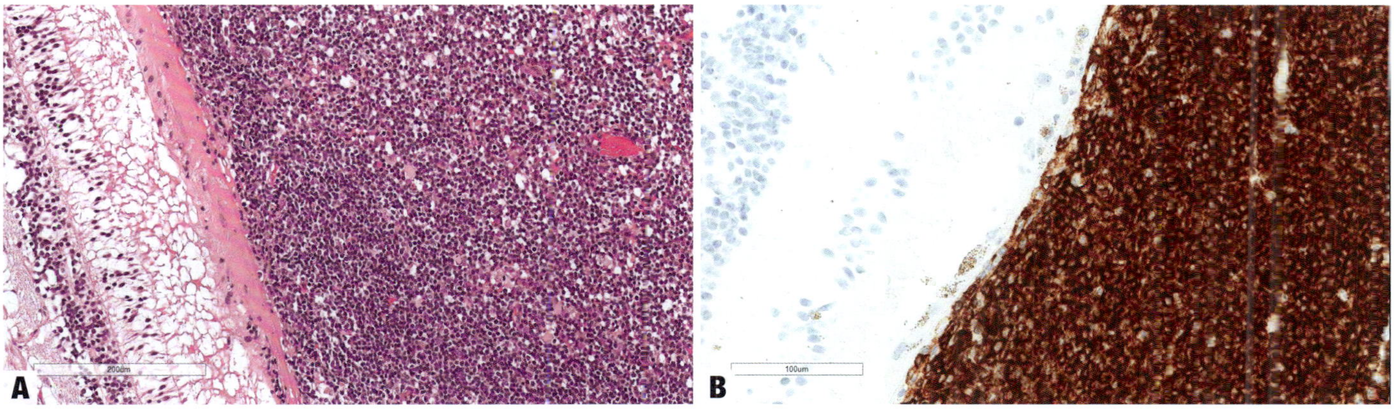

Fig. 10.09 Extranodal marginal zone B-cell lymphoma. **A** Primary choroidal lymphoma in relation to the retina and Bruch membrane. **B** Tumour cells express CD20.

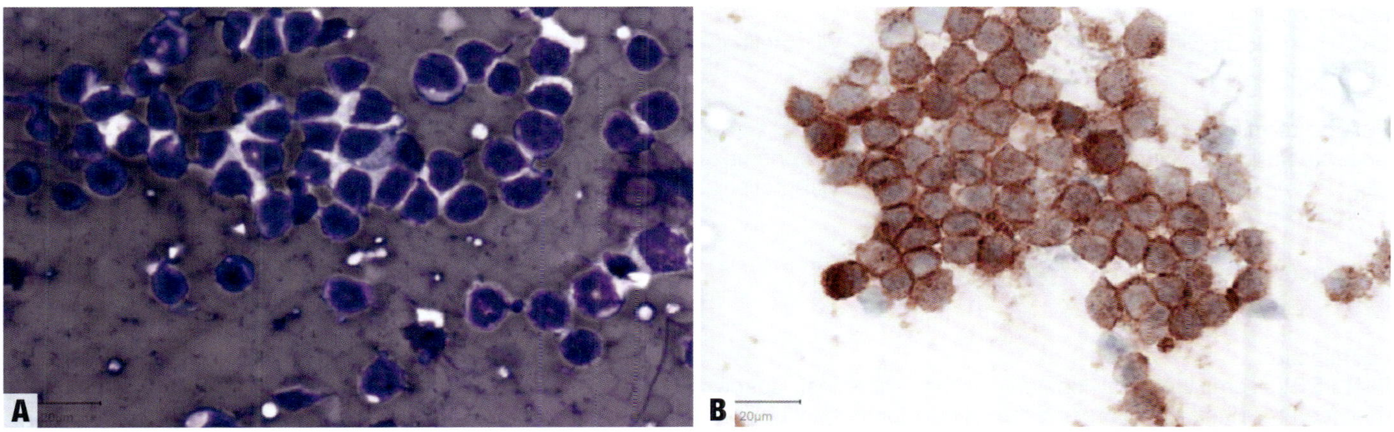

Fig. 10.10 Primary choroidal lymphoma. Intraocular biopsy of extranodal marginal zone B-cell lymphoma. **A** Small to medium-sized cells resembling centrocytes, with moderate amounts of pale cytoplasm, mild nuclear contour irregularities, and inconspicuous nucleoli (Giemsa). **B** Tumour cells are positive for CD79a.

Histopathology

In enucleation specimens, PCL shows diffuse infiltration of choroidal tissue by lymphoid cells that are small to medium sized with morphology similar to that of extranodal marginal zone lymphoma, typically with expansion of small centrocyte-like lymphocytes and varying numbers of plasmacytoid and monocytoid cells {683,2099,679,677,680,1585}. Lymphoid follicles with germinal centres are often present and may be variably colonized by neoplastic cells. The infiltrate may extend to the ciliary body, iris, and/or subconjunctival tissue, or even through the Bruch membrane, disrupting and infiltrating the retinal pigment epithelium.

Immunohistochemistry

Neoplastic cells express pan–B-cell markers (CD20, CD79a, PAX5), and are BCL2+, IgM+, CD43+/–, CD5–, CD23–, cyclin D1–, and CD10–, and show a low Ki-67 proliferation index.

Differential diagnosis

The main differential diagnosis is reactive lymphoid proliferation, which may require immunophenotyping and clonality studies, in addition to histopathology examination. Secondary infiltration of the choroid by systemic B-cell lymphomas (large B-cell and other small B-cell lymphomas) requires exclusion. The differential diagnosis also includes uveal effusion syndrome, sarcoidosis, choroidal metastasis, and amelanotic choroidal melanoma.

Cytology

Choroidal fine-needle biopsy shows a monomorphic population of small atypical B cells with the above immunoprofile.

Diagnostic molecular pathology

Diagnostic molecular pathology includes immunoglobulin gene rearrangement studies.

Essential and desirable diagnostic criteria

Essential: diffuse infiltrate of small to medium-sized lymphoid cells in the choroidal tissue; expression of B-lineage markers; exclusion of systemic lymphoma with secondary ocular involvement.

Desirable: demonstration of light chain monotypia or clonal immunoglobulin gene rearrangement.

Staging

Not applicable

Prognosis and prediction

PCL responds well to low-dose radiotherapy, and the prognosis is good. Unlike in primary vitreoretinal lymphoma, there is no involvement of the CNS.

Primary vitreoretinal large B-cell lymphoma

Coupland SE
Chan ASY

Definition

Primary vitreoretinal large B-cell lymphoma (PVR-LBCL) is the most common aggressive lymphoma that arises in the eye and is frequently accompanied by involvement of the CNS.

ICD-O coding

9680/3 Vitreoretinal lymphoma

ICD-11 coding

2A81 & XH86B5 Diffuse large B-cell lymphoma & Vitreoretinal lymphoma

Related terminology

Acceptable: primary vitreoretinal diffuse large B-cell lymphoma.
Not recommended: primary intraocular lymphoma; vitreoretinal lymphoma.

Subtype(s)

None

Localization

PVR-LCBLs are typically located in the subretinal space (between the photoreceptors and the retinal pigment epithelium overlying the Bruch membrane). Tumour cells are also found around vessels in the retina as well as scattered in the vitreous. With advanced disease, the tumour infiltrates the aqueous, forming deposits on the cornea's posterior surface (keratic precipitates). PVR-LCBL may involve the vitreous without retinal invasion in 15% of cases {3155}. Optic nerve involvement is infrequent {677,3171,3261}.

Clinical features

PVR-LBCLs develop insidiously, typically mimicking other conditions, and thus causing delays in diagnosis. These lymphomas are bilateral in 60–80% of cases and may occur independently or concurrently. Patients present with blurred or decreased vision, floaters, chronic intermediate or posterior uveitis (masquerade syndrome), retinal haemorrhage, and/or serous retinal detachment. Vitreous haze is the most common clinical finding and is characterized by larger vitreous cells that are less dense than those seen in vitritis and which may be arranged in sheets or aligned along vitreous fibrils in an aurora borealis (or string-of-pearls) pattern. A creamy yellow coloured subretinal pigment epithelial accumulation of lymphoma cells is characteristic of PVR-LBCL and may facilitate earlier diagnosis. The cells in the subretinal pigment epithelial space may resolve spontaneously, with their disappearance leaving a retinal pigment epithelium defect, producing a characteristic image on fluorescein angiography. Less commonly, PVR-LBCL may cause ischaemic retinopathy {677,2602,3171,3155,3261}.

Patients with concurrent involvement may have focal neurological deficits (50–80%) as well as headache, nausea, and cranial neuropathies; neuropsychiatric symptoms are common {2877,2452}.

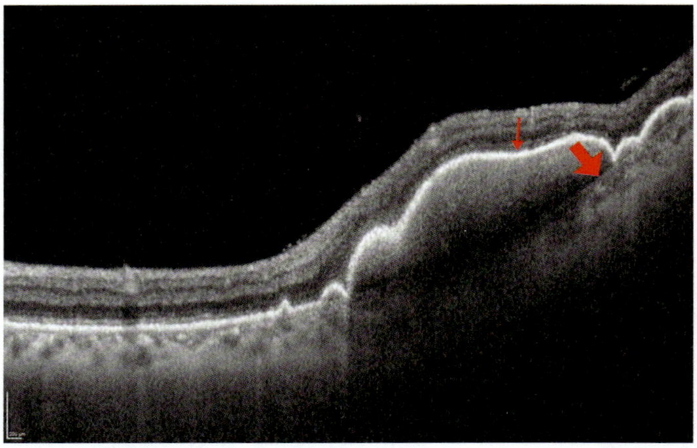

Fig. 10.11 Primary vitreoretinal large cell B-cell lymphoma. An optical coherence tomography image through the yellow subretinal deposits shows their variably sized deposits located beneath the retinal pigment epithelium (thin red arrow) and above the Bruch membrane (thick red arrow).

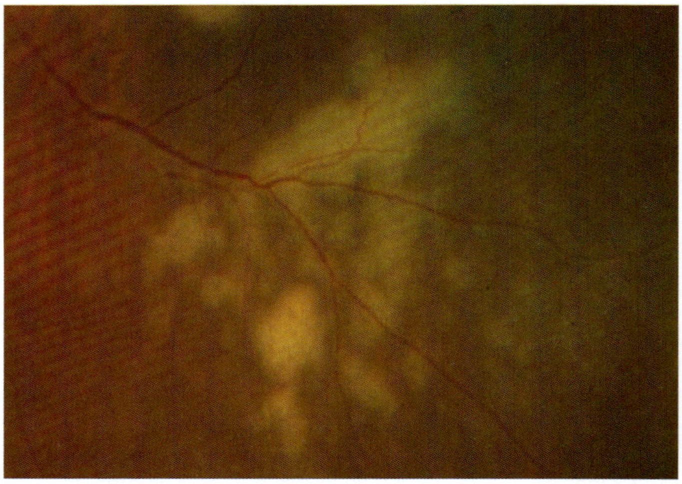

Fig. 10.12 Primary vitreoretinal large cell B-cell lymphoma. Colour fundus photography shows the creamy yellow subretinal deposits typically seen in vitreoretinal lymphoma.

Imaging

Ophthalmic imaging studies, although not specific for the diagnosis, usually provide initial clues regarding the diagnosis of PVR-LBCL. The localized spotty hypofluorescence and hyperfluorescence (a leopard skin–like appearance) on fundus fluorescein angiography or indocyanine green angiography, and focal hyperreflections on optical coherence tomography resulting from the subretinal infiltration can all enable a clinical diagnosis of suspected lymphoma to be made {936, 3171,3155,2547}. Fundus autofluorescence imaging showing hyperautofluorescence has been useful for monitoring of recurrences in known PVR-LBCL cases {3155,3261}.

Epidemiology

PVR-LCBLs represent 1% of all ocular malignancies, with an incidence of 0.47 cases per 100 000 population. The incidence has increased over the last two decades. PVR-LCBL occurs in patients in the fifth to seventh decades of life, with a median age of 58 years. Globally, there is a slight female predominance (M:F ratio 2:3), although this varies between studies {677,1703,1920,2602,3155}.

Etiology

Unknown

Pathogenesis

Like those of other LBCLs arising in immune-privileged sites (i.e. primary diffuse large B-cell lymphoma [DLBCL] of the CNS and primary testicular LBCL; see the *Haematolymphoid tumours* volume {3594}), PVR-LBCL cells demonstrate features corresponding to germinal-centre B cells that have undergone a prolonged germinal-centre reaction with evidence of ongoing somatic hypermutation in their rearranged IG genes {682,293,379}.

PVR-LBCL preferentially rearranges the IGHV4-34 gene segment, which is implicated in autoimmune diseases, in 55% of cases {682,293}. Like other immune-privileged LBCLs, these tumours possess common genetic alterations that enable immune escape and downregulation of specific immune reactions {2709,1544,1543,380,379}.

PVR-LBCLs demonstrate concordant *MYD88* p.L265P and *CD79B* mutations {2603,378,1335,3704,1890,379}, which are probably acquired at an early stage of lymphomagenesis {523}. The genomic signature resembles the C5/MCD/MYD88 signature found in DLBCL-NOS {378,528,1828,3645,379}.

Other mutations include those in *PIM1* (71%), *IGLL5* (52%), *TBL1XR1* (48%), and *ETV6* (45%) {379}.

At the chromosome level, translocations tend to involve the IGH and *BCL6* genes {1890}. Genetic imbalances are frequent, particularly 9p21/*CDKN2A* deletions (75%) {379,241,1890}.

Macroscopic appearance

Enucleation samples are occasionally received for PVR-LBCL; these are only seen in advanced cases where no definitive diagnosis could be reached via vitrectomy or aqueous tap, and the patients have complete painful vision loss. Such specimens usually demonstrate a detached, necrotic, and haemorrhagic retina with dense vitreous strands.

Histopathology

Microscopic examination of chorioretinal biopsy specimens and enucleated eyes reveals atypical lymphocytes in PVR-LBCL in the vitreous and neural retina, and/or beneath the retinal pigment epithelium. The highly characteristic subretinal pigment epithelial infiltrates (of variable thickness) consist of neoplastic B cells accumulating anterior to the Bruch membrane, which acts as a barrier to their infiltration into the choroid. There is perivascular accumulation of atypical lymphocytes in PVR-LBCL cases with the appearance of ischaemic retinopathy often with occlusion of retinal vessels.

Immunophenotyping

This can be undertaken by flow cytometry, immunocytology on cytospins of fluid samples, or immunohistology of cell blocks {726,3614,948,3155}. The neoplastic B cells of PVR-LBCL are positive for CD79a, CD20, PAX5, BCL2, BCL6, IRF4 (MUM1), and IgM, and have a high Ki-67 index {686,948}. Staining for EBV-encoded small RNA (EBER) is negative.

Although vitrectomy specimens are often paucicellular, they can be sufficient for the detection of light chain monotypia by flow cytometry immunophenotyping {726,3614}.

Differential diagnosis

PVR-LBCL can mimic both infectious (e.g. cytomegalovirus retinitis and acute retinal necrosis) and non-infectious uveitides. Ocular disorders that disrupt the retinal pigment epithelium (e.g. adult vitelliform dystrophy, drusenoid pigment epithelium detachment, and confluent drusen) and diseases infiltrating the optic nerve (e.g. sarcoidosis and leukaemia) should also be excluded. Vitreoretinal lymphoma secondary to systemic DLBCL {2831}, or T/NK-cell lymphoma {2096,2115,1540} may also occur.

Finally, extremely rare PVR lymphomas of T-cell lineage have been reported {676,472,527,1069} and these must be considered in the differential diagnosis of vitrectomy specimens with T-cell–rich infiltrates that may show atypia.

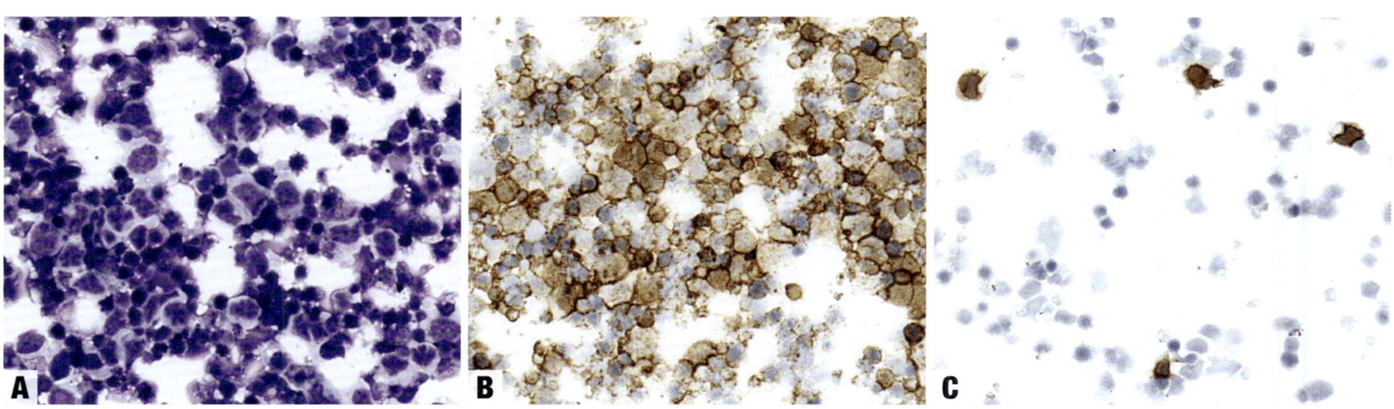

Fig. 10.13 Primary vitreoretinal large cell B-cell lymphoma. **A** Large malignant lymphocytes with pleomorphic, hyperchromatic nuclei and prominent nucleoli in a background of inflammatory cells. **B** Immunocytology staining with CD79a, highlighting the dominance of the neoplastic B-cell population within the vitrectomy sample. **C** Comparative CD3 immunocytochemistry of a vitrectomy sample, showing that only a few reactive T-cells are seen.

Cytology

Vitreous cytological examination is commonly used to diagnose PVR-LBCL. The atypical lymphoid cells are generally medium-sized to large cells with a condensed chromatin and prominent nucleoli. The nuclei are often irregular in shape, with finger-like projections. The neoplastic lymphocytes are usually admixed with reactive inflammatory cells. In some cases, small, mature T lymphocytes predominate and can mask the presence of neoplastic B cells. PVR-LBCL cells are typically friable, with numerous apoptotic bodies; therefore, vitreous samples often contain abundant lytic cell remnants, often within macrophages; together their presence is highly suggestive of PVR-LBCL {2196,2666,177}.

Diagnostic molecular pathology

Clonality analysis of IG genes enables the differentiation of LBCL from reactive inflammatory lesions. In rare cases where a PVR T-cell lymphoma is suspected, clonality analysis of TR genes is also of value.

MYD88 and *CD79B* hotspot mutations are highly recurrent in PVR-LBCL and offer diagnostic value especially when the number of cells is limited {378,1335,175,3273,3276,379,3549}.

Essential and desirable diagnostic criteria

Essential: LBCL primarily confined to the vitreous or retina at presentation; exclusion of secondary involvement by systemic DLBCL.

Desirable: post–germinal-centre B-cell phenotype (CD20+, CD79a+, IRF4+, BCL6+, CD10−); demonstration of a high Ki-67 growth fraction; demonstration of B-cell clonality; detection of mutant *MYD88* and/or *CD79B*.

Staging

This follows the Lugano lymphoma staging system {574}; however, it is key that examination of the contralateral eye and brain imaging should be undertaken {948}.

Prognosis and prediction

The treatment and prognosis for PVR-LBCL are very much dependent on disease extent – i.e. ocular only (unilateral or bilateral), with or without involvement of the brain. Generally, patient survival is very poor {948}. Treatment protocols vary, and usually include intravitreal injections of methotrexate and/or rituximab, rituximab-based systemic chemotherapy, radiotherapy, and haematopoietic stem-cell transplantation {713,1121,3261}.

Extranodal marginal zone lymphoma

Rasmussen PK
Ferry JA
Hindsø TG
Mulay K

Definition
Extranodal marginal zone lymphoma (EMZL) is an indolent B-cell lymphoma with features that recapitulate normal mucosa-associated lymphoid tissue. EMZL can arise primarily in ocular adnexal structures, or, less often, as secondary involvement at other sites.

ICD-O coding
9699/3 Extranodal marginal zone lymphoma

ICD-11 coding
2A85.3 & XH1V99 Extranodal marginal zone B-cell lymphoma, primary site excluding stomach or skin & Extranodal marginal zone lymphoma of mucosa-associated lymphoid tissue

Related terminology
Acceptable: mucosa-associated lymphoid tissue (MALT) lymphoma of the conjunctiva, lacrimal gland, and lacrimal sac.

Subtype(s)
None

Localization
Ocular adnexal EMZL most frequently involves the orbit, followed by the conjunctiva and lacrimal gland. Lacrimal sac and eyelid involvement are uncommon {1341,966}. More than one ocular adnexal site can be involved. Involvement is usually unilateral (85% and 89%, respectively, in two series) {1341,966}.

Clinical features
Clinical presentation depends on the ocular adnexal structure involved. Orbital and lacrimal gland EMZLs often present with a mass causing proptosis and displacement of the eyeball {2430,3490,2860,1341}. Conjunctival EMZL typically presents with a pink-coloured mass, which is often described as a salmon patch {1719,3281}, whereas EMZL of the eyelid often presents with a palpable mass of the eyelid {3249}. Systemic symptoms are rare.

Epidemiology
About 8% of all extranodal lymphomas arise in the ocular adnexa {1032}, and EMZL is the most common subtype of ocular adnexal lymphoma {2430,2860,3076,1555,1381,52,2076,231}. The incidence of ocular adnexal EMZL is low although reported to be increasing {1353}. There is a female predominance reported, ranging from 52% to 75% of cases {966,1341,2347}. EMZL often affects patients in their fifties or sixties {966,1341,2347,1381}. Children are rarely affected.

Etiology
EMZL is thought to arise from acquired MALT, which develops because of an underlying chronic inflammatory stimulus. In most cases that stimulus is unknown, but a small number of patients have an underlying autoimmune disease {966} or IgG4-related disease {354} and a subset have infection with *Chlamydia psittaci*. Some of the latter have shown regression of lymphoma with antibiotics; however, there is substantial geographical variation with respect to the proportion of patients with underlying *Chlamydia* infection {833,958,960,2578}.

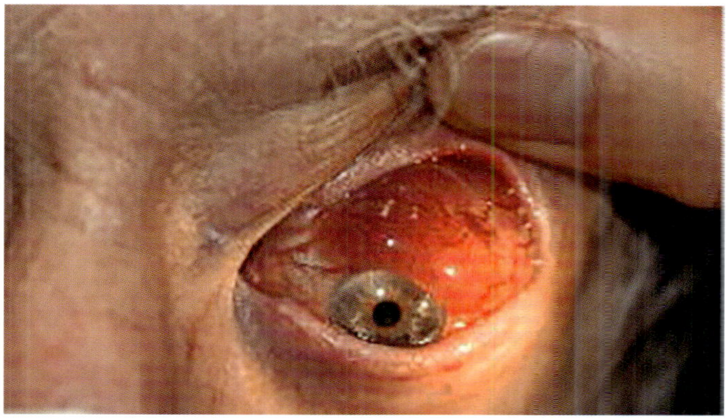

Fig. 10.14 Extranodal marginal zone lymphoma. A salmon-coloured tumour mass of the upper bulbar conjunctiva.

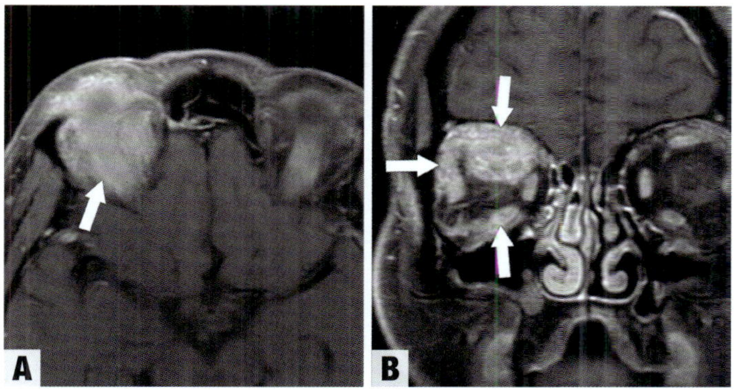

Fig. 10.15 Extranodal marginal zone lymphoma. Axial (**A**) and coronal (**B**) T1-weighted postcontrast MRI shows an intraconal and extraconal right orbital mass with extraocular muscle involvement (arrows).

Pathogenesis
Trisomy of chromosomes 3 and 18 is common in EMZL of various sites; other genetic changes occur at highly variable frequencies. There are several different MALT lymphoma–associated translocations associated with NF-κB activation {834,3691}; among them t(14;18)(q32;q21) (IGH::*MALT1*) occurs in approximately one quarter of ocular adnexal EMZLs while the others are very uncommon {3219}. EMZL of the ocular adnexa shows biased usage of certain immunoglobulin genes, resulting in expression of autoreactive B-cell receptor {3765,703,3444}. Autoantigens then trigger chronic B-cell activation, with resulting complex molecular events including the canonical NF-κB pathway activation, promoting

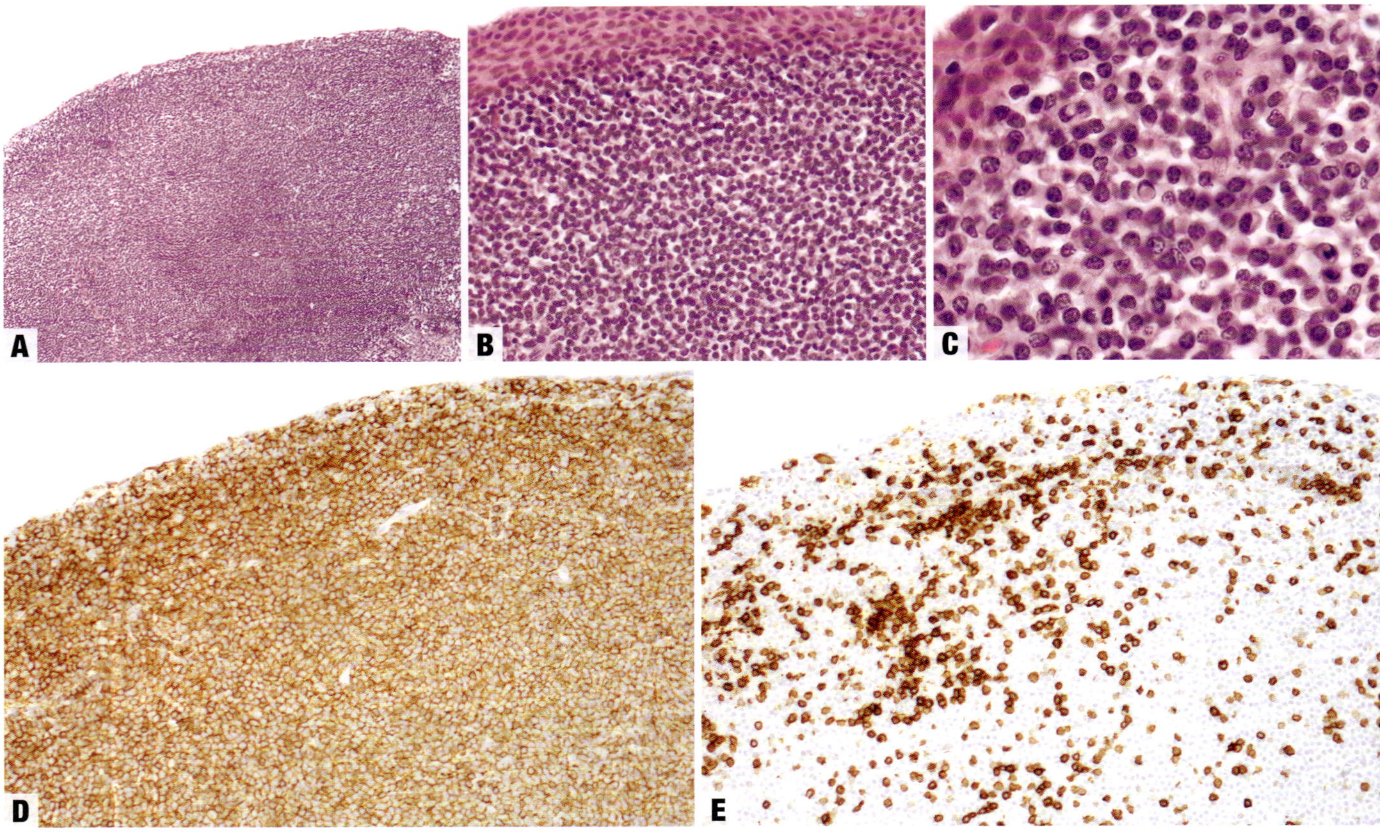

Fig. 10.16 Extranodal marginal zone lymphoma involving conjunctiva. **A** Numerous small lymphoid cells obliterate the normal stroma and invade the overlying conjunctival epithelium. **B** In this area, there is a broad layer of plasma cells, some with Dutcher bodies. **C** Numerous subepithelial plasma cells, some with Dutcher bodies, are seen (oil immersion). **D** An immunostain for CD20 shows diffuse staining of most lymphocytes, including many of those invading the epithelium. **E** An immunostain for CD5 shows staining of small numbers of T cells; B cells are CD5-negative.

lymphomagenesis. *TNFAIP3* is a negative regulator of the canonical NF-κB pathway; it is frequently inactivated by mutation and/or deletion in ocular adnexal EMZL. Alterations of *TNFAIP3* are often associated with IGHV4-34 B-cell receptor, possibly leading to cooperation in NF-κB activation {1361,526,2260}.

Macroscopic appearance

See *Clinical features*, above.

Histopathology

Sections show a vaguely nodular and diffuse proliferation of small lymphocytes and marginal zone B cells which have oval to slightly irregular nuclei, dark chromatin, absent nucleoli, and a moderate amount of pale cytoplasm. Plasma cells, ranging from few to abundant, are commonly seen and in some cases contain Dutcher bodies. A few large lymphoid cells may be admixed. Among cases involving the lacrimal gland, lymphoepithelial lesions are uncommon. Sclerosis is usually absent. In rare cases there is amyloid deposition {966}. Remnants of reactive lymphoid follicles are often identifiable.

Immunohistochemistry

Immunophenotyping typically shows CD20+, CD19+, CD5−, CD10−, BCL6−, BCL2+, CD43−/+, and cyclin D1− B cells. IgM expression is much more common than IgG or IgA expression. Monotypic immunoglobulin light chain expression is demonstrated by flow cytometry. Paraffin section immunohistochemistry commonly demonstrates plasma cells expressing monotypic cytoplasmic immunoglobulin, particularly in cases with numerous plasma cells. Fragmented, CD21+ or CD23+ follicular dendritic cell meshworks consistent with remnants of reactive follicles are usually present {966}.

Differential diagnosis

EMZL can be distinguished from reactive hyperplasia by a sheet-like or permeative infiltration of CD20+ B cells, effacement of architecture, monotypic plasma cells, and monoclonal immunoglobulin gene rearrangements. Other mature B-cell lymphomas (such as follicular lymphoma, mantle cell lymphoma, and chronic lymphocytic leukaemia) can be excluded by lack of CD10, BCL6, CD5, cyclin D1, and LEF1 expression. EMZL with prominent follicular colonization may mimic follicular lymphoma; the presence of an appreciable extrafollicular component of B cells, lack of extensive expression of follicular centre markers (particularly CD10) within and outside follicles {2585}, and absence of *BCL2* gene translocation may support the former. Distinction between EMZL and lymphoplasmacytic lymphoma can be very difficult. Bone marrow and lymph node involvement at presentation, high titre IgM paraproteinaemia, frequent Dutcher bodies, and NP_002459.2 *MYD88* (p.L265P) mutation would favour the latter. Rare cases of EMZL show extensive plasma cell differentiation, mimicking plasmacytoma, but the presence of a component of CD20+ B cells as well as presentation in a typical MALT site would favour the former.

Cytology

Not relevant

Diagnostic molecular pathology

Gene rearrangement studies may be helpful to detect clonal B-cell populations in cases in which light chain restriction is not demonstrable.

Essential and desirable diagnostic criteria

Essential: architectural effacement by a small to medium-sized proliferation of CD5− and CD10− B lymphoid cells; exclusion of other small B-cell lymphomas.

Desirable: demonstration of light chain restriction in lymphoid cells or plasma cells, or clonal immunoglobulin gene rearrangement; remnants of underlying reactive lymphoid follicles.

Staging

The TNM staging system is used to stage primary ocular adnexal EMZL {139}.

Prognosis and prediction

The prognosis for ocular adnexal EMZL is favourable, with a reported 10-year disease-specific survival of primary ocular adnexal EMZL of 93% in a large multicentre study of 689 patients {1341}. Older age, secondary disease, relapse, and higher TNM stage are predictors of a worse prognosis {1341}. Ocular adnexal EMZL can be treated effectively with local radiation therapy, with excellent local control {1341,3415, 2582,3080,2566}. Relapse is common, however, with 5- and 10-year relapse-free survival of 67% and 36% in one series. Most relapses occur in other extranodal sites and less often in lymph nodes. Large cell transformation is uncommon {965} and is associated with more aggressive disease.

Chapter 10

Follicular lymphoma

Hindsø TG
Ferry JA
Mulay K
Rasmussen PK

Definition
Follicular lymphoma (FL) is a B-cell neoplasm of germinal-centre B cells, composed of centrocytes and/or large transformed cells and centroblasts, usually with a pattern that is at least partially follicular.

ICD-O coding
9690/3 Follicular lymphoma

ICD-11 coding
2A80.Z Follicular lymphoma, unspecified

Related terminology
Not applicable

Subtype(s)
None

Localization
Ocular adnexal FL most frequently involves the orbital soft tissue, conjunctiva, and lacrimal gland {2670,966}. Involvement of more than one ocular adnexal site can occur, although patients usually have unilateral disease {2670,966}.

Clinical features
The predominant clinical signs are an enlarging mass of the ocular adnexal soft tissue and displacement of the eyeball {2670,2860}.

Epidemiology
The frequency of FL varies among studies. FL in one series accounts for 23% of ocular adnexal lymphomas, whereas in other series FL makes up 5–13 % of cases {966,681,2191, 1381,1353}. Secondary ocular adnexal FL is relatively common. In these patients the lymph nodes are the most common primary site. Most patients are middle-aged to older adults, often in their fifties or sixties, with a female predominance {2670,966}.

Etiology
Unknown

Pathogenesis
The cell of origin is a germinal-centre B cell.

The t(14;18)(q32;q21) translocation juxtaposes the *BCL2* oncogene with the IGH locus, placing *BCL2* under transcriptional control of immunoglobulin enhancers, leading to constitutive overexpression of the antiapoptotic *BCL2*, and is seen in as many as 80% of all FLs {2672}; genetic features of ocular adnexal FL have not been widely studied. *TP53* mutations and *MYC* rearrangements have been reported in high-grade cases {2860}.

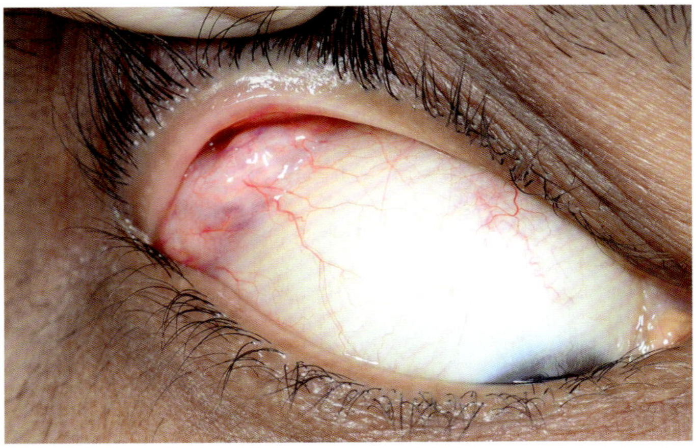

Fig. 10.17 Follicular lymphoma. Protruding tumour in the lateral upper fornix in a patient with follicular lymphoma of the right lacrimal gland.

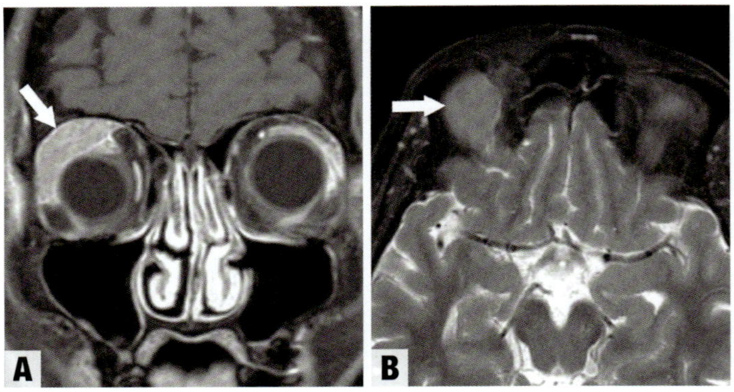

Fig. 10.18 Follicular lymphoma. **A** Coronal T1-weighted postcontrast MRI shows a mass in the superotemporal right orbit (arrow) with mass effect upon an inferomedially displaced globe. **B** Axial T2-weighted MRI with fat saturation shows a homogeneously isointense appearance of the mass (arrow).

Macroscopic appearance
The cut surface of tissues involved by FL may display a vaguely nodular pattern.

Histopathology
FL is characterized by closely packed, usually uniform follicles lacking polarization and often displaying a back-to-back arrangement. They are composed of an admixture of centrocytes and centroblasts, and uncommonly consist entirely of centrocytes or centroblasts. Centrocytes are small cells with scant cytoplasm and cleaved, twisted, indented, elongated, angulated nuclei having inconspicuous nucleoli and less dense chromatin. Centroblasts are large cells with round to oval nuclei, vesicular chromatin, and one to three small, peripheral nucleoli. Except in grade 3 FL, mitoses are infrequent. Tingible-body

macrophages are absent or scant. Mantle zones may be thin or even absent.

Patterns {2670,3594}:

- Follicular (follicular pattern in > 75% of the sample)
- Follicular and diffuse (follicular pattern in 25–75% of the sample)
- Focally follicular / predominantly diffuse (follicular pattern in < 25% of the sample)
- Diffuse (absence of follicular areas) patterns.

Grading

Grading of classic FL (FL composed of centrocytes with a variable admixture of centroblasts) is currently considered optional. FL composed of solid aggregates of centroblasts is diagnosed as follicular large B-cell lymphoma {3594}.

Immunohistochemistry

The neoplastic B cells express the pan–B-cell markers CD19, CD20, CD22, CD79a, PAX5, and monotypic surface immunoglobulin, which is most often IgM. Germinal centre markers expressed include CD10, BCL6, GCET1, GCET2 (HGAL), LMO2, AID, MEF2B, and stathmin {1672,2175,2063}. BCL2 expression helps in the distinction from reactive follicles. However, BCL2 expression may be absent in a subset of FLs, especially follicular large B-cell lymphoma {25}. The Ki-67 labelling index tends to correlate with the proportion of centroblasts.

Differential diagnosis

Differential diagnosis includes follicular hyperplasia (including in IgG4-related disease) and other small B-cell lymphomas. In the differential with follicular hyperplasia, crowded, poorly delineated follicles with a relatively monotonous composition expressing BCL2 and having a low proliferation index favour FL, as does the presence of centrocytes expressing germinal centre markers outside follicles. Hyperplastic follicles are typically well delineated, with intact mantles, are not crowded, and are composed of cells of a range of sizes with polarization, lacking BCL2, and having a high proliferation index.

Extranodal marginal zone lymphoma with follicular colonization can mimic FL but is composed of CD5– and CD10– B cells, and any residual reactive germinal centre cells have the immunophenotype of reactive follicles (BCL2–, high proliferation index). Small lymphocytic lymphoma / chronic lymphocytic leukaemia with prominent proliferation centres can mimic FL but is CD5+, lacks cells with the angulated nuclei of centrocytes, and lacks germinal centre markers.

Cytology

Not applicable

Diagnostic molecular pathology

Immunoglobulin heavy and light chain gene rearrangement in FL allows the distinction from follicular hyperplasia.

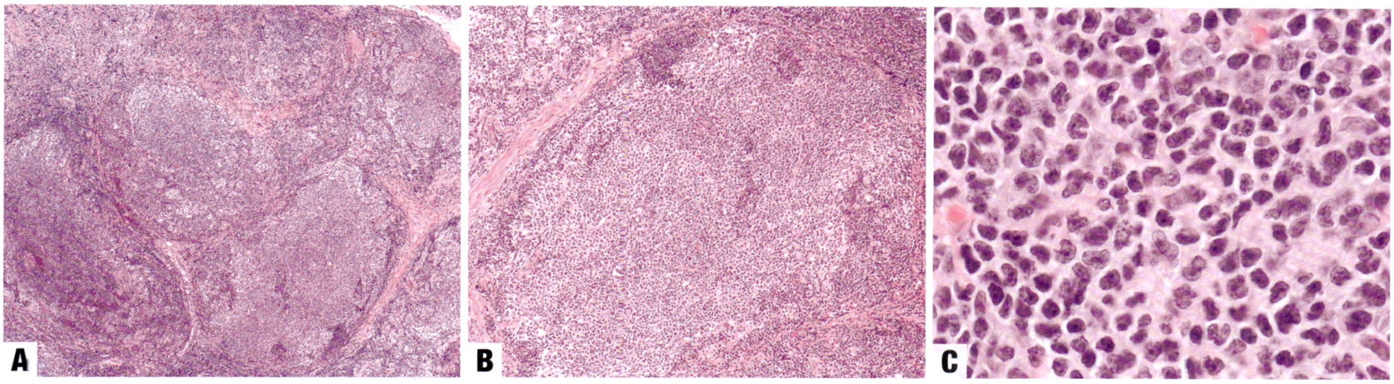

Fig. 10.19 Classic follicular lymphoma, orbital soft tissue. **A** Low-power view shows crowded, poorly delineated follicles replacing normal tissue. **B** This neoplastic follicle has a monotonous composition, lacks polarization, and has an attenuated mantle. **C** High-power view shows a predominance of centrocytes with angulated nuclei and only rare large cells.

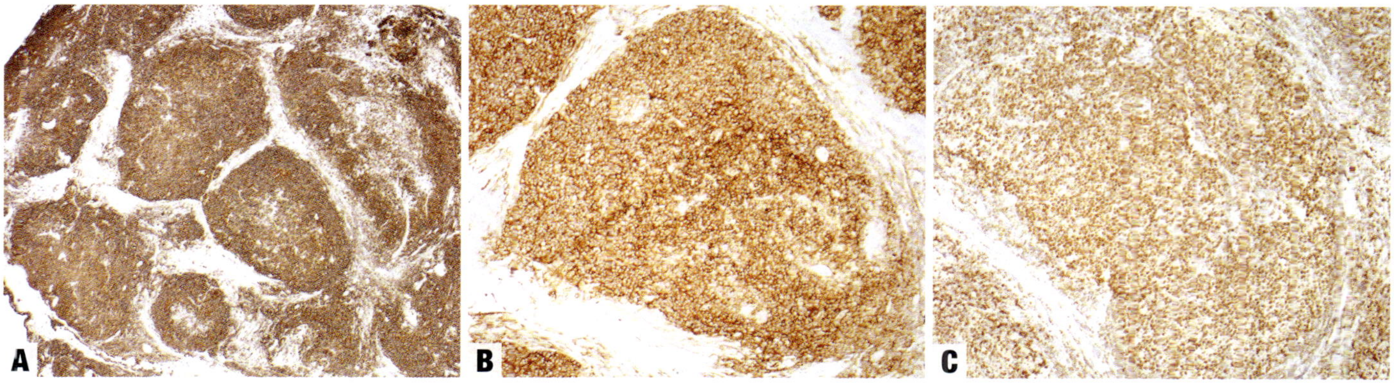

Fig. 10.20 Classic follicular lymphoma, orbital soft tissue. **A** An immunostain for CD20 shows numerous B cells in a follicular pattern. **B** CD10 is positive in the neoplastic B cells. **C** The neoplastic cells express BCL2.

BCL2::IGH fusion or *BCL2* rearrangement analysis can help distinguish FL from follicular hyperplasia and other small B-cell lymphomas.

Essential and desirable diagnostic criteria

Essential: B-cell lymphoma with an admixture of centrocytes and/or centroblasts / large transformed cells; germinal centre immunophenotype, with positivity of markers such as CD10, BCL6, MEF2B, GCET1, GCET2, or LMO2.

Desirable: an at least partly follicular pattern; BCL2 rearrangement.

Staging

The TNM staging system is used to stage primary ocular adnexal FL {139}. Most patients with primary ocular adnexal FL have disease localized to the ocular adnexa {965}.

Prognosis and prediction

Ocular adnexal FL is a relatively indolent disease. The 10-year disease-specific survival has been reported from 69% to 91% {2670}. Relapses are common, most often to lymph nodes but also to a variety of extranodal sites. Large cell transformation is uncommon and may be associated with a more aggressive course {965}. External beam radiation (EBRT) in the mid-20 Gy range results in excellent disease control in localized lesions {2671,2598,1191,1036} and some recent studies have demonstrated that a dosage as low as 4 Gy can be effective {1895,2557}. Patients with widespread symptomatic disease are treated with various regimens of immunochemotherapy {1334,2281}. Neither Ann Arbor staging nor Eastern Cooperative Oncology Group (ECOG) performance status has shown predictive values in ocular adnexal FL {2670}.

Mantle cell lymphoma

Krishna Y
Ferry JA
Heegaard S
Rasmussen PK

Definition

Mantle cell lymphoma (MCL) is a mature B-cell neoplasm arising from the mantle zone of lymphoid follicles, and is typically composed of small to medium-sized monomorphic cells expressing CD5, SOX11, and cyclin D1. It is associated with translocations involving CCND family genes, most commonly *CCND1*.

ICD-O coding

9673/3 Mantle cell lymphoma
9673/3 Cyclin D1–positive mantle cell lymphoma
9673/3 Cyclin D1–negative mantle cell lymphoma

ICD-11 coding

2A85.5 Mantle cell lymphoma

Related terminology

Not recommended: mantle zone lymphoma; centrocytic lymphoma; malignant lymphoma, lymphocytic intermediate differentiation.

Subtype(s)

Cyclin D1–positive mantle cell lymphoma; cyclin D1–negative mantle cell lymphoma

Localization

Ocular adnexal MCL may involve the eyelid, conjunctiva/caruncle, orbit, and the lacrimal gland and its drainage system. The conjunctiva and orbit are most frequently involved {966,2669, 1748}.

Clinical features

Patients present with symptoms related to an ocular adnexal mass. Bilateral manifestation is relatively common, and often more than one ocular adnexal site is involved {966,1748,491}. Most patients have systemic disease at diagnosis, such that the ocular manifestation is secondary {966,1748,491}. Only a few cases arise at these sites as a primary MCL.

Epidemiology

MCL is the fourth most common subtype of ocular adnexal lymphoma and accounts for 5–11% of all ocular adnexal lymphomas {1353,966,2669,681}. Most patients are elderly with a median age of 60–70 years, with a significant male predominance {966,2669,1748,491,2428}.

Etiology

Unknown

Pathogenesis

The t(11;14)(q13;q32) chromosomal translocation is the genetic hallmark and primary event in the pathogenesis of cyclin D1–positive MCL, present in ≥ 95% of cases {3251,1933,3449}. *CCND1* rearrangement results in overexpression of the cell-cycle regulatory protein cyclin D1 {3251,733,734}. Other translocations involving *CCND1* and immunoglobulin light chain genes occasionally occur {2779}. In most MCLs, the translocation is acquired at the precursor B-cell stage mediated by recombination-activating enzymes, but t(11;14) occurs in mature B cells via activation-induced cytidine deaminase in a small subset of cases {2330}. Secondary mutations and chromosomal aberrations are frequent and play important roles in disease progression {2779,1934}.

SOX11 also plays an important oncogenic role in MCL. It is involved in multiple signalling pathways, including B-cell differentiation, and modulating the lymphoma microenvironment, cell-cycle progression, mobility/migration, and apoptosis {284, 2469,3463}.

Cyclin D1–negative MCLs lack *CCND1* rearrangements and therefore expression of cyclin D1 {1045,1102}. Approximately half of these cases harbour rearrangements of *CCND2* and the remaining cases have other genetic alterations leading to expression of cyclin D2 or cyclin D3 {1054,2825,2095}. No cases have been reported to date in the ocular adnexa.

Macroscopic appearance

MCL usually presents as a smooth, pinkish mass.

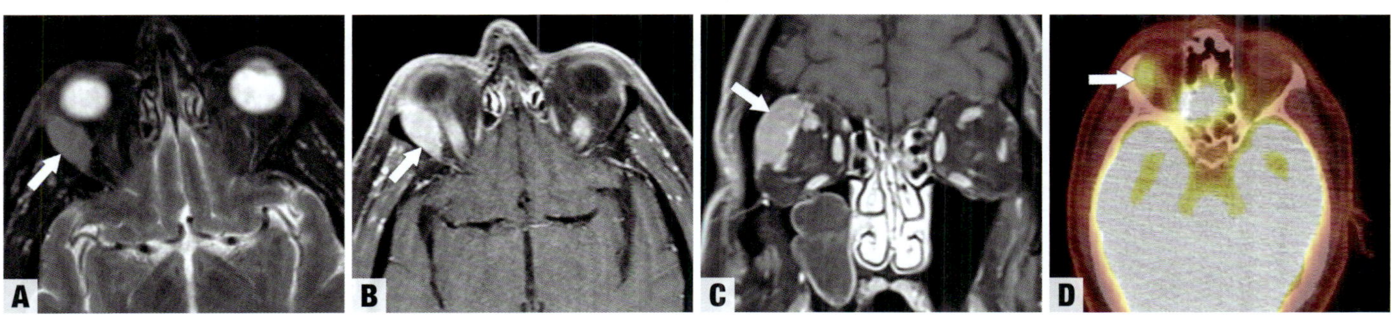

Fig. 10.21 Mantle cell lymphoma. **A** Axial T2-weighted MRI with fat saturation shows a homogeneously isointense right superotemporal orbital mass (arrow). **B,C** Axial and coronal T1-weighted postcontrast MRI shows homogeneous enhancement of the mass (arrows). **D** Axial 18F-FDG PET-CT shows FDG avidity of the mass (arrow).

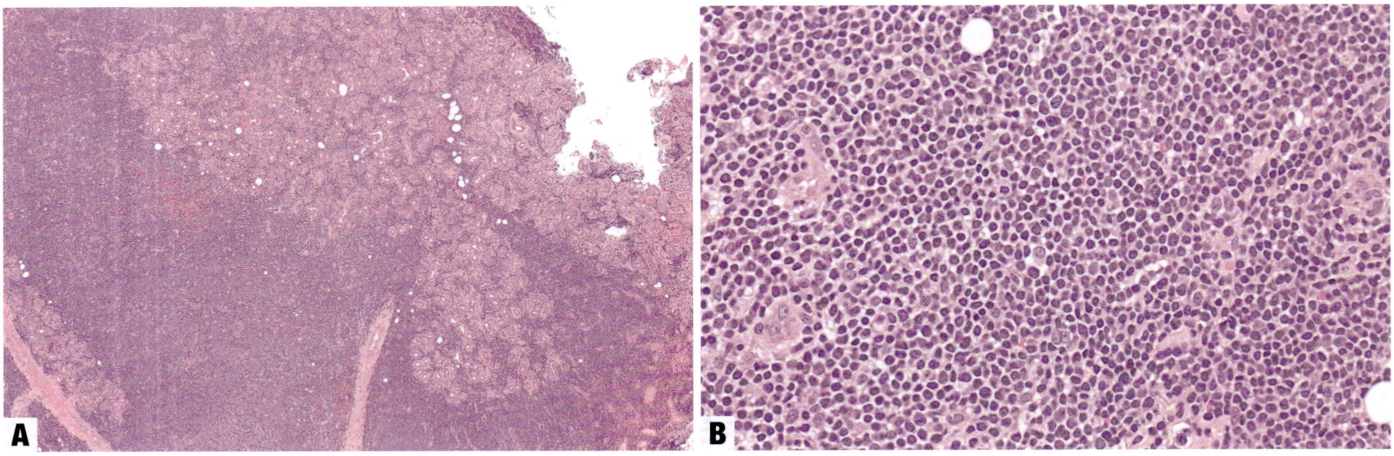

Fig. 10.22 Mantle cell lymphoma involving orbital tissue and the lacrimal gland. **A** A highly cellular and diffuse proliferation, sparing the glands, is seen at low magnification. **B** The proliferation comprises small to medium-sized lymphoid cells with oval to irregular nuclei, inconspicuous nucleoli, and scant cytoplasm. Occasional pale dendritic histiocytes are observed.

Histopathology

MCL is typically composed of a vaguely nodular or diffuse proliferation of small to medium-sized lymphoid cells with oval to irregular nuclei, inconspicuous nucleoli, and scant cytoplasm. Scattered epithelioid histiocytes may be admixed. Rare cases of the blastoid pattern are described, characterized by medium-sized cells with fine chromatin and distinct nucleoli, with frequent mitotic figures, resembling lymphoblastic lymphoma {966,2669}.

Immunohistochemistry

Neoplastic cells are typically positive for B antigens (CD20, CD19, PAX5), and IgM+, sIg+, cIg−, CD5+, CD10−, BCL6−, BCL2+, CD43+, CD23−, cyclin D1+, and SOX11+; often with CD21+ and CD23+ follicular dendritic cell meshworks. The λ light chain is more often expressed than the κ. The follicular dendritic cell staining correlates with architectural nodularity. The Ki-67 index is variable, but it is high in the blastoid and pleomorphic patterns {966,2669}.

Differential diagnosis

This includes other small to medium-sized B-cell lymphomas that can express cyclin D1, such as plasma cell myeloma, which also can have *CCND1* rearrangements, as well as neoplasms that do not carry *CCND1* rearrangements, such as chronic lymphocytic leukaemia (weakly in proliferation centres), diffuse large B-cell lymphoma, and hairy cell leukaemia. In the case of pleomorphic and blastoid patterns of MCL, these must be differentiated from diffuse large B-cell lymphoma, lymphoblastic lymphoma, and Burkitt lymphoma, among others.

Cytology

MCL is rarely diagnosed on the basis of FNAB alone.

Diagnostic molecular pathology

Diagnostic molecular pathology is not usually needed; in unusual cases, demonstration of *CCND1* rearrangement or *CCND1*::IGH translocation and an extended immunohistochemistry panel are recommended to exclude lymphomas that can express cyclin D1 (see *Differential diagnosis*). In the absence of cyclin D1 expression and *CCND1* rearrangements, cyclin D1–negative MCL may be confirmed by testing for *CCND2* translocations. *TP53* mutation analysis may help to define a high-risk MCL cohort {1372,210}.

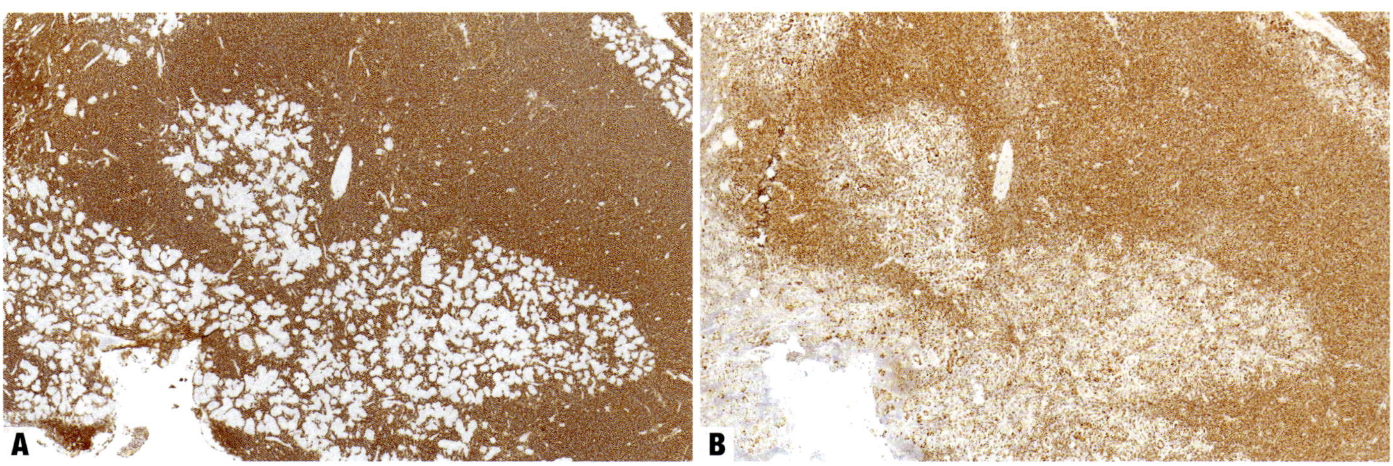

Fig. 10.23 Mantle cell lymphoma. **A** CD20 immunohistochemistry highlighting the density and diffuse spread of the neoplastic mantle cell lymphoma B cells. **B** Cyclin D1 is expressed by the neoplastic B cells, confirming the diagnosis of mantle cell lymphoma.

Essential and desirable diagnostic criteria

Essential: lymphoma cells of B lineage (CD20-positive and usually CD5-positive); morphology of classic pattern (monomorphic and centrocyte-like) or, less often, blastoid pattern morphology; cyclin D1–positive and/or detection of *CCND1* rearrangement, almost always.

Desirable: SOX11 expression (if cyclin D1 is negative, SOX11 staining is essential); expression of monotypic light chain.

Staging

Staging is performed according to the Lugano criteria {574}. For the rare primary MCL arising in the ocular adnexa, the American Joint Committee on Cancer (AJCC) TNM (eighth edition) staging system can be used {3590,3476,3248,2675}.

Prognosis and prediction

MCLs of the ocular adnexa have a worse prognosis than other small B-cell ocular adnexal lymphomas, with 3-year and 5-year disease-specific survival rates of 72% and 38%, respectively {1748,1353}, and 3-year and 5-year overall survival rates of 65% and 34%, respectively {1748}. However, new immunochemotherapeutic regimens with/without autologous stem-cell transplantation have improved survival {3095}

Factors associated with outcome for MCL in general include age, performance status, CNS involvement at diagnosis, stage, serum B2M, serum LDH, morphology (classic vs blastoid pattern), MCL International Prognostic Index (MIPI), Ki-67 (above vs below 30%), p53 expression by immunohistochemistry, and *TP53* mutation and/or deletion {1370,1371,1372,210,692,1733}.

Chronic lymphocytic leukaemia / small lymphocytic lymphoma

Chevez-Barrios P
Verdijk RM

Definition

Chronic lymphocytic leukaemia / small lymphocytic lymphoma (CLL/SLL) is a mature small B monomorphic cell neoplasm coexpressing CD5 and CD23. A B-cell (monoclonal) count of ≥ 5 × 10^9/L cells with characteristic CLL morphology and phenotype in the peripheral blood should be found. SLL applies to cases with a circulating CLL cell count of < 5 × 10^9/L and proven nodal, splenic, or other extramedullary involvement, such as ophthalmic sites.

ICD-O coding

9823/3 Chronic lymphocytic leukaemia / small lymphocytic lymphoma

ICD-11 coding

2A82.0 Chronic lymphocytic leukaemia or small lymphocytic lymphoma

Related terminology

Acceptable: B-cell chronic lymphocytic leukaemia / small lymphocytic lymphoma.

Subtype(s)

None

Localization

For ophthalmic locations, lesions are usually in the posterior pole of the eye (choroid, retina, optic nerve, sclera) and orbital tissues {2860,759}.

Clinical features

Clinical presentations are divided into asymptomatic, symptomatic, and Richter transformation. Clinical features depend on the site of infiltrations but are most frequently bilateral. The main symptoms are visual acuity disturbance, ocular pain, and ophthalmoplegia. Swelling of the lacrimal glands and/or eyelids may be seen in less than half of the patients. Ophthalmic symptoms are usually isolated; < 10% of patients with ophthalmic involvement present with systemic symptoms such as weight loss. On examination, the retina and vitreous may have perivascular infiltrates, haemorrhage, aneurysms, and tortuosity of vessels with neovascularization. Creamy infiltrates in the choroid with secondary retinal pigment epithelium changes and retinal serous detachments may present if the choroid is involved. Posterior scleritis–type presentation may be seen in posterior scleral / episcleral involvement. Ocular involvement in CLL patients is diverse:

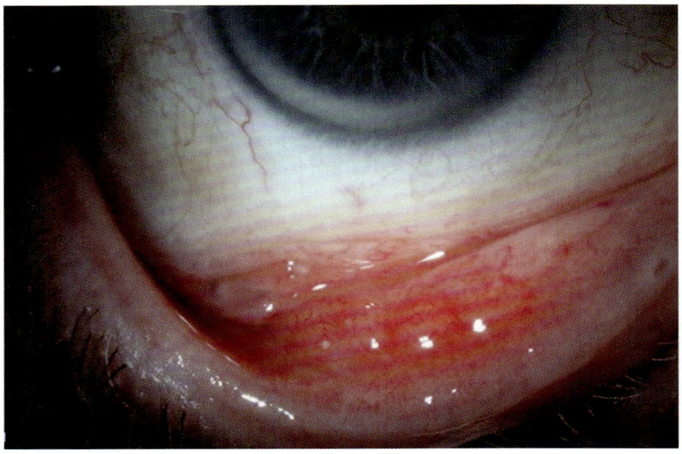

Fig. 10.24 Chronic lymphocytic leukaemia / small lymphocytic lymphoma. Small lymphocytic lymphoma involving the conjunctiva.

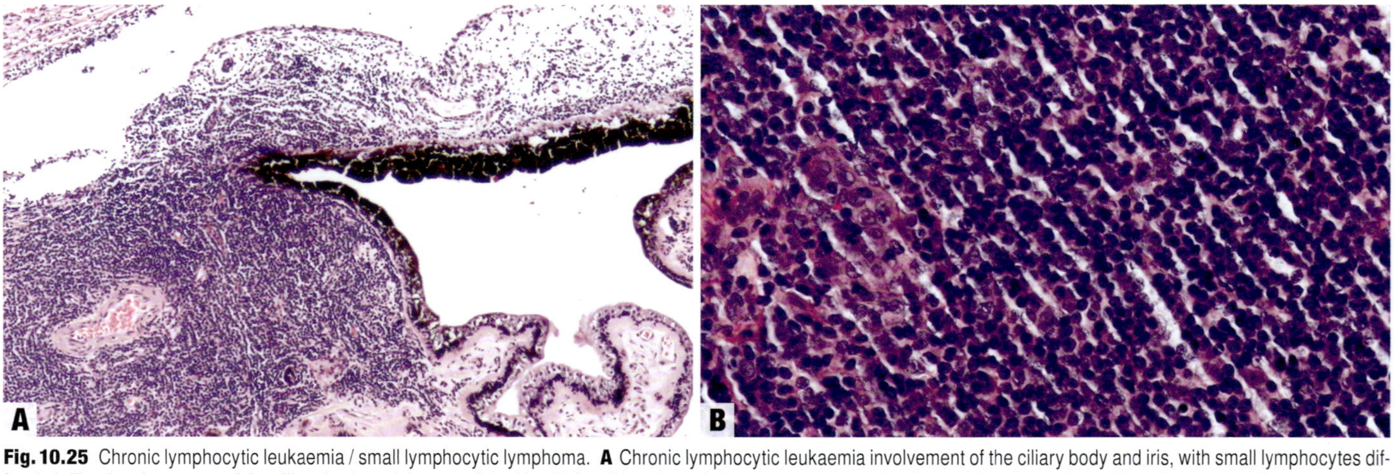

Fig. 10.25 Chronic lymphocytic leukaemia / small lymphocytic lymphoma. **A** Chronic lymphocytic leukaemia involvement of the ciliary body and iris, with small lymphocytes diffusely infiltrating the stroma of the ciliary body and the root of the iris. **B** Small lymphocytic lymphoma in the lacrimal sac with molecularly confirmed monoclonal immunoglobulin rearrangement.

secondary to CLL infiltration (more than half), followed by lymphoma, and least common by infection, and others. CLL infiltration is mostly bilateral, whereas lymphoma is usually unilateral. Optic neuropathy is always secondary to CLL infiltration {3428,759}.

Epidemiology

CLL/SLL is the most common leukaemia in fair-skinned people and is more frequent in men than women. Ocular involvement is rare (30–70%), has a median patient age of 65 years, and is most often seen after patients have a CLL diagnosis rather than as a first symptom of CLL. Usually, ophthalmic symptoms appear after 3 years of CLL follow-up. CLL in these patients is mostly stable, followed by progressive disease, with Richter transformation the least common {759}.

Etiology

The etiology is essentially unknown; family members of patients with CLL have a 5- to 8-fold increased risk of CLL {3225}.

Pathogenesis

The cellular origin of CLL/SLL remains unclear; however transcriptomic and epigenetic analyses suggest that CLL/SLL cells most closely resemble antigen-experienced, memory-like B cells {1787,2405}. CLL/SLL could derive from normal B cells differentiating via follicular or extrafollicular maturation pathways, reflected by the presence or absence of somatic hypermutation, respectively {2376,892}.

For more details, refer to the related section in the *Haematolymphoid tumours* volume {3594}.

Table 10.03 Overview of the most relevant prognostic and predictive markers in chronic lymphocytic leukaemia (CLL) (continued on next page)

Parameter	Frequency	Prognostic impact	Predictive impact	Comment
del(17p) and/or *TP53* mutation (~60% of cases carry both del(17p) and *TP53* mutation) {466}	del(17p) 4–8% and *TP53* mutation 5–12% in early-stage CLL {466} del(17p) 5–8% and *TP53* mutation 8–12% at start of first-line therapy {3742,3211,976,3643} 40–50% in relapsed and refractory CLL {466}	Strong negative prognostic impact on PFS and OS without therapy and with CIT, less adverse impact with targeted therapy (BTK and BCL2 inhibitors) {3211,466}	Predictive for poor response and shorter response duration, PFS, and OS with CIT, as compared with longer response duration, PFS, and OS with BTK and BCL2 inhibitors {466}	Repeated testing at relapse is recommended Associated with a higher risk of RT
Complex karyotype: defined as ≥ 3 or ≥ 5 aberrations	15% detectable by chromosome banding analysis {240}	Independent negative prognostic impact in most studies, particularly for ≥ 5 aberrations in *TP53*-wildtype cases {240,1903}	Not clear, because the predictive impact is also dependent on involved chromosomal and genetic abnormalities; limited evidence from prospective trials	Strong correlation with *TP53* aberrations, but still an independent prognostic factor The optimal definition with respect to defining a number of chromosomal aberrations is unclear The role of involved chromosomal and genetic abnormalities beyond *TP53* is to be evaluated {240}
IGHV status: U-CLL with ≥ 98% identity vs M-CLL with < 98% identity	~30% U-IGHV in early-stage CLL {661} 50–75% U-IGHV in advanced stages {719,1236,3211}	U-IGHV: negative prognostic impact on PFS and OS without therapy and with CIT, less adverse impact with targeted therapy (BTK and BCL2 inhibitors) {1425,977,446,121}	U-IGHV: predictive for shorter response duration, PFS, and OS with CIT, as compared with longer response duration, PFS, and OS with BTK and BCL2 inhibitors	No repeated testing, because IGHV gene somatic hypermutation status does not change over time
***BTK* mutation**	None in BTK-inhibitor-treatment–naïve patients {928,1851}; 23–57% of relapsed CLLs on ibrutinib had *BTK* mutations after a median of 3 years {1536,2624}; 60–80% of ibrutinib-resistant CLLs had *BTK* mutations, which were retrospectively detectable at a median of 8–9 months (range: 3–18 months) before clinical progression {55,3642,1851}	Not tested as an independent parameter	Predictive for progression on therapy with covalent BTK inhibitors within the subsequent 3–18 months {3642}	No routine testing so far

CIT, chemoimmunotherapy; CLL, chronic lymphocytic leukaemia; M-CLL, CLL with mutated IGHV status; OS, overall survival; PFS, progression-free survival; RT, Richter transformation; U-CLL, CLL with unmutated IGHV status; U-IGHV, unmutated IGHV.

Table 10.03 Overview of the most relevant prognostic and predictive markers in chronic lymphocytic leukaemia (CLL) (continued)

Parameter	Frequency	Prognostic impact	Predictive impact	Comment
***PLCG2* mutation**	13% of relapsed CLLs after 3 years on ibrutinib had *PLCG2* mutations in addition to *BTK* mutations {2624} 6% of ibrutinib-resistant CLLs had a sole *PLCG2* mutation, and 13% had *PLCG2* and BTK mutation {3642}	Not tested as an independent parameter	Predictive for progression on therapy with (covalent and non-covalent) BTK inhibitors {3642}	No routine testing so far
***BCL2* mutation**	45–47% of patients with venetoclax-resistant CLL have detectable *BCL2* mutations {362,2004}	Not tested as an independent parameter	Predictive for progression on venetoclax monotherapy {362,2004}	No routine testing so far
Serum B2M	Elevated in 34% of patients with CLL {1425,466}	Independent negative prognostic factor {1425}	None	
≥ 15% prolymphocytes in peripheral blood	Unclear, possibly as high as 33% {2163}	Not tested	Not tested	
Bone marrow infiltration pattern with proliferation centres	Unclear	Not tested	Not tested	Some correlation with *TP53* aberration and complex karyotype {1072}
Large confluent proliferation centres in lymph node	As high as 23% in advanced CLL {1117}	Not tested	Not tested	Expanded proliferation centres (broader than a 20× field) and high proliferation (either > 2.4 mitoses per proliferation centre or Ki-67 > 40% per proliferation centre) are associated with poor prognosis and defined as accelerated CLL {1117}

CIT, chemoimmunotherapy; CLL, chronic lymphocytic leukaemia; M-CLL, CLL with mutated IGHV status; OS, overall survival; PFS, progression-free survival; RT, Richter transformation; U-CLL, CLL with unmutated IGHV status; U-IGHV, unmutated IGHV.

Macroscopic appearance

Macroscopic appearance is dependent on the location of the lesions.

Histopathology

CLL infiltrates are usually diffuse in ophthalmic locations because of the absence of normal lymphoid tissue. Typically, CLL is composed of small lymphocytes with clumped chromatin, occasional small nucleoli, and scant cytoplasm, and rarely plasmacytoid cells. Mitotic count is extremely low.

Immunohistochemistry

CLL/SLL cells express pan–B-cell markers (CD19, CD20, CD79a, and PAX5), CD5, and CD23, and are negative for CD10 and other germinal centre markers. As many as 95% of cases express LEF1, which is rarely expressed in other small B-cell lymphomas {2176, 2174,3280}. Usually, cyclin D1 and SOX11 are negative.

Differential diagnosis

Differential diagnosis includes chronic non-granulomatous uveitis and inflammations, and other small cell non-Hodgkin B-cell lymphomas.

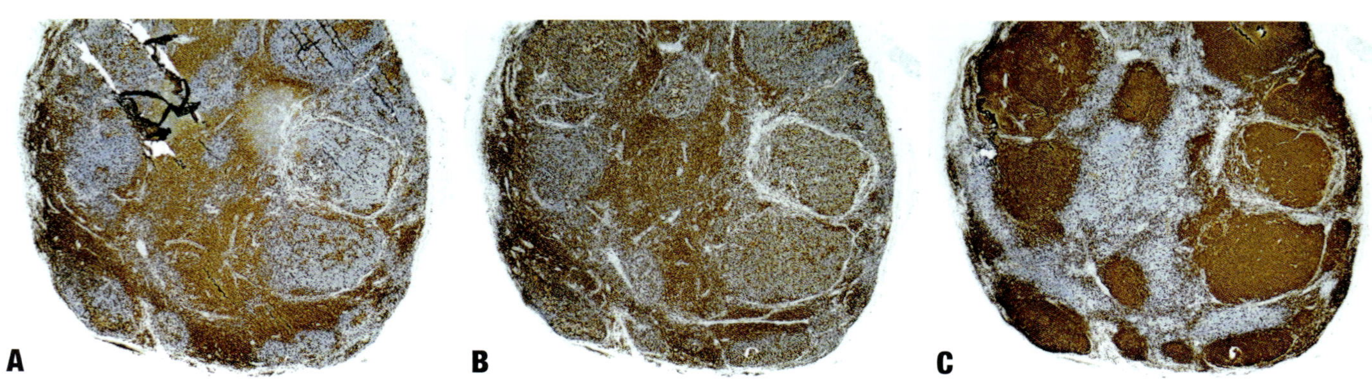

Fig. 10.26 Chronic lymphocytic leukaemia / small cell lymphoma. Small lymphocytic lymphoma involving the lacrimal sac. **A** CD3 is expressed by numerous reactive T cells. **B** CD5 is expressed by the tumour cells. **C** CD20 is expressed by the small tumoural lymphocytes.

Cytology

Cytology is often performed on vitreous specimens with opacities to exclude reactive inflammation versus lymphoma. Cytology of vitreous aspirates/washings or from FNA of a uveal lesion may disclose the presence of CLL/SLL with or without large B-cell (Richter syndrome) transformation. Cytological features may show abundant cellularity of small slightly atypical lymphocytes that are CD20+ and CD5+. In reactive chronic non-granulomatous vitritis, the infiltrate is usually scant and predominantly CD3+/CD20−. In cases of transformation to diffuse large B-cell lymphoma, these cells are seen as the predominant component in patients with a history of CLL/SLL. Vitrectomy specimens containing haemorrhage in patients with CLL may contain the neoplastic lymphocytes but it is not possible to exclude tissue involvement versus circulating CLL cells in the blood from the haemorrhage {2831}.

Diagnostic molecular pathology

The most commonly detected cytogenetic aberrations are deletion of 13q and deletion of 11q, followed by deletion of 17p/*TP53*, and less frequently trisomy 12. Absence of recurrent cytogenetic abnormalities such as deletions of 6q and rearrangements of *BCL2* or *BCL3* with IGH may be seen {115}.

Essential and desirable diagnostic criteria

Essential: classic morphology of CLL cells and absolute B-cell count > 5×10^9/L; flow cytometry (on peripheral blood and/or bone marrow aspirate samples) showing expression of CD19, CD5, CD20, and CD23 (variable) and weakly expressed monotypic light chain; histopathology/immunohistochemistry (on bone marrow cell clot/core biopsy, and biopsies of lymph node or other tissue samples) demonstrating CD20+/weak+, CD5+/weak+, CD23 (variable) expression, and no expression of cyclin D1 (weak positivity in a subset of cells in proliferation centres is allowed).

Desirable: flow cytometry is positive for CD200, ROR1, and CD43 with absence of FMC7, CD79b (can be weakly positive), CD10, and CD81 expression; histopathology/immunohistochemistry is positive for CD23, LEF1, CD43, and IRF4 (MUM1) (proliferation centres) with absence of CD10 and SOX11 expression.

For recommended investigations for prognosis/prediction, see Table 10.03 (p. 345) {3594}.

Staging

For CLL, the Rai and Binet systems are used {3594}. The stage of SLL is determined with the Lugano modifications to the Ann Arbor system {574}.

Prognosis and prediction

In general, for systemic involvement of CLL there are two clinical (Rai and Binet) prognostic systems based on physical examination findings and cell blood counts. Molecular genetics prognosis is based on the following: deletion of 13q is associated with indolent disease, trisomy 12 and absence of recurrent cytogenetic abnormalities are associated with an intermediate prognosis {810,1232}, while deletion of 11q and deletion of 17p/*TP53* and rearrangements of *BCL3* and/or IGH are associated with a more aggressive course and reduced overall survival {933}. A comprehensive, international prognostic score (CLL International Prognostic Index) integrates genetic, biological, and clinical variables to identify distinct risk groups of CLL patients {1425,115}. Furthermore, IGHV-mutated CLL/SLLs (50–70%) and unmutated CLL/SLLs (30–50%) show different kinetics with respect to proliferation and, therefore, have different time-to-therapy and time-to-relapse profiles with time-limited chemotherapy-based regimens {719, 1236}.

In a systematic review of 123 cases of patients with ophthalmic involvement associated with CLL, the patients with ocular involvement had an overall poor prognosis, with a third of the patients having died from the disease within 3 years, and a quarter having partial or total visual loss. Eye infections were associated with the poorest prognosis (almost half died from the disease), with a 6-month median survival {759}.

Diffuse large B-cell lymphoma

Krishna Y
Edward DP
Verdijk RM

Definition

Diffuse large B-cell lymphoma (DLBCL) NOS is a lymphoma consisting of medium-sized to large B cells with a diffuse growth pattern. This is a morphologically and molecularly heterogeneous entity that does not meet the diagnostic criteria for specific large B-cell lymphoma neoplasms.

ICD-O coding

9680/3 Diffuse large B-cell lymphoma
9680/3 Diffuse large B-cell lymphoma, centroblastic subtype
9684/3 Diffuse large B-cell lymphoma, immunoblastic subtype
9680/3 Diffuse large B-cell lymphoma, anaplastic subtype
9680/3 Diffuse large B-cell lymphoma, germinal-centre B-cell subtype
9680/3 Diffuse large B-cell lymphoma, activated B-cell subtype
9680/3 Diffuse large B-cell lymphoma with *MYC* and *BCL6* rearrangements

ICD-11 coding

2A81.Z Diffuse large B-cell lymphoma, NOS

Related terminology

None

Subtype(s)

Morphological subtypes: diffuse large B-cell lymphoma, centroblastic subtype; diffuse large B-cell lymphoma, immunoblastic subtype; diffuse large B-cell lymphoma, anaplastic subtype; other rare variants

Molecular subtypes: germinal-centre B-cell subtype (GCB); activated B-cell subtype (ABC)

Genetic subtype: diffuse large B-cell lymphoma with *MYC* and *BCL6* rearrangements

Localization

Ocular adnexal DLBCL may occur in the eyelid, conjunctiva, orbital soft tissues, and lacrimal system. The orbit is most frequently affected (~50% of cases) {3476,2313,3490,3590}. Often the lesion extends into adjacent ocular adnexal structures.

Clinical features

Patients usually present with a unilateral rapidly expanding orbital mass; it may be asymptomatic or some (~30%) experience pain or irritation {2313}.

Epidemiology

DLBCL accounts for 5–15% of ocular adnexal lymphomas and is the third most common lymphoma subtype in the ocular adnexa. Most patients are about 70 years old, with a slight female predominance {3476,684,966,1353,2313}.

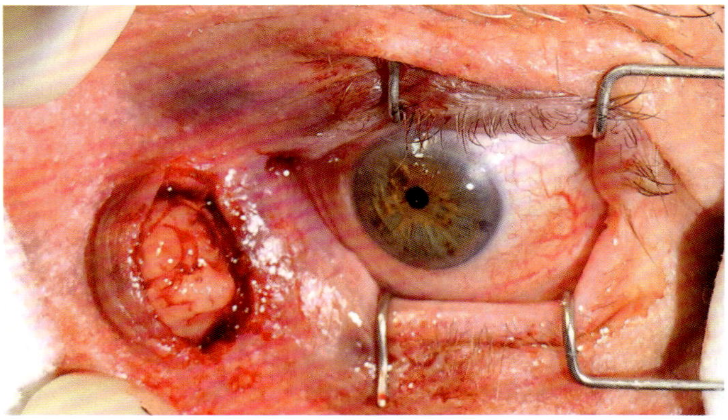

Fig. 10.27 Diffuse large B-cell lymphoma. Perioperative photograph of a lacrimal gland mass.

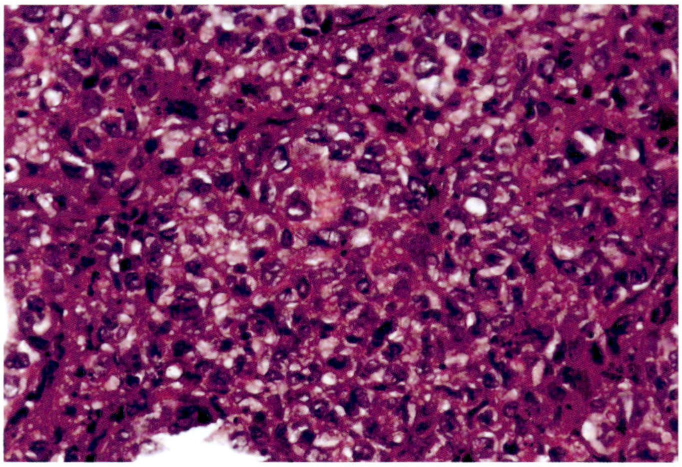

Fig. 10.28 Diffuse large B-cell lymphoma in lacrimal gland. Diffuse effacement of the lacrimal gland by large atypical cells is seen.

Etiology

Two thirds of ocular adnexal DLBCLs are primary, but one third are associated with secondary systemic involvement {3476, 2313}. Although DLBCL-NOS typically arises de novo, it may represent transformation from an underlying known or occult indolent B-cell lymphoma, such as a follicular or marginal zone lymphoma. No predisposing risk factors are known.

Pathogenesis

In contrast to the eyelid, conjunctiva, and lacrimal gland, normal orbital soft tissue has long been considered an extralymphatic site since it lacks lymphatics or lymphoid tissue {3476,3437}. Therefore, it remains unclear where the originating precursor neoplastic B cells arise and expand in DLBCL.

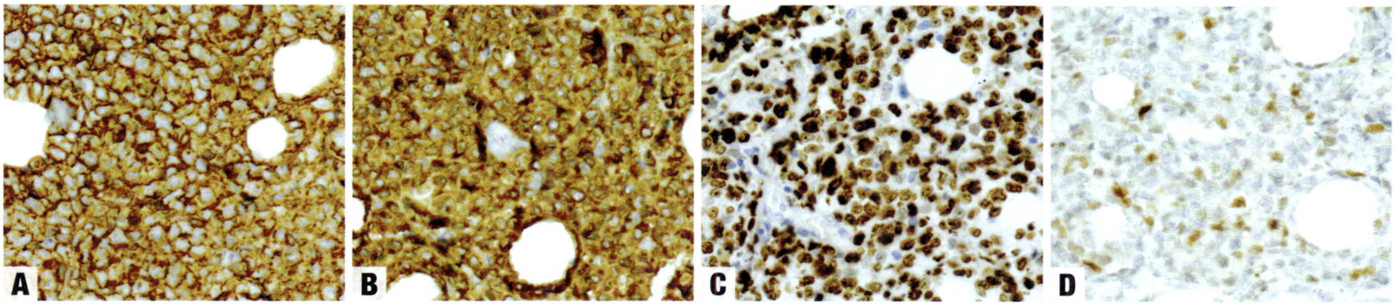

Fig. 10.29 Diffuse large B-cell lymphoma. **A** Tumour cells express CD20. **B** Tumour cells express CD79a. **C** Staining with MIB1 shows a high proliferative index in the tumour cells. **D** A subset of tumour cells express MYC.

DLBCL-NOS can be largely divided into two different molecular groups: GCB-like (31%) and ABC (69%) {2771,2313}; however, 15–30% of DLBCLs cannot be classified definitively.

Macroscopic appearance

The cut surface of the tumour reveals a lobulated salmon-coloured mass.

Histopathology

Ocular adnexal DLBCL shows diffuse effacement of normal architecture and comprises large non-cohesive cells with large vesicular nuclei with multiple irregular eosinophilic nucleoli and atypical mitoses.

Immunophenotype

Ocular adnexal DLBCLs are CD20+. However, CD20 may be negative in biopsies taken after rituximab treatment. Alternative B-cell markers such as CD19, CD22, CD79a, and/or PAX5 should be employed to confirm B-cell differentiation and support the differential diagnosis. Ki-67 is > 50%. The tumour has few reactive T cells.

Immunohistochemical surrogates have been developed for subtyping of DLBCL-NOS according to cell of origin. The Hans algorithm is popular and uses three markers (CD10, BCL6, IRF4) to distinguish the GCB versus non-GCB subtypes {1247}.

Differential diagnosis

The differential diagnosis includes non-haematological malignancies, such as metastatic poorly differentiated carcinoma, metastatic melanoma, and seminoma, and less frequently other haematolymphoid malignancies with a dispersed monotonous pattern such as Burkitt lymphoma; histiocytic sarcoma; myeloid sarcoma; and some cases of Hodgkin lymphoma {687}.

Cytology

Cytology is not suited for the diagnosis of orbital inflammatory disease or haematolymphoid disease.

Diagnostic molecular pathology

Clonality analysis may help to demonstrate the clonal B-cell population.

MYD88 and *CD79B* missense mutations may be identified in 30–70% and 10% of ocular adnexal DLBCLs, respectively {471, 1718}. The ABC-subtype DLBCLs are enriched for BCR pathway mutations such as in *MYD88* (mostly p.L265P), *CD79B*, *PIM1*, and *PRDM1* {2504}.

High-grade B-cell lymphoma with *MYC* and *BCL2* and/or *BCL6* rearrangements may be encountered in 16% of ocular adnexal DLBCLs {1718}. EBV positivity is rare {3395,3317}. Cases displaying an isolated *MYC* rearrangement or dual rearrangements of *MYC* and *BCL6* do fall within the spectrum of DLBCL-NOS; if a *MYC* or a simultaneous *MYC* and *BCL6* rearrangement is detected, it should be reported as "DLBCL-NOS with *MYC* or *MYC* and *BCL6* rearrangement" {899,2928,2896}.

Essential and desirable diagnostic criteria

Essential: large B-cell lymphoma with diffuse or vaguely nodular growth pattern; mature B-cell phenotype; exclusion of any other class of large B-cell lymphoma with ocular adnexal involvement; exclusion of immunodeficiency / dysregulation-related settings.

Desirable: cell-of-origin subtyping; demonstration of a clonal B-cell population or an *MYD88* mutation when histology is not definitive; reporting of isolated *MYC* or dual *MYC* and *BCL6* rearrangements; absence of EBV-associated markers; cytogenetic testing.

Staging

In primary ocular adnexal DLCBL, disease-specific mortality is significantly associated with TNM T category {2313,51}. However, for all such DLBCLs, Lugano staging appears to be superior {2313,51}.

Prognosis and prediction

Younger age (below 60 years) and total resection are associated with increased survival {51}. The ABC subtype of DLBCL-NOS has an inferior outcome in response to standard therapies when compared with the GCB subtype. In ocular adnexal DLBCL, outcomes between the two subtypes are similar {2313}. Ocular adnexal DLBCLs with *MYD88* and *CD79B* mutations are associated with a poor prognosis {1718}. Concurrent high expression of BCL2 and MYC in DLBCL (dual expressers) carries an adverse prognosis {1718,1164,1529,3192,1363}.

Chapter 10

Plasmacytoma

Mittal R
Esmaeli B
Vemuganti GK

Definition

Plasmacytoma of the bone or soft tissues of the orbit is an isolated neoplasm of clonal plasma cells without evidence of plasma cell (multiple) myeloma (PCM/MM).

ICD-O coding

9731/3 Plasmacytoma of bone
9734/3 Extramedullary plasmacytoma
9731/3 Solitary plasmacytoma of bone

ICD-11 coding

2A83.2 Solitary plasmacytoma

Related terminology

Acceptable: extramedullary plasmacytoma; plasmacytoma of bone.
Not recommended: osseous plasmacytoma; plasma cell tumour; primary extramedullary plasmacytoma; solitary extramedullary plasmacytoma.

Subtype(s)

Extramedullary plasmacytoma (EMP); solitary plasmacytoma of bone

Localization

Isolated or primary plasmacytoma of the orbit/adnexa is very rare. It can present as a soft tissue mass or as an osseous lesion. Superotemporal orbit involvement is the commonest {448,2917}, but it can also present as a lacrimal gland mass or as isolated rectus muscle involvement {2807}. It may rarely involve the conjunctiva and eyelid {123,3725}.

Clinical features

Plasmacytoma usually presents in elderly people, with a male preponderance; however, the reported age range is 18–81 years. Symptoms and signs include orbital mass, proptosis, eyelid swelling, conjunctival mass, diplopia, pain, ptosis, and motility restrictions {3406}.

Imaging

Orbital imaging (CT and MRI) features a homogeneous to heterogeneous unencapsulated extraconal mass of altered signal intensity, commonly with bony changes including bone remodelling and hyperostosis. It may involve the lacrimal gland and mould around the orbital structures. It may be associated with involvement of orbital/skull/frontal bones along with intracranial extension {2957,1398,123}.

Epidemiology

Primary plasmacytoma of the orbit/adnexa is extremely rare; however, secondary involvement from a pre-existing or subsequently diagnosed multiple myeloma or secondary invasion from an upper respiratory tract / sinonasal EMP or from osseous plasmacytoma of facial bones is relatively common {123,401, 3406,3333}.

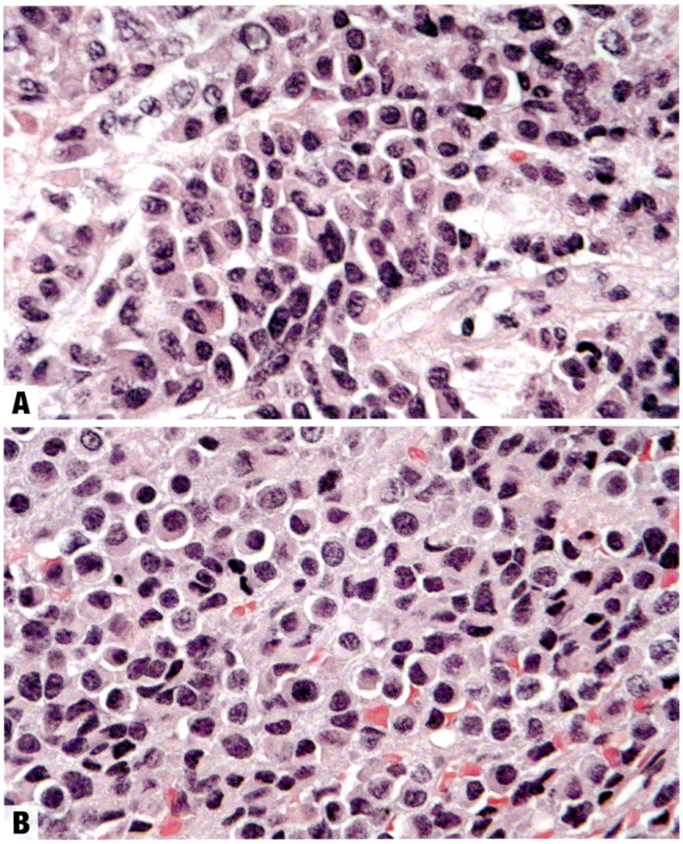

Fig. 10.30 Secondary plasma cell myeloma / plasma cell neoplasm. **A** Sheets of mature-appearing plasma cells with eccentric nuclei with clockwork chromatin, in a patient with known myeloma and an orbital mass. **B** Immature-appearing plasma cells with higher N:C ratios and with some prominent nucleoli, in a patient with known myeloma and an orbital mass. Some mature-appearing plasma cells are also present.

Etiology

The etiology is unknown, although in 10% of EMP cases, EBV has been detected in immunocompetent patients {46,1986, 3462}, and some reports of plasmacytoma show association with ongoing inflammation, trauma, or chronic hepatitis C infection {401}.

Pathogenesis

Solitary EMP and PCM/MM are closely related {338,656}. However, studies show that solitary EMPs are cytogenetically less identical when compared with extramedullary disease (EMD) in PCM/MM {335,975,1786} and have comparatively fewer cytogenetic aberrations.

Macroscopic appearance

These are unencapsulated, greyish-pink masses that are soft, fleshy, to gelatinous in appearance.

Histopathology

The tumour consists of sheets of plasma cells with varying differentiation. The neoplastic plasma cells might appear mature with the presence of binucleated and multinucleated forms, Russell bodies, and Dutcher bodies. Immature plasma cells (plasmablastic or anaplastic features) exhibit a higher N:C ratio, dispersed chromatin, and prominent nucleoli. Poorly differentiated lesions with a predominant population of plasmablastic cells are infrequent in solitary plasmacytoma as compared with EMD in PCM/MM {975}.

Immunohistochemistry

Tumour cells are positive for CD138, CD38, and IRF4 (MUM1) with restriction of κ or λ light chains. EBV may be rarely positive in plasmacytoma {1986,2332}. Unlike PCM/MM and multiple myeloma with EMD, solitary plasmacytoma universally lacks cyclin D1, and may rarely express CD56 {975,1786}. The proliferation index is usually low, but may show marked variation (1–90%).

Differential diagnosis

The main differential diagnosis includes B-cell non-Hodgkin lymphoma with extensive plasma cell differentiation, lymphoplasmacytic lymphoma, and plasmablastic lymphoma, which may require immunohistochemistry, immunophenotyping, and clonality determination. Melanoma and poorly differentiated carcinoma might need to be excluded in cases of plasmacytoma with anaplastic features. Clonality determination helps to exclude orbital inflammatory diseases with plasma cell predominance.

In EBV-positive plasmacytoma, it is mandatory to exclude plasmablastic lymphoma, which has a high Ki-67 proliferative index (often > 60%) {137} and is usually associated with an immunocompromised state. When a clear distinction may be difficult, a descriptive diagnosis such as plasmablastic neoplasm indeterminate between plasmablastic lymphoma and anaplastic plasmacytoma is allowed.

The differential diagnosis from multiple myeloma depends on bone marrow sampling: < 10% clonal plasma cells is required to ascertain the diagnosis of plasmacytoma.

Cytology

On cytological preparations, small bland plasma cells or plasma cells with atypia are seen. Cases of isolated EMP tend to be more differentiated than cases of PCM/MM with EMD {3202}.

Diagnostic molecular pathology

EMPs are closely related to PCM/MM on cytogenetic evaluation. However, the distribution of IGH translocation partners might be different with notable absence of t(11;14) {338}. Clonal immunoglobulin gene rearrangement may assist in cases with ambiguous clonality by light chain immunohistochemistry, in situ hybridization, or flow cytometry.

Essential and desirable diagnostic criteria

Essential: biopsy-proven clonal plasma cell neoplasm of bone/soft tissue; no clonal B-cell proliferation; no physical or radiological evidence of any other plasma cell tumour; no evidence of end-organ damage (hypercalcaemia, renal insufficiency, anaemia, and bone lesions [CRAB]) due to plasma cell neoplasm; < 10% clonal plasma cells on non-targeted bone marrow sampling; plasmacytomas with no marrow involvement must be distinguished from those with minimal (< 10%) marrow involvement.

Staging

Extensive evaluation is required to exclude PCM/MM or the presence of plasmacytoma elsewhere in the body.

There is no staging system for plasmacytoma; however, patients should be evaluated for PCM/MM with a complete blood count, serum creatinine and calcium, serum and urine protein electrophoresis, serum free light chains, radiological evaluation {2643,456}, and bone marrow aspiration/biopsy with flow cytometry and/or immunohistochemistry.

Prognosis and prediction

EMP is usually indolent, in contrast to PCM/MM with EMD. When compared with EMP, solitary plasmacytoma of bone has a worse prognosis with increased rates of progression to PCM/MM, although there might not be a significant difference in overall survival. Minimal bone marrow plasmacytosis (< 10%), abnormal serum free light chain ratio, and persistent serum monoclonal protein after radiation therapy might serve as poor prognostic indicators {456}.

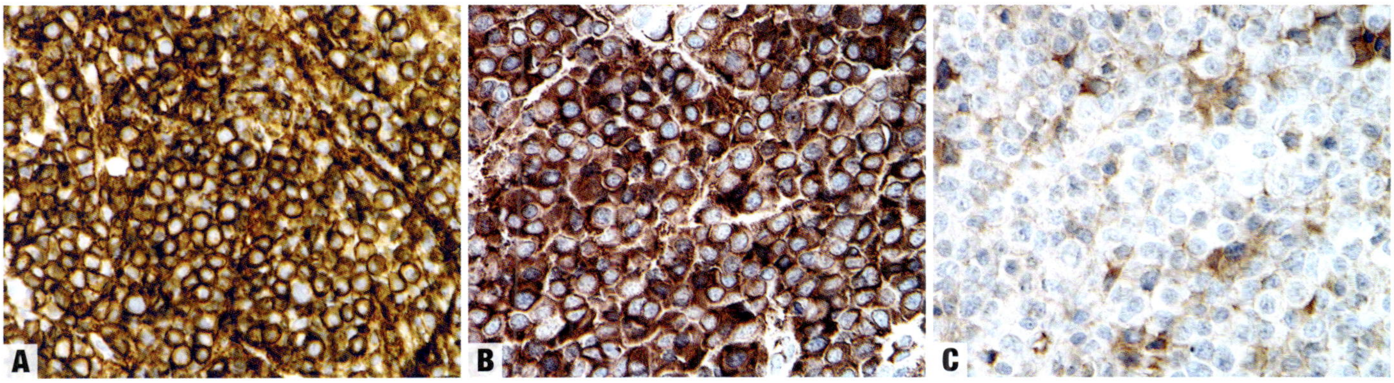

Fig. 10.31 Secondary plasma cell myeloma involving orbit. **A** The atypical plasma cells are positive for CD138. **B** The atypical plasma cells show κ light chain restriction. **C** Only a few tumour cells show expression of lambda light chain.

CD30-positive lymphoproliferative disorders

Krishna Y
Mittal R

Definition

Primary cutaneous CD30+ lymphoproliferative disorders (CD30+ LPD) include lymphomatoid papulosis (LyP) and primary cutaneous anaplastic large cell lymphoma (C-ALCL). LyP is characterized by self-healing but recurrent papulonodular skin lesions, atypical CD30-positive T cells by histology, and an excellent prognosis. C-ALCL is composed of large cells with an anaplastic, pleomorphic, or immunoblastic cytomorphology; > 75% of the tumour cells express CD30.

ICD-O coding

9718/1 Lymphomatoid papulosis
9718/3 Primary cutaneous anaplastic large cell lymphoma

ICD-11 coding

2B03.0 & XH40C0 Primary cutaneous CD30-positive anaplastic large cell lymphoma & Primary cutaneous CD30+ T-cell lymphoproliferative disorder
2B03.1 & XH40C0 Lymphomatoid papulosis & Primary cutaneous CD30+ T-cell lymphoproliferative disorder
2B03.0 & XH3400 Primary cutaneous CD30-positive anaplastic large cell lymphoma & Mature T- and NK-cell lymphomas
2B03.1 & XH3400 Lymphomatoid papulosis & Mature T- and NK-cell lymphomas

Related terminology

Acceptable: ocular adnexal T-cell lymphoma.

Subtype(s)

Cutaneous anaplastic large cell lymphoma and lymphomatoid papulosis

Localization

Ocular adnexal CD30+ LPDs typically arise in the eyelid skin, with C-ALCL found to affect mostly the upper eyelid {678,684, 3249,3248}. They may be primary but are usually secondary to systemic involvement.

Clinical features

Ocular adnexal CD30+ LPDs usually present with unilateral erythema and/or ulceration and swelling of the eyelid, or masses with or without pain, foreign body sensation, or tearing {684, 1353,3249,3248,2428}.

LyP papulonodular lesions have a typical waxing and waning course with different stages of evolution coexisting, and may show partial or complete regression, but relapse is common. LyP may persist for months or several years {3609,292,3248, 3249,749}.

C-ALCL may present with a solitary eyelid-skin nodule often with ulceration {292,1966,3249,3248}. Like LyP, it can show partial or complete regression but relapse is common.

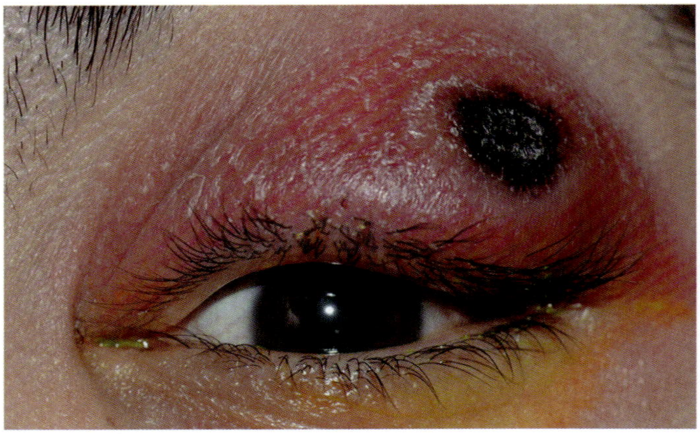

Fig. 10.32 Primary cutaneous anaplastic large cell lymphoma. A 27-year-old male patient with an erythematous poorly defined left upper eyelid nodule with a central eschar.

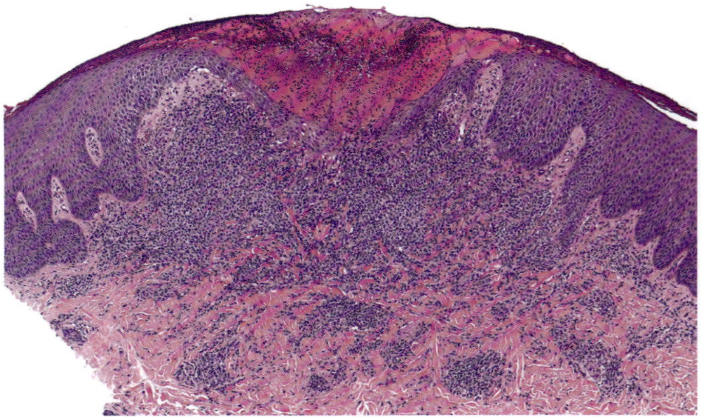

Fig. 10.33 Lymphomatoid papulosis. Wedge-shaped infiltrate of atypical lymphoid cells beneath an ulceration.

Epidemiology

The majority of ocular adnexal T-cell lymphomas (OATCLs) are secondary to systemic disease or direct extension. Primary OATCLs constitute much less than 1% of ocular adnexal lymphomas. Subtypes and their frequency are different for the eyelid compared with the rest of the ocular adnexa, where they are extremely rare.

CD30+ LPDs are the second most common cutaneous T-cell lymphoma with mycosis fungoides being the most common.

LyP most often affects young adults (median age 35–45 years), but children may also be affected, and has a female preponderance {2385,3608,292,749,3249,3248,1966}.

C-ALCL generally occurs in people aged > 50 years (median age 60 years), but children can also be affected, and shows male predominance, similarly to other OATCLs {292,3248,3249, 3607,678,684,3476,2428}.

Etiology

The etiology is unknown. Atopy and staphylococcal superantigens have been pathogenetically linked to LyP {1562}.

A viral etiology has been suggested, but no association has been established {3554,412,1563,1648}. Endogenous retroviral elements have been detected, but their etiological role is unclear {1647,1868}.

Pathogenesis

CD30+ LPDs generally lack the translocation t(2;5) and *ALK* expression, unlike systemic ALCL {753}. Also described are *DUSP22* downregulation; the *NPM::TYK2* translocation; STAT mutations and oncogenic fusion transcripts activating the JAK/STAT pathway; and other frequent chromosomal aberrations including 7q3 gains, and 6q16-21 and 13q34 losses {3517,1833,3655,3442,3465,3248,2122}. *SATB1* is expressed in the vast majority of LyP cases {3240}.

Clonal TR rearrangements have been demonstrated in some LyP cases and associated lymphomas {604,744,64,3248,2428}.

Refer to the fifth-edition *Haematolymphoid tumours* volume {3594}.

Macroscopic appearance

See *Clinical features*, above.

Histopathology

There are six histological subtypes (A–E and 6p25.3 rearrangements) of LyP with distinct histological and/or genetic features {3609,678,292,3608,891,1650,2809,1649,1599}. Broadly, they may comprise diffuse infiltration of small to medium- or large-sized atypical lymphocytes with cerebriform nuclei; occasional large cells (centroblasts, immunoblasts, or Reed–Sternberg-like cells); and scattered plasma cells, eosinophils, neutrophils, and histiocytes.

C-ALCL shows anaplastic lymphocytes with round / oval / irregularly shaped nuclei, prominent nucleoli, and abundant cytoplasm. Similarly to LyP, ulcerating lesions with mixed inflammatory cells are also common {444,678,292,2104,2511,3607}.

Epidermotropism may be present in both proliferations. Lymphovascular invasion is rare.

Immunohistochemistry

Atypical lymphoid cells express CD30 and have an activated CD4+ and/or CD8+ T-cell phenotype depending on subtype. C-ALCL has frequent expression of cytotoxic markers including CD56, TIA1, and granzyme B, and variable loss of CD2, CD3, CD5, and CD7 {678,292,391,1807,2103,3607}. CD15 is expressed in approximately 40% of cases {299,3556}. Tumour cells are negative for B-cell–associated antigens.

Differential diagnosis

C-ALCL and LyP can show significant overlapping histological and phenotypic features among themselves, and also with other cutaneous or systemic TCLs.

Clinicopathological correlation is essential to differentiate LyP not only from these lymphomas, but also from a wide variety of infectious and inflammatory skin diseases that can contain substantial numbers of CD30+ cells {1199,1646,3581}.

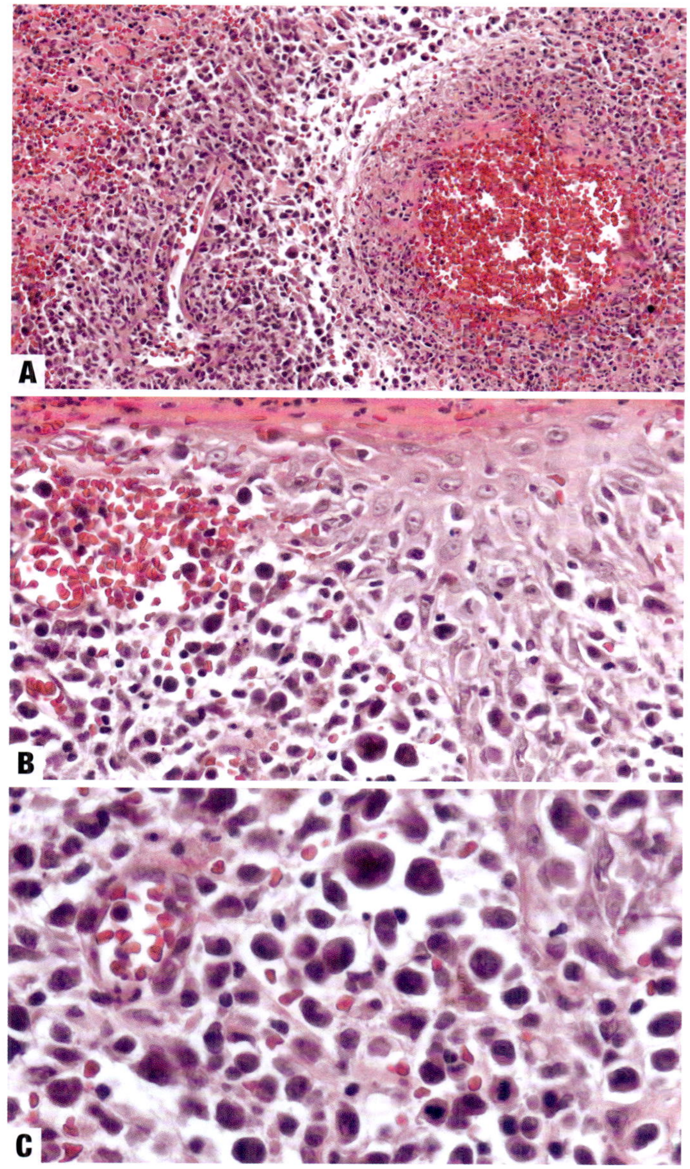

Fig. 10.34 Primary cutaneous anaplastic large cell lymphoma. **A** Angiocentric pattern, associated with necrosis. **B** Epidermotropism is observed. **C** Atypical medium-sized to large lymphocytes with irregular nuclear contours and folds, focally prominent nucleoli, and scant to moderate amounts of cytoplasm, along with brisk mitotic figures and apoptotic bodies.

The term "borderline lesions" refers to cases in which, despite careful clinicopathological correlation, a definite distinction between primary C-ALCL and LyP cannot be made at diagnosis, but evolution of clinical presentation during follow-up discloses whether such patients have C-ALCL or LyP {292,3608,3607,2517}.

Cytology

Not relevant

Diagnostic molecular pathology

Clonal TR gene rearrangements may be detected in C-ALCL and in some LyP cases.

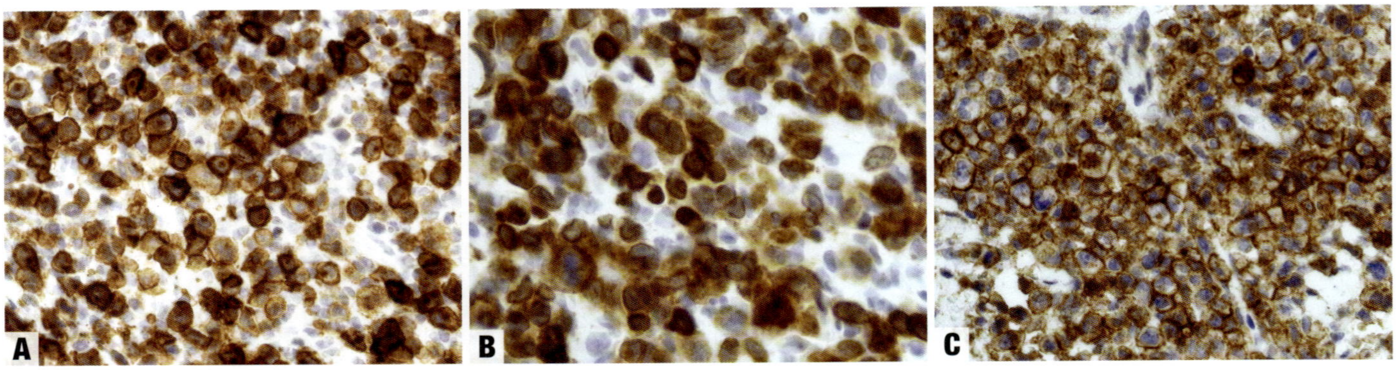

Fig. 10.35 Primary cutaneous anaplastic large cell lymphoma. **A** Tumour cells are positive for CD30. **B** Tumour cells are positive for CD3. **C** Tumour cells are positive for CD4.

Essential and desirable diagnostic criteria

Essential: atypical lymphoid cells expressing CD30 (> 75% of tumour cells in C-ALCL) and T-cell markers; for LyP: a waxing and waning papulonodular rash with spontaneous regression; exclusion of mycosis fungoides; exclusion of reactive process; for C-ALCL: clonal T-cell population; lymphoid cells with anaplastic, pleomorphic, or immunoblastic morphology; no waxing and waning lesions (exclude LyP); exclusion of mycosis fungoides and other TCLs.

Desirable: for LyP: detection of monoclonal rearrangement of TR genes may be helpful in select cases (especially in subtype A).

Staging

LyP: In patients with the typical clinical presentation and no indication of extracutaneous disease on physical examination or blood tests, there is no need for further staging {1651,300}.

C-ALCL: The TNM classification system for primary cutaneous lymphomas other than mycosis fungoides is applied {1701}.

Prognosis and prediction

CD30+ LPDs have a favourable prognosis with absent or low mortality and therefore exclusion of other TCLs is essential to avoid overtreatment.

LyP can have an increased risk (15–50%) of a second lymphoma, particularly mycosis fungoides and C-ALCL, and some non-haematological malignancies, such as cutaneous squamous cell carcinoma, melanoma, and organ-based malignancies. Long-term follow-up is advised owing to increased risk of associated lymphomas {1651,3608,3541,3602,292,749,664,1966,729,24,2161}.

For C-ALCL, worse outcomes are associated with extensive skin lesions on the legs or age > 60 years {300,1966,2900,3633,2851,1353,3249,678,3248}.

T-cell lymphomas

Krishna Y
Auw-Haedrich C
Verdijk RM

Definition
Ocular adnexal T-cell lymphomas (OATCL) are a family of extranodal mature non-Hodgkin lymphomas. They can be primary but are usually secondary to systemic involvement.

ICD-O coding
Code according to lymphoma type.

ICD-11 coding
Code according to lymphoma type.

Related terminology
Acceptable: mature T-cell lymphoma; peripheral T-cell lymphoma.

Subtype(s)
Not applicable

Localization
OATCL may arise in the eyelid, conjunctiva/caruncle, orbital soft tissues, and lacrimal system. The eyelid skin particularly and orbit are the most frequently involved sites {966,678,684,3248}.

Clinical features
Depending on subtype and site, OATCLs usually present with unilateral erythema and/or ulceration and swelling (eyelid), masses with/without foreign body sensation or tearing, proptosis and/or diplopia, and reduced vision {966,684,1353,3248, 2428}.

Epidemiology
OATCLs account for < 1–3% of all ocular adnexal lymphomas. The relative frequencies of the various T-cell lymphoma types in the eyelid are different than in the rest of the ocular adnexa, where T-cell lymphomas are extremely rare. Mycosis fungoides, peripheral T-cell lymphoma (PTCL) NOS, anaplastic large cell lymphoma, γ/δ T-cell lymphoma, and adult T-cell leukaemia/lymphoma have been described in the orbit. Mycosis fungoides is the most common type, followed by PTCL-NOS. They generally occur in patients aged > 50 years and show male predominance. Only lymphomatoid papulosis has female preponderance. However, some mycosis fungoides, cutaneous anaplastic large cell lymphomas, and acute T-cell lymphoblastic leukaemias/lymphomas of the eyelid have been reported in much younger patients {1496,678,684,3476,3248,2428}.

Etiology
The majority of OATCLs are secondary to systemic disease or correspond to a direct extension {678}. Primary OATCLs constitute much less than 1% of ocular adnexal lymphomas overall {2141,684,966,3476}. Causes remain unclear.

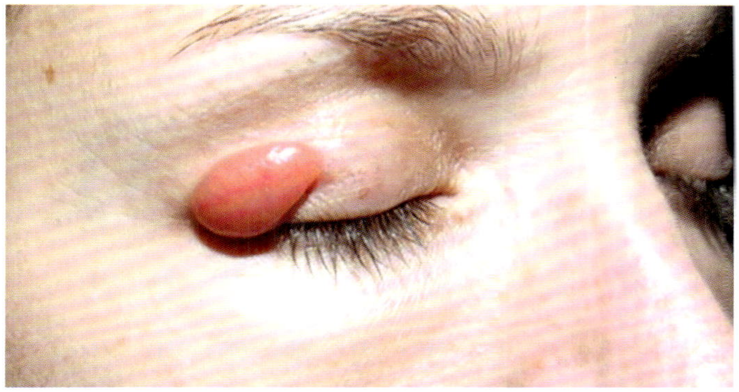

Fig. 10.36 Primary cutaneous T-cell lymphoma involving eyelid. A 35-year-old female patient, otherwise healthy, with a pink, painless mass at the lateral edge of her right upper lid.

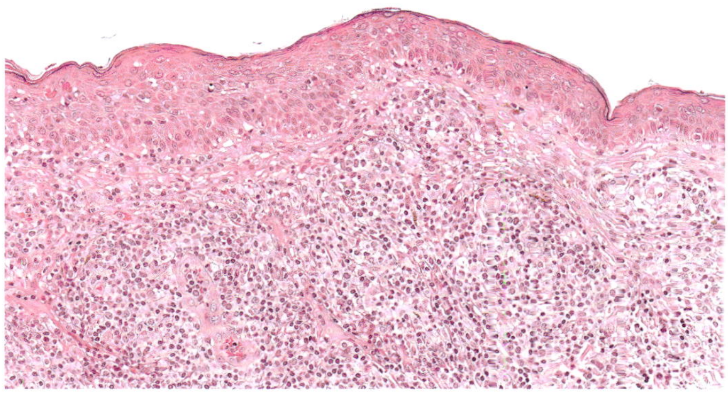

Fig. 10.37 Primary cutaneous T-cell lymphoma. Histology of the upper lid nodule shown in Fig. 10.36. Small to medium-sized atypical CD4+ T cells (also CD3+ and CD2+, not shown) with monoclonal rearrangement of the TR genes.

Pathogenesis
EBV has been associated with PTCL and anaplastic large cell lymphoma, whereas human T-cell lymphotropic virus type 1 has been linked with adult T-cell leukaemia/lymphoma {3131, 64,3248,2428}.

Macroscopic appearance
OATCLs present as ulcerated or papular lesions on eyelid skin and elsewhere in the orbit as a smooth, pinkish mass.

Histopathology
Depending on subtype, OATCLs comprise diffuse infiltration of lymphocytes that are small to medium sized with atypical, irregular nuclei, and scattered plasma cells, eosinophils, histiocytes, and occasional large cells (centroblasts, immunoblasts, or Reed–Sternberg–like cells). Remnants of reactive follicles, small blood vessels, and/or fibrous bands may be seen.

Immunohistochemistry

T-cell–associated antigens (CD3, CD5, CD4, CD8) are positive, with a CD4 predominance, and other markers including CD30, CD56, ALK-1, TIA1, and granzyme B may be positive depending on subtype. Ki-67 is high (60–70%). Tumour cells are negative for B-cell–associated antigens. EBV / EBV-encoded small RNA (EBER) in situ hybridization may be positive, depending on the lymphoma type.

Differential diagnosis

Differential diagnosis includes reactive processes, or any B-cell lymphoma in which infiltrates may be enriched in reactive T cells.

Cytology

FNAB is not recommended for the diagnosis of lymphomas or inflammatory processes of the ocular adnexa.

Diagnostic molecular pathology

Detection of clonal TR gene rearrangements may help in the diagnosis. Refer to the *Haematolymphoid tumours* volume {3594}. It is likely that OATCLs, especially in eyelid skin, share similar genetic aberrations to their counterparts in other locations but these are difficult to confirm owing to their rarity.

Essential and desirable diagnostic criteria

Essential: T-cell lymphoma (confirmatory immunohistochemistry); exclusion of B-cell lymphoma; exclusion of reactive process.

Desirable: demonstration of clonal T-cell population; cell-of-origin subtyping; cytogenetics; EBV-associated markers (depending on type).

Staging

The American Joint Committee on Cancer (AJCC) and eighth-edition TNM staging systems better predict outcome and are preferred over the Ann Arbor staging system for primary ocular adnexal lymphoma {3590,3476,3248,2675}.

Prognosis and prediction

Tumour type is the most important prognostic indicator. Primary OATCLs generally have a good disease-specific survival, especially those of the eyelid, whereas conjunctival T-cell lymphomas have a poorer prognosis. Secondary and high-stage disease are predictors of poorer prognosis. Most OATCLs are secondary manifestations of systemic disease and thus carry a poor prognosis with higher rates of recurrence and relapse {1353,3249,678,3248}.

Extranodal NK/T-cell lymphoma

Krishna Y
Auw-Haedrich C
Verdijk RM

Definition

Extranodal NK/T-cell lymphoma (ENKTL) is an extranodal lymphoma of NK or T-cell lineage, characterized by vascular damage and destruction, prominent necrosis, cytotoxic phenotype, and association with EBV.

ICD-O coding

9719/3 Extranodal NK/T-cell lymphoma

ICD-11 coding

2A90.6 Extranodal NK/T-cell lymphoma, nasal type

Related terminology

Acceptable: extranodal NK/T-cell lymphoma, nasal type.
Not recommended: angiocentric lymphoma; lethal midline granuloma; malignant midline reticulosis; polymorphic reticulosis.

Subtype(s)

None

Localization

Ocular adnexal (OA) ENKTL usually arises from secondary spread from the paranasal sinuses or nasal cavity but metastasis from cutaneous or systemic disease is possible. It may involve the eyelid, conjunctiva/caruncle, orbital soft tissues, and lacrimal system. The orbit and lacrimal gland are most frequently involved. Intraocular and CNS involvement may occur in advanced cases. Primary orbital involvement without evidence of nasal mucosal involvement is rare {678,620,3639, 3476,893,2015,1241}.

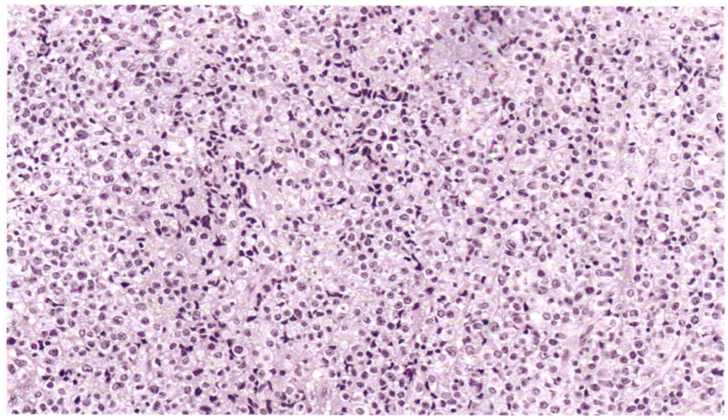

Fig. 10.38 Primary sinonasal extranodal NK/T-cell lymphoma that involved the orbit. A diffuse infiltration of medium-sized to large atypical lymphoid cells is observed.

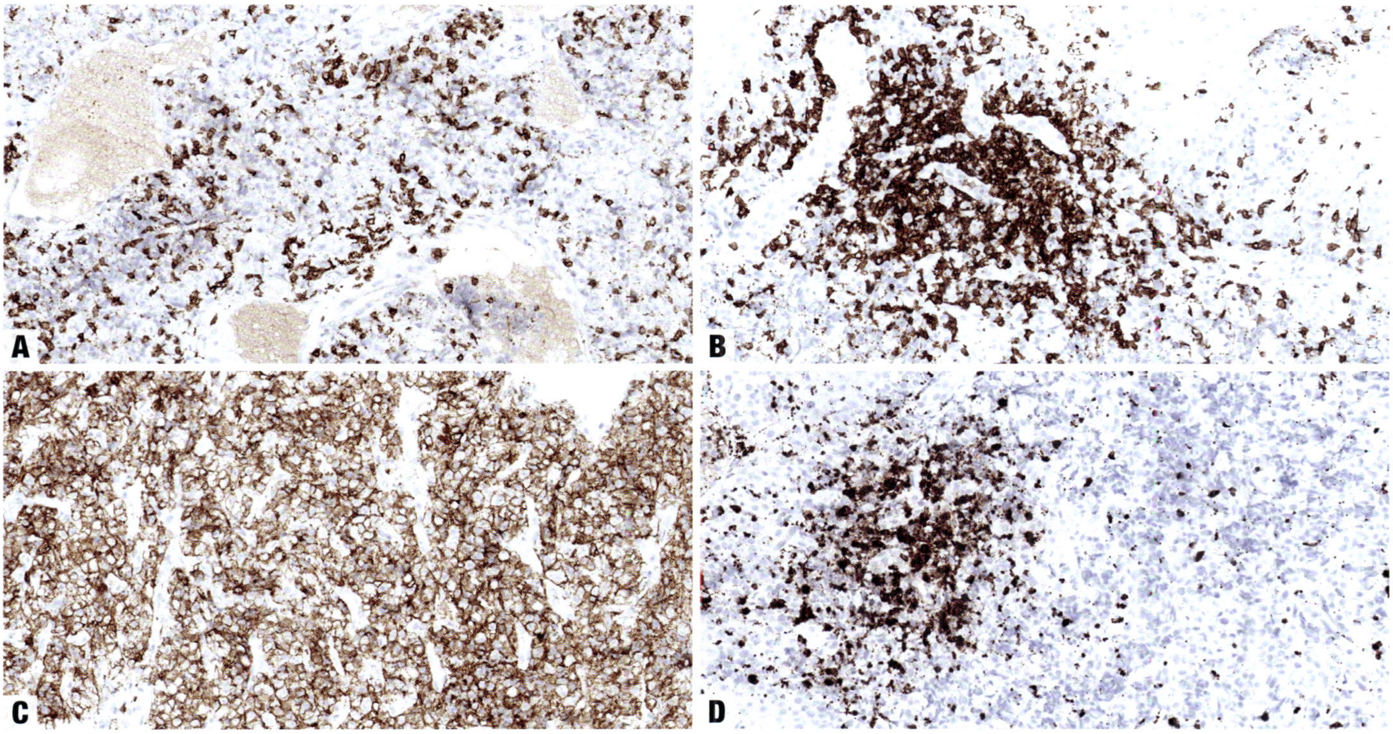

Fig. 10.39 Primary sinonasal extranodal NK/T-cell lymphoma that involved the orbit. The tumour cells show variable expression of the T-cell markers CD2 (**A**) and CD8 (**B**). The cells are uniformly positive for CD56 (**C**), and many tumour cells also stain positive for granzyme B (**D**) and TIA1 (not shown).

Table 10.04 Differential diagnosis of extranodal NK/T-cell lymphoma (ENKTL)

Disease entity	Major distinguishing features vs ENKTL
EBV-positive nodal T- and NK-cell lymphoma	Predominant nodal localization of disease Coagulative necrosis and angioinvasion usually not prominent Neoplastic cells often large (resembling large B-cell lymphoma) Most cases exhibit T-cell rather than NK-cell phenotype
Aggressive NK-cell leukaemia	Predominately involves peripheral blood and bone marrow Prominent constitutional symptoms Always of NK-cell lineage by definition (whereas ENKTL comprises neoplasms of NK- or T-cell lineage)
Subcutaneous panniculitis-like T-cell lymphoma	In the skin, preferential infiltration of subcutaneous tissue with sparing of the dermis Often CD8+, CD56–, TCRαβ+ EBV–
Primary cutaneous gamma-delta T-cell lymphoma	Expression of TCRγδ by definition (contrasting with its extreme rarity in ENKTL) Usually EBV–
Systemic EBV-positive T-cell lymphoma of childhood	Paediatric and adolescent age group Presentation with systemic disease, including hepatosplenomegaly Lymphoid cells show T-cell phenotype
Monomorphic epitheliotropic intestinal T-cell lymphoma	Most commonly monomorphic infiltrate of medium-sized lymphoid cells (contrasting with the usually polymorphic infiltrate of ENKTL) Necrosis uncommon Often CD8+ (which is very uncommon in ENKTL) EBV–
Indolent NK-cell lymphoproliferative disorder of the gastrointestinal tract	Small lesion(s) in the gastrointestinal tract Usually superficial and non-destructive growth Medium-sized lymphoid cells with distinct eosinophilic cytoplasmic granules Always of NK-cell lineage by definition (whereas ENKTL comprises neoplasms of NK- or T-cell lineage) EBV–
Lymphomatoid granulomatosis	Predominant sites are lung, brain, kidney, and skin (all except skin uncommonly involved in ENKTL) Atypical cells are of B-cell lineage EBV+ in B cells
Granulomatosis with polyangiitis (Wegener granulomatosis)	Serum positive for cytoplasmic antineutrophilic cytoplasmic antibodies (c-ANCAs) or myeloperoxidase antibodies Poorly formed granulomas and microabscesses Necrotizing vasculitis involving arterioles, small arteries, and veins Lack of atypical lymphoid cell infiltrate Lack of lymphoid population with NK-cell or aberrant T-cell immunophenotype EBV–
Acute EBV-positive cytotoxic T-cell lymphoid hyperplasia of upper aerodigestive tract	Children and young adults Acute onset of symptoms, often including fever Atypical lymphoid infiltrate usually CD5+ and CD56– Complete remission within 1 month without cytotoxic therapy

Clinical features

OA-ENKTL may present as proptosis and/or diplopia with limited ocular motility, reduced vision, pain, and chemosis. Nasal cavity involvement may present as nasal blockage and epistaxis {678,620,3639,893,2015,2428,1241}.

Epidemiology

OA-ENKTL accounts for < 1–2% of all OA lymphomas. It is prevalent in eastern Asia and in the Indigenous peoples of Central and South America, although cases in White populations are documented. It generally occurs in people aged > 50 years, but has been reported in younger patients, and shows male predominance {1496,678,684,3248,173,1400,3476}.

Etiology

ENKTL is strongly associated with EBV infection, which is present in a clonal episomal form with a type II latency pattern, and shows a 30 bp deletion in the *LMP1* gene {893,519,179,518,880,2625,2576,1592,2258,3656,3594}.

ENKTL can occur in immunosuppressed patients, including after transplantation {1820,1368,3385}. Other risk factors include lifestyle and environmental factors, with increased risk reported among farmers and pesticide users {3658}.

Pathogenesis

A variety of complex genomic alterations have been reported, with region deletion 6q21-25 at chromosome 6q being the most common {2346,1392,2377}. In the 6q21 region, several tumour suppressor genes, including *PRDM1*, *ATG5*, *AIM1*, *HACE1*, and *FOXO3*, have been identified {1429,1616,570}. Recurrent mutations have also been reported in the JAK/STAT pathway genes (*STAT3*, *JAK3*, *STAT5B*), epigenetic regulators (*BCOR*, *KMT2D*, *ARID1A*, *EP300*), tumour suppressor genes (*TP53*, *MGA*), and RNA helicase (*DDX3X*) {2626,1767,1896,1520,3594}.

Macroscopic appearance

OA-ENKTL presents as a fleshy mass often with haemorrhage, necrosis, and/or ulceration.

Histopathology

OA-ENKTL shows diffuse infiltration of variably sized atypical lymphoid cells with an angiocentric-angiodestructive growth pattern and coagulative necrosis; scattered apoptotic bodies and a heavy admixture of small lymphocytes, plasma cells, eosinophils, and histiocytes; and numerous abnormal mitoses.

Immunohistochemistry

Neoplastic cells are CD2+, cytoplasmic CD3ε+, CD56+, CD43+, and CD8+/–; and positive for cytotoxic markers (TIA1, granzyme B, and perforin). They are usually negative for other NK- and T-cell antigens (CD16, CD57, surface CD3, CD4, CD5).

EBV-encoded small RNA (EBER) in situ hybridization positivity is essential.

Differential diagnosis

EBV-negative extranodal cytotoxic T-cell lymphoma is classed as PTCL-NOS.

See Table 10.04 {3594}.

Cytology

Not relevant

Diagnostic molecular pathology

In situ hybridization for EBER is positive in the majority of tumour cells. TR gene rearrangement studies may be performed for select problematic cases {3262}.

Essential and desirable diagnostic criteria

Essential: extranodal infiltration by lymphoma cells with variable morphology; NK/cytotoxic T-cell phenotype; EBER-positive.

Desirable: angiocentric-angiodestructive growth; necrosis.

Staging

The Lugano system is used to stage systemic ENKTL {574}.

For primary OA-ENKTL, the American Joint Committee on Cancer (AJCC) and eighth-edition TNM staging systems better predict outcome and are preferred over the Ann Arbor staging system {3590,3476,3248,2675}.

Prognosis and prediction

With systemic chemoradiotherapy, the 5-year overall survival rate in early stage disease is 54% {1637,1022,1907}. Patients > 60 years, advanced systemic disease, and higher levels of circulating EBV DNA have a significantly worse prognosis {1637, 1022,1973}.

Chapter 10

Myeloid sarcoma

Krishna Y
Mittal R

Definition
Myeloid sarcoma (MS) is a tumour mass involving any anatomical site other than bone marrow (i.e. extramedullary) that effaces tissue architecture and is composed of myeloid blasts, with or without maturation.

ICD-O coding
9930/3 Myeloid sarcoma

ICD-11 coding
2A60.39 Myeloid sarcoma

Related terminology
Not recommended: chloroma; granulocytic/monocytic sarcoma; myeloblastoma; myelocytoma; chloroleukaemia.

Subtype(s)
None

Localization
Ocular adnexal MS (OA-MS) mainly arises in the orbital soft tissue where it moulds around the orbital structures. It may rarely involve the eyelid skin, conjunctiva, and lacrimal drainage system {41,2674,1210,2597,2428,122}.

Clinical features
OA-MS is reported in 2–9% of patients with acute myeloid leukaemia (AML) at diagnosis or relapse. It can rarely precede AML onset. MS may also be a manifestation of secondary AML transformation from myelodysplastic neoplasms, myeloproliferative neoplasms, or myelodysplastic/myeloproliferative neoplasms {2554,1210,3213,238}. De novo isolated MS with morphologically normal bone marrow is rare, occurring in about 1% of AML patients {1210,285,2,2680}.

OA-MS usually presents with unilateral proptosis and diplopia with/without pain, eyelid swelling, chemosis, and/or exposure keratopathy {3073,41,2674,2597,2428,122}.

Epidemiology
MS is more common in children and young adults (median age 7–12 years) but can occur at any age, with a slight male preponderance {3073,41,2674,1210,2597,2428,122,2680}.

Etiology
The etiology is similar to that of AML. The reasons for homing and clustering outside the haematopoietic system as an extramedullary mass are still unknown. OA-MS may originate from an involved area of adjacent bone/periosteum {961,2674,1210}. Adhesion molecules (e.g. ITGA7), chemokine receptor/ligand interactions, and extracellular matrix interactions are suggested as being involved {925,3735,1750}.

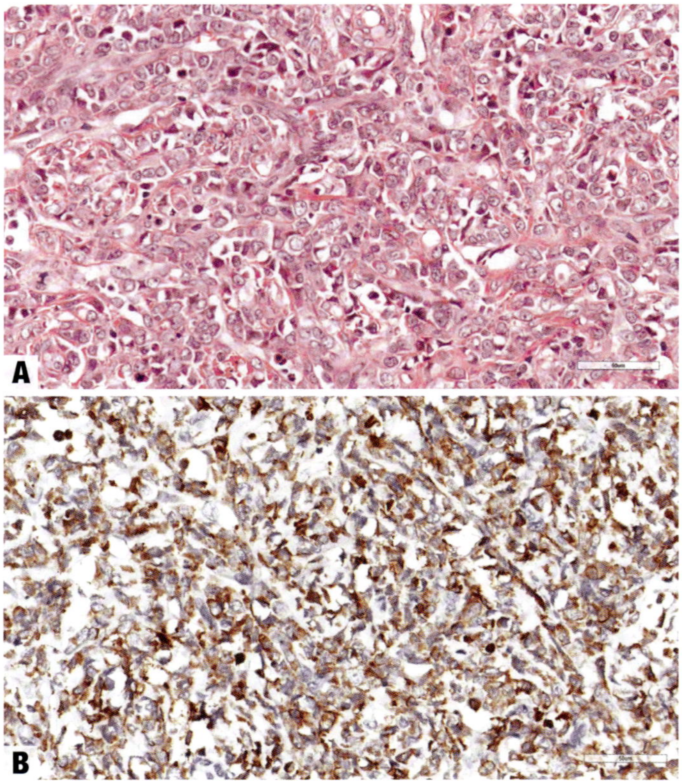

Fig. 10.40 Extramedullary myeloid sarcoma. **A** Sheets of large neoplastic cells with round nuclei, irregular nuclear contours, fine blastic chromatin, and conspicuous nucleoli. **B** The neoplastic cells are strongly positive for myeloperoxidase, supporting the diagnosis of myeloid sarcoma.

Pathogenesis
MS shares similar molecular abnormalities with AML, including t(8;21) (*RUNX1*::*RUNX1T1*), inv(16) (*CBFB*::*MYH11*), trisomy 4 and 8, monosomy 7, and deletions of 5q and 20q {2554,3761}. Some of these aberrations may be associated with particular involved sites, with t(8;21) often involving the orbital region in children {2554,710,3761}.

Other molecular abnormalities include gene mutations in *NPM1*, *KMT2A*, and *FLT3*-ITD, and in RAS pathway (~50%) and epigenetic pathway genes, and signalling, transcription, and tumour suppressor genes {2506,1620,597,1166,2}.

Refer to the fifth-edition *Haematolymphoid tumours* volume {3594}.

Macroscopic appearance
The tumour presents as a diffuse infiltration and enlargement of the involved site with a fish-flesh grey/white cut surface, or as a green mass due to myeloperoxidase expressed by granulocytic cells.

Histopathology

MS diffusely effaces tissue architecture and comprises neoplastic cells as islands or cords or in a single-file pattern, with intervening delicate fibrous stroma. Brisk mitoses, spotty necrosis, and crush artefacts are frequently noted {2674}. Tumour cells are intermediate-sized to large, with scant to moderate amounts of pale or eosinophilic cytoplasm, round-oval nuclei with irregular membranes, fine (blastic) chromatin, and usually small nucleoli {2554,3761,3613}. Tumours may exhibit granulocytic (eosinophilic myelocytes and metamyelocytes), monocytic (cells with folded nuclei promonocytes), or myelomonocytic differentiation.

Immunophenotype

Tumour cells express CD13, CD33, CD43, CD68, and myeloperoxidase; CD45 is positive in 60% of cases. Tumour cells are CD34+ and KIT+ in tumours with an immature granulocytic profile, whereas they are CD34− in tumours with a mature profile. CD11b, CD11c, CD15, CD64, KIT (~30%), and lysozyme are expressed in tumours with immature monocytic cells / monoblasts, whereas expression of CD14, CD68, and CD163 is variable in those with a mature monocytic profile {2775,559, 2554,3073,41,3613,1629,2597,122}. CD61 and glycophorin A are expressed in tumours with megakaryocytic and erythroid differentiation, respectively. MS may express B-cell, T-cell, or NK-cell markers, such as CD19, CD7, and CD56, respectively. CD123, CD99, and TdT (weak) can be expressed in subsets {2554,3613}.

Differential diagnosis

Differential diagnosis includes lymphoblastic lymphomas, small blue round cell tumours, histiocytic/dendritic neoplasms, orbital cellulitis {3073,2847,3613,3235,1678,41,2674,1210,2597,2428, 122}, and extramedullary haematopoiesis {1038,2554,2432}.

Cytology

Not relevant

Diagnostic molecular pathology

Detection of MS is equivalent to a diagnosis of AML {3613, 3764}. Comprehensive evaluation is needed for correct classification, prognostication, and therapy planning.

Essential and desirable diagnostic criteria

Essential: effacement of tissue architecture by a mass comprising myeloblasts of varying maturation; positive expression of granulocytic and/or monocytic markers by tumour cells.

Desirable: complete workup, including cytogenetic and molecular analyses, is suggested in patients with de novo MS.

Staging

Evaluation of peripheral blood and bone marrow for AML or other myeloid neoplasms (myelodysplastic neoplasms, myeloproliferative neoplasms, or myelodysplastic/myeloproliferative neoplasms) is essential.

Prognosis and prediction

Recommended therapy for MS is AML-type chemotherapy, guided by targets identified by cytogenetic and molecular analyses, as per the National Comprehensive Cancer Network (NCCN). Identification of specific genetic aberrations improves diagnosis and prognostication, and provides therapeutic targets. Radiotherapy can be used in select cases.

The prognosis for patients with MS may be similar {2290,392, 1893}, better {3388,1893,285,2}, or worse {2554,3583,1136} when compared with that for patients with AML and their mutation profiles. Patients with isolated MS appear to have a better prognosis and longer remission.

Juvenile xanthogranuloma

Alkatan H
van Halteren AGS

Definition

Juvenile xanthogranuloma (JXG) is a clonal expansion of non–Langerhans cell histiocytes in the skin or mucosa that share a dermal macrophage phenotype with a favourable outcome, except in rare cases with systemic dissemination.

ICD-O coding

9749/1 Juvenile xanthogranuloma

ICD-11 coding

2B31.0 Juvenile xanthogranuloma

Related terminology

Acceptable: disseminated juvenile xanthogranuloma.
Not recommended: nevoxanthoendothelioma.

Subtype(s)

None

Localization

JXGs are generally confined to the skin, with a predilection for the head and neck, upper trunk, and proximal extremities {756,1501,3154,1116,2836,523,2840}. Ocular sites are the commonest extracutaneous sites for JXG compared with the lungs, brain, and spleen {1034,2444}. JXG can affect the eyelids, orbit, iris, conjunctiva/corneal sclera, choroid, retina, and optic nerve {3770,3584,1687,750,2844,1284,1338,1816,2241, 1530}. The most affected ocular sites are the iris, eyelid, and conjunctiva {3770,2836,105}.

Clinical features

Iris lesions are usually nodular and can often be missed clinically until the child presents with spontaneous hyphaema, often associated with increased intraocular pressure. Complications include corneal blood staining, recurrent bleeding, and secondary glaucoma {2479,2836}. Eyelid lesions can present as solitary or multiple yellowish painless nodules or dome-shaped papules; they can be complicated by fibrosis leading to eyelid retraction and lagophthalmos {105}. Choroidal JXG presents as a mass lesion, may result in vitreous opacities, and can be confused clinically with a malignant tumour {2844,2836}. Orbital JXG can present either as a primary soft tissue tumour or as secondary extension {3012}. Conjunctival JXG presents as a pinkish mass with or without redness. Giant JXGs have been described {3493}. Less than 5% of JXGs are systemic {756,1501,3154}.

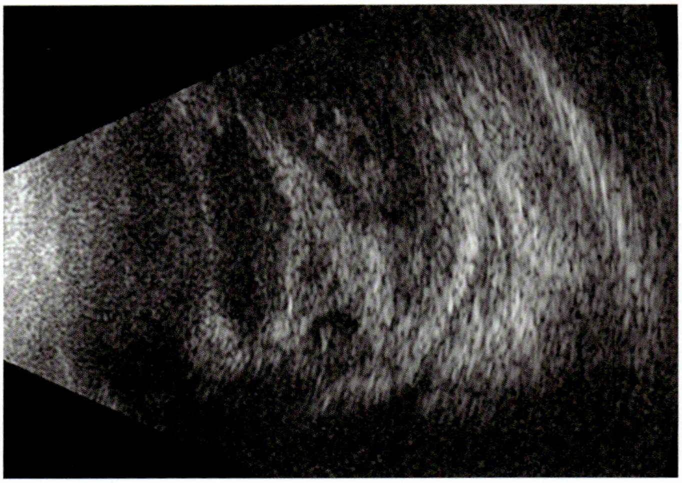

Fig. 10.41 Juvenile xanthogranuloma. Ultrasound biomicroscopy (B-scan) of a case of juvenile xanthogranuloma involving the left eye choroid with adjacent vitreous opacities mimicking intraocular malignancy.

Epidemiology

JXG is rare, with a frequency of about 1 per 1 million children {756,3154}. More than 70% of JXGs arise in the first year of life

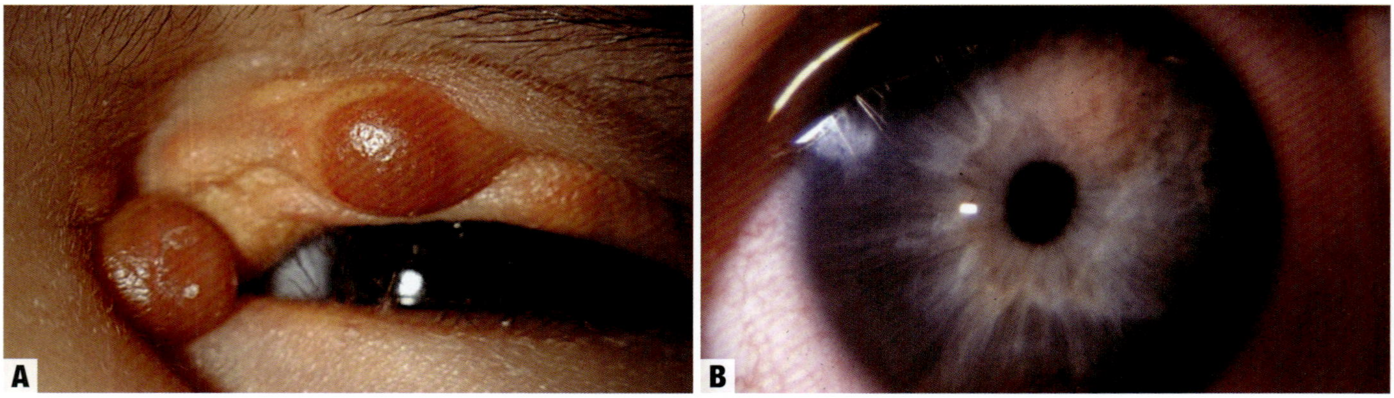

Fig. 10.42 Juvenile xanthogranuloma. **A** The clinical appearance of yellowish-red round juvenile xanthogranuloma lesions affecting the upper lid and the skin of the medial canthus. **B** Juvenile xanthogranuloma involving the iris.

(20–35% congenital) and show a male predilection (M:F ratio 1.4:1) {1501,2130,1430}. JXG is very rare in adults.

Ocular lesions occur in about 0.3–10% of children with cutaneous JXG {523,1606}. Most of the non-congenital JXGs (40–70%) manifest during infancy {1322} with a median age of onset of 5 months {756}. Median age at presentation of ophthalmic JXG varies depending on the location but ranges from 0.5 to 2.5 years {2836}. In a recent series, a higher median age (~6 years) was reported {105}.

Etiology

The etiology is unknown. JXG may occur in patients affected by neurofibromatosis type 1 (NF1) {464}; whether there is a higher prevalence of juvenile myelomonocytic leukaemia in NF1 patients affected by JXG is debated {3777,1979,1034,2322,3154}. JXG is also reported in Wiskott–Aldrich syndrome {3378}. Occurrence of JXG in monozygotic twins may suggest genetic transmission {3271,848}.

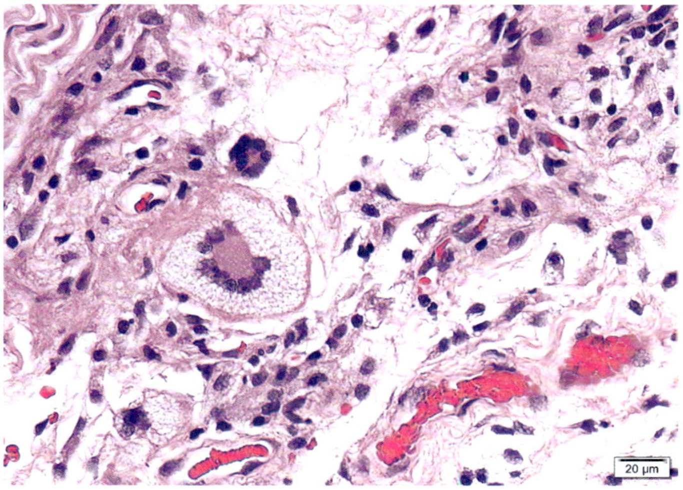

Fig. 10.43 Juvenile xanthogranuloma. Typical Touton giant cell.

Pathogenesis

Pathogenetic mechanisms in JXG are poorly understood. Expression of fascin and factor XIIIa supports a histogenetic link with dermal macrophages {2130}. MAPK/ERK pathway alterations play a pathogenetic role in JXG {847}. Activating mutations of *NRAS*, *KRAS*, *ARAF*, *MAP2K1*, and *CSF1R*, along with *RNF11::BRAF* fusion and *NTRK1* fusions have been reported {2512,848,792,3300,509,2546}. *PIK3CD* mutations, identified in a few cases, suggest a pathogenetic role of the PI3K pathway in some JXGs {510,112}.

Macroscopic appearance

Excised soft tissue masses are usually firm and greyish to brownish in colour, with a smooth outer surface and yellowish cut surface {2286}.

Histopathology

Cutaneous and mucosal JXGs are unencapsulated, circumscribed lesions composed of histiocytes with a dermal macrophage phenotype, which typically spare the epidermis/epithelium {3727,2130}. Their histopathological appearance is related to the duration of inflammation. In recently formed lesions, histiocytes are intermixed with lymphocytes, plasma cells, and to a lesser extent eosinophils, and they may show elongated morphology {1034}. In mature, well-developed lesions, the histiocytes are typically foamy with characteristic Touton giant cells (showing a ring of nuclei surrounded by foamy cytoplasm) observed in 85% of cases {1034,1322,756,2479}. Touton giant cells are less prevalent in intraocular JXG compared with in cutaneous lesions {2499,2479}. Fibroblasts and fibrosis are dominant features in late-stage JXG lesions {1322,2479}.

Immunohistochemistry

JXG-associated histiocytes are positive for CD163, CD68, CD14, lysozyme, factor XIIIa, fascin, vimentin, and CD4, but lack positivity for CD1a and CD207 (langerin) {896,2130}. S100 staining should be negative or weak {756,1160,105}. Staining for ALK is negative.

Differential diagnosis

These include Langerhans cell histiocytosis, ALK-positive histiocytosis, epithelioid fibrous histiocytoma, and Erdheim–Chester disease {1847,2814,2546,1160,1653}. Orbital inflammation in adolescents and adults can be due to IgG4-related

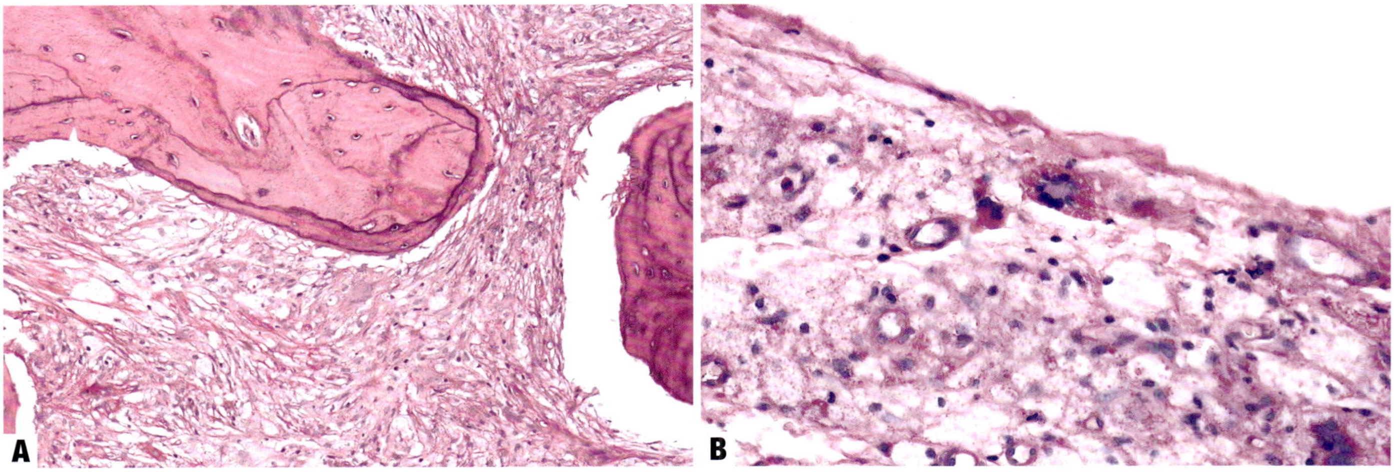

Fig. 10.44 Juvenile xanthogranuloma. **A** Histiocytic infiltration of bone in a case of orbital juvenile xanthogranuloma (PAS stain). **B** Characteristic Touton giant cell in juvenile xanthogranuloma (PAS stain).

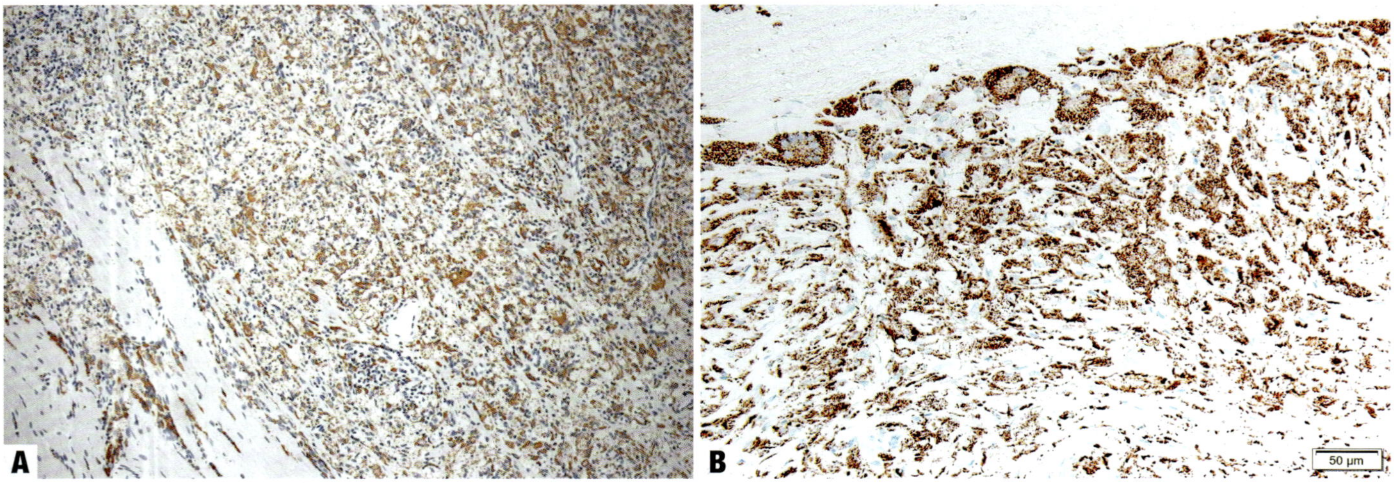

Fig. 10.45 Juvenile xanthogranuloma. **A** The histiocytes showing reactivity with CD68 stain in a case of juvenile xanthogranuloma. **B** Non-Langerhans histiocytes expressing reactivity to CD68.

xanthogranulomatous disease {1304,3479}. Necrobiotic xanthogranulomas also present as eyelid or anterior orbital lesions {3479,1687}.

Cytology

Cytological features in JXG can be difficult to differentiate from other histiocytic lesions that share the presence of foamy histiocytes and Touton giant cells, but immunocytochemistry may help {1930,247}, together with molecular analysis and the exclusion of typical clinical features associated with Erdheim–Chester disease. In choroidal JXG, FNAB may be useful to establish the diagnosis and rule out malignant tumours {2844,2836}.

Diagnostic molecular pathology

Not relevant in typical cases

Essential and desirable diagnostic criteria

Essential: circumscribed lesion comprising histiocytes (commonly foamy) lacking significant nuclear pleomorphism, with immunophenotype of dermal macrophage (CD68 / CD163 / factor XIIIa); background comprising admixed diverse inflammatory cells and fibroblasts; negativity of histiocytes for CD1a, CD207, and ALK.

Desirable: Touton giant cells; low number of IgG4+ plasma cells; clinical exclusion of Erdheim–Chester disease.

Staging

Not relevant

Prognosis and prediction

JXG has an excellent prognosis: cutaneous and mucosal lesions often resolve spontaneously, possibly leaving an atrophic scar. Surgical excision is indicated in eyelid and orbital JXG in cases of functional limitation {896} and should be curative {1108,1256,1430, 1627}. Conjunctival lesions can be treated by different modalities including the use of steroids {2241,2836}. Ocular JXG may be complicated by glaucoma, uveitis, or visual impairment {2025,502}.

A comprehensive clinical assessment should be undertaken in patients with JXG who are suspected to have systemic involvement. Ophthalmic or intracranial JXG can be part of systemic JXG presentation.

Treatment with clofarabine, cladribine, and combined cytarabine with cladribine has been used in patients with systemic JXG with variable response {3098,2130}. Treatment with targeted kinase inhibition is also a newer option for those for whom conventional treatment does not work {874,2130,2546}.

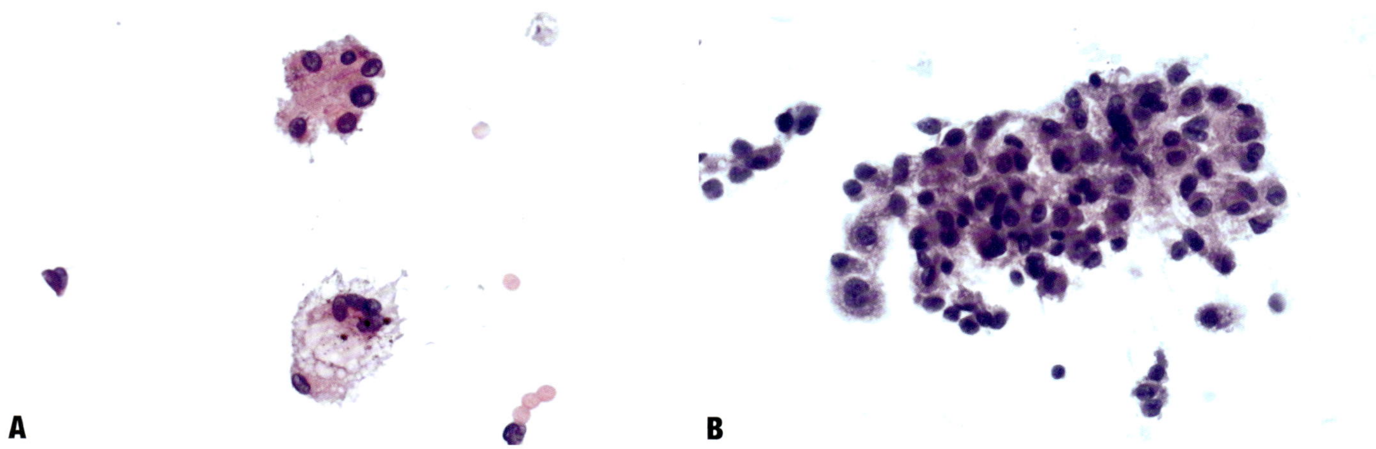

Fig. 10.46 Juvenile xanthogranuloma. **A** FNA showing characteristic Touton cells in a mild inflammatory background. **B** FNA reveals aggregates of histiocytes.

Rosai–Dorfman disease

Alkatan H
Eberhart CG
van Halteren AGS

Definition

Rosai–Dorfman disease (RDD) is a histiocytic disorder characterized by nodal or extranodal accumulation of large S100-positive macrophage-like histiocytes commonly displaying emperipolesis.

ICD-O coding

9749/3 Rosai–Dorfman disease

ICD-11 coding

EK92 Histiocytoses of uncertain malignant potential

Related terminology

Acceptable: Rosai–Dorfman–Destombes disease.
Not recommended: sinus histiocytosis with massive lymphadenopathy.

Subtype(s)

None

Localization

RDD most frequently involves lymph nodes, particularly in the cervical region. Extranodal disease occurs in 43% of cases. Ophthalmic manifestations occur in 10–30% of cases {1021, 598,17,2351}, and include unilateral or bilateral soft tissue masses in the orbit, eyelids, lacrimal glands, extraocular muscles, conjunctiva, or cornea {17,2351,1687}. Intraocular RDD can present as choroidal masses {1021,2243,2564}. Isolated ophthalmic RDD is extremely rare {1021,1020,2101,130}.

Clinical features

The typical presentation is that of painless, slow-growing lymphadenopathy, with accompanying B symptoms in one third of patients, or symptoms related to involved extranodal sites {1020,17}. A painless soft tissue mass and/or proptosis are the commonest clinical manifestations of orbital RDD. Other symptoms include reduced vision, restricted motility, ptosis, pain, compressive optic neuropathy, and diplopia {1021,130}. The presentation of cutaneous RDD is variable, typically that of painless, multiple, reddish-brown papules, nodules, or plaques, often reaching a large size of 300 mm {708,1763}, though single nodules are also common. This cutaneous RDD has its own unique clinical and epidemiological characteristics {431}.

Clinical associations are recognized: familial RDD, classic RDD, extranodal RDD, neoplasia-associated RDD; and immune disease–associated RDD {895}.

Imaging may show destruction of surrounding bones including the nasal cavity and paranasal sinuses {130,17}. RDD presenting in the sella region is often accompanied by visual changes and diabetes insipidus {3751}. Epibulbar masses, uveitis, and papilloedema have also been reported {1021,2243,2564}.

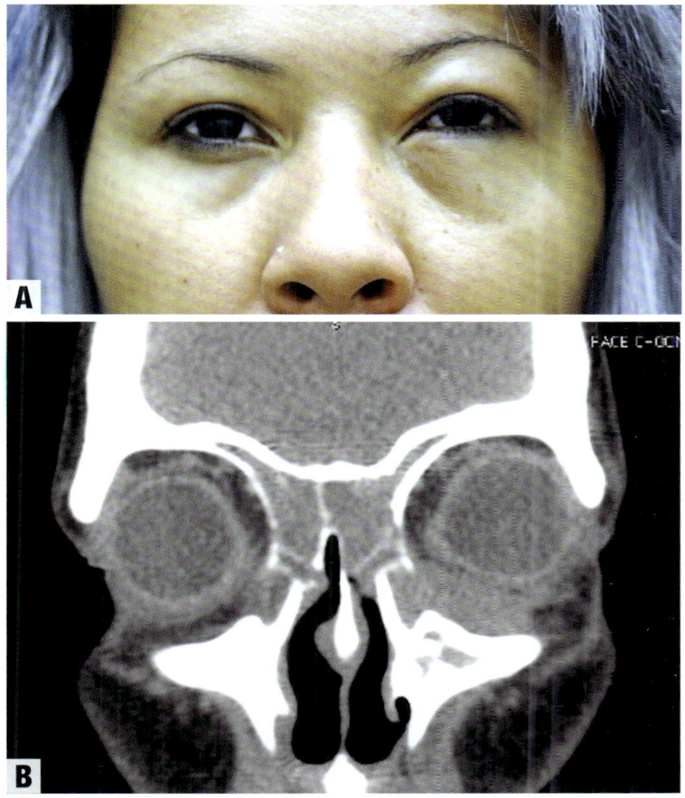

Fig. 10.47 Rosai–Dorfman disease. **A** A case of Rosai–Dorfman disease in a female patient presenting at the age of 32 years with left proptosis and superior displacement of the left globe due to an inferomedial orbital mass. **B** Coronal CT of the orbits in the same patient showing a left inferomedial orbital mass with involvement of the ethmoidal sinuses.

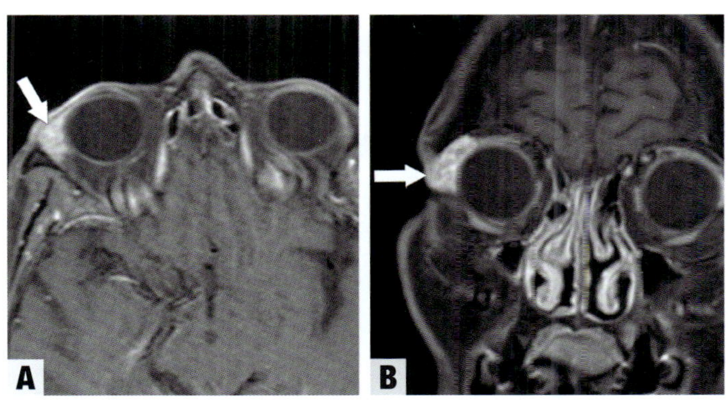

Fig. 10.48 Rosai–Dorfman disease. Axial (**A**) and coronal (**B**) T1-weighted post-contrast MRI shows a heterogeneously enhancing lesion in the right lacrimal gland and superotemporal right orbit (arrows).

Epidemiology

The global incidence of RDD is unknown; the annual prevalence in the USA is 1:200 000 {17}. It affects children and young adults

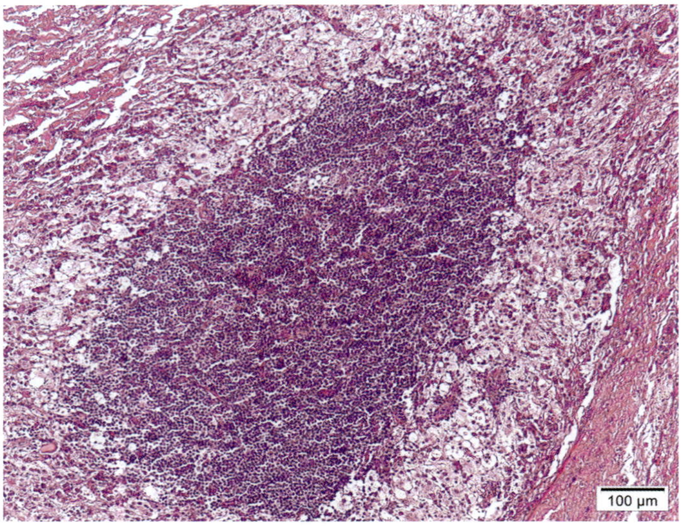

Fig. 10.49 Rosai–Dorfman disease. A mixed infiltrate of histiocytes with abundant vacuolated cytoplasm and lymphocytes.

(mean age: 20 years) with a slight male predilection (58% of cases) {1020}. In other series, the median age was 40–42 years {598,130}. RDD is more common among individuals of African descent {1818}. Asian people are more likely to present with cutaneous eyelid lesions {3543}.

Etiology

The etiology is unknown. An infectious etiology has been suggested with a possible role of parvovirus B19 {2156} and retroviruses like HIV {2253}. Neoplasia-associated RDD (including RDD mixed with malignant histiocytosis, Langerhans cell histiocytosis [LCH], or Erdheim–Chester disease [ECD]) can also occur {895}. Rare inherited conditions predispose to familial RDD, including germline mutations in *SLC29A3* (H syndrome / Faisalabad histiocytosis) or *FAS* (*TNFRSF6*) (autoimmune lymphoproliferative syndrome) {2272,2247,2082}.

Pathogenesis

In contrast to LCH {3654} and ECD, the cell of origin that gives rise to histiocytes accumulating in RDD lesions is unknown {849}. Monocytes derived from a myeloid-committed progenitor cell have been suggested as an immediate precursor {847}. Approximately 50% of cases carry gain-of-function mutations in the MAPK/ERK pathway, including *KRAS*, *NRAS*, *MAPK21*, *ARAF*, *CSF1R*, and rarely *BRAF* p.V600E, suggesting that at least a proportion of cases of RDD represent a neoplastic disorder {792,2945,2117,1073,1445,508}. Their differentiation trajectory and susceptibility to inflammatory factors seems critically dependent on this MAPK signalling {458,793}.

Macroscopic appearance

Grossly, lesions are rubbery with a lobulated surface, which is usually covered by a smooth capsule {2131,3467}.

Histopathology

RDD typically shows a mixed infiltrate of histiocytes displaying abundant or vacuolated cytoplasm, large nuclei but no xanthomatous features, lymphocytes, and variable numbers of plasma cells with or without Russell bodies {3467,1020}. While emperipolesis (lymphocytophagocytosis) with lymphocytes being typically phagocytized {2131} is classic for RDD, Touton giant cells should be absent {1160}.

Immunohistochemistry

Histiocytes classically express S100, which highlights the emperipolesis, CD14, CD163, CD68, factor XIIIa, fascin, and OCT2 {2678}, but not CD1a or CD207 (langerin) {2132,130}. While cyclin D1 and phosphorylated ERK are often positive {2678}, mitotic figures are rare and the proliferation index is low {2131,1020}. Cytoplasmic BRAF (VE1) is rarely positive; however, ALK and NTRK should be negative {1160}.

Differential diagnosis

Orbital mass: differential diagnosis includes ECD, LCH, adult-onset xanthogranuloma, juvenile xanthogranuloma, necrobiotic xanthogranuloma, and malignant histiocytosis {17,2949}.

Eyelid swelling: differential diagnosis includes LCH, ECD, adult-onset xanthogranuloma, and adult-onset asthma and periocular xanthogranuloma {1687}.

Lesions in iris, lacrimal glands, cornea, conjunctiva, extraocular muscles, choroid: differential diagnosis includes adult-onset xanthogranuloma, juvenile xanthogranuloma, ECD, malignant histiocytosis {1687}.

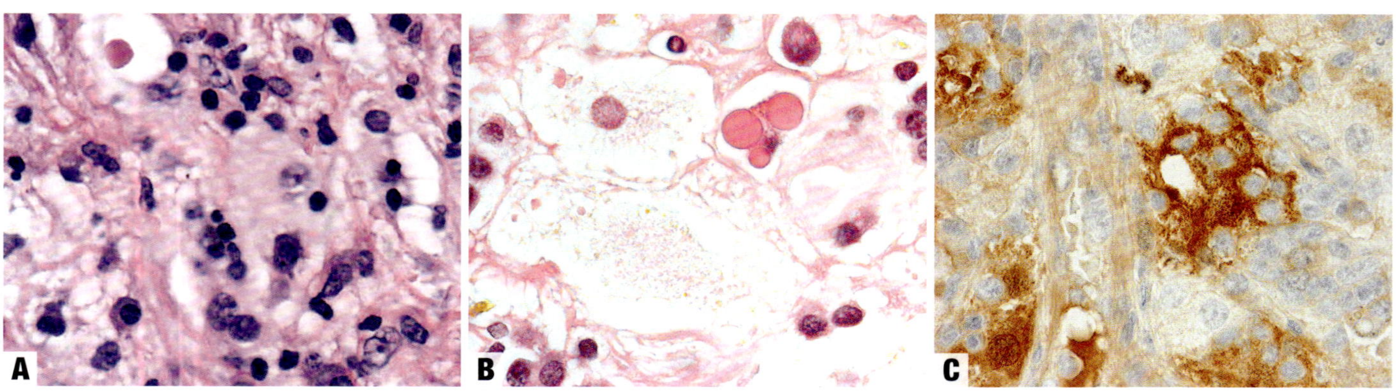

Fig. 10.50 Rosai–Dorfman disease. **A** Biopsy in a case of Rosai–Dorfman disease showing a collection of histiocytes, lymphocytes, plasma cells (with Russell body), and typical emperipolesis. **B** Rosai–Dorfman disease infiltrate showing features of emperipolesis and Russell bodies. **C** The histiocytes in Rosai–Dorfman disease express reaction to S100 stain. Note the lymphocytes that are engulfed by the macrophage in the centre of the photo.

Cytology

Demonstration of sheets of large histiocytes preferably displaying emperipolesis {2644} is seen with FNAC.

Diagnostic molecular pathology

Histiocytes expressing MAPK pathway–activating molecular alterations, in particular *KRAS* and *MAP2K1* mutations, are found in a significant proportion of patients {847}. Mutations in *BRAF* (including *BRAF* p.V600E), *ARAF*, and *CSF1R* are rare {17, 431,1160}. For suspected familial RDD, workup should include *SLC29A3* and *FAS* germline mutation analysis {2247,2272, 2082}. However, these are not readily available as routinely performed analyses on a common basis. At the same time, these are highly relevant to the etiology and pathogenesis and thus prove to be helpful in the differential diagnosis {431}.

Essential and desirable diagnostic criteria

Essential: large histiocytes with round nuclei, prominent nucleoli, and abundant pale cytoplasm, often with emperipolesis; abundant plasma cells in the background; positive immunostaining for S100, which also highlights the emperipolesis.

Desirable: coinfiltrating lymphocytes, and plasma cells; in diagnostically challenging cases, expression of OCT2 and cyclin D1, in the absence of CD1a, CD207, and ALK expression; MAPK pathway mutations.

Staging

Not applicable

Prognosis and prediction

Diagnostic evaluation should include assessment of disease extent by PET-CT or other anatomical imaging, as well as evaluation for conditions known to be associated with RDD. Orbital involvement should be investigated by gadolinium-enhanced MRI {17}. Published case series are too limited to describe the prognosis for ophthalmic RDD. Treatment should be tailored to the individual clinical situation. Extranodal RDD, including orbital manifestation, responds poorly to steroids alone {17}. Recurrence and/or progression of orbital RDD after surgery may necessitate chemotherapy {2243,130,17} or combined chemotherapy and radiation therapy {2043}. Some refractory extranodal RDD cases have been successfully treated with a MEK inhibitor {1445,793}.

Erdheim–Chester disease

Salomao DR
van Halteren AGS

Definition

Erdheim–Chester Disease (ECD) is a clonal haematopoietic neoplasm characterized by accumulation of mature histiocytes, usually involving several organs, associated with inflammation and fibrosis.

ICD-O coding

9749/3 Erdheim–Chester disease

ICD-11 coding

2B31.Y & XH1VJ3 Other specified histiocytic or dendritic cell neoplasms & Erdheim–Chester disease

Related terminology

Not recommended: lipogranulomatosis; lipoid granulomatosis; polyostotic sclerosing histiocytosis.

Subtype(s)

None

Localization

ECD is a multisystem disease and can affect virtually any organ, including bone, while lymph nodes, spleen, and liver are generally spared {1160,646,896}. Periocular, orbital, and retro-orbital manifestations are common {1160,1258,328,1687}. Extraorbital extension to the pituitary gland or cavernous sinus may occur {824}. Rare ophthalmic localizations include the conjunctiva, cornea, extraocular musculature, and lacrimal glands, and subretinal or choroidal infiltration {9,3269,397}.

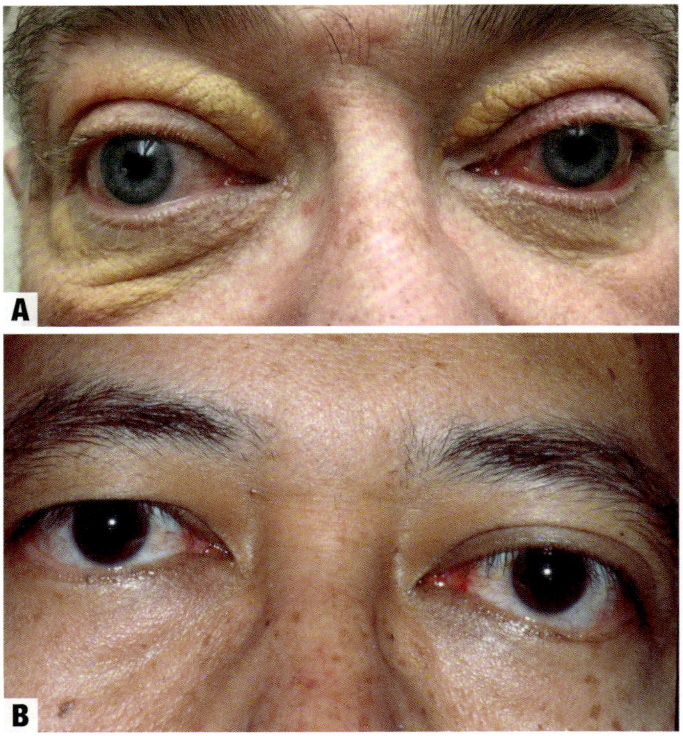

Fig. 10.51 Erdheim–Chester disease. **A** Clinical photograph shows bilateral proptosis and lid xanthelasma. **B** Clinical photograph shows left eye proptosis resulting from the presence of an orbital mass.

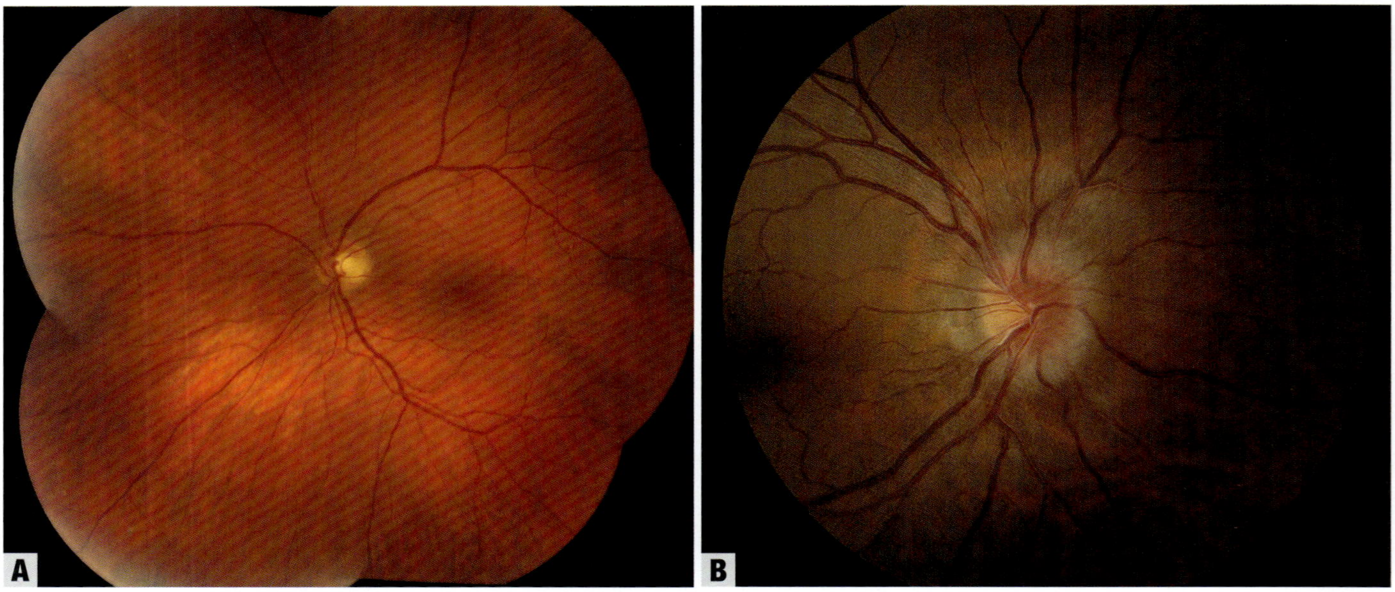

Fig. 10.52 Erdheim–Chester disease. **A** Left eye fundus photograph shows choroidal folds resulting from a posterior orbital mass compressing the globe. **B** A right eye fundus photograph shows choroidal folds and papilloedema secondary to the presence of a posterior orbital mass compressing the globe.

Clinical features

ECD may be asymptomatic, but more often patients present with systemic symptoms with fatigue, fever, and/or site-related symptoms, most of which are considered to be related to the inflammation, and fibrosis associated with histiocytic infiltration of the tissues. Visual abnormalities occur in < 5% of patients {3269}. Ocular motility disturbances, exophthalmos, and retro-orbital pain are typically associated with diffuse infiltration of retro-orbital soft tissues affecting intraconal and extraconal compartments {1160,328}. Vision loss {2183} can result from posterior visual pathway involvement or optic nerve compression. Other manifestations include anterior uveitis, vitritis, optic disc oedema, eyelid oedema, choroidal infiltration, recurrent serous retinal detachment, retinal drusen-like deposits, and retinal pigment epithelial changes {1591}. ECD can also present as periocular yellowish plaques (xanthelasma).

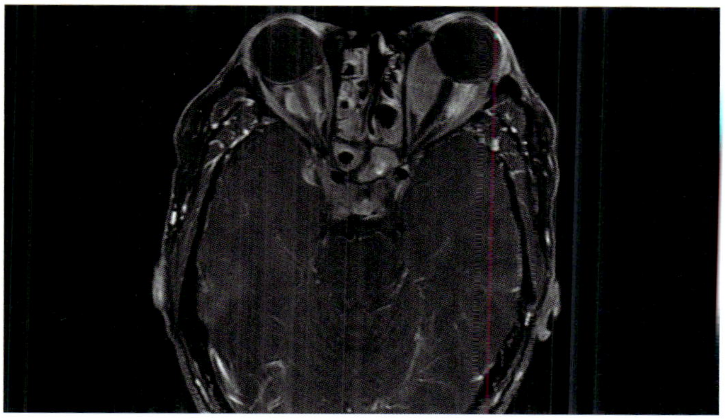

Fig. 10.53 Erdheim–Chester disease. MRI with contrast shows bilateral, well-demarcated, intraconal masses surrounding each optic nerve.

Imaging

Imaging includes 18F-FDG PET-CT of the entire body or 99mTc bone scanning; CT and MRI (with contrast) for evaluation of the pituitary gland and orbital or CNS involvement {1258,1160, 1717}; and fundus fluorescein angiography and optical coherence tomography imaging to assess choroidal infiltration and intraocular disease progression {3269}.

Epidemiology

ECD is a rare but probably underdiagnosed disease; the actual incidence is unknown. It predominantly affects middle-aged men. Rare paediatric cases have been reported {3223,2460, 3315}.

Etiology

ECD is a clonal neoplastic disorder without known genetic predisposition {1257,792,848}. It is marked by xanthomatous histiocytes of monocyte/macrophage lineage expressing MAPK pathway–activating genetic alterations {895,2460,1257}. An underlying clonal haematopoiesis has been described in 42% of cases {641,375}, which is significantly higher than that in the age-related general population.

Pathogenesis

The detection of oncogenic *RAF* or *RAS* mutations in bone marrow CD34+ cells and circulating offspring cells points to early haematopoietic stem/progenitor cells as histiocyte precursor cells {849,2221,641}. *MAPK* mutations seem to favour the generation of myeloid cells with an intrinsic hyperinflammatory phenotype {2251}. Monocytes coexpressing clonal haematopoiesis-associated mutations are found in many ECD patients. Sequential acquisition of driver mutations may lead to development of secondary myeloid neoplasms/malignancies {849,641,2484,3404,1652}.

Macroscopic appearance

Biopsies are usually firm and fibrotic. Periorbital skin biopsies are yellowish in colour.

Histopathology

Sheets of xanthomatous (foamy) and lipid-laden histiocytes admixed with lymphoplasmacytic infiltrate are seen. Fibrosis and multinucleated giant cells (Touton giant cells) are frequent {2460}. The proliferative index is usually low.

Histopathological findings of ECD do not discriminate between ECD and xanthogranulomatous-type histiocytoses. The most typical picture is an infiltrate of foamy macrophages, associated with Touton giant cells, lymphocytes, plasma cells, and neutrophils {895,2460}. In xanthelasma, Touton cells are more abundant in ECD than in other etiologies {543}. Tissue fibrosis is frequently observed and may predominate, leading to a misdiagnosis of a reactive fibroinflammatory process. Admixed Langerhans cell histiocytosis may be present in the

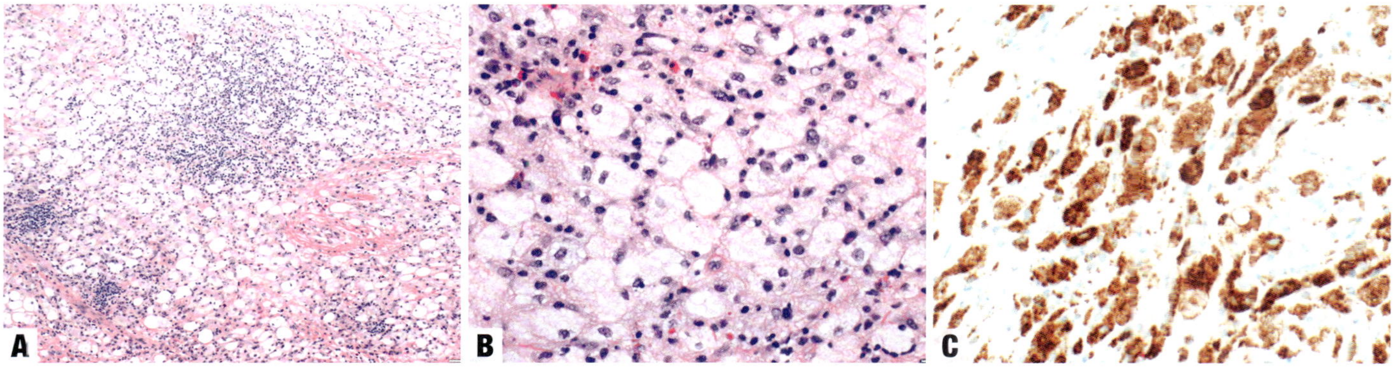

Fig. 10.54 Erdheim–Chester disease. **A** Sheets of xanthomatous (foamy) and lipid-laden histiocytes admixed with lymphoplasmacytic infiltrate in a fibrotic background. **B** Numerous foamy histiocytes characterized by ample finely vacuolated cytoplasm and small nuclei. **C** Tumour cells are positive for BRAF p.V600E immunohistochemistry, indicating the presence of *BRAF* mutations.

same biopsy or other tissues, in cases of mixed histiocytosis {1328,377,543,1258,1160,328,1942}. Occasionally, a morphological and immunophenotypical overlap with Rosai–Dorfman disease or with reticulohistiocytosis may be seen {2679,376}.

Immunohistochemistry

Histiocytes express CD68, CD163, CD14, factor XIIIa, fascin, and phosphorylated ERK, but are negative for CD1a, langerin (CD207) {1160,3578,849}, and OCT2 {2682,2678}. S100 is usually weak or negative. Emperipolesis is rare {847,1160}.

Differential diagnosis

Differential diagnosis includes Rosai–Dorfman disease, Langerhans cell histiocytosis, adult-onset xanthogranuloma, juvenile xanthogranuloma, necrobiotic xanthogranuloma {3128,1285, 1208}, adult-onset asthma and periocular xanthogranuloma {1687}, non-malignant xanthelasma, metastatic tumours {2150}, and malignant histiocytosis {17,2949,1687}.

Cytology

Not clinically relevant

Diagnostic molecular pathology

MAPK pathway–activating somatic mutations are common and may aid in diagnosis and treatment {896}. Half of patients carry *BRAF* p.V600E mutations {895,847}, which are associated with retro-orbital involvement {646}. Negative staining with VE1 {2814} should be confirmed by molecular testing as variant allele frequency may be low.

Essential and desirable diagnostic criteria

Essential: collections of bland, foamy histiocytes in the appropriate clinical and radiological context.
Desirable: MAPK pathway–activating somatic mutations.

Staging

Not relevant

Prognosis and prediction

Usually, there is progressive disease with a variable prognosis and substantial mortality, depending on the organs involved and response to therapy. 18F-FDG PET-CT imaging is used for assessment of disease extent and response evaluation {1160}. CNS involvement is an independent predictor of death {1258}. Patients with ECD obtain clinical benefit with interferon alfa-2a or pegylated interferon alfa {1160,896}. However, in recent years, MAPK pathway alterations have been recognized and targeted therapies with kinase inhibitors are frequently used {1259,640}. Note that these drugs have been registered for use in this context in just a few countries. BRAF or MEK targeted therapy significantly increases 5-year overall survival from 43% to 83% {1160,792}. Approximately 10–15% of ECD cases co-develop an additional haematological malignancy, negatively affecting prognosis.

Langerhans cell tumours

McKelvie PA
Salomao DR
van Halteren AGS

Definition

Langerhans cell neoplasms are clonal proliferations of myeloid dendritic cells expressing a Langerhans cell phenotype (CD1a and CD207 expression). Langerhans cell histiocytosis (LCH) usually follows a benign clinical course. Langerhans cell sarcoma (LCS) is an aggressive malignant neoplasm of Langerhans cell immunophenotype with high-grade cytological features.

ICD-O coding

9751/1 Langerhans cell histiocytosis, NOS
9751/3 Langerhans cell histiocytosis, disseminated
9756/3 Primary Langerhans cell sarcoma
9756/3 Secondary Langerhans cell sarcoma (following or associated with another haematological neoplasm)

ICD-11 coding

2B31.2 Langerhans cell histiocytosis
2B31.3 Langerhans cell sarcoma

Related terminology

Langerhans cell histiocytosis

Not recommended: Langerhans cell granulomatosis; histiocytosis X; eosinophilic granuloma; Hand–Schüller–Christian disease (multifocal); Letterer–Siwe disease (disseminated or visceral involvement).

Langerhans cell sarcoma

Acceptable: malignant histiocytoses of Langerhans phenotype.
Not recommended: malignant histiocytosis X.

Subtype(s)

Langerhans cell histiocytosis

None

Langerhans cell sarcoma

Primary malignant histiocytoses of Langerhans subtype; secondary malignant histiocytoses (after or associated with another haematological neoplasm) of Langerhans subtype

Table 10.05 Main presentation of Langerhans cell neoplasms

Langerhans cell histiocytosis	
Single system	*One organ system involved*
Unifocal	Skin, bone,[a] subcutis, lymph node, and less frequently thyroid and pituitary stalk
Multifocal	Skin, bone[a]
Isolated pulmonary disease	
CNS[c]	
Multisystem	*More than two organ systems involved*
With or without risk organ involvement[b]	Skin, bone,[a] lymph node, pituitary stalk, and less frequent involvement of gastrointestinal tract, thymus, or lungs
Langerhans cell sarcoma	
Unifocal or locoregional	Skin,[d] lymph node, and less frequently affecting lungs, bone, liver, spleen, gastrointestinal tract, bone marrow, or brain {1376}
Advanced stage disseminated disease	

[a]Osteolytic lesions presenting in the skull base and/or orbit-forming bones are designated as CNS-risk lesions. These lesions can be unifocal or part of multifocal bone or multisystem presentation {1838}. According to current standard treatment {1056}, systemic therapy is indicated for paediatric patients with single-system multifocal bone disease, multisystem disease, and isolated CNS-risk lesions to limit the risk of late effects / permanent consequences including diabetes insipidus {2322} and neurodegenerative Langerhans cell histiocytosis {1280,915,1320,1838}. [b]Involvement of liver, spleen, or bone marrow, or a combination thereof, is associated with increased mortality risk {2741,1056}. [c]Clinical neurodegeneration may present in the presence or absence of tumorous brain lesions {1320}. [d]Skin lesions affect underlying soft tissues {2755}.

Localization

LCH can affect many organ systems (see Table 10.05), but most frequently presents in bone as osteolytic lesions with or without soft tissue extension {2741,2711}. Ophthalmic presentation can be solitary or part of a multisystem presentation {1838}. Orbital LCH usually manifests as a unilateral, extraconal

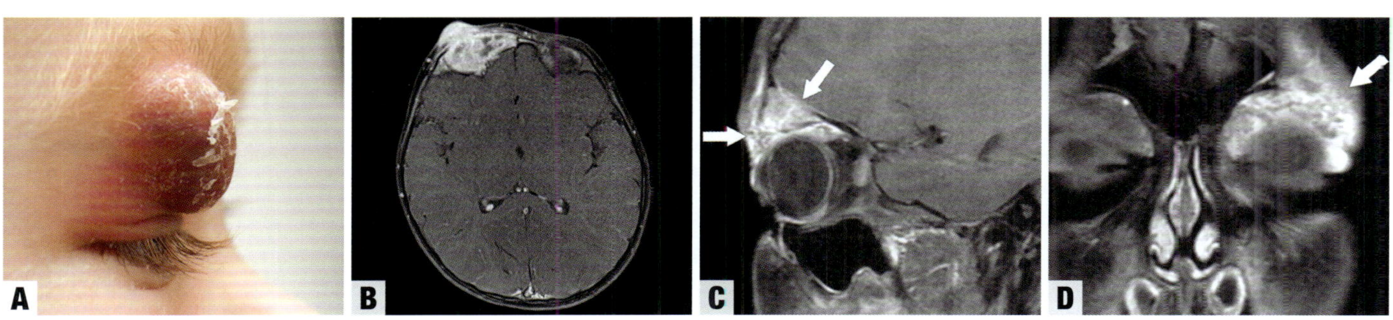

Fig. 10.55 Langerhans cell histiocytosis. **A** Clinical photograph showing an infant presenting with an orbital mass with notable soft tissue extension. **B** Axial T1-weighted MRI of the same case. **C,D** Sagittal and coronal T1-weighted post-contrast MRI shows tumour involving the left frontal bone, eyelid, and periorbital soft tissues (arrows).

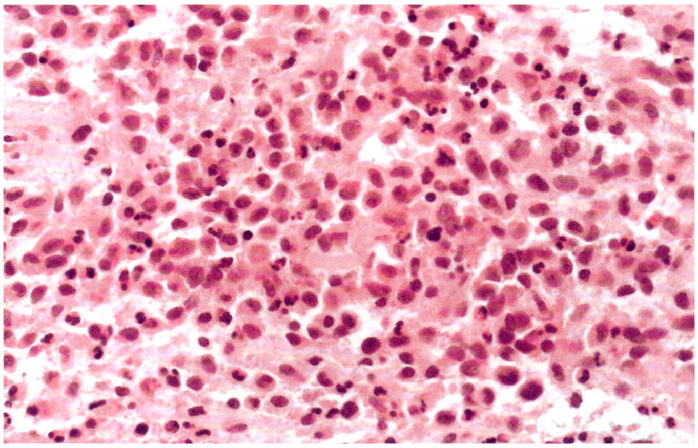

Fig. 10.56 Langerhans cell histiocytosis. Typical Langerhans cell histiocytosis with large cells with bean-shaped and grooved nuclei and an admixture of leukocytes including neutrophils and eosinophils.

lesion, affecting the roof and lateral orbital wall with or without intracranial extension {1838} and eyelid involvement. Less-common ophthalmic sites include the extraocular muscles, lacrimal gland, and periocular skin without orbital bone involvement {1983,2569}. Iris, conjunctival, and choroid involvement have also been reported {2569,1687}. Presentation of LCS in periocular tissues is extremely rare {1201}.

Clinical features

Common symptoms of ophthalmic LCH include eyelid swelling, exophthalmos, palpable orbital mass, pain, limited eye movement, visual dysfunction, uveitis, and retinal vasculitis {3648, 3665,1687}. LCS generally presents with rapid growth and local invasion, and symptoms/signs vary with the site involved.

Imaging

Gadolinium-enhanced MRI is advised to investigate histiocytosis lesions in the orbit {17}. Fundus fluorescein angiography and optical coherence tomography imaging can be used to assess choroidal infiltration and intraocular disease {3269}.

Epidemiology

LCH incidence ranges from 2.6 to 8.9 cases per 1 million children under 15 years of age with an M:F ratio of 1.2:1 {124, 1220,2832}. Incidence in adults is 1–2 cases per 1 million {192,2255}. Orbital involvement occurs in 8% of children with skull lesions {1838}.

LCS is very rare with a reported incidence of 2 per 100 million {2343,3304}. Almost all cases present in adults, with a median age of 50 years {1376}.

Etiology

Unknown

Pathogenesis

LCHs are clonal neoplastic disorders of haematopoietic origin {316,2221,1894,3654} and are marked by Langerhans cell–like histiocytes frequently expressing MAPK pathway–activating somatic mutations {316,847,849,2221,3654,111,1945,2130,896} evidenced by near universal phosphorylated ERK expression. *BRAF* p.V600E is the most prevalent molecular alteration, followed by hotspot mutations affecting *MAP2K1* or exon 12 of *BRAF* and more rarely *ARAF*, *ERBB3*, *NRAS*, and *KRAS* {847, 111,1654,1546}.

LCS is a clonal disease with unknown cell of origin. A subset shows MAPK pathway mutation, including *KRAS* and infrequently *BRAF* p.V600E {3651,2106,2287}, and a few others including deletions in *CDKN2A* and *TP53*, and *PTEN* mutation {2106,3651}. Secondary LCS has been associated with follicular lymphoma {3585,3077}, chronic lymphocytic leukaemia {2946, 3651,565}, and T-lymphoblastic leukaemia {1652}, and shares clonality / molecular aberration with the original haematological neoplasm, suggesting transdifferentiation {1892,1698,609}. Progression is not well documented in primary (de novo) LCS {494,895}.

Macroscopic appearance

The macroscopic appearance varies with site of involvement from bony to fibrotic to soft haemorrhagic lesions.

Histopathology

LCH shows aggregates of large oval or epithelioid histiocytes (10–25 microns) with folded or grooved nuclei and abundant eosinophilic (pale-pink) cytoplasm, fine chromatin, and inconspicuous nucleoli. Nuclear features are usually bland; mitotic figures can be brisk. LCH lesions typically display an inflammatory infiltrate composed of eosinophils, lymphocytes, and other myeloid cells, including monocytes, myeloid dendritic cells, neutrophils, and osteoclastic-type multinucleated giant cells

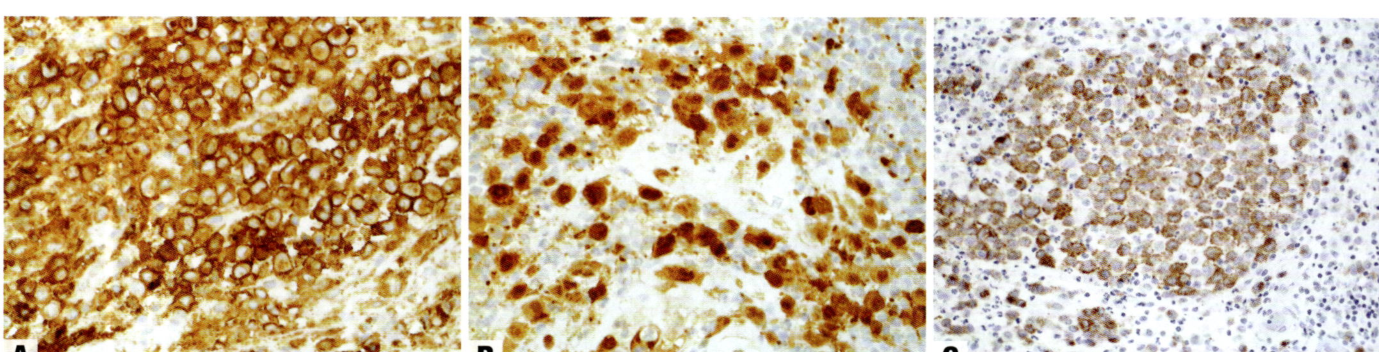

Fig. 10.57 Langerhans cell histiocytosis. **A** CD1a shows strong surface reactivity with a perinuclear dot. **B** S100 shows cytoplasmic and nuclear staining in the Langerhans cells. **C** CD207 (langerin) shows granular and cytoplasmic staining.

{847,3654,1160} also found in non-osseous lesions {698}. No emperipolesis is noted {1160}. The proliferation index with Ki-67 is usually < 10%. Birbeck granules with a tennis-racket shape can be demonstrated on ultrastructural examination {2555}.

LCS is characterized by overtly malignant pleomorphic cells with a high N:C ratio, clumped chromatin, conspicuous nucleoli, and occasional nuclear grooves. A high mitotic count and atypical mitoses are classic features.

Immunohistochemistry

LCH histiocytes display membranous or perinuclear CD1a staining and a granular/cytoplasmic pattern with CD207 (langerin) staining. S100 reactivity is also seen. Both S100 and CD207 patterns are often discordant with CD1a {1945}. A variable number of LCH cells display cytoplasmic phosphorylated ERK and nuclear cyclin D1{297}. Some cells may display staining of CD68 {3654}, but not of other macrophage markers (CD163, factor XIIIa, or fascin).

LCS cells are positive for CD1a, CD207 (langerin), and S100, which might be focal. Reactivity for vimentin, CD68, fascin, factor XIIIa, cyclin D1, and HLA-DR has been reported {2343, 2755}. An assessment of staining should be made on high-grade atypical cells.

Differential diagnosis

See Table 10.05 (p. 371).

For LCH, this includes other histiocytic lesions involving orbital, periocular, or intraocular sites such as Rosai–Dorfman disease, Erdheim–Chester disease, and juvenile/adult-onset xanthogranuloma {3128,1285,1208,1687}.

For LCS, differential diagnosis includes malignant histiocytosis {17,2949,1687}. The histological features often overlap with those of other histiocytic malignancies, including those of the histiocytic, interdigitating, and indeterminate cell types. Some cases may have an atypical immunophenotype, with overlapping dendritic and macrophage phenotypes, defying strict classification of either LCS or histiocytic sarcoma {895}.

Cytology

Definitive diagnosis on cytological specimens is difficult {2545, 572}.

Diagnostic molecular pathology

Properly validated immunohistochemistry (VE1 antibody specific for BRAF p.V600E) may be used in conjunction with nucleic acid–based assays detecting the *BRAF* c.1799T>A mutation encoding BRAF p.V600E {2814,2348,243,3654} and other molecular alterations of the MAPK pathway.

Essential and desirable diagnostic criteria

Langerhans cell histiocytosis

Essential: large round to oval histiocytes with grooved to convoluted nuclei and Langerhans cell phenotype (CD1a+, CD207+/–) in the correct histological/anatomical context.

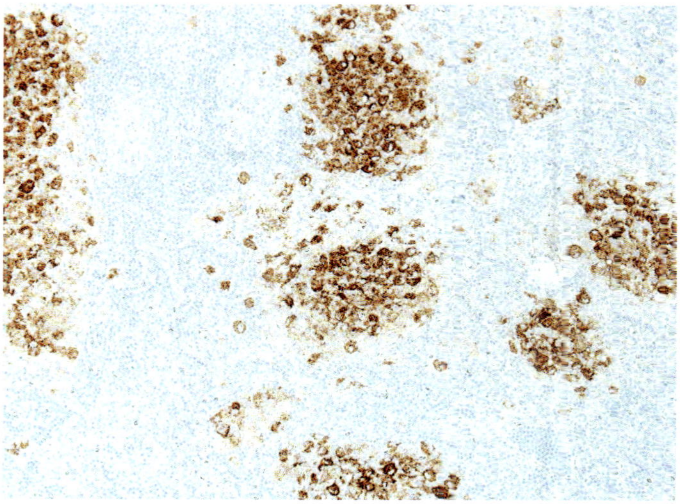

Fig. 10.58 Langerhans cell sarcoma. Strong diffuse cytoplasmic reactivity for BRAF p.V600E in the neoplastic cells.

Desirable: mutation analysis in the MAPK pathway, with sensitive testing for low-frequency allele detection.

Langerhans cell sarcoma

Essential: pleomorphic histiocytes with high-grade cytology, increased mitoses, and immunoreactivity for CD1a, S100, and CD207, any of which can be focal

Desirable: clinical evidence of rapid tumour progression; molecular alteration, preferably in the MAPK pathway.

Staging

Not relevant

Prognosis and prediction

Clinical evaluation and therapy decisions are based on the number and type of affected tissues assessed by PET-CT or MRI imaging of the entire body {1160,2741,1133,1279}.

LCH, except for a disseminated presentation affecting, among others, the spleen, liver, and/or bone marrow (MS-RO+, i.e. multisystem, risk organ involvement), has excellent survival rates. BRAF inhibitors have been shown to induce durable responses in MS-RO+ patients testing positive for refractory BRAF p.V600E {814,1894,1288,3682,3684}. Patients co-presenting with haemophagocytic lymphohistiocytosis have significantly poorer survival {556,3287}.

The prognosis for LCS depends on clinical presentation with a high (50%) mortality risk for patients with disseminated disease; the median survival is 19 to 27 months {2555,3304,1376}. Multimodality treatment (surgery combined with chemotherapy and/or radiotherapy) seems more effective {1996,2287}. Bone marrow transplantation is an additional option for patients with disseminated disease {1376}. More localized disease confers a survival advantage if complete surgical excision can be achieved {1376,1455}.

Xanthelasma

Laver NM
van Halteren AGS

Definition
Xanthelasma are benign, subcutaneous, localized lesions composed of foamy histiocytes and Touton giant cells with a variable degree of lipid deposition in the absence of a metabolic disorder.

ICD-O coding
None

ICD-11 coding
9A06.4 Xanthelasma of eyelid

Related terminology
Acceptable: xanthomatous lesions.
Not recommended: histiocytomas; non–Langerhans cell histiocytosis.

Subtype(s)
Xanthoma

Localization
Xanthelasma involves the eyelids.

Clinical features
Xanthelasma appears as flat or minimally elevated yellow lesions commonly in the medial aspect of the eyelids; the lesions are often bilateral and symmetrical {2339}.

A tuberous xanthoma is an elevated and nodular xanthelasma. These appear as solitary or multiple, placoid or papular lesions of the eyelids, more probably associated with hyperlipidaemia types II and III {1702}.

Epidemiology
Xanthelasma has a reported incidence of 0.56–1.5% and represents approximately 6% of eyelid lesions {776}. The age of onset varies from 15 to 75 years with a peak between the fourth and fifth decades of life {1452}. It is unclear if there is a female predilection.

Xanthomas may occur in individuals of any age and show no sex predilection. In xanthoma disseminatum, there is a male predilection and the age of onset is < 25 years in as many as a third of cases {776}.

Etiology
The etiology is unknown. Xanthelasma and xanthoma are not true neoplasms but are reactive developmental or inflammatory lesions {1766}.

Pathogenesis
The pathogenesis is unknown. The inflammatory milieu in xanthelasma is considered analogous to the early stages of cardiac atherosclerotic plaque formation {1159}.

Macroscopic appearance
See *Clinical features*.

Histopathology
Xanthelasma shows focal collections of lipid-laden histiocytes distributed mainly around blood vessels and adnexal structures in the eyelid dermis with chronic inflammatory cells and fibrosis.

Tuberous xanthomas are more deeply located in the dermis and display foamy histiocytes, Touton giant cells, extracellular cholesterol deposits, chronic inflammation, and fibrosis.

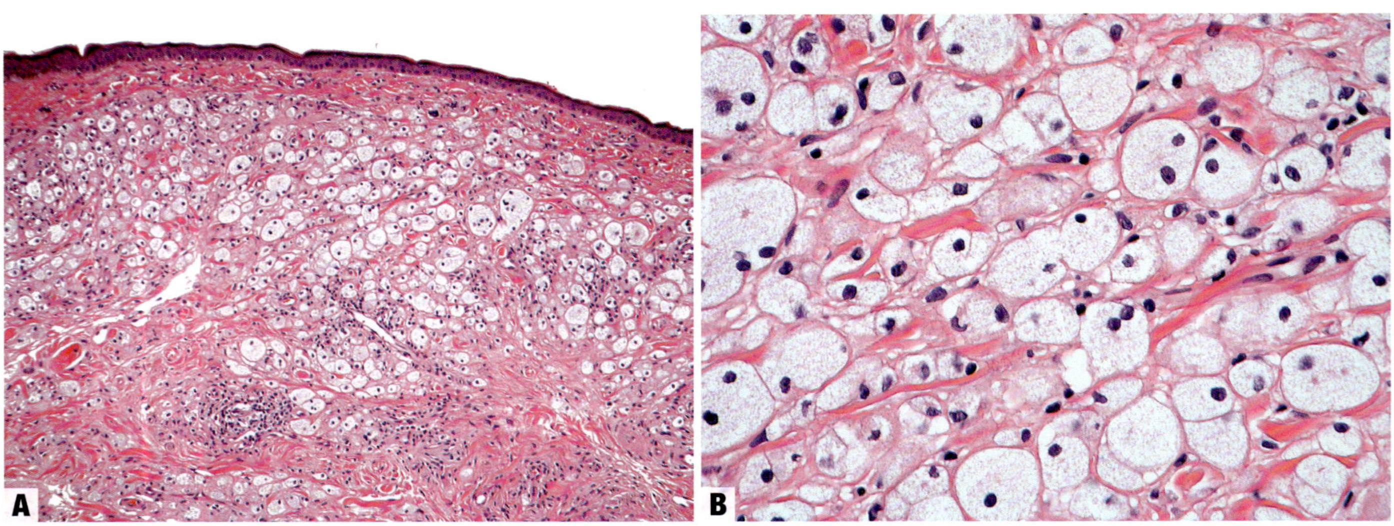

Fig. 10.59 Xanthelasma. **A** Eyelid skin comprising collections of foamy histiocytes in the dermis, associated with some patchy collections of lymphocytes around the vessels. Note how the foamy histiocytes peter out towards the deeper aspect of the biopsy. **B** Higher-power image showing the frothy/foamy cytoplasm of the histiocytes and small bland nuclei.

Immunohistochemistry

The foamy histiocytes typically express CD68, CD163, and factor XIIIa, but lack CD21, CD35, S100, CD1a, and Birbeck granules {1163,1208}.

Differential diagnosis

This includes necrobiotic xanthogranuloma, Erdheim–Chester disease and adult-onset xanthogranuloma with periocular xanthogranuloma {3044,895}, Langerhans cell histiocytosis, Rosai–Dorfman disease, and crystal-storing histiocytosis (see related sections).

A clinicopathological correlation may be necessary for challenging cases.

Cytology

Not relevant

Diagnostic molecular pathology

Not relevant

Essential and desirable diagnostic criteria

Essential: yellowish plaque or flat lesion around the eyelids; presence of lipid-laden histiocytes, giant cells, and chronic inflammatory cells.

Staging

Not relevant

Prognosis and prediction

The lesions are benign and are commonly observed. Surgical excision for larger lesions or cosmetic reasons may be considered

Chapter 10

Adult orbital xanthogranulomatous disease

Laver NM
van Halteren AGS

Definition

Adult orbital xanthogranulomatous disease (AOXGD) is a group of rare orbital and ocular adnexal disorders within the spectrum of non–Langerhans cell histiocytoses.

ICD-O coding

None

ICD-11 coding

None

Related terminology

Acceptable: non–Langerhans cell histiocytosis; xanthogranuloma; adult-onset xanthogranuloma.
Not recommended: histiocytomas.

Subtype(s)

Based on clinical features and systemic associations, four subtypes are identified: adult-onset xanthogranuloma (AOX); adult-onset asthma and periocular xanthogranuloma (AAPOX); necrobiotic xanthogranuloma (NBX); and Erdheim–Chester disease (ECD).

Localization

AOXGD involves the subconjunctiva, eyelids, and subcutaneous periocular regions, and the orbit. Very occasionally, the corneal limbus can be affected {1766}.

Clinical features

These vary considerably according to the subtype of AOXGD.

AOX may present as a solitary xanthogranulomatous eyelid or orbital lesion {1711,3128,782}.

AAPOX presents with lesions like those of AOX but is associated with late-onset asthma. In addition, it may be associated with IgG4-related disease and some cases may show reactive lymphadenopathy or lymphoma {205,1357,1992,3199,1163, 2480,782}.

NBX is one of the most frequently reported subtypes of AOXGD and is characterized by the presence of necrobiosis in adnexal and frequently accompanying skin lesions {3128}. Systemic findings include monoclonal gammopathy and associated haematological malignancies {3128,864,1337,782}.

ECD is a lymphohistiocytic disorder of the orbit, often with systemic infiltration, affecting the long bones and visceral organs such as the lungs and heart. The orbital lesions in ECD tend to have a more diffuse involvement than the other subtypes of AOXGD. Because of the extensive involvement and the progressive and therapy-resistant lesions, ECD is the most devastating subtype (see *Erdheim–Chester disease*, p. 368).

Epidemiology

AOXG tends to affect patients ranging from 30 to 85 years of age with no significant sex prevalence {782}.

Etiology

Unknown

Pathogenesis

Pathogenesis is unclear: it is debated whether histiocytosis is of a reactive or neoplastic nature. Multiple mutations including the *BRAF* p.V600E mutations and those in the *MAP2K1* (*MEK1*), *MAP2K2* (*MEK2*), *ARAF*, *KRAS*, and *NRAS* genes in the MAPK pathway have been found in patients with histiocytic and related disorders including ECD, AAPOX, and juvenile xanthogranuloma {1257,2460,2208}.

Macroscopic appearance

See *Clinical features*, above.

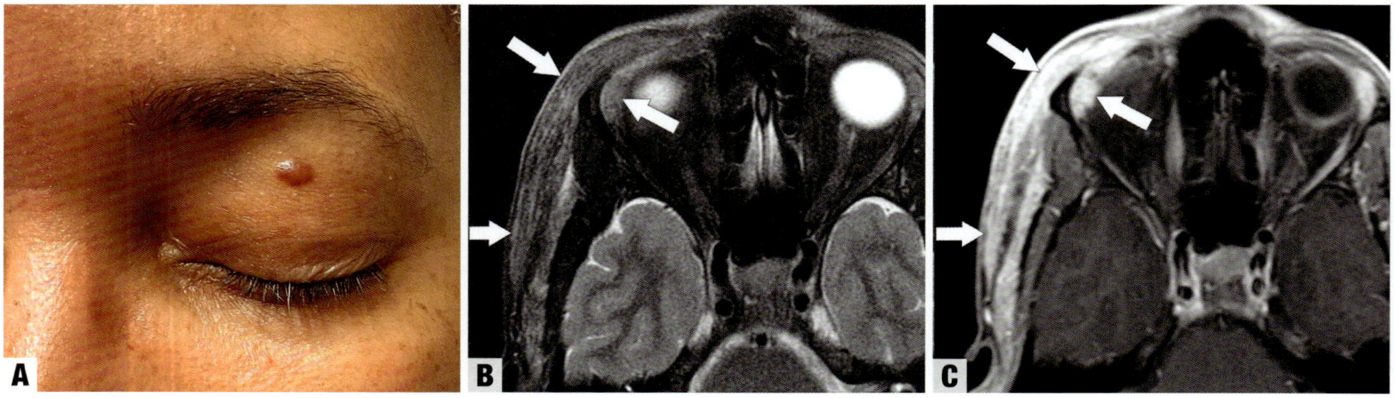

Fig. 10.60 Adult xanthogranuloma. **A** Circumscribed nodular xanthogranuloma involving the eyelid in an adult. **B** Axial T2-weighted MRI with fat saturation shows an isointense to hypointense lesion in the right temporal and periorbital soft tissues with involvement of the right upper eyelid and lacrimal gland (arrows). **C** Axial T1-weighted postcontrast MRI shows homogeneous enhancement of the lesion (arrows).

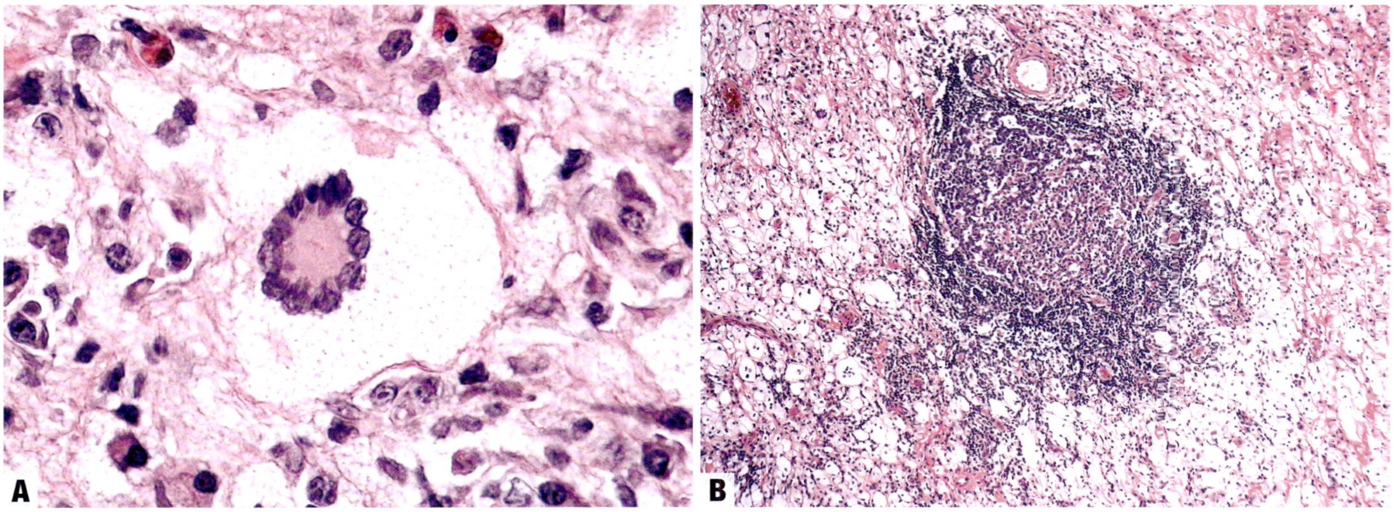

Fig. 10.61 Adult xanthogranuloma. **A** A classic Touton giant cell in orbital xanthogranuloma, with a dense eosinophilic central cytoplasm and a ring of nuclei, surrounded by foamy cytoplasm. **B** Xanthomatized histiocytes with foamy cytoplasm and reactive lymphoid aggregate.

Histopathology

All AOXGD subtypes share common histopathological features characterized by sheets of mononuclear foamy histiocytes (xanthoma cells) infiltrating the orbicularis muscles and the orbital tissue, accompanied by variable numbers of dispersed and/or aggregates of lymphocytes, plasma cells, and Touton giant cells. These infiltrating xanthoma cells often have small round nuclei and abundant clear or vacuolated cytoplasm. The cellular population usually abuts the surface epidermis or conjunctival epithelium, but a grenz zone may be present {1663,782}.

In AAPOX, scattered lymphoid follicles with variable reactive germinal centres can be observed {1663}.

In NBX, the lesions show necrobiosis, which can vary in extent.

For ECD, see *Erdheim–Chester disease* (p. 368).

Immunohistochemistry

The foamy histiocytes typically express CD68, CD163, and factor XIIIa, but lack CD21, CD35, S100, CD1a, and Birbeck granules {1163,1208}.

Differential diagnosis

The AOXGDs must be differentiated from each other because these diseases share similar histological patterns but differ in their systemic associations and overall prognosis.

Other entities such as Langerhans cell histiocytosis, Rosai–Dorfman disease, and crystal-storing histiocytosis as well as non-Hodgkin lymphoma and IgG4+ disease must be excluded (see related sections).

Infectious diseases must be also ruled out.

Cytology

A definitive diagnosis of any of the AOXGD subtypes is difficult to achieve with cytological smears.

Diagnostic molecular pathology

Molecular analyses are relevant in some ECDs, AAPCX with *BRAF* mutations having been described {1257,2460,2203}.

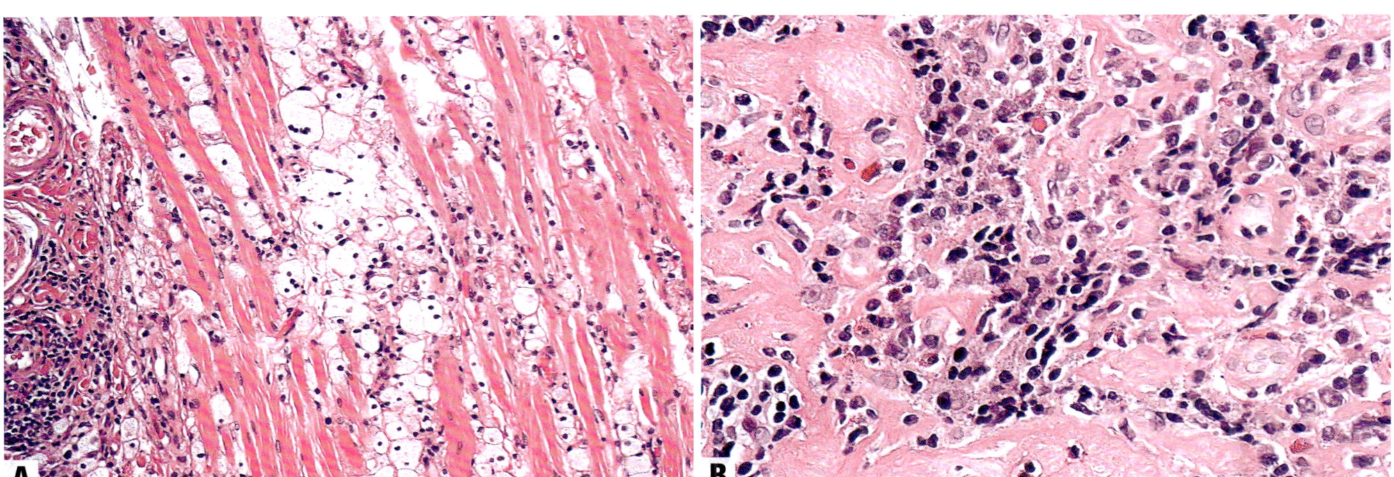

Fig. 10.62 Adult xanthogranuloma. **A** Xanthomatized histiocytes percolating between extraocular muscle fibres. **B** Plasma cells, lymphocytes, and eosinophils in a more sclerotic area of orbital xanthogranuloma.

Essential and desirable diagnostic criteria

Essential: presence of lipid-laden histiocytes, giant cells, and chronic inflammatory cells; for AAPOX: a setting of late-onset asthma; for NBX: foci of necrobiosis are required; for ECD: see *Erdheim–Chester disease* (p. 368).

Desirable: immunohistochemical profile of normal histiocytes and appropriate clinical setting to rule out other histiocytic disorders; *BRAF* mutation analysis or immunohistochemistry.

Staging

Since the prognosis and associated systemic diseases vary between the AOXGD subtypes, a thorough diagnostic workup is warranted. Staging is particularly relevant in those AOXGDs where an additional underlying non-Hodgkin lymphoma or monoclonal gammopathy may be present, the NBX may be multifocal, and systemic IgG4+ is suspected; ECD may or may not be present.

Prognosis and prediction

The AOXGDs differ significantly in their prognoses. Owing to their rarity, optimal treatment guidelines have not been established. Surgical debulking and steroids might be sufficient therapy for patients with AOX. Patients with AAPOX, NBX, and ECD need systemic therapy, with ECD being the most devastating subtype of non–Langerhans cell histiocytosis and having the poorest prognosis. Treatment targeted against *BRAF* or MAPK mutations have been shown effective in various histiocytic disorders and might indicate a possible role for targeted therapy in the treatment of AOXGD.

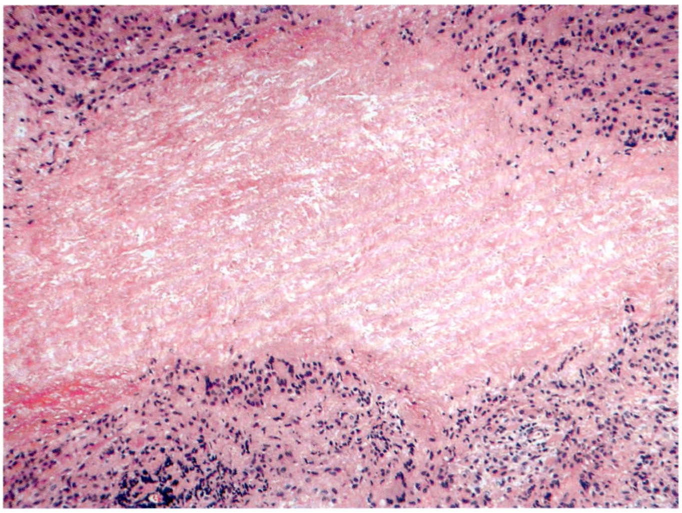

Fig. 10.63 Necrobiotic xanthogranuloma involving the orbit. Necrobiotic collagen and giant cells at the edge of the necrobiotic tissue.

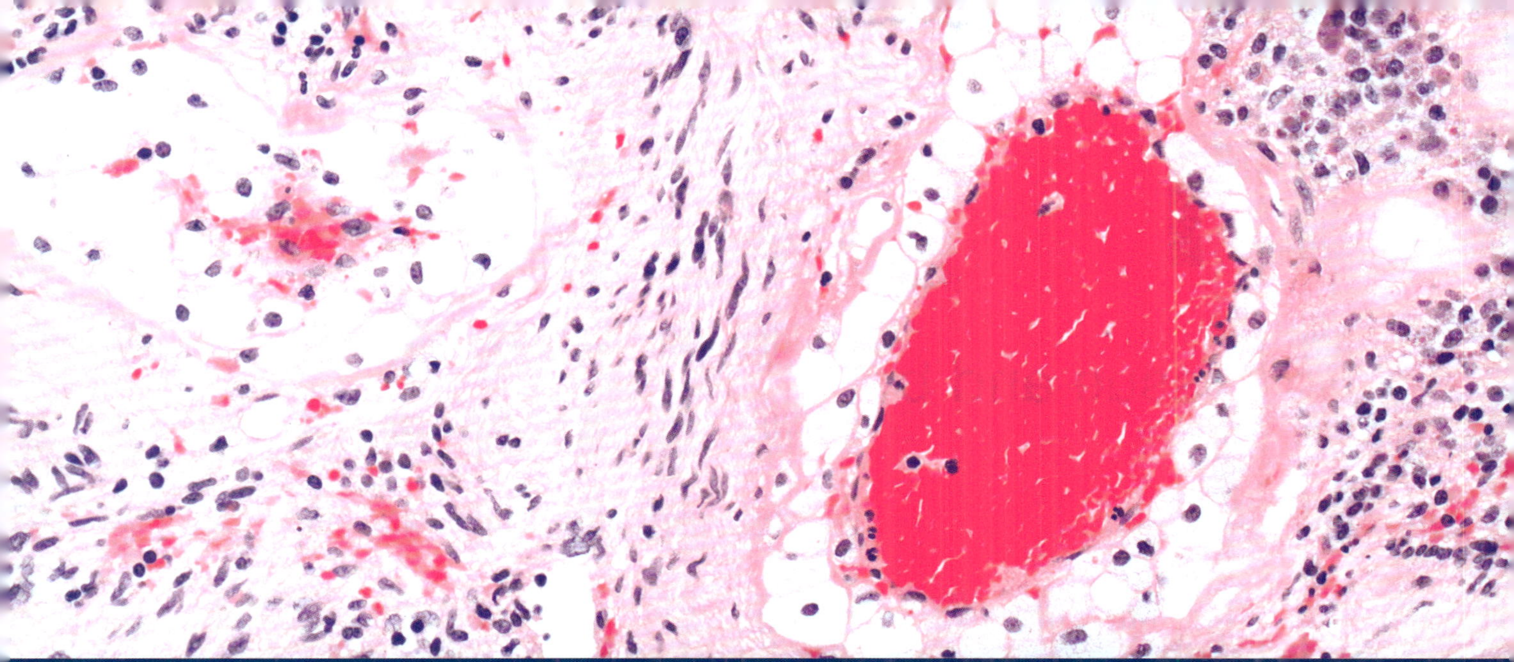

11

Soft tissue and bone tumours

Edited by: Cree IA, Grossniklaus HE, Hodge JC, Lazar AJ, Milman T, Rodríguez-Reyes AA, Vemuganti GK, Verdijk RM, White VA

(continued on next page)

11

Soft tissue and bone tumours (continued)

Soft tissue and bone tumours: Introduction

Milman T
Grossniklaus HE
Hodge JC
Lazar AJ
Rodríguez-Reyes AA
Verdijk RM
White VA

A variety of soft tissue tumours arise in the eye and ocular adnexal tissues (eyelids, conjunctiva, and orbit). The most significant change from the fourth edition of the classification is to combine all soft tissues of the eye and ocular adnexa in a single chapter. The neoplasms that are most commonly encountered or have a characteristic presentation are discussed in detail. For others not specifically discussed here, the fifth edition of the *Soft tissue and bone tumours* volume

Table 11.01 Types and frequency of orbital tumours with an emphasis on soft tissue tumours (continued on next page)

	All ages combined						Adults				Children					
Author	Verdijk {3480}		Shields {3069}		Ohtsuka {2418}		Demirci {773}		Alsamalah {120}		Shields {3026}		Alkatan {99}		Bajaj {233}	
Data collection time frame	1987–2012		1971–2002		1981–2002		1974–2000		2000–2017		1962–1983		2000–2013		1991–2000	
Lesion category[a]	***N***	**%**[b]	***N***	**%**	***N***	**%**	***N***	**%**	***N***	**%**	***N***	**%**	***N***	**%**	***N***	**%**
Soft tissue tumours total	105	17%	243	30%	40	19%	23	14%	45	43%	30	15%	44	42%	54	51%
Fibrous, fibroblastic total	13	2%	15	2%	3	2%	3	2%	4	4%	0	0%	4	4%	1	1%
Solitary fibrous tumour	3	< 1%	2	< 1%	2	1%	3	2%	4	4%	0	0%	1	1%	0	0%
Fibrous histiocytoma	3	< 1%	6	1%	0	0%	0	0%	0	0%	0	0%	0	0%	1	1%
Myofibroma	0	0%	2	< 1%	0	0%	0	0%	0	0%	0	0%	0	0%	0	0%
Angiofibroma	2	< 1%	2	< 1%	0	0%	0	0%	0	0%	0	0%	0	0%	0	0%
Nodular fasciitis / proliferative myositis	2	< 1%	2	< 1%	0	0%	0	0%	0	0%	0	0%	0	0%	0	0%
Fibromatosis	2	< 1%	0	0%	0	0%	0	0%	0	0%	0	0%	3	3%	0	0%
Fibrosarcoma	0	0%	1	< 1%	1	< 1%	0	0%	0	0%	0	0%	0	0%	0	0%
IMT	1	< 1%	0	0%	0	0%	0	0%	0	0%	0	0%	0	0%	0	0%
Adipocytic total	3	< 1%	3	< 1%	0	0%	0	0%	2	2%	0	0%	0	0%	0	0%
Lipoma	1	< 1%	2	< 1%	0	0%	0	0%	0	0%	0	0%	0	0%	0	0%
Liposarcoma	2	< 1%	1	< 1%	0	0%	0	0%	2	2%	0	0%	0	0%	0	0%
Skeletal muscle	8	1%	35	4%	2	1%	0	0%	0	0%	10	5%	11	11%	29	28%
Rhabdomyosarcoma family	8	1%	35	4%	2	1%	0	0%	0	0%	10	5%	11	11%	29	28%
Smooth muscle	2	< 1%	0	0%	0	0%	0	0%	2	2%	0	0%	0%	0%	0	0%
Leiomyoma	1	< 1%	0	0%	0	0%	0	0%	0	0%	0	0%	0	0%	0	0%
Leiomyosarcoma	1	< 1%	0	0%	0	0%	0	0%	2	2%	0	0%	0	0%	0	0%
Peripheral nerve sheath total	17	3%	21	3%	11	5%	0	0%	13	13%	3	1%	7	7%	4	4%
Schwannoma	3	< 1%	14	2%	7	3%	0	0%	9	9%	1	< 1%	NA	NA	2	2%
Neurofibroma	12	2%	6	1%	2	1%	0	0%	4	4%	2	1%	NA	NA	2	2%
MPNST	1	< 1%	1	< 1%	0	0%	0	0%	0	0%	0	0%	NA	NA	0	0%
Granular cell tumour	1	< 1%	0	0%	2	1%	0	0%	0	0%	0	0%	NA	NA	0	0%

AVM, arteriovenous malformation; CVM, cavernous venous malformation; IMT, inflammatory myofibroblastic tumour; LVM, lymphatic-venous malformation; MPNST, malignant peripheral nerve sheath tumour; NA, not available.
[a]Excluded for consistency: histiocytic-dendritic neoplasms, inflammatory, infectious, traumatic (haematoma), structural (varix, fistula, deformity, high myopia, herniated fat), degenerations, lacrimal gland, amyloid deposits. [b]All percentage values are rounded to the nearest whole number. [c]Both malformations and neoplastic lesions are included because of the inconsistent use of terminology before the 2018 International Society for the Study of Vascular Anomalies (ISSVA) classification {1436}. [d]Florid reactive lymphoid hyperplasia and lymphomas grouped for consistency.

Chapter 11

Table 11.01 Types and frequency of orbital tumours with an emphasis on soft tissue tumours (continued from previous page, continued on next page)

	All ages combined						Adults				Children					
Author	Verdijk {3480}		Shields {3069}		Ohtsuka {2418}		Demirci {773}		Alsamalah {120}		Shields {3026}		Alkatan {99}		Bajaj {233}	
Data collection time frame	1987–2012		1971–2002		1981–2002		1974–2000		2000–2017		1962–1983		2000–2013		1991–2000	
Lesion category[a]	***N***	**%**[b]	***N***	**%**	***N***	**%**	***N***	**%**	***N***	**%**	***N***	**%**	***N***	**%**	***N***	**%**
Vascular total[c]	57	9%	168	21%	24	11%	20	12%	23	22%	16	8%	17	16%	18	18%
Cavernous haemangioma / CVM	37	6%	77	9%	18	9%	15	9%	20	19%	2	1%	NA	NA	5	5%
Haemangioma NOS	0	0%	0	0%	0	0%	0	0%	0	0%	0	0%	NA	NA	0	0%
Lymphangioma/LVM	5	1%	54	7%	3	1%	4	2%	1	1%	4	2%	NA	NA	7	7%
Capillary haemangioma / infantile haemangioma	7	1%	36	4%	3	1%	0	0%	0	0%	10	5%	NA	NA	1	1%
Epithelioid haemangioma	1	< 1%	0	0%	0	0%	0	0%	0	0%	0	0%	0	0%	0	0%
Masson tumour	1	< 1%	1	< 1%	0	0%	1	1%	0	0%	0	0%	NA	NA	0	0%
Vascular malformation / AVM	6	1%	0	0%	0	0%	0	0%	2	2%	0	0%	NA	NA	5	5%
Perivascular tumours	2	< 1%	0	0%	0	0%	0	0%	0	0%	0	0%	0	0%	0	0%
Tumours of uncertain derivation	1	< 1%	1	< 1%	0	0%	0	0%	1	1%	1	< 1%	1	1%	2	2%
Epithelioid sarcoma	1	< 1%	0	0%	0	0%	0	0%	0	0%	0	0%	1	1%	0	0%
Alveolar soft part sarcoma	0	0%	1	< 1%	0	0%	0	0%	0	0%	1	< 1%	0	0%	2	2%
Undifferentiated/ unclassified sarcoma	0	0%	0	0%	0	0%	0	0%	1	1%	0	0%	0	0%	0	0%
Tumours of orbital bone total	25	4%	22	3%	6	3%	0	0%	1	1%	3	1%	3	3%	4	4%
Osteogenic total	8	1%	9	1%	2	1%	0	0%	0	0%	0	0%	0	0%	0	0%
Osteosarcoma	1	< 1%	5	1%	0	0%	0	0%	0	0%	0	0%	0	0%	0	0%
Osteoma	7	1%	4	< 1%	2	1%	0	0%	0	0%	0	0%	0	0%	0	0%
Chondrogenic	8	1%	0	0%	0	0%	0	0%	0	0%	1	< 1%	2	2%	0	0%
Fibrous, fibroblastic total	8	1%	10	1%	2	1%	0	0%	0	0%	2	1%	1	1%	0	0%
Fibrous dysplasia	7	1%	7	1%	2	1%	0	0%	0	0%	0	0%	NA	NA	0	0%
Ossifying fibroma	1	< 1%	3	< 1%	0	0%	0	0%	0	0%	2	1%	NA	NA	0	0%
Vascular tumours of bone	0	0%	0	0%	0	0%	0	0%	1	1%	0	0%	0	0%	0	0%
Osteoclast-rich giant cell tumours	0	0%	1	< 1%	1	< 1%	0	0%	0	0%	0	0%	0	0%	0	0%
Ewing sarcoma	1	< 1%	2	< 1%	1	< 1%	0	0%	0	0%	0	0%	0	0%	4	4%

AVM, arteriovenous malformation; CVM, cavernous venous malformation; IMT, inflammatory myofibroblastic tumour; LVM, lymphatic-venous malformation; MPNST, malignant peripheral nerve sheath tumour; NA, not available.

[a]Excluded for consistency: histiocytic-dendritic neoplasms, inflammatory, infectious, traumatic (haematoma), structural (varix, fistula, deformity, high myopia, herniated fat), degenerations, lacrimal gland, amyloid deposits. [b]All percentage values are rounded to the nearest whole number. [c]Both malformations and neoplastic lesions are included because of the inconsistent use of terminology before the 2018 International Society for the Study of Vascular Anomalies (ISSVA) classification {1436}. [d]Florid reactive lymphoid hyperplasia and lymphomas grouped for consistency.

Table 11.01 Types and frequency of orbital tumours with an emphasis on soft tissue tumours (continued)

	All ages combined						Adults				Children					
Author	Verdijk {3480}		Shields {3069}		Ohtsuka {2418}		Demirci {773}		Alsamalah {120}		Shields {3026}		Alkatan {99}		Bajaj {233}	
Data collection time frame	1987–2012		1971–2002		1981–2002		1974–2000		2000–2017		1962–1983		2000–2013		1991–2000	
Lesion category[a]	***N***	**%**[b]	***N***	**%**	***N***	**%**	***N***	**%**	***N***	**%**	***N***	**%**	***N***	**%**	***N***	**%**
Other lesions total	481	79%	549	67%	161	78%	140	85%	59	57%	168	84%	57	55%	47	45%
Haematolymphoid[d]	124	20%	132	16%	104	50%	56	34%	29	28%	6	3%	5	5%	4	4%
Cysts	112	18%	70	9%	16	8%	6	4%	6	6%	130	65%	47	45%	12	11%
Optic nerve / meningeal	60	10%	101	12%	10	5%	10	6%	2	2%	6	3%	1	1%	9	9%
Melanocytic	16	3%	11	1%	0	0%	0	0%	0	0%	0	0%	0	0%	0	0%
Miscellaneous	13	2%	3	< 1%	0	0%	0	0%	3	3%	17	8%	2	2%	0	0%
Secondary	120	20%	141	17%	23	11%	48	29%	16	15%	9	4%	0	0%	21	20%
Metastatic	36	6%	91	11%	8	4%	20	12%	3	3%	0	0%	2	2%	1	1%
Total orbital tumours	611	100%	814	100%	207	100%	163	100%	105	100%	201	100%	104	100%	105	100%

AVM, arteriovenous malformation; CVM, cavernous venous malformation; IMT, inflammatory myofibroblastic tumour; LVM, lymphatic-venous malformation; MPNST, malignant peripheral nerve sheath tumour; NA, not available.

[a]Excluded for consistency: histiocytic-dendritic neoplasms, inflammatory, infectious, traumatic (haematoma), structural (varix, fistula, deformity, high myopia, herniated fat) degenerations, lacrimal gland, amyloid deposits. [b]All percentage values are rounded to the nearest whole number. [c]Both malformations and neoplastic lesions are included because of the inconsistent use of terminology before the 2018 International Society for the Study of Vascular Anomalies (ISSVA) classification {1436}. [d]Florid reactive lymphoid hyperplasia and lymphomas grouped for consistency.

Table 11.02 Types and frequency of orbital bone tumours

Author	**Selva {2914A}**		**Jorgensen {1544A}**	
Data collected	**Primary orbital bone tumours at one institution**		**Survey of literature: tumours of orbital bone invading the orbit**	
Data collection time frame	**1976–1998**		**1966–2016**	
Lesion category[a]	***N***	**%**[b]	***N***	**%**
Osteogenic total	14	39%	102	77%
Osteoma	11	31%	77	58%
Osteoblastoma	0	0%	16	12%
Osteosarcoma	3	8%	9	7%
Chondrogenic total	4	11%	30	23%
Osteochondroma/enchondroma	1	3%	0	0%
Chondrosarcoma	3	8%	30	23%
Fibrous, fibroblastic total	13	36%	0	0%
Fibrous dysplasia	11	31%	0	0%
Ossifying fibroma	1	3%	0	0%
Vascular tumours of bone	1	3%	0	0%
Haemangioma	1	3%	Unknown	Unknown
Osteoclast-rich giant cell tumours	2	6%	0	0%
Aneurysmal bone cyst	2	6%	0	0%
Giant cell tumour of bone	0	0%	0	0%
Ewing sarcoma	3	8%	Unknown	0%
Total orbital bone tumours	**36**	**100%**	**132**	**100%**

[a]Excluded for consistency: histiocytic-dendritic neoplasms; haematolymphoid; inflammatory/pseudoinflammatory; hormone, metabolism, or trauma related. [b]All percentage values are rounded to the nearest whole number.

Chapter 11

Table 11.03 Types and frequency of eyelid tumours with an emphasis on soft tissue tumours

Author	Gundogan {1200}		Deprez {776}		Banerjee {248}		Yu {3721}	
Data collection time frame	2008–2012		1989–2007		1996–2016		2002–2015	
Lesion category[a]	*N*	%[b]	*N*	%	*N*	%	*N*	%
Soft tissue tumours total	33	2%	112	2%	34	8%	243	12%
Fibrous, fibroblastic total	1	< 1%	9	0%	0	0%	5	< 1%
Fibrous histiocytoma/ dermatofibroma	1	< 1%	9	< 1%	0	0%	5	< 1%
Adipocytic total	4	0%	3	0%	0	0%	0	0%
Lipoma	4	< 1%	2	< 1%	0	0%	0	0%
Angiolipoma	0	0%	1	0%	0	0%	0	0%
Skeletal muscle	0	0%	0	0%	0	0%	0	0%
Smooth muscle	0	0%	0	0%	0	0%	0	0%
Peripheral nerve sheath total	10	1%	17	< 1%	24	5%	14	1%
Schwannoma	0	0%	0	0%	0	0%	3	< 1%
Neurofibroma	5	< 1%	4	< 1%	24	5%	6	< 1%
Solitary circumscribed neuroma	3	< 1%	10	< 1%	0	0%	3	< 1%
Traumatic neuroma	2	< 1%	3	< 1%	0	0%	2	< 1%
Vascular total[c]	18	1%	83	2%	10	2%	112	6%
Cavernous haemangioma / cavernous venous malformation	4	< 1%	18	0%	2	0%	37	2%
Lymphangioma / lymphatic-venous malformation	0	0%	0	0%	3	1%	0	0%
Capillary haemangioma / infantile haemangioma	14	1%	32	1%	5	1%	45	2%
Arteriovenous malformation	0	0%	28	1%	0	0%	30	2%
Others	0	0%	5	< 1%	0	0%	0	0%
Tumours of uncertain derivation	0	0%	0	0%	0	0%	0	0%
Other total	1389	98%	5129	98%	409	92%	1733	88%
Epidermal	908	64%	3704	71%	146	33%	900	46%
Adnexal	202	14%	579	11%	161	36%	162	8%
Melanocytic	279	20%	846	16%	102	23%	671	34%
Total eyelid tumours	**1422**	**100%**	**5241**	**100%**	**443**	**100%**	**1976**	**100%**

[a]Excluded for consistency: haematolymphoid, inflammatory, infectious, traumatic (haematoma), metastatic. [b]All percentage values are rounded to the nearest whole number. [c]Both malformations and neoplastic lesions are included because of the inconsistent use of terminology before the 2018 International Society for the Study of Vascular Anomalies (ISSVA) classification {3557}.

{3598} provides a more detailed account of each soft tissue tumour. This chapter provides the key etiological, pathogenetic, diagnostic, and prognostic information on each neoplasm with an emphasis on site-specific characteristics. Mesenchymal neoplasms of the eye and ocular adnexa are uncommon. Soft tissue and bone tumours make up 20–30% and 1–3% of all orbital tumours, respectively (see Table 11.01, p. 381, and Table 11.02, p. 383) {3069,2418,3580,1296}. Soft tissue tumours account for 2–12% of all eyelid tumours and 3–4% of all conjunctival tumours (see Table 11.03 and Table 11.04) {1200,776,248,3721,2968,2527}.

Collectively, vascular lesions predominate in all age groups, followed by tumours of peripheral nerve sheath and fibrocytic lineage, and rhabdomyosarcoma in children {773,120,3026, 99,233,2968,1200,776,3721}. However, the collated data on the frequency of soft tissue and bone tumours in the eye and ocular adnexa are limited by the usage of old terminology and the uneven application of more modern immunohistochemical and molecular diagnostic methods for definitive characterization. This is particularly relevant in the categorization of fibroblastic lesions (e.g. solitary fibrous tumour), adipocytic lesions (e.g. herniated subconjunctival orbital fat vs spindle

Table 11.04 Types and frequency of conjunctival tumours with an emphasis on soft tissue tumours

Author	Shields {2968}		Pellerano {2527}	
Data collection time frame	**1974–2015**		**2010–2018**	
Lesion category[a]	***N***	**%**[b]	***N***	**%**
Soft tissue tumours total	154	4%	4	3%
Fibrous, fibroblastic total	15	< 1%	0	0%
Fibrous histiocytoma	9	< 1%	0	0%
Fibroma	5	< 1%	0	0%
Others	1	< 1%	0	0%
Adipocytic total	8	< 1%	0	0%
Lipoma	8	< 1%	0	0%
Skeletal muscle	0	0%	0	0%
Smooth muscle	0	0%	0	0%
Peripheral nerve sheath total	5	< 1%	0	0%
Schwannoma	1	< 1%	0	0%
Neurofibroma	4	< 1%	0	0%
Vascular total[c]	117	3%	4	3%
Cavernous haemangioma / cavernous venous malformation	5	< 1%	0	0%
Lymphangioma	0	0%	3	2%
Capillary haemangioma / infantile haemangioma	26	1%	0	0%
Arteriovenous malformation	11	< 1%	0	0%
Lymphangiectasia	42	1%	0	0%
Telangiectasia	18	< 1%	0	0%
Kaposi sarcoma	15	< 1%	0	0%
Haemangioma NOS	0	0%	1	< 1%
Perivascular	1	< 1%	0	0%
Tumours of uncertain derivation	7	< 1%	0	0%
Myxoma	7	< 1%	0	0%
Others	3587	96%	130	97%
Choristomatous	101	3%	7	5%
Epithelial	824	22%	66	49%
Melanocytic	2590	69%	57	43%
Secondary	66	2%	0	0%
Metastatic	6	0%	0	0%
Total conjunctival tumours	**3740**	**100%**	**134**	**100%**

[a]Excluded for consistency: histiocytic-dendritic neoplasms, inflammatory, infectious, degenerative, traumatic (haematoma), structural (herniated fat), lacrimal gland, amyloid deposits. [b]All percentage values are rounded to the nearest whole number. [c]Both malformations and neoplastic lesions are included because of the inconsistent use of terminology before the 2018 International Society for the Study of Vascular Anomalies (ISSVA) classification {3557}.

cell / pleomorphic lipoma), and sarcomas {3598}. In addition to their diagnostic value, cytogenetic and molecular techniques are increasingly important in guiding targeted therapies for various soft tissue and bone tumours {2213,2723}.

This volume follows the International Society for the Study of Vascular Anomalies (ISSVA) classification of vascular anomalies with separation into tumours and malformations {1436}. Cavernous vascular malformations, venous malformations, and arteriovenous malformations are discussed in Chapter 9: *Tumours of the orbit*, where they occur most commonly. Occasionally malformations may involve the retina, conjunctiva, or eyelid as part of a larger malformation that also involves the orbit – these lesions are not discussed further in this chapter. Retina and choroidal haemangiomas have not been classified by ISSVA and it is uncertain at this time if they are neoplasms or malformations; these lesions are summarized in Table 11.05 (p. 386).

Table 11.05 Vascular anomalies with no equivalent International Society for the Study of Vascular Anomalies (ISSVA) nomenclature

Entity	Clinical features	Pathological findings	Additional features
Cavernous haemangioma of the retina (RCH)	RCH is typically unilateral and asymptomatic, discovered on routine examination Some lesions may be associated with vision loss due to macular subretinal fluid or haemorrhage, vitreous haemorrhage with secondary vitreoretinal traction, and hyphaema with secondary glaucoma {3548,3033}	RCH is composed of grape-like clusters of dilated thin-walled interconnected vascular spaces lined by a continuous non-fenestrated endothelial lining {1078,2187,3548} Occasional areas of partially organized thrombus may be present The adjacent retina may exhibit gliosis	RCH can be sporadic or coexist with familial cerebral cavernous malformation (CCM) and cutaneous vascular malformations It is seen primarily in the White population with an even sex distribution; although RCH is believed to be a congenital lesion, the median age at presentation is 21 years {3548} 5% of patients with familial CCM also have RCH {1823}
Circumscribed choroidal haemangioma (CCH)	CCH typically presents in the fourth to sixth decades of life with loss of vision, metamorphopsia, and visual field defects CCH in patients < 20 years of age is associated with worse visual acuity {711} Subretinal fluid accumulation is seen in 64–80% of cases Cystoid macular oedema and retinal haemorrhage can occur {2915} On ultrasonography, CCH demonstrates high internal reflectivity and acoustic solidity CCH shows hyperfluorescence in all phases on intravenous fluorescein angiography and early hyperfluorescence with the washout phenomenon on indocyanine green angiography MRI demonstrates a choroidal mass that is hyperintense to vitreous on T1-weighted images and hyperisointense on T2-weighted images with contrast enhancement {2915}	Tumours are unilateral, orange-red, round, and well circumscribed, with a predilection for the superotemporal quadrant close to the macula The average basal diameter is 7.2 mm and the average height is 2.4 mm {1795} Choroidal haemangioma is composed of various proportions of dilated (cavernous) or capillary-sized thin-walled vascular channels lined by flat endothelial cells with scant intervening stroma {3618} CCH has sharply demarcated pushing margins that compress adjacent normal choroid {3618} Associated histopathological features include dilated draining vortex veins, retinal pigment epithelial hyperplasia, chorioretinal adhesions, and serous (exudative) retinal detachment	In CCH, *GNAQ* mutations occur in Q209, similar to those seen in intraocular melanocytic naevi and melanomas {1876}
Choroidal capillary malformation (CM) / diffuse choroidal haemangioma (DCH) (See also *Sturge–Weber syndrome*, p. 501)	DCH occurs in the setting of Sturge–Weber syndrome (SWS) in 20–70% of cases {2713,3103,3237}, usually ipsilateral to the facial CM (naevus flammeus) and presents as a diffuse, poorly defined red-orange mass involving > 50% of the choroid {1310} DCH remains asymptomatic early in childhood with a later increase in choroidal thickness with ageing Vision loss occurs from refractive error (hyperopic shift), overlying retinal changes, exudative retinal detachment, and secondary glaucoma {2713}	DCH appears as an unencapsulated collection of thin-walled, variably sized vascular channels Secondary changes include retinal pigment epithelial alteration, subretinal fibrosis, serous (exudative) retinal detachment, and sequelae of paediatric glaucoma (buphthalmos) {1310,3618}	In DCH, *GNAQ* mutations involve the R183 codon, similarly to other Sturge–Weber syndrome–associated capillary malformations {3079}

High-resolution MRI with and without gadolinium is recommended for evaluation of most soft tissue orbital tumours. CT, using 0.6–1 mm slices after contrast, is the imaging modality of choice for evaluating calcifications and osseous orbital lesions. Ultrasound and optical coherence tomography are valuable diagnostic imaging modalities for ocular soft tissue tumours {2608}. Although cytology-based techniques are employed with increasing frequency in the diagnosis of intraocular and orbital tumours, incisional and excisional biopsies remain standard methods for pathological diagnosis of soft tissue tumours {3604,1604}. Cytology-based diagnosis is particularly challenging for vascular malformations, cystic lesions, fibrous bone lesions, and lesions localized to the orbital apex {3604,1604, 45}. Currently, the grading system of the French Fédération Nationale des Centres de Lutte Contre le Cancer (FNCLCC) Sarcoma Group is the preferred system for grading of sarcomas

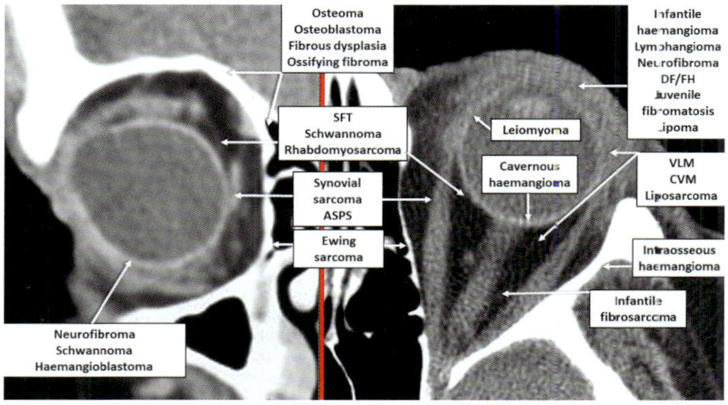

Fig. 11.01 Distribution of soft tissue and bone tumours in the eye and ocular adnexa. Both vascular malformations and neoplastic lesions are included because of the inconsistent use of terminology before the 2018 International Society for the Study of Vascular Anomalies (ISSVA) classification. ASPS, alveolar soft part sarcoma; CVM, cavernous venous malformation; DF, dermatofibroma; FH, fibrous histiocytoma; SFT, solitary fibrous tumour; VLM, venolymphatic malformation (lymphatic-venous malformation).

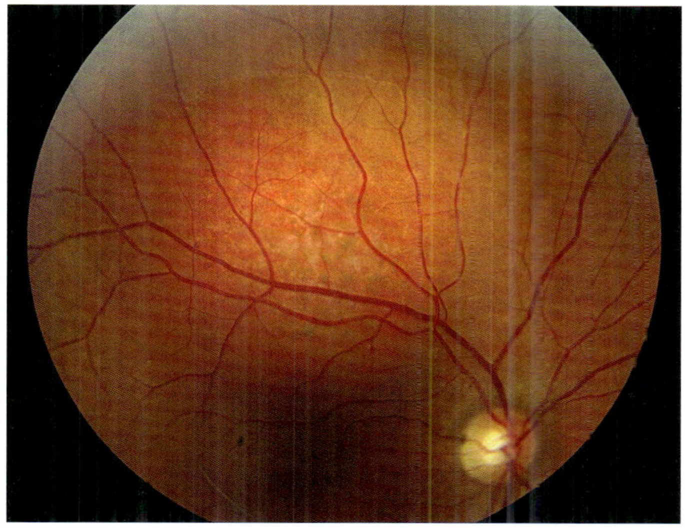

Fig. 11.02 Choroidal haemangioma. Fundus photograph showing a circumscribed choroidal haemangioma.

of the orbit {3377}. The ophthalmic site-specific staging system developed by the Union for International Cancer Control (UICC) and American Joint Committee on Cancer (AJCC) is the main staging system used for orbital sarcomas {2795}.

In this chapter, rare benign and malignant fibroblastic and myofibroblastic tumours of the ocular adnexa are summarized in Table 11.01 (p. 381). Some of these lesions have predilection for the eyelid, such as fibrous hamartoma of infancy, while others, such as myxofibrosarcoma, primarily involve deep orbital tissues. The epidemiology, microscopic features, and biological behaviour of these tumours are generally similar to the non-ocular counterparts {3598}. Some tumours, such as dermatofibroma of the eyelid, may demonstrate site-specific morphological differences {8}. Dermatofibrosarcoma protuberans is the most common of these rare entities and is described in greater detail.

Conjunctival stromal tumour and ocular surface fibroma

Mudhar HS
Herwig-Carl MC

Definition

Conjunctival stromal tumour (COST) is a benign lesion composed of spindle-shaped cells with pseudonuclear inclusions and multinucleated cells, in a variably myxoid stroma, with scattered mast cells.

Ocular surface fibroma (OSF) is a benign tumour composed of a collagen-rich stroma, bland spindle cells, and scattered mast cells.

ICD-O coding

None

ICD-11 coding

2F36.Y & XH2E97 Other specified benign neoplasm of eye or ocular adnexa & Stromal tumour, benign

2F36.Y & XH8E66 Other specified benign neoplasm of eye or ocular adnexa & Fibroma, NOS

Related terminology

Acceptable: for OSF: epibulbar subconjunctival fibroma; epibulbar fibroma; tarsal fibroma.

Subtype(s)

None

Localization

COST and OSF typically involve the bulbar conjunctiva and less frequently the palpebral conjunctiva {1329,2092,2296}.

Clinical features

Patients with COST and OSF may report a foreign body sensation and mild ocular injection {1329,2296}. COST and OSF are typically well circumscribed. Both tumours can be white, yellow, pink, or reddish in colour. COST is typically soft, cystoid, or gelatinous in appearance {1329}.

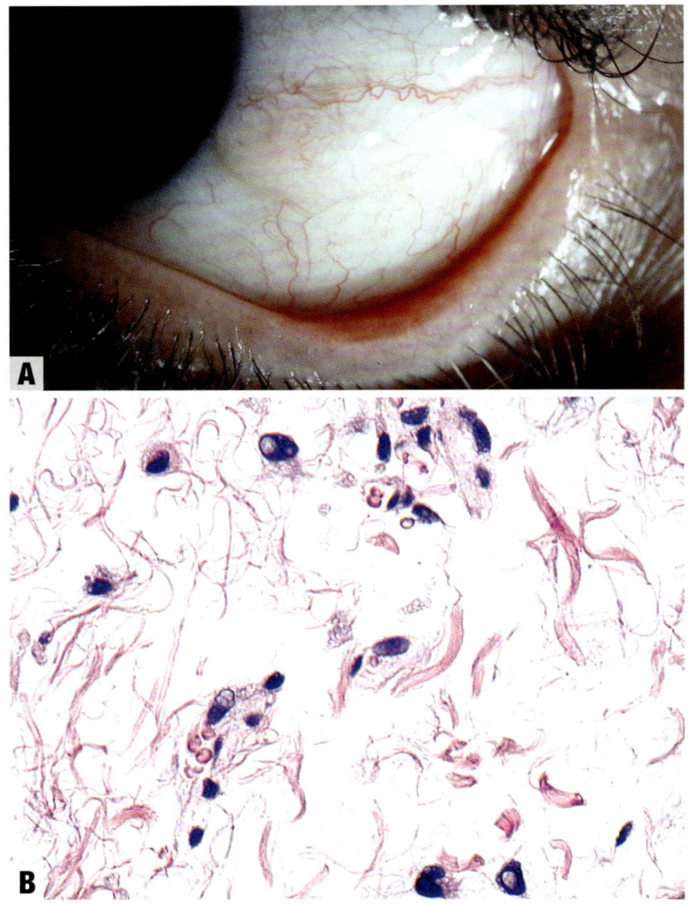

Fig. 11.03 Conjunctival stromal tumour. **A** A gelatinous translucent lesion of the temporal conjunctiva in a 52-year-old woman. **B** A loose myxoid matrix, wiry collagen, and cells with nuclear pseudoinclusions.

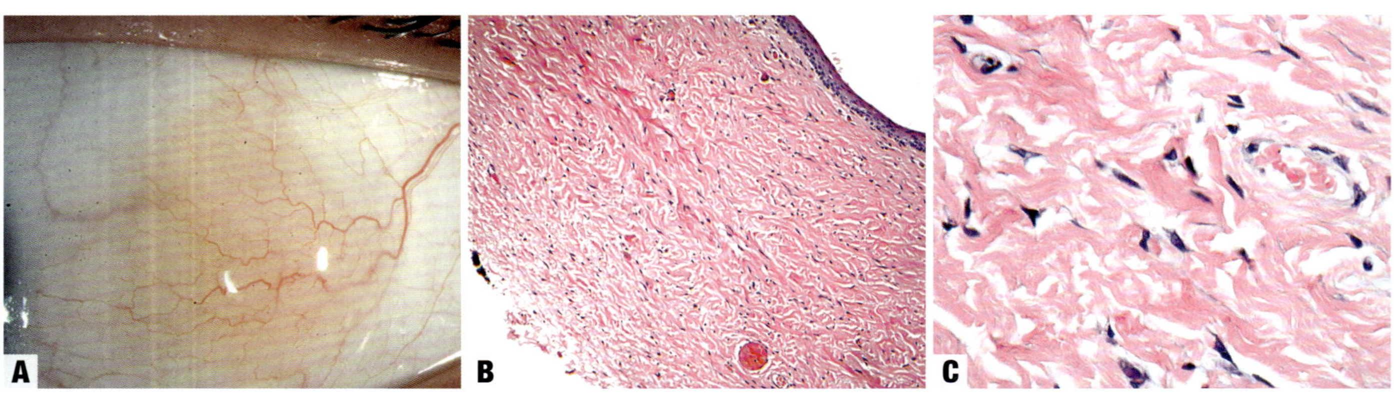

Fig. 11.04 Ocular surface fibroma. **A** External photograph of the left eye showing a circumscribed, pink, translucent temporal bulbar mass beneath conjunctival epithelium. **B** A collagen-rich lesion in the conjunctival substantia propria is observed. **C** Non-atypical spindle and stellate cells, with inconspicuous nucleoli and delicate basophilic cytoplasm, embedded in the collagen-rich stroma, are seen.

Epidemiology

COST and OSF have been observed in patients between the second and eighth decades of life. Patients with COST are younger than those with OSF (mean: 47 vs 78 years). COST has no sex predilection, while OSF has a male predilection {1329,214,2217}.

Etiology

The etiology of OSF and COST is unknown, but appears to be reactive in nature {1329,2296}.

Pathogenesis

The conjunctival substantia propria, Tenon capsule, and tarsal plate contain CD34-positive resident fibroblasts and factor XIIIa–positive dendritic cells that are the mucosal equivalent of dermal-skin dermal dendrocytes. It is speculated that in a likely inflammatory setting, these resident CD34-positive and factor XIIIa–positive cells undergo reactive proliferation with elaboration of the associated stromal response {2296}.

Macroscopic appearance

See *Clinical features*.

Histopathology

COST is composed of variably myxoid stroma and can contain variable wiry to ropy collagen, with loosely arranged spindle-shaped cells. The spindle cells exhibit pseudonuclear inclusions. Multinucleated cells in a floret-like configuration are present {1329,214}. There are usually no mitotic figures. Scattered aggregates of lymphocytes and histiocytes may be present. Scattered mast cells may be seen.

COST histochemistry: The stroma in most cases stains positively with Alcian blue / colloidal iron {1329,214}.

COST immunohistochemistry: The spindle cells are positive for CD34 {1329}, PRKAR1A {2217}, factor XIIIa {2217}, and RB1 {2217}. There may be scattered CD68-positive histiocytes.

OSF is composed of evenly distributed, similar-appearing spindle cells and dendritic cells, with delicate basophilic

Table 11.06 Histological differential diagnosis of conjunctival stromal tumour and ocular surface fibroma

Diagnosis	Histological features	Immunohistochemistry	Molecular pathology	References
Conjunctival stromal tumour	Myxoid stroma; wiry to ropy collagen; bland spindle cells with pseudonuclear inclusions; multinucleated floret-like cells	Spindle cells: CD34+, PRKAR1A+, RB1+ Dendritic cells: factor XIIIa+ Negative for S100, SMA, desmin	None	{1329,214, 2217}
Ocular surface fibroma	Collagenous stroma with mast cells; bland spindle cells; some occasional plumper spindle cells with very occasional pseudonuclear inclusions	Spindle cells: CD34+ Dendritic cells: factor XIIIa+ Negative for S100, melan-A, SMA, desmin	None	{1326,1477, 538,2296}
Conjunctival myxoma (Carney complex)	Abundant myxoid stroma; mostly stellate cells; predominantly fibrillary collagen	Stellate cells: CD34+, can be PRKAR1A– Some cases have factor XIIIa+ cells Negative for S100, SOX10, SMA	Mutations in *PRKAR1A* gene in 1 case recorded	{2217}
Fat-free spindle cell lipoma and pleomorphic lipoma	Ropy collagen and myxoid stroma with mast cells Spindle cell lipoma has short, stubby spindle cells with uniform elongated nuclei and bipolar eosinophilic cytoplasm; some cases show cytoplasmic vacuolation; spindle cells are usually arranged in short fascicles in a school-of-fish pattern, sometimes with nuclear palisading Pleomorphic lipoma has pleomorphic spindle cells and multinucleated floret-like giant cells, which have peripheral radially placed hyperchromatic nuclei around central deeply eosinophilic cytoplasm	Spindle cells: CD34+ For other soft tissue sites: RB1 loss	No available molecular data in conjunctiva For other soft tissue sites: demonstration of loss of the *RB1* locus	{2931,1929, 557,704,271}
Neurofibroma	May be solitary, diffuse, or plexiform; haphazard proliferation of spindle Schwann cells and fibroblasts, with mast cells present; degenerative atypia of cells can be seen; myxomatous stroma can be present; pseudomeissnerian corpuscles may be present; axons permeate the lesion	Spindle cells: patchy variable S100+ Axons: neurofilament+	No available molecular data in conjunctiva	{1582}
Solitary fibrous tumour	Tapering spindle and ovoid/rounded cells; wiry interstitial collagen investing between individual spindle cells; multinucleated tumour giant cells can be present around pseudovascular spaces in giant cell–rich solitary fibrous tumour	Spindle and multinucleated cells: CD34+, STAT6+ Negative for SMA, S100, melan-A, desmin	No available molecular data in conjunctiva	{2516,1283, 3166,2300, 2414}
Fibrous histiocytoma	Spindle to pleomorphic cells with conspicuous storiform to vaguely spindled architecture and a variably prominent collagenous or fibrous background	Spindle and pleomorphic cells: factor XIIIa+, CD68+, CD163+, α1-antitrypsin+ Negative for CD34	No available molecular data in conjunctiva	{1474,1742, 363,490,[illegible]474, 3168,3333}

cytoplasm, in a collagen-rich matrix that is wiry/ropy to keloid-like {1326,1477,538,2296}. In some cases, the spindle cells are plumper and can occasionally harbour pseudonuclear inclusions {2296}. The spindle cells show no to minimal nuclear pleomorphism. No mitotic figures are present and multinucleated cells are not present. There are scattered evenly distributed mast cells. Occasional aggregates of chronic inflammatory cells are present at the periphery of the lesion.

OSF histochemistry: The stroma is negative for Alcian blue.

OSF immunohistochemistry: The spindle cells (including the plumper ones) are CD34-positive. There are scattered factor XIIIa–positive dendritic cells and some cases can show scattered CD68-positive histiocytes {2296}.

The spindle cells of COST and OSF are negative for S100, SMA, and desmin {1329,2296}.

It is likely, given some histological similarity (presence of pseudonuclear inclusions) and immunohistochemical overlap (CD34+, factor XIIIa+), that COST and OSF may represent a continuum, with COST being myxoid paucicollagenous and OSF being collagen rich {2296}.

Differential diagnosis

For the histological differential diagnosis, see Table 11.06 (p. 389).

Cytology

Not relevant

Diagnostic molecular pathology

Not relevant

Essential and desirable diagnostic criteria

Conjunctival stromal tumour

Essential: bland spindle cells with pseudonuclear inclusions, multinucleated cells in floret-like configuration, and myxoid stroma with wiry or ropy non-compact collagen.

Desirable: stroma that stains positive with Alcian blue / colloidal iron; factor XIIIa+ dendritic cells; CD34 positivity.

Ocular surface fibroma

Essential: bland spindle cells, collagen-rich matrix, and scattered mast cells.

Desirable: presence of factor XIIIa+ dendritic cells; CD34 positivity.

Staging

Not relevant

Prognosis and prediction

There are no reported cases of malignant change or metastasis. Recurrence has been described rarely {214,2296}.

Fibrous histiocytoma

Mudhar HS

Definition

Fibrous histiocytoma is a common benign mesenchymal tumour consisting of a combination of fibroblasts, myofibroblasts, reactive dendritic cells, and macrophages in between collagen bundles.

ICD-O coding

8831/0 Deep fibrous histiocytoma
8832/0 Classic dermatofibroma
8832/0 Cellular dermatofibroma
8832/0 Aneurysmal dermatofibroma
8832/0 Atypical dermatofibroma

ICD-11 coding

2F23.0 Dermatofibroma

Related terminology

Acceptable: dermatofibroma (skin).

Subtype(s)

Eyelid: deep fibrous histiocytoma; classic dermatofibroma; cellular dermatofibroma; aneurysmal dermatofibroma; atypical dermatofibroma
Conjunctiva: none

Localization

Fibrous histiocytoma of the ocular area is mostly located within the bulbar conjunctiva and limbus {3123}. The next commonest site is the upper eyelid skin (dermatofibroma) {8}. Very rare sites include the caruncle {3123}, lacrimal sac {594}, and uveal tract (choroid) {1845}. While the orbit was thought to be a common site {1005}, most of these cases are judged to be orbital solitary fibrous tumours {311,1053}.

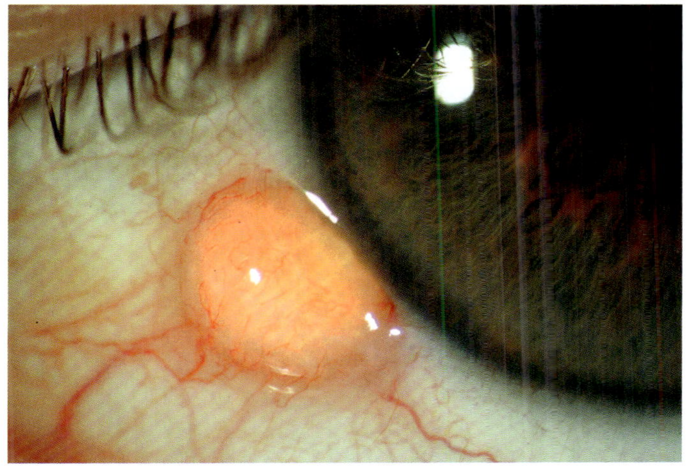

Fig. 11.05 Fibrous histiocytoma of the limbal conjunctiva. A nodular yellowish tumour.

Clinical features

Eyelid: Most lesions occur on the upper eyelid as a painless nodule that can be white, yellow, skin coloured, or reddish {8}.

Conjunctiva: Most cases comprise a painless, yellowish to tan-coloured, dome-shaped mass, often lacking a feeder vessel at the base, but sometimes with vascularization over the surface {3123,198,1686,1742,1354}.

Epidemiology

Eyelid: The age range is 5–68 years with an equal sex distribution {8}.

Conjunctiva: Fibrous histiocytoma is rare, accounting for only 0.2% of all conjunctival tumours {2972}. The age of onset ranges from infancy to the eighth decade of life (mean age: 31 years), with a male preponderance {3123}.

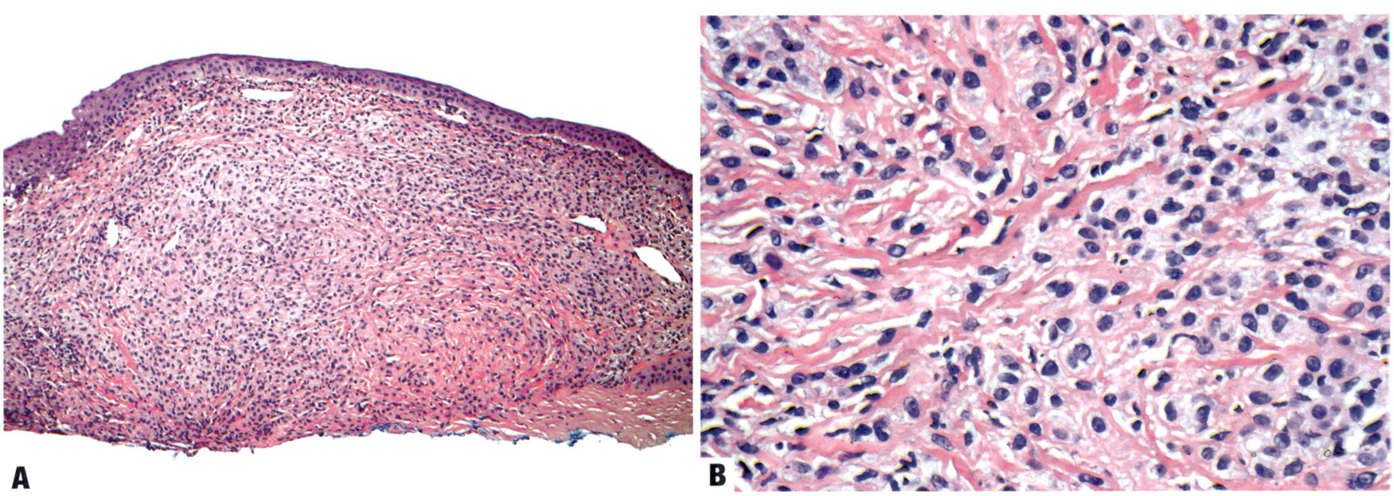

Fig. 11.06 Fibrous histiocytoma of the limbal conjunctiva. **A** Expansion of the stroma is seen. **B** The stroma is expanded by plump spindle cells.

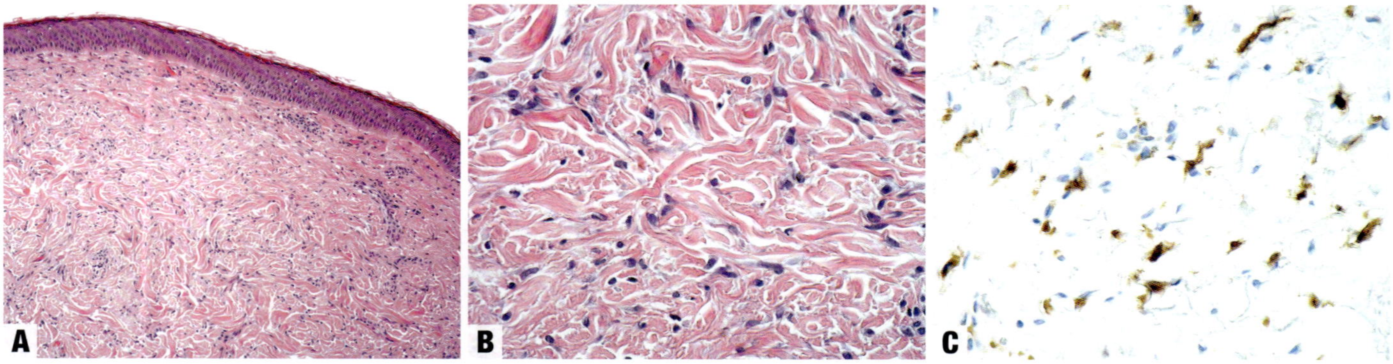

Fig. 11.07 Fibrous histiocytoma involving eyelid. **A** A fibrocollagenous lesion in the dermis without epidermal hyperplasia is observed. **B** The tumour comprises bland spindle, ovoid, and triangular fibroblast-like cells between coarse collagen. **C** Factor XIIIa-positive reactive dendrocytes are seen within the tumour.

Etiology

Unknown

Pathogenesis

In non-eyelid skin, recurrent gene fusions involving protein kinase C isoforms (*PRKCA*, *PRKCB*, and *PRKCD*) with various genes encoding membrane-associated proteins (e.g. *LAMTOR1*, *PDPN*, *CD63*, and KIRREL) have been identified in a minority of cases {3537,2565,1510,2475}. These data provide proof of the neoplastic, clonal nature of dermatofibroma (see the related section in the *Skin tumours* volume {3597}), which is lacking for conjunctival and eyelid fibrous histiocytoma.

Macroscopic appearance

See *Clinical features*.

Histopathology

The usual histology is a reticular dermis–based, poorly defined, polymorphous population of cells, comprising spindled to rounded neoplastic cells with surrounding dermal dendrocytes and macrophages {470}. There are characteristic collagen balls in the lesion. A storiform growth pattern may be seen. The epidermis is usually hyperplastic {302,3090,3737}. Early lesions are cellular and older lesions appear more fibrotic with fewer macrophages. Lipidized tumour contains histiocytes with vacuolated cytoplasm {1439}. Because of the relative lack of reticular dermis from eyelid skin, some cases of eyelid-skin dermatofibroma deviate from the classic appearance and show histological variance. Some cases are well defined, basophilic, and cellular, lack peripheral collagen trapping (collagen balls), lack a zone of collagen separating the tumour from the epidermis, and do not exhibit overlying epidermal hyperplasia {8}. These differences are thought to reflect an origin within the papillary dermis rather than from the reticular dermis {8}. For further details on cutaneous subtypes, refer to the related section in the *Skin tumours* volume {3597}.

The histology of conjunctival and limbal fibrous histiocytomas is very similar to that described above, with classic and other morphological patterns {3339,1686}, with some cases being lipidized {88}.

Immunohistochemistry

There are no specific markers for ocular fibrous histiocytoma {3182}. CD68 and CD163 stain in interspersed histiocytes. SMA stains in the myofibroblastic component. Factor XIIIa stains in interspersed reactive dendritic cells {363,490,1474,3168}.

Differential diagnosis

Differential diagnosis includes nodular episcleritis, juvenile xanthogranuloma, spindle cell carcinoma, and solitary fibrous tumour {363,490,2522}.

Cytology

Not relevant

Diagnostic molecular pathology

Not clinically relevant

Essential and desirable diagnostic criteria

Essential: combination of fibroblasts, myofibroblasts, reactive dendritic cells, and macrophages in between collagen bundles.

Desirable: supportive immunohistochemical data.

Staging

Not relevant

Prognosis and prediction

Complete excision is usually curative, with no recurrence {3123, 1474,1595,1686,3168}.

Nodular and proliferative fasciitis, proliferative myositis

Stagner AM
Grossniklaus HE
Rodriguez FJ
Wang WL

Definition

Nodular fasciitis is a rapidly growing, self-limited or transient fibroblastic/myofibroblastic neoplasm composed of plump spindled cells arranged in a tissue culture–like architectural pattern, and usually harbouring a *USP6* rearrangement.

ICD-O coding

8828/0 Nodular fasciitis
8828/0 Proliferative fasciitis
8828/0 Proliferative myositis

ICD-11 coding

FB51.2 & XH5LM1 Pseudosarcomatous fibromatosis & Nodular fasciitis
FB51.2 & XH6JX7 Pseudosarcomatous fibromatosis & Proliferative fasciitis
FB51.Y & XH87F9 Other specified fibroblastic disorders & Proliferative myositis

Related terminology

Not recommended: pseudosarcomatous fasciitis; pseudosarcomatous fibromatosis.

Subtype(s)

Proliferative fasciitis/myositis; intravascular and cranial fasciitis (probably not applicable to ocular adnexa)

Localization

Typical nodular fasciitis arises from superficial fascia and extends into the subcutis; it may also be intramuscular or dermal {2160,754} and usually arises in the upper extremities, trunk, and head and neck. Within the ocular adnexa, nodular fasciitis most commonly develops in the anterior periorbital tissues including eyelids and canthi, or as episcleral nodules; deep orbital lesions also occur {1009,2710,658,172}.

Proliferative fasciitis is very rare, but has been described a handful of times in the orbit, with 1 epibulbar case reported {280,2534,1459}.

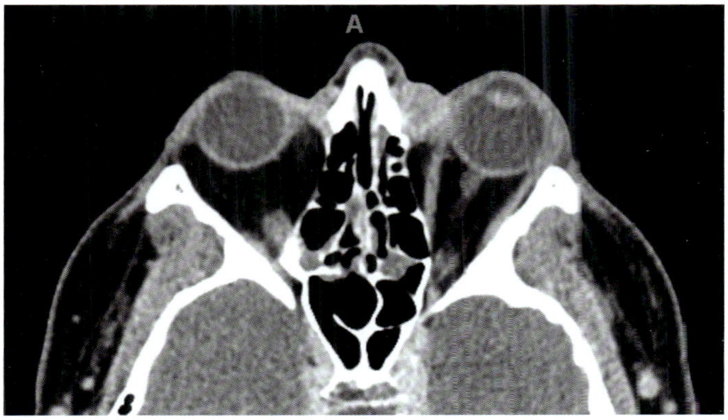

Fig. 11.08 Nodular fasciitis of the orbit. Axial CT demonstrates a circumscribed mass in the region of the left lacrimal sac.

Clinical features

Nodular fasciitis of the ocular adnexa is a rapidly growing (over weeks to months) epibulbar, anterior periorbital, or orbital mass that is typically well circumscribed, but may be poorly defined within the orbit. CT and MRI demonstrate an enhancing mass rarely associated with bone remodelling {658}. Epibulbar lesions may mimic nodular episcleritis {2105}. Lesions are usually < 10 mm on the epibulbar surface, and < 30 mm in the orbit {1009}.

Proliferative fasciitis is very rare in this location {2534,1459}.

Proliferative myositis of the ocular/periocular tissues has not been documented.

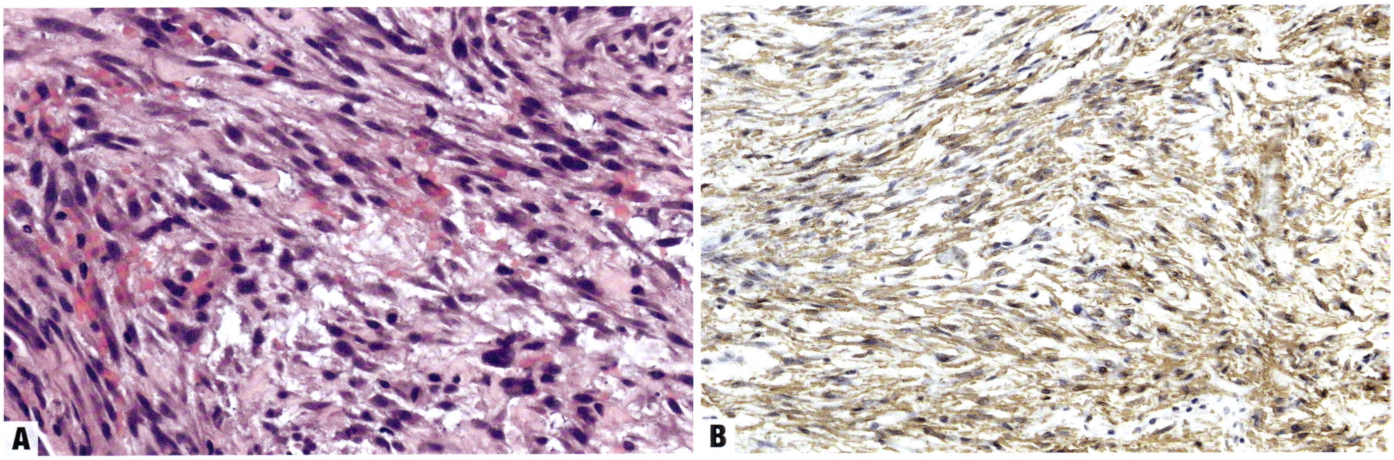

Fig. 11.09 Nodular fasciitis. **A** Discohesive spindle cells in a tissue culture–like arrangement and myxoid stroma with extravasated erythrocytes are seen. **B** Spindle cells express SMA at the periphery of the cytoplasm (tram-track pattern), compatible with myofibroblastic proliferation.

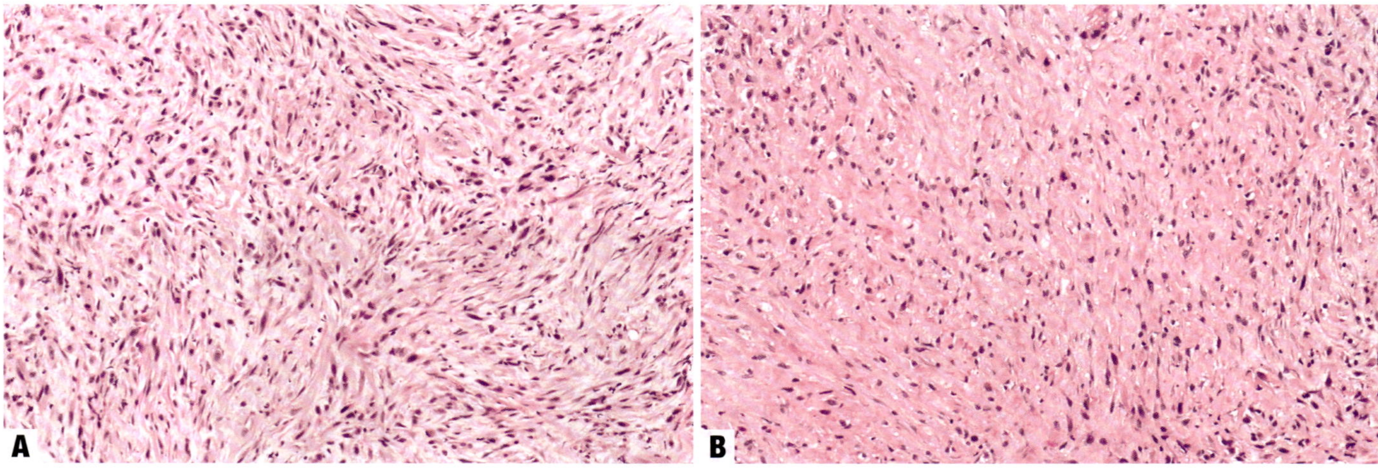

Fig. 11.10 Nodular fasciitis. **A** Feathery, plump spindled cells with conspicuous mitotic activity in a tissue culture–like arrangement. **B** A hypocellular area with myxoid stroma.

Epidemiology

Nodular fasciitis is rare in the orbit and ocular adnexa. This lesion occurs in all age groups but is more prevalent in young adults; a quarter of cases occur in children and orbital lesions are more common in children.

Etiology

Historically these were postulated to be incited by trauma; currently the etiology is unknown.

Pathogenesis

Recurrent *USP6* gene rearrangements have been reported in about 70% of cases {2508}, including in nodular fasciitis of the orbit {172}.

Macroscopic appearance

The lesions are typically a well-circumscribed, unencapsulated mass with a myxoid cut surface.

Histopathology

Nodular fasciitis is composed of plump spindle and stellate cells (fibroblasts and/or myofibroblasts) without overt cytological atypia. Mitotic activity can be frequent, without atypical mitoses. Cellularity often varies. Feathery tissue culture–like areas with myxoid stroma are characteristic, often with extravasated red blood cells, but more cellular areas can form fascicles and sometimes have a storiform pattern. Stroma can be myxoid with microcystic-like changes and/or collagenous or keloidal-like. Osteoclastic giant cells and chronic inflammatory cells can be present.

Proliferative fasciitis and proliferative myositis contain plump myofibroblastic/fibroblastic spindle cells similar to those in nodular fasciitis and also demonstrate large ganglion-like cells with rounded nuclei, prominent nucleoli, and abundant amphophilic to basophilic cytoplasm {616}. The ganglion cells can be variably distributed and usually have one nucleus, but may be multinucleated. Proliferative myositis may contain metaplastic bone.

Immunohistochemistry

SMA and MSA expression in a tram-track pattern is characteristic but not specific for these lesions. The ganglion-like cells are often negative for actins {884,2008}.

Cytology

Cytologically, nodular fasciitis features bland spindle cells with bipolar and dendritic processes, ovoid nuclei, and occasional small nucleoli in a tissue culture–like arrangement, and variably myxoid stroma {1631}.

Diagnostic molecular pathology

Diagnostic molecular pathology is not always necessary, but in uncommon sites such as the ocular adnexa, *USP6* rearrangement may be confirmatory {2508,1849}.

Essential and desirable diagnostic criteria

Essential: for nodular fasciitis: loose intersecting fascicles of plump myofibroblasts in a tissue culture–like arrangement, variably myxoid stroma, and extravasated erythrocytes; for proliferative fasciitis and myositis: myofibroblastic/fibroblastic proliferation with ganglion-like cells and variable myxoid stroma.

Desirable: USP6 rearrangement in select cases.

Staging

Not applicable

Prognosis and prediction

Surgical excision is usually undertaken for diagnostic and therapeutic purposes, particularly given the common clinical concern for malignancy. Recurrence in large series outside the ocular adnexa is very rare after excision {315}. An orbital case has been successfully treated with intralesional steroids {1659}. Since periorbital involvement is relatively rare, specific data regarding recurrence is not available in the orbit / ocular adnexa {3054,172}.

Solitary fibrous tumour

Alkatan H
Demicco EG
Rodriguez FJ
Smith SC

Definition

Solitary fibrous tumour (SFT) is a fibroblastic neoplasm characterized by a prominent, branching, dilated (staghorn) vasculature and a *NAB2::STAT6* rearrangement.

ICD-O coding

8815/1 Solitary fibrous tumour, NOS
8815/0 Solitary fibrous tumour, benign
8815/3 Solitary fibrous tumour, malignant
8815/1 Fat-forming (lipomatous) solitary fibrous tumour
8815/1 Giant cell–rich solitary fibrous tumour
8815/3 Dedifferentiated solitary fibrous tumour

ICD-11 coding

2F7C & XH7E62 Neoplasms of uncertain behaviour of connective or other soft tissue & Solitary fibrous tumour, NOS
2B5Y & XH1HP3 Other specified malignant mesenchymal neoplasms & Solitary fibrous tumour, malignant

Related terminology

Not recommended: haemangiopericytoma; giant cell angiofibroma; benign solitary fibrous tumour.

Subtype(s)

Fat-forming (lipomatous) solitary fibrous tumour; giant cell–rich solitary fibrous tumour; dedifferentiated solitary fibrous tumour

Localization

Orbital SFT can affect intraconal and extraconal spaces {3151, 103}. Other periocular sites include the lacrimal gland, lacrimal sac, conjunctiva, sclera, and eyelids {1684,1214}. Fat-forming SFT has been reported in the orbit {1195,935,2563}, while giant cell–rich SFT is more common in periorbital soft tissue {768, 3165,875,3291}.

Clinical features

The clinical presentation depends on the location of the tumour. The commonest presentation is periorbital fullness, orbital mass (with or without proptosis), globe displacement, limitation of extraocular motility, diplopia, ptosis, and blurred vision {1684, 1053,103}. Intraconal and orbital apex tumours may cause optic disc oedema, afferent pupillary defect, and choroidal folds {357, 103}. MRI has value in the diagnosis and delineation of soft tissue involvement in SFT, while CT is important in detecting bone involvement {3676}. The tumour is isointense with homogeneous appearance on T1-weighted MRI and shows a well-defined isodense enhancing mass with contrast on CT {3676,103}.

Epidemiology

Orbital SFT is most common in the mid-forties {1792,103,3268} and is rare in childhood {2706,768}. Sex distribution has been variably reported between being equally distributed and having a male predilection with an M:F ratio of 3:1 {1792,3151,103}.

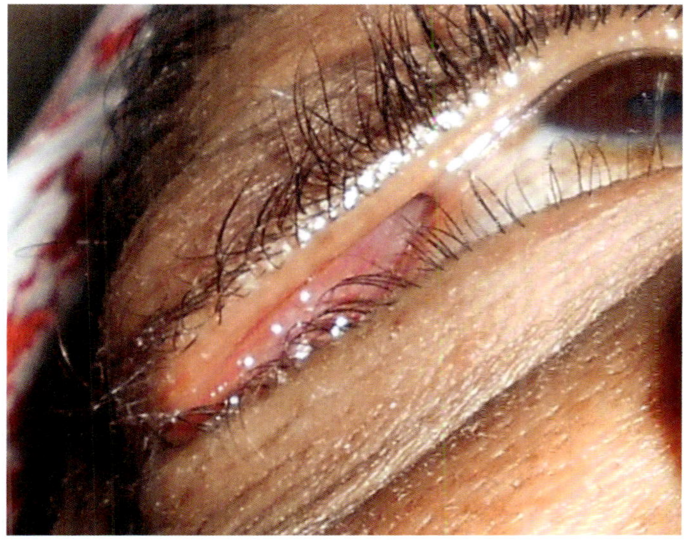

Fig. 11.11 Solitary fibrous tumour. The clinical appearance of an anterior orbital solitary fibrous tumour in a patient presenting with a right upper lid mass and downward/inward globe displacement.

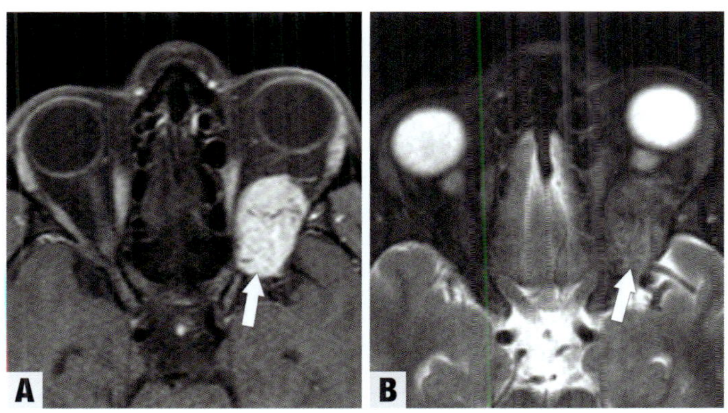

Fig. 11.12 Solitary fibrous tumour. **A** Axial T1-weighted postcontrast MRI shows an enhancing mass (arrow) in the superior left orbit. Punctate and linear hypointense areas in the mass suggest the presence of vessels. **B** Axial T2-weighted MRI shows a hypointense appearance of the mass (arrow).

Etiology

Unknown

Pathogenesis

SFT is characterized by a paracentric inversion involving chromosome 12q, resulting in the fusion of the *NAB2* and *STAT6* genes {590,2244,2731}. The fusion protein is thought to drive

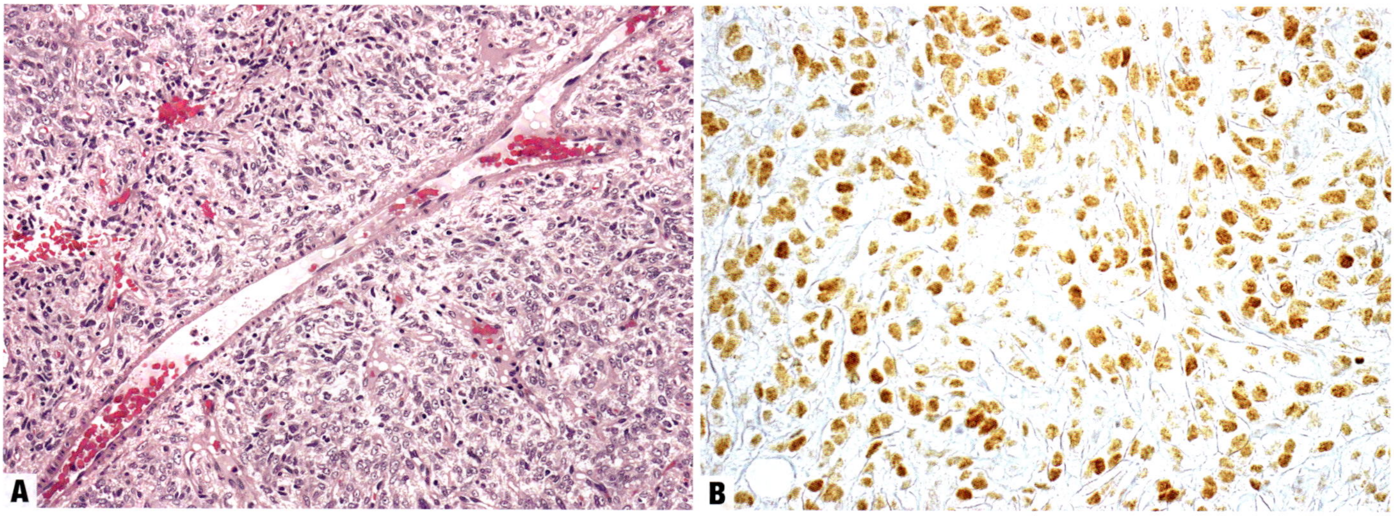

Fig. 11.13 Solitary fibrous tumour. **A** Patternless arrangement of spindle cells in a collagenous stroma with a branching, staghorn-like vascular channel. **B** Diffuse and strong nuclear expression of STAT6 by the tumour cells.

tumorigenesis via feed-forward activation of the EGR1 pathway {2731}.

Macroscopic appearance

Grossly, SFTs are usually partially encapsulated and well circumscribed, and exhibit a whitish, multinodular firm cut surface with possible myxoid areas and/or haemorrhage {3151,3291}.

Histopathology

SFT has a variable histopathological appearance showing hypocellular to hypercellular areas of proliferating ovoid to spindle cells with patternless arrangement, separated by collagen fibres of variable thickness (keloid type in classic SFTs) with a storiform pattern {103,3291}. Cell pleomorphism and multinucleated giant cells (giant cell–rich SFT) occur in a subset of cases {757}. The stroma contains thin-walled and hyalinized branching staghorn-shaped blood vessels {3291}. Hyalinized stroma is also reported {103}. Dedifferentiated SFTs show transition to a high-grade sarcoma {2431}.

Table 11.07 Three-variable and modified four-variable risk models for the prediction of metastatic risk in solitary fibrous tumours {763,764}

Risk factor	Cut-off point	Points assigned	
		3-variable model	4-variable model
Patient age in years	< 55	0	0
	≥ 55	1	1
Mitoses/mm² (mitoses/10 HPF)	0 (0)	0	0
	0.5–1.5 (1–3)	1	1
	≥ 2 (≥ 4)	2	2
Tumour size in mm	0–49	0	0
	50–99	1	1
	100–149	2	2
	≥ 150	3	3
Tumour necrosis	< 10%	n/a	0
	≥ 10%	n/a	1
Risk	Low	0–2 points	0–3 points
	Intermediate	3–4 points	4–5 points
	High	5–6 points	6–7 points

HPF, high-power field; n/a, not applicable

Immunohistochemistry

STAT6 is the most sensitive immunohistochemical marker {2893, 822,3291,1095}. Other markers may be used in combination if STAT6 immunohistochemistry is not available: CD34 (expressed in 81–95% of cases), BCL2 (expressed in > 90% of cases), and CD99, which is less sensitive {3291}.

Differential diagnosis

In the ocular adnexa this includes peripheral nerve sheath tumours, leiomyoma, nodular fasciitis, adipocytic tumours, and synovial sarcoma (see related sections).

Cytology

Cytopathology has limited value in the evaluation of SFT (accurate and specific in 9% of cases). Therefore, positivity of STAT6 is essential for diagnosis, particularly in small specimens {3288, 3525}.

Diagnostic molecular pathology

NAB2::STAT6 fusions are pathognomonic of SFT, but the detection of fusion types is difficult without multiplexed sequencing assays. STAT6 immunohistochemistry is a sensitive and specific surrogate for all fusions {822,1757,2893}.

Essential and desirable diagnostic criteria

Essential: spindled to ovoid cells arranged around a branching and hyalinized vasculature; variable stromal collagen deposition; STAT6 expression by immunohistochemistry.

Desirable: demonstration of a *NAB2::STAT6* fusion (in select cases).

Staging
Risk stratification models are preferred over anatomical staging {763,764}.

Prognosis and prediction
The most widely used models for metastatic risk of thoracic and extrathoracic SFTs (see Table 11.07) incorporate mitotic count ($\geq$ 2 mitoses/mm^2), patient age ($\geq$ 55 years), tumour size, and necrosis to classify SFTs into low-, intermediate-, and high-risk groups {763,764,2694}. Staining of p53 and a higher proliferation index using Ki-67 (> 5%) are associated with a worse prognosis {1053,3671}. Ocular adnexal SFT carries a relatively high risk of regional recurrence (~25%) and a low risk of distant metastasis (~2%), which can occur many years after initial surgery {3330}. Thus, long-term follow-up is recommended {3268, 2540,2961,3681}.

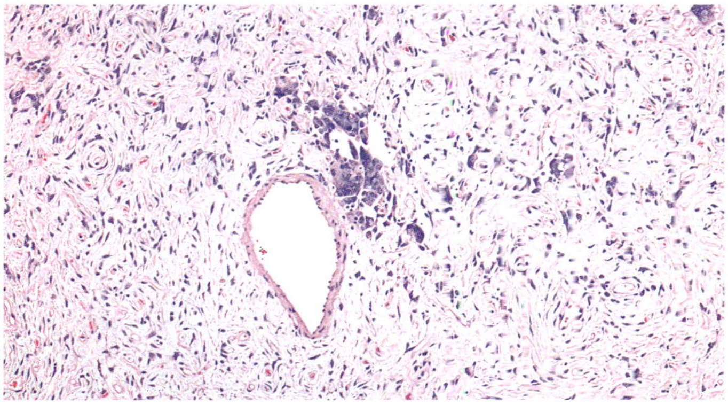

Fig. 11.14 Solitary fibrous tumour. Low-magnification histopathological appearance of a giant cell–rich solitary fibrous tumour.

Inflammatory myofibroblastic tumour

Rodriguez FJ
Ng T
Yamamoto H

Definition
Inflammatory myofibroblastic tumour (IMT) is a distinctive neoplasm of low metastatic potential composed of myofibroblastic and fibroblastic spindle cells accompanied by an inflammatory infiltrate of plasma cells, lymphocytes, and/or eosinophils.

ICD-O coding
8825/1 Inflammatory myofibroblastic tumour

ICD-11 coding
2B53.Y & XH66Z0 Other specified fibroblastic or myofibroblastic tumour, primary site & Myofibroblastic tumour, NOS

Related terminology
Not recommended: inflammatory pseudotumour.

Subtype(s)
None

Localization
In the ocular/periocular region, the orbit is a favoured site, and the lacrimal gland may also be involved {390,3220}.

Clinical features
Symptoms and signs of orbital IMT include proptosis, ptosis, diplopia, visual loss, swelling, and pain {3220,2572,777}.

Epidemiology
IMT has a wide age distribution (0 to 81 years). No consistent sex predilection is observed {569,2435}.

Etiology
Unknown

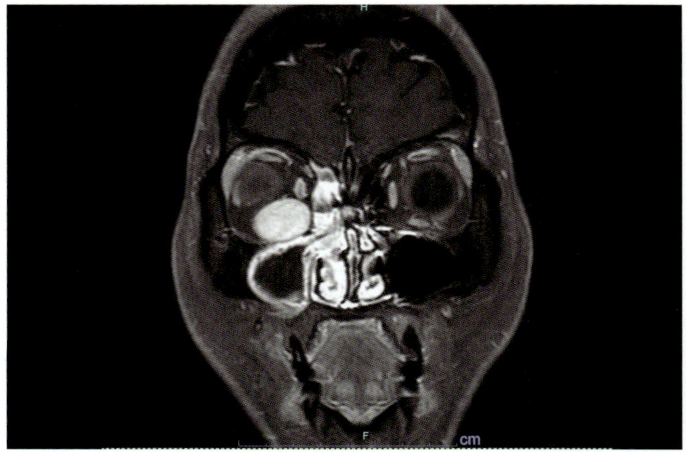

Fig. 11.15 Inflammatory myofibroblastic tumour. Gadolinium-enhanced T1-weighted MRI.

Pathogenesis
As many as 60% of tumours have an *ALK* gene (2p23) rearrangement with a wide variety of fusion partners. Among head and neck IMTs, *ALK* fusion with *TIMP3* has been most commonly detected, and *ROS1* fusion is seen rarely {3707,1661}.

Macroscopic appearance
The tumours are usually < 50 mm, firm, and fleshy with a tan-white whorled to myxoid cut surface, occasionally showing haemorrhage and calcification.

Histopathology
Three principal patterns may coexist: a myxoid fasciitis or granulation tissue–like pattern, a hypercellular spindle-cell pattern, and a hypocellular fibrous (fibromatosis-like) pattern {638,

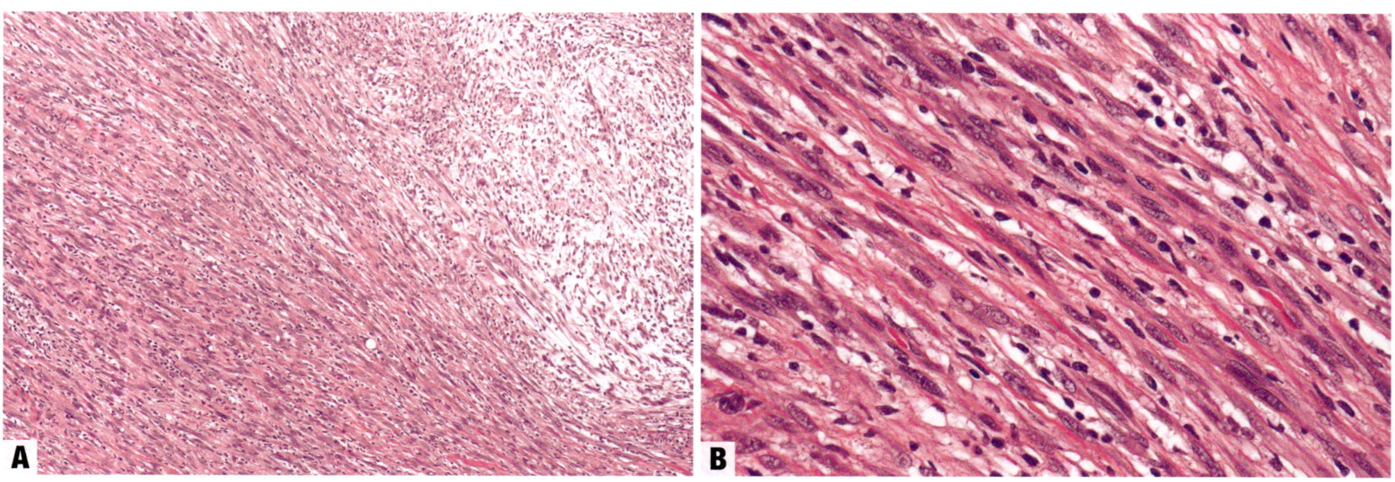

Fig. 11.16 Inflammatory myofibroblastic tumour. **A** Spindle tumour cells proliferate in a background of collagenous and myxoid stroma. **B** Spindle tumour cells are admixed with lymphocytes and plasma cells.

637,252}. The spindle cells associate with a variable inflammatory infiltrate and fibromyxoid stroma {638,637,252}. Necrosis is infrequent. Mitotic activity is variable but generally low {638, 1289,637}.

Immunohistochemistry

Most IMTs, especially in patients < 40 years of age, express ALK, correlating with *ALK* gene rearrangements {606,3667,1835}. ROS1 may show cytoplasmic reactivity in *ROS1*-rearranged IMT {3667,1367}. The spindle cells generally show a patchy, variable reactivity for SMA, MSA, calponin, and desmin, with focal keratin reactivity in 30% of cases {638,252}.

Differential diagnosis

Differential diagnosis of IMT depends on the predominant histological pattern and includes idiopathic orbital inflammatory disease, IgG4-related disease, and nodular fasciitis (see related sections).

Cytology

The cytology of IMT features bland spindle cells with oval nuclei and small nucleoli, occasionally with ganglion-like cells, in a background of lymphocytes and plasma cells {3212,2956}.

Diagnostic molecular pathology

Molecular assays for *ALK*, *ROS1*, and other gene rearrangements may be used, particularly if targeted therapy is being considered {3667,586,1995}.

Essential and desirable diagnostic criteria

Essential: loose or compact proliferation of spindle cells with myofibroblastic differentiation; fibrous or myxoid stroma; associated chronic inflammatory cell infiltrate.

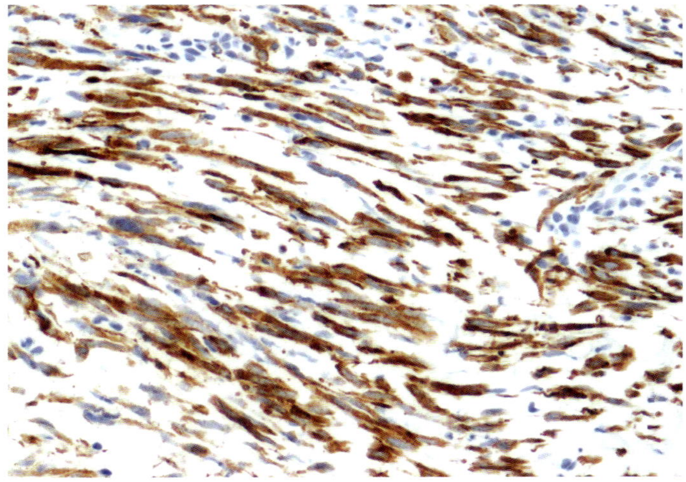

Fig. 11.17 Inflammatory myofibroblastic tumour. Spindle tumour cells show diffuse cytoplasmic positivity with ALK immunohistochemistry.

Desirable: demonstration of ALK or ROS1 expression by immunohistochemistry; rearrangement of *ALK* or other implicated receptor tyrosine kinase genes (in select cases).

Staging

Not clinically relevant

Prognosis and prediction

The natural history of IMT is variable. Overall, approximately 25% of IMTs recur, related to anatomical site and resectability {1289, 1835,3767,638}. Most patients with IMT remain recurrence-free after surgery with or without steroids {2559}. Targeted therapies (i.e. ALK inhibitors) may improve the outcome {2235,3323,1995}.

Dermatofibrosarcoma protuberans

Mittal R
Rodriguez FJ
Verdijk RM

Definition
Dermatofibrosarcoma protuberans (DFSP) is a locally aggressive fibroblastic neoplasm with a cellular storiform appearance and carries a *COL1A1::PDGFB* or related fusion.

ICD-O coding
8832/1 Dermatofibrosarcoma protuberans
8833/1 Pigmented dermatofibrosarcoma protuberans
8832/3 Fibrosarcomatous dermatofibrosarcoma protuberans
8832/1 Myxoid dermatofibrosarcoma protuberans
8832/1 Dermatofibrosarcoma protuberans with myoid differentiation
8832/1 Plaque-like dermatofibrosarcoma protuberans

ICD-11 coding
2B53.Y & XH4QZ8 Other specified fibroblastic or myofibroblastic tumour, primary site & Dermatofibrosarcoma, NOS
2B53.Y & XH5CT4 Other specified fibroblastic or myofibroblastic tumour, primary site & Pigmented dermatofibrosarcoma protuberans
2B53.Y & XH9V92 Other specified fibroblastic or myofibroblastic tumour, primary site & Dermatofibrosarcoma protuberans, fibrosarcomatous

Related terminology
Not recommended: Bednar tumour.

Subtype(s)
Pigmented DFSP; fibrosarcomatous DFSP; myxoid DFSP; DFSP with myoid differentiation; plaque-like DFSP

Localization
Periocular DFSP most commonly arises in the superficial periocular skin and secondarily involves deeper orbital soft tissues and the nasolacrimal system {1713,1150,405,901,434}. Primary orbital DFSP is extremely rare {907,2636,2876}. Advanced tumours can involve bone, paranasal sinuses, and the cranial cavity {273,2953}.

Clinical features
Signs and symptoms include a nodular or multinodular painless mass, often with a history of indolent but persistent growth, sometimes with rapid enlargement, proptosis, ptosis, epiphora, and decreased visual acuity {907}.

Epidemiology
DFSP is very rare in the orbit/adnexa with < 20 reported cases with a wide age range (26–72 years) {907}.

Etiology
Most of these tumours occur sporadically.

Pathogenesis
DFSP is commonly characterized by a reciprocal linear translocation or supernumerary rings involving chromosomes 17 and 22, leading to fusion transcripts that place the *PDGFB* gene under the control of the *COL1A1* promoter {3125,2843,3099}.

Macroscopic appearance
DFSP lesions may appear as plaque-like or nodular/multinodular masses with a firm grey-white cut surface.

Histopathology
Classic DFSP is characterized by a storiform, cartwheel, whorled, or fascicular arrangement of monomorphic, cytologically uniform slender spindle cells containing plump or elongated wavy nuclei. Mitotic activity is low. Inflammatory cells may be scant to absent. Rare cases may show prominent vessels, granular cell change, prominent nuclear palisading, and Verocay body formation {3289,3566}. Rarely DFSP can show myoid components, prominent myxoid change {1041,2690}, giant cells, pigmented cells {846}, and fibrosarcomatous areas {2177, 1142,5}. Exceptionally, transformation to pleomorphic sarcomatous areas has been reported {2177,3250}.

Immunohistochemistry
Tumour cells stain positively for CD34 and may express EMA {3732,3587}. Fibrosarcomatous areas in a DFSP can show loss of CD34 expression {2177}. Tumour cells in myoid nodules and bundles stain strongly for SMA {462}.

Differential diagnosis
This includes dermatofibroma, which is more polymorphous and lacks the infiltrative pattern and diffuse CD34 positivity of DFSP. Spindle cell melanoma, spindle cell carcinoma, and leiomyosarcoma may be excluded by appropriate immunohistochemical stains (see also *Invasive cutaneous melanoma*, p. 147, *Leiomyosarcoma*, p. 416, and *Squamous cell carcinoma of the eyelid*, p. 102).

Cytology
Not clinically relevant

Diagnostic molecular pathology
Detection of the *COL1A1::PDGFB* fusion can help in diagnosis of challenging cases; however, cases with cryptic fusions {1603,1437} and alternative fusions involving *PDGFD* are also reported {702,798}.

Essential and desirable diagnostic criteria
Essential: a storiform architecture and uniform spindle-cell morphology; diffusely infiltrative growth; expression of CD34.
Desirable: *COL1A1::PDGFB* gene fusion or rarely alternative *PDGFD* rearrangements (in select cases).

Staging

The American Joint Committee on Cancer (AJCC) or Union for International Cancer Control (UICC) TNM system can be applied for fibrosarcomatous DFSP.

Prognosis and prediction

DFSP is characterized by locally aggressive growth and frequent, often repeated local recurrences unless widely excised {1150,907,405}. Distant metastases from periocular DFSP have not been documented {907}. DFSP arising in non-ocular sites can rarely metastasize to the lungs. Tyrosine kinase inhibitors have been used as adjuvant and palliative agents in locally advanced periocular DFSP {3694,2953}.

Chapter 11

Angiomyxoma

Kashyap S
Howitt BE
Milman T

Definition
Angiomyxoma is a benign mesenchymal tumour comprising spindle or stellate cells and thin-walled arborizing vessels in a myxoid stroma.

ICD-O coding
8841/0 Angiomyxoma
8841/0 Cutaneous myxoma (superficial angiomyxoma)
8841/0 Aggressive angiomyxoma

ICD-11 coding
2F7C & XH9HK9 Neoplasms of uncertain behaviour of connective or other soft tissue & Angiomyxoma
2E84.0 & XH58A9 Benign fibrogenic or myofibrogenic tumour of skin & Superficial angiomyxoma
2F7C & XH4V74 Neoplasms of uncertain behaviour of connective or other soft tissue & Deep angiomyxoma

Related terminology
Acceptable: for superficial angiomyxoma: cutaneous myxoma; for deep angiomyxoma: aggressive angiomyxoma.

Subtype(s)
Superficial angiomyxoma; deep (aggressive) angiomyxoma

Localization
Superficial angiomyxomas occur in the conjunctiva {2600} and eyelids {3726,3724}; deep angiomyxomas occur in the soft tissues of the orbit {232,1332}.

Clinical features
Eyelid angiomyxomas present as multinodular, polypoid, or pedunculated slow-growing dermal/subcutaneous masses involving the eyelid margin {3724,84,3726}. In the conjunctiva, they appear as well-circumscribed, fleshy masses {2600}. Orbital angiomyxomas present with proptosis and visual disturbances {232,1332}.

Epidemiology
Angiomyxomas arise in patients across a wide age range, but predominantly in the third to fifth decades of life {3726,2600,84, 232,1332}, with no sex predilection.

Etiology
The etiology is unknown. Multiple superficial angiomyxomas may be seen in Carney complex, an autosomal dominant syndrome with germline mutation in *PRKAR1A* encoding a PKA subunit {3491}.

Pathogenesis
Angiomyxomas of the eye region have not been reported to be associated with Carney complex, although it is suspected that *PRKAR1A* inactivation may play a role in the pathogenesis of sporadic tumours given the lack of protein expression on immunohistochemistry in 80% of cases {668,1225}.

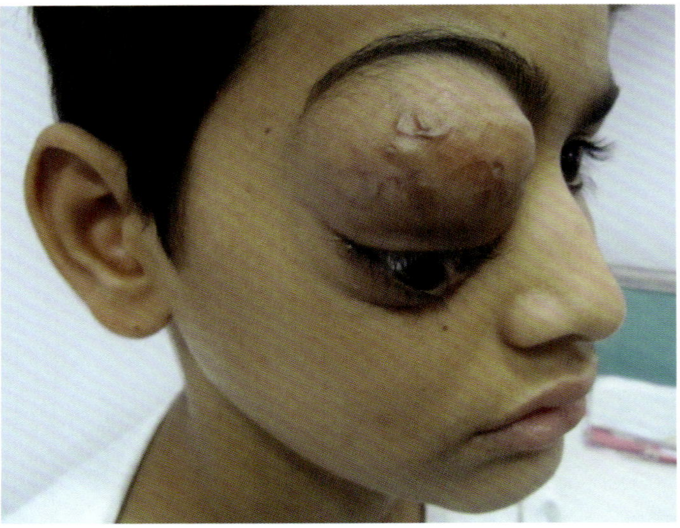

Fig. 11.18 Angiomyxoma. Inferior displacement of the globe in a young boy.

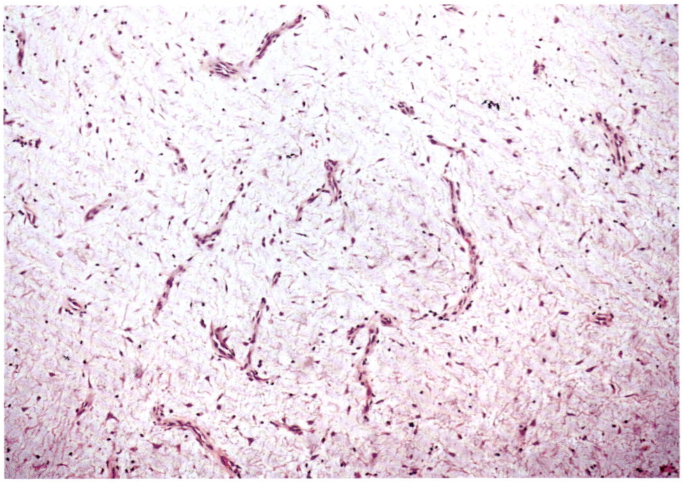

Fig. 11.19 Superficial angiomyxoma. The tumour is composed of spindle-shaped to stellate cells in a myxoid background with thin-walled capillaries.

Macroscopic appearance
Angiomyxomas form poorly circumscribed, lobulated masses with a gelatinous surface {3726,232}.

Histopathology
Superficial angiomyxomas are poorly circumscribed, forming lobules separated by collagenous septa, composed of spindle-shaped to stellate cells with bland ovoid nuclei in an abundant

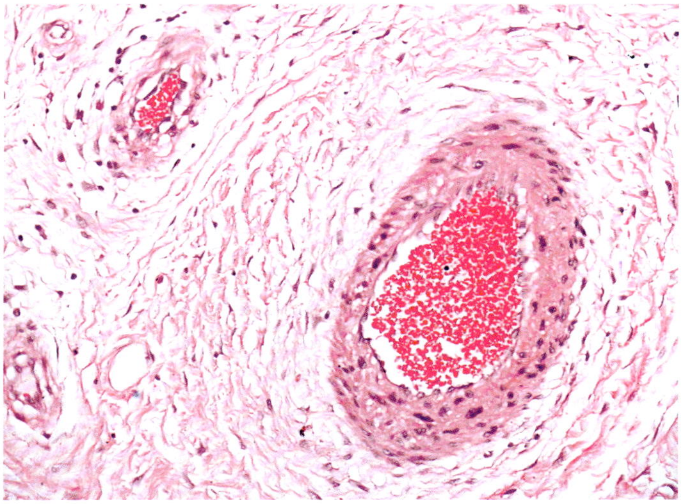

Fig. 11.20 Deep angiomyxoma. An example of a deep angiomyxoma showing thick-walled blood vessels.

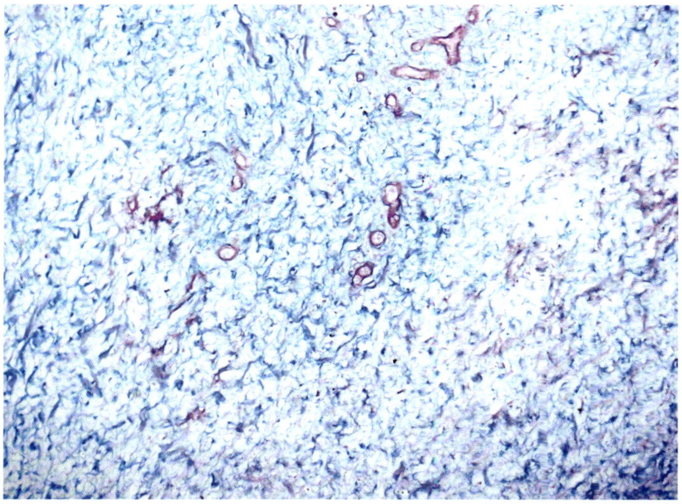

Fig. 11.21 Angiomyxoma. Alcian blue / PAS staining of the lesion demonstrates abundant myxoid material.

myxoid and variably collagenous stroma {3726,232,2600}. Thin-walled non-arborizing vessels are prominent {2217,3726, 1332}. Stromal neutrophils may be seen {3724,84}.

Deep angiomyxomas have increased cellularity and thick-walled vessels showing medial hypertrophy and perivascular hyalinization {232}.

Immunohistochemistry

Tumour cells express vimentin and CD34, and are negative for S100, desmin, SMA, and cytokeratins {3726}. There is loss of PRKAR1A expression, particularly in Carney complex–associated lesions {2217}.

Differential diagnosis

The differential diagnosis includes nerve sheath myxoma (S100 positive) {1198}.

Cytology

Not relevant

Diagnostic molecular pathology

Not clinically relevant

Essential and desirable diagnostic criteria

Essential: hypocellular, myxoid, lobulated tumour; bland stellate to spindle-shaped cells; non-arborizing capillary-like vasculature.

Staging

None

Prognosis and prediction

Complete excision with wide margins is recommended {2600, 232}. There is frequent recurrence (30–40%) due to infiltrative growth and the inability to excise completely, requiring prolonged follow-up {113,84,1332,232}.

Benign lipomatous tumours

Mendoza P
Fritchie KJ
Mishra DK

Definition
Benign lipomatous tumours are a family of benign tumours composed of mature adipocytes comprising lipoma, angiolipoma, and spindle cell / pleomorphic lipoma (SCL/PL).

ICD-O coding
8850/0 Lipoma, NOS
8861/0 Angiolipoma, NOS

ICD-11 coding
2E80.Z Benign lipomatous neoplasm, unspecified
2E80.0Y Lipoma, other specified site
2E80.0Y & XH3C77 Lipoma, other specified site & Angiolipoma, NOS
2E80.0Y & XH30M7 Lipoma, other specified site & Pleomorphic lipoma
2E80.0Y & XH4E98 Lipoma, other specified site & Spindle cell lipoma

Related terminology
None

Subtype(s)
None

Localization
Lipomas have been described in the eyelid, orbital fat, and extraocular muscles {3197,2423,2436,2933,1692,1378}. SCL/PLs have been reported in the orbital fat and conjunctiva {3375, 3348,2226,1929}. Angiolipomas have been described in the subcutis and anterior orbit {488,91,947}.

Clinical features
Lipomas are slow growing and often asymptomatic. Progressive enlargement may cause proptosis, globe displacement, or diplopia. They are unilateral in > 60% of cases {720} in contrast to prolapsed orbital fat, which is frequently bilateral.

Imaging
CT demonstrates a well-circumscribed, non-enhancing mass with homogeneous low attenuation displacing but not infiltrating adjacent structures. On MRI, T1-weighted images show a mass isointense to fat and hypointense to muscle, whereas T2-weighted images show lipomas to be hyperintense to muscle.

Epidemiology
The true incidence of these tumours is unknown, because of incomplete immunohistochemical and molecular characterization of nearly all previously reported cases. Most previously reported orbital lipomas and SCL/PLs may in fact have been misdiagnosed herniated orbital fat (especially when bilateral) and atypical lipomatous tumour / well-differentiated liposarcoma {720,603,1473,2144,3375}. Some reported cases of conjunctival SCL/PL may in fact have been misdiagnosed conjunctival stromal tumour {2226,1929}.

Etiology
Unknown

Pathogenesis
Cytogenetic abnormalities are found in as many as 75% of lipomas, most often affecting the 12q13-q15 region. Chromosomal rearrangements of 12q target the *HMGA2* gene. The pathogenesis of lipomas is related to expression of the HMGA2 protein, which plays a role in the development of the mesodermal lineage during embryogenesis {1944}.

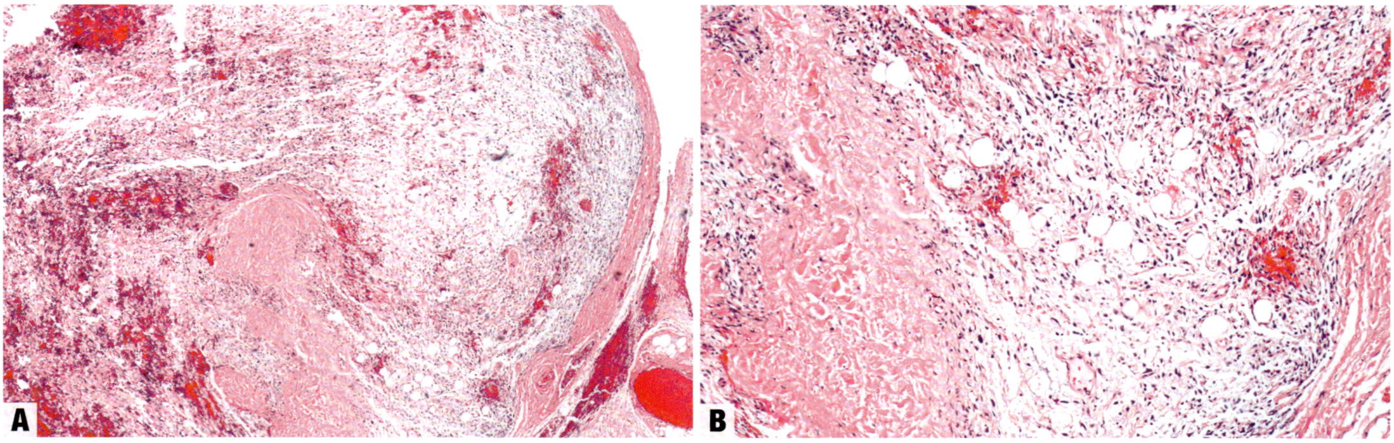

Fig. 11.22 Spindle cell / pleomorphic lipoma of the orbit. **A** Mature adipocytes within a spindle cell tumour are seen. **B** The tumour is composed of a triad of mature adipocytes, bland spindle cells, and rope-like collagen fibrils.

Macroscopic appearance

Lipomas are soft, well-circumscribed, encapsulated, lobulated, yellow-tan lesions, while angiolipomas are usually encapsulated and yellow to reddish. The cut surface of SCL/PL may be yellow or grey-white, or myxoid. Extensively myxoid tumours can be gelatinous.

Histopathology

Lipoma: Lipomas are composed of lobules of mature adipocytes often separated by thin bands of fibrous tissue. The adipocytes are uniform but may demonstrate slight variation in size and shape compared with normal fat.

Angiolipoma: Angiolipomas contain mature adipose tissue with a proliferation of small-calibre vessels most prominent at the periphery and may have variable amounts of intravascular thrombi.

SCL/PL: SCL is composed of variable amounts of mature adipocytes, bland spindle cells, and ropy collagen. PL has similar features to SCL but also contains pleomorphic and multinucleated floret-like giant cells. Adipocytes with intranuclear vacuoles (Lochkern cells) and lipoblasts may occasionally be observed.

Immunohistochemistry

Lesional adipocytes are HMGA2-positive, which helps the distinction from normal adipose tissue {823}.

Neoplastic SCL/PL spindle cells express CD34 with loss of nuclear RB1 expression {557,1944,2880}.

Differential diagnosis

The differential diagnosis mainly includes herniated orbital fat and atypical lipomatous tumour / well-differentiated liposarcoma.

Cytology

Lipomas show adipocytes with a single lipid droplet and flattened nucleus on aspiration. SCL/PLs also show uniform spindle cells and eosinophilic collagen fibres, while PL may also contain multinucleated giant cells.

Diagnostic molecular pathology

Lipoma: The presence of cytogenetic abnormalities in chromosome 12 {2436} distinguishes these lesions from prolapsed orbital fat, which has no copy-number alterations {3184}, and the absence of *MDM2* amplification may be tested when lesions are deep and recurrent, or have equivocal atypia or concerning clinical or radiological features {629}.

SCL/PL: Deletion of 13q14 with loss of the *RB1* gene and the absence of *MDM2* amplification can be helpful in select cases (see above).

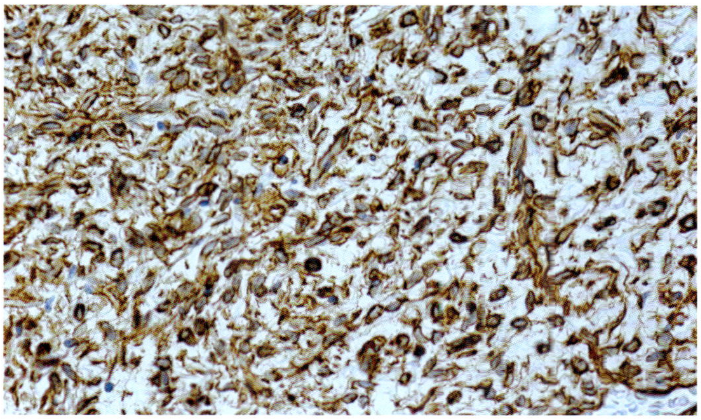

Fig. 11.23 Spindle cell / pleomorphic lipoma of the orbit. This tumour stains strongly for CD34.

Essential and desirable diagnostic criteria

Essential: for lipoma: circumscribed mass; relatively uniform proliferation of mature adipocytes; absence of hyperchromatic stromal cells within thickened fibrous septa; for angiolipoma: mature fat with clusters of capillaries that have variable amounts of intravascular thrombi; for SCL/PL: mature adipose tissue, spindle cells, and ropy collagen; PLs also contain floret-like multinucleated cells.

Desirable: for lipoma and SCL/PL: absence of *MDM2* amplification in challenging cases.

Staging

Not applicable

Prognosis and prediction

While the definitive treatment for benign lipomatous tumours is surgical excision, observation may be a reasonable alternative for these indolent lesions. The prognosis is excellent. Recurrence is rare even after subtotal resection {3348,2933,3375}.

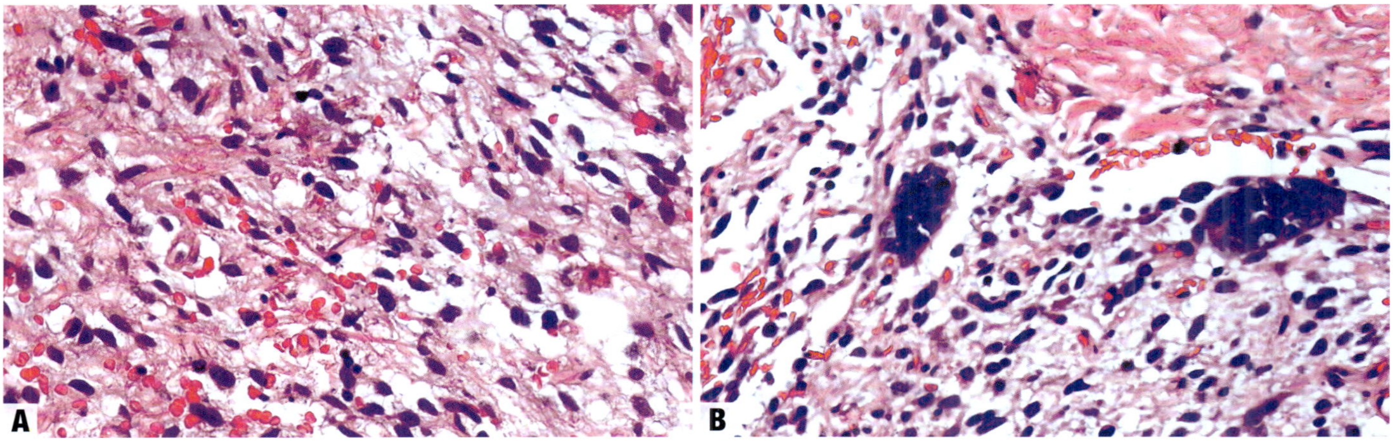

Fig. 11.24 Spindle cell / pleomorphic lipoma of the orbit. **A** The lesion contains a proliferation of spindle-shaped cells with bland nuclei. **B** The lesion may contain multinucleated cells.

Malignant adipocytic tumours

Roberts F
Billings SD
Grossniklaus HE
Mendoza P
Ng T

Definition

Liposarcomas are a family of malignant tumours with adipocytic differentiation, including atypical lipomatous tumour / well-differentiated liposarcoma (ALT/WDLPS), dedifferentiated liposarcoma (DDLPS), myxoid liposarcoma (MLPS), and pleomorphic liposarcoma.

ICD-O coding

8850/1 Atypical lipomatous tumour
8851/3 Liposarcoma, well-differentiated
8858/3 Dedifferentiated liposarcoma
8852/3 Myxoid liposarcoma
8854/3 Pleomorphic liposarcoma

ICD-11 coding

2B5H Well-differentiated lipomatous tumour, primary site
2B59.Y Liposarcoma, other specified primary site

Related terminology

Not recommended: atypical lipoma; round cell liposarcoma.

Subtype(s)

None

Localization

Malignant adipocytic tumours usually involve the intraconal or superior extraconal orbital fat.

Clinical features

Symptoms and signs are related to mass effect and include eye displacement, diplopia, and optic nerve compression {1593}. Imaging usually demonstrates a heterogeneous soft tissue mass. Rarely, liposarcoma may present with muscle thickening and calcification {3078}.

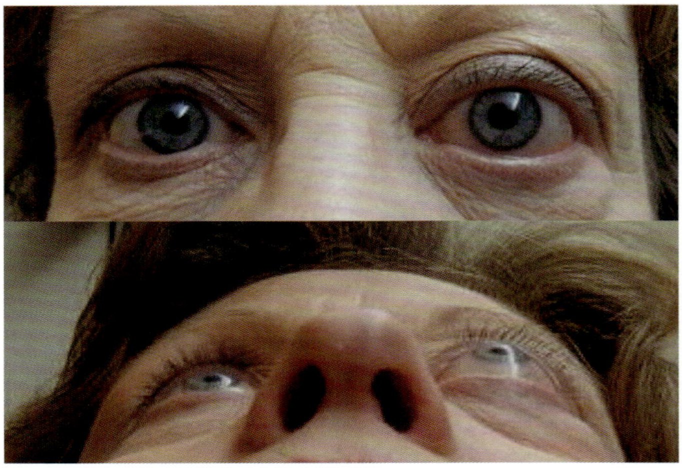

Fig. 11.25 Atypical lipomatous/well-differentiated liposarcoma of the orbit. Clinical appearance shows left proptosis.

Epidemiology

Primary orbital liposarcoma is rare, accounting for < 1% of orbital tumours, usually presenting in the fifth to sixth decades of life (range: 11–69 years) without sex predilection {1593,3553}. The majority (~43%) are ALT/WDLPS {1593} and pleomorphic liposarcoma (~9%) and DDLPS (~8%) are less frequent {3553, 3672,149}. The incidence of myxoid liposarcoma is difficult to estimate as many reported cases may correspond to myxoid change in ALT/WDLPS {2514}.

Etiology

The etiology of these tumours is unknown.

ALT/WDLPS may be associated with Li–Fraumeni syndrome, but nearly all cases are sporadic, and the etiology is unknown.

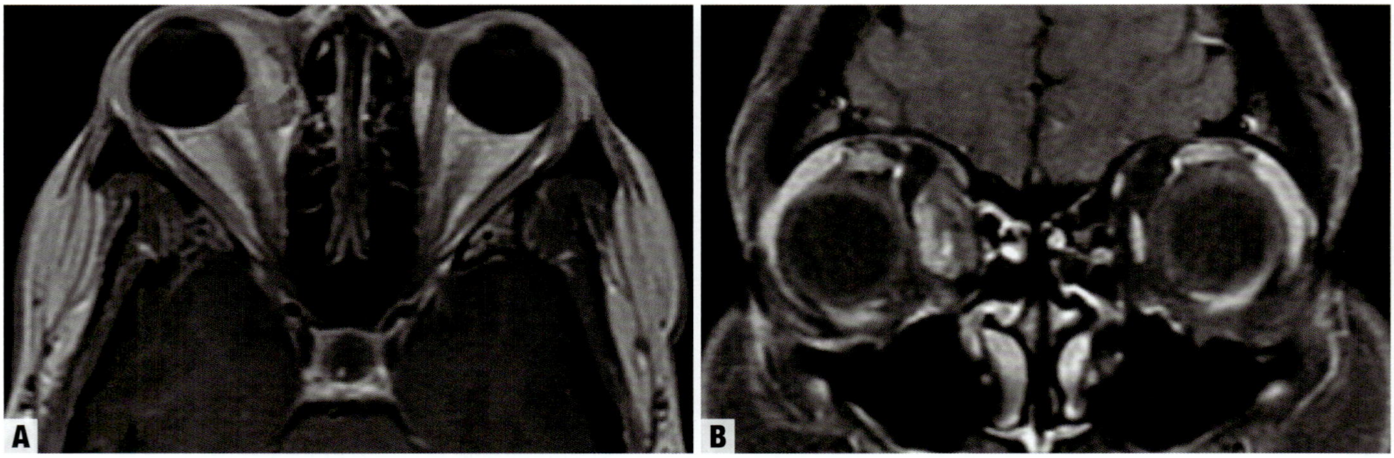

Fig. 11.26 Atypical lipomatous tumour / well-differentiated liposarcoma of the orbit. **A,B** MRI shows right anterior medial orbital mass.

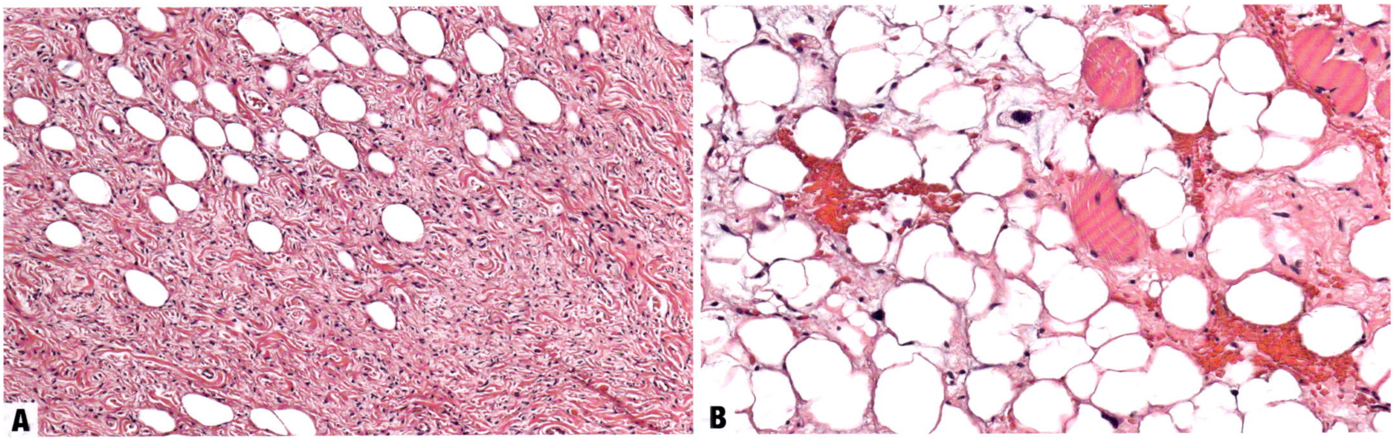

Fig. 11.27 Atypical lipomatous tumour / well- differentiated liposarcoma involving orbit. **A,B** This lesion was initially interpreted as spindle cell lipoma, recurred a decade later, and showed *MDM2* and *CDK4* amplification by FISH in both the original and recurrent tumours.

Pathogenesis

ALT/WDLPSs and DDLPSs are characterized by a supernumerary ring containing a neocentromere and giant marker chromosomes {2514,3334} containing amplified genes from the 12q14-15 region, including *CDK4*, *HMGA2*, *YEATS4*, *TSPAN31*, *FRS2*, and *MDM2* {2514,3334}. However, *MDM2* (12q15) is the main driver gene. Overexpression of MDM2 from genomic amplification inactivates p53 by targeting degradation and inhibiting p53-mediated transcription.

Most MLPSs have a t(12;16)(q13;p11) rearrangement, generating a *FUS*::*DDIT3* fusion transcript; a t(12;22)(q13;q12) rearrangement generating an *EWSR1*::*DDIT3* fusion transcript is present in 2–5% of cases {3334}. DDIT3 is a DNA binding transcription factor which blocks adipocytic terminal differentiation. *FUS* and *EWSR1* provide promoter sequences. Other genomic events include *TERT* promoter mutations (~50%) and P13K/mTOR pathway activating mutations (~20%) {1808,3371}.

The molecular profile of pleomorphic liposarcoma resembles that of pleomorphic undifferentiated sarcoma rather than ALT/WDLPS or myxoid liposarcoma {3545}.

Macroscopic appearance

ALT/WDLPS may closely resemble normal fat or may appear whiter with a fibrous cut surface. Dedifferentiated areas can appear tan or grey and may have areas of necrosis.

MLPS can have a gelatinous or myxoid appearance.

Pleomorphic liposarcoma usually appears white to yellow, sometimes with myxoid areas and necrosis.

Histopathology

ALT/WDLPS can be divided into three main morphological patterns – adipocytic or lipoma-like, sclerosing, and inflammatory – although more than one pattern can coexist. There is variation in cell size and nuclear atypia in adipocytes and stromal cells. In sclerosing tumours there is a collagenous stroma containing scattered bizarre stromal cells. In the inflammatory pattern, chronic inflammatory cells can obscure the adipocytic nature of the tumour, but atypical stromal cells are an important diagnostic feature. Lipoblasts are sparse or absent in all patterns {1593}.

DDLPS has a transition from ALT/WDLPS to a dedifferentiated sarcoma, which is usually high-grade, resembling pleomorphic sarcoma or myxofibrosarcoma {1695}.

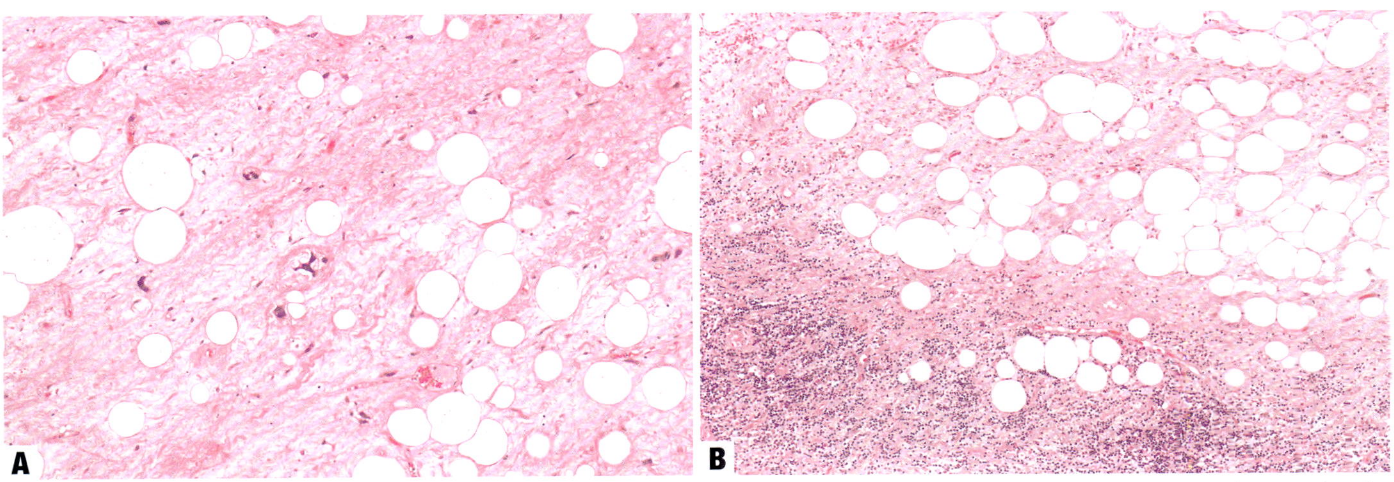

Fig. 11.28 Atypical lipomatous tumour / well-differentiated liposarcoma. **A** The image shows the sclerosing pattern featuring a fibrous background with adipocytes of varying sizes. Within the fibrous tissue there are scattered cells with atypical nuclei. **B** The image shows the inflammatory pattern featuring a fibrous background with adipocytes of varying sizes. Inflammatory infiltrate partially obscures atypical cells within the fibrous tissue.

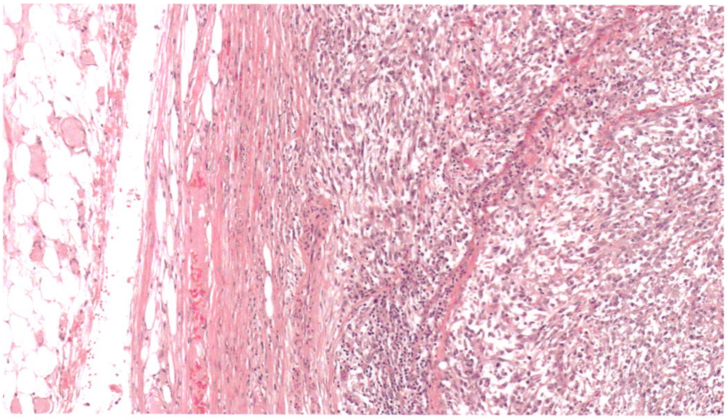

Fig. 11.29 Dedifferentiated liposarcoma. A high-grade spindle cell sarcoma has arisen within an atypical lipomatous tumour / well-differentiated liposarcoma.

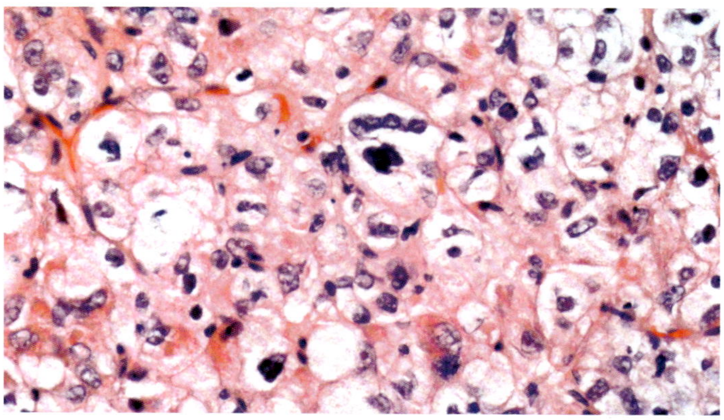

Fig. 11.30 Pleomorphic liposarcoma. There is a background of pleomorphic sarcoma with scattered pleomorphic lipoblasts.

Low-grade MLPS has abundant myxoid stroma with a characteristic chicken-wire vascular pattern and very few lipoblasts. High-grade lesions have transition to round cell morphology with high-grade nuclei and increased mitoses. The characteristic vascular network is often obscured.

Pleomorphic liposarcoma has varying proportions of pleomorphic lipoblasts on a background of pleomorphic undifferentiated sarcoma.

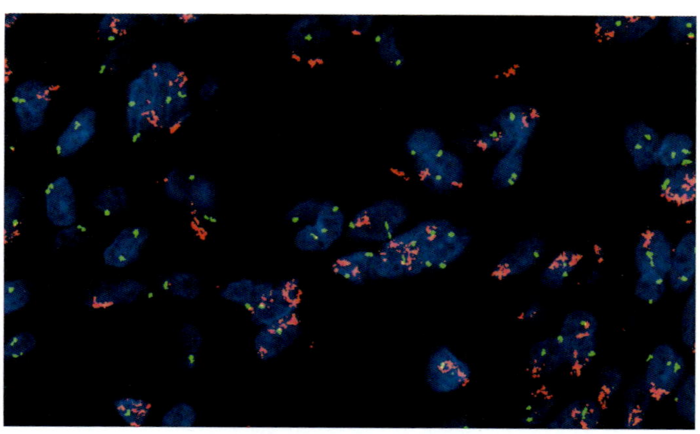

Fig. 11.31 Atypical lipomatous tumour / well-differentiated liposarcoma. FISH for *MDM2* amplification status shows two green CEP12 signals located on the centromere of chromosome 12 and the red *MDM2* signals located on the long arm of the same chromosome. There is amplification of *MDM2* relative to CEP12.

Immunohistochemistry

MDM2 and/or CDK4 positivity is seen in most cases of ALT/WDLPS and DDLPS {3598}.

Differential diagnosis

ALT/WDLPS need to be distinguished from herniated orbital fat and spindle cell / pleomorphic lipoma (see *Benign lipomatous tumours*, p. 404).

Cytology

Not clinically relevant

Diagnostic molecular pathology

Diagnostic molecular pathology includes:

- for ALT/WDLPS and DDLPS: detection of amplification of *MDM2* (and/or *CDK4*)
- for MLPS: demonstration of *FUS::DDIT3* or *EWSR1::DDIT3*
- for pleomorphic liposarcoma: absence of *MDM2* amplification.

Essential and desirable diagnostic criteria

Atypical lipomatous tumour / well-differentiated liposarcoma

Essential: variation in adipocytic size with nuclear atypia in stromal cells or adipocytes.

Desirable: MDM2 and/or CDK4 nuclear expression or detection of *MDM2* and/or *CDK4* amplification.

Dedifferentiated liposarcoma

Essential: abrupt transition from WDLPS to pleomorphic tumour.

Desirable: MDM2 and/or CDK4 nuclear expression or detection of *MDM2* and/or *CDK4* amplification.

Myxoid liposarcoma

Essential: myxoid stroma with a chicken-wire vascular pattern and variable numbers of lipoblasts.

Desirable: demonstration of *FUS::DDIT3* or *EWSR1::DDIT3* fusion transcripts.

Pleomorphic liposarcoma

Essential: pleomorphic sarcoma with variable numbers of pleomorphic lipoblasts.

Staging

The American Joint Committee on Cancer (AJCC) and the Union for International Cancer Control (UICC) TNM system for soft tissue sarcoma of the head and neck and orbit is applied.

Prognosis and prediction

Given the small numbers of cases in the literature, it is difficult to accurately predict the outcome of orbital liposarcomas.

ALT/WDLPS tends to remain localized and does not metastasize except when it undergoes dedifferentiation (~10%) and the overall prognosis is good. DDLPS is a more aggressive tumour, but it has been suggested that the orbital location may offer a better outcome in terms of local control and survival mainly owing to early presentation. The outcomes of orbital MLPS and pleomorphic liposarcoma are difficult to determine owing to the small number of well-characterized cases with sufficient follow-up {1593,382,1705}.

Rhabdomyosarcomas

Bahrami A
Agaram NP
Dry SM
Honavar SG
Stagner AM

Definition

Rhabdomyosarcoma is a group of malignant mesenchymal tumours with skeletal muscle differentiation, which consists of four types: embryonal rhabdomyosarcoma (ERMS), alveolar rhabdomyosarcoma (ARMS), spindle cell / sclerosing rhabdomyosarcoma, and pleomorphic rhabdomyosarcoma. Ectomesenchymoma consists of rhabdomyosarcoma intermixed with ganglionic/neuroblastic components.

ICD-O coding

8910/3 Embryonal rhabdomyosarcoma
8920/3 Alveolar rhabdomyosarcoma
8912/3 Spindle cell rhabdomyosarcoma
8901/3 Pleomorphic rhabdomyosarcoma
8921/3 Ectomesenchymoma

ICD-11 coding

2B55.Y & XH83G1 Rhabdomyosarcoma, other specified primary site & Embryonal rhabdomyosarcoma, NOS
2B55.Y & XH7099 Rhabdomyosarcoma, other specified primary site & Alveolar rhabdomyosarcoma
2B55.Y & XH7NM2 Rhabdomyosarcoma, other specified primary site & Spindle cell rhabdomyosarcoma
2B55.Y & XH5SX9 Rhabdomyosarcoma, other specified primary site & Pleomorphic rhabdomyosarcoma, NOS
2B55.Y & XH0S12 Rhabdomyosarcoma, other specified primary site & Ectomesenchymoma

Related terminology

Not recommended: sarcoma botryoides.

Subtype(s)

None

Localization

Ocular rhabdomyosarcoma can develop within the orbit, conjunctiva, eyelid, or uveal tract (iris, ciliary body). The most common location is the orbit, with a predilection for the superior nasal quadrant {3052,1605}.

Clinical features

Proptosis of rapid onset, eyelid swelling, and blepharoptosis are the main presenting features of orbital rhabdomyosarcoma {3017}. A rapidly growing conjunctival mass is the characteristic presentation of conjunctival rhabdomyosarcoma {3052}.

Epidemiology

Orbital rhabdomyosarcoma makes up approximately 10% of all rhabdomyosarcoma cases {3017}. ERMS and ARMS are the predominant types, and ERMS accounts for the vast majority. Patients with ERMS are typically children < 10 years in age, whereas those with ARMS are most often adolescents and young adults {1754,3052,1605}. Pleomorphic and spindle cell / sclerosing rhabdomyosarcoma of primary eye/periocular origin are exceedingly rare {2259} (see the fifth-edition *Soft tissue and bone tumours* volume {3598}). Primary ocular/periocular ectomesenchymoma is also uncommon, with only a few case reports in the literature; most patients are infants or children {1000,2668}.

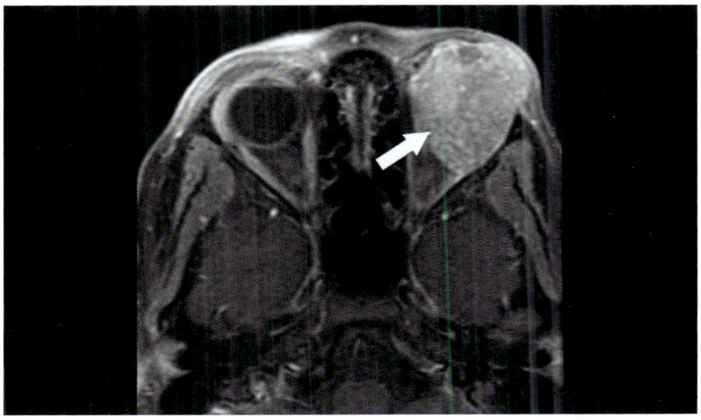

Fig. 11.32 Rhabdomyosarcoma. Axial T1-weighted postcontrast MRI shows a heterogeneously enhancing mass in the superior left orbit (arrow).

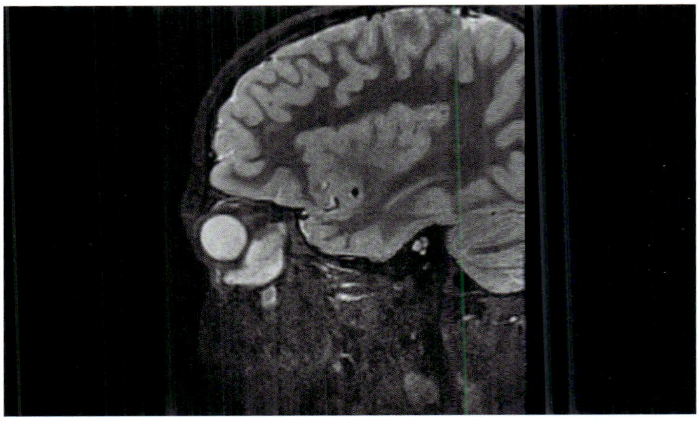

Fig. 11.33 Embryonal rhabdomyosarcoma. Sagittal MRI demonstrates a homogeneously enhancing extraconal mass in the inferior orbit.

Etiology

Most cases of rhabdomyosarcoma are sporadic, but certain genetic conditions can increase the risk, particularly for ERMS, such as Li–Fraumeni syndrome (germline *TP53* mutation) or RASopathies (e.g. neurofibromatosis–Noonan syndrome) {601,1224,1550}.

Pathogenesis

ERMS commonly harbours whole-chromosome gains (of 2, 8, 11, 12, 13, and/or 20) and losses (of 10 and 15), and loss of

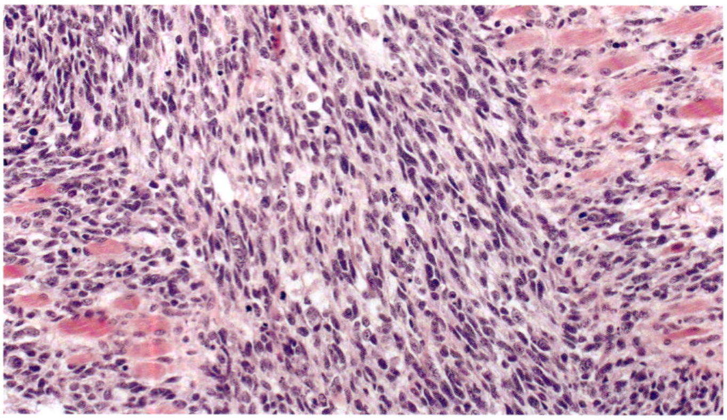

Fig. 11.34 Eyelid embryonal rhabdomyosarcoma. A cellular malignant neoplasm composed of mitotically active undifferentiated spindle cells which infiltrate skeletal muscle.

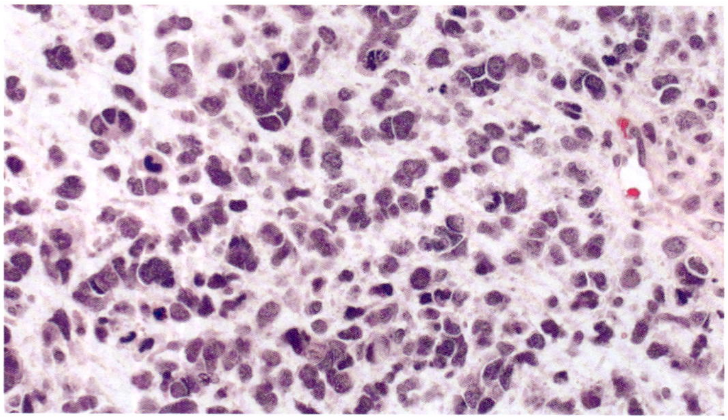

Fig. 11.35 Anaplastic embryonal rhabdomyosarcoma. Embryonal rhabdomyosarcoma with anaplastic features characterized by pronounced nuclear pleomorphism and large atypical mitotic figures.

heterozygosity at 11p15.5. Mutations in the RAS pathway (*NRAS*, *KRAS*, *HRAS*, *NF1*, *FGFR4*), the PI3K pathway (*PTEN*, *PIK3CA*), or the cell-cycle regulatory genes (*FBXW7*, *CTNNB1*) are frequent in ERMS {2962,2963,3145,37}.

In ARMS, t(2;13) or t(1;13) rearrangement produces *PAX3::FOXO1* or *PAX7::FOXO1* fusion genes, encoding transcription factors that activate the *PAX3* and/or *PAX7* target genes {263,728,1060,3145}.

Ectomesenchymoma shares molecular similarities with ERMS and frequently carries *HRAS* mutations {1390}.

Macroscopic appearance

Most lesions present as poorly circumscribed, soft, fleshy, gelatinous masses with a pale-tan cut surface. Botryoid ERMS has a grape-like polypoid appearance.

Histopathology

ERMS consists of atypical primitive round and spindle-shaped tumour cells set in a variably myxoid background. Large differentiated rhabdomyoblasts with bright eosinophilic cytoplasm can be observed. Mitotic figures are often numerous, and necrosis can be seen. Botryoid ERMS grows as a submucosal polypoid mass with a cambium layer (cellular aggregates beneath the surface). Anaplastic ERMS is recognized by pronounced nuclear pleomorphism and/or enlarged atypical mitoses {2618}.

ARMS is composed of monomorphic small round to ovoid cells with scant cytoplasm organized into an alveolar architectural pattern or arranged in solid sheets and nests.

Ectomesenchymoma has features of ERMS intermixed with ganglioneuroblastomatous elements.

Immunohistochemistry

All types of rhabdomyosarcomas express desmin, myogenin, and MYOD1 {2278}. Myogenin expression tends to be more diffuse in ARMS than in ERMS.

Cytology

Not clinically relevant

Diagnostic molecular pathology

Demonstration of *PAX::FOXO1* fusion is particularly useful for classification of rhabdomyosarcoma with a round cell phenotype.

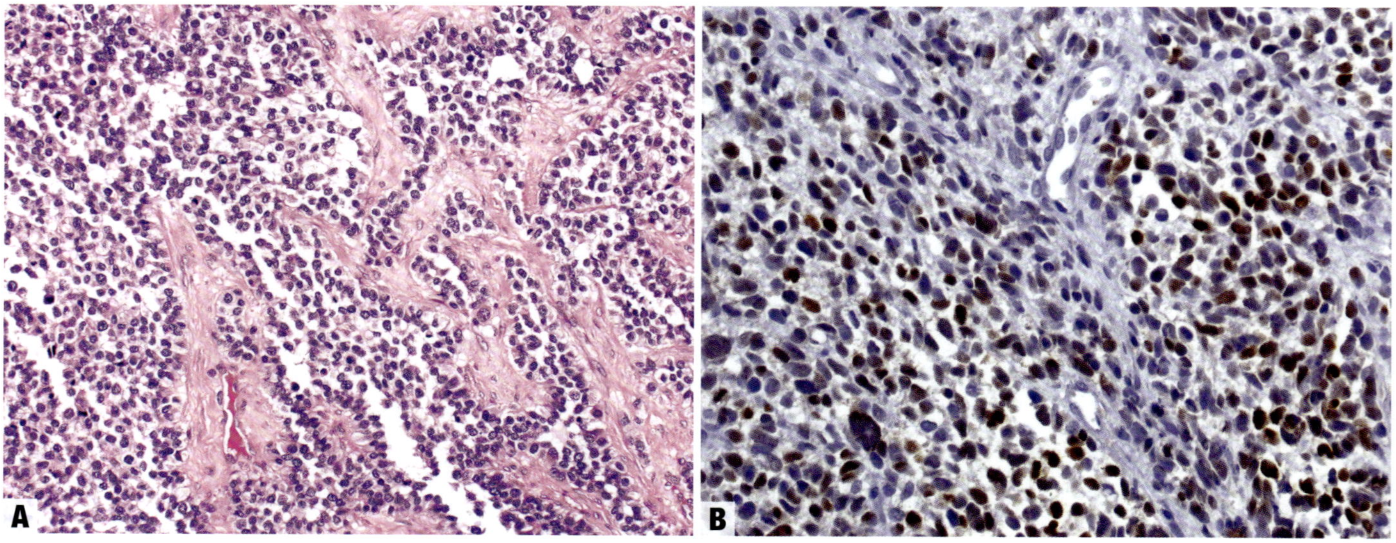

Fig. 11.36 Orbital alveolar rhabdomyosarcoma. **A** A malignant small round cell neoplasm with a prominent alveolar growth pattern characterized by nests of tumour cells with central discohesion. **B** Diffuse nuclear expression of myogenin in neoplastic cells.

Essential and desirable diagnostic criteria

Embryonal rhabdomyosarcoma

Essential: mitotically active, primitive spindle to round cells; alternating cellular and myxoid areas; heterogeneous myogenin expression.

Desirable (in select cases): absence of *PAX3*, *PAX7*, or *FOXO1* rearrangement in tumours morphologically reminiscent of ARMS.

Alveolar rhabdomyosarcoma

Essential: malignant small blue round cell neoplasm; homogeneous myogenin expression; *PAX3*, *PAX7*, or *FOXO1* rearrangement.

Ectomesenchymoma

Essential: composite ERMS with neuroblastic elements; immunolabelling for desmin or myogenin and synaptophysin.

Staging

Staging for paediatric rhabdomyosarcoma is based on the Intergroup Rhabdomyosarcoma Study Group (IRSG) system. The orbit is a favourable site, and tumours confined to the orbit are considered stage I {2045,3145}.

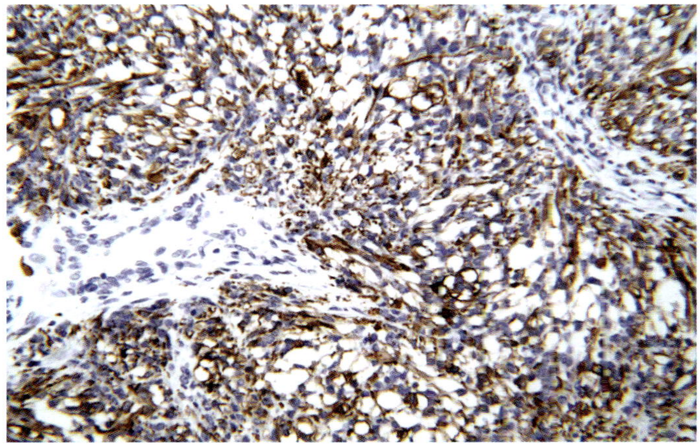

Fig. 11.37 Orbital embryonal rhabdomyosarcoma. Neoplastic cells diffusely express desmin.

Prognosis and prediction

Patients with ocular ERMS have excellent outcomes {1754,855, 3017}. The prognosis is worse for patients with anaplastic ERMS and *FOXO1* fusion–positive ARMS {1753,3145,195 672,2213}.

Leiomyoma

Subramanian K
Billings SD
Watanabe R

Definition
Leiomyoma is a benign tumour of smooth muscle.

ICD-O coding
8890/0 Leiomyoma

ICD-11 coding
2F36.Y & XH4CY6 Other specified benign neoplasm of eye or ocular adnexa & Leiomyoma, NOS

Related terminology
None

Subtype(s)
None

Localization
Leiomyomas have been reported in the orbit, eyelid {1532,1401, 1899}, conjunctiva {32,269,2493,403}, and caruncle {1299}, and intraocularly in the iris, ciliary body, and choroid (see *Mesectodermal leiomyoma*, p. 414). Orbital leiomyomas may be located in any area of the orbit, including the orbital apex with intracranial extension, or inferior orbit with extension into the paranasal sinuses {2358,176,2181,322,1469,1204,1803,3600}.

Clinical features
Orbital leiomyomas may cause proptosis, diplopia, deviation of the globe, and pain {176,2358,1803,1421}. There may be swelling of the eyelids, conjunctiva {32}, and caruncle {1299} with limited ocular motility.

Epidemiology
There are < 25 cases of documented orbital leiomyoma {176, 3644,2181,3438,950,3675,1421,2920}. The mean age is 38 years (range: 3–74 years) and there is a slight male predominance. There are 4 cases of conjunctival leiomyomas {32,269,2493,403}, 1 of caruncular leiomyoma {1299}, and 3 of eyelid leiomyomas {1532, 1401,1899}.

Etiology
Not known

Pathogenesis
Orbital leiomyoma is thought to arise from the smooth muscle cells of orbital vessels or from Müller muscle cells {1468}.

Macroscopic appearance
Orbital leiomyomas are usually firm, well circumscribed but unencapsulated, and lobulated; cut sections typically show a firm, whorled, white surface with solid areas, sometimes with calcification {176,1204}.

Histopathology
Ocular leiomyomas are composed of intersecting fascicles of spindled cells with blunt-ended cigar-shaped nuclei and eosinophilic cytoplasm. There is no atypia or necrosis.

Immunohistochemistry
Spindle cells are positive for SMA, desmin, and h-caldesmon, and negative for S100 {176,1204,950}.

Differential diagnosis
Other benign spindle cell tumours that occur in the orbit should be considered, such as neurofibroma, schwannoma, and solitary fibrous tumour {1204}.

Cytology
No information has been reported on orbital leiomyoma.

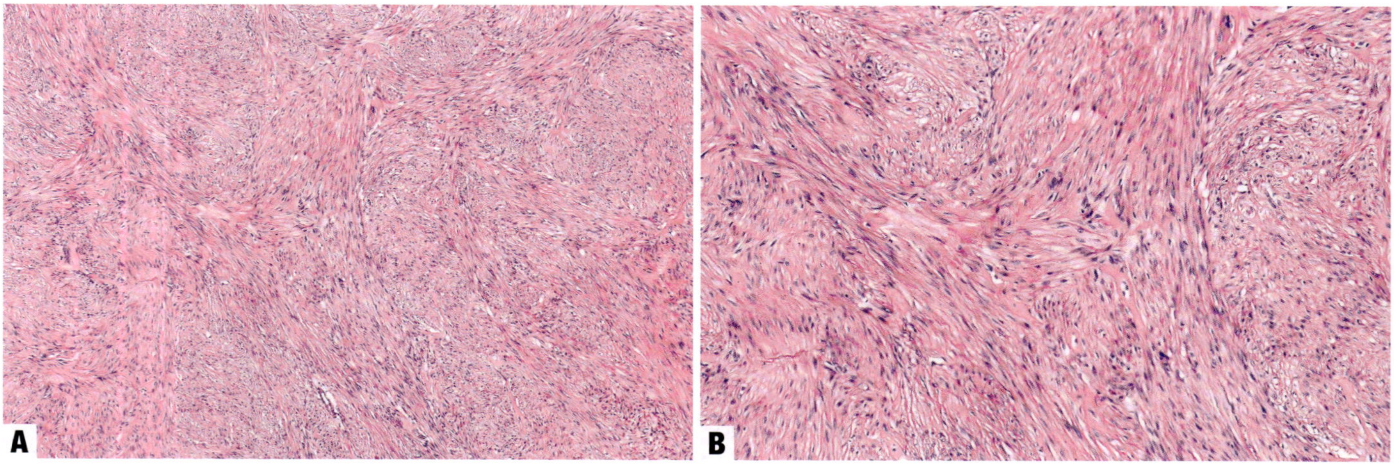

Fig. 11.38 Leiomyoma. **A,B** Intersecting fascicles of spindled cells with blunt-end cigar-shaped nuclei and eosinophilic cytoplasm.

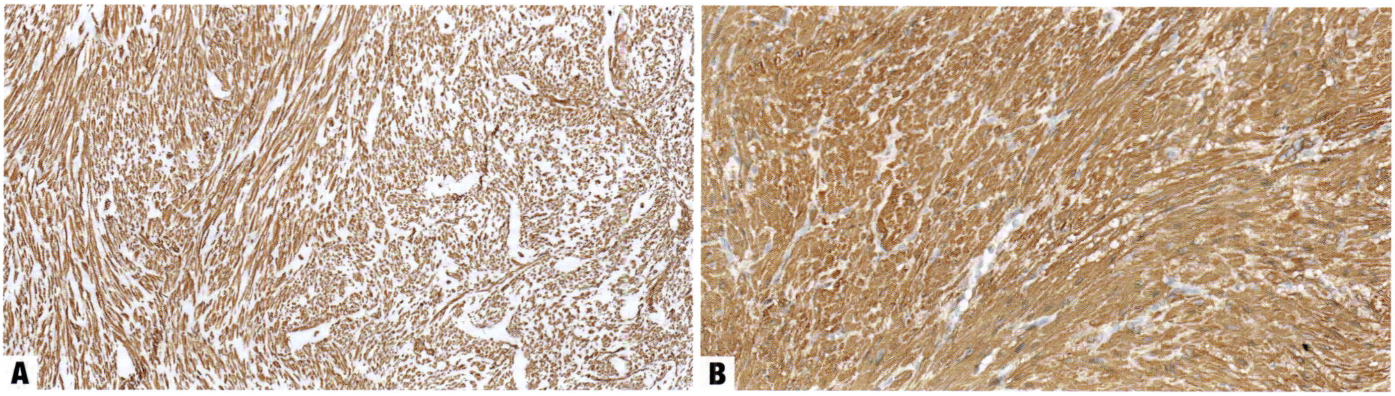

Fig. 11.39 Leiomyoma. **A,B** Expression of desmin (**A**) and expression of SMA (**B**) are characteristic features.

Diagnostic molecular pathology

Not clinically relevant

Essential and desirable diagnostic criteria

Essential: morphology of intersecting fascicles of spindled cells with blunt-ended cigar-shaped nuclei and eosinophilic cytoplasm; no atypia or necrosis.

Desirable: expression of SMA, h-caldesmon, and desmin; no staining for HMB45, cytokeratin, or S100.

Staging

Not clinically relevant

Prognosis and prediction

Orbital leiomyomas are benign, but there can be destruction of the orbital bone {3675} and local recurrence due to incomplete removal {2841,176,1468,1803}. Two reported cases developed intracranial extension {1803,1468}, and one case transformed to a malignant sarcoma possibly due to radiotherapy {1468}.

Mesectodermal leiomyoma

Mudhar HS
Alkatan H
Billings SD
Odashiro AN
Sinard J

Definition

Mesectodermal leiomyoma is a benign tumour arising from the neural crest–derived ciliary body muscle, with hybrid smooth muscle and neural features.

ICD-O coding

8890/0 Mesectodermal leiomyoma

ICD-11 coding

2F36.2 & XH4CY6 Benign neoplasm of ciliary body & Leiomyoma, NOS

Related terminology

None

Subtype(s)

None

Localization

Mesectodermal leiomyoma occurs in the suprauveal space and is probably unique to the ciliary body, whereas mesodermal leiomyomas have been described in the iris and choroid {3356}.

Clinical features

The tumour mass is characteristically dome shaped and yellow to orange in colour with intrinsic vascularity, but can be darkly pigmented and may block transillumination {3352,2696}. It may also be asymptomatic and found incidentally, cause anterior staphyloma, or present differently if ring shaped {2622,1871, 3397}. Acute presentation due to rapid growth is possible with loss of vision, lens opacification and/or displacement, glaucoma, and retinal detachment {1688,95}.

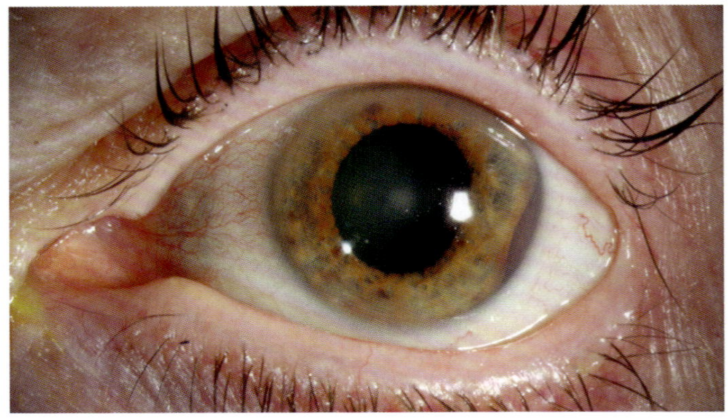

Fig. 11.40 Mesectodermal leiomyoma. A clinical photograph of the left eye shows a ciliary body mesectodermal leiomyoma. A pink mass is seen laterally with displacement of the iris.

Epidemiology

There is no known race predilection. Mesectodermal leiomyoma typically affects women in their reproductive age (second to fourth decades of life) but has been reported in postmenopausal women as well {2622,1688}.

Etiology

Unknown

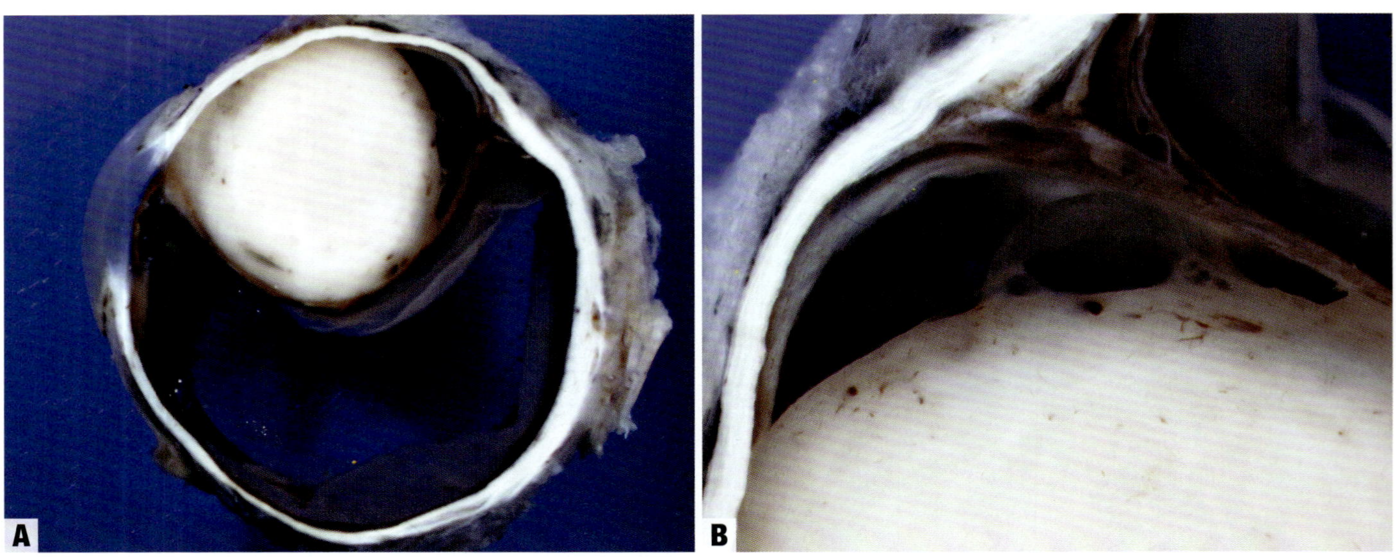

Fig. 11.41 Mesectodermal Leiomyoma. **A** A macroscopic image of an enucleation specimen shows a ciliary body mesectodermal leiomyoma. It has a solid whorled cut surface and is present in a suprauveal location, with its base against the sclera. **B** A higher-power image of the macroscopic appearance of a mesectodermal leiomyoma is shown. Note the suprauveal location, with the solid white leiomyoma abutting the sclera on the left and lifting off the pigmented choroid superiorly.

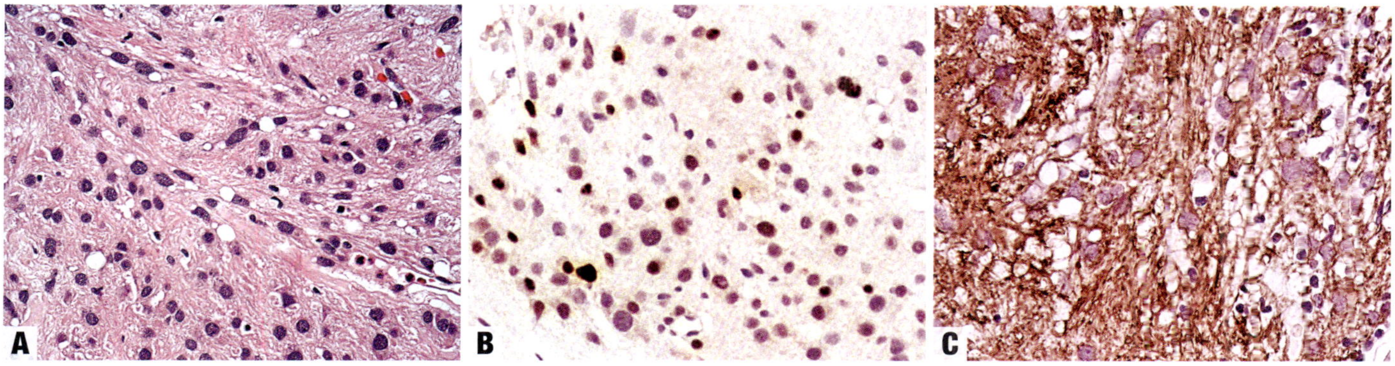

Fig. 11.42 Mesectodermal Leiomyoma. **A** H&E showing spindle cells with fibrillary eosinophilic cytoplasm containing oval, granular nuclei, some of which are indented by cytoplasmic paranuclear vacuoles. **B** Immunohistochemical demonstration of nuclear PR positivity in some of the lesional cells. **C** Cytoplasmic SMA positivity of the tumour

Pathogenesis

Mesectodermal leiomyomas are thought to arise from the ciliary body muscle, which is of neural-crest origin {1466,3257}, explaining the characteristic microscopic appearance of both muscular and neural features.

Macroscopic appearance

The tumour is usually a well-demarcated, round to oval solid mass. The cut surface is typically non-pigmented and grey to white or yellow, with a soft to firm consistency. The tumours reportedly range from 4 to 22 mm in greatest diameter, with most cases not exceeding 10 mm {1761}.

Histopathology

Mesectodermal leiomyoma is composed of spindle- to epithelioid-shaped cells with abundant fibrillar eosinophilic cytoplasm containing round to oval, finely granular, slightly pleomorphic nuclei {360,1466,3589}. Perinuclear cytoplasmic vacuoles are often seen {3257}. Scattered melanocytes can be present {3257}.

Immunohistochemically, this tumour is positive for SMA, MSA, caldesmon, calponin, and desmin {447,1761,76,3059}, and can express CD56 and NSE {1836,2408,1761,1419}. It is negative for GFAP, S100, HMB45, and melan-A {1836,2408,1761}. Some cases express nuclear sex hormone receptors {2622,95}.

Transmission electron microscopy shows myofilaments with fusiform densities, characteristic of smooth muscle, and fibrillary cytoplasmic processes containing myofilaments with fusiform densities arranged in a neurogenic pattern {1466,3257}. Some cases show skeinoid fibres {465}.

The differential diagnosis includes ciliary body melanocytic naevus, ciliary body melanoma, neurofibroma, and schwannoma. These can be distinguished from mesectodermal leiomyoma by attention to cytological features and a judicious immunohistochemical panel.

Cytology

Cell blocks from FNAs demonstrate uniform cells with oval nuclei and abundant eosinophilic cytoplasm {1708}.

Diagnostic molecular pathology

There are no studies on the molecular pathology of this tumour.

Essential and desirable diagnostic criteria

Essential: morphology of spindle-shaped cells with abundant fibrillar eosinophilic cytoplasm containing round to oval nuclei positive SMA, MSA, caldesmon, calponin, and desmin; negative melanocytic markers.

Desirable: expression of neural markers such as CD56 and NSE.

Staging

Not clinically relevant

Prognosis and prediction

The tumour is usually slowly progressive and complete local resection is generally successful in treating accessible tumours. However, enucleation may be necessary in advanced cases {3763,95,532,1688,3397}. There is a low risk of recurrence but follow-up is recommended {2494,3763}.

Leiomyosarcoma

Mishra DK
Dry SM
Ng T

Definition
Leiomyosarcoma (LMS) is a malignant mesenchymal neoplasm of smooth muscle origin.

ICD-O coding
8890/3 Leiomyosarcoma

ICD-11 coding
2B58.Y & XH7ED4 Leiomyosarcoma, other specified primary site & Leiomyosarcoma, NOS

Related terminology
None

Subtype(s)
None

Localization
Ocular LMS is rare, with few cases described arising from the soft tissue of the conjunctival stroma {3591,1193,2337,2257, 738} or the orbit {1468,3625,3600,1373,1949,3695,1417,547}.

Clinical features
Conjunctival lesions present as a raised, fleshy, pale to hyperaemic growth that may extend from fornix to limbus. Orbital lesions present as painless mass lesions, occasionally with proptosis {3695}.

Epidemiology
Ocular LMS is very rare, has a male predilection, and arises across a wide age range with a peak incidence in the seventh decade of life {3591,1193,1655,2925,2337,2257,3518,738}.

Etiology
Risk factors include hereditary retinoblastoma, radiation exposure, and Li–Fraumeni syndrome {3470,2410,415,1093,1006}.

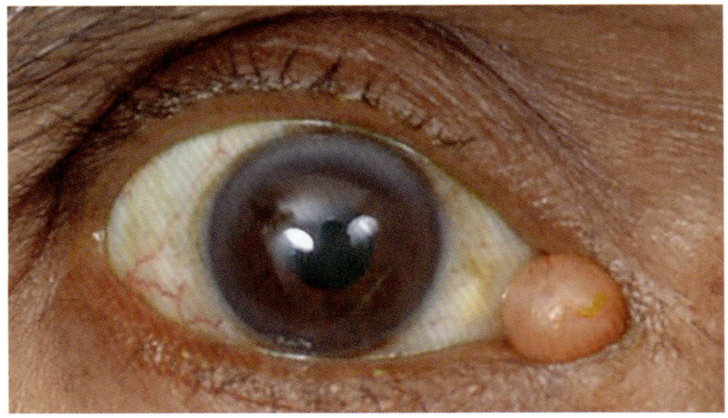

Fig. 11.43 Conjunctival leiomyosarcoma. Clinical image showing a nodular pink growth in the caruncle.

Pathogenesis
Soft tissue LMSs display extensive genomic instability, including chromothripsis and whole-genome duplication in subsets of cases {614}, with a modest burden of somatic mutations and substantial mutation heterogeneity {469,614}. Recurrent DNA copy-number alterations include losses involving the tumour suppressors *PTEN* (10q23.31), *RB1* (13q14.2), and *TP53* (17p13.1), as well as amplification of *MYOCD* at 17p12, which encodes a smooth muscle–specific transcriptional coactivator {887,2055,3547,1749,3677,1110,469,614}. Ocular LMSs have yet to be investigated.

Macroscopic appearance
LMSs appear soft, fleshy, and red to pink in colour. Areas of necrosis may be seen.

Histopathology
LMSs are cellular tumours containing spindle to cigar-shaped cells with moderate eosinophilic cytoplasm arranged in fascicles, sheets, and bundles. Nuclear pleomorphism is typically

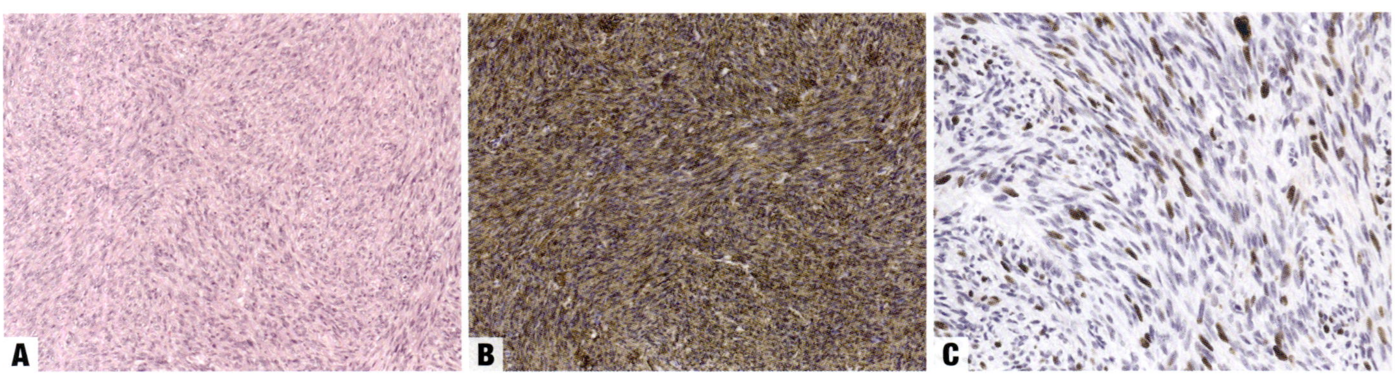

Fig. 11.44 Conjunctival leiomyosarcoma. **A** The tumour is composed of spindle cells arranged in bundles and fascicles with scattered mitotic activity. **B** Spindle neoplastic cells exhibiting strong immunoreactivity with SMA antibodies. **C** Spindle neoplastic cells display a high Ki-67 index.

found easily, although it may be absent or focal in some cases. Mitotic figures are generally abundant, including atypical forms. Giant cells may be seen.

For further details, see the related section in the *Soft tissue and bone tumours* volume of this series {3598}.

Immunohistochemistry

Tumour cells are positive for at least one smooth muscle marker (i.e. SMA, MSA, desmin, or caldesmon) in all cases, and most cases are positive for two or more. LMS may be positive, often focally, for cytokeratins, EMA, and CD34. LMSs are negative for S100 and MYOD1.

Cytology

Cytological features have not been described for ocular leiomyosarcomas.

Diagnostic molecular pathology

Not relevant

Essential and desirable diagnostic criteria

Essential: fascicles of spindle cells with variable pleomorphism; positivity for SMA, MSA, desmin, or caldesmon by immunohistochemistry.

Staging

Not applicable

Prognosis and prediction

Conjunctival LMSs have a favourable prognosis perhaps due to their small size and early stage at presentation {738}. A minority of orbital LMSs show local recurrence and rare cases develop metastasis {547}.

Schwannoma

Rodriguez FJ
Cummings TJ
McKelvie PA
Perry A

Definition
Schwannoma is a benign nerve sheath tumour composed entirely or nearly entirely of differentiated neoplastic Schwann cells.

ICD-O coding
9560/0 Schwannoma
9560/0 Cellular schwannoma
9560/0 Plexiform schwannoma
9560/0 Epithelioid schwannoma
9560/0 Microcystic/reticular schwannoma

ICD-11 coding
2A02.3 & XH98Z3 Benign neoplasm of cranial nerves & Schwannoma, NOS

Related terminology
Not recommended: neurilemoma.

Subtype(s)
Cellular schwannoma; plexiform schwannoma; epithelioid schwannoma; microcystic/reticular schwannoma

Localization
Common sites of origin are peripheral nerves in the skin and subcutaneous tissues of the head and neck. The most frequent location for schwannomas of the orbit is the superior or superomedial aspect of the orbit, where probably they originate from the supratrochlear or supraorbital branches of the ophthalmic division of the trigeminal nerve {3551}. Other ocular and periocular locations are relatively rare but examples involving the conjunctiva {536}, caruncle {1047}, choroid {3712}, and ciliary body {2774} have been recognized.

Clinical features
Schwannomas are slow-growing tumours, often appearing as asymptomatic masses or incidental findings on imaging studies. Painful schwannomas may be associated with schwannomatosis.

Epidemiology
More than 90% of schwannomas are solitary and sporadic, including those developing in the orbit, a minority of which are associated with neurofibromatosis type 2 (NF2) {487}. Schwannomas affect people of all ages, but the peak incidence is in the fourth to sixth decades of life. There is no known sex or race predisposition.

Etiology
The etiology of most sporadic schwannomas is unknown, although there is an established increased incidence associated with prior irradiation {2754,2590}. There is an association with NF2 or schwannomatosis in some cases.

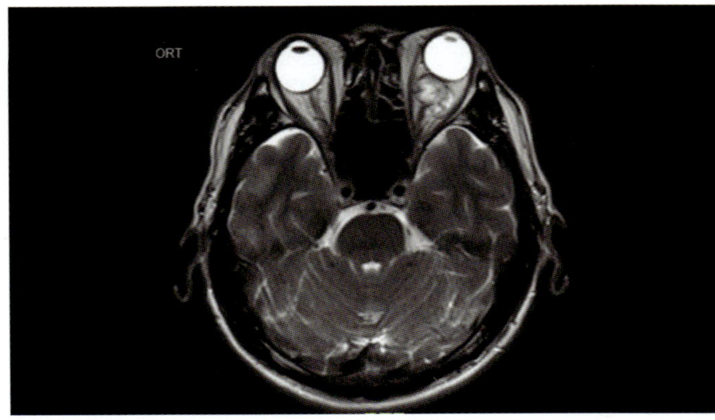

Fig. 11.45 Orbital schwannoma. Axial T2-weighted image demonstrating a well-circumscribed left orbital mass with a histological diagnosis of schwannoma.

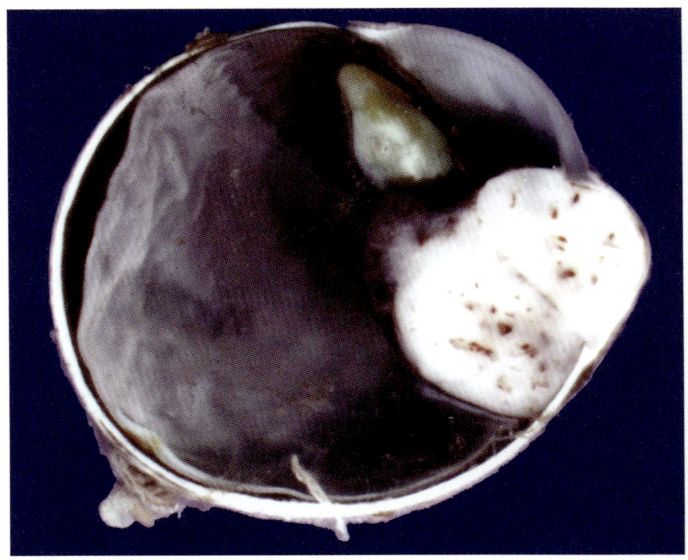

Fig. 11.46 Ciliary body schwannoma. The tumour effaces the iris, expanding into the anterior chamber, with associated scleral thinning and lens subluxation; its cut surface is solid and white, punctuated by blood vessels.

Pathogenesis
A causal relationship exists between schwannoma tumorigenesis and loss of expression of merlin (also called NF2 or schwannomin), the growth inhibitory protein product of the *NF2* tumour suppressor gene located at 22q12.2 {3200}. *NF2*-inactivating mutations have been detected in approximately 50–75% of sporadic cases {1446,1863,2413,1281}. Underlying genetic events are predominantly frameshift and nonsense mutations, with loss of the remaining wildtype allele on chromosome 22. Other common mutations involve the *LATS1*, *LATS2*, *ARID1A*, *ARID1B*, and

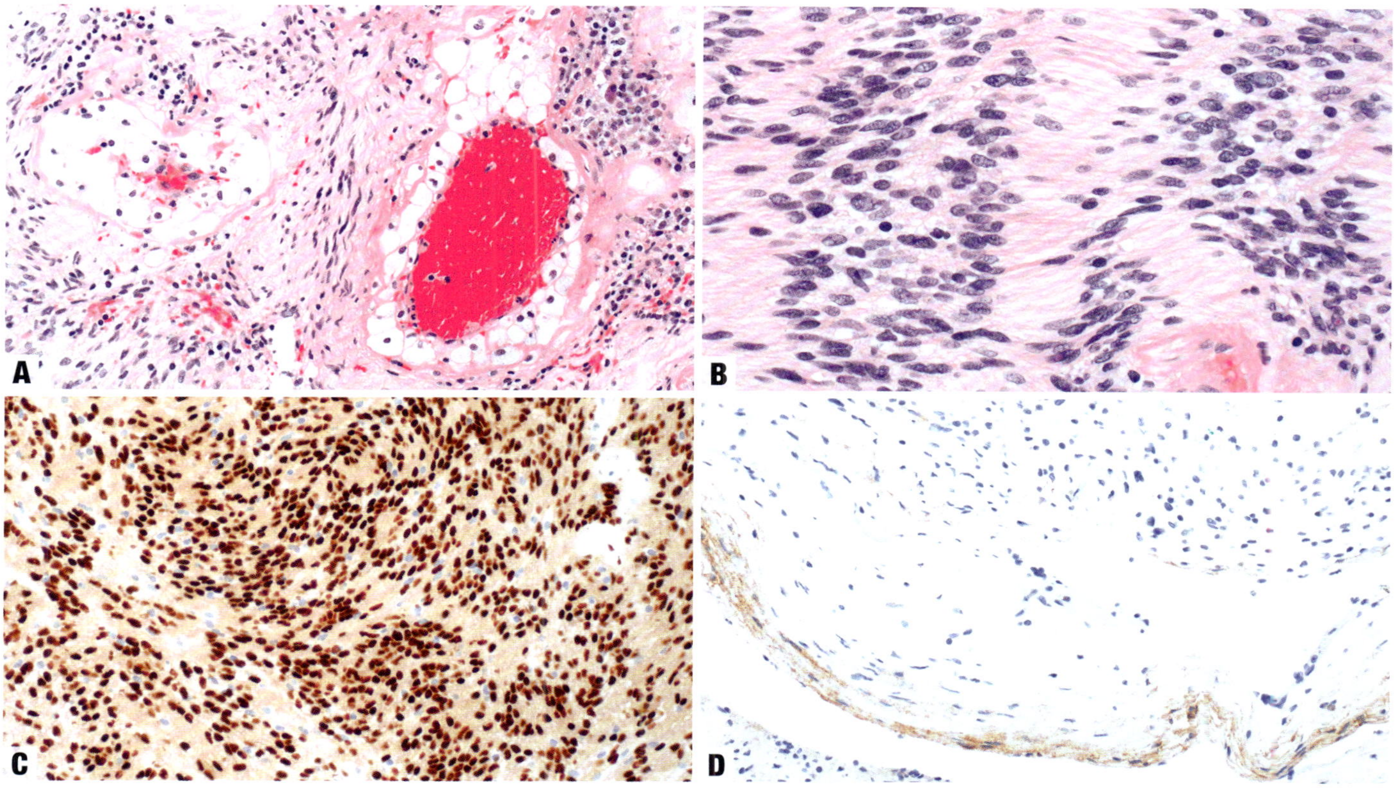

Fig. 11.47 Orbital schwannoma. **A** Frequent degenerative changes in schwannomas include hyalinized vessels, haemosiderin deposition, and foamy macrophages. **B** Verocay bodies are important diagnostic features of schwannoma, identifiable as palisades of neoplastic Schwann cells around anucleate zones. **C** As with S100, SOX10 expression is consistently present in schwannomas of all sites, but it is a pure nuclear stain. **D** EMA immunoreactivity is limited to the periphery / capsular area in schwannomas at all sites, including orbital examples.

DDR1 genes, whereas a recurrent in-frame *SH3PXD2A*::*HTRA1* fusion is found in roughly 10% of cases {2413,44}.

Multiple schwannomas are a feature of NF2 and schwannomatosis, both of which can also occur in mosaic or segmental forms {351,1642}.

Macroscopic appearance

Schwannomas are mainly solitary and globoid, with a smooth surface. Fewer than half of all schwannomas have an evident attached nerve, which is most often small and draped over the tumour capsule. A capsule may be absent in tumours involving head and neck sites, including the orbit. Sectioned tumours reveal firm, light-tan, glistening tissue, interrupted by white/yellow areas and/or patches of haemorrhage.

Histopathology

Conventional schwannoma is usually an encapsulated spindle cell tumour composed nearly entirely of well-differentiated

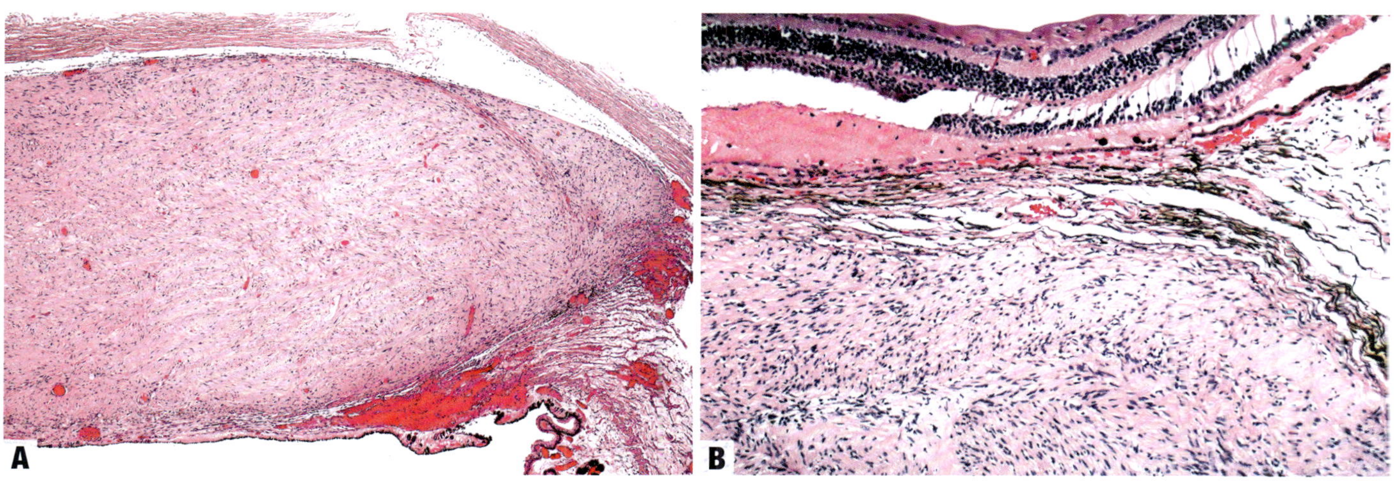

Fig. 11.48 Choroidal schwannoma. **A** Schwannomas form well-circumscribed but unencapsulated intraocular masses. **B** An intimate association with the choroid is typical of intraocular schwannomas.

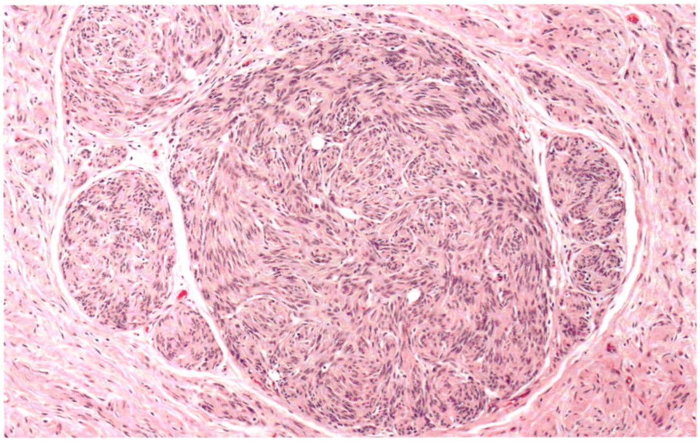

Fig. 11.49 Orbital plexiform schwannoma. Schwann cell morphology is present at intermediate magnification in this plexiform schwannoma arising in the orbit.

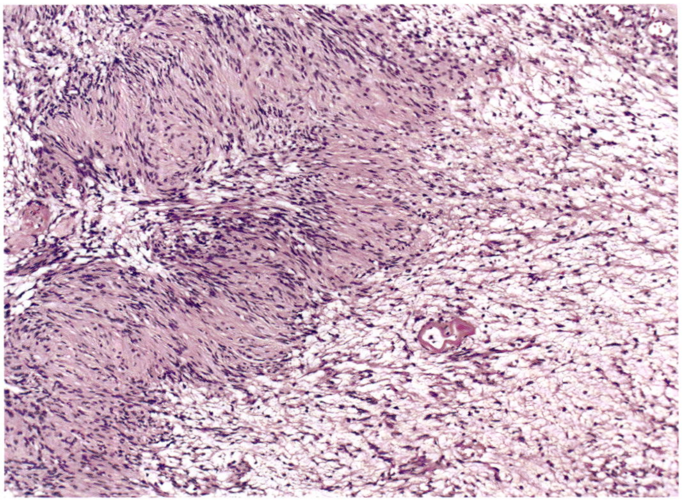

Fig. 11.50 Schwannoma of the conjunctiva. Schwannomas are characterized by the Antoni A pattern (at the left side of the field) and the looser Antoni B pattern (at the right side of the field).

Schwann cells. Schwannomas have a broad morphological range. The large majority are biphasic tumours with compact areas (Antoni A tissue) showing occasional nuclear palisading (Verocay bodies), alternating with loosely arranged foci (Antoni B tissue). Cells of Antoni A tissue have eosinophilic cytoplasm, no discernible cell borders, and normochromic, elongated, tapered nuclei. Cytoplasmic nuclear inclusions, nuclear pleomorphism, and mitotic figures may be seen. Palisading (Verocay bodies) takes the form of parallel rows of Schwann cell nuclei separated by their aligned cell processes. Antoni B tissue commonly contains a cobweb-like network of tumour processes with collections of lipid-laden histiocytes and thick-walled, hyalinized blood vessels. Lymphoid aggregates are often present in a subcapsular distribution or at the periphery in unencapsulated tumours.

Diffuse staining for S100 in the cell nuclei and cytoplasm, which is more prominent in Antoni A areas than in Antoni B areas, is found in all tumours and subtypes. Similarly, SOX10 immunoreactivity is usually extensive {2394,1600}. Expression of GFAP is less frequent and more variable. Staining for neurofilament protein is helpful in identifying entrapped intratumoural axons, found in many sporadic schwannomas, albeit most often at their periphery {2352}. EMA highlights perineurial cells in the capsule, if present.

Scattered atypical to bizarre-appearing nuclei, a feature that is often considered degenerative, have been designated ancient change. Benign hybrid nerve sheath tumours with schwannoma components have been reported in the orbit but they appear rare {1919}.

Cellular schwannoma is composed exclusively or predominantly of Antoni A tissue and is devoid of Verocay bodies. The tumours most commonly involve large nerves and nerve plexuses at paravertebral sites and in the mediastinum, retroperitoneum, and pelvis {3637,3593,2525}. Sinonasal schwannomas are often of the cellular subtype and may be locally aggressive with orbital extension {1269}.

Plexiform schwannoma, which can be conventional or cellular, often arises in skin or subcutaneous tissue, growing as thinly encapsulated plexiform or multinodular tumours {305, 984}. Less frequently, these tumours can occur in the deep soft tissues {38} and occasionally in the orbit {305,3747}.

Epithelioid schwannoma and microcystic/reticular schwannoma are rare subtypes that typically do not involve the orbit.

Other patterns: Although most syndrome-associated schwannomas are not histologically distinguishable from their sporadic counterparts, several clinicopathological clues may indicate a setting of NF2 or schwannomatosis: young patient age, multiple tumours, extensive longitudinal involvement of a nerve, a discontinuous or multinodular growth pattern, and a mosaic SMARCB1 immunostaining pattern (an admixture of positive and negative nuclei) {2509,463}. Some schwannomas feature predominantly small blue round cells, and may or may not have structures resembling Homer Wright rosettes or giant rosettes, which surround collagen fibres resembling those of low-grade fibromyxoid sarcoma; these cases are often referred to as neuroblastoma-like, although they lack increased proliferative activity and show a typical schwannoma immunoprofile {1777}. Another rare pitfall is a schwannoma with neuromelanin-like pigment accumulation that is positive on Fontana–Masson staining. Nevertheless, the histology is otherwise typical of schwannoma, and the tumour cells are negative for more-specific melanocytic markers, such as HMB45 {1048}; therefore, these should not be equated with the more aggressive, Carney complex / PRKAR1A–associated malignant melanotic nerve sheath tumour (previously termed "melanotic schwannoma").

Cytology

Aspirate smears of schwannoma typically yield cohesive syncytial fragments of spindle cells {555}. Within the fragments, variably wavy and bent tumour cell nuclei with tapered edges and elongate cytoplasm are seen. Nuclear pleomorphism or degenerative atypia and intranuclear inclusions may be seen. Schwannomas may be difficult to distinguish from other spindle cell neoplasms on cytological preparation alone, and their diagnosis requires correlation with core biopsy and/or immunohistochemical staining {54}.

Diagnostic molecular pathology

Loss of chromosome 22q and/or mutation of *NF2* in schwannomas are frequent but nonspecific molecular alterations. Schwannomas exhibit a distinct DNA methylation pattern {478, 2750,1755,44}.

Essential and desirable diagnostic criteria

Essential: histopathology of schwannoma, such as Antoni A or Antoni B areas.

Desirable: extensive S100 or SOX10 expression; Verocay bodies; subcapsular lymphocytes; hyalinized blood vessels; lack of a lattice-like pattern of CD34 staining; loss of SMARCB1 (INI1) expression (epithelioid schwannoma), or a mosaic pattern of SMARCB1 (INI1) expression (syndrome-associated schwannoma).

Staging

Not clinically relevant

Prognosis and prediction

Schwannomas are benign and do not usually recur if treated by gross total resection. Cellular and plexiform examples are least amenable to total removal and sometimes can only be debulked. Malignant transformation of conventional schwannoma is extremely rare, and not a feature in orbital examples.

Neurofibroma

Stemmer-Rachamimov AO
Cummings TJ
Perry A
Rodriguez FJ

Definition

Neurofibromas are benign peripheral nerve sheath tumours composed of mature neoplastic Schwann cells intermixed with non-neoplastic cell types and extracellular matrix.

ICD-O coding

9540/0 Neurofibroma
9550/0 Plexiform neurofibroma
9540/0 Solitary neurofibroma
9540/0 Diffuse neurofibroma
9541/0 Melanotic neurofibroma

ICD-11 coding

2F3Z & XH87J5 Benign neoplasms except of mesenchymal origin, of unspecified site & Neurofibroma, NOS
2F24 & XH87J5 Benign cutaneous neoplasms of neural or nerve sheath origin & Neurofibroma, NOS
2F36.0 & XH87J5 Benign neoplasm of choroid & Neurofibroma, NOS
2F36.Y Other specified benign neoplasm of eye or ocular adnexa

Related terminology

Acceptable: orbitofacial neurofibroma.

Subtype(s)

Plexiform neurofibroma; solitary neurofibroma; diffuse neurofibroma; melanotic neurofibroma

Localization

Orbitofacial neurofibroma occurs in the conjunctival stroma, the subcutaneous layer of the eyelid, and the orbit. In the choroid, diffuse/multifocal choroidal involvement is typical, and there is a predilection for the posterior pole {3423}. Associated involvement of small ciliary nerves is variable.

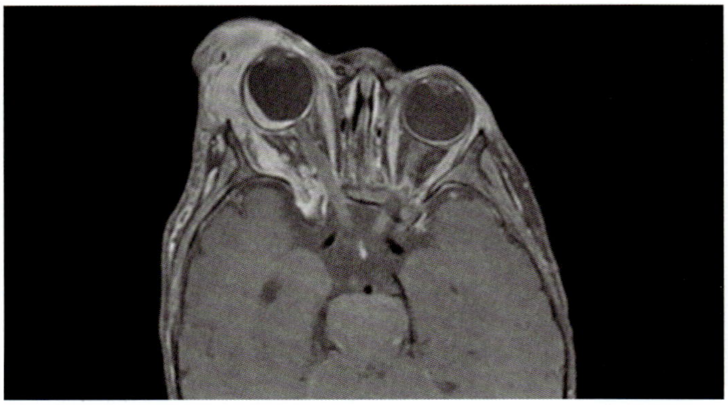

Fig. 11.51 Neurofibroma of the conjunctiva. T1-weighted MRI showing a plexiform tumour involving the orbit, eyelid, and conjunctiva.

Clinical features

Orbital neurofibroma can manifest as proptosis and optic nerve compression.

Neurofibromas of the conjunctiva may be solitary, diffuse, or extension of a plexiform type {1582}. Plexiform neurofibromas involving the orbit, eyelid, and facial structures (orbitofacial neurofibromas) occur predominantly in paediatric patients with neurofibromatosis type 1 (NF1) and may cause significant visual loss and disfigurement {2458}. These tumours are often more aggressive and have a unique methylation profile {194}.

Recent studies using modern imaging techniques (MRI, indocyanine green angiography, infrared fundus autofluorescence, and optical coherence tomography) suggest that choroidal neurofibroma is common in NF1 and choroidal abnormalities have

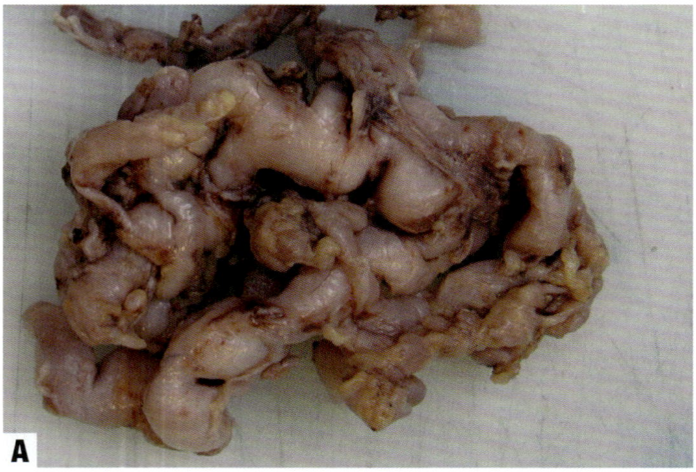

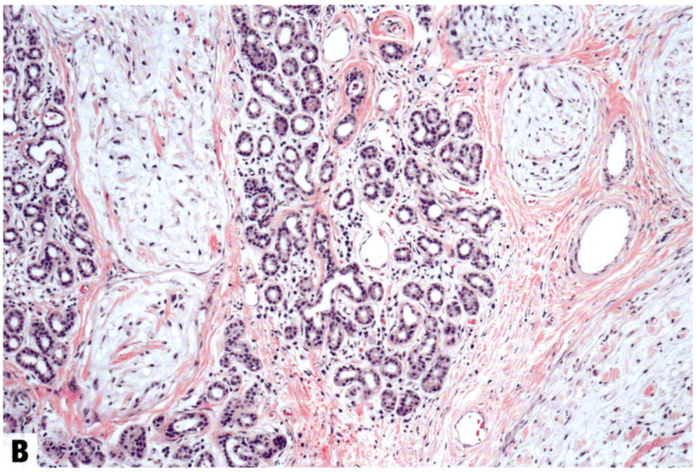

Fig. 11.52 Plexiform neurofibroma. **A** Macroscopic impression of plexiform neurofibroma of the orbit at grossing. **B** Plexiform neurofibroma infiltrating the lacrimal gland.

recently been added as a diagnostic criterion for the disease {3423,3497,3686,1905}.

Epidemiology

Solitary conjunctival neurofibromas are rare. In one large series of 1643 conjunctival tumours, only one neurofibroma was found {2972}. Plexiform neurofibromas of the eyelid and orbit, which are typically associated with NF1 (MIM number 162200), may extend to involve the conjunctiva {430}.

In patients with NF1, choroidal lesions (which include neurofibromas) develop in paediatric patients and appear to increase in frequency with age.

Etiology

Conjunctival, eyelid, choroidal, and orbital neurofibromas may arise owing to underlying NF1, but most are sporadic {350}.

Pathogenesis

Plexiform neurofibromas occur mainly in the context of NF1, in association with inactivation and allelic loss in Schwann cells of both copies of the *NF1* gene at chromosome 17q {653}.

Macroscopic appearance

Five macroscopic forms are distinguished: localized/nodular cutaneous, diffuse cutaneous, localized/nodular intraneural, plexiform intraneural, and massive diffuse soft tissue neurofibroma. Localized cutaneous neurofibromas can have a variety of gross appearances, including flat, sessile, globular, and pedunculated, whereas plexiform tumours involve multiple fascicles imparting a rope-like or bag-of-worms appearance; diffuse neurofibromas typically form large plaques {2447}.

Histopathology

Neurofibroma is characterized by a haphazard proliferation of Schwann cells and specialized fibroblasts {1582}. Mast cells are often present. Tactile-like structures (pseudomeissnerian corpuscles) may be seen. Degenerative nuclear atypia may occur. A mucinous or myxomatous extracellular matrix is often present, with other regions featuring wavy collagen resembling shredded carrots. Neurofibroma shows patchy, variable immunoreactivity for S100 and SOX10 in the Schwann cell component and a reticular pattern of CD34 positivity in the fibroblastic element. Axons permeate the lesion and are highlighted by immunohistochemical staining for neurofilament protein. In some cases, the tumour is composed of neurofibroma component and another component of a schwannoma or a perineurioma, to which the term "hybrid tumour" is applied. Hybrid tumours of neurofibroma/schwannoma are associated with the neurofibromatoses (NF1, NF2, and schwannomatosis). Neurofibromas/perineuriomas are often associated with NF1.

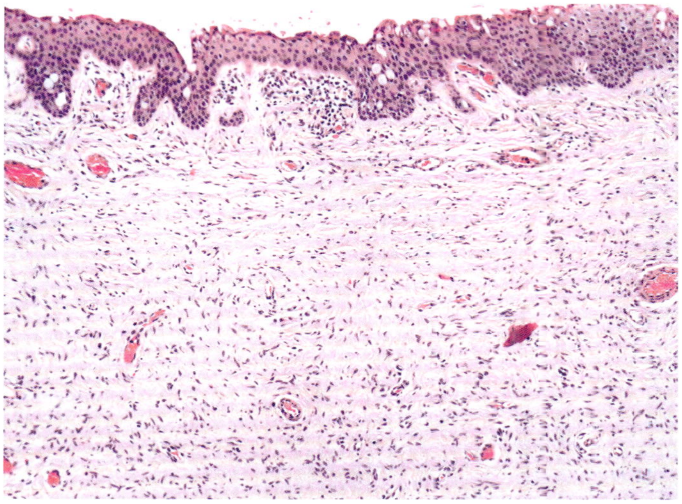

Fig. 11.53 Neurofibroma of the conjunctiva. Conjunctival epithelium with goblet cells is visible at the top of the figure.

In the uveal tract, histopathology often reveals diffuse thickening by a proliferation of Schwann cells, fibroblasts, and choroidal melanocytes. This thickening is massive in some cases; parts of the choroid may be several times as thick as the sclera. The lesion may contain ovoid bodies that resemble tactile corpuscles, ultrastructurally composed of Schwann cells arranged in lamellae {1814}. Ganglion cells are a normal constituent of the choroid, but when numerous and probably neoplastic, the tumour is classified as a ganglioneuroma {3638,3085}.

In the conjunctiva, the differential diagnosis includes traumatic neuroma, mucosal neuroma associated with multiple endocrine neoplasia type 2B, solitary circumscribed neuroma, schwannoma, low-grade malignant peripheral nerve sheath tumour, perineurioma, and myxoma {536}.

Cytology

Intraoperative smears and FNA specimens are often paucicellular owing to the increased collagen stroma in neurofibromas.

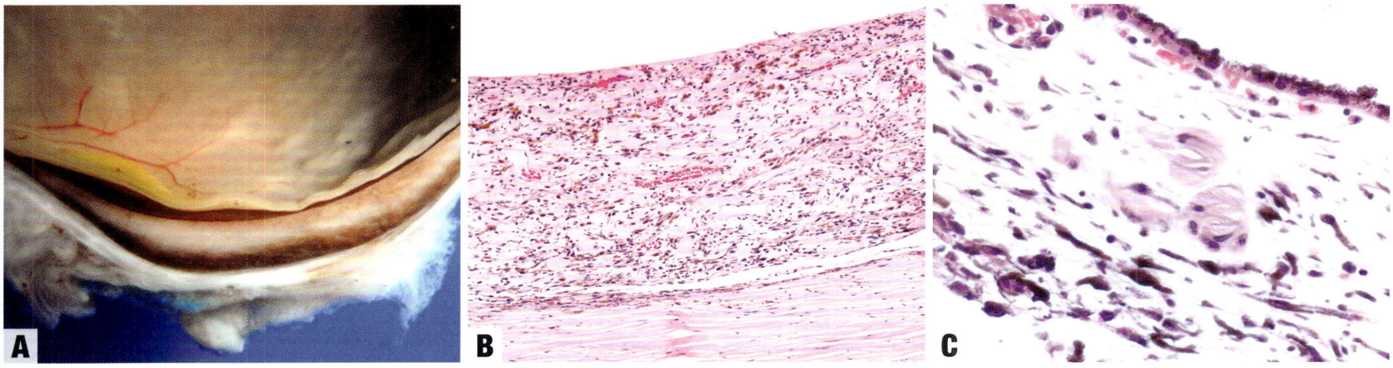

Fig. 11.54 Neurofibroma of the choroid. **A** Neurofibromatosis type 1. Uveal neurofibromas typically cause diffuse expansion of the choroid. **B** Diffuse expansion of the choroid by a proliferation of Schwann cells. **C** Ovoid bodies resembling Meissner (tactile) corpuscles are composed of concentric Schwann cell processes.

Nevertheless, the presence of a mucin-rich background and small spindled cells with thin, wavy nuclei can provide diagnostic clues.

Diagnostic molecular pathology

Molecular analyses do not have an established role in the diagnosis of neurofibroma. However, chromosomal copy-number profiling may be helpful for the evaluation of atypical neurofibroma / atypical neurofibromatous neoplasm of uncertain biological potential; see the section in the *Soft tissue and bone tumours* volume of this series {3598} on neurofibroma (*CDKN2A* and/or *CDKN2B* deletion) and its differentiation from malignant peripheral nerve sheath tumour (complex highly rearranged genome). Of note, conventional dermal and plexiform neurofibromas, atypical neurofibroma / atypical neurofibromatous neoplasm of uncertain biological potential, and malignant peripheral nerve sheath tumour all exhibit distinct DNA methylation profiles {2750}.

Essential and desirable diagnostic criteria

Essential: infiltrative, low-cellularity spindle cell neoplasm associated with a variably myxoid to collagenous stroma.

Desirable: S100 positivity in the Schwann cell population, with CD34 highlighting a lattice-like stromal component.

Staging

Not applicable

Prognosis and prediction

Solitary lesions can be excised. Plexiform lesions are difficult to remove and scarring and recurrences may occur. Malignant transformation is rare.

Diffuse uveal tract abnormalities are typically found incidentally during histopathological examination of blind, painful, buphthalmic eyes enucleated from patients with NF1.

Solitary circumscribed neuroma

Rodriguez FJ
Ferguson PM

Definition
Solitary circumscribed neuroma (SCN) is a benign nodular proliferation of nerve fibres with Schwann cells predominating over axons, showing a strong predilection for the face.

ICD-O coding
9570/0 Solitary circumscribed neuroma
9570/0 Plexiform solitary circumscribed neuroma

ICD-11 coding
2F24 & XH90Y8 Benign cutaneous neoplasms of neural or nerve sheath origin & Solitary circumscribed neuroma

Related terminology
Acceptable: palisaded neuroma; palisaded encapsulated neuroma; palisaded and encapsulated neuroma.

Subtype(s)
Plexiform solitary circumscribed neuroma

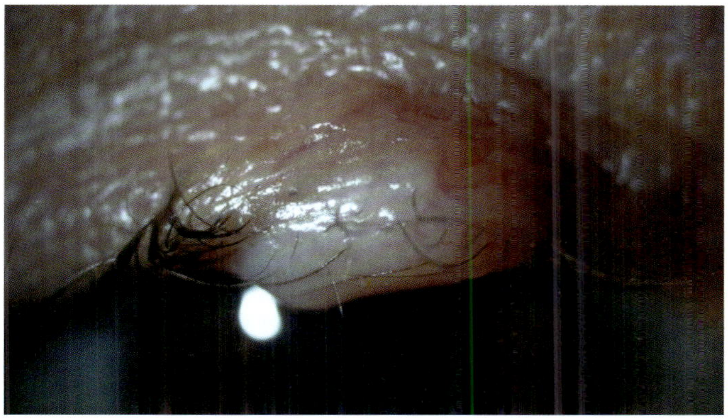

Fig. 11.55 Solitary circumscribed neuroma. Solitary circumscribed neuroma involving the eyelid.

Localization
The skin of the face hosts approximately 90% of SCNs with many lesions arising near mucocutaneous junctions or in oral

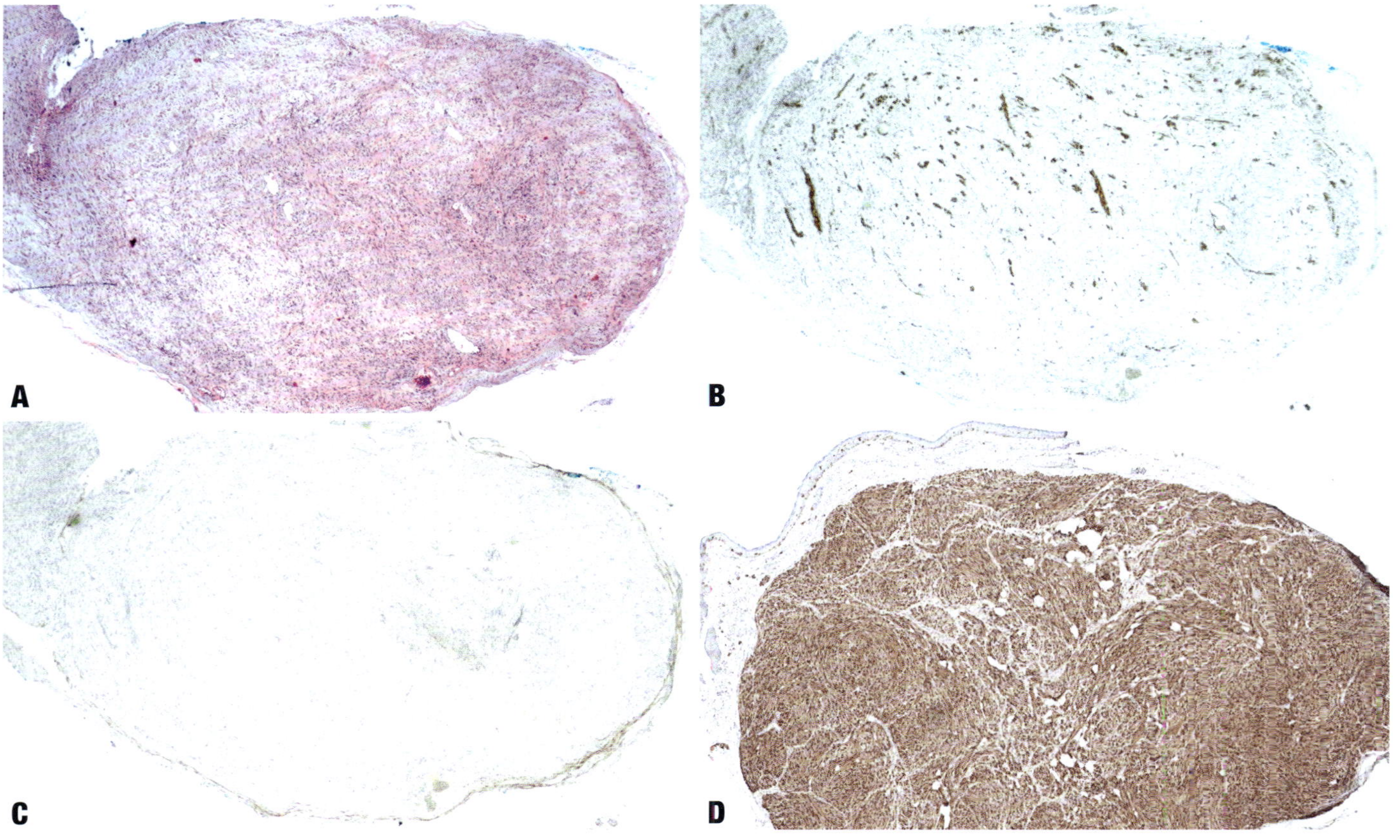

Fig. 11.56 Solitary circumscribed neuroma. **A** Solitary circumscribed neuromas form well-circumscribed nodules evident at low magnification. **B** Neurofilament protein highlights a high axonal density in solitary circumscribed neuroma, a usual feature that distinguishes it from schwannoma. **C** Perineurial cells at the periphery are typically highlighted with EMA. **D** The lesion shows diffuse S100 expression.

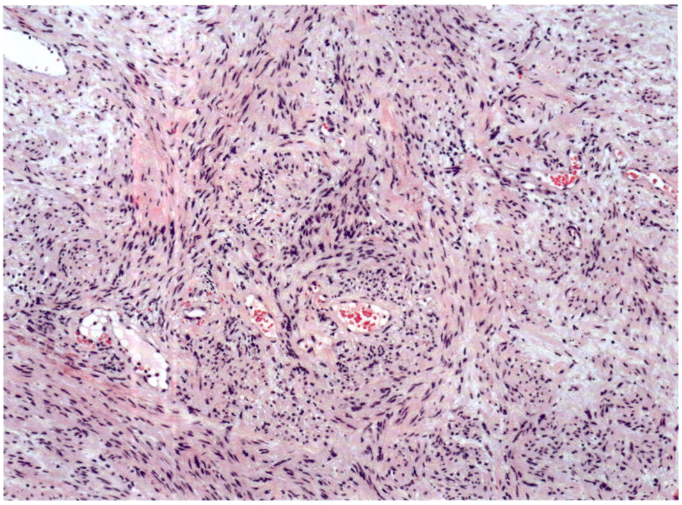

Fig. 11.57 Solitary circumscribed neuroma. Solitary circumscribed neuromas are characterized by a predominant content of Schwann cells.

mucosa {1778}. They may involve the upper or lower eyelids {838,2189,3245,2277} but involvement of the palpebral conjunctiva is very rare {1434}.

Clinical features

SCN usually presents as a slow-growing, firm, painless, circumscribed dermal-based nodule. In the eyelid the main clinical differential diagnosis is basal cell carcinoma. SCN is mostly solitary, but rare examples of multiple SCNs have been reported with no evidence of any associated systemic disease {1964}.

Epidemiology

SCN is most common in the fifth to seventh decades of life, but it can occur in patients of any age without a sex predilection. In the periocular region, SCN accounts for only about 2% of nerve sheath tumours {3747} but represented half (5 of 10 cases) of non-syndromic peripheral nerve sheath tumours developing in the eyelid in one study {3187}.

Etiology

Unknown

Pathogenesis

SCN is a benign tumour of nerve fibres with slow growth over many years and is unrelated to trauma {983}.

Macroscopic appearance

SCN usually presents as a circumscribed dermal-based nodule with a firm, pale-grey cut surface, < 10 mm in diameter.

Histopathology

SCN is a circumscribed dermal-based tumour composed of bland spindle-shaped cells with wavy nuclei in a background of hyalinized collagen. The cells often form well-developed fascicles, and some palisading of nuclei within the tumour is characteristically present. A thin perineurial-derived fibrous capsule may surround the lesion, but it is often incomplete at the superficial aspect. Artefactual clefting is a frequent finding, and extension into the subcutis may be present on occasion {2685}. No cytological atypia is present and mitoses are inconspicuous. The spindle cells are strongly and diffusely positive for S100. Neurofilament protein staining typically identifies the presence of small axons within the tumour {189}. Perineurial cells in the capsule stain for EMA, claudin-1, and GLUT1 {1778}. Occasionally, SCNs may have a multinodular or plexiform growth pattern {1531,190}.

Cytology

FNA of SCN shows a nonspecific paucicellular pattern of bland spindle cells.

Diagnostic molecular pathology

No diagnostic molecular findings have been described.

Essential and desirable diagnostic criteria

Essential: circumscribed cutaneous lesion of Schwann cell–rich fascicles of nerve fibres with or without partial encapsulation.
Desirable: S100 positivity with focal neurofilament protein staining; the peripheral capsule is highlighted by perineurial markers (EMA, GLUT1).

Staging

Not clinically relevant

Prognosis and prediction

SCN is a benign neoplasm with no metastatic potential.

Granular cell tumour

Reis-Filho JS
Rodriguez FJ

Definition
Granular cell tumour is a benign neuroectodermal tumour with Schwann cell differentiation composed of epithelioid cells with abundant lysosome-rich granular eosinophilic cytoplasm.

ICD-O coding
9580/0 Granular cell tumour
9580/3 Granular cell tumour, malignant

ICD-11 coding
2E89.1 & XH09A9 Benign tumours of uncertain differentiation, soft tissue & Granular cell tumour, NOS
2B5F.2 & XH90D3 Sarcoma, not elsewhere classified of other specified sites & Granular cell tumour, malignant

Related terminology
Not recommended: Abrikossoff tumour; granular cell myoblastoma; granular cell schwannoma; granular cell nerve sheath tumour.

Subtype(s)
Granular cell tumour, malignant

Localization
Granular cell tumours typically affect the skin and mucosa {2020,1826}. They are often solitary lesions, but 7–29% of patients may display multiple lesions {2612}. In the eye, these tumours are preferentially observed in the soft tissues of the orbit, particularly involving the extraocular muscles {1105}.

Clinical features
Granular cell tumours generally present as slow-growing and painless solitary lesions resulting in worsening proptosis, diplopia, and restriction of movement, given the predilection for an extraocular muscle location {2705,264}. Pain and signs of optic nerve involvement are rare {264}.

Epidemiology
Granular cell tumours of the orbit have a mode of incidence in the fifth and sixth decades of life, with an equal distribution between men and women {264}. The malignant form is exceedingly rare.

Etiology
Granular cell tumours are predominantly sporadic, but there are reports of the occurrence of these tumours in the context of Bannayan–Riley–Ruvalcaba syndrome {2065}, neurofibromatosis type 1 {2020}, Watson syndrome, LEOPARD syndrome (multiple lentigines, electrocardiographic conduction abnormalities, ocular hypertelorism, pulmonic stenosis, abnormal genitalia, retardation of growth, and sensorineural deafness) {2887} and neurofibromatosis–Noonan syndrome {245,2647}.

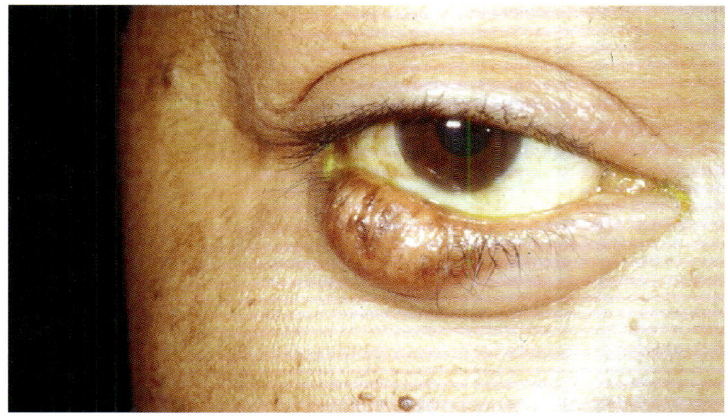

Fig. 11.58 Granular cell tumour. A localized tumour on the eyelid margin.

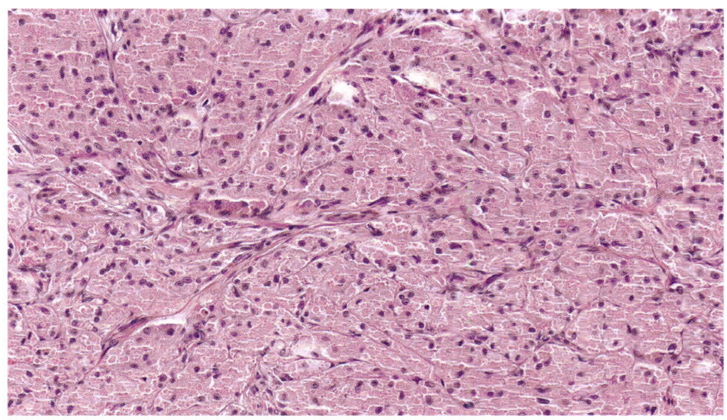

Fig. 11.59 Granular cell tumour. An example from the eyelid showing granular eosinophilic cytoplasm.

Pathogenesis
Whole-exome and targeted sequencing analyses of these cancers have revealed loss-of-function mutations affecting *ATP6AP1* and *ATP6AP2*, which encode accessory components of the vacuolar H+ ATPase {2486}, and less frequently loss-of-function mutations affecting other genes encoding other components of the vacuolar H+ ATPase {2907,1023}. Loss of function of *ATP6AP1* and *ATP6AP2* has been shown to be oncogenic and causative of the intracytoplasmic accumulation of early and recycling endosomes, which confer the characteristic granular eosinophilic cytoplasm of granular cell tumours and are pathognomonic {2486}.

Macroscopic appearance
Granular cell tumours are uninodular and firm homogeneous masses, tan to white in colour {2833,264}.

Histopathology
Granular cell tumours display an infiltrating growth pattern with poorly defined borders. The tumours are composed of sheets,

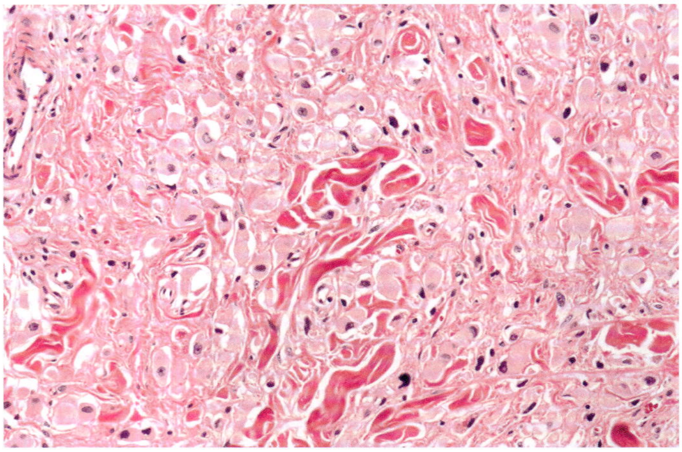

Fig. 11.60 Granular cell tumour. An example infiltrating the extraocular muscle.

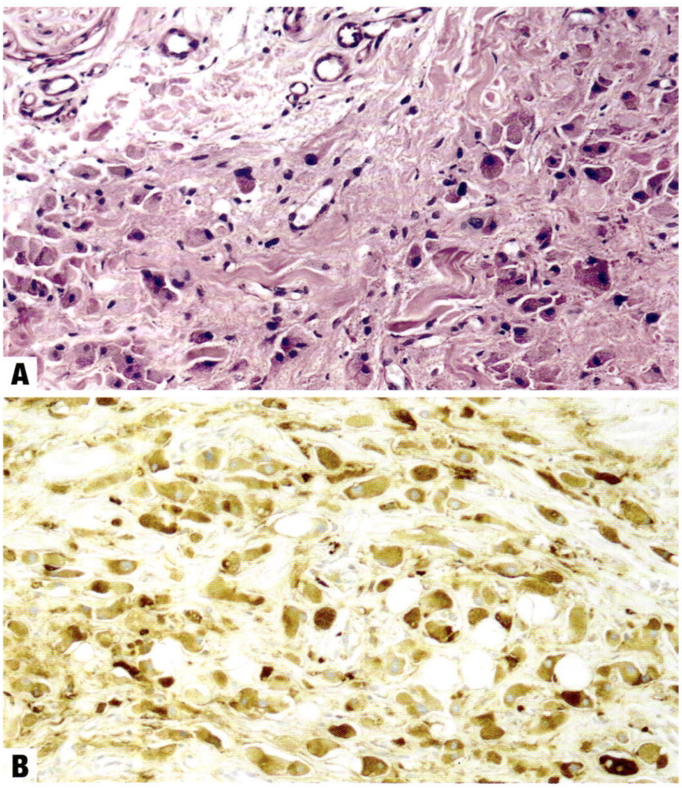

Fig. 11.61 Granular cell tumour. **A** PAS staining showing diastase-resistant positivity in granular cell tumour. **B** S100 positive staining in granular cell tumour.

nests, and trabeculae of epithelioid to polygonal cells with abundant cytoplasm containing many eosinophilic PAS-positive/diastase-resistant cytoplasmic granules. Nuclei are usually centrally located, ranging from small and uniform to larger and vesicular with prominent nucleoli {2440,2020,931}. Mitotic figures are generally scant. The exceedingly rare malignant granular cell tumour may display increased cellularity, prominent spindling, a high N:C ratio, marked pleomorphism, increased mitotic activity, and necrosis {931,2354,2020}.

Immunohistochemistry

Granular cell tumours display strong and diffuse expression of S100, SOX10, inhibin, and calretinin {1600,1300,2020}. CD68, CD63 (NKI/C3 clone), and NSE can also be positive, probably owing to nonspecific reactivity with the abundant lysosomal granules {2020}. TFE3 and MITF expression, in the absence of rearrangements of these genes, is common {2885,1975,1126}, whereas HMB45 is consistently negative {1126,2020}. CD163 is negative, a useful marker separating granular cell tumours from histiocytic disorders.

Cytology

Useful cytological features for a diagnosis of granular cell tumours include discohesive cells, abundant granular cytoplasm, a low N:C ratio, and bland nuclei {2773,2222,1775}. Carcinomas (in particular apocrine carcinomas) and histiocytic processes should be excluded.

Diagnostic molecular pathology

Not clinically relevant

Essential and desirable diagnostic criteria

Essential: nests, sheets, and trabeculae of large epithelioid to polygonal cells with abundant granular cytoplasm.

Desirable: diffuse strong expression of S100 and SOX10.

Staging

Not relevant unless malignant

Prognosis and prediction

The treatment for most granular cell tumours of the orbit is wide surgical excision with complete removal, which is often curative {264}. Malignant granular cell tumours may require more aggressive approaches, including chemotherapy and radiation therapy, given the risk of distant metastatic dissemination in as many as 50% of cases {2020}.

Malignant peripheral nerve sheath tumour

Stemmer-Rachamimov AO
Edward DP
Nielsen GP
Perry A
Rodriguez FJ

Definition

Malignant peripheral nerve sheath tumour (MPNST) is a malignant spindle cell tumour often arising from a peripheral nerve or a pre-existing benign nerve sheath tumour, or in a patient with neurofibromatosis type 1 (NF1) and often showing limited Schwannian differentiation.

ICD-O coding

9540/3 Malignant peripheral nerve sheath tumour
9542/3 Epithelioid malignant peripheral nerve sheath tumour

ICD-11 coding

2B5E & XH2XP8 Malignant nerve sheath tumour of peripheral nerves or autonomic nervous system, primary site & Malignant peripheral nerve sheath tumour
2B5E & XH4V81 Malignant nerve sheath tumour of peripheral nerves or autonomic nervous system, primary site & Malignant peripheral nerve sheath tumour, epithelioid
2B5E & XH2VV8 Malignant nerve sheath tumour of peripheral nerves or autonomic nervous system, primary site & Malignant peripheral nerve sheath tumour with rhabdomyoblastic differentiation

Related terminology

Not recommended: malignant schwannoma; neurofibrosarcoma; neurogenic sarcoma; malignant perineurioma.

Subtype(s)

Epithelioid malignant peripheral nerve sheath tumour

Localization

The most common locations are the trunk and extremities followed by the head and neck area {1875,839,837}.

Clinical features

MPNSTs typically present in people between 20 and 50 years of age, with younger ages for NF1-associated tumours. Patients present with proptosis and displacement of the globe. There may be associated neuropathic symptoms such as paraesthesia and pain {1856}.

Epidemiology

Orbital MPNST is rare accounting for < 1 in 1000 orbital biopsies {3480} and < 1 orbital case in 100 MPNSTs {3478}.

Etiology

Some cases are associated with NF1 (~50%) or radiation (~10%) {996}.

Pathogenesis

MPNSTs have complex karyotypes and frequent concurrent inactivating mutations involving three pathways: *NF1*, *CDKN2A* and/or *CDKN2B*, and PRC2 core components (*EED* or *SUZ12*) {1901,747,3746,2530}. As many as 80% of high-grade MPNSTs exhibit complete loss of PRC2 activity and complete loss of H3 p.K27me3 on immunohistochemistry {2595,1901,2866}. Epithelioid MPNSTs are molecularly distinct, characterized by frequent *SMARCB1* gene inactivation {2865}.

Macroscopic appearance

Most MPNSTs are > 50 mm. Intraneural tumours show fusiform enlargement of the involved nerve. MPNST shows a tan-white, fleshy cut surface, often with haemorrhage and necrosis.

Histopathology

MPNST shows interlacing fascicles of spindle-shaped cells, often with alternating hypercellular and hypocellular areas. A haemangiopericytoma-like vascular pattern is characteristic, and denser perivascular growth is common. There are often areas of geographical necrosis and high mitotic activity. Nuclei are hyperchromatic and spindled to serpentine, while the cytoplasm is pale and eosinophilic. Occasional cases show prominent pleomorphism. Approximately 15% of MPNSTs show heterologous differentiation, which may be rhabdomyoblastic (triton tumour), osseous, cartilaginous, or vascular, as well as epithelial (glandular or squamous).

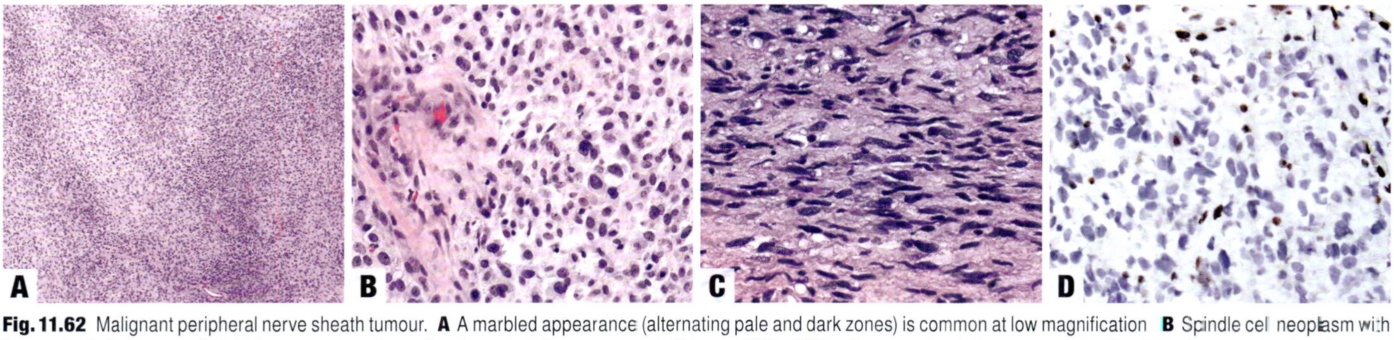

Fig. 11.62 Malignant peripheral nerve sheath tumour. **A** A marbled appearance (alternating pale and dark zones) is common at low magnification. **B** Spindle cell neoplasm with frequent mitotic figures. **C** A high-power view shows the characteristic wavy nuclei. **D** Loss of H3 p.K27me3 expression in tumour nuclei, with retained expression in entrapped non-neoplastic elements.

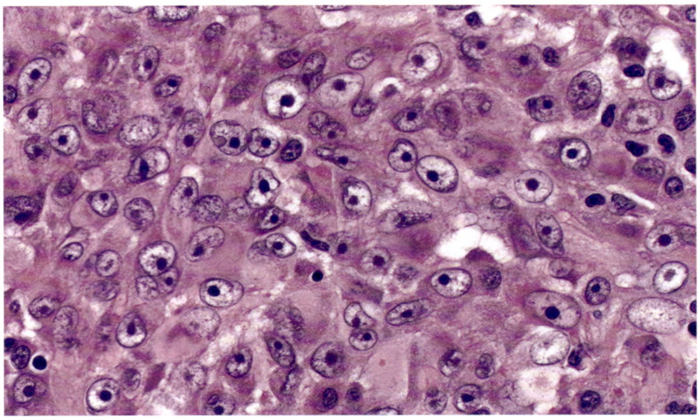

Fig. 11.63 Epithelioid malignant peripheral nerve sheath tumour. The cells are epithelioid with eosinophilic cytoplasm and large nuclei with prominent nucleoli, mimicking a melanoma.

Box 11.01 Diagnostic criteria for conventional malignant peripheral nerve sheath tumour

Essential:

Histopathologically consistent malignant spindle cell tumour in a patient with NF1[a] **OR** in a pre-existing neurofibroma

OR

Malignant spindle cell tumour associated with a peripheral nerve **AND** no more than focal/patchy S100/SOX10 expression **AND** no *SS18*::SSX (*SSX1*, *SSX2*, or *SSX4*) fusion gene present

OR

Malignant spindle cell tumour associated with a peripheral nerve **AND** evidence of PRC2 inactivation (molecularly or via loss of H3 p.K28me3 [K27me3] immunostaining)

OR

Tumour with features of ANNUBP in a patient with NF1, but with a mitotic count of ≥ 1.5–4.5 mitoses/mm² (3–9 mitoses/10 HPF of 0.51 mm in diameter and 0.20 mm² in area)

OR

Unresolved lesion with the methylation profile of MPNST

Desirable:

Loss of H3 p.K28me3 (K27me3)

Loss of neurofibromin (NF1) expression

ANNUBP, atypical neurofibromatous neoplasm of uncertain biological potential; HPF, high-power field; MPNST, malignant peripheral nerve sheath tumour; NF1, neurofibromatosis type 1.

[a]In the setting of NF1, a diagnosis other than conventional MPNST demands strong molecular evidence (e.g. detection of a fusion gene pathognomonic of another tumour type).

MPNSTs show limited staining for S100 (< 50% of tumours), SOX10 (< 70%), and GFAP (20–30%) {1594}. Complete loss of staining for H3 p.K27me3 is seen in 50–80% of all MPNSTs, with loss being more frequent in high-grade and radiation-induced than NF1-associated MPNST {2524,2595,2866,2454}.

Differential diagnosis from melanoma (especially desmoplastic melanoma) can be challenging as there is overlap of histological and immunohistochemical features. Also, with melanoma being more common in the head and neck than MPNST, some of the reported MPNSTs in the past were, in fact, melanomas {2737}.

Epithelioid MPNST is composed of epithelioid cells with abundant eosinophilic cytoplasm, sometimes embedded in an abundant myxoid or hyalinized stroma {1862}. It is not associated with NF1 and rarely arises ex schwannoma {1523}. Unlike conventional MPNST, epithelioid MPNST shows strong and diffuse staining for S100 and SOX10, with retained H3 p.K27me3 and loss of SMARCB1 expression {2865}.

Diagnostic criteria have been proposed to distinguish atypical neurofibroma, cellular neurofibroma, atypical neurofibromatous neoplasm of uncertain biological potential, and low-grade and high-grade MPNST in NF1 patients {2198}.

The main differential diagnosis at this site is with melanoma and solitary fibrous tumour.

Cytology

Not clinically relevant

Diagnostic molecular pathology

In diagnostically challenging cases, DNA methylation profiling can identify a specific tumour signature of MPNST {1756}. Other supporting molecular data include mutations in *NF1* and *SUZ12* or *EED*.

Essential and desirable diagnostic criteria

See Box 11.01.

Staging

Not clinically relevant

Prognosis and prediction

MPNST shows aggressive behaviour with poor prognosis. Adverse prognostic factors include a tumour size > 50 mm, local recurrence, positive surgical margins, and high-grade morphology (including triton tumour). Patients with NF1-associated MPNST appear to have a worse prognosis than patients with sporadic tumours {1875}. Epithelioid MPNSTs are less aggressive {1523}.

Masson tumour

Maktabi A
Laver NM

Definition

Masson tumour is a benign vascular lesion composed of endothelial proliferation, usually within the blood vessel.

ICD-O coding

None

ICD-11 coding

2F2Y Other specified benign cutaneous neoplasms

Related terminology

Acceptable: intravascular papillary endothelial hyperplasia.

Not recommended: intravascular angiomatosis; vegetant intravascular haemangioendothelioma.

Subtype(s)

Primary (pure) Masson tumour; secondary (mixed) Masson tumour; extravascular Masson tumour

Localization

Masson tumour rarely affects periocular tissues. The eyelids are most commonly involved, followed by the orbit and conjunctiva {2044}.

Clinical features

Eyelid and conjunctival lesions usually present as a painless, slow-growing, solid or cystic, red-purple vascular mass {2044}. Orbital lesions may present with proptosis.

Imaging

MRI demonstrates a well-circumscribed homogeneously enhancing mass, which is isointense on T1-weighted imaging and hyperintense on T2-weighted imaging {830}.

Epidemiology

It is estimated that Masson tumour accounts for approximately 2% of all benign and malignant vascular tumours of the skin and subcutaneous tissues {940}. This lesion has no clear sex, age, or race predilection. There is a wide age distribution, ranging from 9 months to 80 years {940,2044}.

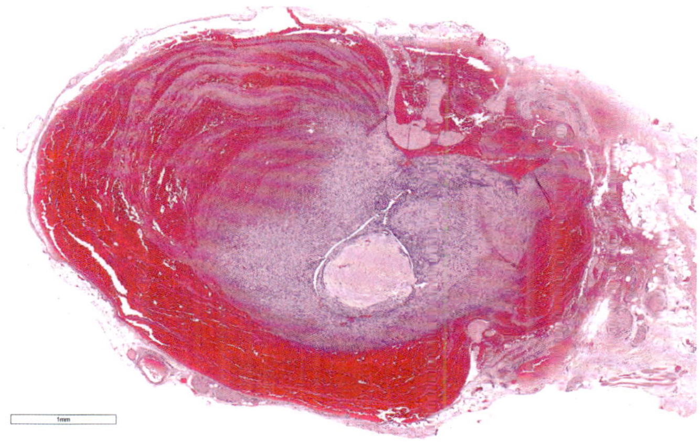

Fig. 11.64 Masson tumour. Vascular proliferation in a background of organizing haemorrhage within a dilated varix.

Etiology

Masson tumour is currently believed to be a reactive lesion, associated with organized thrombus formation and recanalization within a dilated vascular space, pre-existing vascular abnormality, or haematoma {1694}.

Pathogenesis

Vascular proliferation may be driven by thrombus-induced hypoxia, as supported by the upregulation of HIF-1α and VEGF expression in the proliferating vascular endothelium {1694, 795}.

Macroscopic appearance

The lesion appears grossly as a circumscribed red-purple mass with a cystic component.

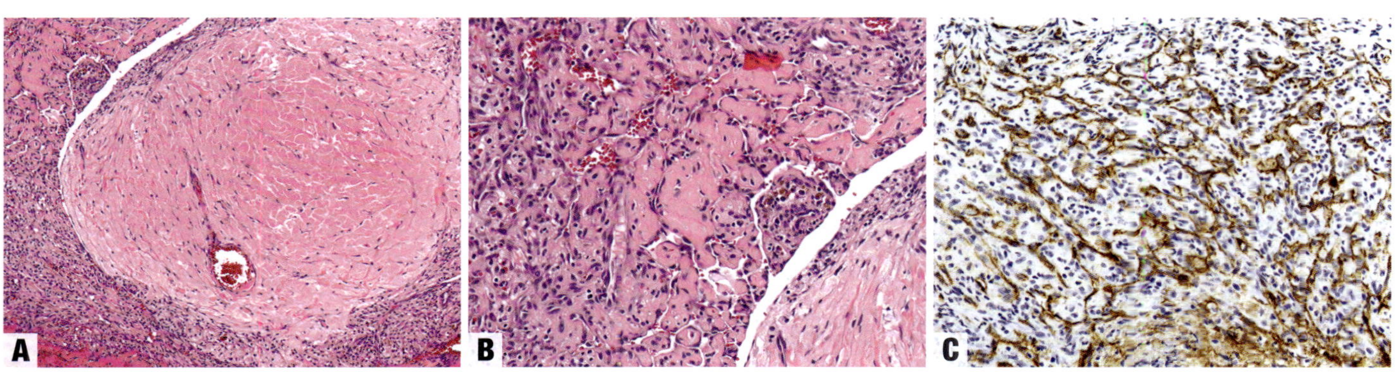

Fig. 11.65 Masson tumour. **A** Higher magnification demonstrates a thrombus with partial recanalization and vascular proliferation. **B** The lesion is composed of papillary and interconnecting fibrous trabeculae lined by a single layer of endothelial cells. **C** The flattened endothelial cells express CD31.

Histopathology

Masson tumour is a circumscribed lesion composed of papillary, interconnecting fibrous trabeculae lined by a single layer of flattened or plump endothelial cells in a background of fibrin thrombi. Primary lesions are observed within a dilated normal vascular channel, most frequently a vein. Secondary lesions arise as focal changes in the setting of a pre-existing vascular abnormality, such as a vascular malformation. A third, rare, subtype appears as an extravascular papillary endothelial proliferation in an organizing haematoma {2044,1272}.

Immunohistochemistry (generally not required for diagnosis) demonstrates positivity of lesional cells for CD31, CD34, ERG, and SMA {3679}.

Differential diagnosis

An absence of infiltrative margins, significant nuclear atypia, frequent mitotic figures, and necrosis help distinguish Masson tumour from angiosarcoma {830,630,1008}.

Cytology

Not relevant

Diagnostic molecular pathology

Not relevant

Essential and desirable diagnostic criteria

Essential: circumscribed papillary lesion lined by benign endothelial cells with hyalinized cores in a background of an organizing haematoma/thrombus.

Desirable: intravascular location.

Staging

Not applicable

Prognosis and prediction

The lesion is benign with no documented malignant transformation. Complete excision is curative {2044}. Orbital lesions can be rarely associated with visual loss from optic nerve compression {940}.

Infantile haemangioma

Calonje JE
Colmenero I
Farmer J
Mudhar HS

Definition
Infantile haemangioma (IH) is a benign vascular tumour characterized by a rapid proliferative phase during infancy followed by gradual involution.

ICD-O coding
9131/0 Infantile haemangioma

ICD-11 coding
2E81.2Y & XH3U29 Other specified benign vascular neoplasms of infancy or childhood & Capillary haemangioma

Related terminology
Not recommended: capillary haemangioma; juvenile haemangioma; strawberry naevus; capillary-cavernous haemangioma; infantile haemangioendothelioma.

Subtype(s)
None

Localization
IH most commonly involves the skin of the upper eyelid / orbit and less frequently the conjunctiva, sclera, and iris {3296,3046,2729,307}.

Clinical features
IH appears soon after birth as a distinct or diffuse red mass and undergoes rapid growth (up to 2 years), with most tumours involuting by 48 months {3046,2427}. Approximately 20% of children have additional non-periocular haemangiomas {117}.

Epidemiology
IHs have a female predilection and more common in White populations and premature infants {117}. This lesion accounts for 1–5% of all ocular adnexal tumours {3069,2968,3721,1296}, 40–80% of all vascular eyelid tumours {1200,3721}, and 15–20% of vascular conjunctival tumours {3046,2968}.

Etiology
The etiology of IH is not well understood. Germline genetic variants and familial clustering have been reported as risk factors {493}.

Pathogenesis
IH is caused by the uncontrolled proliferation of clonally expanded vascular endothelial cells {398}. Causative genes have not been described. Hypoxia has been postulated to play a role in the pathogenesis of IH, supported by the demonstration of GLUT1, IGF2, VEGF-A, and HIF1α in endothelial cells {742,2721,828}. Immunophenotypic similarity to placental microvessels has raised a theory that IH may result from embolization of placental cells or stem cells differentiating towards placental vascular cells {2402}.

Macroscopic appearance
IH usually occurs as a lobulated vascular-appearing mass.

Histopathology
IH in the proliferative stage is composed of capillary-sized vascular channels lined by plump endothelial cells intermixed with pericytes, arranged in lobules around larger vessels. In the regressive stages, the lobules are progressively replaced by fibrosis.

Immunohistochemistry
Endothelial cells express GLUT1, CD31, ERG and CD34 and lack staining with D2-40 {1486}.

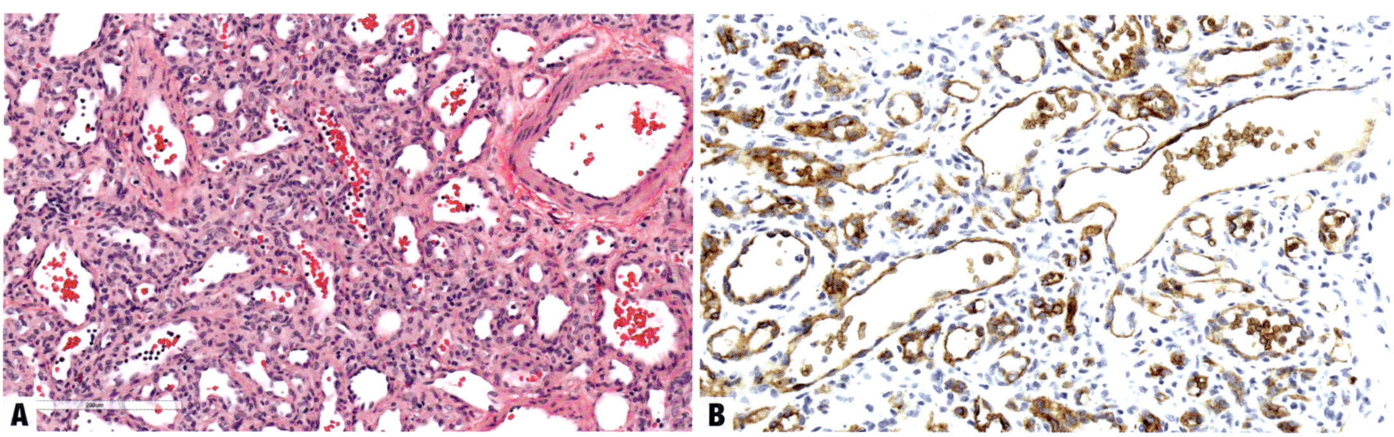

Fig. 11.66 Infantile haemangioma. **A** Higher magnification highlights plump endothelial cells lining the small-calibre vascular channels. **B** Vascular endothelium strongly and diffusely expresses GLUT1. Note GLUT1 expression in the red blood cells, an internal positive control.

Differential diagnosis
Congenital non-progressive haemangiomas and lobular capillary haemangioma (see related section) are distinguished from IH based on clinicopathological correlation and GLUT1 immunohistochemistry.

Cytology
Not clinically relevant

Diagnostic molecular pathology
Not relevant

Essential and desirable diagnostic criteria
Essential: proliferative stage: lobules of capillaries each of which is surrounded by a layer of pericytes; regressive stage: fibrous tissue replacing capillary lobules.
Desirable: endothelial cells are GLUT1-positive.

Staging
Not relevant

Prognosis and prediction
IH involutes spontaneously; some lesions can be associated with amblyopia from compression of the eyeball and obscuration of vision. Eyelid lesions respond to oral and topical propranolol {3459,1248}.

Lobular capillary haemangioma

Calonje JE
Colmenero I
Farmer J
Mudhar HS

Definition

Lobular capillary haemangioma (LCH) is a benign vascular cutaneous and mucosal neoplasm that consists of a proliferation of capillaries with a lobular architecture.

ICD-O coding

9131/0 Lobular capillary haemangioma

ICD-11 coding

2F26 Lobular capillary haemangioma

Related terminology

Not recommended: pyogenic granuloma.

Subtype(s)

None

Localization

LCH occurs in the eyelid, the conjunctiva, and, less frequently, the sclera {3186,291}.

Clinical features

LCH presents as a rapidly growing (weeks to months), circumscribed, lobular, red, occasionally ulcerated, vascular mass {1467,399,1136,291,3186}.

Epidemiology

LCH of the periocular region is rare. This tumour occurs without appreciable sex predilection in adults at a median age of 40 years {3186,291}.

Etiology

The etiology of LCH is not well understood. Conjunctival LCH has been occasionally associated with pregnancy {2908}. Non-periocular LCH has been associated with vascular malformations and biological agents (retinoids and BRAF inhibitors) {699, 924,1316,1683}.

Pathogenesis

LCH may be driven by *FLT4* and the nitric oxide pathway {1135}. *BRAF*, *KRAS*, *HRAS*, *NRAS*, *GNA11*, and *GNA14* mutations have been reported in cutaneous LCH {2533,1176,1946}, suggesting that MAPK signalling activation may be involved in the pathogenesis of some lesions.

Macroscopic appearance

See *Clinical features*.

Histopathology

LCH consists of lobular arrangements of numerous capillary-sized vessels lined by proliferating endothelial cells {3046}. Each vascular channel is surrounded by a layer of pericytes.

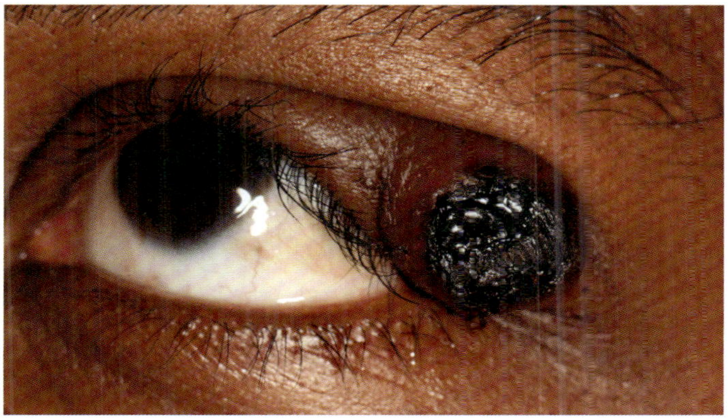

Fig. 11.67 Lobular capillary haemangioma of the eyelid skin. A dome-shaped ulcerated nodule in the upper eyelid in a 35-year-old man.

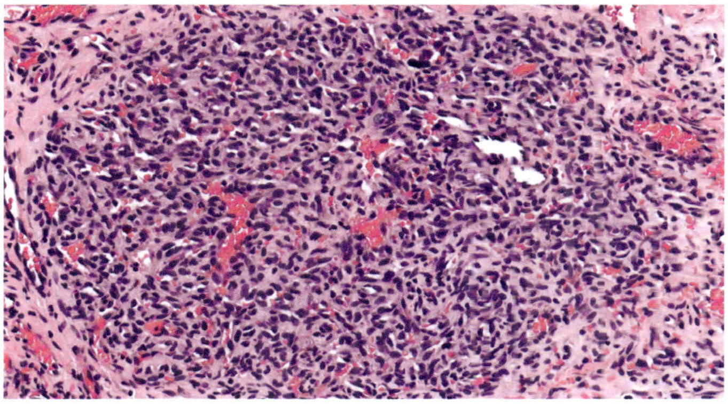

Fig. 11.68 Lobular capillary haemangioma of the eyelid skin. Lobular proliferation of small vascular channels.

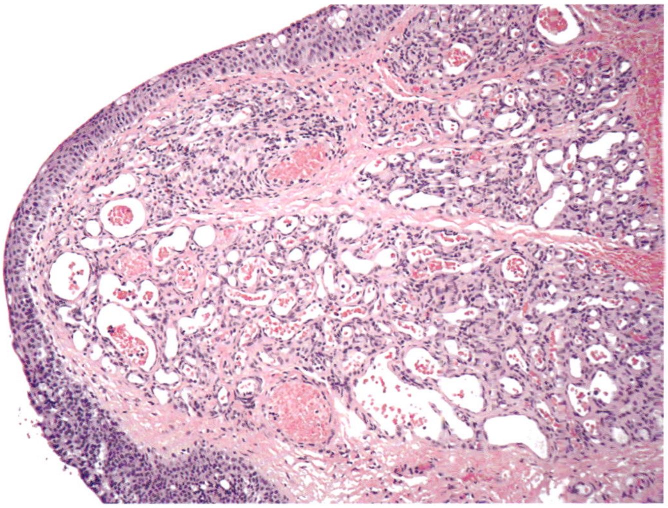

Fig. 11.69 Lobular capillary haemangioma of the conjunctiva. Lobules of capillary-sized vessels of varying canalization in the conjunctival substantia propria.

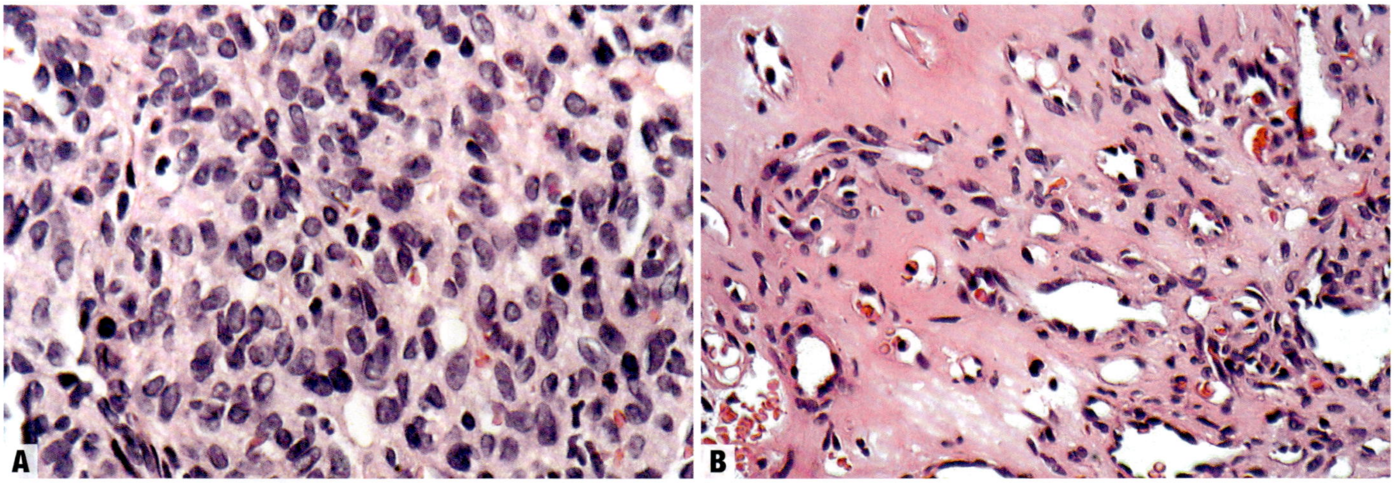

Fig. 11.70 Lobular capillary haemangioma of the conjunctiva. **A** A solid area of vascular endothelial proliferation with minimal canalization. **B** Sclerotic focus in lobular capillary haemangioma.

The overlying epithelium/epidermis is often thinned and frequently ulcerated. There may be oedema and inflammation in the area of ulceration where, in addition, granulation tissue–like changes may be seen. The lobular arrangement of the lesion and relatively scant inflammatory infiltrate in the non-ulcerated region distinguish LCH from the exuberant granulation tissue in the conjunctiva (a lesion termed conjunctival pyogenic granuloma by clinicians) {3186,291}.

Immunohistochemistry

Endothelial cells express CD31, ERG, and CD34, and are negative for GLUT1 and on staining with D2-40 {3186}.

Cytology

Not clinically relevant

Diagnostic molecular pathology

Not clinically relevant

Essential and desirable diagnostic criteria

Essential: lobular proliferation of capillaries associated with oedematous stroma.

Desirable: endothelial cells are GLUT1-negative.

Staging

Not relevant

Prognosis and prediction

Periocular LCH is successfully treated with complete excision {3186,291}.

Lymphangiectasia

Mudhar HS
Alkatan H
Colmenero I
Thway K

Definition
Lymphangiectasia is a bulbar conjunctival dilation of developmentally normal lymphatic channels, produced as a result of degenerative, inflammatory, iatrogenic, or neoplastic etiologies, leading to either focal or diffuse lymphatic channel dilation.

ICD-O coding
None

ICD-11 coding
9A61.40 Vascular abnormalities of conjunctiva

Related terminology
None

Subtype(s)
None

Localization
Lymphangiectasia affects the bulbar conjunctiva.

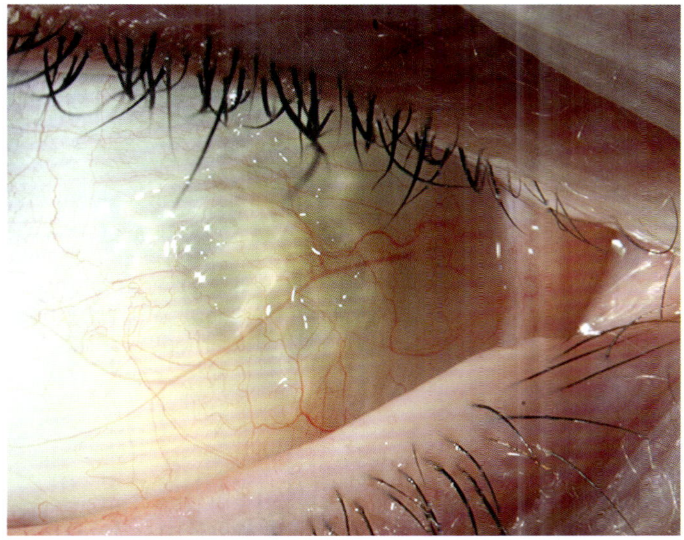

Fig. 11.71 Conjunctival lymphangiectasia. Lymphangiectasis of the medial conjunctiva showing a multiloculated, clear cystic lesion.

Clinical features
Lymphangiectasia presents with ocular surface irritation {3579}. Most lesions involve the temporal bulbar conjunctiva. A common comorbidity is pterygium {3579}. If blood is present in the dilated lymphatics, it is termed lymphangiectasia haemorrhagica {1984}.

Epidemiology
Lymphangiectasia accounts for 1% of all conjunctival lesions and 5–8% of all conjunctival cystic lesions {1181,2357,3319}. In the largest series of conjunctival vascular lesions, lymphangiectasia accounts for 19% of 140 cases, with a male predilection {3046,3579}.

Etiology
Lymphangiectasia can be induced by IgE-mediated ocular surface allergies, degenerative lesions (especially pterygium and conjunctivochalasis), other inflammatory or local neoplastic diseases, organ transplant rejection, or scarring from ocular trauma, surgery, and radiotherapy {1181,3579,1660,1271}. There is also association with Fabry disease {3130} and hereditary transthyretin amyloidosis {1286,443}.

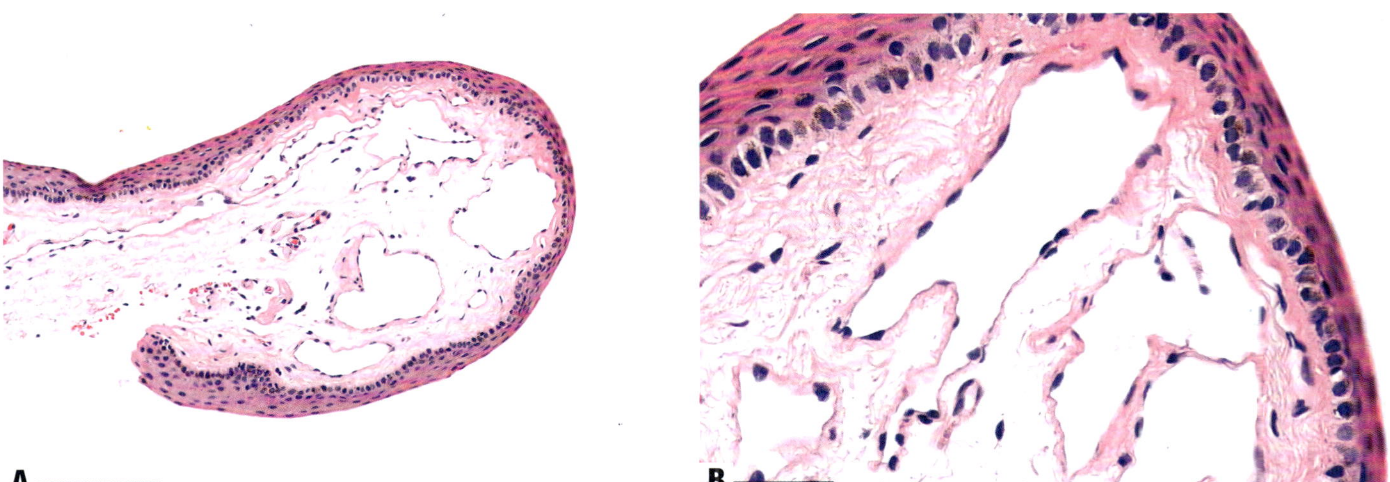

Fig. 11.72 Conjunctival lymphangiectasia. **A** Dilation of conjunctival lymphatic channels, with surrounding oedematous substantia propria. **B** Higher magnification showing flattened endothelial cells lining the fibrous wall of an ectatic lymphatic channel.

Pathogenesis

Lymphangiectasia is caused by the obstruction of normal lymphatic channels by local perilymphatic scarring or distal obstruction {3579}. Lymphangiectasia haemorrhagica is caused by abnormal communications between conjunctival lymphatics and the deep conjunctival venous plexus {1984}, with retrograde flow into the lymphatics.

Macroscopic appearance

See *Clinical features*.

Histopathology

Developmentally normal lymphatic channels are dilated and lined by flattened endothelial cells that stain positive with D2-40. The dilated channels may contain proteinaceous material and lymphocyte clusters. The surrounding stroma may be oedematous, fibrotic, and chronically inflamed {3579,1049}. The overlying conjunctival epithelium may show squamous metaplasia and/or keratinization {3579}. In lymphangiectasia haemorrhagica conjunctivae, blood will be seen in the lumen {1984}.

Cytology

Not relevant

Diagnostic molecular pathology

Not clinically relevant

Essential and desirable diagnostic criteria

Essential: dilation of normal lymphatic channels, lined by flattened endothelial cells.

Desirable: establishing a cause of the secondary lymphatic dilation (e.g. degenerative, inflammatory, iatrogenic, neoplastic); immunohistochemical expression of CD31 and CD34 and staining with D2-40 in the endothelial cells.

Staging

Not clinically relevant

Prognosis and prediction

Asymptomatic lesions can be observed. Symptomatic cases can be locally excised {2159,3180,3228,3579} with a low risk of recurrence. Other modalities include cryotherapy, diathermy, and argon laser {1029,217,1984}.

Epithelioid haemangioma

Mittal R
Proia AD
Wang J

Definition

Epithelioid haemangioma (EH) is a benign vascular neoplasm composed of well-formed capillary-sized vessels lined by plump epithelioid endothelial cells in a variable background of chronic inflammation containing numerous eosinophils.

ICD-O coding

9125/0 Epithelioid haemangioma
9125/0 Cellular epithelioid haemangioma
9125/0 Atypical epithelioid haemangioma

ICD-11 coding

2E81.0Y & XH10T4 Neoplastic haemangioma of other specified site & Epithelioid haemangioma

Related terminology

Not recommended: angiolymphoid hyperplasia with eosinophilia; histiocytoid haemangioma.

Subtype(s)

Cellular epithelioid haemangioma; atypical epithelioid haemangioma

Localization

EH can involve the eyelid skin and superficial and deep orbital soft tissues {2429,220,2306,3210}.

Clinical features

Clinical signs and symptoms are related to the mass effect, and include eyelid fullness, ptosis, globe displacement/proptosis, and ocular motility restriction {220,2306}. The lesion can be either poorly defined or well circumscribed on imaging {220, 2306}.

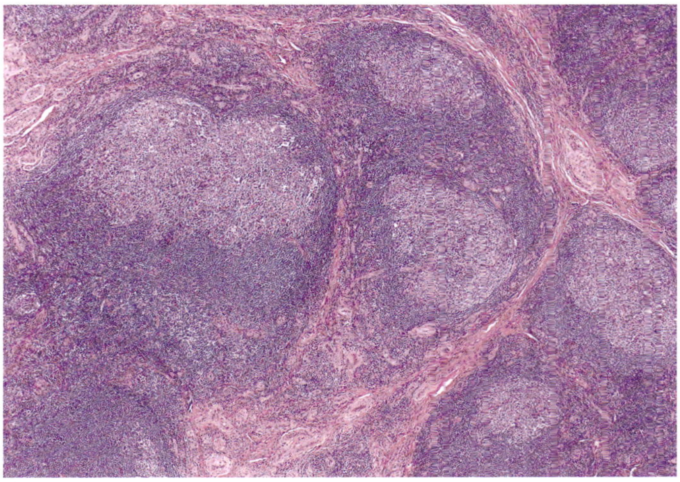

Fig. 11.73 Epithelioid haemangioma. Prominent lymphoid follicles and intervening vascular proliferation are observed.

Epidemiology

EH may occur at any age (reported range 11–86 years) with a peak incidence in the fourth decade of life {220,2306}. There is no significant sex predilection {2306,220}.

Etiology

Unknown

Pathogenesis

EH is characterized by recurrent fusions involving the *FOS* or *FOSB* genes in as many as one half of cases {168,1391}. *FOS*-negative and *FOSB*-negative tumours may harbour an alternative *GATA6*::*FOXO1* fusion {169}.

Macroscopic appearance

Grossly, EH is circumscribed and nodular or multinodular.

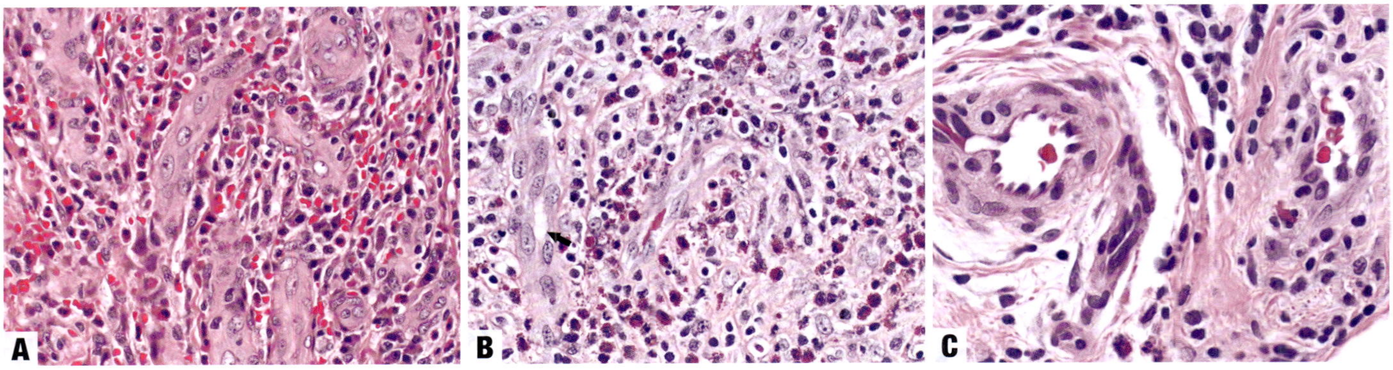

Fig. 11.74 Epithelioid haemangioma. **A** High-power view shows proliferating vessels with epithelioid endothelial cells with abundant eosinophilic cytoplasm, round or oval nuclei, small nucleoli in some cells, and a lack of vascular lumina. The stroma has a mixture of mononuclear leukocytes and eosinophils. **B** Endothelial cells may have large cytoplasmic vacuoles (arrow), so-called blister cells. This orbital tumour has numerous stromal eosinophils. **C** Endothelial cells lining larger-calibre vessels may protrude into the lumen with a tombstone pattern, as in this lacrimal gland tumour.

Histopathology

EH typically manifests as a lobular or multinodular proliferation of small vessels, frequently surrounding a central small artery with more mature vessels at the periphery of the lobules {967, 904,3416}. The endothelial cells have a distinctive appearance with an abundant eosinophilic cytoplasm, large rounded nuclei, and a central nucleolus, and are associated with a pericytic layer. The endothelial cells may contain large cytoplasmic vacuoles (blister cells) and may protrude into the lumen with a tombstone pattern {967,904,2137}. A variably intense infiltrate of lymphocytes with occasional lymphoid follicles, eosinophils, and plasma cells is noted in an oedematous stroma {3416,967}. Mitotic figures are rare {967}.

Immunohistochemistry

The endothelial cells express CD31, FLI1, ERG, and to a lesser extent CD34 {967,1391}. Expression of cytokeratin and EMA may be noted focally {2406,3474}. Expression of FOSB may be helpful in distinguishing from malignant epithelioid vascular tumours {1405}.

Cytology

Not relevant

Diagnostic molecular pathology

Diagnostic molecular pathology includes evaluation for *FOS* or *FOSB* gene rearrangements in some cases {1980,1391,2445}.

Essential and desirable diagnostic criteria

Essential: lobular vascular proliferation of epithelioid endothelial cells with abundant eosinophilic cytoplasm and enlarged round nuclei; stroma with chronic inflammation and eosinophils.

Desirable: demonstration of FOSB expression or rearrangements of the *FOS* and/or *FOSB* genes may be useful in a subset of cases.

Staging

Not relevant

Prognosis and prediction

Complete surgical excision is the treatment of choice, but lesions may recur {31,220}. Oral propranolol has been used in several reported recurrent or incompletely excised orbital lesions in young children {2284,2133}.

Haemangioblastoma

Grossniklaus HE
Tihan T

Definition

Haemangioblastoma of the retina is a vascular tumour defined by unique stromal cells that have characteristic histological, immunohistochemical, and molecular features (e.g. *VHL* alterations).

ICD-O coding

9161/1 Haemangioblastoma

ICD-11 coding

2F36.Y & XH6810 Other specified benign neoplasm of eye or ocular adnexa & Haemangioblastoma

Related terminology

Not recommended: von Hippel's tumour; retinal capillary haemangioma; angiomatosis retinae; angioblastoma.

Subtype(s)

None

Localization

Haemangioblastomas usually occur in the retina, where they are most common in the temporal quadrants {3105}. Lesions can be located in association with the optic disc (juxtapapillary) or within the retina elsewhere (extrapapillary) {3605}. Haemangioblastomas can also occur in the optic nerve head, retrobulbar optic nerve {583,2193,3105}, and rarely in the orbit {2113}.

Clinical features

Small retinal haemangioblastomas appear as flat or slightly raised clumps of capillary-sized vessels. Juxtapapillary lesions have a similar appearance, but they often have an indistinct margin where they abut the optic nerve, and they are often associated with serous retinal detachment. Larger haemangioblastomas are elevated, and lipid exudate surrounds the lesion because of vascular leakage. The dense capillary plexus acts as a shunt, causing the feeding artery and draining vein to become dilated, resulting in a very characteristic clinical appearance. Larger haemangioblastomas often also have a fibrotic so-called glial component, and the overlying vitreous may become adherent to the lesion. Vascular leakage may progress to the point of exudative retinal detachment, with the vitreous adhesion providing a tractional component to the detachment. A small proportion of

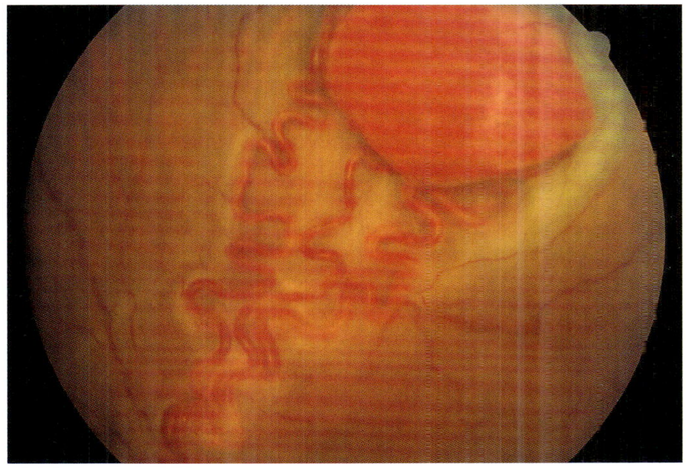

Fig. 11.75 Haemangioblastoma of the retina. This large retinal haemangioblastoma is elevated and contains very prominent feeder vessels and surrounding lipid exudate.

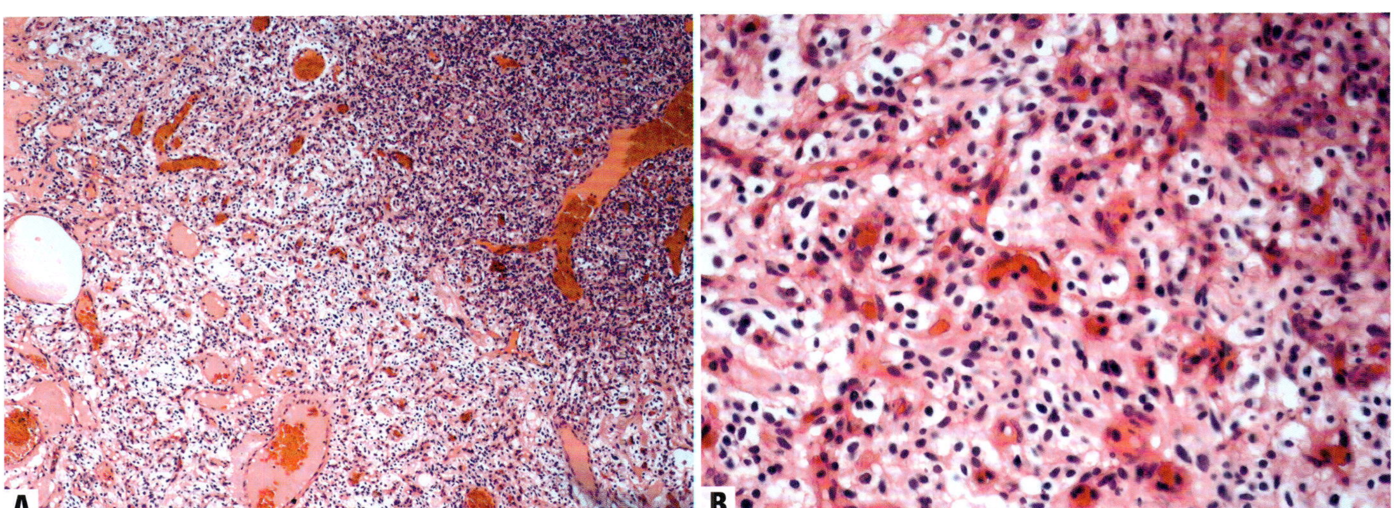

Fig. 11.76 Haemangioblastoma of the retina. **A** A low-magnification photomicrograph of a retinal haemangioblastoma shows numerous stromal cells and capillary-sized vessels. **B** A high magnification of a retinal haemangioblastoma shows the foamy/clear cytoplasm of stromal cells and numerous small vascular channels.

patients develop retinal neovascularization {583}. In the most extreme cases, progressive exudative retinal detachment can lead to phthisis bulbi.

Epidemiology

Retinal haemangioblastomas can occur sporadically or as part of von Hippel–Lindau syndrome (VHL) along with CNS haemangioblastomas (see *Von Hippel–Lindau syndrome*, p. 499). Sporadic tumours are generally solitary and unilateral, whereas haemangioblastomas occurring in VHL are frequently multiple with bilateral involvement. The median patient age at diagnosis of sporadic cases has been reported to be about 40 years, and older than those with VHL, which typically arises within the second decade of life {3105,337}. There is equal sex distribution {583,3105}. Approximately 50% of patients with *VHL* mutations develop retinal haemangioblastoma {583}.

Etiology

Retinal haemangioblastomas occur in 45% of patients with partial deletions, simple missense mutations, or nonsense mutations of the *VHL* gene at chromosome 3p25.3; they are much less common in patients with complete deletion of the *VHL* gene, occurring in only 9% {583}. In VHL, there is a germline defect in one copy of the gene; random loss of the normal allele (loss of heterozygosity) predisposes patients to developing haemangioblastomas (see *Von Hippel–Lindau syndrome*, p. 499). In sporadic cases, presumably there is somatic loss of both copies of the *VHL* gene, resulting in a similar but solitary tumour {583,2878}.

Pathogenesis

VHL is a tumour suppressor gene, encoding VHL protein, which has many different functions (see *Von Hippel–Lindau syndrome*, p. 499). VHL protein is lost in the stromal cells of the tumour {516}, leading to upregulation of HIF1 and angiogenic factors, including VEGF. Tumorigenesis in VHL has been suggested to parallel haemangioblast formation and differentiation in the embryo {3081,596,1123}.

Macroscopic appearance

The tumours may appear as well-circumscribed reddish-orange masses sometimes associated with a dilated, tortuous feeding artery {712,3107}.

Histopathology

Haemangioblastomas demonstrate two components: stromal cells with hyperchromatic nuclei and abundant pink to clear foamy cytoplasm with fine vacuoles; and capillary-sized vascular channels. Small clusters of angiomesenchymal cells, called tumourlet cells, have also been described {515}. Some haemangioblastomas may exhibit extramedullary haematopoiesis, but this feature is more common in extraocular tumours. The stromal cells and tumourlet cells may express CD133, a marker present on haematopoietic, endothelial, and neural progenitor cells. Only the stromal cells harbour alterations in the *VHL* gene; these alterations are not present in the vascular or glial components {516}. This observation suggests that only the stromal cells are truly neoplastic cells {515}. The neoplastic stromal cells frequently express inhibin {1347,2238}, which has been considered as one of the key diagnostic features. In addition stromal cells may express aquaporin and cytoplasmic brachyury, and stain positive with D2-40 {3264,266}. Negative staining for PAX2, PAX8, RCCm, and EMA helps exclude metastatic renal cell carcinoma {482}. Proliferation markers typically show very low indices.

Cytology

Not clinically relevant

Diagnostic molecular pathology

Demonstration of a *VHL* germline sequence variant is desirable to confirm VHL.

Essential and desirable diagnostic criteria

Essential: a non-infiltrative tumour composed of large multivacuolated and lipidized stromal cells in a rich capillary network; AND one of the following: focal or strong immunopositivity for inhibin in stromal cells OR loss or inactivation of the *VHL* gene OR clinical diagnosis of VHL disease.

Staging

No currently accepted staging system is recognized.

Prognosis and prediction

The disease phenotype depends on the type of germline mutation present in the *VHL* gene (see *Von Hippel–Lindau syndrome*, p. 499). Treatment has been reported to correlate with tumour size, location, degree of exudation, presence of retinal detachment, and associated fibrotic or haemorrhagic changes {3605}. The prognosis for vision in patients with VHL is good: the majority of patients retain 20/20 (or better) vision in at least one eye {583,3605}. Laser therapy and cryotherapy are effective treatments for small to medium-sized intraocular haemangioblastomas that do not involve the optic nerve. Surgical resection of unresponsive and large retinal haemangioblastomas is becoming increasingly common, with good visual outcomes {2878,3605}. Treatment of haemangioblastomas involving the optic nerve remains challenging. In terms of systemic morbidity and overall survival in VHL, the prognosis depends on the treatment of the other associated pathologies such as cerebellar haemangioblastoma and renal cell carcinoma.

Angiosarcoma of soft tissue

Flucke U
Thway K

Definition

Angiosarcoma (AS) is a rare aggressive sarcoma that recapitulates features of endothelial cells.

ICD-O coding

9120/3 Angiosarcoma

ICD-11 coding

2B56.Y & XH6264 Angiosarcoma, other specified primary site & Haemangiosarcoma

Related terminology

Not recommended: haemangiosarcoma; lymphangiosarcoma; malignant haemangioendothelioma; malignant angioendothelioma.

Subtype(s)

None

Localization

AS associated with ultraviolet (UV) radiation occurs in skin, mainly of the scalp and face, including the eyelids. Deep periocular tissues can be involved secondarily or as a primary process {2218}.

Clinical features

AS usually presents as a rapidly growing haemorrhagic mass or plaque. Symptoms are site-dependent, including visual loss and ptosis {2218}.

Epidemiology

Periocular AS is rare {608}. Eyelid AS typically presents about the seventh decade of life {2218}. Primary orbital AS has a wide age distribution with a median age of 24 years {2188}.

Etiology

UV or other radiation exposure is a risk factor. The etiology is unknown for de novo tumours {3568,1209,2464}.

Pathogenesis

The pathogenesis of AS is complex, heterogeneous, and subtype specific. Altered genes include *TP53*, *KDR*, *PLCG1*, *ASXL1*, *PIK3CA*, *COL19A1*, *LPPRC*, *CACNA1S*, *GRIN2A*, *NOTCH2*, and *PTPRB*. Genes affecting the MAPK pathway may be involved. *MYC* and *FLT4* amplification are mainly reported in radiation-induced AS. A high mutation burden is reported in head and neck AS {1209,2464,290,2319,3568}.

Macroscopic appearance

AS is diffuse or (multi)nodular, haemorrhagic and spongy or more solid and fleshy, often with necrosis. Small lesions can be subtle.

Histopathology

The spectrum of AS ranges from well to poorly differentiated lesions. Features can vary within a single neoplasm. Poorly defined variably formed anastomosing vascular channels dissect local tissues, with variable, occasionally predominant solid growth. Atypical spindle or epithelioid endothelial cells are usually multilayered with enlarged, often hyperchromatic nuclei and frequently distinct nucleoli. Pleomorphism can be striking. Mitotic figures, haemorrhage, and necrosis are more frequent in less-differentiated tumours {987}.

Immunohistochemistry

The most reliable immunohistochemical markers are CD31 (strong cytoplasmic and membranous staining) and ERG in combination, with variable CD34. Most ASs also stain with D2-40.

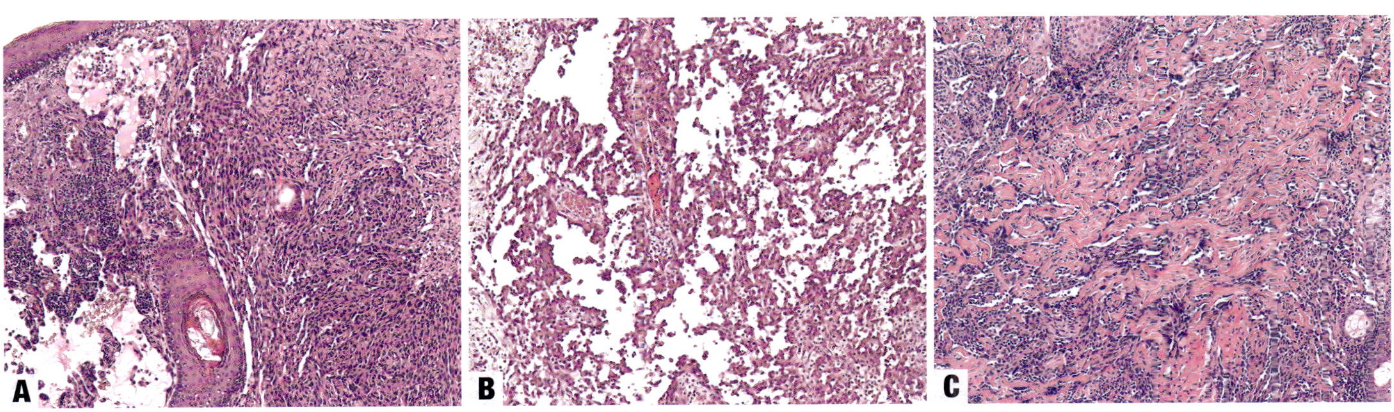

Fig. 11.77 Angiosarcoma. **A** Cutaneous tumour showing dissecting irregular vascular channels with atypical endothelial cells is seen. **B** This lesion consists of an irregular network of poorly defined vessels lined by epithelioid endothelial cells. **C** This skin tumour is characterized by connected dissecting slit-like vessels with pleomorphic endothelial cells.

Differential diagnosis

Loss of pericytic layers by α-SMA distinguishes AS from benign vascular lesions. AS with keratin expression can mimic carcinomas {987}.

Cytology

Cytology demonstrates loosely cohesive clusters and dispersed atypical often oval to spindled cells with pleomorphic variably hyperchromatic nuclei, nucleoli, and mitotic and apoptotic figures. Sometimes cytoplasmic vacuoles are seen {2813}.

Diagnostic molecular pathology

MYC amplification may support the diagnosis of irradiation-induced AS and to a lesser extent (40%) UV-associated AS {2179,3087}.

Methylation profiling can be helpful in discriminating AS from other (vascular) lesions {1756}.

Essential and desirable diagnostic criteria

Essential: at least focal vasoformative growth; multilayering of endothelial cells in a morphologically well-differentiated neoplasm; nuclear atypia, increased mitoses; CD31 and ERG positivity.

Staging

Staging is not recommended as the aggressive nature of AS does not align with soft tissue staging systems.

Prognosis and prediction

AS of soft tissue is highly aggressive. Five-year overall survival is about 25–50% {987,2464,1834}.

Glomus tumour

Dickson BC
Specht CS

Definition

Glomus tumour is a mesenchymal neoplasm showing differentiation analogous to perivascular cells of the glomus body.

ICD-O coding

8711/0 Glomus tumour, NOS
8711/1 Glomus tumour of uncertain malignant potential
8711/3 Glomus tumour, malignant

ICD-11 coding

2F36.Y & XH47J2 Other specified benign neoplasm of eye or ocular adnexa & Glomus tumour, NOS
2D0Y & XH21E6 Other specified malignant neoplasms of eye or ocular adnexa & Glomus tumour, malignant

Related terminology

None

Subtype(s)

Glomangioma; symplastic glomus tumour; malignant glomus tumour

Localization

Tumours may arise in the soft tissue or bone {2875,348,40}. The orbit and eyelid are rarely involved {1522,1512}.

Clinical features

Pain is a common manifestation {2135}. Eye tumours may present with blindness and/or proptosis {1246,522}.

Epidemiology

Glomus tumours rarely involve the eye; they have been reported in children and adults, with no clear sex predilection {1512,1246, 3412}.

Etiology

Most tumours are sporadic. A minority result from a germline *GLMN* {422} or *NF1* mutation {1732,408}.

Pathogenesis

Sporadic non-ophthalmic tumours frequently harbour gene fusions involving *NOTCH1*, *NOTCH2*, or *NOTCH3*, with multiple potential partners (e.g. *MIR143*, *CARMN*) {2283,40,1119}; fusions are less common in malignant tumours {40}. A minority have mutations of *BRAF* {511,1601} or *KRAS* {511}. The molecular pathogenesis appears to vary based on anatomical location. These molecular features are based on non-ophthalmic tumours; however, there is no reason to suspect a difference from those arising elsewhere in the body.

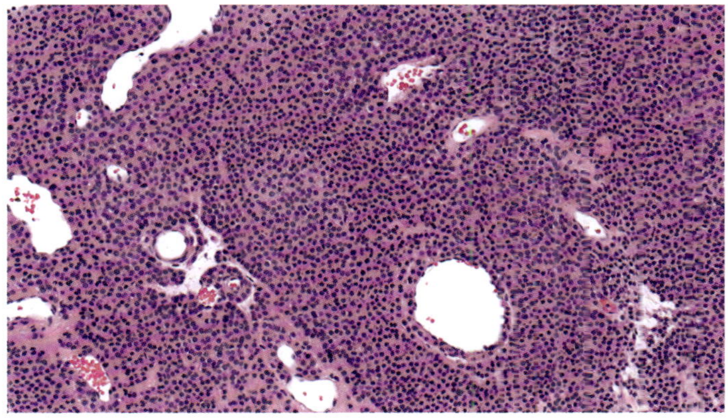

Fig. 11.78 Glomus tumour. A conventional glomus tumour with sheets of polygonal cells with monomorphic central nuclei is seen.

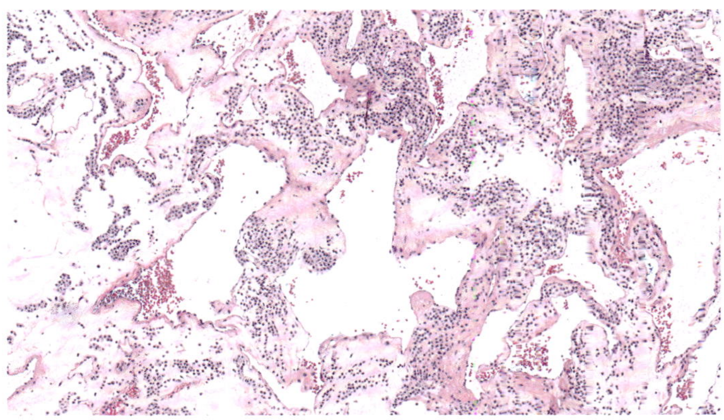

Fig. 11.79 Glomangioma. The tumour shows ectatic vascular spaces lined by multiple layers of glomus cells.

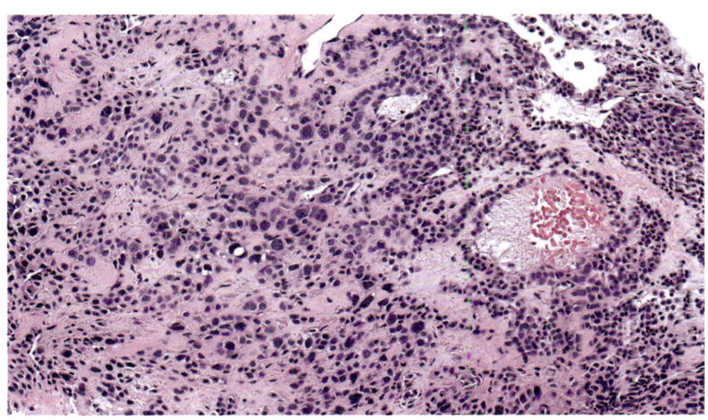

Fig. 11.80 Symplastic glomus tumour. This example shows marked nuclear atypia but absent mitotic activity.

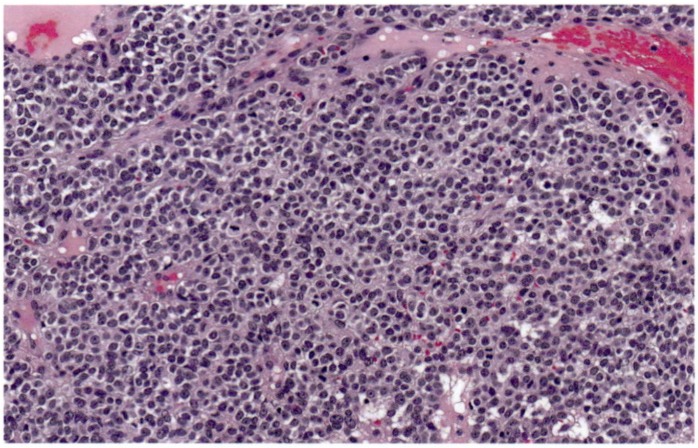

Fig. 11.81 Malignant glomus tumour. This tumour was positive for the *MIR143::NOTCH1* fusion.

Macroscopic appearance

Tumours are typically small and circumscribed. They may appear purple-blue, and solid or cystic {1885}.

Histopathology

Morphologically tumours are composed of sheets of round to polygonal cells. The cytoplasm is eosinophilic to amphophilic with well-defined membranes. The nuclei are centrally located, round to ovoid, and monomorphic; mitotic activity is inconspicuous. Tumours have a delicate capillary-sized vasculature. The intervening stroma may be myxoid to collagenous; glomangioma is additionally characterized by ectatic and branching vascular spaces. Symplastic tumours contain marked nuclear pleomorphism, but no mitotic activity. Malignant tumours are classified based on: (1) atypical mitotic figures, (2) nuclear pleomorphism and high mitotic activity, or (3) size > 20 mm and deep anatomical location {998}.

Immunohistochemistry is typically positive for SMA and h-caldesmon, with variable staining for desmin and CD34.

Cytology

Not clinically relevant

Diagnostic molecular pathology

NOTCH family rearrangement or *BRAF* or *KRAS* mutation, in the appropriate clinical and histomorphological context, may be diagnostically helpful.

Essential and desirable diagnostic criteria

Essential: sheets of round-polygonal cells with well-defined cell borders, and monomorphic round central nuclei.

Desirable: immunoreactivity for SMA or h-caldesmon; NOTCH family rearrangement or mutations involving *BRAF* or *KRAS* in malignant tumours.

Staging

Not clinically relevant

Prognosis and prediction

Conventional glomus tumours are benign. Malignant tumours are locally aggressive with the potential for metastasis {998, 3636}.

Myopericytoma, including myofibroma

Ng T
Dickson BC
Irion LCD

Definition
Myopericytoma is a perivascular myoid neoplasm on a continuum with myofibroma.

ICD-O coding
8824/0 Myofibroma
8824/1 Multicentric myofibromatosis
8824/0 Myopericytoma

ICD-11 coding
2F36.Y & XH2HE9 Other specified benign neoplasm of eye or ocular adnexa & Myopericytoma
2F36.Y & XH0953 Other specified benign neoplasm of eye or ocular adnexa & Myofibroma

Related terminology
None

Subtype(s)
Myofibroma; myofibromatosis; infantile myofibromatosis

Localization
Ophthalmic myopericytoma usually arises in the dermis or subcutis of the eyelid {2280}, and rarely the orbit {1351,2280, 3699}. Paediatric myofibroma may involve orbital or periorbital sites, with frequent involvement of periorbital bones and the skull base, particularly in the setting of infantile myofibromatosis {2353,3521,1958,840,2980,2734,2327}.

Clinical features
Tumours usually occur as a painless mass, sometimes with ptosis or eye displacement {2327}.

Epidemiology
Solitary cases predominate in adults, with a male predominance {2178}; multifocal myofibromatosis arises in paediatric patients, most often at birth or in the first 2 years of life, and has a female predominance {615,1958}.

Etiology
Infantile myofibromatosis is familial, with reports of both autosomal dominant {1416,2824,3148} and recessive {2350} inheritance.

Pathogenesis
PDGFRB mutations are common {1406,34}, with germline mutations seen in familial cases {581,2089}. Cellular myofibromas may demonstrate recurrent *SRF* rearrangement {171,3246,1602}.

Macroscopic appearance
Myopericytomas are usually circumscribed, firm, and homogeneous. Orbital cases of infantile myofibroma average 30 mm (range: 2–100 mm) with frequent bone destruction {2327}.

Histopathology
Myopericytomas are unencapsulated, circumscribed, variably cellular, nodular lesions composed of myoid spindle cells concentrically arranged around prominent vasculature {2178}. Myofibromas are similar but often demonstrate a biphasic pattern, with central hypercellularity showing plump immature-appearing spindle cells, and peripheral nodular growth showing variable hyalinization {2327}. "Cellular myofibroma/myopericytoma" refers to hypercellular and hyperproliferative lesions with infiltrative growth but lacking frankly malignant features including pleomorphism or necrosis {171}; these have not been described in ophthalmic cases.

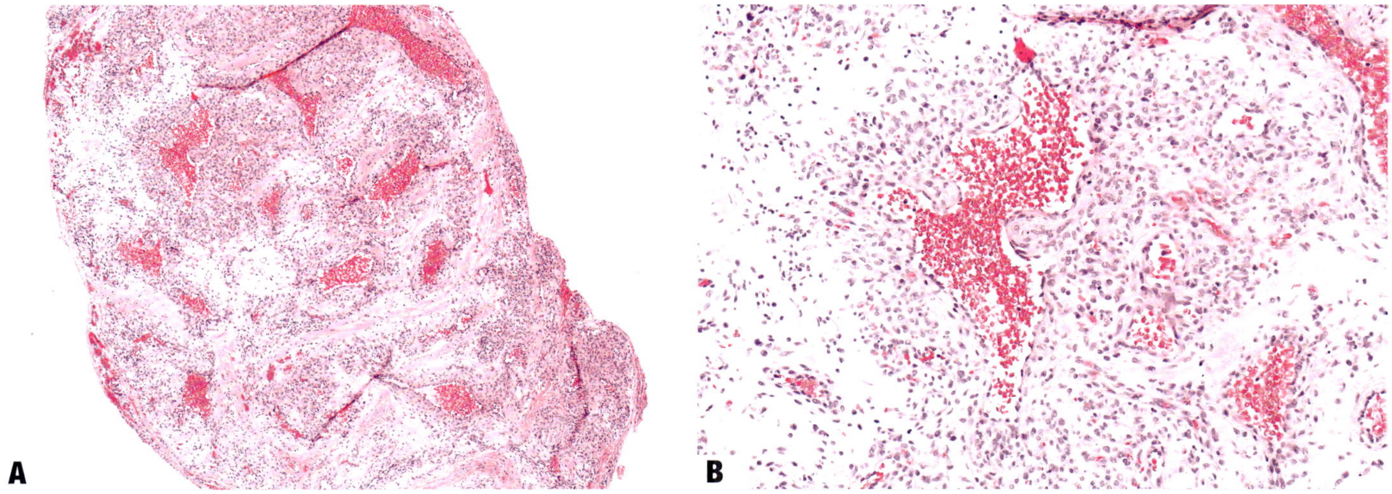

Fig. 11.82 Myopericytoma. **A** Scanning magnification of this well-circumscribed cutaneous lesion of the eyelid shows the characteristic concentric perivascular arrangement of tumour cells. **B** High-power view shows cytologically bland myoid spindle cells.

Myopericytomas/myofibromas express SMA and are often negative for desmin (except *SRF*-rearranged lesions). H-caldesmon may be expressed by both, although less consistently in myofibromas.

Cytology

Cytology is not reported for ophthalmic cases.

Diagnostic molecular pathology

PDGFRB point mutations or *SRF* rearrangement can be diagnostically supportive in the appropriate context.

Essential and desirable diagnostic criteria

Essential: for myopericytoma: bland myoid spindle cells with perivascular concentric growth; for myofibroma: biphasic pattern with immature hypercellular areas surrounded by a less cellular myoid population.

Desirable (in select cases): SMA immunopositivity; *PDGFRB* point mutations or *SRF* rearrangements.

Staging

Not relevant

Prognosis and prediction

Myopericytomas are clinically indolent, although the rare *SRF*-rearranged tumours can behave aggressively {3246}. Solitary myofibromas likewise have an excellent prognosis, with frequent spontaneous regression; occasionally they recur locally after incomplete excision. Cases of multicentric myofibromatosis, particularly those with visceral involvement, have a significantly worse outcome {2327}.

PEComa

Subramanian K
Doyle LA
Larque AB

Definition

PEComas are mesenchymal neoplasms composed of perivascular epithelioid cells (PECs) – distinctive epithelioid cells closely associated with blood vessel walls which express both melanocytic and smooth muscle markers.

ICD-O coding

8714/0 Perivascular epithelioid tumour, benign
8714/3 Perivascular epithelioid tumour, malignant

ICD-11 coding

2F36.Y & XH4CC6 Other specified benign neoplasm of eye or ocular adnexa & Perivascular epithelioid tumour, benign
2B5F.2 & XH9WD1 Sarcoma, not elsewhere classified of other specified sites & Perivascular epithelioid tumour, malignant

Related terminology

Acceptable: angiomyolipoma; epithelioid angiomyolipoma.
Not recommended: clear cell myomelanocytic tumour; clear cell sugar tumour.

Subtype(s)

Perivascular epithelioid tumour, malignant

Localization

PEComas may arise in orbital soft tissues as intraconal or extraconal masses {1440,2336,68,1216,968,2001,3457,2436,1947,188}, in the choroid {1070} and ciliary body {1153,1052}, or superficially involving the eyelid or canthus {806,1052,1070}. Metastatic PEComa to the orbit has also been reported {3403}.

Clinical features

PEComas in and around the eye usually present as slow-growing masses {1070}. Less frequent symptoms include proptosis {3457,68,2336}, lid swelling {806,1052}, and loss of vision with intraocular tumours {1153}.

Epidemiology

PEComas arising in orbital/periorbital locations are very rare; 19 cases have been reported in the literature. The age range at presentation for ophthalmic PEComas is broad (2–54 years), and there is a slight male predilection.

Etiology

Most PEComas are sporadic, but a small subset is associated with tuberous sclerosis {371,1001,1366}. One PEComa arising in the eyelid was associated with tuberous sclerosis {806}.

Pathogenesis

Loss of heterozygosity involving the *TSC2* locus and resulting in activation of the mTOR pathway occurs in most sporadic and tuberous sclerosis–associated tumours {2470}. Deletion of 16p, the location of the *TSC2* gene, indicates the oncogenetic relationship of PEComas and angiomyolipomas as *TSC2*-linked neoplasms. *TP53* mutations have been identified in 63% of *TSC2*-mutated PEComas {39}. A small subset of PEComas harbour *TFE3* gene fusions, which correlate with strong nuclear immunoreactivity for TFE3 {185}. The most common fusion partner with *TFE3* is *SFPQ* (*PSF*) {2664,3275,39}. *DVL2*::*TFE3* and *NONO*::*TFE3* gene fusions have also been identified in PEComa arising in soft tissue {188}. *TFE3*-rearranged PEComa lacks *TSC2* mutations / loss of heterozygosity and thus appears to be pathogenetically distinct {39,2048}. *NONO*::*TFE3* fusions have been reported in one canthal and two orbital PEComas {968,188,1070}. *PRCC*::*TFE3* fusion was reported in a choroidal PEComa {1070}.

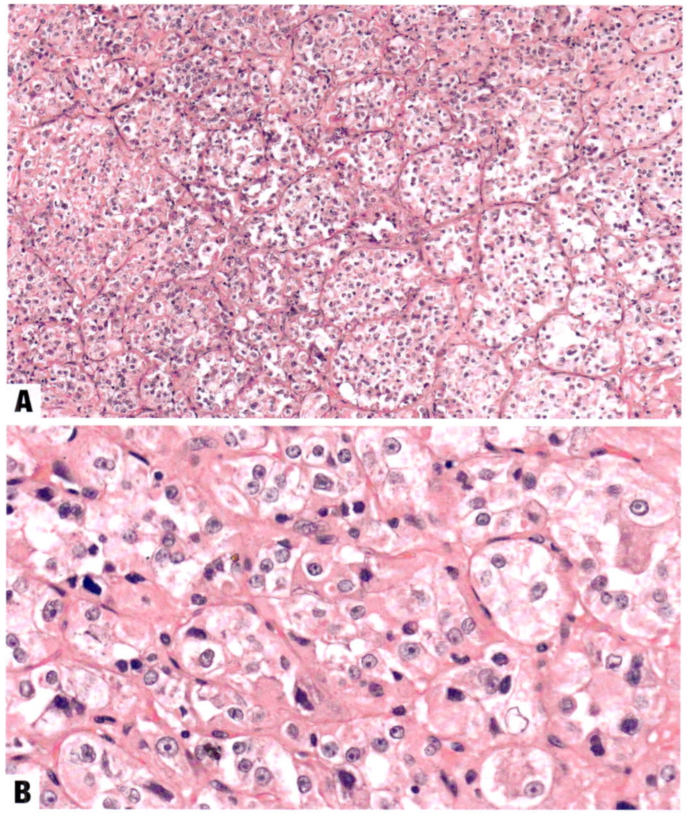

Fig. 11.83 PEComa. **A** Nested and solid alveolar growth patterns are observed. **B** A nested growth pattern of polygonal and epithelioid cells is seen. The cells have large oval nuclei with prominent nucleoli. The cytoplasm is abundant, eosinophilic, and granular.

Macroscopic appearance

PEComas are well circumscribed with a firm or fleshy cut surface, and are brown-yellow in colour. Orbital tumours can have ulceration or haemorrhage {3403}.

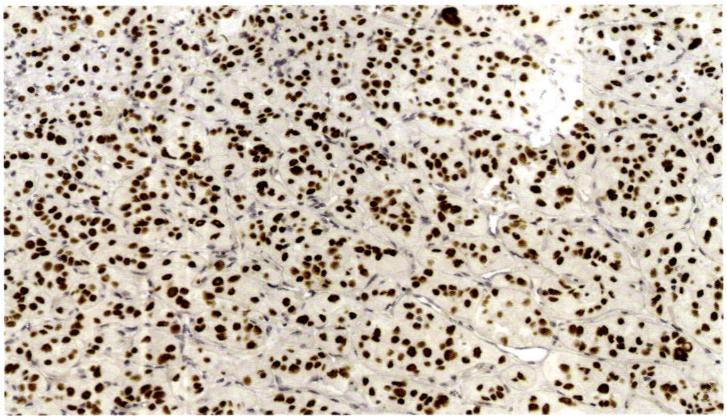

Fig. 11.84 PEComa. Diffuse and strong nuclear expression of TFE3 in tumour cells.

Histopathology

PEComas typically show a nested growth pattern and are composed of epithelioid or spindled cells, or a mix thereof. Most orbital PEComas have an epithelioid cytomorphology with abundant granular eosinophilic or clear cytoplasm and round nuclei with small nucleoli. The nests are surrounded by thin-walled capillaries. PEComa usually shows a distinctive perivascular pattern of growth, with tumour cells radially arranged around vessels, replacing the vessel wall and approaching the endothelium. Hyalinization of the tumour stroma may be present {2336}.

Malignant PEComas generally show variable degrees of nuclear atypia/pleomorphism, mitotic activity, and necrosis {68, 3403,3457}.

Immunohistochemistry

PEComas characteristically express both melanocytic markers, such as HMB45 (the most sensitive immunomarker), melan-A, and MITF, and muscle markers, such as SMA, desmin, and caldesmon {999,1366,821,301,2038}. Expression of melanocytic markers is more common in epithelioid than spindled tumour cells. Desmin and h-caldesmon are often less extensively positive than SMA {1366}. Some tumours lack expression of muscle markers {999}.

Approximately 15% of cases show strong nuclear staining for TFE3 {188,1001,821,185}. PEComas with *TFE3* rearrangement tend to occur in younger patients, have a prominent alveolar growth pattern and epithelioid morphology, and often lack expression of smooth muscle markers {188,2048,2664,39}.

Differential diagnosis

In the orbit, the differential diagnosis of PEComa includes alveolar soft part sarcoma, paraganglioma, and melanoma.

Cytology

Cytology has not been reported for primary cases. Cytological features in 1 case metastatic to the orbit showed epithelioid cells with prominent nucleoli in a haemorrhagic background and an absence of melanin pigmentation {3403}.

Diagnostic molecular pathology

For cases with strong TFE3 protein expression, identification of *TFE3* gene rearrangement or a corresponding fusion gene can help confirm the diagnosis.

Essential and desirable diagnostic criteria

Essential: epithelioid and/or spindle cells with granular eosinophilic to clear cytoplasm; nested, trabecular, or sheet-like architecture with frequent perivascular orientation; variable coexpression of melanocytic and smooth muscle markers.

Desirable: TFE3 expression if smooth muscle markers are negative.

Staging

Not clinically relevant

Prognosis and prediction

While there is limited data specific to ophthalmic PEComa, across all anatomical sites, clinically malignant PEComas are typically large (> 50 mm); show marked nuclear atypia and pleomorphism, conspicuous mitoses, necrosis, and infiltrative margins {1001,301,355}; and pursue an aggressive clinical course. The most common metastatic sites are the liver, lymph nodes, lungs, and bone.

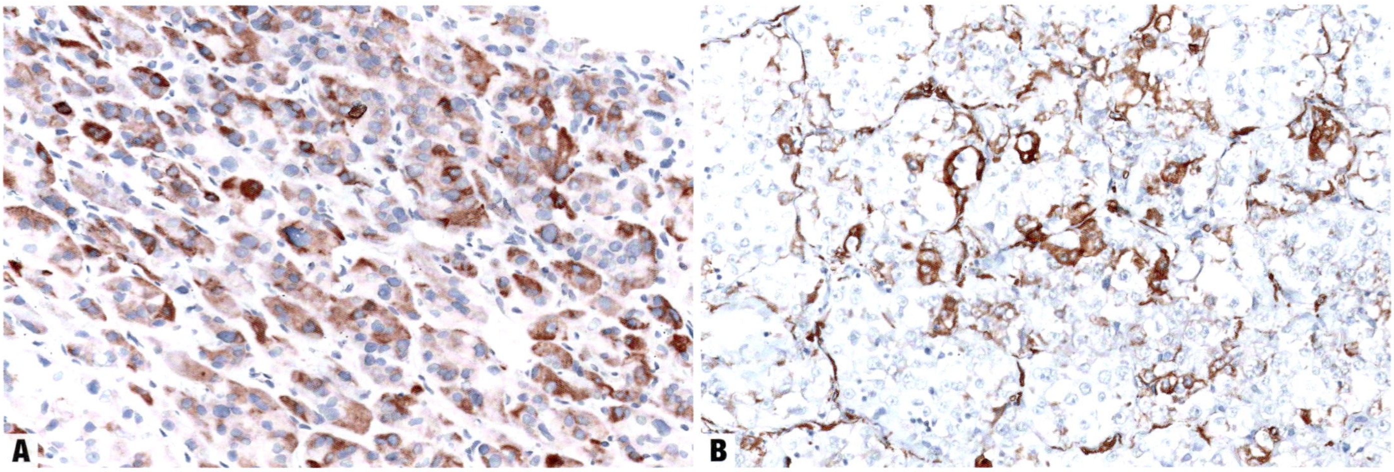

Fig. 11.85 PEComa. **A** HMB45 immunohistochemical expression in the cytoplasm of tumour cells. **B** SMA immunohistochemistry focally expressed in perivascular epithelioid cells.

Epithelioid sarcoma

Nielsen TO
Oda Y

Definition

Epithelioid sarcoma is a malignant soft tissue tumour with hybrid mesenchymal and epithelial morphological and immunophenotypic features.

ICD-O coding

8804/3 Epithelioid sarcoma
8804/3 Classic epithelioid sarcoma
8804/3 Proximal epithelioid sarcoma

ICD-11 coding

2B5F.2 & XH4F96 Sarcoma, not elsewhere classified of other specified sites & Epithelioid sarcoma

Related terminology

None

Subtype(s)

Classic epithelioid sarcoma (also known as conventional or distal epithelioid sarcoma); proximal epithelioid sarcoma

Localization

Epithelioid sarcomas have been reported in the extraconal soft tissues of the orbit.

Clinical features

Patients typically present with a mass which may cause globe displacement depending on location.

Epidemiology

Epithelioid sarcomas account for < 1% of soft tissue sarcomas {1505}, and < 1% of epithelioid sarcomas present in head and neck sites {3647}. In the orbit, 6 primary cases and 1 metastatic case have been reported {3592,108,1632}. Patient age ranged from infancy to 87 years.

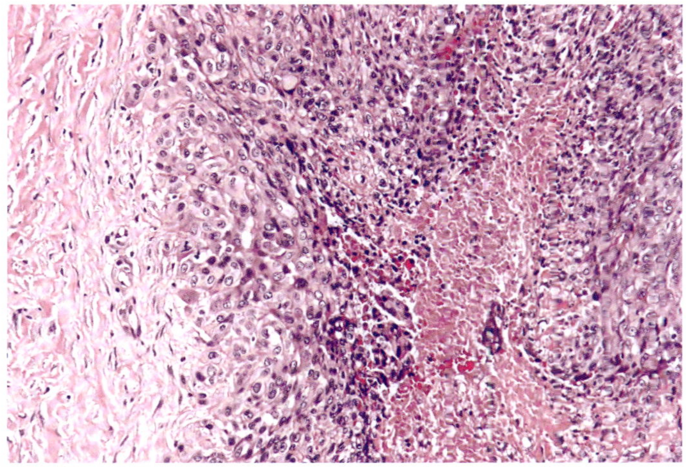

Fig. 11.86 Classic/conventional epithelioid sarcoma. Granulomatous nodule composed of polygonal epithelioid cells, accompanied by central necrosis.

Etiology

Unknown

Pathogenesis

The fundamental oncogenic driver event in epithelioid sarcoma is loss of *SMARCB1*, leading to dysfunction of the BAF chromatin-remodelling complex, which alters cellular differentiation {2329}. The background genome shows complex mutational changes without additional consistent driver events {1493}.

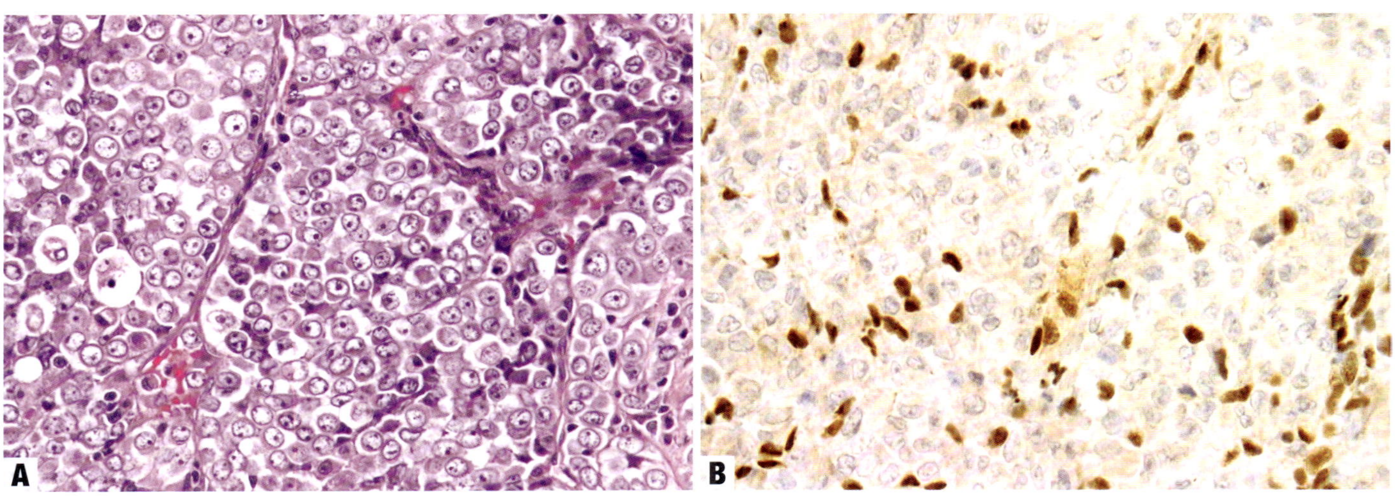

Fig. 11.87 Proximal epithelioid sarcoma. **A** A sheet-like arrangement of poorly differentiated carcinoma-like epithelioid cells with enlarged nuclei and prominent nucleoli. **B** There is loss of expression of SMARCB1 (INI1) in the nuclei of neoplastic tumour cells with retention in stromal and vascular nuclei.

Macroscopic appearance

Epithelioid sarcomas in sites deep to skin form multinodular masses tracking along fascial planes. Cut surfaces show solid grey areas with foci of necrosis and haemorrhage. Orbital cases have ranged from 20 to 45 mm.

Histopathology

Classic epithelioid sarcoma shows plump spindle cells with prominent eosinophilic cytoplasm blending into areas of larger more polygonal epithelioid cells, forming infiltrative, irregular sheets that frequently surround areas of necrosis in a pseudogranulomatous fashion {542}. Nuclei exhibit comparatively mild atypia, with vesicular chromatin and nucleoli. Mitotic activity is low. The proximal subtype displays sheet-like growth with only focal necrosis and is composed of more purely epithelioid carcinoma–like cells {1270}. These have enlarged nuclei and prominent nucleoli, often with rhabdoid cytoplasm. Both subtypes have been reported in the orbit.

Immunohistochemistry

Epithelioid sarcoma cells coexpress epithelial (keratins, EMA) and mesenchymal (vimentin, CD34) markers. Most useful is loss of SMARCB1 (INI1) {1365}, a feature relatively specific to this disease {35}.

Differential diagnosis

This includes granulomatous processes, carcinomas, and epithelioid vascular tumours.

Cytology

Cytology is not reported for ophthalmic cases.

Diagnostic molecular pathology

Panel sequencing may detect mutations inactivating *SMARCB1* {1632}.

Essential and desirable diagnostic criteria

Essential: epithelioid to spindled cytomorphology, with infiltrative growth; positivity for keratins, EMA, and vimentin; loss of expression of SMARCB1 (INI1).

Staging

The American Joint Committee on Cancer (AJCC) or Union for International Cancer Control (UICC) TNM system may be used.

Prognosis and prediction

Epithelioid sarcoma is an aggressive disease with a significant risk of local recurrence and nodal and systemic metastases. Five-year survival is about 70% but may be lower in orbital cases. Treatment generally requires exenteration supported by radiation therapy. Chemotherapy provides limited benefit but EZH2 inhibitors have shown activity in phase II studies {1158,128}.

Synovial sarcoma

Milman T
Stagner AM
Suurmeijer AJH

Definition

Synovial sarcoma (SS) is a spindle cell mesenchymal neoplasm showing variable epithelial differentiation and characterized by a specific *SS18*::SSX fusion gene.

ICD-O coding

9040/3 Synovial sarcoma, NOS
9041/3 Monophasic synovial sarcoma
9043/3 Biphasic synovial sarcoma
9040/3 Poorly differentiated synovial sarcoma

ICD-11 coding

2B5A.Y Synovial sarcoma, other specified primary site
XH9B22 Synovial sarcoma, NOS

Related terminology

Not recommended: synovioma; synovial cell sarcoma; synoviosarcoma.

Subtype(s)

Monophasic synovial sarcoma; biphasic synovial sarcoma; poorly differentiated synovial sarcoma

Localization

Most SS cases (73%) arise in the extremities and 7% in the head and neck {218}. Primary ocular adnexal SS has been described in the epibulbar region, anterior orbit, and intraconal space, where the tumour is frequently adherent to extraocular muscles. Bone destruction is uncommon {3190}. Secondary involvement of the orbit by metastatic SS can occur rarely {3622}.

Clinical features

SS can present insidiously with pain, proptosis, periorbital swelling, and diplopia {1100 3190}. Imaging generally reveals a circumscribed mass with occasional calcification {3190}.

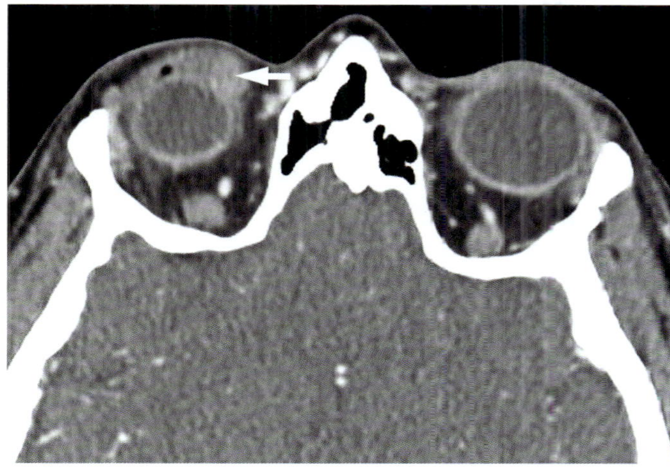

Fig. 11.88 Synovial sarcoma. Axial CT demonstrates a circumscribed weakly enhancing mass in the superomedial orbit (arrow).

Epidemiology

Overall, SS has an even sex distribution and can occur at any age. Over 50% of cases present in adolescents and young adults {218}. Ocular adnexal SS is rare, has a female predilection, and occurs at a mean age of 25 years {1100}.

Etiology

There are no known predisposing factors, although rarely SS has been reported after radiotherapy {1325}.

Pathogenesis

In nearly all cases, SS bears a unique chromosomal t(X;18)(p11;q11) translocation, in which *SS18* on chromosome 18 is fused to an SSX gene on the X chromosome, resulting in the oncogenic *SS18*::SSX fusion gene {818,1539,267}. The fusion protein may block mesenchymal differentiation by various

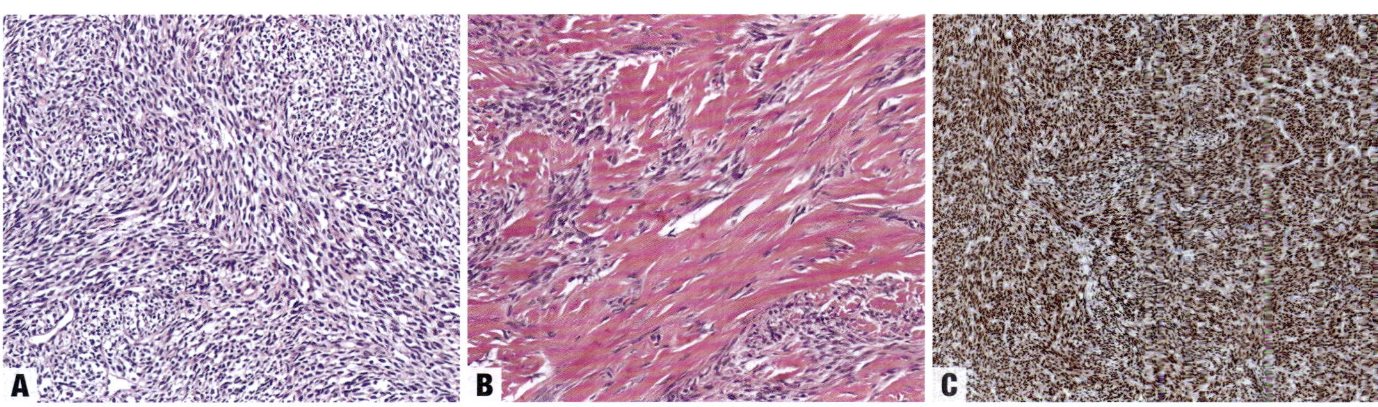

Fig. 11.89 Synovial sarcoma, monophasic. **A** Cellular fascicles of monotonous spindle cells with nuclear overlapping and scant collagenous matrix. **B** Spindle cells in a coarsely collagenous, hyalinized stroma. **C** Strong diffuse nuclear staining with *SS18*::SSX-specific antibody.

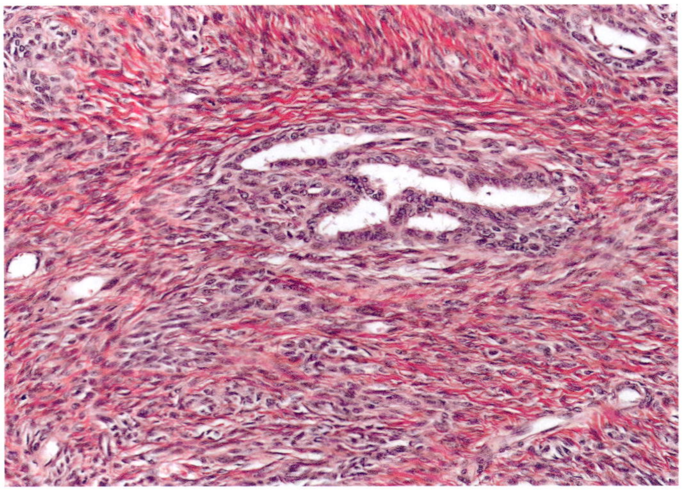

Fig. 11.90 Synovial sarcoma, biphasic. Cuboidal epithelial cells arranged in glands and nests set in a background of a spindle cell sarcoma.

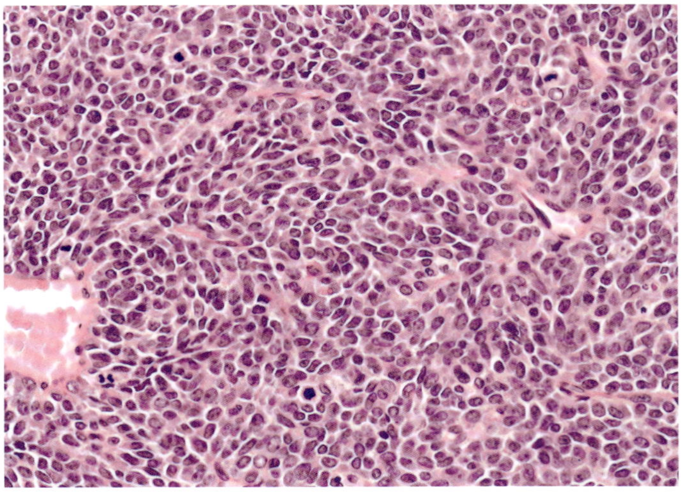

Fig. 11.91 Synovial sarcoma, poorly differentiated. Small round hyperchromatic cells with brisk mitotic activity.

epigenetic mechanisms, which include binding and displacing native SS18 in the SWI/SNF chromatin-remodelling complex {1564}. See the fifth-edition *Soft tissue and bone tumours* volume {3598} for additional details.

Macroscopic appearance

SS demonstrates a yellow-tan to grey cut surface with occasional foci of necrosis, calcification, and haemorrhage {2213}.

Histopathology

There are three main histological patterns of SS: monophasic (most common), biphasic (as many as one third of cases), and poorly differentiated.

Monophasic SS is composed of uniform spindle cells with ovoid hyperchromatic, frequently overlapping nuclei, inconspicuous nucleoli, and sparse cytoplasm, arranged in cellular sheets and fascicles. There may be areas of dense fibrosis and myxoid change. A staghorn-shaped vascular pattern may be observed. Foci of calcification and/or ossification are identified in as many as one third of SS cases {3335}.

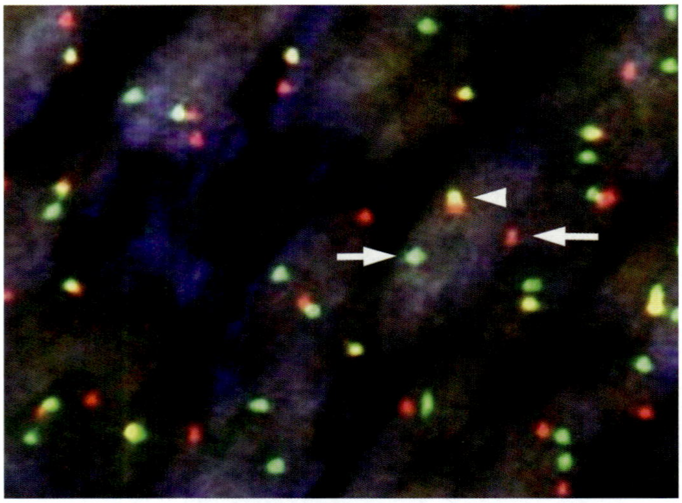

Fig. 11.92 Synovial sarcoma. FISH with *SS18* break-apart probes shows a yellow signal corresponding to the closely apposed red and green signals (arrowhead) indicative of the absence of *SS18* rearrangement (wildtype allele). The widely separated red and green signals (arrows) correspond to separation of *SS18* gene loci, indicative of *SS18* gene rearrangement.

Biphasic SS contains epithelial and spindle-cell components in varying proportions. The epithelial cells of SS have ovoid vesicular nuclei with pale eosinophilic cytoplasm and occasional keratinization, and are arranged in nests and cords {3335}.

Poorly differentiated SS can feature small round hyperchromatic cells, reminiscent of Ewing family tumours, or fascicular spindle cells, reminiscent of malignant peripheral nerve sheath tumour {3335}. Severe nuclear atypia, necrosis, and brisk mitotic activity can be seen {1194}.

Immunohistochemistry

Immunohistochemistry with the *SS18*::SSX fusion–specific antibody and the C-terminus SSX-specific antibody shows strong diffuse nuclear staining in SS with high (> 95%) sensitivity and specificity {253}. TLE1 shows diffuse nuclear staining in as many as 95% of SS cases, but can be expressed in histological mimics, including malignant peripheral nerve sheath tumour and solitary fibrous tumour. Most SS lesions express CD99 and BCL2. Epithelial cells in biphasic SS express EMA and cytokeratins. S100 and SMA are variably expressed {2529}. SMARCB1 (INI1) and H3 p.K27me3 may be partially or completely lost in a subset of SS cases {1758,2325}.

Cytology

SS may show clusters of and single round, oval, and spindle cells with pericapillary arrangement and occasionally pink background stroma. Glandular formation or epithelial components may be seen in biphasic SS {3752}. Conclusive diagnosis requires molecular confirmation {3453}.

Diagnostic molecular pathology

Approximately two thirds of SS lesions carry an *SS18*::*SSX1* fusion, one third carry *SS18*::*SSX2*, and a few carry *SS18*::*SSX4* {818,136}. *SSX1* fusions with *SS18L1*, *EWSR1*, *MN1*, and *NEDD4* are rare {3708,187}. Detection of *SS18*::SSX fusion by either molecular assay or immunohistochemistry should be performed in all SS cases when possible {1437}.

Essential and desirable diagnostic criteria

Essential: monomorphic small blue / spindle cell sarcoma showing variable epithelial/glandular differentiation; diffuse, strong nuclear immunoreactivity for TLE1.

Desirable: diffuse, strong nuclear immunoreactivity for SS18::SSX fusion protein OR demonstration of an *SS18*::SSX gene fusion.

Staging

The Union for International Cancer Control (UICC) or American Joint Committee on Cancer (AJCC) TNM system may be used.

Prognosis and prediction

The overall survival for patients with SS is 138 months, with 5-, 10-, and 20-year survival rates of 59%, 51%, and 43%, respectively {218}. SS can metastasize to lungs, bone, and regional lymph nodes. Unfavourable prognostic factors include higher tumour stage at the time of presentation, size > 50 mm, higher French Fédération Nationale des Centres de Lutte Contre le Cancer (FNCLCC) grade, non-extremity site, and older age {1194,3308,218}. The specific *SS18* partner does not appear to significantly alter prognosis {1830,1194}.

Alveolar soft part sarcoma

Odashiro AN
Jambhekar NA
Mulay K
Vemuganti GK

Definition

Alveolar soft part sarcoma (ASPS) of the orbit, similarly to those at other sites, is a high-grade tumour of uncertain histogenesis having a distinctive alveolar arrangement of epithelioid tumour cells and characterized by the der(17)t(X;17)(p11.2;q25) rearrangement resulting in the *ASPSCR1::TFE3* gene fusion.

ICD-O coding

9581/3 Alveolar soft part sarcoma

ICD-11 coding

2B5F.2 & XH8V95 Sarcoma, not elsewhere classified of other specified sites & Alveolar soft part sarcoma

Related terminology

None

Subtype(s)

None

Localization

ASPS of the orbit is located close to the extraocular muscles, sometimes intraconal, in the medial part of the orbit, supraorbital, or involving the eyelid {3550,1303,2308}.

Clinical features

ASPS presents as a slowly progressive, painless proptosis of the eye with eyelid swelling and dilatation of conjunctival vessels, but rarely compressing the optic nerve {3550}. Radiologically, the tumours are well-circumscribed ovoid masses, isodense or hypodense on CT {3336}. MRI demonstrates intermediate signal intensity and marked enhancement {2129}.

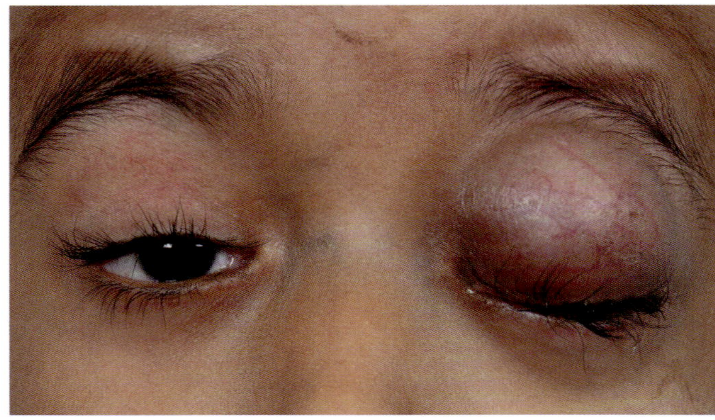

Fig. 11.93 Alveolar soft part sarcoma. Orbital alveolar soft part sarcoma in a 7-year-old boy presenting with progressive left upper eyelid swelling of 2 months' duration.

Epidemiology

While ASPS is rare, representing 0.5–0.9% of all soft tissue sarcomas, orbital involvement by the tumour is relatively frequent. Although any age group may be affected, peak occurrence is in the third decade of life {1303}.

Etiology

The etiology is unknown. No cases have reported in association with a history of irradiation or a germline cancer predisposition syndrome.

Pathogenesis

The *ASPSCR1::TFE3* translocation appears to be the initiating genetic event in ASPS {1831}, defined by a specific alteration, der(17)t(X;17)(p11.2;q25). This translocation results in fusion of the *TFE3* transcription factor gene (from Xp11.2) with *ASPSCR1*

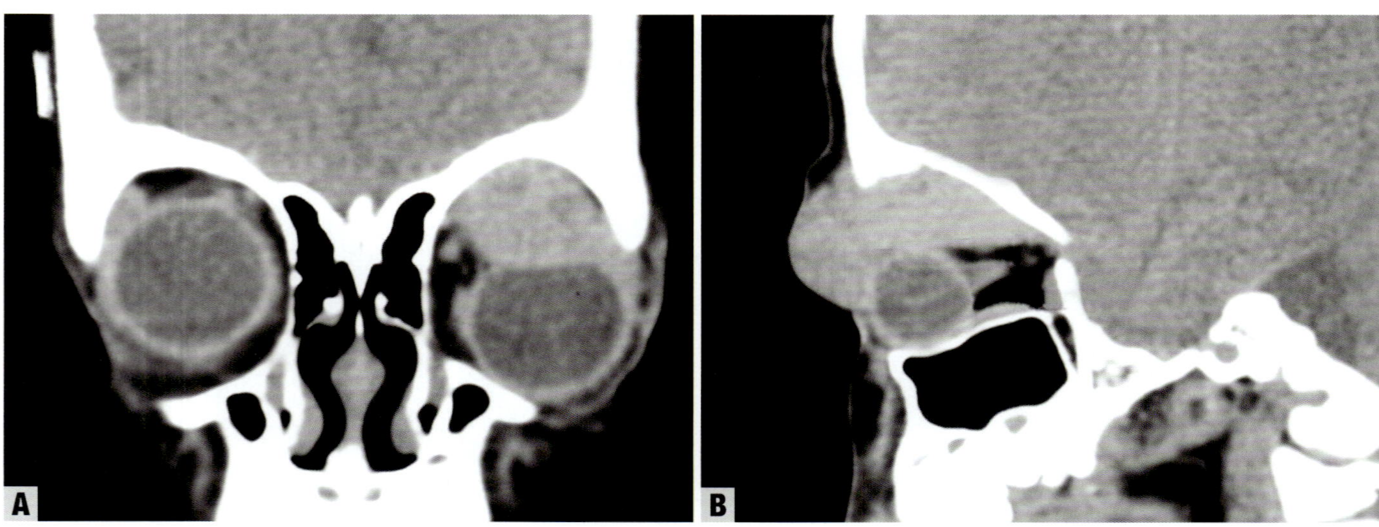

Fig. 11.94 Orbital alveolar soft part sarcoma. **A,B** CT showed a hyperdense orbital mass extending to the apex and indenting the globe.

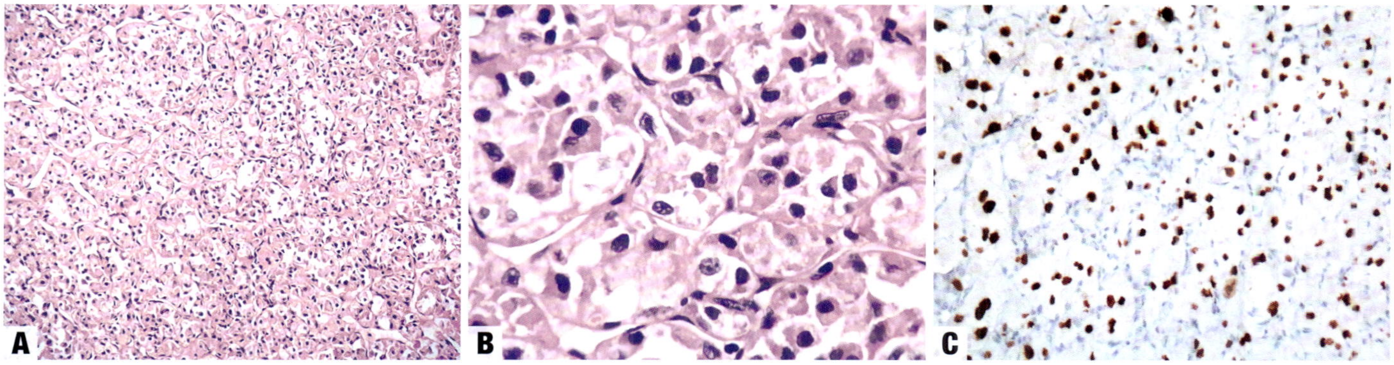

Fig. 11.95 Alveolar soft part sarcoma. **A** Organoid arrangement of tumour cells with central discohesion giving alveolar soft part sarcoma its characteristic alveolar pattern with a rich sinusoidal network separating the nests from each other. **B** Large, polygonal cells of alveolar soft part sarcoma with distinct cell borders, eosinophilic granular cytoplasm, and central vesicular nuclei having prominent nucleoli, admixed with rhabdoid cells having eccentric nuclei. **C** Tumour cells showing strong nuclear staining for TFE3.

(also known as *ASPL*) at 17q25.3 {1831}. The *ASPSCR1::TFE3* fusion protein localizes to the nucleus, causing c-Met activation of c-Met signalling. Depending on the *TFE3* intron involved in the genomic rearrangement, *ASPSCR1::TFE3* fusion transcripts can differ by the presence or absence of one additional exon of *TFE3*.

Macroscopic appearance

Tumours vary from 20 to 50 mm (median 34.5 mm) {732,3550,92,2407,1303,545}. They are usually circumscribed, but can be invasive {3550,1303,2036,2308,2767}. The tumours are often soft, and vary from grey or yellow to tan and reddish in colour. The centre of larger lesions often shows haemorrhage or necrosis {3550,1303,2036,2308,2767}.

Histopathology

Microscopy often shows an organoid or nest-like pattern with central discohesion resulting in the characteristic alveolar pattern with a rich sinusoidal vascular network seen throughout the tumour separating the nests from each other. Solid and haemangiopericytoma-like patterns may be encountered focally in many tumours. Cells are large and polygonal with well-defined cell borders, eosinophilic granular cytoplasm, a rounded central or eccentric vesicular nucleus, and a prominent nucleolus. Vascular invasion is very common. Cytoplasmic clearing, rhabdoid cells, a pseudoglandular pattern, and cystic change with myxoid material may be seen {2695,1541}. Many tumours show intracytoplasmic rod-like/rhomboid crystalline structures in a sheaf-like or stacked configuration {2695,932}. These crystals may be irregular, are PAS-positive/diastase resistant, and are immunoreactive for MCT1 and CD147 {1829,3396,1409}. Glycogen is usually present.

Immunohistochemistry

ASPS shows immunoreactivity for TFE3 (nuclear), cathepsin K (100%), and CD147 (100%). Immunoreactivity for S100, calretinin, desmin, and NSE is variable {997,186,2929,3610,2030,513}.

Cytology

In cytological preparations, smears reveal large cells, mostly single and granular, which may have vacuoles {3524,2929}.

Diagnostic molecular pathology

Detection of the fusion transcript *ASPSCR1::TFE3* {1443,1350,3610} may be diagnostically helpful. This gene fusion is also seen in paediatric renal cell carcinomas {184[illegible]}.

Essential and desirable diagnostic criteria

Essential: organoid/nesting pattern of polygonal cells; rich sinusoidal capillary network; diffuse, nuclear TFE3 expression by immunohistochemistry.

Desirable: intracytoplasmic crystals; demonstration of *TFE3* gene rearrangement or *ASPSCR1::TFE3* fusion.

Staging

The Union for International Cancer Control (UICC) or American Joint Committee on Cancer (AJCC) TNM system can be used.

Prognosis and prediction

Local recurrence is seen in 18.6–47.7% of orbital ASPSs {3550}. Metastasis can occur long (as long as 6 years) after the initial diagnosis and most commonly affects lungs, brain, and bones {2308}.

Chapter 11

Osteoma

Cleven AHG
Bredella MA
Rogozhin DV

Definition
Osteoma is a benign tumour arising on the surface of bone and is composed primarily of lamellar mature cortical-type bone. The term "bone island" is used when an osteoma develops within the medullary cavity.

ICD-O coding
9180/0 Osteoma

ICD-11 coding
2E83.Z & XH4818 Benign osteogenic tumours of unspecified site & Osteoma, NOS

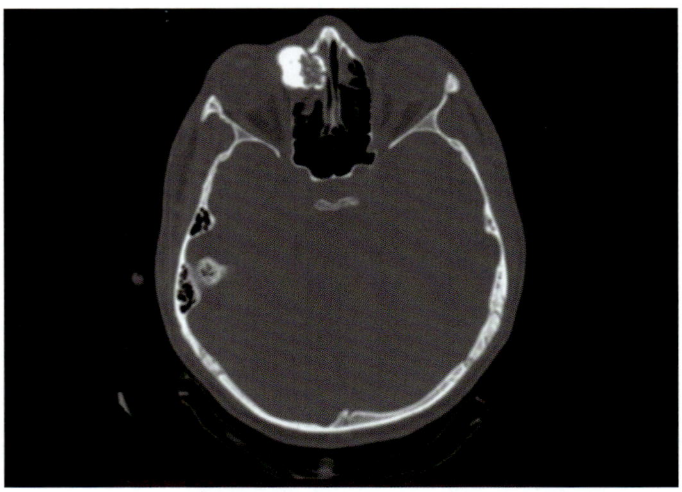

Fig. 11.96 Osteoma. Osteoma of the right medial wall of the orbit is seen. Axial CT shows a prominent dense bone tumour with sharp borders. The surrounding tissues appear intact.

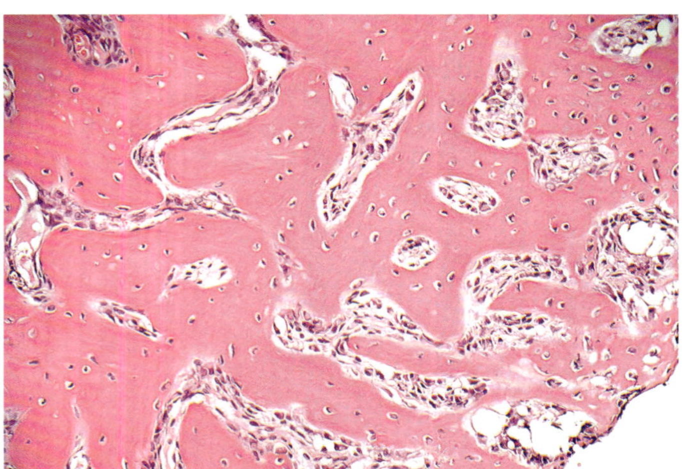

Fig. 11.97 Osteoma. Compact mature lamellar/cortical-type bone.

Related terminology
Not recommended: ivory exostosis; parosteal osteoma.

Subtype(s)
None

Localization
Osteomas predominantly affect craniofacial bones formed by membranous ossification {1858}.

Clinical features
Osteomas are usually slow growing and asymptomatic {1858}. On radiological imaging, osteomas are round, dense, well-defined ivory-like lesions which are attached to the underlying bone without cortical invasion. The presence of multiple osteomas suggests the diagnosis of Gardner syndrome {3242}, which is a subtype of familial adenomatous polyposis.

Epidemiology
Since osteomas commonly represent incidental findings, their actual prevalence is difficult to determine but has been reported to reach 6.4% in select case series {1883}.

Etiology
The etiology of sporadic cases is unknown.

Pathogenesis
Most osteomas develop sporadically and a small subset of cases is associated with Gardner syndrome, a phenotypic variant of familial adenomatous polyposis caused by mutations in the *APC* gene resulting in aberrant activation of the WNT/β-catenin signalling pathway. In 61.1% of sporadic osteomas, hotspot mutations in the *CTNNB1* gene (encoding β-catenin) were found {279}.

Macroscopic appearance
Osteomas arise on the surface of the bone and are typically well-circumscribed tumours with a broad attachment to the underlying bone.

Histopathology
Osteomas are predominantly composed of mature lamellar/cortical-type bone and can be divided histologically into compact and (less frequent) spongious subtypes.

Cytology
Not clinically relevant

Diagnostic molecular pathology
Not clinically relevant

Essential and desirable diagnostic criteria

Essential: bone tumour with compatible imaging; tumour arises on the surface of bone or within the medullary cavity; tumour composed of lamellar/cortical-type bone.

Staging

Not clinically relevant

Prognosis and prediction

Asymptomatic cases generally do not require treatment and follow an indolent clinical course; symptomatic cases can be conservatively excised.

Osteoblastoma

Cleven AHG
Amary F
Dubovy SR

Definition
Osteoblastoma is a locally aggressive bone-forming tumour, generally > 20 mm.

ICD-O coding
9200/1 Osteoblastoma

ICD-11 coding
2E83.Z & XH4316 Benign osteogenic tumour of unspecified site & Osteoblastoma, NOS

Related terminology
Acceptable: epithelioid osteoblastoma.
Not recommended: pseudomalignant osteoblastoma; aggressive osteoblastoma.

Subtype(s)
None

Localization
In more than one third of cases the spine is affected. The craniofacial bones, including the orbit, are affected in < 5% of cases {1077,1535,2162}.

Clinical features
The presenting symptom is frequently pain and/or swelling {2003,1077}. In the orbit, this may include exophthalmos, hearing or visual loss, diplopia, and nasal obstruction {2162,1077}.

On radiographs and CT, osteoblastomas present as lytic lesions > 20 mm, frequently with surrounding reactive sclerosis {1059}.

Epidemiology
Osteoblastomas represent < 1% of primary bone tumours {318,2003}. The peak incidence is between the second and third decades of life. In general, the M:F ratio is 2:1 {318, 2003}; however, in the orbit the reported sex distribution is equal {1077}.

Etiology
Unknown

Pathogenesis
Rearrangement of *FOS* is present in 87% of osteoblastomas {980,278}, and in a smaller percentage of cases *FOSB* rearrangement has been detected {980}. *FOS* rearrangements can be detected using an antibody against the FOS N-terminus, which results in nuclear immunoreactivity in the osteoblastic cells {278,133,1850}.

Macroscopic appearance
Not clinically relevant

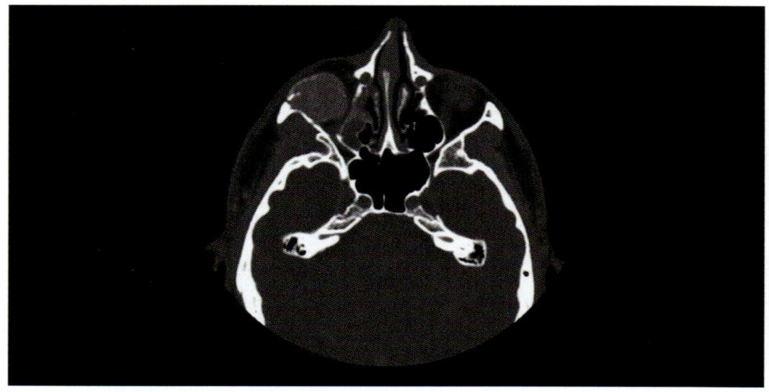

Fig. 11.98 Osteoblastoma. Axial bone algorithm CT image showing a heterogeneous dense mass with incomplete peripheral ossification arising from the lateral wall of the right orbit.

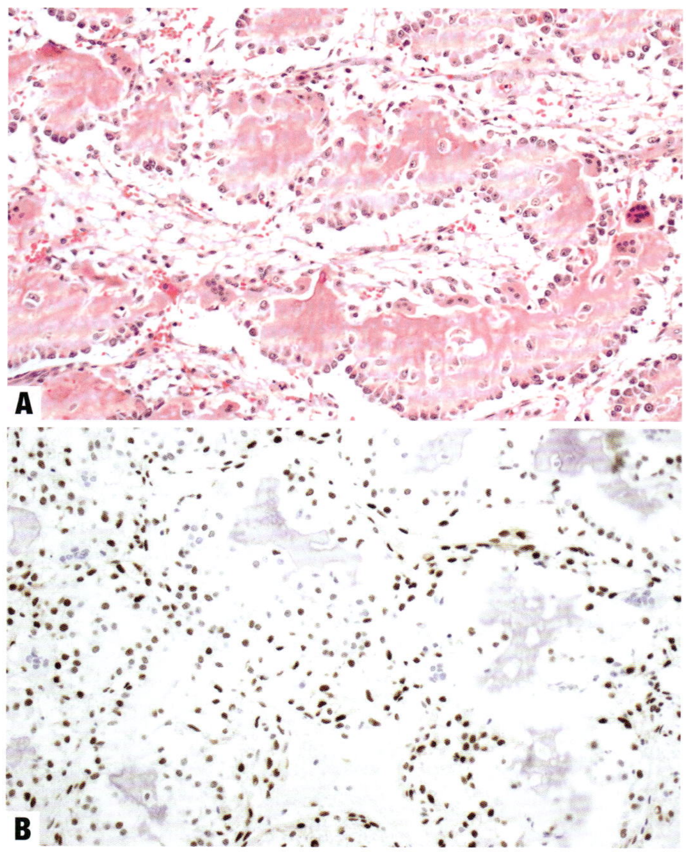

Fig. 11.99 Osteoblastoma. **A** Interconnecting trabeculae of woven bone rimmed by osteoblasts in a richly vascularized fibroblastic stroma. **B** Nuclear expression of FOS (c-FOS) in the lesional cells highlighting the osteoblastic cells.

Histopathology
Osteoblastomas are characterized by interconnecting, delicate, woven bone trabeculae, rimmed by a single layer of polygonal

osteoblasts {2003}. The stroma is loose and usually richly vascularized, with dilated capillary-type blood vessels. Destructive host bone permeation and atypical mitotic figures should not be seen. The differential diagnosis includes sino-orbital osteoma with osteoblastoma-like features.

Cytology

Not clinically relevant

Diagnostic molecular pathology

FOS gene rearrangement or rarely *FOSB* gene rearrangement is found in the majority of osteoblastomas {980}.

Essential and desirable diagnostic criteria

Essential: bone-forming tumour composed of trabeculae of woven bone rimmed by plump osteoblasts in a vascularized stroma; absence of host bone permeation; compatible radiological features of a > 20 mm lesion with well-defined tumour borders

Staging

Not clinically relevant

Prognosis and prediction

The prognosis is good, but recurrences are described in as many as 23% of cases {318}, more frequently in patients in which complete excision has not been achieved, and this can be challenging at this location {318}.

Osteosarcoma

Hogendoorn PCW
Baumhoer D
Cates JMM
Rogozhin DV
Zambrano E

Definition

Osteosarcoma is a high-grade sarcoma in which the tumour cells produce bone. A rare low-grade type exists called low-grade central osteosarcoma (LGCOS), which is a low-grade malignant bone-forming neoplasm that originates within the intramedullary cavity and consists of fibroblastic tumour cells with low-grade nuclear atypia and well-formed neoplastic bony trabeculae.

ICD-O coding

9180/3 Osteosarcoma, NOS
9183/3 Telangiectatic osteosarcoma
9185/3 Small cell osteosarcoma
9187/3 Low-grade central osteosarcoma

ICD-11 coding

2B51.Z Osteosarcoma of bone or articular cartilage of unspecified sites
2B51.Z & XH5CL5 Osteosarcoma of bone or articular cartilage of unspecified sites & Telangiectatic osteosarcoma
2B51.Z & XH4EZ4 Osteosarcoma of bone or articular cartilage of unspecified sites & Small cell osteosarcoma
2B51.Z & XH7N84 Osteosarcoma of bone or articular cartilage of unspecified sites & Low-grade central osteosarcoma

Related terminology

Acceptable: for low-grade central osteosarcoma: well-differentiated intramedullary osteosarcoma.

Subtype(s)

Subtypes of high-grade osteosarcoma: telangiectatic osteosarcoma; small cell osteosarcoma

Localization

Osteosarcoma is much more common in the extremities, but the orbit may rarely be involved.

Clinical features

There is usually a relatively short history of a painful, enlarging mass and occasionally restricted movement of the eye.

Epidemiology

Osteosarcoma is the most common primary high-grade sarcoma of the skeleton, but presentation in the orbital bones without a history of irradiation is very uncommon. A bimodal age distribution is known but most cases develop between 14 and 18 years and a second smaller peak occurs in older adults.

LGCOS is rare, accounting for 1–2% of all osteosarcomas. It most commonly affects young adults, with a peak incidence in the third decade of life {1815}. There is a mild female predilection {2890,3709}.

Etiology

Ionizing irradiation used in the treatment of retinoblastoma is the strongest risk factor for developing secondary osteosarcoma and appears to be dose dependent. It tends to develop in areas with lower potentially mutagenic doses at the margins of the radiation field.

Pathogenesis

The pathogenesis and cell of origin of osteosarcoma are unknown, though mesenchymal stem cells have been suggested in murine models. Many potential driver genes have been identified {288}. Although these mutations occur early in disease development, it seems likely that chromothripsis caused by an unknown trigger initiates chromosomal instability and subsequent tumour development {288}. Amplification of 12q13-q15 involving *MDM2* and *CDK4* is common in low-grade osteosarcoma {1291,3292,842}. *MDM2* amplification is maintained in high-grade progression. A small subset of LGCOSs lack *MDM2* amplification.

Macroscopic appearance

Osteosarcoma presents itself as a destructive mass with destruction of the cortex. The cut surface is heterogeneous, depending on the type and degree of mineralization of the predominant matrix. Most tumours are tan-white and in high-grade cases they may show areas of necrosis. The telangiectatic subtype shows a haemorrhagic multicystic appearance.

Histopathology

High-grade osteosarcoma has a broad histomorphological spectrum. Essential to the diagnosis is the identification of neoplastic bone formation. The tumour grows with a permeative pattern, replacing the marrow space and encasing and eroding pre-existing trabeculae. The neoplastic cells typically demonstrate severe anaplasia and pleomorphism, and they may be fusiform, plasmacytoid, or epithelioid. Neoplastic cells often become small and normalized in appearance (mimicking benign osteocytes) when surrounded by bone matrix. Mitotic activity is usually brisk, and abundant atypical mitotic figures are often present, which are useful in the differential diagnosis of benign mimics.

Bone matrix is eosinophilic on H&E-stained sections if unmineralized and basophilic/purple if mineralized, and it may have a pagetoid appearance imparted by haphazardly deposited cement lines. Distinguishing unmineralized matrix (osteoid) from other eosinophilic extracellular materials such as collagen or compacted fibrin matrices may be difficult and subjective. High-grade osteosarcoma may have different histological patterns. Currently, there is no relationship between histological patterns, treatment, and prognosis {1277}.

High-grade osteosarcoma commonly contains varying amounts of neoplastic cartilage and/or fibroblastic components;

on the basis of the predominant matrix, they are subdivided into osteoblastic (76–80%), chondroblastic (10–13%), and fibroblastic (10%) patterns {1277}. In osteoblastic osteosarcoma, neoplastic bone is the principal matrix and varies from thin, lace-like trabeculae to compact bone. When the latter is pronounced, the tumour is designated as a sclerosing osteosarcoma.

In telangiectatic osteosarcoma, the tumour is composed of blood-filled or empty cystic spaces closely simulating an aneurysmal bone cyst. The septa show variable thickness and are populated by pleomorphic cells showing substantial nuclear hyperchromasia. Atypical mitoses are easily identified. Osteoid formation is usually focal and confluent but may be absent in a biopsy. The septa also contain osteoclast-type giant cells.

Small cell osteosarcoma is composed of small cells with scant cytoplasm, associated with osteoid production. Nuclei are round to oval and the chromatin may be fine to coarse; mitoses can easily be found. Particular care must be taken to distinguish osteoid from fibrin deposits that may be seen among Ewing sarcoma cells.

Low-grade central osteosarcoma is composed of mildly to moderately cellular fascicles of spindle cells with mild nuclear atypia in a fibrous stroma. These are admixed with a neoplastic bone component, often with a parallel arrangement. Permeation of host bone is invariably present. Cortical destruction with soft tissue infiltration may also be present. Mitotic activity is low. In 10–36% of cases, the tumour may progress to high-grade sarcoma.

Cytology

Not clinically relevant

Diagnostic molecular pathology

No specific diagnostic molecular pathology tests are available for high-grade osteosarcoma. Testing for *MDM2* amplification is helpful to differentiate low-grade osteosarcoma from benign mimics. Unlike fibrous dysplasia, LGCOS lacks *GNAS* mutation {2828}. The lack of *MDM2* amplification cannot exclude the diagnosis of LGCOS.

Essential and desirable diagnostic criteria

High-grade osteosarcoma

Essential: bone tumour with compatible imaging; bone production by tumour cells; permeative and destructive growth pattern.

Desirable: tumour cells with high-grade atypia; atypical mitotic figures frequently present.

Low-grade osteosarcoma

Essential: bone tumour with compatible imaging; intramedullary location; predominantly fibroblastic osteosarcoma with mild nuclear atypia and well-formed neoplastic bony trabeculae.

Desirable: *MDM2* amplification.

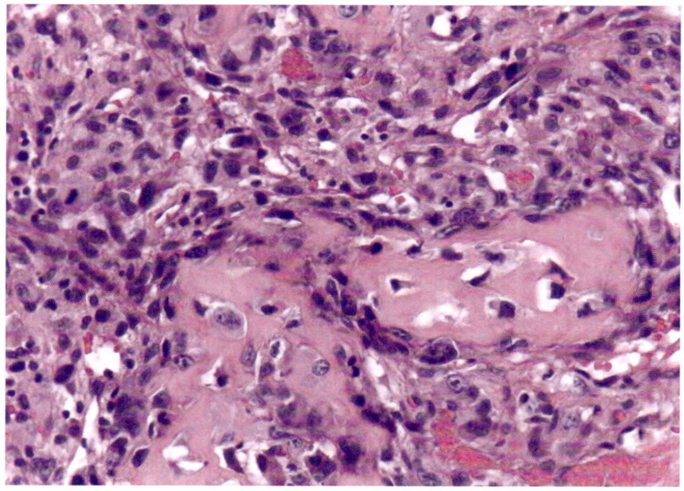

Fig. 11.100 Orbital osteosarcoma. Tumour cells with high-grade atypia with accompanying neoplastic bone formation.

Staging

The eighth edition of the Union for International Cancer Control's (UICC) *TNM classification of malignant tumours* stages osteosarcoma of the skull and facial bones on the basis of the greatest tumour dimension (≤ 80 mm is T1; > 80 mm is T2) and discontinuous involvement of the primary bone site (T3). The eighth edition of the American Joint Committee on Cancer's *AJCC cancer staging manual* stages osteosarcoma arising in the craniofacial bones on the basis of the presence or absence of distant metastasis, histological grade, and greatest tumour dimension (≤ 80 mm or > 80 mm).

Prognosis and prediction

Aggressive local growth and rapid haematogenous dissemination characterize the clinical course. Pulmonary metastases are the most frequent sites of systemic disease. High-grade osteosarcoma is treated with preoperative and postoperative chemotherapy; local control is achieved via surgical resection with wide margins. Radiation can be used for unresectable tumours if not the cause of the tumour {2720}. The use of chemotherapy has a dramatic impact on outcome {163,701}. Patients presenting with metastatic or recurrent disease have a survival rate of < 30% {1565,605}. The histological response to neoadjuvant chemotherapy remains one of the most important prognosticators of overall and disease-free survival {163, 701}. A good response is usually defined as ≥ 90% necrosis {2835,495}.

LGCOS has a good prognosis when widely resected, with a metastatic rate of < 5% and 5-year and 10-year overall survival rates of 90% and > 80%, respectively {2046,602,1815}. The tumour invariably recurs after curettage and incomplete excision.

Chondroma

Demicco EG
Bovée JVMG
Lee NG
Wenig BM

Definition

Orbital chondroma is a benign chondrocytic neoplasm, producing hyaline or myxoid cartilage, and arising periosteally or in orbital soft tissue.

ICD-O coding

9220/0 Chondroma

ICD-11 coding

2E89.1 & XH0NS4 Benign tumours of uncertain differentiation, soft tissue & Chondroma, NOS

Related terminology

Acceptable: chondroma of soft parts; extraskeletal chondroma; periosteal chondroma.

Not recommended: juxtacortical chondroma.

Subtype(s)

None

Localization

Orbital chondromas arise in the superomedial orbit in the vicinity of the trochlea, which is the only cartilaginous structure found normally in the orbit {1516,1559,1265,3266,926}.

Clinical features

Tumours are solitary and present as a painless firm mass in the superomedial orbit. Ptosis and restrictive strabismus have been reported {3266,1265,1559}.

Epidemiology

Orbital chondroma is extremely rare, accounting for 1 of 645 orbital masses in one survey {3025}. Of 3 reported cases in the English-language literature, all included male patients, aged 9–27 years {1559,1265,3266}.

Etiology

Unknown

Pathogenesis

Genetic analysis of orbital chondroma has not been performed. Location in the region of the trochlea suggests an origin from residual chondroid progenitor cells in this area.

Cytogenetic analyses of limited numbers of soft tissue chondromas of other sites reveal variable aberrations, including rearrangements of 12q13-q15 and trisomy 5. In a set of tumours with rearrangements of 12q13-q15, a truncated or full-length *HMGA2* transcript was found {413,2930,3267,705, 3230}. In about 50% of the cases, *FN1* gene rearrangements were reported, with *FGFR1* and *FGFR2* as fusion partners {134}. Periosteal chondromas may harbour mutations in *IDH1* {135}.

Macroscopic appearance

Orbital chondroma is a 10–20 mm, well-circumscribed, nodular, solid greyish-bluish-white mass. Myxoid/cystic change may be present.

Histopathology

The tumour is composed of lobules of well-formed hyaline and/or myxoid cartilage delineated by fibrous septa. Chondrocytes are arranged in clusters and reside within lacunar spaces or float in a flocculent myxoid matrix. The nuclei are usually small, round, and dark, but may be enlarged with fine or coarse chromatin and small nucleoli, and exhibit mild pleomorphism. Coarse calcifications and endochondral ossification may be present {3266}. Mitotic activity is absent or very low and abnormal mitotic figures are not observed. If periosteal, there should be no invasion of the underlying cortex.

Cytology

Not clinically relevant

Diagnostic molecular pathology

Not clinically relevant

Essential and desirable diagnostic criteria

Essential: soft tissue mass composed of well-delineated cartilage nodules; matrix is hyaline or myxoid and may calcify; chondrocytes show limited atypia and no or little mitotic activity.

Staging

Not clinically relevant

Prognosis and prediction

Marginal excision is curative. Recurrence has not been reported, although experience is limited.

Mesenchymal chondrosarcoma

Subramanian K
Fanburg-Smith JC
Odashiro AN

Definition

Mesenchymal chondrosarcoma is a high-grade, malignant, biphasic, primitive mesenchymal tumour with a well-differentiated, organized hyaline cartilage component.

ICD-O coding

9240/3 Mesenchymal chondrosarcoma

ICD-11 coding

2B50.Z & XH8X47 Chondrosarcoma of bone or articular cartilage of unspecified sites & Mesenchymal chondrosarcoma

Related terminology

None

Subtype(s)

None

Localization

Mesenchymal chondrosarcoma occurs in the orbital bones and soft tissues {3399,109}; it can be adherent to the optic nerve or entirely intraneural {228,1969,1324}. It may also involve the lacrimal gland {1709} and the lid {2748}.

Clinical features

Orbital mesenchymal chondrosarcoma presents with non-specific symptoms such as proptosis, ptosis, diplopia, loss of vision, and pain {2409,69,1626}.

Epidemiology

Approximately 50 cases of primary orbital mesenchymal chondrosarcoma have been reported {1134,707,2409}. There is a predilection for the second and third decades of life and for women, although mesenchymal chondrosarcoma also occurs in young children {109,3399}.

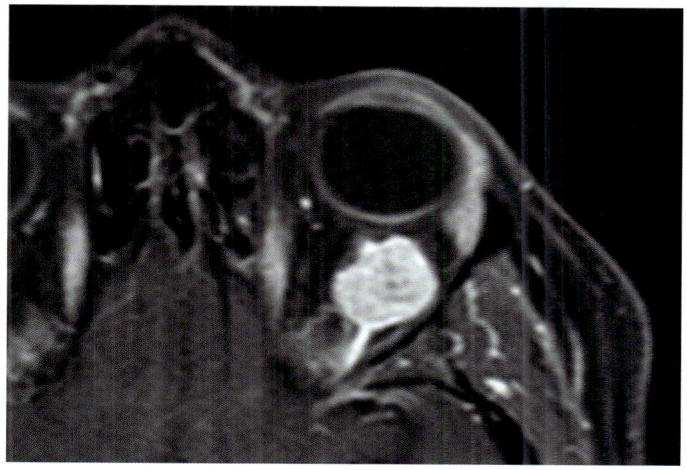

Fig. 11.101 Orbital mesenchymal chondrosarcoma. T1-weighted postcontrast fat saturation MRI shows a left orbital conus mass. The two components are subtle with mostly a solid enhancing (round cell component) appearance with subtle flecks of heterogeneous density (cartilage component).

Etiology

Unknown

Pathogenesis

Mesenchymal chondrosarcoma arises from immature cartilage precursors and develops via *HEY1::NCOA2* fusion {2614}. The fusion of *HEY1* at 8q21.13 and *NCOA2* at 8q13.3 results in the *HEY1::NCOA2* fusion gene, which appears to play a role in extraskeletal mesenchymal chondrosarcoma {3544,876}. *IRF2BP2::CDX1* fusion is reported in a single case of mesenchymal chondrosarcoma {876}. However, not much information on fusion genes is available on orbital mesenchymal chondrosarcomas.

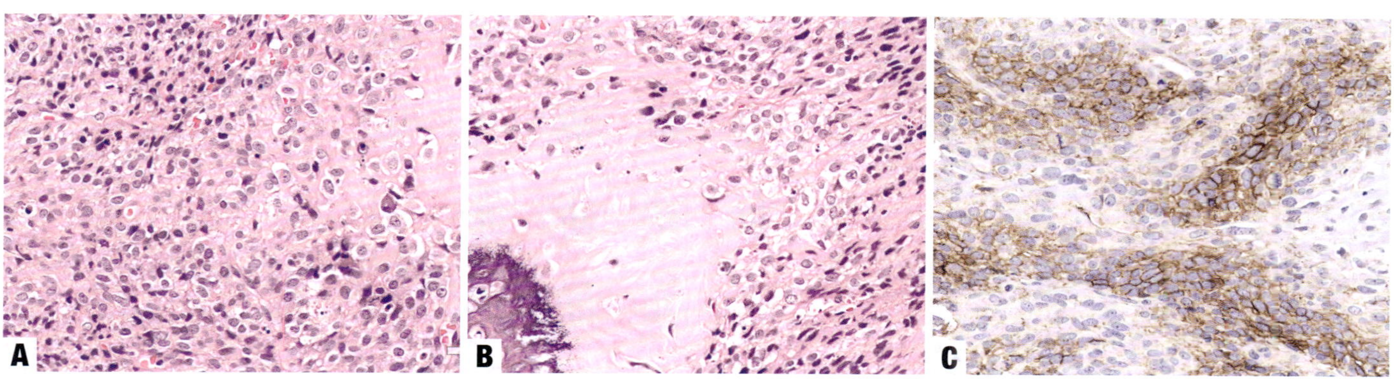

Fig. 11.102 Mesenchymal chondrosarcoma. **A** An eosinophilic matrix mimicking osteoid cells and the mesenchymal tumour cells is shown. **B** The tumour shows a biphasic component. The cartilage component of the tumour and primitive mesenchymal cells composed of round and spindle cells are seen. **C** Membrane positivity of CD99 in the tumour cells and negativity in the cartilage component is seen.

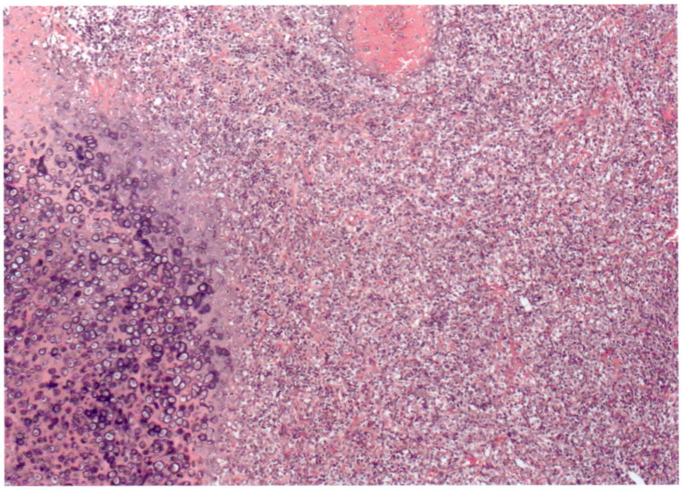

Fig. 11.103 Mesenchymal chondrosarcoma. The cartilage component of the tumour and a mesenchymal component made of undifferentiated small round or spindled cells are seen.

Macroscopic appearance

The tumour is lobulated and well defined, and contains areas of cartilage, calcification, and haemorrhage {2834,1134,1444}.

Histopathology

Mesenchymal chondrosarcoma reveals two components: foci of well-differentiated hyaline cartilage that have a zonal appearance as endochondral ossification {929,930} and a mesenchymal tumour composed of undifferentiated small round or spindled cells with a high N:C ratio. These two areas can be indistinct or separated. Areas of necrosis and brisk mitotic activity may be observed. There is almost always a distinctive haemangiopericytoma-like vascular pattern in the mesenchymal portion of the tumour {2834,1444}.

Immunohistochemistry

While immunostains are not specific, SOX9 and focal S100 are often positive in the round cells. CD99 can be positive. The tumour is usually negative for CD34, cytokeratin, EMA, and muscle markers. NKX3-1 (coding gene located at 8p21.1) immunohistochemistry expression in variable {3710,3252,564}.

Differential diagnosis

Orbital mesenchymal chondrosarcoma diagnosis is challenging if the biopsy sample is small and there is no cartilage component. The main differential diagnoses for the round cell tumour component include synovial sarcoma, Ewing sarcoma, and other round cell tumours, and if the tumour shows spindle cells,

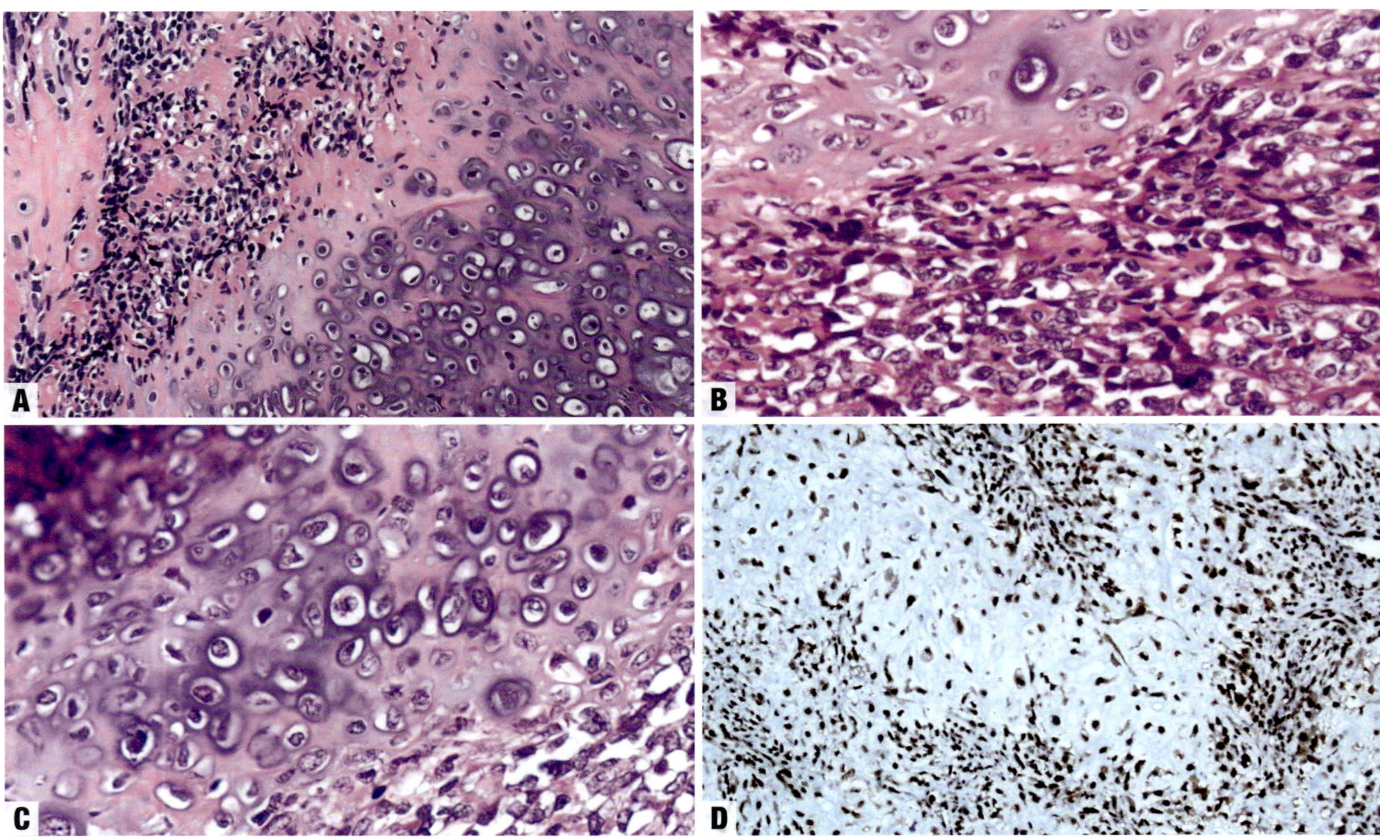

Fig. 11.104 Mesenchymal chondrosarcoma. **A** A case of orbital mesenchymal chondrosarcoma with transition from a round cell component to a cartilage component, with resting chondrocytes at the interface. **B** A different case of orbital mesenchymal chondrosarcoma, with the same transition from a round cell component to a cartilage component, with resting chondrocytes at the interface. **C** A round cell to matrix transition with the matrix exhibiting a zonal endochondral ossification-like progression of cartilage to bone/ mineralization is seen. At the interface between the round cells and cartilage on the lower right are resting, then proliferative, then hypertrophic chondrocytes, with ossification/ mineralization at the upper left. **D** This master regulator of chondrogenesis, SOX9, stains in both round cells and cartilage, indicating that the primitive round cell component is composed of immature cartilage-phenotype cells.

then synovial sarcoma and malignant solitary fibrous tumour have to be considered {109}.

Cytology

There is a biphasic appearance of medium-sized cells, oval to spindled in CNS tumours, that have a high N:C ratio and basophilic extracellular matrix {3372,929,930}.

Diagnostic molecular pathology

Detection of a *HEY1::NCOA2* fusion {3544,876} may be helpful in the diagnosis.

Essential and desirable diagnostic criteria

Essential: presence of both a cartilage component and the undifferentiated small round to spindled cells.

Desirable: staghorn vasculature; round cells positive for SOX9 and focal S100; detection of a *HEY1::NCOA2* fusion gene.

Staging

Mesenchymal chondrosarcoma of the orbit is staged according to the TNM system described by the American Joint Committee on Cancer (AJCC), based on the tumour size, involvement of lymph nodes, and presence of metastases.

Prognosis and prediction

Overall, the prognosis for orbital mesenchymal chondrosarcoma is reported to be slightly better than that of other locations {109}. Local recurrence and distant metastasis can occur several years after treatment and, therefore, a long follow-up is indicated {3757,1324,2409}.

Fibrous dysplasia

Rodríguez-Martínez HA
Bertin H
Cates JMM
Roberts F
Salomao DR

Definition

Fibrous dysplasia is a benign bone neoplasm characterized by the proliferation of clonal fibrous tissue of osteoprogenitor cell origin capable of producing only woven bone. It may involve one or multiple bones.

ICD-O coding

8818/0 Fibrous dysplasia
8818/0 Monostotic fibrous dysplasia
8818/0 Polyostotic fibrous dysplasia

ICD-11 coding

FB80.0 Fibrous dysplasia of bone

Related terminology

Acceptable: craniofacial fibrous dysplasia (extending across more than one bone).
Not recommended: liposclerosing myxofibrous tumour; fibrocartilaginous dysplasia.

Subtype(s)

Monostotic fibrous dysplasia; polyostotic fibrous dysplasia

Localization

Fibrous dysplasia can involve any bone. The more frequent locations are the craniofacial bones, femurs, and ribs. In 631 Mayo Clinic cases, 297 (47%) involved craniofacial bones; excluding 66 (11%) mandibular lesions, the remaining 231 (37%) cases were located in other craniofacial bones {3454}. The percentage of lesions originating in orbital bones is probably unknown.

Clinical features

Fibrous dysplasia usually produces radiolucent images, except cranial and mandibular lesions, which generate radiopaque images because of a more sclerotic bone composition {2730}. Polyostotic fibrous dysplasia is frequently unilateral, and can arise in the orbit. It may be associated with McCune–Albright syndrome (multiple endocrine dysfunctions, precocious puberty, and café-au-lait spots). In the craniofacial skeleton, fibrous dysplasia usually involves the mandible, but can also involve the orbital, nasal, and/or intracranial regions, as well as the paranasal sinuses. When it arises in the orbital region, patients typically present with pain, proptosis, and altered ocular motility.

Epidemiology

Fibrous dysplasia accounts for 7% of bone tumours. Monostotic fibrous dysplasia represents about 75–80% of all cases and affects adolescents and young adults {1118,2635}. Polyostotic fibrous dysplasia makes up about 20–25% of cases, usually affects young children, and has a female predilection.

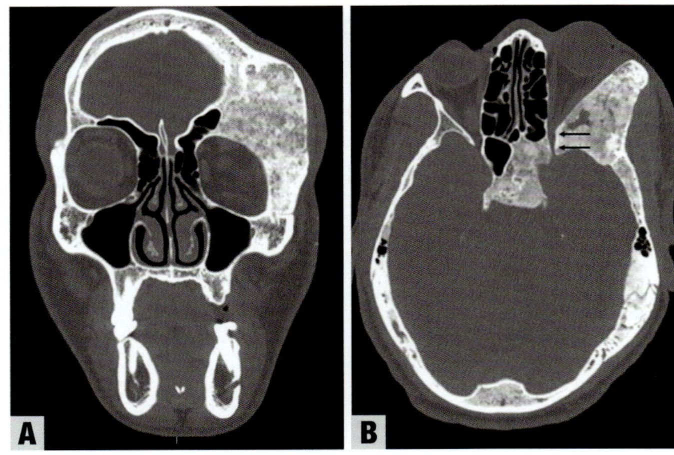

Fig. 11.105 Fibrous dysplasia, CT. **A** Polyostotic fibrous dysplasia affecting periorbital bones. **B** Polyostotic fibrous dysplasia showing narrowing of the optic canal (arrows).

Polyostotic fibrous dysplasia is associated with McCune–Albright syndrome in approximately 25% of cases and with Mazabraud syndrome in < 1% {2715,2708,2730}. Fibrous dysplasia remains quiescent in adults.

Etiology

Fibrous dysplasia is caused by activating missense mutations in the *GNAS* gene; mutations arise in postzygotic somatic cells {643,2083,2821,2730}. Normally, activation of G protein stimulates WNT/β-catenin signalling, which inhibits the terminal maturation/differentiation of osteoprogenitor cells {1670}. The presence of karyotypic abnormalities and clonality for *AR* (*HUMARA*) confirms that fibrous dysplasia is neoplastic in nature {2200}. However, the actual factor(s) triggering these changes remain(s) unknown.

Pathogenesis

Riminucci et al. {2715} showed that spindle cells are actually preosteogenic cells, rather than fibroblasts. Kashima et al. {1619} confirmed the expression of periostin, a marker of intramembranous ossification, in the fibrous component. Fibrous dysplasia is the result of the maturation arrest of osteoprogenitor cells that are capable of forming woven bone {2684}. Cells in fibrous dysplasia may also secrete FGF23 leading to hypophosphataemia. An excess of growth hormone is associated with the expansion of craniofacial fibrous dysplasia. Moreover, lesions may grow during pregnancy {2730}.

Fibrous dysplasia is caused by postzygotic activating missense mutations in the *GNAS* gene (20q13.32), encoding the alpha subunit of the stimulatory G protein ($G_s\alpha$). *GNAS* activating mutations are detected in 50–70% of cases; p.R201H and p.R201C are the most common {1897}.

Macroscopic appearance

Fibrous dysplasia is a tan-grey lesion that expands the host bone, with a firm to gritty consistency {3093}. Cystic degeneration is common; grossly identifiable chondroid nodules are exceptional. When cartilage is present (a rare event), it often stands out as sharply circumscribed, blue-tinged, translucent material {3414}.

Histopathology

Most cases show varying extents of fibrous and osseous components. Cases involving the craniofacial bones are often more osteogenic and may show extensive areas of psammomatous or cementum-like bone {3126}. The fibrous component consists of variable cellular tissue with banal spindled fibroblastic-like cells. Mitoses are very rare. The pattern of bone deposition is irregular, with curvilinear trabeculae of woven (or rarely lamellar) bone, lacking obvious osteoblastic rimming. Pagetoid type ossification (interconnecting thickened trabeculae and scant intervening fibrous tissue), foci of hyaline cartilage, hyalinization, haemorrhage, cystic degeneration, aneurysmal bone cyst–like changes, osteoclastic resorptions, and xanthomatous change may be present {2708}.

Differential diagnosis

This includes osteofibrous dysplasia {2821}, non-ossifying fibroma, aneurysmal bone cyst, and low-grade central osteosarcoma.

Cytology

Not relevant

Diagnostic molecular pathology

Diagnostic molecular pathology is not clinically relevant in most cases, though *GNAS* mutation analysis may be helpful occasionally – especially when fibrous dysplasia may be confused histologically with low-grade central osteosarcoma.

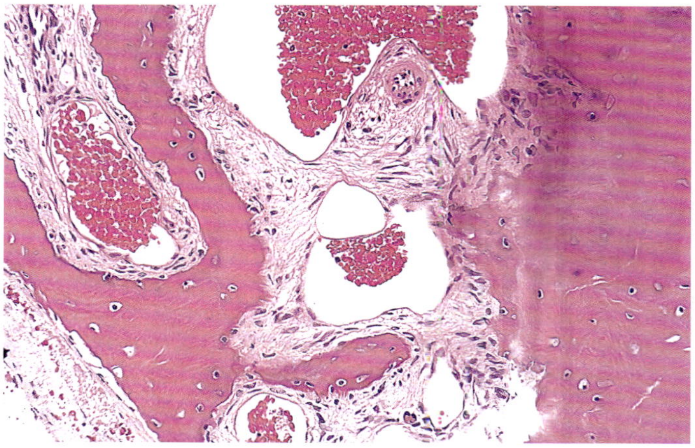

Fig. 11.106 Fibrous dysplasia. Trabeculae of woven bone without peripheral osteoblasts.

Essential and desirable diagnostic criteria

Essential: bone tumour with compatible imaging; osseous component composed of irregular, curvilinear trabeculae of woven bone without conspicuous osteoblastic rimming; fibrous component composed of bland fibroblastic cells.

Desirable (in select cases): detection of activating missense mutation in *GNAS*.

Staging

Not relevant

Prognosis and prediction

Surgical excision or debulking is the treatment of choice. An orbital location habitually precludes complete resection. Recurrence depends on tumour size and the structures involved, such as the optic nerve or CNS elements. The incidence of recurrence rates for orbital tumours is not available. Metastases do not occur, although rare cases can undergo sarcomatous transformation, mostly to osteogenic sarcoma (70%), fibrosarcoma (20%), or undifferentiated sarcoma {2708}.

Chapter 11

Haemangioma of bone

Flucke U
Righi A

Definition

Haemangioma of bone (HA-B), including epithelioid haemangioma (EH), is a benign vascular tumour infrequently involving the calvarium or facial bone including the orbit. It is genetically characterized by a fusion gene and can be locally aggressive.

ICD-O coding

9120/0 Haemangioma
9125/0 Epithelioid haemangioma

ICD-11 coding

2E81.0Y & XH5AW4 Neoplastic haemangioma of other specified site & Haemangioma, NOS
2E81.0Y & XH10T4 Neoplastic haemangioma of other specified site & Epithelioid haemangioma

Related terminology

Acceptable: intraosseous haemangioma.

Subtype(s)

Epithelioid haemangioma of bone (EH-B)

Localization

The craniofacial skeleton including the orbit can be affected {815,1138,2586,3307,3393}. Lesions can be multifocal {1404, 3652,3393}.

Clinical features

Lesions grow slowly and are often asymptomatic. They can present as a swelling/mass and can cause a range of symptoms including pain, displacement (with proptosis and diplopia), ophthalmoparesis, and epiphora {815,1138,3307}.

Imaging shows an expansile, often lobulated lesion with a polka-dot pattern that is hyperintense on MRI {3652,1404}.

Epidemiology

HA-Bs are relatively common and often incidental findings. They can be found at any age. Lesions often present in adulthood. The spine is the most common site followed by the craniofacial bones. The orbit is very rarely affected {2586,3307,1404,989}.

EH-B is rare, involving orbital bone exceptionally {3652,2586}.

Etiology

Unknown

Pathogenesis

HA-Bs are fusion gene–driven tumours, of which the genetic drivers are:

- for HA-B: *EWSR1::NFATC1* or *EWSR1::NFATC2* {2437,178,1404}
- for EH-B: *FOS* or *FOSB* rearrangements with variable partners (e.g. *ZFP36::FOSB*, *WWTR1::FOSB*, *FOS::LMNA*, and *FOS::VIM)* {2712,3393}.

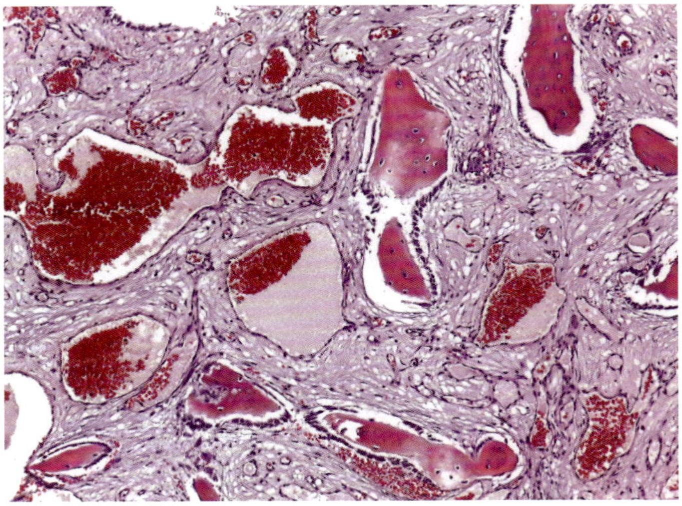

Fig. 11.107 Haemangioma of bone. This is characterized by thin-walled irregular dilated vessels surrounded by a cellular stroma.

Macroscopic appearance

These lesions are situated in the medullary cavity with a sponge-like haemorrhagic appearance and a delineated sclerotic border {1404}.

Histopathology

HA-B shows variable thin- and thick-walled vessels of different calibre without remarkable endothelial lining. A stromal reaction can be prominent. A vascular malformation can be difficult to differentiate.

EH-B is distinguished by a lobular architecture of well-formed vessels with a pericytic cuff. In the centre of the lesion, the plump monomorphic epithelioid cells are sometimes tightly packed. There is a zonation pattern with peripheral maturation. The eosinophilic cytoplasm may possess vacuoles. Cellular atypia and necrosis can be confused with a malignant tumour {1404,3393,2712}.

Immunohistochemistry

Immunohistochemistry accentuates the organoid vasculature by highlighting the endothelial cells with CD31, CD34, ERG, and FLI1 staining. Pericytes / smooth muscle cells express αSMA {1404,987}.

In EH-B, FOS or FOSB is positive {2712}.

Cytology

Not relevant

Diagnostic molecular pathology

HA-B: *EWSR1::NFATC1 or EWSR1::NFATC2*

EH-B: *FOS* or *FOSB* rearrangement with variable fusion partners

Essential and desirable diagnostic criteria

Essential: bone (orbit) as primary site; compatible radiology; for HA-B: thin-walled blood vessels lined by a single layer of non-atypical endothelial cells; for EH-B: large epithelioid endothelial cells with densely eosinophilic cytoplasm.

Desirable: detection of a fusion gene (see *Diagnostic molecular pathology*); for EH-B: lobular architecture with distinct vasoformation; FOS and FOSB positivity by immunohistochemistry.

Staging

Not relevant

Prognosis and prediction

The prognosis is excellent. Recurrences are rare. Multifocality should not be interpreted as metastases {815,1138,3307,3652, 1404}.

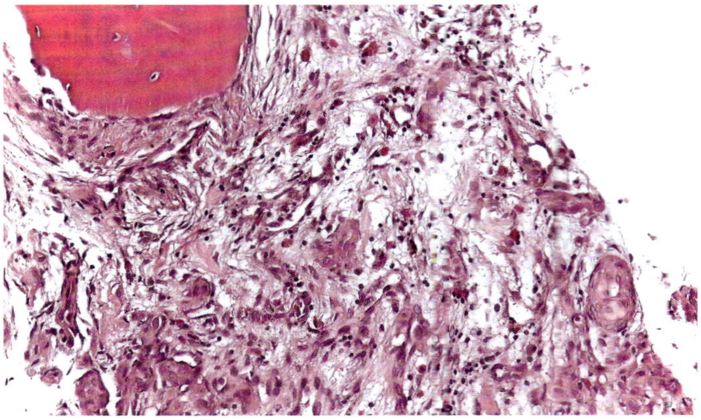

Fig. 11.108 Epithelioid haemangioma of bone. The well-formed vascular channels are lined by plump epithelioid endothelial cells.

Chapter 11

Epithelioid haemangioendothelioma

Flucke U
Tanas MR

Definition

Epithelioid haemangioendothelioma (EHE) is a fusion gene–driven sarcoma composed of epithelioid cells with endothelial differentiation.

ICD-O coding

9133/3 Epithelioid haemangioendothelioma
9133/3 Epithelioid haemangioendothelioma with *WWTR1::CAMTA1* fusion
9133/3 Epithelioid haemangioendothelioma with *YAP1::TFE3* fusion

ICD-11 coding

2B5Y & XH9GF8 Other specified malignant mesenchymal neoplasms & Epithelioid haemangioendothelioma

Related terminology

Not recommended: malignant epithelioid haemangioendothelioma.

Subtype(s)

Epithelioid haemangioendothelioma with *WWTR1::CAMTA1* fusion; epithelioid haemangioendothelioma with *YAP1::TFE3* fusion

Localization

Lesions can occur in the orbit (bone, soft tissue), skin, and lacrimal gland {3734,1716,1494,2014,3394}.

Clinical features

Patients present with a slowly growing mass, which is sometimes painful owing to vascular occlusion. Other symptoms are site- and size-dependent including proptosis, dystopia, and visual loss. There is a propensity for lymph node metastases. Multifocal disease may occur {987,2483,3734}.

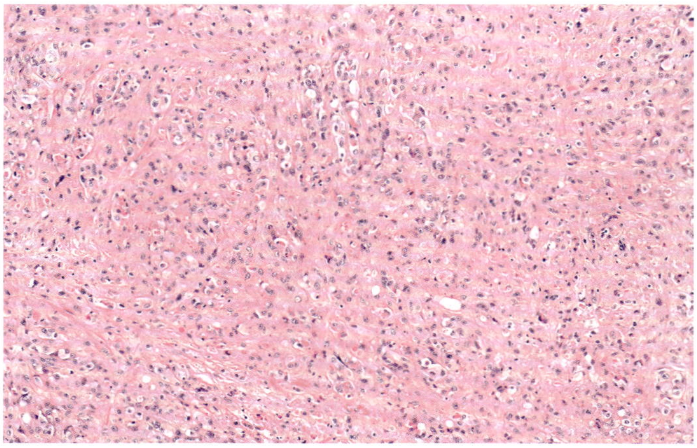

Fig. 11.109 Epithelioid haemangioendothelioma. The tumour is characterized by nests of, or loosely arranged, epithelioid endothelial cells forming subtle lumina. The mainly rounded nuclei are slightly pleomorphic. There is a collagenous background.

Epidemiology

Patient age ranges from childhood to elderly people; young to middle-aged adults are mainly affected {432,990,987,2483}.

Etiology

Unknown

Pathogenesis

As a specific driver genetic alteration, the *WWTR1::CAMTA1* fusion gene occurs in most EHEs (~90%) {2167,905,3279,3278}. Remaining cases display a *YAP1::TFE3* fusion gene {170,990}. The chimeric transcription factors are oncogenic owing to diminished negative regulation by the Hippo pathway {3278,2898,827,3254} and recruitment of epigenetic modifiers {2184}.

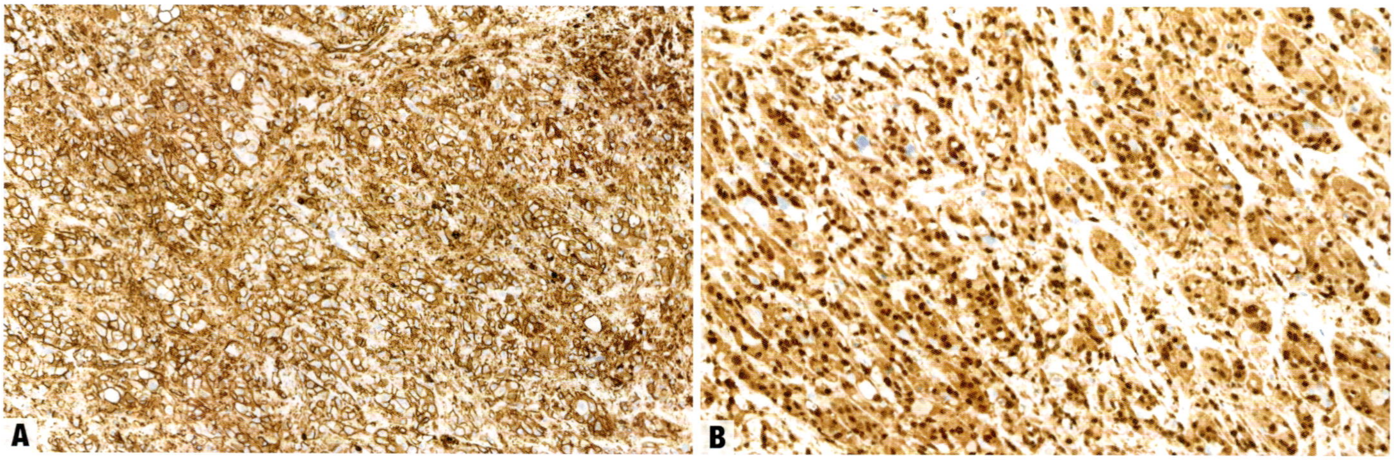

Fig. 11.110 Epithelioid haemangioendothelioma. **A** CD31 is membranous and expressed in the cytoplasm. **B** Diffuse expression of ERG.

Macroscopic appearance

EHE presents as a (multi)nodular mass with a pale, solid cut surface, sometimes with haemorrhage {990}.

Histopathology

Epithelioid-, spindle-, and histiocytoid-appearing endothelial cells with minimal cytological atypia are arranged in short cords and strands in a myxohyaline stroma. They show abundant hyaline cytoplasm with subtle intracytoplasmic lumina. Striking nuclear atypia is seen in approximately 30% of tumours. Clusters of epithelioid and spindle cells with round to ovoid nuclei and occasional vacuolated cytoplasm with signet ring–cell appearance are observed. Binucleated and multinucleated cells may occur. Mitotic activity is usually low {1509,778}. Multicellular vascular channels can be present in individual cases and are reported to be more prominent in lesions associated with *YAP1::TFE3*.

Immunohistochemistry

CD31 and ERG are consistently expressed. CAMTA1 and TFE3 are expressed depending on the fusion gene present {3577, 170,905,990,987,2483,778}.

Cytology

Not relevant

Diagnostic molecular pathology

Identification of a *WWTR1::CAMTA1* or *YAP1::TFE3* fusion helps distinguish EHE from other tumours.

Essential and desirable diagnostic criteria

Essential: strands, cords, and nests of epithelioid, spindle, and histiocytoid cells with usually minimal cytological atypia, glassy cytoplasm, and subtle intracytoplasmic lumina; myxohyaline background; positivity for CD31 and ERG.

Desirable: occasionally well-formed vessels (EHE with *YAP1::TFE3*); positivity for CAMTA1 or TFE3, and/or detection of the related fusion gene.

Staging

The Union for International Cancer Control (UICC) and American Joint Committee on Cancer (AJCC) TNM8 staging system for soft tissue sarcoma of the trunk and extremities is used.

Prognosis and prediction

Most cases are indolent. There is a risk of metastatic disease and a significant mortality rate (as high as 45%) {987,2483,778}.

Angiosarcoma of bone

Flucke U
Thway K

Definition
Angiosarcoma of bone (AS-B) is a highly aggressive sarcoma with endothelial differentiation. It is extremely rare in the orbit.

ICD-O coding
9120/3 Angiosarcoma

ICD-11 coding
2B56.Y & XH6264 Angiosarcoma, other specified primary site & Haemangiosarcoma

Related terminology
None

Subtype(s)
None

Localization
The orbit and adjacent cranial structures can be affected, with extension into the cranium, organs, and external soft tissue {1993}. AS-B can be multifocal {1404}.

Clinical features
AS-B usually presents as a rapidly growing mass with symptoms depending on the site, including visual disorders (e.g. diplopia), exophthalmia, chemosis, ptosis, and pain/headache {1993}.

Radiographically, AS-B appears lytic and aggressive with poorly defined borders and frequent cortical destruction with extraosseous spread {1404}.

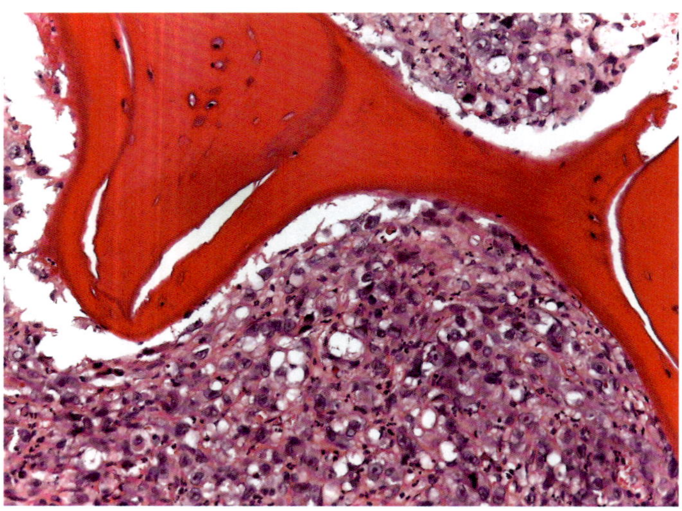

Fig. 11.111 Angiosarcoma of bone. There are sheets of atypical epithelioid cells forming subtle lumina. The tumour cells have enlarged nuclei with prominent nucleoli.

Epidemiology
AS-B is rare (< 1% of malignant bone tumours) with the orbit one of the least frequent sites {1404,1993}. Primary AS from other sites exceptionally metastasizes to the orbit {1274}. AS-B typically affects elderly people {1404}.

Etiology
The etiology is mostly unknown, but radiation therapy can be causative {2236,1993}.

Pathogenesis
The pathogenesis is complex with karyotypic and genetic heterogeneity with overlap with AS at other sites. *MYC* amplification is not necessarily associated with previous radiation therapy {1404,3475}.

Macroscopic appearance
AS-B is typically haemorrhagic, friable, and destructive, with poorly defined borders and commonly extraosseous extension {1404}.

Histopathology
Primary AS-Bs usually show epithelioid morphology with a diffuse and permeative growth pattern. Spindle cell tumours are less frequent, and in this case metastasis from elsewhere needs to be ruled out {1404,3473}.

Appearances range from relatively well to poorly formed vascular channels with variable solid growth and heterogeneity within a single neoplasm. Atypical (mainly epithelioid) endothelial cells show enlarged often hyperchromatic nuclei and frequently distinct nucleoli. Mitoses, haemorrhage, and necrosis are more frequent in less-differentiated tumours.

Immunohistochemistry
AS expresses CD31, ERG, and FLI1. There is often variable cytokeratin expression in tumours with epithelioid morphology, which can lead to confusion with metastatic carcinoma {1404, 987,3473}.

Differential diagnosis
This includes metastatic carcinoma, epithelioid haemangioendothelioma, pseudomyogenic (epithelioid sarcoma–like) haemangioendothelioma, epithelioid haemangioma, Kaposi sarcoma, and melanoma {1404}.

Cytology
Not clinically relevant

Diagnostic molecular pathology
Not clinically relevant

Essential and desirable diagnostic criteria

Essential: bone as primary site; microscopically, at least focally, vasoformative appearance and/or immunohistochemical expression of endothelial markers; prominent nuclear atypia and readily observed mitoses.

Staging

The Union for International Cancer Control (UICC) and American Joint Committee on Cancer (AJCC) TNM8 staging system for soft tissue sarcoma of the trunk and extremities is used.

Prognosis and prediction

The prognosis is very poor, and site and stage dependent {1404}, with general 5-year overall survival for skeletal AS < 40%. Cases may be managed by surgery, chemotherapy, radiotherapy, or a combination thereof {1404}.

Aneurysmal bone cyst

Agaram NP
Bredella MA

Definition

Aneurysmal bone cyst (ABC) is a destructive, expansile neoplasm of bone composed of multiloculated blood-filled cystic spaces and with a potential for local recurrence.

ICD-O coding

9260/0 Aneurysmal bone cyst

ICD-11 coding

FB80.6 Aneurysmal bone cyst

Related terminology

Not recommended: giant cell reparative granuloma of small bone; giant cell lesion of small bones.

Subtype(s)

None

Localization

ABC can affect any bone, but usually arises in the metaphysis of long bones, especially the femur, tibia, and humerus, and the posterior elements of vertebral bodies. Rarely, the bones surrounding the orbit may be involved {3526,3720}.

Clinical features

The most common signs and symptoms are pain and swelling, which are rarely secondary to fracture. In the orbit, the common signs and symptoms include proptosis, ophthalmoplegia, and exophthalmos. Radiographically, ABC presents as a lytic eccentric, expansile mass with well-defined margins. Most tumours contain a thin shell of subperiosteal, reactive bone. CT shows a cystic, expansile, and radiolucent tumour. MRI studies show internal septa and the characteristic fluid-fluid levels {1780,3482}.

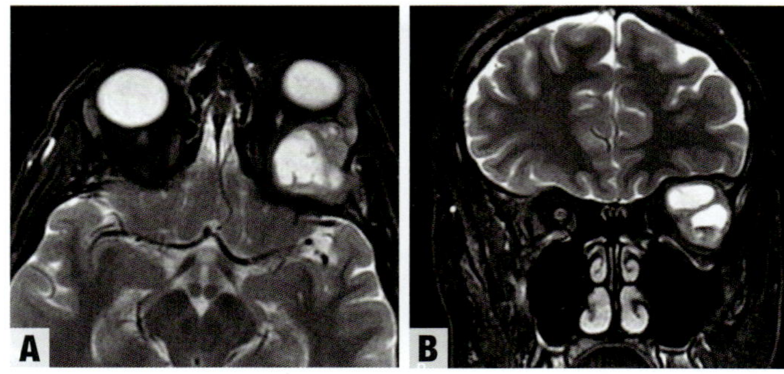

Fig. 11.112 Aneurysmal bone cyst. Fat-suppressed T2-weighted MRI showing a multicystic lesion with fluid-fluid levels. **A** Axial plane. **B** Coronal plane.

Epidemiology

ABC affects all age groups but is most common during the first two decades of life (80%). Both sexes are equally affected {2093,3482}. The estimated annual incidence is 0.15 per 1 million {1912}.

Etiology

Unknown

Pathogenesis

ABC most commonly shows the translocation t(16;17)(q22;p13) {706,2424,2478,2542,2894} leading to the fusion of *CDH11* with *USP6*, with resultant upregulation of *USP6* transcription {2424, 2425}. *USP6* rearrangements are found in approximately 70% of primary ABCs but not in secondary ABC {2426}. While the most frequent *USP6* fusion partner is *CDH11* (30%), others include *THRAP3* (*TRAP150*), *CNBP* (*ZNF9*), *OMD*, *COL1A1*, *CTNNB1*, *STAT3*, *FOSL2*, *EIF1*, *SPARC*, *PAFAH1B1*, *USP9XI*, and *RUNX2* {2425,3555,2909,1215,349}.

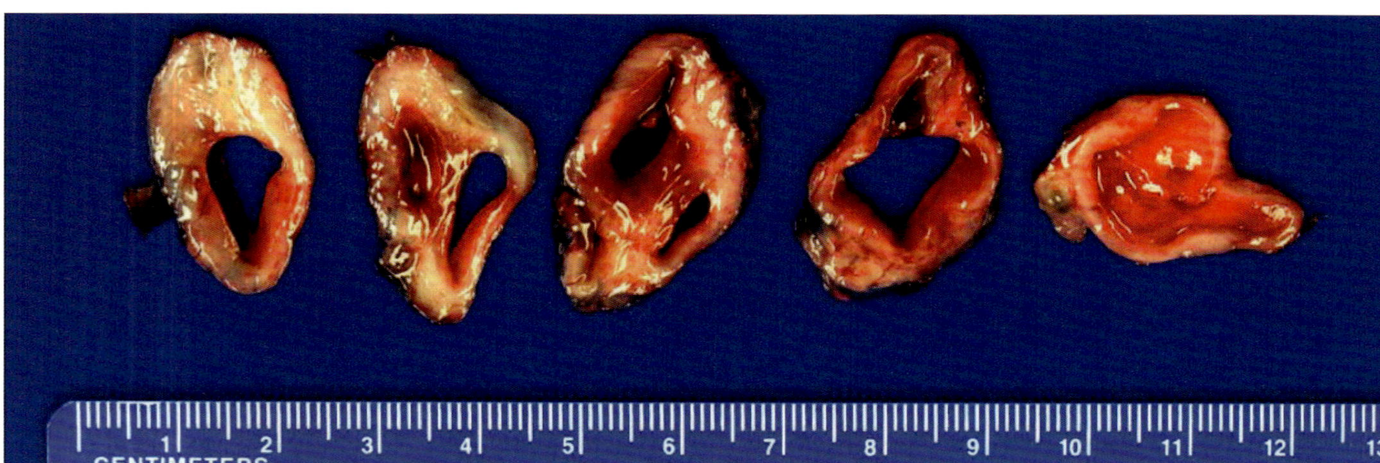

Fig. 11.113 Aneurysmal bone cyst. Gross image of a resected specimen from the retro-orbital bone showing multiple haemorrhagic cystic spaces with intervening septations.

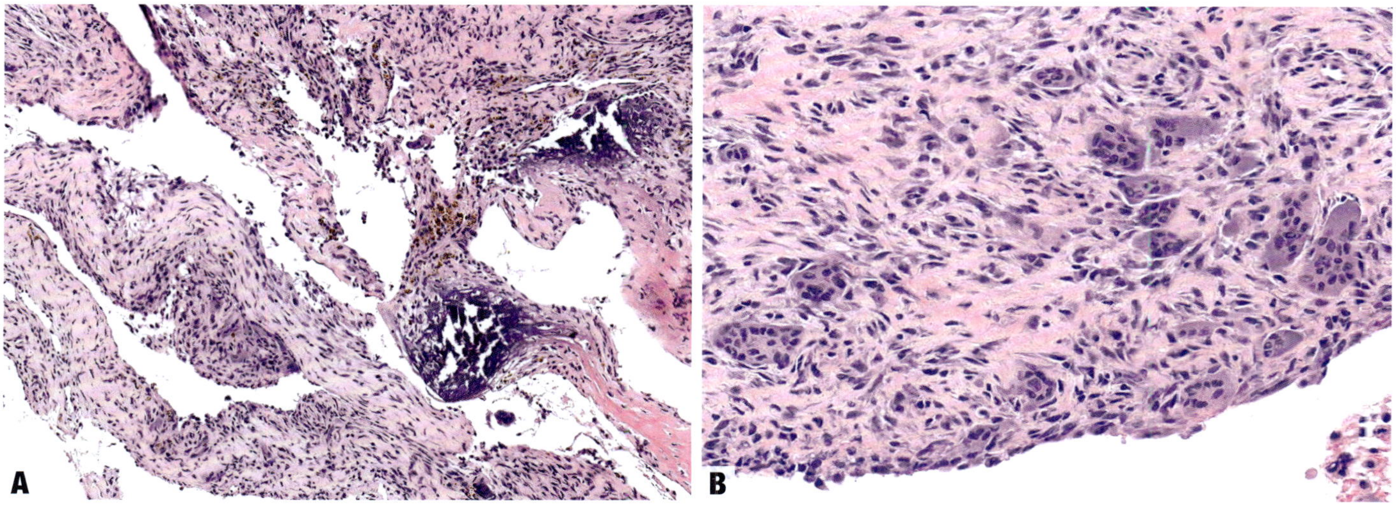

Fig. 11.114 Aneurysmal bone cyst. **A** Microscopic image showing cyst wall with multiple septations. Cyst wall showing lack of distinctive cell lining and composed of spindle cells with scattered osteoclast-like giant cells, haemorrhage, haemosiderin pigment deposition and areas of so-called blue bone. **B** Cyst wall composed of fibroblast-like spindle cells and osteoclast-like giant cells.

Macroscopic appearance

Grossly, ABC is well defined and multiloculated, and composed of blood-filled cystic spaces separated by tan-white, gritty septa. Solid areas can be seen.

Histopathology

ABC is well circumscribed and composed of blood-filled cystic spaces separated by fibrous septa, which are composed of a moderately dense cellular proliferation of bland fibroblasts, with scattered, multinucleated, osteoclast-like giant cells and reactive woven bone rimmed by osteoblasts. In about one third of cases, the bone is basophilic and has been termed "blue bone", although its presence is not diagnostic. Mitoses are commonly present and can be numerous; however, atypical forms are absent. Necrosis is rare unless there has been a pathological fracture. The solid pattern of ABC has the same components and is very similar to giant cell lesion of small bones {320,2846}. Primary ABC accounts for approximately 70% of all cases, while secondary ABCs may develop in association with other benign neoplasms, most commonly giant cell tumour of bone, osteoblastoma, chondroblastoma, and fibrous dysplasia {1780,2093,3482}.

Differential diagnosis includes ABC-like areas consequent to haemorrhagic changes, associated with benign and, less frequently, malignant bone tumours (formerly termed "secondary aneurysmal bone cyst") {1780,2093,3482}. Telangiectatic osteosarcoma may mimic ABC on imaging and macroscopically, but microscopically malignant cells within fibrous septa are seen

Cytology

Not clinically relevant

Diagnostic molecular pathology

USP6 gene rearrangement can be detected by FISH study using break-apart probes, or by next-generation sequencing.

Essential and desirable diagnostic criteria

Essential: radiology: multicystic lesion with fluid-fluid levels; histology: cyst wall composed of fibroblasts, osteoclast-like giant cells, haemosiderin pigment, and new bone formation; molecular: *USP6* gene rearrangement.

Staging

Not relevant

Prognosis and prediction

ABC is a potentially locally recurrent neoplasm. The recurrence rate after curettage is variable (20–70%). Spontaneous regression after incomplete removal is very unusual

Giant cell tumour of bone

Flanagan AM
Proia AD

Definition

Giant cell tumour of bone is a locally aggressive and rarely metastasizing neoplasm composed of neoplastic mononuclear stromal cells with a monotonous appearance admixed with macrophages and osteoclast-like giant cells.

ICD-O coding

9250/1 Giant cell tumour of bone
9250/1 Conventional giant cell tumour of bone
9250/3 Malignant giant cell tumour of bone
9250/3 Dedifferentiated giant cell tumour of bone

ICD-11 coding

2F7B & XH4TC2 Neoplasms of uncertain behaviour of bone or articular cartilage & Giant cell tumour of bone, NOS
2B5Y & XH0492 Other specified malignant mesenchymal neoplasms & Giant cell tumour of bone, malignant

Related terminology

Not recommended: osteoclastoma; benign fibrous histiocytoma.

Subtype(s)

Conventional giant cell tumour of bone; malignant giant cell tumour of bone; dedifferentiated giant cell tumour of bone

Localization

Most lesions occur predominantly in the bones around the knee, sited in the epiphysis. Orbital tumours usually arise from the frontal bone {3487,1590,3284,3701,1981} and may rarely arise in the temporal bone {1891}.

Clinical features

Signs and symptoms are not specific for giant cell tumour but are similar to any space-occupying lesion in the orbit and include a visible mass, proptosis, eyelid oedema, diplopia, eyelid erythema, and neurological sequelae such as hearing loss, changes in vision acuity, and facial changes due to nerve compression.

Imaging

Imaging does not exhibit specific diagnostic features for a giant cell tumour. It is an osteolytic lesion without a sclerotic well-defined rim. The surrounding cortical bone is thinned.

Epidemiology

Giant cell tumour of orbital bone is rare {1891,3701}. In the most common sites, the peak incidence is between the ages of 20 and 45 years, with approximately 10% of cases occurring in the second decade of life {85}. There are several reports in the old literature of giant cell tumour in children of 10 years or younger but these may represent other pathologies.

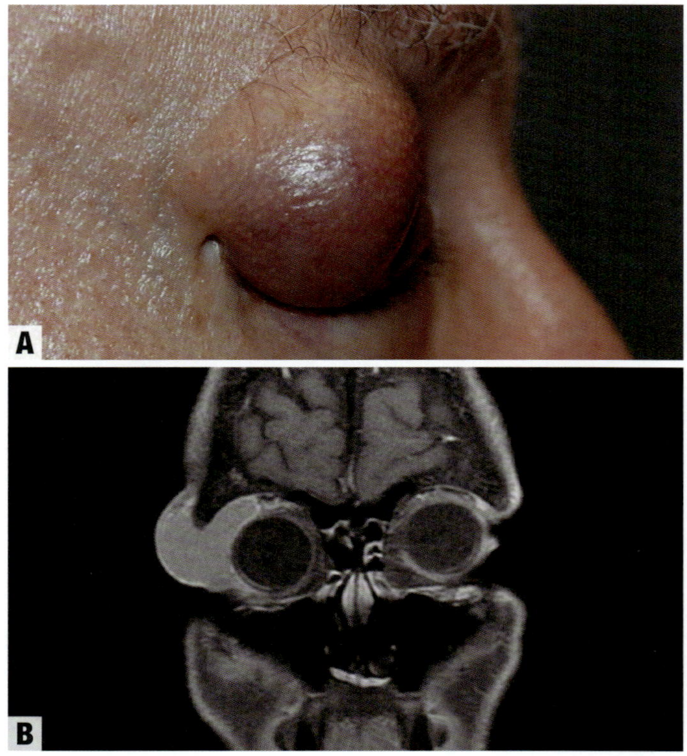

Fig. 11.115 Giant cell tumour of bone. Lateral view (**A**) and coronal T1-weighted MRI with contrast (**B**) of a recurrent right orbital giant cell tumour.

Etiology

Giant cell tumour, defined by the presence of a histone (*H3-3A*) gene sequence variant, is a sporadic disease the cause of which is unknown, other than in phaeochromocytoma/paraganglioma and giant cell tumour syndrome, which is brought about by an early postzygotic event {3350,3349}. Giant cell tumour–like tumours that occur associated with pagetic bone disease do not harbour the *H3-3A* SNV but are associated with specific germline alterations, namely in *ZNF687* {807} and *PFN1* {3567}.

Pathogenesis

There is limited literature with respect to the presence of an *H3-3A* mutation in giant cell tumour of orbital bone {1891,3701}. The pathogenic changes are driven by the oncohistone *H3-3A* gene by altering the epigenome and transcriptome and disrupting the physiological differentiation of the osteoprogenitor {1673,1456,2011}.

Macroscopic appearance

The macroscopic appearance of giant cell tumour of the orbit is not reported but probably shows features typical of giant cell tumour elsewhere in the body (see the fifth-edition *Soft tissue and bone tumours* volume {3598}).

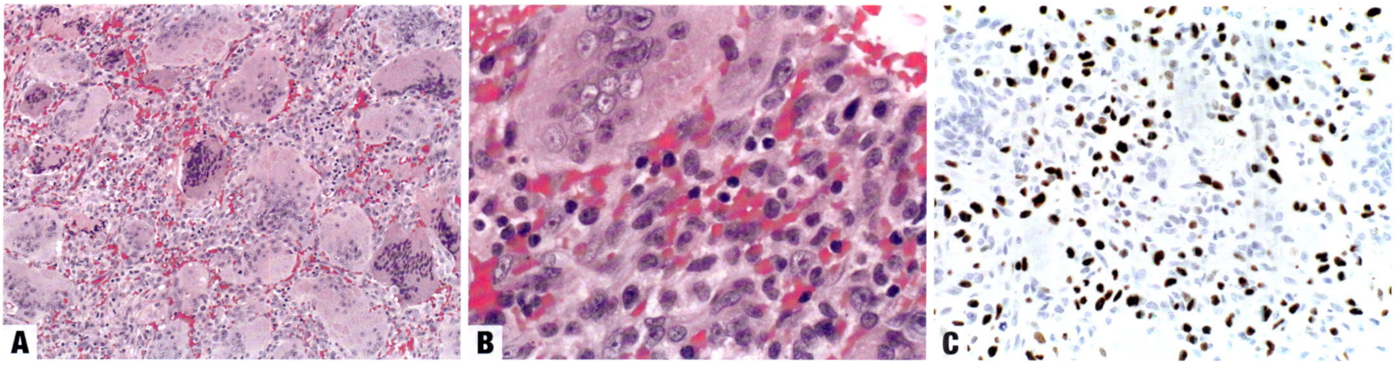

Fig. 11.116 Giant cell tumour of bone. **A** Typical features of a giant cell tumour are seen, showing a predominance of osteoclast-like giant cells with interspersed mononuclear neoplastic cells. **B** A high-power view shows nuclear atypia of the neoplastic mononuclear cells with irregular nuclear profiles and moderate-sized to large nucleoli in some cells. **C** H3.3 p.G34W immunoreactivity of atypical stromal cells is present in a large majority of giant cell tumours of bone. It is often absent in patients with a predisposing genetic syndrome such as Paget disease of bone, Gorlin–Goltz syndrome, and Jaffe–Campanacci syndrome.

Histopathology

A conventional giant cell tumour is characterized by abundant large osteoclasts containing as many as 100 nuclei set amid the neoplastic monotonous mononuclear cell population harbouring the *H3-3A* mutation. Mitotic figures may be copious but atypical forms are not present. Ischaemic necrosis may be present. Scattered enlarged mononuclear cells may be present and should not be interpreted as malignant.

Denosumab treatment of giant cell tumour shows significantly reduced numbers of osteoclasts and bone formation {1120, 404}. The features may raise concern of malignancy {3624}

Malignancy in giant cell tumour arises simultaneously or subsequent to a conventional benign giant cell tumour with an *H3-3A* mutation and may occur subsequent to radiotherapy. It can show a variety of histological features. The conventional malignant tumour is an osteoclast-rich tumour but the neoplastic tumour exhibits highly atypical cells and commonly atypical mitotic figures.

The dedifferentiated malignant giant cell tumour is defined, like dedifferentiated chondrosarcoma and liposarcoma, by the presence of a biphasic tumour including a conventional benign component of a giant cell tumour abruptly delineated from a non-osteoclast–rich tumour exhibiting a spindle cell sarcoma NOS or osteosarcomatous features. Generally, this component is high-grade but may have low-grade morphology {132,979}. Malignancy in giant cell tumour may be associated with loss of the *H3-3A* mutation {3711,979}.

Immunohistochemistry

H3.3 p.G35W (G34W) immunoreactivity is a reliable indicator of the presence of the mutation {132,3666}. Antibodies are not employed clinically for other H3.3 p.G35 SNVs.

Differential diagnosis

Other osteoclast-rich tumours include primary and secondary aneurysmal bone cyst, giant cell reparative granuloma {553}, chondroblastoma, and the recently identified giant cell tumour–like lesion with *MGA2::NCOR2* fusion, although not as yet reported in the orbit {2473}, as well as germline lesions including cherubism and neurofibromatosis–Noonan syndrome, and brown tumour of hyperparathyroidism {3526}. The malignant subtype can mimic a telangiectatic osteosarcoma. Giant cell tumour of orbital bone must be differentiated from giant cell tumour of soft tissue, which also arises rarely in the orbit and has been characterized recently by a recurrent *HMGA2::NCOR2* fusion gene and immunoreactivity for AE1/AE3 {6,2639,2640,36}.

Cytology

Not clinically relevant

Diagnostic molecular pathology

A driver gene mutation is detected in the neoplastic stromal cell population in as many as 96% of giant cell tumours {132, 289,2412,632,1664,3666}, 90% of which are represented by the H3.3 p.G35W (G34W) sequence variant. Other H3.3 p.G35 variants are uncommon {289,2412,2589}. Detection of the mutation does not distinguish between conventional and malignant giant cell tumours.

Loss of the *H3-3A* variant in an undifferentiated or osteosarcomatous component of a conventional giant cell tumour which harbours an *H3-3A* mutation represents a dedifferentiated giant cell tumour {979,132}. Failure to detect H3.3 p.G35 mutation should prompt testing for alterations characteristic of giant cell tumour mimics.

Essential and desirable diagnostic criteria

Essential: bone tumour compatible with imaging; unusually large osteoclasts and a mononuclear cell population without atypia in the conventional subtype.

Desirable: skeletally mature individuals; detection of H3.3 p.G35 (G34) mutated cells.

Staging

Not relevant

Prognosis and prediction

A multidisciplinary approach to surgical treatment is recommended in view of the potential complications including ocular morbidity, orbital compartmental syndrome, and facial disfigurement.

Surgical resection is the recommended treatment. Recurrence rates vary depending on whether a wide resection (7%) or more limited surgery (60%) is undertaken. Radiotherapy is generally restricted to inoperable tumours {2007}. Denosumab can be used for reducing tumour size thereby facilitating surgical treatment; it also reduces pain {554,2007}.

Ewing sarcoma

de Álava E
Bahrami A

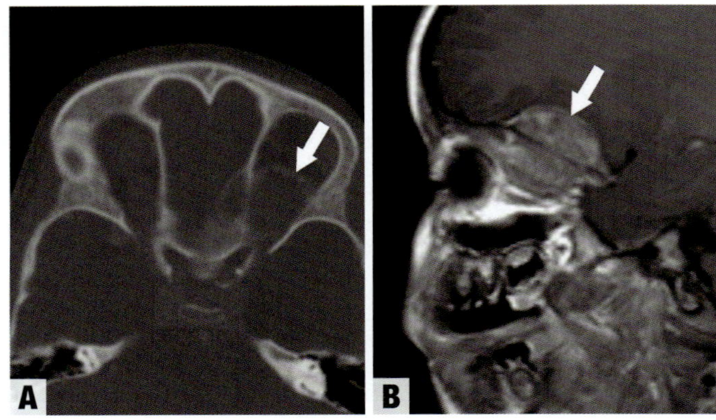

Fig. 11.117 Ewing sarcoma. **A** Axial CT, bone window shows bony sclerosis in the left orbit (arrow) and skull base associated with the Ewing sarcoma. **B** Sagittal T1-weighted postcontrast MRI shows a heterogeneously enhancing mass arising from the left orbital roof with extension into the orbit and intracranial compartment (arrow).

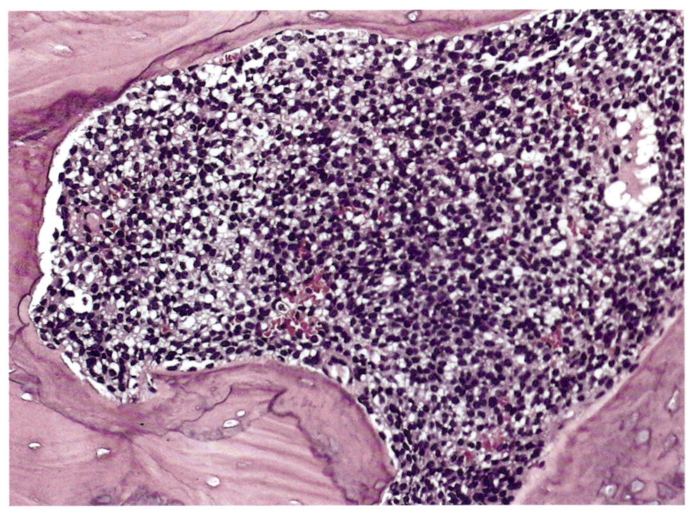

Fig. 11.118 Ewing sarcoma of bone. Notice the dark and uniform nuclei and cleared-out cytoplasms, due to glycogen deposits.

Definition

Ewing sarcoma of the orbital bone is a small round cell sarcoma containing a fusion between one FET family gene (usually *EWSR1*) and one ETS family gene (most often *FLI1*).

ICD-O coding

9364/3 Ewing sarcoma

ICD-11 coding

2B52.Y Ewing sarcoma of bone or articular cartilage of other specified sites

Related terminology

Not recommended: (peripheral) primitive neuroectodermal tumour.

Subtype(s)

None

Localization

Ewing sarcoma of the orbital area is more likely to arise from orbital bone (83%) than soft tissue (17%) {1576}. Extraorbital extension occurs in most patients and is mainly intracranial.

Clinical features

The most common presenting complaints were proptosis and upper eyelid swelling in the largest reported series {1576}.

Epidemiology

Ewing sarcoma of the orbit occurs most commonly in children and young adults {1576}.

Etiology

The majority of cases are sporadic. Although germline mutations (in *BRCA1*, for example) have been detected {1190}, their pathogenetic roles remain unclear.

Pathogenesis

Most tumours harbour a t(11;22)(q24;q12) translocation {3401, 212}, resulting in *EWSR1::FLI1* fusion {1190}. The second most common translocation is t(21;22)(q22;q12), which results in *EWSR1::ERG* fusion {1190}.

Macroscopic appearance

The cut surface of untreated Ewing sarcoma specimens is greyish-white and soft, and it frequently includes areas of haemorrhage and necrosis.

Histopathology

Tumours consist of a monotonous population of small round cells arranged in sheets or solid aggregates, separated by fibrous septa. Focal rosettes are sometimes present. Cells have round nuclei, coarse chromatin, small nucleoli, and scant eosinophilic or clear cytoplasm. Mitotic activity is brisk and necrosis is common.

Immunohistochemistry

There is diffuse, strong, membranous CD99 expression and nuclear FLI1 expression. NKX2-2 has a higher specificity than CD99 {2021}. Focal positivity with broad-spectrum cytokeratins is common. Desmin, myogenin, and MYOD1 are negative.

Cytology

Not clinically relevant

Diagnostic molecular pathology

All cases of Ewing sarcoma harbour a FET::ETS fusion. Genetic confirmation is often required for Ewing sarcoma diagnosis. The most common Ewing sarcoma fusion (present in ~85% of cases) is *EWSR1::FLI1*. The second most common is *EWSR1::ERG* in about 10% of cases. The remaining cases have alternative translocations that join either *EWSR1* or *FUS* (which, along with *TAF15*, form the FET family) to other ETS family members.

Essential and desirable diagnostic criteria

Essential: small round cell morphology; strong CD99 membranous expression.

Desirable: strong and diffuse NKX2-2 expression; detection of a FET::ETS fusion.

Staging

The American Joint Committee on Cancer (AJCC) and Union for International Cancer Control (UICC) TNM systems can be applied.

Prognosis and prediction

The prognosis for Ewing sarcoma has improved considerably with current multimodal therapy, with a 65–70% cure rate for localized disease. However, metastatic and early relapsing tumours have a poor prognosis, with a 5-year survival rate of < 30%. The presence of metastases appears to be the main prognostic factor. Other prognostic factors include the anatomical location of the tumour, tumour volume, and the patient's age {1190}. Complete pathological response to neoadjuvant chemotherapy is a favourable prognostic factor {70}. There are currently no other prognostic markers in widespread use.

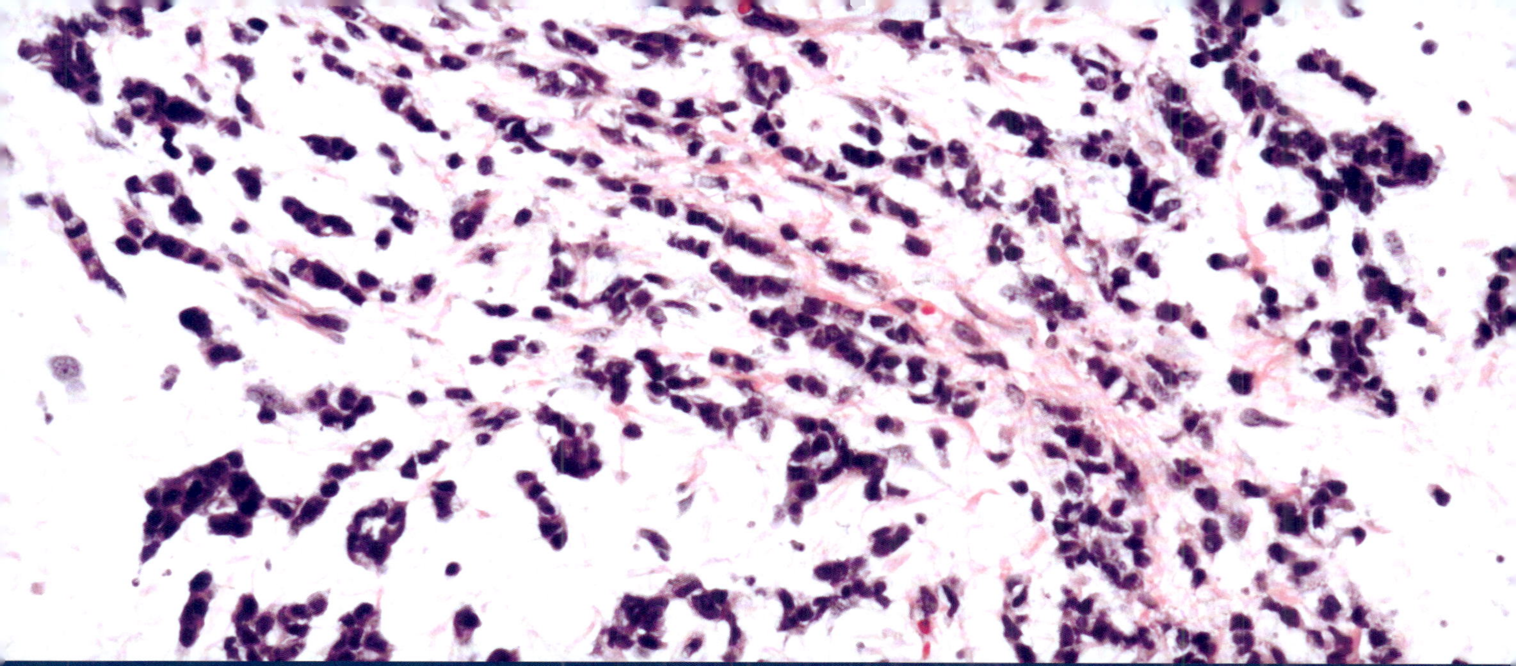

12

Metastases to the eye and surrounding structures

Edited by: Cree IA, Esmaeli B, White VA

Metastases to ocular adnexal structures
Metastases to intraocular structures

Metastases to the eye and surrounding structures: Introduction

Esmaeli B
White VA

Orbital metastases are estimated to occur in < 5% of patients with cancer, although this may be an underestimation given that in patients with end-stage cancer the presence of orbital metastasis maybe underrecognized {48,882}. The incidence of orbital metastases has increased in the past few decades given that patients with cancer are living longer as newer treatments have led to improved survival {1014}. Most often the diagnosis of orbital metastases is made in a patient with a previous known history of cancer, but in a minority of cases, orbital symptoms are the first sign of widely metastatic cancer, and in an even smaller number of cases, the orbit is the only identifiable anatomical site of metastasis. An orbital biopsy may be indicated to confirm the diagnosis and give access to tissue for analysis in case potential targeted therapy or immunotherapy is contemplated, helping treatment selection.

In a cohort of 118 patients with orbital metastasis treated at a tertiary cancer centre in a recent period, the most common types of cancer that metastasized to the orbit were breast carcinoma followed by cutaneous melanoma and lung carcinoma.

The usual presenting signs and symptoms of orbital metastasis are proptosis, diplopia, droopy eyelid, orbital pain, and optic nerve compression. Multidisciplinary management of orbital metastasis using a combination of chemotherapy, targeted therapy, immunotherapy, palliative radiation therapy, and surgery can help improve quality of life {882,1014}.

Metastases to ocular adnexal structures

Verdijk RM
Mudhar HS

Definition

Metastases to the ocular adnexal structures are malignancies that originate from a distant organ site or are from a discontinuous primary tumour elsewhere in the periorbital area.

ICD-O coding

Code according to the originating tumour type.

ICD-11 coding

Code according to the originating tumour type.

Related terminology

None

Subtype(s)

None

Localization

Metastases involve the ocular adnexal structures, which comprise the eyelids, conjunctiva, orbit, lacrimal gland, and lacrimal drainage system (see Table 12.01).

Clinical features

Patients with ocular adnexal metastases can present with a discrete mass. The clinical features are dependent on the exact adnexal structure involved. Metastases to the eyelid may present with diffuse eyelid oedema or a discrete mass {333}. Metastases to the conjunctiva may present with a red eye, foreign body sensation, or tearing {1715}. Orbital and lacrimal gland metastases may present with ptosis, increased retrobulbar resistance, diplopia, reduced eye movement, and proptosis {882}. Lacrimal sac metastases present with symptoms typical of acquired nasolacrimal duct obstruction, including epiphora, epistaxis, and a palpable mass with or without pain {3516}. They are typically initially diagnosed clinically as either chronic dacryocystitis or a primary malignancy {3623}. Metastases are fast growing and usually unifocal. Most patients with ocular adnexal metastasis have concurrent metastases to adjacent ocular adnexal as well as non-ocular sites {1715, 2972}. Metastases may also manifest as the first sign of a primary tumour.

CT and MRI show a soft tissue mass in the ocular adnexa and orbit, which may show bony erosion. Almost all ocular adnexal metastases evaluated by MRI show some degree of enhancement with contrast agents. The diagnosis is made on the basis of a thorough history, ocular examination, general physical assessment looking for a primary neoplasm and other metastases, orbital CT or MRI, and open biopsy or FNAB. Biopsy is necessary to confirm that the lesion is a metastatic tumour and not a primary tumour or a simulating lesion such as idiopathic orbital inflammation.

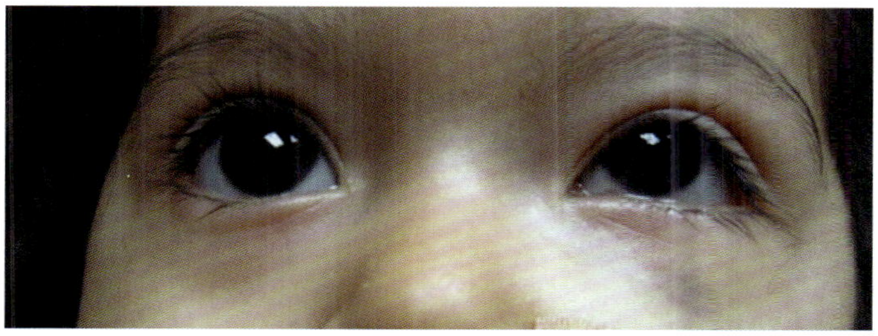

Fig. 12.01 Metastatic neuroblastoma to orbit. Clinical photograph of a child with metastatic neuroblastoma with a metastatic focus in the inferior left orbit and the typical periorbital echymosis.

Table 12.01 Metastases to ocular adnexal structures

	Eyelid	Conjunctiva	Orbit	Lacrimal gland	Lacrimal sac
Studies (*n*)	3	1	3	1	7
Cases (*n*)	66	13	301	23	7
Location					
Breast (%)	30%	38%	44%	39%	14%
Lung (%)	5%	23%	11%	0%	29%
Melanoma (%)	22%	15%	8%	0%	14%
Kidney (%)	8%	0%	6%	13%	14%
Prostate (%)	2%	0%	7%	0%	0%
Gastrointestinal tract (%)	8%	0%	5%	4%	0%
Other (%)	26%	15%	14%	43%	29%
Unknown (%)	3%	8%	4%	4%	0%
References	{2059,2714,333}	{2972}	{882,2005,1076A}	{1180A}	{1180A}

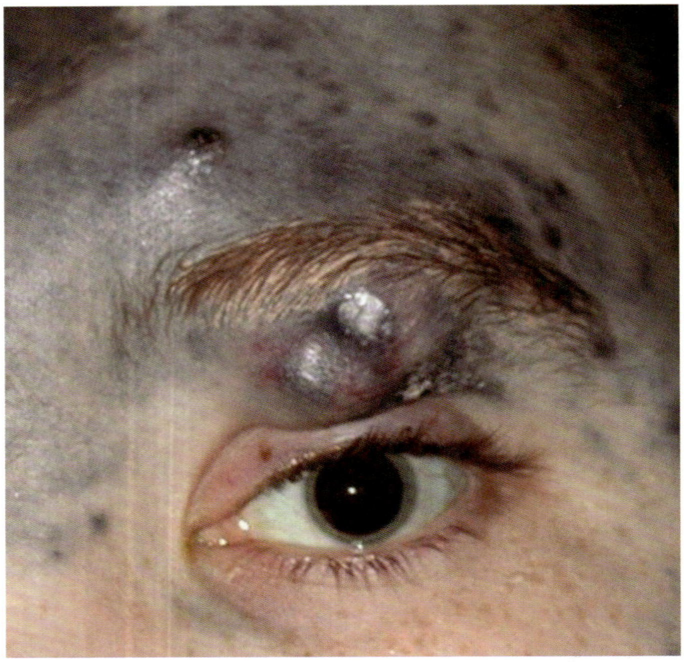

Fig. 12.02 Cutaneous melanoma metastatic to eyelid. Clinical photograph of a patient with metastatic cutaneous melanoma with multiple metastases in the periocular skin and eyelid area.

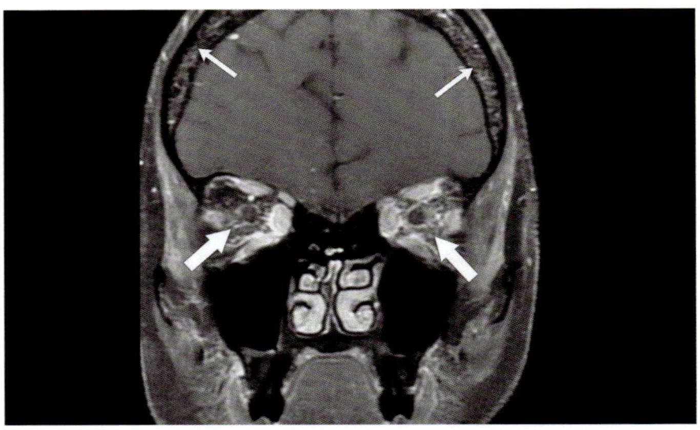

Fig. 12.03 Metastatic breast carcinoma. Coronal T1-weighted postcontrast MRI shows infiltrative tumour in the orbits bilaterally (large arrows). Diffuse enhancing calvarial metastases are also present (small arrows).

Epidemiology

Metastases account for < 1% of all ocular adnexal tumour pathology specimens {333,1181,1715,2968,2972,3510,3480}. Metastatic tumours to the ocular adnexa generally occur in older individuals and there may be a slight preponderance of women over men. Apart from the orbit and eyelid, reports of other specific ocular adnexal metastases are mainly anecdotal case reports; no comprehensive series have been published. Series reports on the tissue specificity of metastasis to the orbit often mention fat, muscle, and bone, but rarely mention the lacrimal gland {61,1141} or conjunctiva. Several factors may result in underestimation of the true incidence; for example, patients with small lesions may remain asymptomatic, and the eye and ocular adnexa are not part of standard autopsy protocols.

Etiology

The most frequent primary origins of tumours metastatic to the ocular adnexa as reported in the literature are summarized in Table 12.01 (p. 485). For metastases to the ocular adnexa, metastatic breast carcinoma is the most common, followed by lung carcinoma, renal cell carcinoma, and metastatic cutaneous melanoma. In contrast, a recent report on 118 patients from a US tertiary cancer centre found the most frequent primary tumour metastatic to the orbit to be breast carcinoma, followed by cutaneous melanoma, lung carcinoma, thyroid carcinoma, renal cell carcinoma, and neuroendocrine carcinoma {882}. However, any tumour type has the potential to metastasize to the ocular adnexa. It is also important to note that most series are based on a mainly White population. A literature-based series on 128 orbital metastases in the Japanese population, for example, showed that metastases from the liver and stomach are seen more frequently in Japan than in the USA and Europe {138}.

Uveal and conjunctival melanoma and sebaceous carcinoma can recur in the ocular adnexa, often several years after initial treatment {2073,2228,2676}. It is sometimes unclear whether such recurrence results from direct extension or metastatic seeding. For involvement of the ocular adnexa by lymphoma or leukaemia, see the specific sections on haematolymphoid tumours in Chapter 11: *Soft tissue and bone tumours*.

Pathogenesis

Pathogenesis is dependent on the primary tumour involved.

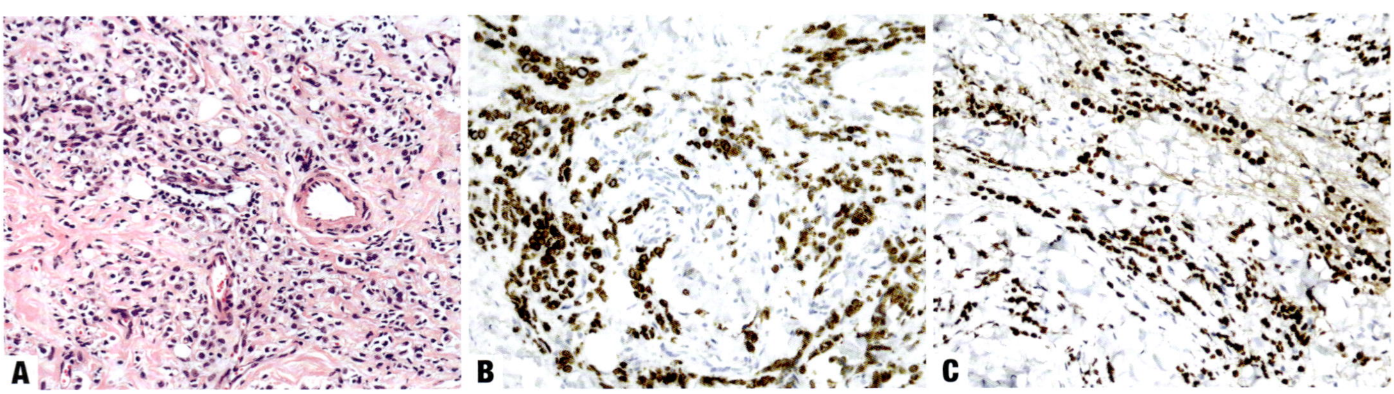

Fig. 12.04 Lobular breast carcinoma metastatic to the eyelid. **A** An eyelid tumour in a 68-year-old female patient with a metastasis from occult lobular breast carcinoma is seen. **B** CK7 positivity is seen. **C** Staining for ER is strongly positive.

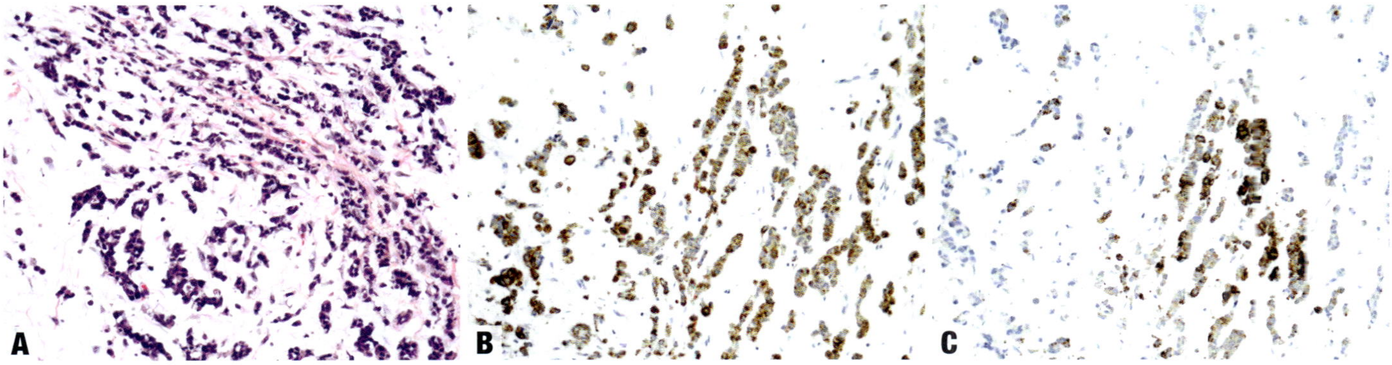

Fig. 12.05 Prostate adenocarcinoma metastatic to the orbit. **A** An orbital tumour in a 77-year-old male patient with extensive metastatic prostate carcinoma. **B** There is strong pankeratin staining. **C** PAP staining is positive.

Macroscopic appearance

The macroscopic appearance depends on the origin of the metastasis; it may be fibrous with metastatic breast carcinoma or fleshy with haemorrhage in renal cell carcinoma and neuroendocrine tumours (carcinoids). Metastases can be yellow, red, or brown, depending on the nature of the primary tumour.

Histopathology

Generally, metastases retain (to some extent) the histological pattern and cytological characteristics of the primary tumour. Immunohistochemistry is a valuable tool for distinguishing between primary and metastatic neoplasms. No marker is entirely specific; therefore, the use of a carefully constructed panel of markers is important {1273,1789}.

Cytology

Cytological features generally resemble those of the primary tumour.

Diagnostic molecular pathology

DNA methylation profiling {2267} and RNA expression profiling {1245} are promising potential tools for the identification of primary tumour origin in the future.

Essential and desirable diagnostic criteria

If known primary malignancy

Essential: concurrence of the histological appearance of the metastasis with the histology of the original primary malignancy.

Desirable: immunohistochemical confirmation of primary site.

If no known primary malignancy

Essential: tumour with malignant cytology and other features of malignant tumours (destruction of anatomy, necrosis, vascular channel invasion, etc.); assessment must distinguish primary malignancy of an adnexal site from metastasis using a combination of clinical history, imaging modalities, histopathology, immunohistochemistry, and molecular assessment.

Staging

Stage according to the originating tumour type.

Prognosis and prediction

The prognosis for metastatic disease is highly dependent on tumour type and stage. The decision to treat with irradiation, chemotherapy, and/or adjuvant targeted therapies may be facilitated by specific immunohistochemical and molecular findings, such as hormone receptor expression and *ERBB2* amplification status in breast carcinoma.

For a discrete eyelid metastasis, surgical resection might be a reasonable treatment option, albeit palliative in nature. Radiation therapy at a palliative dose and/or systemic treatments for cancer such as targeted therapy, immunotherapy, or chemotherapy can also be considered for the management of ocular adnexal metastasis.

Metastases to intraocular structures

Mudhar HS
Sagoo MS
Verdijk RM

Definition

Metastases are malignant tumours that originate from a distant organ site and deposit at any intraocular structure.

ICD-O coding

Code according to the originating tumour type.

ICD-11 coding

Code according to the originating tumour type.

Related terminology

None

Subtype(s)

None

Localization

Intraocular metastases involve the choroid (90%), ciliary body (2%), iris (8%), and retina, optic disc, vitreous, and/or lens capsule (< 1–4%) (see Table 12.02).

Clinical features

In the choroid, metastases occur as yellow-coloured tumour(s) with subretinal fluid and surface retinal pigment epithelial changes (leopard spotting). B-scan ultrasound shows a high echogenicity mass (80%) and optical coherence tomography shows an irregular ("lumpy bumpy") choroidal surface (64%). In the iris, metastases produce a pale nodule in the iris stroma; in the ciliary body, metastasis is rare but occurs as a mass. Retinal, vitreous, and lens capsule metastases are frequently pigmented tumours originating from cutaneous melanoma. Optic disc metastasis is often associated with adjacent choroidal metastasis and can present with optic disc swelling {2981}.

Epidemiology

Postmortem studies have recorded a prevalence of intraocular metastases in patients who have died from disseminated malignancy in 2–10% of cases {71,1513,359,964,883,2366}, as opposed to living patients, for whom the prevalence is 2–7% {2112}. The uvea is the commonest site for intraocular metastases {3016,964,3203,1031,3067,2984,181,1764}. Uveal metastases are seen in all age groups. The mean patient age is 60 years {2967}, there is a female predilection (64% female, 36% male) {2967}, and a predominance in White people (88% White people vs 12% non-White people) {2967}. Unilateral metastases are more common than bilateral (76% unilateral, 24% bilateral) {3016}. In 67% of cases, the primary tumour is diagnosed before the metastasis {3024}.

Etiology

The primary sites from which metastatic malignancies arise are in the following order of frequency: breast (37%), lung (27%),

Table 12.02 Frequency of different types of metastatic tumours at different intraocular locations

Intraocular structure	Metastatic tumours (in order of frequency)	Reference
Iris	Breast carcinoma Lung carcinoma Skin melanoma Renal carcinoma Oesophageal carcinoma	{3024,2984}
Ciliary body and choroid	Breast carcinoma Lung carcinoma Renal carcinoma Gastrointestinal tract carcinoma Skin melanoma Lung carcinoid Prostate carcinoma Thyroid carcinoma Pancreatic carcinoma	{3024}
Lens capsule	Skin melanoma	{1207,396,3163,2510, 2621}
Vitreous	Skin melanoma Breast carcinoma	{1207,1644,1024,396, 2561,3730,1087}
Retina	Skin melanoma Lung carcinoma Gastrointestinal tract carcinoma Breast carcinoma	{2459,3000,2645, 3285}
Optic disc	Breast carcinoma Lung carcinoma Gastrointestinal tract carcinoma Renal carcinoma Prostate carcinoma	{3072}

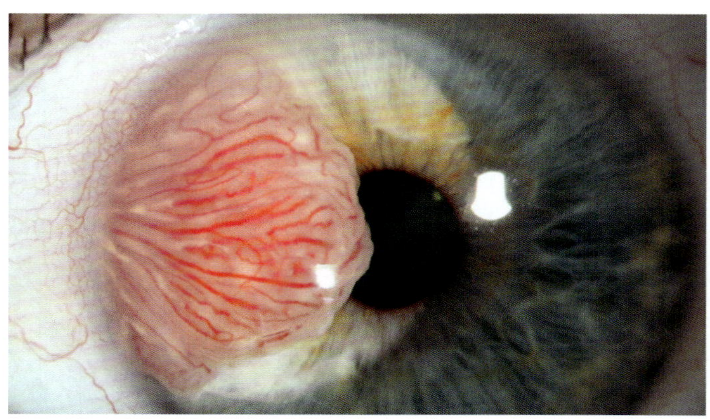

Fig. 12.06 Iris metastasis from endometrial carcinoma. A highly vascularized, pink, metastatic deposit in the iris from endometrial carcinoma.

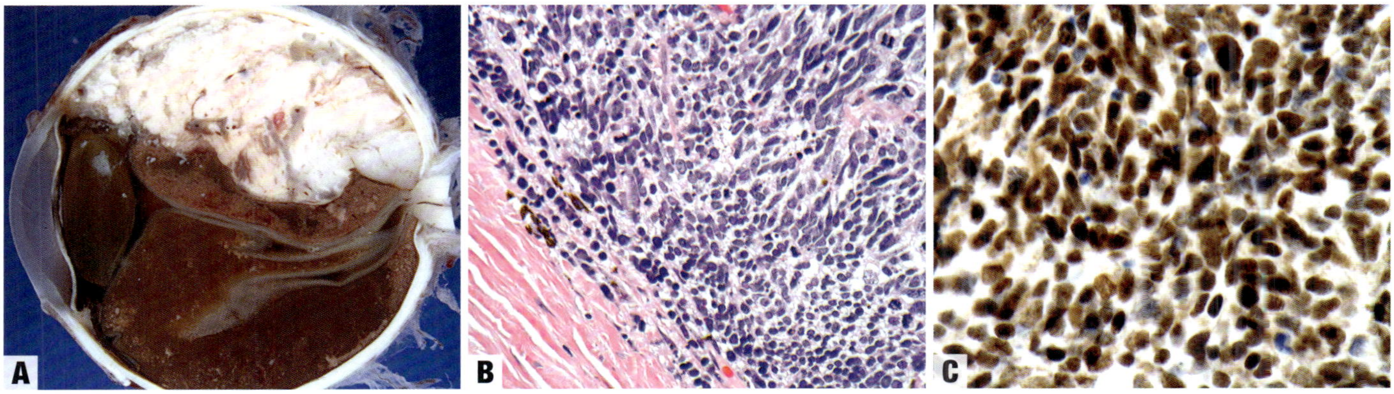

Fig. 12.07 Choroidal metastasis from small cell lung carcinoma. **A** A macroscopic photo of an enucleation specimen reveals a partly necrotic, chalky white, extensive metastasis in the superior choroid. There is associated subretinal haemorrhage and a funnel retinal detachment. Histology showed metastatic small cell carcinoma consistent with origin from lung. **B** The sclera is at the lower left. The upper right shows the metastatic small cell lung carcinoma completely effacing the choroid, with tumour directly apposed to the sclera. **C** The metastatic small cell carcinoma is positive for thyroid transcription factor 1 (TTF1) (nuclear).

kidney (4%), gastrointestinal tract (4%), skin (cutaneous melanoma) (2%), lung (carcinoid, neuroendocrine tumours [NETs]) (2%), prostate (2%), thyroid (1%), pancreas (1%), and other (3%).

Table 12.02 summarizes the various intraocular locations with their commonest metastatic malignancies.

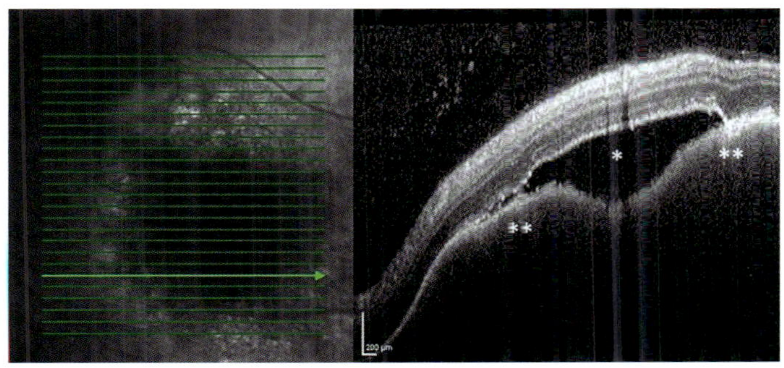

Fig. 12.08 Metastases to intraocular structures. Optical coherence tomography of a choroidal metastasis shows subretinal fluid (single asterisk) with choroidal tumour that has a lumpy-bumpy profile (double asterisk).

Pathogenesis

The mechanism by which metastases reach the intraocular compartment is via haematogenous dissemination. The choroid is highly vascularized, with 80–85% of the blood flow to the eye dedicated to the choroid {1855}. The choroid has the highest metastatic efficiency index of any organ and is involved in 8–10% of metastatic cases {2127,3575}. Most metastases occur in the postequatorial choroid, thought to be due to the rich vascular supply from the posterior ciliary arteries {964}, which may explain why metastases are rare in the anterior uvea (iris and ciliary body).

Macroscopic appearance

See *Clinical features*.

Histopathology

Generally, metastases retain (to some extent) the histological, immunohistochemical, and molecular pattern characteristic of the primary tumour. Anterior chamber metastases may be associated with the following histological changes: iris rubeosis, chronic iridocyclitis, angle closure, features of chronic glaucoma (loss of retinal ganglion cells and retinal atrophy), and haemorrhage {963}. Choroidal metastases are usually well defined on enucleation specimens with a sharp demarcation with unaffected choroid. They may be necrotic and/or associated with chronic scleritis, serous retinal detachment, and subretinal haemorrhage.

Cytology

Cytology is performed in only a small number of cases with suspected intraocular tumours (2.5% of patients) {3063,2994},

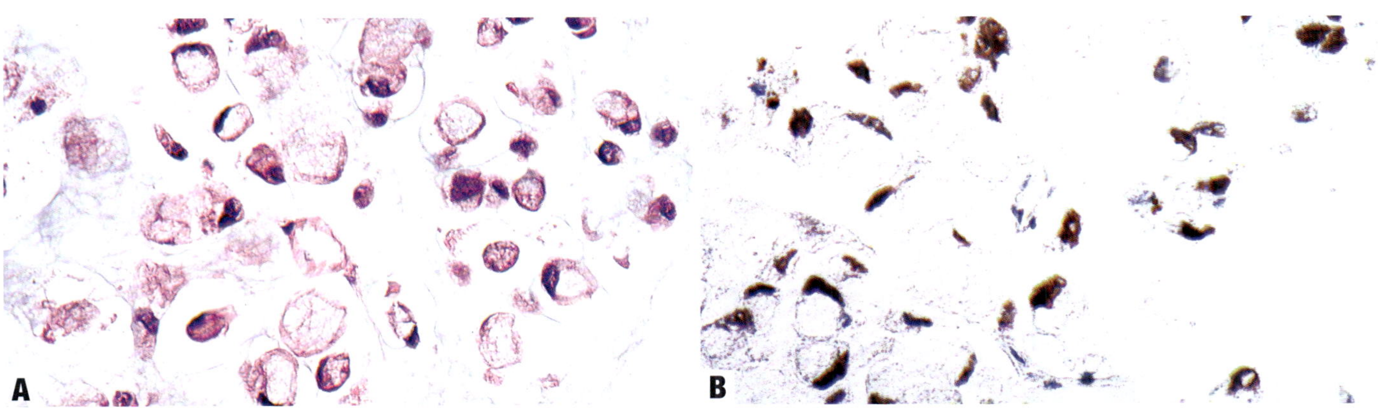

Fig. 12.09 Choroidal metastasis from gastric signet-ring cell adenocarcinoma. **A** FNAC specimen of a choroidal mass shows metastatic signet-ring cell adenocarcinoma consistent with origin from the stomach. **B** The metastatic gastric signet-ring cell adenocarcinoma is positive for nuclear CDX2.

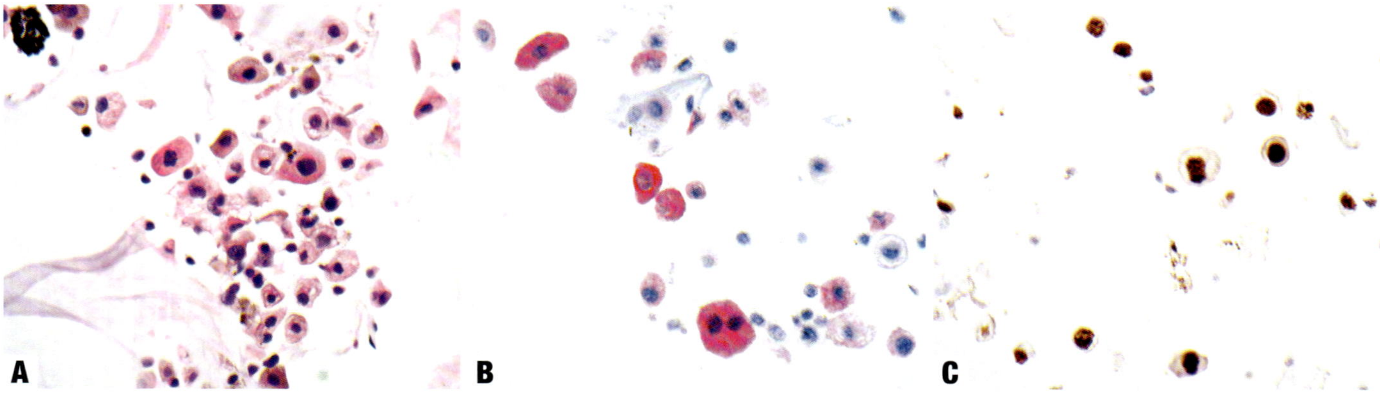

Fig. 12.10 Vitreous metastasis from skin melanoma. **A** Atypical cells, some containing melanin, are seen in this vitreous aspiration biopsy. There was a history of previous invasive skin melanoma. **B** The vitreous metastatic skin melanoma is immunohistochemically positive for melan-A (red chromogen). **C** The vitreous metastatic skin melanoma is immunohistochemically positive for nuclear SOX10 (brown chromogen).

where the differential lies between a primary uveal melanoma and a metastasis, and to confirm a metastasis when the primary is already known. The cytological confirmation of an intraocular metastasis can be the primary presentation in about a third of cases, therefore playing a critical role in diagnosing metastatic disease and establishing a primary malignant site {3067,207, 1596}. Metastatic carcinomas are usually cohesive, which is a reflection of epithelial differentiation, whereas uveal melanomas are dispersed individual cells, with less nuclear atypia. An immunohistochemical panel including cytokeratins and melanocytic markers can greatly assist in this distinction if the cytological features are equivocal.

Diagnostic molecular pathology

The diagnostic molecular pathology depends on the primary neoplasm.

Essential and desirable diagnostic criteria

In cases of histopathologically confirmed systemic primary malignancy

Essential: malignant histological/cytological features on an intraocular biopsy / enucleation that match the histopathological features of the systemic malignancy index biopsy.

Desirable: immunohistochemical and molecular features of the intraocular biopsy / enucleation that match the original systemic malignancy.

In cases of no known systemic malignancy

Essential: malignant histological/cytological features on an intraocular biopsy / enucleation with immunohistochemistry and molecular analysis to distinguish a primary intraocular malignancy from a metastasis.

Staging

Stage according to the original tumour type.

Prognosis and prediction

Local tumour control can be achieved by external beam radiotherapy (EBRT), brachytherapy, chemotherapy, immunotherapy, or photodynamic therapy. Survival is dependent on the site of the primary and available treatments; in a series of 1111 patients with uveal metastasis, there was 32% survival at three years and 24% at five years. Favourable prognosis was found in carcinoid (neuroendocrine) tumour cases, and the worst prognosis was found in pancreatic and kidney carcinoma {3024}.

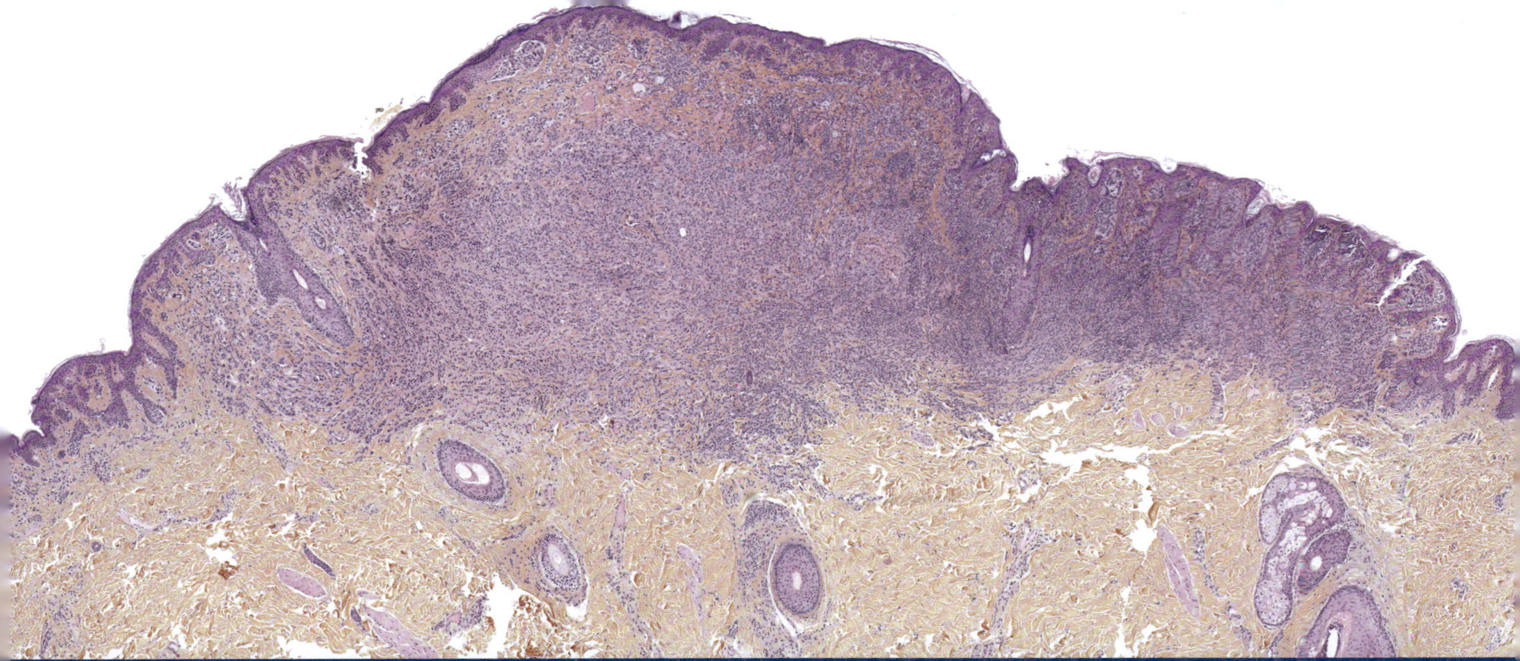

13

Genetic tumour syndromes associated with eye and orbit malignancies

Edited by: Cree IA, Grossniklaus HE, Hodge JC, Lazar AJ

Retinoblastoma syndrome
BAP1 tumour predisposition syndrome
Von Hippel–Lindau syndrome
Sturge–Weber syndrome
Neurofibromatosis type 1
Goldenhar syndrome
Muir–Torre syndrome

Genetic tumour syndromes associated with eye and orbit malignancies: Introduction

Grossniklaus HE
Hodge JC
Lazar AJ

There are numerous genetic tumour predisposition syndromes that may manifest as tumours of the eye (Table 13.01). In this chapter, several of these syndromes have been selected for more in-depth discussion owing to their prominent clinical considerations in the practice of eye pathology. An additional 10 syndromes are listed only in Table 13.01, as they also can have eye tumour findings but are well described in other WHO Classification of Tumours volumes. It is important for ophthalmologists and pathologists to recognize these syndromes as they can be associated with tumours elsewhere in the body, requiring monitoring and early intervention for optimal outcomes.

Retinoblastoma syndrome typically results from inheritance of a single copy pathogenic sequence variant in the tumour suppressor *RB1* gene, which makes all cells in the body susceptible to cancer development through acquiring a somatic

Table 13.01 Tumour syndromes with ophthalmic manifestations (continued on next page)

Disease/phenotype	MIM number	Inheritance	Locus	Gene	Gene/locus MIM number	Select ophthalmic manifestations	Select systemic manifestations
Retinoblastoma syndrome	180200	AD	13q14.2	*RB1*	614041	Retinoblastoma, retinoma, leukocoria, strabismus	Leukaemia, lymphoma, leiomyosarcoma, osteosarcoma
***BAP1* tumour predisposition syndrome**	614327	AD	3p21.1	*BAP1*	603089	Uveal melanoma	Cutaneous melanoma, mesothelioma, renal cell carcinoma, cholangiocarcinoma, basal cell carcinoma
Von Hippel–Lindau syndrome	193300	AD	3p25.3	*VHL*	608537	Retinal haemangioblastoma	Phaeochromocytoma, spinal or cerebellar haemangioblastoma, renal cell carcinoma, hypernephroma, pancreatic cancer
Sturge–Weber syndrome	185300	Early SM	9q21.2	*GNAQ*	600998	Choroidal haemangiomata, glaucoma, naevus flammeus of the eyelid, episcleral tortuous vessels, retinal vascular changes, heterochromia, and retinal pigment epithelium pigment changes	Facial haemangiomata, ipsilateral leptomeningeal angioma
Neurofibromatosis type 1	162200	AD	17q11.2	*NF1*	613113	Optic nerve glioma and Lisch nodules	Neurofibromas (including plexiform), café-au-lait macules, glomus tumours
Goldenhar syndrome (craniofacial microsomia)	164210	AD	11q13.1	*SF3B2*	605591	Epibulbar choristoma or dermoid, colobomas, microphthalmia/anophthalmia, strabismus, cataract, ptosis, microcornea	Facial asymmetry, hypoplasia (mandibular, maxillary, zygomatic arch, and temporal bone), skin tags, auricular malformations, vertebral anomalies
Muir–Torre syndrome	158320	AD	3p22.2 2p21 2p16.3 7p22.1	*MLH1* *MSH2* *MSH6* *PMS2*	120436 609309 600678 600259	Sebaceous neoplasms of the ocular adnexa	Sebaceous neoplasms (carcinoma, epithelioma, and adenoma), colon cancer, duodenal carcinoma, laryngeal carcinoma, benign gastrointestinal and genitourinary tract tumours, malignant gastrointestinal and genitourinary tract tumours, breast cancer

AD, autosomal dominant; SM, somatic mutation

second-hit alteration {1989}. The most common secondary cancer types are leiomyosarcoma in the field of radiation if the retinoblastoma was irradiated and osteosarcoma outside the field of radiation {549}. Retinoblastoma treatment is now so successful in developed countries that secondary cancers more commonly cause death rather than the primary retinoblastoma {549}.

The two-hit scenario for tumour formation occurs in additional syndromes that predispose to eye and other neoplasms: *BAP1* alterations are associated with uveal melanoma in *BAP1* tumour predisposition syndrome {2551}; *VHL* mutations predispose to retinal haemangioblastoma in von Hippel–Lindau syndrome {3455}; and *NF1* mutation in neurofibromatosis type 1 results in optic nerve glioma and Lisch nodules {1039}.

Sturge–Weber syndrome (encephalofacial haemangiomatosis) arises owing to somatic activating mutations of *GNAQ*, or more rarely *GNA11* and *GNB2*, that induce increased blood vessel growth {3696,3456}. This syndrome may include naevus flammeus of the eyelid, episcleral tortuous vessels, glaucoma, diffuse haemangioma of the choroid, retinal vascular changes, heterochromia, and pigmentary changes of the retina pigment epithelium.

Goldenhar syndrome (craniofacial microsomia) is thought to be multifactorial with multiple genetic candidates; most recently, haploinsufficiency of *SF3B2* was found in about 3% of sporadic and about 25% of familial cases {3342}. It probably involves abnormal development of the first and second branchial arches resulting in structural eye anomalies.

Muir–Torre syndrome is a subtype of Lynch syndrome and the dominant form arises from microsatellite instability induced by mutations in the mismatch repair genes *MLH1*, *MSH2*, *MSH6*, or *PMS2* {1415}. Sebaceous neoplasms of the ocular adnexa may rarely occur in people with Muir–Torre syndrome.

Diagnosticians must be familiar with these syndromes so that they are recognized (often after presentation of patients with the corresponding tumour) and managed appropriately.

Table 13.01 Tumour syndromes with ophthalmic manifestations (continued)

Disease/phenotype	MIM number	Inheritance	Locus	Gene	Gene/locus MIM number	Select ophthalmic manifestations	Select systemic manifestations
Cowden syndrome 1	158350	AD	10q23.31	*PTEN*	601728	Trichilemmoma	Palmar keratosis, lipoma, naevi, café-au-lait macules, mucosal papillomas, uterine leiomyoma, colonic polyp, breast fibroadenoma, intraductal papilloma, as well as carcinomas of the breast, uterus, cervix, ovary, thyroid, and other sites
Basal cell naevus syndrome (Gorlin syndrome)	109400	AD	1p34.1 9q22.32 10q24.32	*PTCH2* *PTCH1* *SUFU*	603673 601309 607035	Multiple basal cell carcinomas	Odotogenic keratocyst, ovarian and cardiac fibroma and medulloblastoma
Multiple endocrine neoplasia type 2B syndrome	162300	AD	10q11.21	*RET*	164761	Enlarged corneal nerves	Submucosal neuroma, medullary thyroid carcinoma, adrenal phaeochromocytoma
Familial adenomatous polyposis 1 (Gardner syndrome)	175100	AD	5q22.2	*APC*	611731	Retinal pigment epithelium hamartomas; congenital hypertrophy of retinal pigment epithelium	Colon adenomatous polyposis
Tuberous sclerosis 1 and 2	191100 613254	AD	9q34.13 16p13.3	*TSC1* *TSC2*	605284 191092	Retinal astrocytoma, retinal giant cell astrocytoma, cutaneous angiofibroma	Subependymal giant cell astrocytoma, cortical tubers
Proteus syndrome	176920	SM	14q32.33	*AKT1*	164730	Retinal pigmentary abnormalities	Ovarian cystadenoma, testicular tumours, meningioma, parotid monomorphic adenoma
Carney complex type 1	160980	AD	17q24.2	*PRKAR1A*	188830	Periocular myxomas	Atrial myxoma, endocrine abnormalities, cutaneous lentigines
Peutz–Jeghers syndrome	175200	AD	19p13.3	*STK11*	602216	Melanocytic macule of conjunctiva	Hamartomatous polyps of gastrointestinal tract, hyperpigmented macules of lips
DICER1 pleuropulmonary blastoma familial predisposition syndrome	601200	AD	14q32.13	*DICER1*	606241	Ciliary body medulloepithelioma	Pleuropulmonary blastoma

AD, autosomal dominant; SM, somatic mutation

Retinoblastoma syndrome

Cassoux N
Bechrakis NE
Berry JL
Chevez-Barrios P
Gallie BL
Khetan V
Rojanaporn D

Definition
Retinoblastoma syndrome is a heritable cancer predisposition disorder associated with a germline heterozygous pathogenic *RB1* variant with development of retinoblastoma and other extraocular malignancies.

MIM numbering
180200 Retinoblastoma; RB1

ICD-11 coding
2D02.2 Retinoblastoma

Related terminology
Acceptable: trilateral retinoblastoma; heritable retinoblastoma, familial retinoblastoma, hereditary cancer syndrome.

Subtype(s)
Heritable unilateral and bilateral retinoblastoma; trilateral retinoblastoma – associated with primary intracranial tumour (pineal or suprasellar tumour); second primary non-ocular malignancies

Localization
Retinoblastoma develops in the retina of one or both eyes. In retinoblastoma syndrome, bilateral tumours most frequently occur, although 15% of patients will have unilateral disease. In 5% of affected children, synchronous or metachronous malignant intracranial tumours (pineal or suprasellar) develop. Pineoblastomas occur in retina-like tissue in the pineal gland of the brain. Concurrence of pineoblastomas or primitive neuroectodermal tumours and retinoblastoma is referred to as trilateral retinoblastoma. Pineoblastoma is rare (< 5% of patients with retinoblastoma syndrome) and usually fatal, unlike retinoblastoma of the eye, which is generally curable when diagnosed before extraocular spread {739}. Later in life, patients with retinoblastoma syndrome may develop second primary malignancies (SPM), most frequently in soft tissues (rhabdomyosarcoma), bone (osteosarcoma), endometrium, lung, or skin (melanomas) {3629,1735}. The overall risk of a second tumour is 0.5–1% per year of life {2245}.

Clinical features
MRI of the orbits and brain is performed during the initial diagnosis of intraocular retinoblastoma to exclude extraocular extension (extrascleral and/or optic nerve) and brain involvement with a pineoblastoma. If possible, radiation (including X-ray, CT, and external beam radiation [EBRT]) should be avoided in individuals with heritable retinoblastoma to minimize the lifetime risk of developing late-onset second cancers.

Synchronous trilateral retinoblastoma initial therapy should address both ocular and intracranial disease (see *Retinoblastoma*, p. 197). For pineal tumours, a maximal safe surgical resection is encouraged at diagnosis followed by intensive chemotherapy, often requiring autologous haematopoietic cell rescue. Irradiation can be done using focal radiotherapy on the pineal region (proton beam or stereotactic radiotherapy) associated or not with craniospinal irradiation {7}.

Survivors of heritable retinoblastoma may develop SPM. They should receive counselling and enrolment in long-term survivor programmes that have access to specific screening, follow-up, and treatment.

Epidemiology
The incidence, localization, and type of SPM is retinoblastoma treatment–type dependent. EBRT is especially associated with a 36% cumulative incidence of sarcoma in the irradiation field {1736,549}. Chemotherapy plus EBRT further increases the risk of SPMs {3629}.

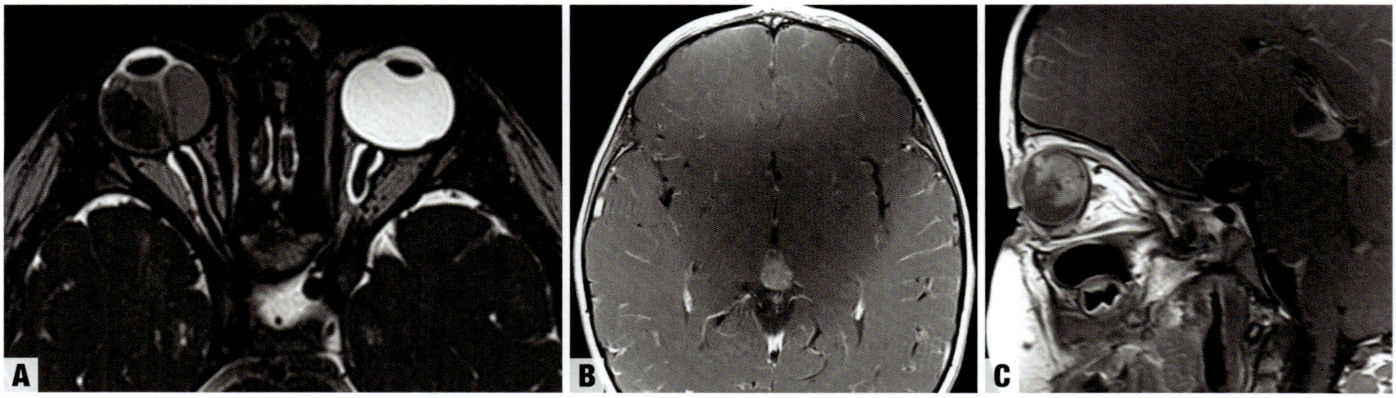

Fig. 13.01 Trilateral retinoblastoma. A 6-month-old patient affected by a trilateral retinoblastoma. **A** Axial T2-weighted MRI showing an advanced intraocular retinoblastoma in the left eye and a small tumour in the temporal quadrant of the right eye. **B** Axial MRI disclosing a pineal tumour. **C** Sagittal MRI showing both the advanced retinoblastoma of the left eye and the pinealoblastoma.

Etiology

Heritable retinoblastoma is caused by a germline pathogenic *RB1* mutation (first hit) followed by a somatic alteration (second hit), and originates from developing retinal cells, probably cone progenitors {3661,3114}. Although this event is required for initiation, it may not be independently sufficient; presumed benign retinal lesions (see *Retinocytoma*, p. 194) also have biallelic *RB1* mutation {801}. Germline pathogenic *RB1* variants are heterogeneous. Low- and regular-penetrance alterations show variation of phenotypic expression for retinoblastoma and for SPM in families {1666}. Patients with somatic mutational mosaicism more often develop a milder phenotype and unilateral retinoblastoma compared with patients with non-mosaic variants {2791}. Large deletions on the q-arm of chromosome 13 including *RB1* and neighbouring genes cause a rare genetic disorder referred to as "13q deletion syndrome". Depending on the localization and the size of the deletion, these patients may show a neurodevelopmental delay, characteristic facial features, organ malformation, and retinoblastoma {2237,755}.

The origin of intracranial (pineal) retinoblastoma, somatic or germline associated, is probably different from other pineal tumours based on divergent DNA methylation profiles, as well as finding common characteristics specifically between intracranial and ocular retinoblastoma (e.g. chromosome 16 loss and 1q gain) {1927,2541}.

Pathogenesis

See *Retinoblastoma* (p. 197).

Macroscopic appearance

Intracranial tumours are poorly demarcated, soft, and friable. Adequacy of surgical resection of intracranial tumours may be defined based on postoperative imaging studies, and the surgical specimen is representative of the amount of tumour resected (see the section on pineoblastoma in the *Central nervous system tumours* volume of this series {1998}).

Histopathology

The histological features of the intracranial tumour in trilateral retinoblastoma are identical to those of retinoblastoma (see *Retinoblastoma*, p. 197). Pineoblastoma is a high-grade embryonal tumour (WHO grade 4) (see the section on pineoblastoma in the *Central nervous system tumours* volume {1998}).

Cytology

Not clinically relevant

Diagnostic molecular pathology

Identification of the specific *RB1* gene variant and genetic counselling should be considered for any patient with retinoblastoma, regardless of laterality or trilateral disease. Inactivation of *RB1* can result from small or large DNA alterations, complex rearrangements such as chromothripsis, loss of heterozygosity, and promoter methylation {1989,2138,725,2707}. Increasingly, next-generation sequencing is used to analyse the exons of *RB1* and determine complex rearrangements {1937,725}. *RB1* RNA analysis may identify pathogenic splice variants caused by deep intronic mutations {811}. Methods such as next-generation sequencing and PCR-based assays can detect mosaic *RB1* variants or promoter methylation {2791,1937,2591}. In addition, capture-based targeted sequencing and relative haplotype dosage analysis of maternal plasma have been used to evaluate fetal *RB1* status for paternal or de novo variants; in a small study, the prenatal diagnosis was 100% concordant with the postdiagnostic result {1097}.

Box 13.01 Diagnostic criteria for familial retinoblastoma

Essential:

Intraocular small blue round cell tumour with typical histopathology and demonstrated germline alteration of the *RB1* gene

OR

Trilateral occurrence of intraocular small blue round cell tumours in both eyes and in the pineal region

Essential and desirable diagnostic criteria

Essential: confirmation of diagnosis from ocular tumour(s); degree of differentiation for intracranial tumours; association with meningeal involvement should be included.

Desirable: demonstration of presence of germline pathogenic variant in *RB1*.

See Box 13.01 for diagnostic criteria for familial retinoblastoma.

Staging

The American Joint Committee on Cancer (AJCC) has developed a clinical and pathological TNM, and new in the eighth edition is the hereditary classification system (cTMNH) for retinoblastoma. The hereditary category includes HX (unknown or insufficient evidence of a germline pathogenic *RB1* gene variant), H0 (normal *RB1* alleles in blood tested), and H1 (bilateral retinoblastoma, trilateral retinoblastoma, patient with family history of retinoblastoma, or molecular definition of germline pathogenic *RB1* gene variant).

Prognosis and prediction

Trilateral retinoblastoma has a poor prognosis. Prognosis is related to age at presentation with children < 6 years of age having the worse outcomes (~6% survival) {71}. The mortality of SPM in patients with heritable retinoblastoma syndrome remains about 50% {1521,3718}.

Current screening recommendations include annual history and physical examination with a focus on bony structures and radiotherapy field, and regular skin examination {3359}. Each tumour type presents at different ages – osteosarcomas (first and second decades of life), soft tissue sarcomas (10–50 years after retinoblastoma diagnosis), and epithelial tumours and melanoma (after the second decade of life). Screening should continue through the life of the patient as they may develop more than one SPM.

BAP1 tumour predisposition syndrome

Santagata S
Abdel-Rahman MH
Cebulla CM
de la Fouchardière A
López-Terrada DH

Definition
BAP1 tumour predisposition syndrome is an autosomal dominant disorder caused by pathogenic germline variants in the *BAP1* tumour suppressor gene. The syndrome is characterized by a predisposition to various tumours, most frequently including uveal melanoma, mesothelioma, cutaneous melanoma, and renal cell carcinoma.

MIM numbering
614327 Tumour predisposition syndrome; TPDS

ICD-11 coding
None

Related terminology
Acceptable: *BAP1* loss familial cancer syndrome; *BAP1* hereditary cancer syndrome.
Not recommended: tumour predisposition syndrome; cutaneous/ocular melanoma, atypical melanocytic proliferations, and other internal neoplasms (COMMON) syndrome.

Subtype(s)
None

Localization
Multiple sites and organ systems are involved, including the eyes {1250,10,1450}, pleura, peritoneum {3311}, skin {3603, 3519}, kidney {2580}, liver {2552}, and meninges {10,2943}.

Clinical features
The median age of tumour onset is younger in people with *BAP1* tumour predisposition syndrome than in the general population. Affected individuals can have multiple types of primary cancers {3532}. Mesotheliomas have substantially different clinical features when arising in *BAP1* tumour predisposition syndrome: they arise 20 years earlier, lack male predominance, and are frequently peritoneal rather than pleural {277,2415,2507}. Histologically distinctive *BAP1*-inactivated naevi/melanocytomas occur in as many as three quarters of germline carriers {1278, 3650}, yet they are not specific for the syndrome {453}. Patients are diagnosed through genetic testing owing to personal or family history of cancer or through identification of cutaneous lesions associated with the syndrome.

Criteria for genetic counselling and testing include (1) a medical history of at least two tumours associated with *BAP1* tumour predisposition syndrome, (2) one tumour associated with *BAP1* tumour predisposition syndrome and a first- or second-degree relative with at least one tumour associated with *BAP1* tumour predisposition syndrome, and/or (3) young age at tumour onset {2638,3532,544}. In the context of these criteria, loss of BAP1 on immunohistochemistry or detection of *BAP1* variants in relevant tumours further supports a need for germline testing {1278,3532}. For uveal melanoma, the youngest age reported is 15 years {3713}. To identify tumours at early stages, screening (including eye examinations, skin examinations, and abdominal MRI) starting 5 years before the earliest reported cancer has been recommended {2638,3195,3532,544}. *BAP1*-inactivated naevi can arise in children, and thus the *BAP1* tumour predisposition syndrome can be diagnosed at a young age.

Epidemiology
The literature reports 141 families with pathogenic null variants (104 unique), and 85% of mutation carriers in these families presented with one or more cancers {3532}. Rare missense variants in the catalytic UCH are associated with a syndromic neurodevelopmental disorder {1817} or *BAP1*-associated cancers. The carrier frequency of germline pathogenic variants is 1 in 19 698 in people without cancer {1607}, and about 1 in 1299 {1388}

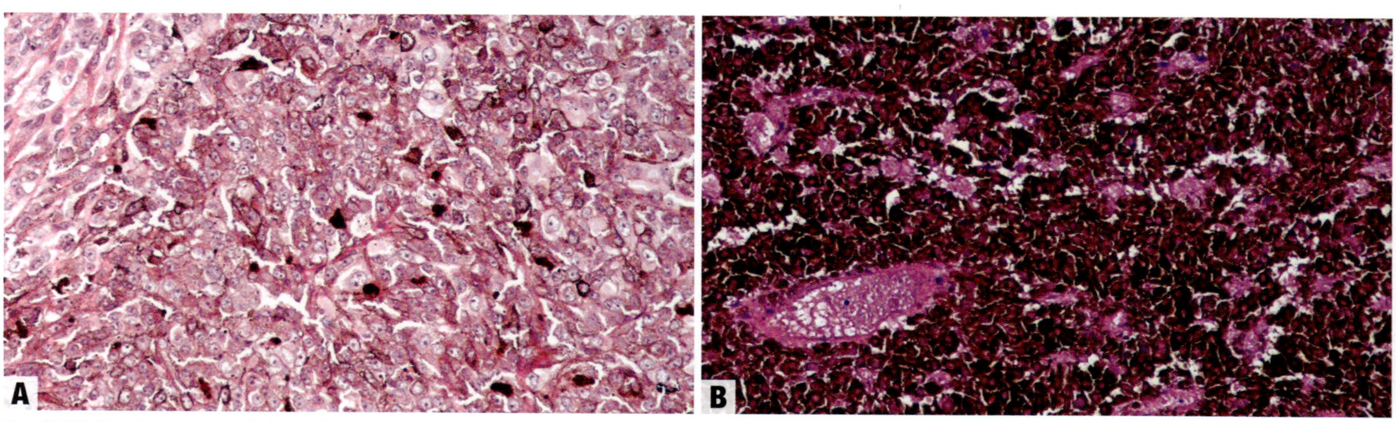

Fig. 13.02 Uveal melanoma. **A** A uveal melanoma from a patient with the c.1938T>A (p.Y646*) nonsense germline *BAP1* mutation is seen. This is a highly vascular tumour with heavily pigmented spindle tumour cells. Large areas of necrosis were observed (not shown). The tumour metastasized to liver and other organs. **B** A uveal melanoma from a patient with the c.799C>T (p.G267*) nonsense germline *BAP1* mutation is seen. Tumour cells were mostly epithelioid. The tumour metastasized to the liver and other organs.

Table 13.02 Frequency of germline and somatic (sporadic) *BAP1* mutations in tumours and occurrence of tumours in non-proband carriers with null *BAP1* variants

Tumour type	Prevalence of germline *BAP1* mutations	Prevalence of somatic *BAP1* mutations	Occurrence of tumours in non-proband carriers with null *BAP1* variants
Uveal melanoma	1–2%	40–45%	15.9%
Mesothelioma	1–2%	23–64%	16.9%
Cutaneous melanoma	< 0.001%	2–3%	12%
Kidney cancer	0.5–1%	10–15%	4.9%
Basal cell carcinoma	< 1%	1–3%	n/a
Hepatocellular carcinoma	0.5%	5%	n/a
Intrahepatic cholangiocarcinoma	1–2%	15–25%	n/a
Meningioma (all)	< 1%	< 1%	n/a

among patients with cancer, suggesting that the syndrome prevalence is underestimated. Two common founder variants, NM_004656.4(*BAP1*):c.1780_1781insT (p.G594Vfs*49) (in Finland) and NM_004656.4(*BAP1*):c.1717del (p.L573Wfs*3) (in the USA), have been identified, with the latter traced back to Swiss origins in the 16th century {480,3532}. The lifetime risk of developing cancer is reported to be as high as 80–100%, with many carriers developing multiple cancers; most families have at least two types of tumours in first- or second-degree relatives {2638,3532}.

BAP1 is the most frequently mutated gene in sporadic mesothelioma {436} and in metastatic uveal melanoma {1250, 10,1450}, but only 1–2% of these *BAP1*-mutant tumours arise in germline carriers {3311,2788,1211,2699}. Although the frequency of *BAP1* germline mutations is low in the overall population of patients with uveal melanoma, the frequency increases to about 20% in patients with familial occurrence {2637}, which is defined as the occurrence of uveal melanoma in two or more members of the same blood line {1450}. The frequency of germline and somatic *BAP1* mutations in various tumour types and the occurrence of those tumours in probands with null variants in *BAP1* are listed in Table 13.02.

Etiology

BAP1 tumour predisposition syndrome is caused by heterozygous pathogenic germline sequence variants, or more rarely deletions, involving the *BAP1* tumour suppressor gene, located at chromosome 3p21.1 {3311}. The mutations are most commonly deleterious nonsense, frameshift, or splice-site alterations that result in a truncated, non-functional protein (null variants), or deleterious missense mutations that interfere with the ubiquitin hydrolase function of BAP1 {2321}. More data are required to evaluate the effect of environmental mutagens (e.g. asbestos, ultraviolet [UV] radiation) on modulating the penetrance of germline mutations. De novo *BAP1* germline mutations are uncommon {3532,544}. Germline homozygous deletion of *BAP1* in mice is lethal in early embryogenesis whereas mice with heterozygous *BAP1* deletion are viable with no obvious anatomical abnormalities, but these mice have a higher frequency of spontaneous tumours and increased risk of mesotheliomas upon asbestos exposure {785,3657,1561}.

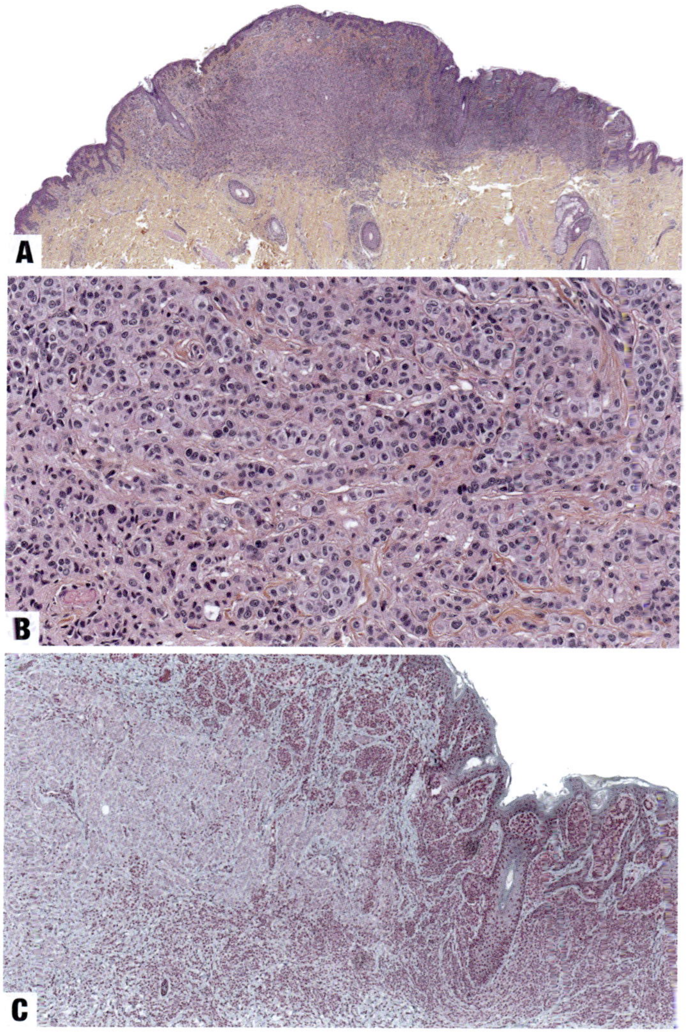

Fig. 13.03 *BAP1*-inactivated naevus. **A** A dermal clone within a common compound naevus (haematoxylin eosin safranin stain). **B** High-power view of a dermal clone made of large unpigmented epithelioid melanocytes with mild atypia (haematoxylin eosin safranin stain). **C** Loss of nuclear expression of BAP1 in the dermal epithelioid clone. Adjacent naevus retains expression.

Pathogenesis

The *BAP1* gene at chromosome 3p21.1 comprises 17 exons encoding a protein with ubiquitin carboxyl hydrolase activity first identified as interacting with BRCA1 {1511}. BAP1 interactors include ASXL1, ASXL2, FOXK1, FOXK2, HCFC1, and YY1, consistent with roles in DNA damage response, transcriptional regulation, cell-cycle regulation, metabolism, inflammatory responses, and lineage differentiation {2944,580,3532,1819}. Nuclear localization and deubiquitination activity are both necessary for BAP1-mediated tumour suppression {3472}.

Macroscopic appearance

The macroscopic appearance of tumours in patients with *BAP1* tumour predisposition syndrome is similar to that of sporadic tumours.

Histopathology

The histopathology of tumours associated with *BAP1* tumour predisposition syndrome is similar to that of their sporadic counterparts.

Cytology

The cytology of tumours associated with *BAP1* tumour predisposition syndrome is similar to that of sporadic tumours.

Diagnostic molecular pathology

BAP1 sequencing and deletion/duplication analysis performed on peripheral blood to identify a germline heterozygous pathogenic mutation confirms the diagnosis of *BAP1* tumour predisposition syndrome. Loss of BAP1 immunoreactivity in tumour nuclei readily identifies deficient tumours; however, concordance between immunohistochemistry and genotyping is high but incomplete {389,1771,2356,3436}.

Essential and desirable diagnostic criteria

Essential: demonstration of germline pathogenic variant in *BAP1*.

Note: No phenotypic diagnostic criteria are associated with *BAP1* tumour predisposition syndrome. Although there are no formal criteria, testing for *BAP1* mutations should be considered in patients with (1) two or more confirmed tumours associated with *BAP1* tumour predisposition syndrome or (2) one confirmed tumour associated with *BAP1* tumour predisposition syndrome and a first- or second-degree relative with a confirmed tumour associated with *BAP1* tumour predisposition syndrome {3195, 3532,2638,2551}. Loss of BAP1 by immunohistochemistry in these tumours can be used to further screen for individuals who need germline testing {937,3532}.

Staging

Stage as appropriate for the tumour type.

Prognosis and prediction

Sporadic *BAP1*-mutant tumours are often more aggressive than corresponding tumours lacking such mutations {1230,334}. The prognosis for germline carriers with tumours is incompletely characterized because most studies of single tumour histology contain few patients with *BAP1* tumour predisposition syndrome. Uveal melanomas arising in *BAP1* tumour predisposition syndrome have increased risk of metastasis {2388,1211}. *BAP1*-mutant meningiomas display aggressive behaviour with frequent recurrences {2943,2944}, although it is unclear whether meningiomas arising in *BAP1* tumour predisposition syndrome have a different prognosis than sporadic *BAP1*-mutant meningiomas. By contrast, patients with germline *BAP1*-related mesothelioma have a better 5-year survival rate (47%) than those with sporadic mesotheliomas (6.7%) {277,2415,2507}.

Von Hippel–Lindau syndrome

Aldape KD
Aronow ME
Kilic E
Singh A

Definition

Von Hippel–Lindau syndrome (VHL) is an autosomal dominant disorder caused by pathogenic germline variants of the *VHL* tumour suppressor gene (located at chromosome 3p25.3) and characterized by the development of haemangioblastoma of the CNS and retina, clear cell renal cell carcinoma (RCC), phaeochromocytoma, pancreatic neuroendocrine tumours, and endolymphatic sac tumours.

MIM numbering

193300 Von Hippel–Lindau syndrome; VHLS

ICD-11 coding

None

Related terminology

None

Subtype(s)

Von Hippel–Lindau syndrome types 1, 2A, 2B, and 2C

Localization

Haemangioblastomas most often involve the retina, cerebellum, and spinal cord (especially paraspinal nerve roots), but they can occur anywhere along the craniospinal axis, including peripheral nerves and even tissues outside the nervous system {3515, 3514,141,820,340,2323}. Endolymphatic sac tumours arise from the vestibular aqueduct and may invade through the temporal bone and into the cerebellopontine angle {1124,832}.

Clinical features

Retinal haemangioblastomas manifest at a mean age of 25 years (earlier than RCC) and thus offer the possibility of an early diagnosis {1869}. CNS haemangioblastomas develop mainly in young adults (mean age: 29 years). They are predominantly located in the cerebellum and next most commonly in the brainstem or spinal cord {816}. Approximately 25% of all cases of CNS haemangioblastoma are associated with hereditary VHL. Key clinical characteristics of VHL-associated versus sporadic haemangioblastoma are presented in Table 13.03.

Renal cysts and clear cell RCCs are typically multifocal and bilateral. Age of onset is 16–67 years with a mean of 37 years (compared with 61 years for sporadic clear cell RCC). Patients with VHL have a 70% chance of developing clear cell RCC by the age of 70 years. Metastatic RCC is the leading cause of death from VHL.

Adrenal phaeochromocytomas arise in 20% of patients with VHL; the mean age at onset is 30 years.

Pancreatic manifestations are predominantly multiple cysts but also neuroendocrine tumours {1782}.

Table 13.03 Clinical characteristics of sporadic versus von Hippel–Lindau syndrome (VHL)-associated haemangioblastoma

Characteristic	Sporadic	VHL-associated
Female sex	41%	56%
Median patient age	44 years (range: 7–82 years)	23 years (range: 7–64 years)
Intracranial location	79%	73%
Spinal location	11%	75%
Multiple haemangioblastomas	5%	65%

Other VHL-associated tumours include endolymphatic sac tumours (associated with hearing loss, tinnitus, and vertigo) and epididymal and broad ligament cystadenomas.

VHL type 1 is characterized by haemangioblastomas and RCCs (phaeochromocytomas are rare or absent), and it is typically caused by *VHL* deletions, truncations, or missense mutations that are predicted to highly disrupt VHL protein expression or function {3455}. VHL type 2 is mainly associated with missense mutations that are less severe in impact on VHL protein expression and function. Type 2A is characterized by haemangioblastomas and phaeochromocytomas (RCCs are rare). Type 2B by haemangioblastomas, RCCs, and phaeochromocytomas; and Type 2C by phaeochromocytomas (haemangioblastomas and RCCs are absent).

Epidemiology

VHL is estimated to have an annual incidence rate of 2.8 cases per 100 000 population.

Etiology

VHL is caused by heterozygous germline pathogenic sequence variants or deletion of *VHL* at chromosome 3p25.3; more than 1000 variants have been identified spread over the three exons and are highly penetrant. Missense mutations are the most common, but nonsense mutations, in-frame deletions/insertions, splice-site mutations, and large/complex deletions also occur {2395}. The heterogeneous clinical manifestations of VHL are a reflection of the diversity of germline mutations.

Pathogenesis

Mutational inactivation of the *VHL* tumour suppressor gene in affected family members is responsible for their genetic susceptibility to tumour development at various organ sites. However, the mechanisms by which the inactivation or loss of VHL protein causes neoplastic transformation are only partly understood {1151}. The cell of origin (haemangioblast, stromal cell) is not well defined, but current evidence points to a developmentally arrested haemangioblast precursor {3513}. Mutations are also common in sporadic haemangioblastomas (occurring in as many as 78% of cases) and ubiquitous in clear cell RCCs.

VHL protein has many different functions, and it is critically involved in protein degradation. A complex of the VHL protein α domain, elongin B, and other proteins has ubiquitin ligase activity, thereby targeting cellular proteins for ubiquitination and proteasome-mediated degradation. The α domain binding site for elongin B is frequently mutated in neoplasms associated with VHL.

VHL protein plays a key role in cellular oxygen sensing by polyubiquitination and proteasomal degradation of hypoxia-inducible factors (HIF1α and HIF2α) {3729,982}. In the absence of functional VHL protein, HIF1α accumulates and activates the transcription of several hypoxia-inducible genes such as *VEGFA* and *EPO*, leading to a pseudohypoxia state characterized by altered expression of genes that drive vascularization, cyst formation, lipid storage, metabolic adaptation, and extramedullary erythropoiesis. Constitutive overexpression of *VEGFA* {3621, 3215} explains the extraordinary vascularization of neoplasms associated with VHL due to increased angiogenesis/vasculogenesis, as well as the formation of cysts due to increased vascular permeability {2022}. Increased erythropoietin expression is common in haemangioblastomas {1788} and is responsible for intratumoural (extramedullary) haematopoiesis and for the paraneoplastic erythrocytosis syndrome that can occur in patients with VHL. HIF-dependent downregulation of carnitine palmitoyltransferase 1A leads to enhanced lipid storage, a characteristic of VHL-dependent tumours {2776}.

Macroscopic appearance

The macroscopic appearance of VHL-associated tumours is similar to that of their sporadic counterparts.

Histopathology

The histopathology of VHL-associated tumours is similar to that of their sporadic counterparts. The three major types of cells of the retinal capillary haemangioblastoma are endothelial cells, pericytes, and stromal cells. The stromal cells are frequently foamy in appearance.

Cytology

The cytology of VHL-associated tumours is similar to that of their sporadic counterparts.

Diagnostic molecular pathology

VHL sequencing and deletion/duplication analysis performed on peripheral blood to identify a germline heterozygous pathogenic mutation confirms the diagnosis of VHL.

Essential and desirable diagnostic criteria

Essential: demonstration of pathogenic germline variant in *VHL* and manifestation of any of the associated neoplasm(s).

Desirable: manifestation of haemangioblastomas of retina and/or CNS and any other associated neoplasm in the absence of a pathogenic germline sequence variant in *VHL*.

Staging

Stage as appropriate for the tumour type.

Prognosis and prediction

The median life expectancy of patients with VHL is 49 years. Outcome is improved by screening that allows earlier detection of malignancies. Clinical surveillance guidance has been published {336,2683}.

Sturge–Weber syndrome

Francis JH
Eberhart CG
Milman T

Definition

Sturge–Weber syndrome (SWS) is a congenital neurocutaneous condition due to a somatic mosaic activating mutation, most often in *GNAQ*, affecting small blood vessels and capillaries. There is no clear evidence that it is hereditary.

MIM numbering

185300 Sturge–Weber syndrome; SWS

ICD-11 coding

LD23 Syndromes with vascular anomalies as a major feature

Related terminology

Acceptable: encephalofacial angiomatosis; encephalotrigeminal angiomatosis; craniofacial angiomatosis.

Subtype(s)

Sturge–Weber syndrome types 1, 2, 3, 4 (see Table 13.04)

Localization

The vascular anomaly (capillary malformation [CM]; see Table 13.04) that characterizes SWS can impact as many as three organ systems, including the eye (choroid, episclera, conjunctiva, anterior segment) {2061,3097}, skin {272,2793}, and brain (leptomeninges) {225,2623,657}.

Clinical features

Choroid CM (diffuse choroidal haemangioma) occurs in 20–70% of SWS patients {3103,3237}. Patients may experience blurry, distorted, or declining vision related to choroidal thickening and secondary retinal and retinal pigment epithelium changes from exudation {454,2659,2581}.

Conjunctival and episcleral CMs appear as red, dilated, tortuous, and elevated vessels {2061,3103,3237}.

Anterior segment abnormalities of eyes with SWS include iris heterochromia and malformations in the anterior chamber angle {2326}. Anterior chamber angle malformations, increased episcleral venous pressure related to CM, and accelerated ageing of the trabecular meshwork are some of the proposed mechanisms for pathogenesis of glaucoma in SWS {2061,1310}.

Cutaneous CM appears as discolouration of the skin, ranging from pink to red to deep purple. It can appear flat, but with time may develop vascular ectasias producing a nodular appearance and superficial blebbing {2798}. The characteristic SWS cutaneous lesion, facial CM (port-wine stain), is usually unilateral and follows the distribution of the first branch of the trigeminal nerve and the embryonic vasculature in this area. SWS-associated CMs less frequently involve the trunk and extremities.

Leptomeningeal CM most commonly involves the parietal and occipital lobes and is best diagnosed by MRI {225}. Venous stasis within the malformation may lead to hypoxia and ischaemia

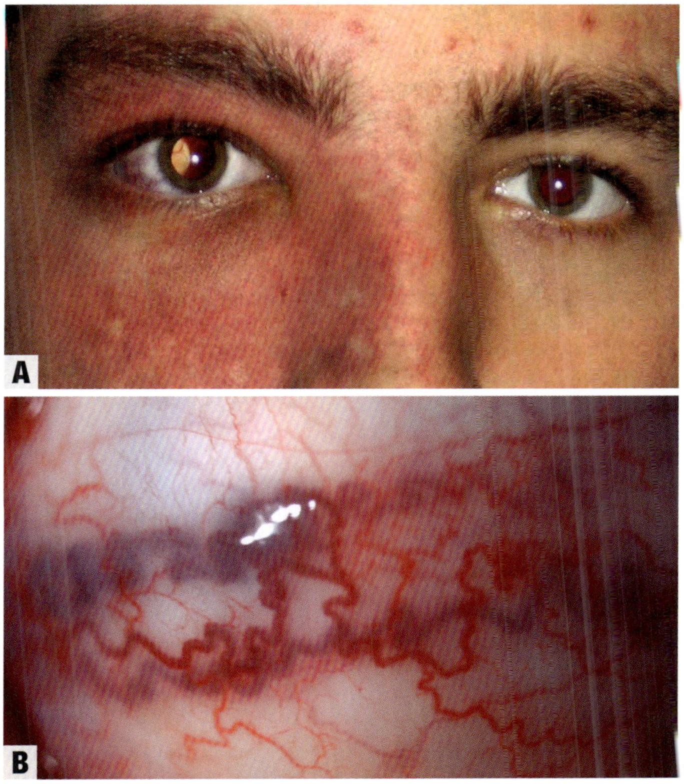

Fig. 13.04 Sturge–Weber syndrome. **A** An external facial photo of Sturge–Weber syndrome is shown. The port-wine stain is a red discolouration of the skin that follows the distribution of the first branch of the trigeminal nerve and the embryonic vasculature in this area. **B** A conjunctival photo of Sturge–Weber syndrome is shown. Conjunctival and episcleral capillary malformations appear as red, dilated, tortuous, and elevated vessels.

Table 13.04 Sturge–Weber syndrome subtypes

Clinical finding	Type 1	Type 2	Type 3	Type 4
Facial capillary malformation	Present	Present	Absent	Present
Leptomeningeal capillary malformation	Present	Absent	Present	Present
Glaucoma	Maybe	Maybe	Maybe	Maybe
Systemic manifestations	Maybe	Absent	Absent	Present

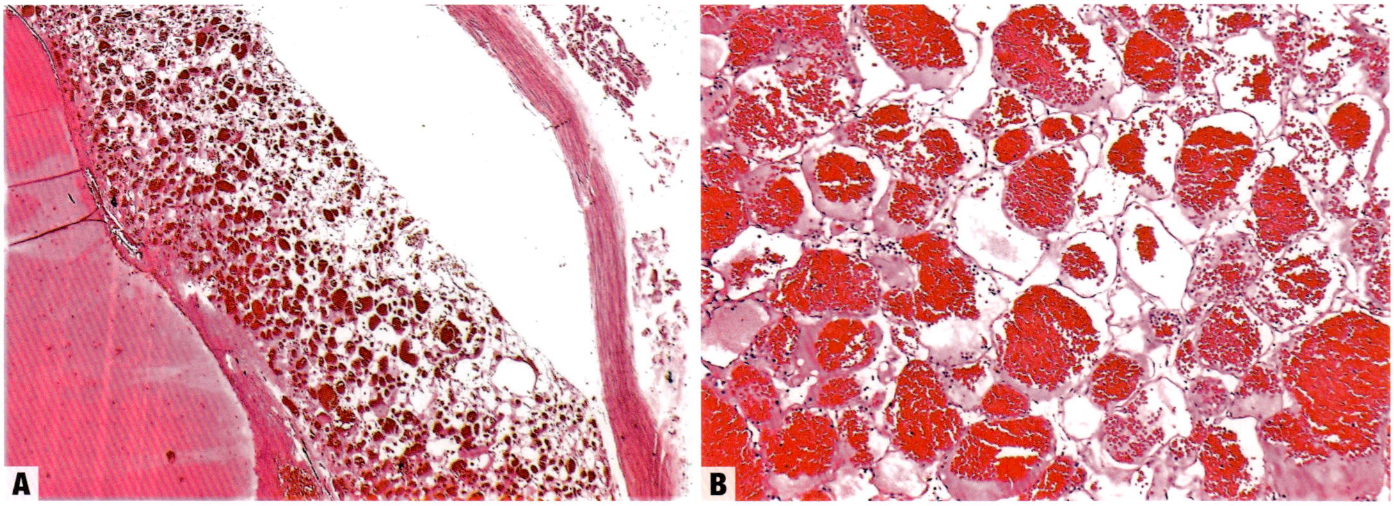

Fig. 13.05 Diffuse choroidal haemangioma / choroidal capillary malformation. **A** The sclera is the collagenous band on the right. On the left is an eosinophilic subretinal exudate. Located between the two, effacing the normal choroidal anatomy, is a diffuse cavernous haemangioma / cavernous venous malformation. **B** A higher-magnification image shows the variably sized vascular channels separated by thin septa.

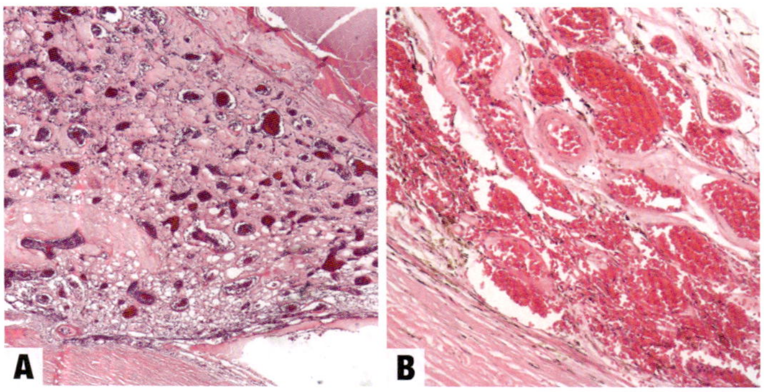

Fig. 13.06 Choroidal haemangioma. **A** This diffuse choroidal haemangioma in Sturge–Weber syndrome is associated with extensive changes to the overlying retinal pigment epithelium and retina. **B** Back-to-back dilated capillary channels in the choroid.

marked by dystrophic calcification and cortical necrosis. Neurological manifestations are variable and include headaches, hemiparesis/hemiplegia, visual field deficits (if involving the occipital cortex), recurrent stroke-like episodes / transient ischaemic attacks, and seizures of varying degrees of severity {657,978,3233}. Cognitive effects are highly variable ranging from unaffected to mild learning disabilities to severe cognitive impairments. Behavioural problems have been reported including attention problems and mood issues {2628}.

SWS is associated with endocrine dysfunction, including central hypothyroidism and an increased risk of growth hormone deficiency {2207}. This presents as childhood growth below the fifth percentile or height significantly below the mean parental height.

Epidemiology

The incidence of SWS is estimated at 1 in 20 000–50 000 births. There is no sex predilection and individuals of any ethnicity or race are affected equally.

Etiology

The congenital vascular anomalies characterizing SWS are due to a gain-of-function somatic mosaic mutation in *GNAQ* at chromosome 9q21.2. Approximately 90% of SWS patients have a specific *GNAQ* variant, NM_002072.5:c.548G>A, predicted to result in p.R183Q, which has been found in affected tissues at a mosaicism level of 1–18% {3079}. This leads to activation of downstream MAPK signalling, resulting in vascular anomalies {3079}. The p.R183Q alteration has also been detected in skin tissue from patients with non-syndromic port-wine stains. Recently, a mosaic activating variant, NM_002067.5:c.547C>T p.(R183C), in *GNA11*, a gene located at chromosome 19p13.3 that is highly homologous to *GNAQ*, was identified in a limited number of SWS cases negative for *GNAQ* p.R183Q; the *GNA11*-mutated cases may have an atypical clinical presentation {3332,2575,812,1542}.

Pathogenesis

SWS is thought to result from aberrant vessel growth and malformations in the skin, eye, and brain due to the effects of somatic mosaic *GNAQ* mutation on the cephalic neural crest during the first trimester {3079}. It is hypothesized that *GNAQ* mutation may affect the G-protein–coupled receptor endothelin, which has important roles in vasculogenesis {3079}. The embryonic stage of development during which mutation occurs may govern whether the malformations are syndromic or not {3079}; non-syndromic port-wine stains may represent a late origin of somatic *GNAQ* mutation in vascular endothelial cells, while mutation in SWS may occur earlier in development in progenitor cells that are precursors to a larger variety of cell types and tissues resulting in a syndromic phenotype.

Macroscopic appearance

Choroid CM appears as a diffusely thickened choroid with variably sized blood-filled vascular channels separated by thin septa, associated with dilated draining vortex veins.

Histopathology

CMs in the choroid, episclera, and conjunctiva appear as unencapsulated collections of thin-walled, variably sized vascular channels. Secondary changes include retinal pigment epithelial alteration, subretinal fibrosis, serous (exudative) retinal detachment, and sequelae of paediatric glaucoma (buphthalmos) {1310,3618}.

Cytology

Not relevant

Diagnostic molecular pathology

GNAQ evaluation is performed using the affected tissue to identify a somatic heterozygous pathogenic sequence variant consistent with the diagnosis of SWS (although not specific for SWS) {3079}.

Essential and desirable diagnostic criteria

Essential: two of three diagnostic criteria: cutaneous facial CM, increased intraocular pressure, and leptomeningeal CM; individuals with leptomeningeal angiomatosis only are considered to have type 3 SWS.

Desirable: demonstration of pathogenic somatic variant in *GNAQ* or related gene in affected tissue.

Staging

Not relevant

Prognosis and prediction

The prognosis and life expectancy for SWS is markedly variable and depends on the location of lesions and their functional impact. The extent of facial cutaneous CM may be predictive of neurological disability {854,730,3227}. Bilateral brain involvement and early onset of intractable seizures before 1 year of life are clinical features associated with worse outcomes. Intellectual disability occurs in approximately half of individuals with SWS and is reportedly severe in a third of patients {2502,3232}. Screening and earlier detection of lesions may be beneficial to patients. Published guidelines for surveillance are available {2798,3731,745}.

Neurofibromatosis type 1

Rodriguez FJ
Midena E
Perry A

Definition

Neurofibromatosis type 1 (NF1) is an autosomal dominant disorder caused by a pathogenic germline variant of *NF1*.

MIM numbering

162200 Neurofibromatosis type 1; NF1

ICD-11 coding

LD2D.10 Neurofibromatosis type 1

Related terminology

Not recommended: Von Recklinghausen disease; peripheral neurofibromatosis.

Subtype(s)

Mosaic neurofibromatosis type 1, including segmental neurofibromatosis type 1; spinal neurofibromatosis; neurofibromatosis–Noonan syndrome; 17q11.2 microdeletion syndrome; orbitofacial neurofibromatosis type 1

Localization

NF1 affects many different cell types and tissues in the body, predominantly localizing to central and peripheral nervous system sites.

Clinical features

Multiple café-au-lait macules are usually present at birth, and increase in number during the first 2 years of life. Skinfold freckling in the axillary, inguinal, and submammary regions occurs in > 80% of adults with NF1. Lisch nodules and skinfold freckling are usually detectable before puberty. Cutaneous neurofibromas typically develop during puberty and are identified in > 85% of adults {1218}. In contrast, plexiform neurofibromas

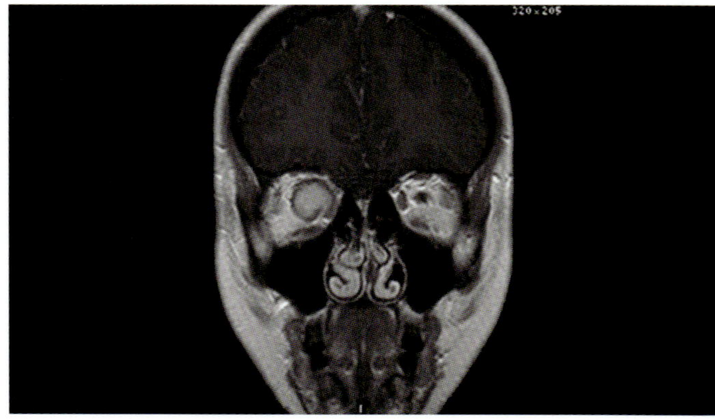

Fig. 13.07 Pilocytic astrocytoma of the optic nerve. Coronal T1-weighted MRI demonstrates an enhancing mass expanding the right optic nerve. The optic nerve is a favoured site for glioma development in patients with neurofibromatosis type 1.

are considered congenital, developing in 30–50% of children with NF1 {2195}. Malignant peripheral nerve sheath tumours (MPNSTs) are extremely uncommon in the periocular tissues {3747}. Lisch nodules are the most common ocular manifestations, usually detected before puberty. Other ocular/orbital manifestations include optic pathway gliomas and sphenoid wing dysplasia {407}. Orbitofacial neurofibromatosis type 1 (OFNF) has been historically studied as a clinical form of NF1 {546}. OFNF is often characterized by progressive, large disfiguring neurofibromas involving the orbit and periorbital tissues, with associated remodelling of adjacent skull bones. Recurrence after excision is relatively high, but tumour growth may stabilize as the individual ages. Progression to MPNST is extremely rare {3747}.

Epidemiology

NF1 has a birth incidence of approximately 1 per 3000 {3419}.

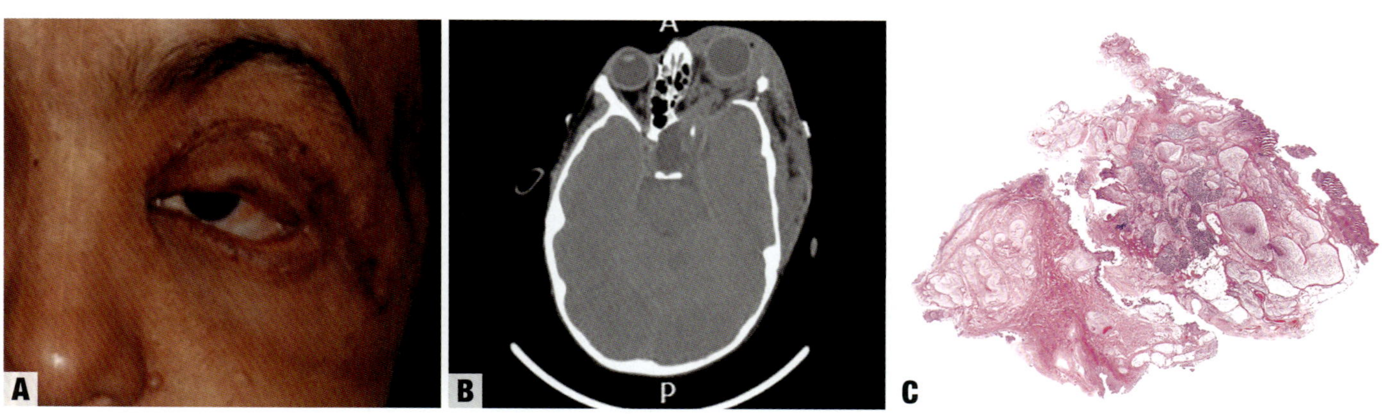

Fig. 13.08 Orbital neurofibromatosis type 1. **A** This unique clinical subtype affects the bone and soft tissues of the orbital region and may result in profound asymmetry. Café-au-lait spots and conventional cutaneous neurofibromas are also present in this patient. **B** This axial CT using bone windows highlights prominent bone remodelling, facial neurofibromatosis, and proptosis associated with a large orbital neurofibroma in a patient with neurofibromatosis type 1. **C** Orbital neurofibromas frequently have plexiform components and may intimately involve ocular adnexa such as the lacrimal gland as in this example.

Etiology

NF1 is a highly penetrant disorder caused by heterozygous pathogenic loss-of-function variants in the tumour suppressor gene *NF1*, located at chromosome 17q11.2 and encoding neurofibromin (NF1) {3529,499,3502}. More than 3000 different disease-causing variants, including deletions and duplications, have been described in *NF1*, most of which are novel and truncate the gene, often through alteration of mRNA splicing {1039}. Half of the individuals with NF1 have unaffected parents and represent de novo mutations.

Pathogenesis

Neurofibromin (NF1) primarily functions as a GAP for RAS proto-oncogenes {1904}. Most NF1 clinical features in germline mutation carriers, including café-au-lait macules, bony abnormalities, and benign tumours, result from complete loss of neurofibromin (NF1) function due to subsequent somatic mutation of the wildtype allele (biallelic *NF1* inactivation), leading to increased RAS and RAS effector (MEK/ERK or AKT/mTOR) signalling. In both neurofibromas and optic pathway gliomas / pilocytic astrocytomas, murine studies have revealed that non-neoplastic (stromal) cells with a heterozygous *NF1* mutation, including mast cells, macrophages, neurons, T cells, and microglia, are critical for tumorigenesis and continued growth.

Novel *NF1* mutations associated with OFNF have been detected in some Chinese families, as well as more severe ocular phenotypes in successive generations (i.e. anticipation) {506}. Differential promoter methylation and expression of the HOX family genes has also been reported in OFNF-associated tumours compared with neurofibromas developing at other sites {194}.

Macroscopic appearance

See individual tumours.

Histopathology

Lisch nodules develop on the anterior face of the iris, where there is usually a dome-shaped plaque of mostly spindle-shaped, cytologically bland melanocytes, arranged haphazardly. Nucleoli are not prominent and mitotic figures are not identified. Nerve sheath tumours in NF1 are predominantly neurofibromas. Recently proposed criteria for atypical neurofibromatous neoplasms of undetermined biological potential are used to describe premalignant or potentially early malignant changes in neurofibromas {2198}. Most MPNSTs in individuals with NF1 are high-grade malignant spindle cell neoplasms with brisk mitotic activity and necrosis, which either develop in a pre-existing plexiform neurofibroma or arise de novo. Optic pathway gliomas are almost always pilocytic astrocytomas.

Cytology

Similar to sporadic counterparts

Diagnostic molecular pathology

Although no mutation hotspots have been identified, a pathogenic *NF1* variant is detected in 95% of people with NF1 {2186}. Nonsense, frameshift, and splice-site mutations, insertions, small deletions or duplications, and larger deletions including whole gene loss all result in *NF1* inactivation. In approximately 5–11% of NF1 cases, a large 17q11.2 microdeletion is identified, in which multiple genes are codeleted along with the *NF1* gene {1641}. Therefore, sequencing and deletion/duplication analysis are used to identify the *NF1* mutation spectrum. Owing to the frequency of mutations in *NF1* affecting splicing, a subset of which are not demonstrable by standard genomic DNA sequencing, cDNA analysis results in a higher mutation detection rate {920}. Karyotype analysis may be considered for mutation-negative cases that have a strong NF1 clinical suspicion as (rarely) *NF1* is disrupted by a translocation or complex cytogenetic abnormality.

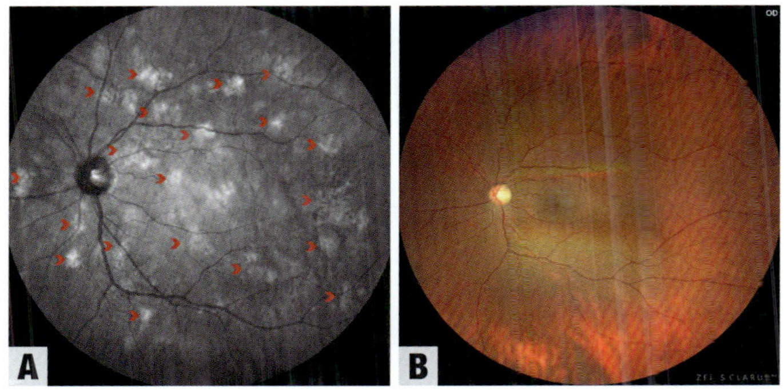

Fig. 13.09 Choroidal abnormalities in neurofibromatosis type 1. **A** A near-infrared image of the posterior pole of a patient affected by neurofibromatosis type 1, showing multiple choroidal abnormalities (red chevrons). **B** The choroidal abnormalities, histologically consisting of variable mixtures of hyperplastic Schwann cells, melanocytes and ganglion cells localized to the choroid, are completely asymptomatic and undetectable by conventional ophthalmoscopy, as shown in this colour fundus image of the same eye. Note that several retinal vascular abnormalities are also present.

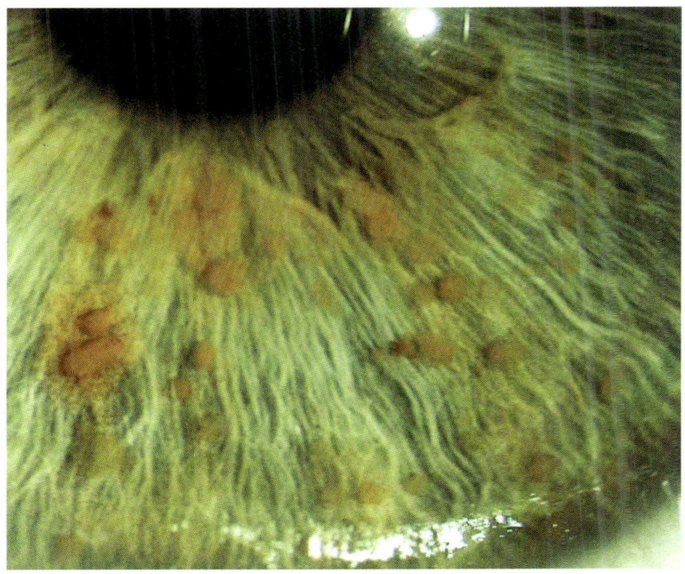

Fig. 13.10 Lisch nodules. Lisch nodules are small hamartomas that involve the anterior surface of the iris and are present in the majority of patients with neurofibromatosis type 1 at some point.

Essential and desirable diagnostic criteria

Essential: a clinical diagnosis of NF1 requires the presence of at least two of the following features:

- six or more café-au-lait macules (> 5 mm diameter in children, > 15 mm in adults)
- axillary/inguinal freckling
- two or more neurofibromas of any type or one plexiform neurofibroma
- optic pathway glioma
- two or more iris hamartomas (Lisch nodules) or two or more choroidal abnormalities
- distinctive bony abnormality (anterolateral bowing of the tibia, pseudarthrosis of a long bone, sphenoid dysplasia)
- heterozygous pathogenic *NF1* variant with a variant allele fraction of 50% in apparently normal tissue
- parent with NF1 (by the above criteria).

These criteria were revised in 2021 {1905}. Of note, there are other conditions with features that overlap with NF1, including Legius syndrome (MIM number 611431), Noonan syndrome {659}, and constitutive mismatch repair deficiency {3226}.

Staging

Staging for NF1-associated MPNSTs is identical to that utilized for their sporadic counterparts.

Prognosis and prediction

Individuals often have a shortened lifespan, mainly due to malignant tumours and cerebrovascular accidents {3419,921,2673}. The standard mortality ratio for many complications is higher in women < 50 years {3419}.

Goldenhar syndrome

Stagner AM
Alkatan H
Eagle RC Jr
Perry A

Definition

Goldenhar syndrome (GS) is a constellation of congenital anomalies due to impaired formation of the face, ears, eyes, and skeletal system, as well as variable abnormalities of internal organs, due to anomalous development of the first and second branchial arches.

MIM numbering

164210 Craniofacial microsomia; CFM

ICD-11 coding

LD2F.16 Otomandibular dysplasia

Related terminology

Acceptable: craniofacial microsomia; oculoauriculovertebral syndrome; otomandibular dysplasia; oculoauriculovertebral dysplasia; facioauriculovertebral sequence; Goldenhar–Gorlin syndrome.

Not recommended: first and second branchial arch syndrome; hemifacial microsomia.

Subtype(s)

None

Localization

GS is unilateral in 70–90% of cases. Epibulbar dermoids are most common at the inferotemporal limbus but may also occur nasally. They may affect the superficial cornea only, involve the full-thickness stroma, or extend through the entire cornea into the anterior chamber. Lipodermoids are more common superotemporally and are less specific for GS. Eyelid colobomas are most frequently located at the junction of the middle and inner thirds of the upper eyelid {3364,2051}.

Clinical features

GS shows variable expressivity; the classic disease phenotypic triad involves mandibular or hemifacial hypoplasia, ocular and auricular malformations, especially limbal dermoids and accessory tragi, and vertebral anomalies, particularly of the cervical spine. CNS malformations and cardiac and urogenital anomalies are variably encountered {364}. The ophthalmological features typically include the upper eyelid with or without intraocular colobomas (6–75%), epibulbar choristoma or dermoid/dermolipoma (30–50%), and less frequently microphthalmia/anophthalmia, strabismus (particularly Duane syndrome), cataract, unequal palpebral fissures, ptosis, decreased corneal sensation, microcornea, and rarely posterior segment abnormalities such as optic nerve hypoplasia {276,1482,73,3115,2079,2060}. Abnormalities of the lacrimal drainage system including nasolacrimal duct obstruction and atresia may cause recurrent dacryocystitis {2060,73}. GS in association with complex choristoma, linear naevus sebaceus syndrome, and/or encephalocraniocutaneous lipomatosis has been reported {73}.

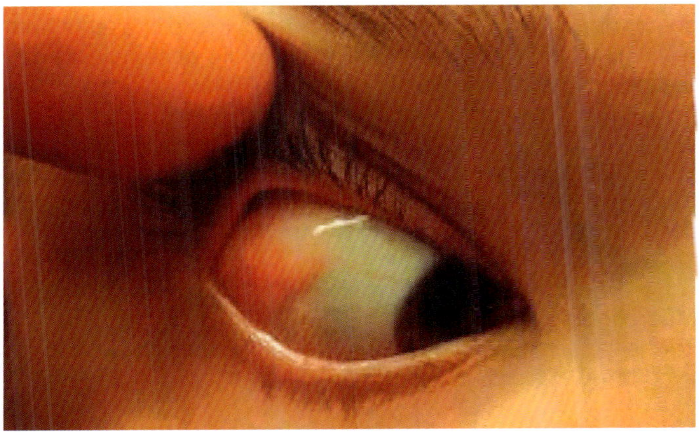

Fig. 13.11 Epibulbar complex choristoma. A 6-year-old girl with Goldenhar syndrome and a superotemporal, smooth, elevated tan-pink to yellowish epibulbar mass.

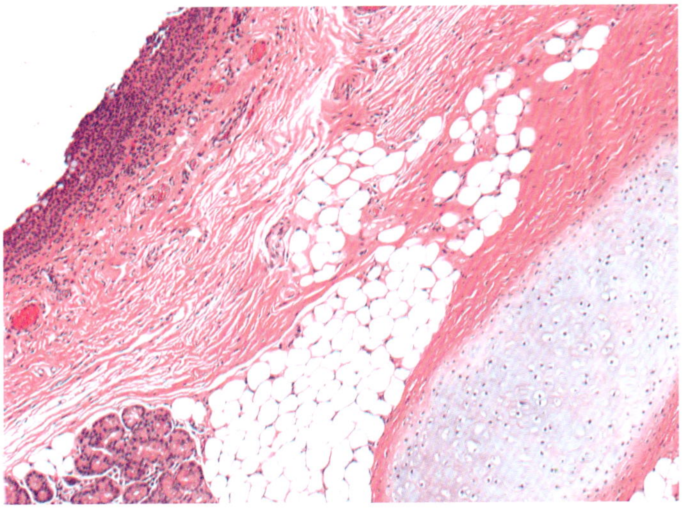

Fig. 13.12 Epibulbar complex choristoma. Beneath the conjunctival epithelium is a dense collagenous stroma containing mature adipose tissue, hyaline cartilage, and lobules of lacrimal gland.

Epidemiology

GS is the second most frequent craniofacial malformation after cleft palate and occurs in about 1:5000 births, although estimations based on specific populations vary widely. Most, but not all large studies show a male predominance {276,3115,2060}

Etiology

GS is typically sporadic and the etiology in most cases is poorly understood. Inheritance typically occurs in an autosomal dominant fashion when a family history is present.

Pathogenesis

GS results from late first trimester abnormal development of structures derived from the first and second branchial arches. Numerous copy-number variants have been detected in patients with clinical GS, including 22q11.2 deletions and 14q22.3 duplications (*OTX2*). SNVs have also been described in various candidate genes, including *MYT1* {3344}. Recently, heterogeneous loss-of-function variants in *SF3B2* at chromosome 11q13.1 have been identified in 25% of patients with a family history of GS and 3% of sporadic cases via whole-exome or whole-genome sequencing of a large cohort; inheritance was dominant with interfamilial and intrafamilial phenotypic variability {3342}. GS is also more common in twins; in infants of mothers with diabetes mellitus; and in children born to mothers with potential disruptions in placental vascularization, including exposure to certain medications, hypertension, and smoking {364}.

Macroscopic appearance

This is the same as in the sporadic tumour types involved in the syndrome.

Histopathology

As in sporadic cases, epibulbar dermoids are composed of dense subepithelial collagen bundles resembling dermal collagen rather than substantia propria. Dermal appendages including pilosebaceous and apocrine/eccrine units are present to varying degrees. Variable amounts of fat can be observed; dermolipomas contain abundant adipose tissue. Complex choristomas composed of particularly lacrimal gland, cartilage, and smooth muscle are also seen {1482, 2058}. Complex choristoma constituted 10.8% of all epibulbar choristomas in one of the series, and GS was found in 38% of these cases, while osseous choristoma was less common (1.7%) and isolated {73}.

Cytology

Not relevant

Diagnostic molecular pathology

Currently, genetic testing is not necessary for diagnosis. While a variety of alterations, including copy-number variants and SNVs, are correlated with the development of the GS phenotype, these findings are not diagnostic or identifiable in many cases.

Essential and desirable diagnostic criteria

Essential: facial asymmetry with preauricular tags; an ocular finding such as epibulbar dermoid or eyelid coloboma.

Note: specific diagnostic criteria are still debated.

Staging

Not relevant

Prognosis and prediction

The majority of patients with GS have normal intelligence and lifespan. Without systemic complications, the prognosis is good. Newborns may experience difficulty in breathing, feeding, and sleeping due to mandibular and other hypoplasias. Eyelid reconstruction may be needed early in life owing to exposure keratopathy and corneal ulceration from eyelid coloboma {3297}. Dermoids and lipodermoids may induce astigmatism or cause direct visual obstruction, leading to amblyopia; early surgical excision may prevent these complications {2051}.

Muir–Torre syndrome

Eiger-Moscovich M
Lazar AJ
Milman T

Definition

Muir–Torre syndrome (MTS) is a rare autosomal dominant disorder defined by the association of cutaneous lesions (sebaceous neoplasms or keratoacanthoma) and Lynch syndrome (LS)-associated visceral malignancies. MTS results from constitutional (germline) pathogenic alterations affecting the DNA mismatch repair genes *MLH1*, *MSH2*, *MSH6*, and *PMS2*.

MIM numbering

158320, Muir–Torre syndrome; MRTES
608456, Familial adenomatous polyposis 2; FAP2

ICD-11 coding

Not available

Related terminology

None

Subtype(s)

None

Localization

Lesions are skin, eyelid, and visceral malignancies (see below).

Clinical features

MTS patients present with cutaneous manifestations which can appear before (22%), concurrent with (6%), or after (56%) the diagnosis of visceral malignancy {62}. The cutaneous manifestations include well-differentiated sebaceous neoplasms, such as sebaceous adenoma and sebaceoma and, less frequently, sebaceous carcinoma and keratoacanthoma, generally in non-periocular skin {445,1527,3119,1517}. Many patients have numerous lesions and/or a family history {2892}.

Visceral malignancies associated with LS (MIM number 120435) include tumours of the colorectum, endometrium, stomach, small bowel, ovary, gallbladder, hepatobiliary tract, pancreas, urinary tract, kidney, brain, and prostate {2248,2249, 3562}. Neoplasms can develop at any age, but often arise in young people. Some develop multiple tumours.

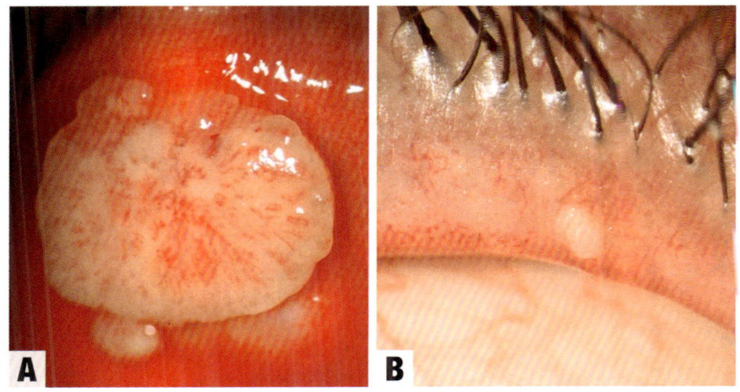

Fig. 13.13 Sebaceous epithelioma (sebaceoma) in a patient with Muir–Torre syndrome. **A** Papillomatous tarsal conjunctival mass. **B** A circumscribed lesion protrudes from the meibomian gland orifice.

Epidemiology

The population incidence of MTS has not yet been determined but the syndrome has been identified in approximately 5–9% of individuals from families with LS {1517,2577,3172}.

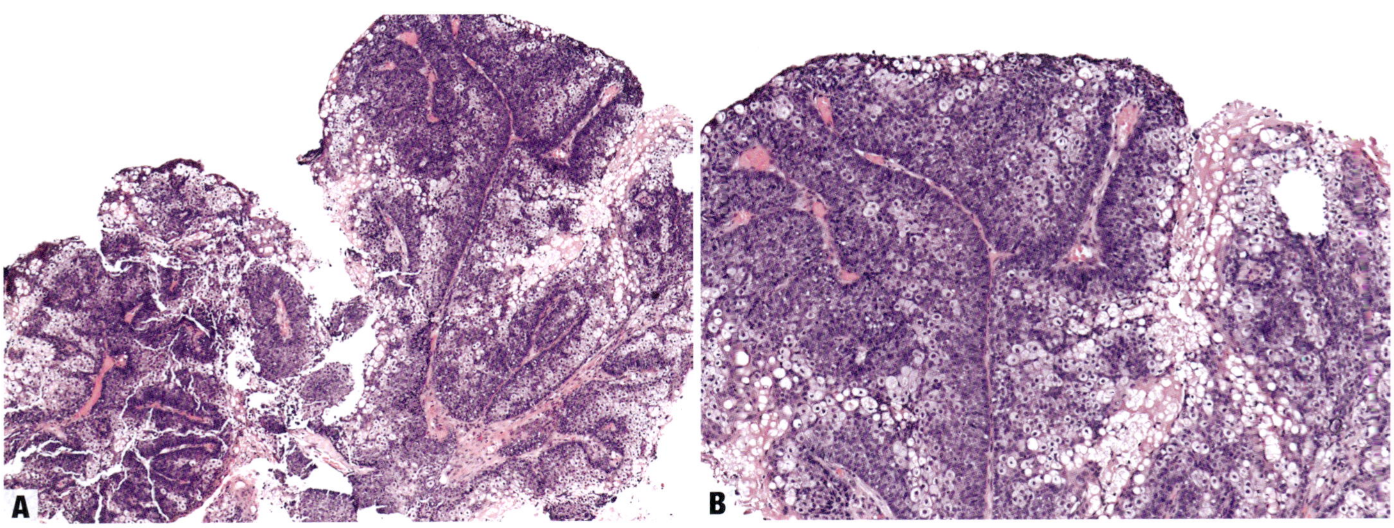

Fig. 13.14 Sebaceous epithelioma (sebaceoma) in a patient with Muir–Torre syndrome. **A** A papillomatous lesion composed of enlarged and haphazardly arranged sebaceous gland lobules with immature sebocytes predominating over mature sebocytes. **B** Lack of normal maturation within the lobules of a sebaceoma.

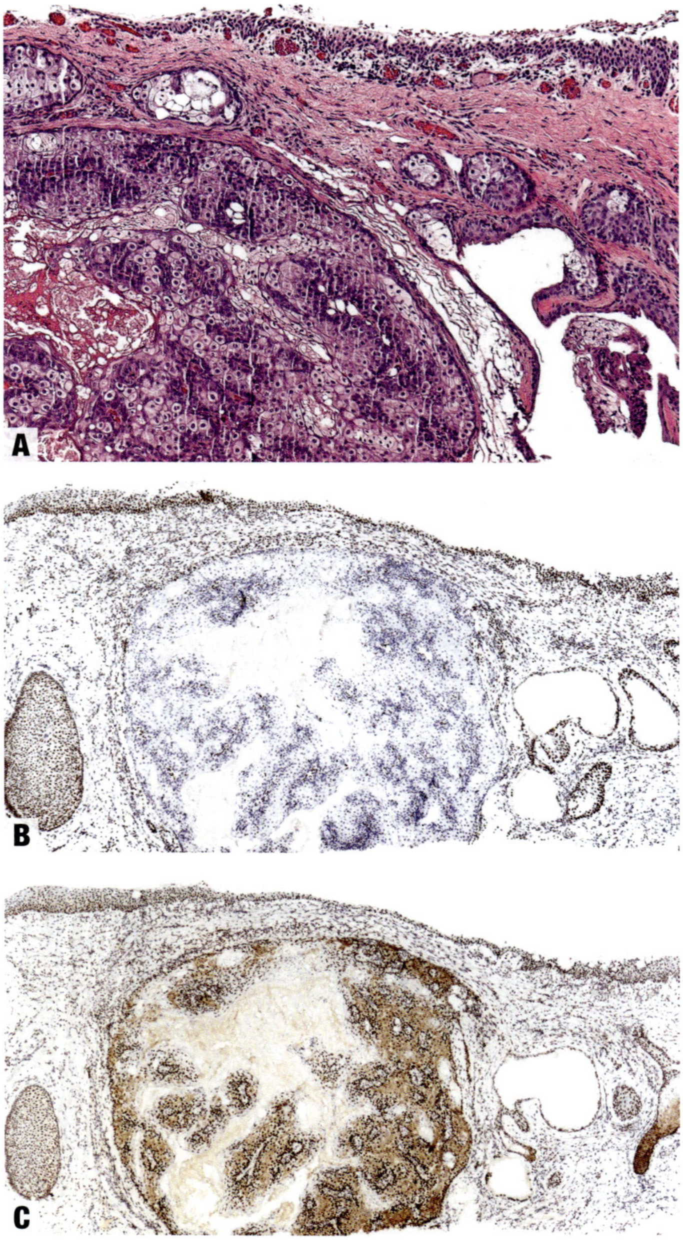

Fig. 13.15 Sebaceous adenoma in a patient with Muir–Torre syndrome. **A** A circumscribed neoplasm is seen, composed of enlarged, irregular sebaceous gland lobules with prominent central holocrine secretion contributing to a cystic architecture. Mature sebocytes predominate over the immature sebocytes when compared with the normal adjacent sebaceous gland lobules. **B** Loss of nuclear MSH2 in the neoplastic cells with preservation of staining in the tumour-infiltrating lymphocytes, adjacent stroma, normal adjacent sebaceous glands, and overlying conjunctival epithelium. **C** Intact nuclear PMS2 in the lesion and the adjacent tissues.

Etiology

The primary cause of MTS is a germline mutation affecting a DNA mismatch repair (MMR) gene: *MLH1*, *MSH2*, *MSH6*, or *PMS2*. Some individuals have deletions involving *EPCAM* (*TACSTD1*) that can silence the neighbouring *MSH2* gene. Based on immunohistochemistry, abnormalities of MSH2 and MSH6 expression are strongly associated with the MTS phenotype, and with *MSH2* mutations in 90% of cases. Most of the remaining cases harbour *MLH1* or *PMS2* abnormalities. An isolated deficiency of *MSH6* or *PMS2* has been documented {1517}. This strongly contrasts with LS, where germline deficits of *MLH1* and *MSH2* have roughly equal incidence. The phenotype of sebaceous neoplasia and visceral malignancy can also be seen in patients with autosomal recessive *MUTYH*-associated adenomatous polyposis (familial adenomatous polyposis 2; MIM number 608456).

A number of environmental and lifestyle factors have been identified as modifiers of LS. Cigarette smoking, increased body mass index, and alcohol consumption are associated with increased risk, whereas acetylsalicylic acid, ibuprofen, multivitamin and calcium supplements, and hormone replacement therapy are associated with a reduction of cancer risk {2477, 3616,2289,58}.

Pathogenesis

The four MMR genes encode proteins that detect and repair errors in base pairing during DNA replication by forming complexes {870}. MLH1 dimerizes with PMS2, while MSH2 dimerizes with MSH6 {1448}. A germline pathogenic sequence alteration in one of the MMR genes followed by a second somatic hit to the remaining wildtype allele {3119} leads to cells becoming mismatch repair deficient. This deficiency has several important consequences. Firstly, mismatch repair–deficient cells escape from the normal control of apoptosis and gain a relative growth advantage {2584}. Secondly, mismatch repair deficiency leads to an increase in the point mutation rate, especially within repetitive stretches of DNA called microsatellites; this manifests as microsatellite instability (MSI). Thirdly, mismatch repair deficiency may also lead to abnormal mismatch repair protein expression, which is identifiable by immunohistochemistry.

Macroscopic appearance

The gross appearance is related to the tumour type and is not distinctive.

Histopathology

The histopathological appearance is related to the tumour type and is not distinctive.

Immunohistochemically, approximately one half to two thirds of unselected sebaceous neoplasms are deficient in MMR proteins {922,1517,3119}. The rates of loss vary: in the head and neck region, adenomas show 30–40% loss, whereas loss in carcinomas in this region is rare. Outside the head and neck region, both adenomas and carcinomas commonly show loss (in > 80% of cases).

MMR immunohistochemistry was found to be comparable to PCR-based MSI testing in LS-associated tumours {3750, 2965}. Nevertheless, the sensitivity and specificity of MMR immunohistochemistry in predicting the underlying gene defect is 85% and 48%, respectively, in sebaceous neoplasms, compared with the sensitivity and specificity values of 92–94% and 88–100%, respectively, in colorectal tumours {2725,2724}. The value of MMR immunohistochemistry and MSI testing is low in periocular sebaceous neoplasms, specifically in sebaceous carcinoma. It is considerably enhanced by testing more than one tumour from the same family and/or individual, especially if the tumours are rare.

Cytology

Not relevant

Diagnostic molecular pathology

Molecular genetic studies on tumour and blood DNA can directly evaluate the MMR gene status {1109}. Since it is established that somatic MMR gene mutations are seen in sebaceous tumours, germline testing for confirmation is preferred {3314}.

Although routine MTS and LS screening is not recommended for periocular sebaceous carcinoma, the Mayo MTS risk score guidelines may be applicable to periocular sebaceous neoplasms {2456,2724,870}. Patients with a score ≥ 2 should be evaluated by MMR immunohistochemistry on colon or endometrial cancer or, when available, by molecular genetic testing {2724}.

Essential and desirable diagnostic criteria

Essential: at least one visceral cancer; neoplasms with evidence of mismatch repair deficiency (by MMR immunohistochemistry or MSI testing); definitive MTS/LS diagnosis involves identification of a germline MMR gene pathogenic mutation.

Desirable: multiple skin sebaceous neoplasms often present.

Staging

Tumours are staged according to Union for International Cancer Control (UICC) TNM8, depending on the tumour type.

Prognosis and prediction

The visceral malignancies of MTS and LS are generally found to have less-aggressive behaviour than their sporadic counterparts {2892}. The periocular cutaneous manifestation is usually of benign well-differentiated sebaceous neoplasms.

Contributors

ABDEL-RAHMAN, Mohamed H.
Ohio State University
202 Wiseman Hall
Columbus OH 43210

AGARAM, Narasimhan P.
Memorial Sloan Kettering Cancer Center
1275 York Ave
New York NY 10065

AGNI, Meghana
Endeavor Health
2650 Ridge Ave
Evanston IL 03766

AL HUSSAINI, Maysa
King Hussein Cancer Center
202 Queen Rania Al-Abdullah St
Amman 11941

ALDAPE, Kenneth D.
National Cancer Institute
10 Center Dr, Building 10, Room 2S235
Bethesda MD 20892

ALKATAN, Hind
King Saud University (College of Medicine)
PO Box 18097
Riyadh 11415

AMARY, Fernanda
Royal National Orthopaedic Hospital
Brockley Hill
Stanmore, Middlesex HA7 4LP

ARONOW, Mary Elizabeth
Massachusetts Eye and Ear
Harvard Medical School
243 Charles St
Boston MA 02114

AUW-HAEDRICH, Claudia
Eye Center Freiburg
Killianstraße 5
79106 Freiburg

BAHRAMI, Armita
Emory University School of Medicine
1364 Clifton Rd NE
Atlanta GA 30322

BARNHILL, Raymond L.
Institut Curie (and Faculty of Medicine, Université Paris Cité)
26 Rue d'Ulm
75005 Paris

BASTIAN, Boris C.*
UCSF Helen Diller Family Comprehensive Cancer Center
1450 3rd St, Box 3116
San Francisco CA 94158-9001

BAUMHOER, Daniel
University Hospital Basel
Schönbeinstrasse 40
4031 Basel

BECHRAKIS, Nikolaos E.
University Hospital Essen
Hufelandstraße 55
45147 Essen

BEENAKKER, Jan-Willem M.*
Leiden University Medical Center
Albinusdreef 2
2333 ZA Leiden

BERRY, Jesse L.
Children's Hospital Los Angeles
University of Southern California
4650 Sunset Blvd, Mail Stop #88
Los Angeles CA 90027

BERTIN, Helios
University Hospital of Nantes
1 Place Alexis-Ricordeau
44093 Nantes

BILLINGS, Steven D.
Cleveland Clinic
9500 Euclid Ave, L25
Cleveland OH 44195

BOVÉE, Judith V.M.G.
Department of Pathology
Leiden University Medical Center
Albinusdreef 2
2333 ZA Leiden

BREDELLA, Miriam
NYU Langone Health and Grossman School of Medicine
227 E 30th St, 743
New York NY 10016

BRENN, Thomas
University of Michigan
NCRC Bldg 35, 2800 Plymouth Rd
Ann Arbor MI 48109-2800

BROUWER, Niels J.
Leiden University Medical Center
Albinusdreef 2
2333 ZA Leiden

CALONJE, Jaime E.
St John's Institute of Dermatology
St Thomas' Hospital
Westminster Bridge Rd
London SE1 7EH

CASSOUX, Nathalie
Institut Curie
26 Rue d'Ulm
75005 Paris

CATES, Justin M.M.
Vanderbilt University Medical Center
1161 21st Ave S, MCN-3322
Nashville TN 37232

CEBULLA, Colleen M.
Ohio State University
915 Olentangy River Rd, Suite 5000
Columbus OH 43212

CHAN, Anita S.Y.*
Singapore National Eye Centre
11 Third Hospital Ave
Singapore 168751

CHEREPANOFF, Svetlana
St Vincent's Hospital Sydney
390 Victoria St
Darlinghurst NSW 2010

CHEVEZ-BARRIOS, Patricia
Houston Methodist Hospital
6565 Fannin St, M227
Houston TX 77030

CHHABLANI, Jay
University of Pittsburgh
200 Lothrop St
Pittsburgh PA 15213

CLEVEN, Arjen H.G.
University Medical Center Groningen
Hanzeplein 1
9713 GZ Groningen

COLMENERO, Isabel
Hospital Infantil Universitario Niño Jesús
Av. de Menéndez Pelayo, 65
28009 Madrid

COUPLAND, Sarah E.*
Institute of Systems, Molecular and Integrative Biology, University of Liverpool
W Derby St, William Henry Duncan Building, 3rd Floor
Liverpool L7 8TX

* Indicates disclosure of interests (see p. 519).

CREE, Ian A.
International Agency for Research on Cancer
25 Av. Tony Garnier, CS 90627
69366 Lyon, CEDEX 07

CUMMINGS, Thomas J.
Duke University Medical Center
PO Box 3712
Durham NC 27710

DALVIN, Lauren A.
Mayo Clinic
200 1st St SW
Rochester MN 55905

DAMATO, Bertil Eric
Moorfields Eye Hospital
162 City Road
London EC1V 2PD

DE ÁLAVA, Enrique
Hospital Universitario Virgen del Rocío-IBiS
University of Seville
Av. Manuel Siurot, s/n
41013 Seville

DE GRAAF, Pim
Amsterdam UMC and
Vrije Universiteit Amsterdam
De Boelelaan 1117
1081 HV Amsterdam

DE KLEIN, Annelies
Erasmus MC
PO Box 2040
3000 CA Rotterdam

DE LA FOUCHARDIÈRE, Arnaud
Centre Léon Bérard
28 Rue Laennec
69008 Lyon

DEBNAM, J. Matthew
University of Texas
MD Anderson Cancer Center
1400 Pressler St, FCT16.5024
Houston TX 77030

DEMICCO, Elizabeth G.*
University of Toronto
Mount Sinai Hospital, 600 University Ave
Toronto ON M5G 1X5

DENTON, Erika R.E.
Norfolk and Norwich University Hospitals
NHS Foundation Trust
Colney Ln
Norwich NR4 7UY

DICKSON, Brendan Craig*
Mount Sinai Hospital
600 University Ave
Toronto ON M5G 1X5

DORSMAN, Josephine C.
Amsterdam UMC
De Boelelaan 1118
1081 HV Amsterdam

DOYLE, Leona A.
University College Dublin
Belfield
Dublin 4

DRY, Sarah M.
University of California, Los Angeles (UCLA)
13-222 CHS, 10833 Le Conte Ave
Los Angeles CA 90095

DUBOVY, Sander R.
Bascom Palmer Eye Institute
900 NW 17th St
Miami FL 33136

DUNCAN, Lyn M.
Massachusetts General Hospital
55 Fruit St, Warren 825
Boston MA 02114

EAGLE, Ralph C. Jr
Wills Eye Hospital
840 Walnut St, Suite 1410
Philadelphia PA 19107

EBERHART, Charles G.
Johns Hopkins University
720 Rutland Ave, Ross Building 558
Baltimore MD 21205

EDEN, Michael
Cambridge University Hospitals
NHS Foundation Trust
Hills Rd
Cambridge CB2 0QQ

EDWARD, Deepak P.
King Khaled Eye Specialist Hospital
and Research Centre
Riyadh

EIGER-MOSCOVICH, Maya
Hadassah Medical Center
Kalman Ya'akov Man St
9112001 Jerusalem

ELDER, David E.
Hospital of the University of Pennsylvania
3400 Spruce St
Philadelphia PA 19104

ELENITSAS, Rosalie
University of Pennsylvania
3600 Spruce St, 2 Maloney Building
Philadelphia PA 19104

ESMAELI, Bita
University of Texas
MD Anderson Cancer Center
1515 Holcombe Blvd, Unit 1488
Houston TX 77030

FANBURG-SMITH, Julie C.
University of Virginia
1215 Lee St, Room 3060
Charlottesville VA 22908

FARMER, James
Queen's University /
EORLA-University of Ottawa
99 University Ave
Kingston ON K7L 3N6

FERGUSON, Peter M.
Royal Prince Alfred Hospital
Missenden Rd, Camperdown
Sydney NSW 2050

FERREIRA, Teresa A.
Leiden University Medical Center
Albinusdreef 2
2333 ZA Leiden

FERRY, Judith A.
Massachusetts General Hospital
55 Fruit St
Boston MA 02114

FIELD, Andrew S.
University of NSW Sydney and
University of Notre Dame Medical Schools
Department of Anatomical Pathology
St Vincent's Hospital Sydney
Victoria St
Darlinghurst, Sydney NSW 2010

FLANAGAN, Adrienne Margaret
Royal National Orthopaedic Hospital
Brockley Hill
Stanmore, Middlesex HA7 4LP

FLUCKE, Uta
Radboud University Medical Center
PO Box 9101
6500 HB Nijmegen

FOLBERG, Robert
Oakland University William Beaumont
School of Medicine
586 Pioneer Dr
Rochester MI 48309

FRANCIS, Jasmine H.
Memorial Sloan Kettering Cancer Center
1275 York Ave
New York NY 10065

* Indicates disclosure of interests (see p. 519).

FRITCHIE, Karen J.
Cleveland Clinic
9500 Euclid Ave
Cleveland OH 44195

FULLEN, Douglas R.
University of Michigan Hospital and
Health Systems - UMHS
NCRC Building 35, Room 36-1221-13
2800 Plymouth Rd
Ann Arbor MI 48109-2800

GALLIE, Brenda L.
Hospital for Sick Children
11 Rose Ave
Toronto ON M4X 1N6

GERAMI, Pedram
Feinberg School of Medicine
Northwestern University
NMH Arkes Family Pavilion, Suite 1600
676 N Saint Clair St
Chicago IL 60611

GILL, Anthony J.
Royal North Shore Hospital
Pacific Hwy
St Leonards NSW 2065

GOLDMAN-LÉVY, Gabrielle
Hôpitaux Universitaires de Genève (HUG)
Rue Gabrielle-Perret-Gentil 4
1205 Geneva

GRAYSON, Wayne
Ampath Laboratories, Johannesburg
and School of Pathology
University of the Witwatersrand
7 York Rd
Parktown 2193

GROSSNIKLAUS, Hans E.
Emory Eye Center
1365 Clifton Rd
Atlanta GA 30322

HEEGAARD, Steffen
Department of Ophthalmology and
Department of Pathology / Eye Pathology
Section
University of Copenhagen
Frederik V's Vej 11
2100 Copenhagen

HEINDL, Ludwig M.
University Hospital Cologne
Kerpener Str 62
50937 Cologne

HERWIG-CARL, Martina C.
Department of Ophthalmology
University Hospital Bonn
Ernst-Abbe-Straße 2
53127 Bonn

HINDSØ, Tine Gadegaard
Rigshospitalet
Copenhagen University Hospital
Blegdamsvej 9
2100 Copenhagen

HODGE, Jennelle C.
Indiana University School of Medicine
975 W Walnut St, IB-354
Indianapolis IN 46202

HOGENDOORN, Pancras C.W.
Leiden University Medical Center
PO Box 9600
2300 RC Leiden

HONAVAR, Santosh G.*
Centre for Sight Eye Hospital
Ashoka Capitol, Road No. 2, Banjara Hills
Hyderabad 500034

HOWITT, Brooke E.
Stanford University School of Medicine
Department of Pathology, L235
300 Pasteur Dr
Stanford CA 94305

HYRCZA, Martin D.*
University of Calgary
Arnie Charbonneau Cancer Institute
Rm 7508, McCaig Tower, 1403 29 St NW
Calgary AB T2N 2T9

IACOB, Codrin E.
New York Eye and Ear Infirmary
of Mount Sinai
310 E 14th St, 3rd Floor
New York NY 10003

IRION, Luciane C. Dreher
Manchester University NHS Foundation Trust
Oxford Rd
Manchester M13 9WL

JAGER, Martine J.
Leiden University Medical Center
PO Box 9600
2300 RC Leiden

JAMBHEKAR, Nirmala A.
Tata Memorial Hospital
4, Aamrai, Arvind
Vishnunagar, Naupada
Thane West 400 602

KALIKI, Swathi
LV Prasad Eye Institute
Road No. 2, Banjara Hills
Hyderabad 500034

KASHYAP, Seema
All India Institute of Medical Sciences
A 1/250, Safdarjung Enclave
New Delhi 110029

KAZAKOV, Dmitry V.
Pathologie Institut Enge
Hottingerstrasse 9
8032 Zürich

KEMPF, Werner
Kempf und Pfaltz Histologische Diagnostik
Affolternstrasse 56
8050 Zürich

KHETAN, Vikas
Flaum Eye Institute
601 Elmwood Ave
Rochester NY 14642

KHOURY, Joseph David
University of Nebraska Medical Center
985900 Nebraska Medical Center
Omaha NE 68198

KIILGAARD, Jens F.
Rigshospitalet
Copenhagen University Hospital
Blegdamsvej 9
2100 Copenhagen

KILIC, Emine
Erasmus MC
Dr Molewaterplein 40
3015 GD Rotterdam

KIVELÄ, Tero
University of Helsinki and
Helsinki University Hospital
Zaidankatu 2 A, PL 225
00029 HUS Helsinki

KRISHNA, Yamini
Royal Liverpool University Hospital
University Hospitals of Liverpool Group
Mount Vernon St
Liverpool L7 8YE

LARQUE, Ana B.
Hospital Clínic de Barcelona
C. de Villarroel, 170
08036 Barcelona

LAVER, Nora Marina
Tufts University School of Medicine,
Tufts Medicine, Tufts Medical Center
800 Washington St, PO Box 6700
Boston MA 02111

LAZAR, Alexander J.
University of Texas
MD Anderson Cancer Center
1515 Holcombe Blvd, Unit 85
Houston TX 77030

LEE, Nahyoung Grace
Harvard Medical School
243 Charles St
Boston MA 02114

* Indicates disclosure of interests (see p. 519).

LEITE, Katia R.M.
University of São Paulo Medical School
Av. Dr. Arnaldo, 455
São Paulo SP 01246-903

LIANG, Zhiyong
Peking Union Medical College Hospital
Chinese Academy of Medical Sciences &
Peking Union Medical College
1 Shuaifuyuan, Wangfujing
Beijing 100730

LOEFFLER, Karin U.
Department of Ophthalmology
University Hospital Bonn
Ernst-Abbe-Straße 2
53127 Bonn

LOKUHETTY, Dilani
International Agency for Research on Cancer
25 Av. Tony Garnier, CS 90627
69366 Lyon, CEDEX 07

LÓPEZ-TERRADA, Dolores H.
Texas Children's Hospital
Baylor College of Medicine
6621 Fannin St, AB1195
Houston TX 77030

MADIGAN, Michele C.
UNSW and University of Sydney
School of Optometry and Vision Science
Room 3.045, Rupert Myers Building North
Sydney NSW 2052

MAEDA, Daichi
Graduate School of Medicine
Kobe University
7-5-1 Kusunokimachi Chuo-ku
Kobe 650-0017

MAKTABI, Azza
King Khaled Eye Specialist Hospital
Ar Rahmaniyah
Riyadh 1234

MARGO, Curtis
Morsani College of Medicine
University of South Florida
USF Eye Pathology
13330 USF Laurel Dr, 4th Floor
Tampa FL 33612

MASSI, Daniela
University of Florence
Viale Gaetano Pieraccini, 6
50139 Florence FI

MATERIN, Miguel A.
Duke University Medical Center
2351 Erwin Rd
Durham NC 27710

McKELVIE, Penelope A.
St Vincent's Hospital Melbourne
PO Box 2900
Fitzroy VIC 3065

MENDOZA, Pia
Wellstar Medical Group
303 Parkway Dr NE
Atlanta GA 30312

MESSINA, Jane L.
Moffitt Cancer Center and Research Institute
12902 USF Magnolia Dr
Tampa FL 33612

MIDENA, Edoardo
Institute of Ophthalmology
Via Nicolò Giustiniani, 2
35128 Padua PD

MIHIC-PROBST, Daniela
University Hospital Zürich
Schmelzbergstrasse 12
8091 Zürich

MILMAN, Tatyana
Wills Eye Hospital, Sidney Kimmel Medical
College – Thomas Jefferson University
840 Walnut St, Suite 1410
Philadelphia PA 19107

MISHRA, Dilip K.
LV Prasad Eye Institute
Kallam Anji Reddy Campus
Road No. 2, Banjara Hills
Hyderabad, Telangana 500034

MITTAL, Ruchi
Bagchi Sri Shankara Cancer Centre and
Research Institute
Bhubaneswar
Odisha 752054

MOCH, Holger
University of Zürich and
University Hospital Zürich
Schmelzbergstrasse 12
8091 Zürich

MOLL, Annette C.
Amsterdam UMC
De Boelelaan 1117
1081 HV Amsterdam

MORI, Taisuke
National Cancer Center Hospital
5-1-1 Tsukiji, Chuo-ku
Tokyo 140-0045

MOULIN, Alexandre
Jules Gonin Eye Hospital
University of Lausanne
Av. de France 15
1004 Lausanne

MUDHAR, Hardeep Singh
National Specialist Ophthalmic
Pathology Service (NSOPS)
Department of Histopathology
E-Floor, Royal Hallamshire Hospital
Glossop Rd
Sheffield S10 2JF

MULAY, Kaustubh
Centre For Sight
Ashoka Capitol Building, 2nd Floor
Road No. 2, Banjara Hills
Hyderabad 500034

NG, Tony*
University of British Columbia
Anatomical Pathology JPN 1416
Vancouver General Hospital
855 W 12th Ave
Vancouver BC V5Z 1M9

NIELSEN, G. Petur
Massachusetts General Hospital
55 Fruit St
Boston MA 02114-2696

NIELSEN, Torsten O.
University of British Columbia
Anatomical Pathology JPN 1401
Vancouver Hospital
855 W 12th Ave
Vancouver BC V5Z 1M9

ODA, Yoshinao
Department of Anatomic Pathology
Graduate School of Medical Sciences
Kyushu University
3-1-1 Maidashi, Higashi-ku
Fukuoka 812-8582

ODASHIRO, Alexandre N.
Centre hospitalier de l'Université de Montréal
Pavillon F - 7e étage
1000 rue Saint-Denis
Montréal QC H2X 0C1

PARIDAENS, Dion
Rotterdam Eye Hospital and Erasmus MC
p/a Schiedamse Vest 180
3011 BH Rotterdam

PE'ER, Jacob
Hadassah Hebrew University Hospital
PO Box 12000
91120 Jerusalem

PEKMEZCI, Melike
University of California, San Francisco
505 Parnassus Ave, M551
San Francisco CA 94143

* Indicates disclosure of interests (see p. 519).

PERRY, Arie
University of California, San Francisco
505 Parnassus Ave, M551
San Francisco CA 94143-0102

PIŽEM, Jože
Faculty of Medicine, University of Ljubljana
Korytkova ulica 2
1000 Ljubljana

PROIA, Alan D.
Duke University Medical Center
DUMC 3712
Durham NC 27710

PUSPANATHAN, Pavitratha
International Agency for Research on Cancer
25 Av. Tony Garnier, CS 90627
69366 Lyon, CEDEX 07

RADVANYI, Francois
Institut Curie
26 Rue d'Ulm
75005 Paris

RAO, Narsing
USC Roski Eye Institute
1450 San Pablo St
Los Angeles CA 90033

RASMUSSEN, Peter Kristian
University of Copenhagen
Nordre Ringvej 57
2600 Glostrup

REIS-FILHO, Jorge Sergio
Memorial Sloan Kettering Cancer Center
1275 York Ave
New York NY 10065

REKHI, Bharat
Tata Memorial Centre, HBNI University
Dr Ernest Borges Rd, Parel
Mumbai, Maharashtra 400012

RIGHI, Alberto
IRCCS, Istituto Ortopedico Rizzoli
Via di Barbiano, 1/10
40136 Bologna BO

ROBERTS, Fiona
Queen Elizabeth University Hospital
Govan Rd
Glasgow G51 4TF

RODRIGUEZ, Fausto J.
David Geffen School of Medicine at UCLA
10833 Le Conte Ave, CHS 18-170B
Los Angeles CA 90095

RODRÍGUEZ-MARTÍNEZ, Héctor A.
Unidad de Investigación en Medicina Experimental
Dr. Balmis 148, Col. Doctores
06720 Mexico City

RODRÍGUEZ-REYES, Abelardo A.
Asociación para Evitar la Ceguera en México, IAP
Calle Vicente Garcia Torres 46
San Lucas, Coyoacán
04030 Mexico City

ROGOZHIN, Dmitrii V.
Russian Children's Clinical Hospital of Pirogov Russian National Research Medical University
Leninskiy Prospekt, 117
Moscow 119571

ROJANAPORN, Duangnate
Ramathibodi Hospital
270 Rama VI Rd
Bangkok 10400

ROOTMAN, Daniel B.
University of California, Los Angeles (UCLA)
300 Stein Plaza
Los Angeles CA 90095

ROUS, Brian
NHS England
Victoria House, Capital Park
Fulbourn, Cambridge CB21 5XA

RUSHING, Elisabeth J.
Medica Laboratories
Hottingerstrasse 9/11
8024 Zürich

SAGIV, Oded
Sheba Medical Center, Tel Aviv University
52621 Ramat Gan

SAGOO, Mandeep S.
UCL Institute of Ophthalmology / Moorfields Eye Hospital
162 City Rd
London EC1V 2PD

SALOMAO, Diva Regina
Mayo Clinic
200 1st St SW
Rochester MN 55905

SANGÜEZA, Omar P.
Wake Forest University School of Medicine
Medical Center Blvd
Winston-Salem NC 27157-1072

SANTAGATA, Sandro
Brigham and Women's Hospital
60 Fenwood Rd, Hale 8002P
Boston MA 02115

SAYED, Shahin
Aga Khan University
PO Box 30270
00100 Nairobi

SCOLYER, Richard A.
Royal Prince Alfred Hospital
Melanoma Institute Australia and University of Sydney
Missenden Rd, Camperdown
Sydney NSW 2050

SINARD, John
Yale Medical School
310 Cedar St
New Haven CT 06510

SINGH, Arun
Cleveland Clinic
9500 Euclid Ave
Cleveland OH 44195

SINGH, Rajendra
Summit Health
1225 McBridge Ave
Woodland Park NJ 07424

SMITH, Steven Christopher
VCU School of Medicine
1200 E Marshall St
Richmond VA 23298

SPECHT, Charles S.
Penn State Health
Milton S. Hershey Medical Center
500 University Dr, PO Box 850
Hershey PA 17033-0850

STAGNER, Anna M.
Massachusetts Eye and Ear
Harvard Medical School
Massachusetts General Hospital
248 Charles St, Room 328
Boston MA 02114

STEMMER-RACHAMIMOV, Anat Olga
Harvard Medical School
Massachusetts General Hospital
55 Fruit St
Boston MA 02114

STRIANESE, Diego
University of Naples Federico II
C.so Vittorio Emanuele, 167
80121 Naples NA

SUBRAMANIAN, Krishnakumar
Vision Research Foundation
No. 41 College Rd, Nungambakkam
Chennai 600006

* Indicates disclosure of interests (see p. 519).

SUURMEIJER, Albert J.H.
University Medical Center Groningen
Hanzeplein 1
9700 RB Groningen

TAN, Kong-Bing
Department of Pathology,
Yong Loo Lin School of Medicine,
National University of Singapore,
and National University Health System
5 Lower Kent Ridge Rd
Singapore 119074

TAN, Puay Hoon
Luma Medical Centre
Mount Elizabeth Medical Centre
3 Mount Elizabeth, #13-01
Singapore 228510

TANAS, Munir R.
University of Iowa
200 Hawkins Dr
Iowa City IA 52242

TETZLAFF, Michael
University of California, San Francisco
1701 Divisadero St, Suite 271
San Francisco CA 94115

THOMPSON, Lester D.R.
Head and Neck Pathology Consultations
22543 Ventura Blvd, Ste 22, PMB1034
Woodland Hills CA 91364

THWAY, Khin
Royal Marsden Hospital /
Institute of Cancer Research
203 Fulham Rd
London SW3 6JJ

TIHAN, Tarik
University of California, San Francisco
505 Parnassus Ave, Room M551
San Francisco CA 94143-0102

TORRELO, Antonio
Hospital Infantil Universitario Niño Jesús
Av. de Menéndez Pelayo, 65
28009 Madrid

VAN DOORN, Remco
Leiden University Medical Center
Albinusdreef 2
2300 RC Leiden

VAN GINDERDEUREN, Rita
University Hospitals Leuven
Herestraat 49
3000 Leuven

VAN HALTEREN, Astrid G.S.
Erasmus University Medical Center
Dr Molewaterplein 40
3015 GD Rotterdam

VEMUGANTI, Geeta K.
LV Prasad Eye Institute
Banjara Hills
Hyderabad, Telangana 500034

VERDIJK, Robert M.
Erasmus University Medical Center and
Leiden University Medical Center
PO Box 2040
3000 CA Rotterdam

VISHNEVSKIA DAI, Vicktoria
Goldschleger Eye Institute, Sheba Medical
Center, Tel Aviv University Faculty of Medicine
Derech Sheba 2
5265601 Ramut Gun

VON HOLSTEIN, Sarah Linea
Rigshospitalet
Copenhagen University Hospital
Blegdamsvej 9
2100 Copenhagen

WANG, Jian
Fudan University Shanghai Cancer Center
270 Dong An Rd
Shanghai 200032

WANG, Wei-Lien
University of Texas
MD Anderson Cancer Center
1515 Holcombe Blvd, Unit 085, Room
B3.4611
Houston TX 77030

WASHINGTON, Mary K.
Vanderbilt University Medical Center
C-3321 MCN
Nashville TN 37232

WATANABE, Reiko
St. Marianna University School of Medicine
2-16-1 Sugao, Miyamae-ku, Kawasaki
Kanagawa 216-8511

WEIS, Ezekiel
University of Alberta
1743 47 Ave SW
Calgary AB T2T 2S2

WENIG, Bruce M.
Moffitt Cancer Center
12902 Magnolia Dr
Tampa FL 33612

WHITE, Valerie A.
University of British Columbia
6200 University Blvd
Vancouver BC V6T 1Z4

WIJESINGHE, Harshima
International Agency for Research on Cancer
25 Av. Tony Garnier, CS 90627
69366 Lyon, CEDEX 07

WOLKOW, Natalie
Massachusetts Eye and Ear
Harvard Medical School
243 Charles St
Boston MA 02114

YAMAMOTO, Hidetaka
Okayama University
2-5-1 Shikata-cho, Kita-ku
Okayama 700-8558

YUN, Sook Jung
Chonnam National University School of
Medicine
160 Baekseo-ro, Dong-gu
Gwangju 61469

ZAMBRANO, Eduardo
University of Pittsburgh Medical Center
UPMC Children's Hospital of Pittsburgh
One Children's Hospital Dr
Pittsburgh PA 15224

ZEMBOWICZ, Artur
DermatopathologyConsultations.com
c/o Harvard Vanguard Medical Associates
152 2nd Ave
Needham Heights MA 02494

* Indicates disclosure of interests (see p. 519).

Declaration of interests

Dr Bastian reports holding US patent #20130102653.

Dr Beenakker reports that his unit at Leiden University benefits from non-monetary support from Philips Healthcare.

Dr Chan reports that her unit at Singapore National Eye Centre benefited from research funding from Menarini Biomarkers Singapore; and holding a patent on "Single cellular diagnosis of primary vitreoretinal lymphoma", licensed to Menarini Biomarkers Singapore Pte Ltd and Singapore Health Services Pte Ltd.

Dr Coupland reports having received personal consultancy fees, in her capacity as an advisor, from Immunocore.

Dr Demicco reports that her unit at the University of Toronto benefited from non-monetary support from Novartis.

Dr Dickson reports that his unit at Mount Sinai Hospital benefits from non-monetary support from Illumina.

Dr Honavar reports being the editor of the Indian Journal of Ophthalmology.

Dr Hyrcza reports that his unit at the University of Calgary benefits from research funding from Bayer Canada.

Dr Ng reports that his unit at the University of British Columbia benefited from non-monetary support from NanoString Technologies.

IARC/WHO Committee for the International Classification of Diseases for Oncology (ICD-O)

BRAY, Freddie
International Agency for Research on Cancer
25 Av. Tony Garnier, CS 90627
69366 Lyon, CEDEX 07

CREE, Ian A.
International Agency for Research on Cancer
25 Av. Tony Garnier, CS 90627
69366 Lyon, CEDEX 07

FERLAY, Jacques
International Agency for Research on Cancer
25 Av. Tony Garnier, CS 90627
69366 Lyon, CEDEX 07

GOLDMAN-LÉVY, Gabrielle
Hôpitaux Universitaires de Genève (HUG)
Rue Gabrielle-Perret-Gentil 4
1205 Geneva

JAKOB, Robert
Classifications and Terminologies
World Health Organization (WHO)
Av. Appia 20
1211 Geneva

KRPELANOVA, Eva
Classifications and Terminologies
World Health Organization (WHO)
Av. Appia 20
1211 Geneva

LOKUHETTY, Dilani
International Agency for Research on Cancer
25 Av. Tony Garnier, CS 90627
69366 Lyon, CEDEX 07

ROUS, Brian
NHS England
Victoria House, Capital Park
Fulbourn, Cambridge CB21 5XA

WATANABE, Reiko
St. Marianna University School of Medicine
2-16-1 Sugao, Miyamae-ku, Kawasaki
Kanagawa 216-8511

ZNAOR, Ariana
International Agency for Research on Cancer
25 Av. Tony Garnier, CS 90627
69366 Lyon, CEDEX 07

Sources

Note: For any figure, table, or box not listed below, the original source is this volume; the suggested source citation is

WHO Classification of Tumours Editorial Board. Eye and orbit tumours. Lyon (France): International Agency for Research on Cancer; 2025. (WHO classification of tumours series, 5th ed.; vol. 13). https://publications.iarc.who.int/660.

TNM staging tables

Brierley JD, Gospodarowicz MK, Wittekind C, editors. TNM classification of malignant tumours. 8th ed. Oxford (UK): Wiley Blackwell; 2017.

Figures

2.01	Auw-Haedrich C; and Eye Center Freiburg
2.02A,B	Mudhar HS
2.03	Auw-Haedrich C
2.04	Mudhar HS
2.05	Auw-Haedrich C
2.06	Mudhar HS; and Paul Johnston, Ophthalmology and Histopathology Departments, Royal Hallamshire Hospital, Sheffield
2.07A,B	Mudhar HS
2.08	Eberhart CG
2.09	Auw-Haedrich C
2.10	Auw-Haedrich C
2.11	Mudhar HS
2.12A	Herwig-Carl MC
2.12B	Mudhar HS
2.13A	Verdijk RM
2.13B	Mudhar HS
2.14	Mudhar HS
2.15A,C	Moulin A
2.15B	Mudhar HS
2.16A,B	Moulin A
2.17	Milman T
2.18A,B	Milman T
2.19	Eagle RC Jr
2.20	Auw-Haedrich C
2.21A,B	Auw-Haedrich C
2.22A,B	Milman T
2.23	Cummings TJ
2.24A,B	Cummings TJ
2.25	Cummings TJ
2.26	Hibba Quhill, Sheffield Ocular Oncology Service, Ophthalmology Department, Royal Hallamshire Hospital, Sheffield
2.27	Mudhar HS
2.28	Mudhar HS
2.29	Mudhar HS
2.30A–C	Ferreira TA
2.31	El-Naggar AK, Chan JKC, Grandis JR, Takata T, Slootweg PJ, editors. WHO classification of head and neck tumours. Lyon (France): International Agency for Research on Cancer; 2017. (WHO classification of tumours series, 4th ed.; vol. 9). https://publications.iarc.who.int/548; and Gichuhi S, Sagoo MS, Weiss HA, et alEpidemiology of ocular surface squamous neoplasia in Africa. Trop Med Int Health. 2013 Dec;18(12):1424–43. PMID:24237784. https //creativecommons.org/licenses/by/4.0/
2.32A–F	El-Naggar AK, Chan JKC, Grandis JR, Takata T, Slootweg PJ, editors. WHO classification of head and neck tumours. Lyon (France): International Agency for Research on Cancer; 2017. (WHO classification of tumours series, 4th ed.; vol. 9). https://publications.iarc.who.int/548.
2.33	Mudhar HS
2.34	Mudhar HS
2.35A–C	Milman T
2.36	Milman T
2.37A,B	Mudhar HS
2.38A,B	Mudhar HS
2.39A–C	Reprinted, with permission from Wolters Kluwer Health, Inc., from: Laird PW, Woodward MA, Williams JG, et al. Cystic benign melanosis of the conjunctiva. Cornea. 2012 Nov;31(11):1273–7. PMID:23044615.
2.40A,B	Eberhart CG
2.41A	Rodríguez-Reyes AA
2.41B,D	Zembowicz A
2.41C	Mudhar HS
2.42	Mudhar HS
2.43	Mudhar HS
2.44	Peter J
2.45A,B	Eberhart CG
2.46A,B	Chevez-Barrios P
2.47	Eagle RC Jr
2.48A,B	Milman T
2.49	Milman T
2.50	Pižem J
2.51A–D	Pižem J
2.52	Pižem J
2.53A–C	Pižem J
2.54A,B	Pižem J
2.55	Margo C
2.56A–C	Milman T
2.57	Coupland SE
2.58A,B	Moulin A
2.59A–C	Ferreira TA
2.60A–C	Moulin A
2.61A–C	Moulin A
3.01A,B	Debnam JM
3.02A–C	Debnam JM
3.03	Eberhart CG
3.04A	Wolkow N
3.04B,C	Stagner AM
3.05A,B	Adel Alsuhaibani, Department of Ophthalmology, College of Medicine, King Saud University, Riyadh
3.06A	Wolkow N
3.06B	Alkatan H
3.07	Eagle RC Jr
3.08A–D	Verdijk RM
3.09	Van Ginderdeuren R
3.10A,B	Verdijk RM
3.11	Van Ginderdeuren R
3.12A,B	Tan KB

3.13	Mihic-Probst D
3.14A,B	Mihic-Probst D
3.15A,B	Auw-Haedrich C; and Eye Center Freiburg
3.16	Mihic-Probst D
3.17A,B	Mihic-Probst D
3.18	Auw-Haedrich C
3.19A,B	Auw-Haedrich C; and Eye Center Freiburg
3.20	Kaliki S
3.21A,B	Debnam JM
3.22A,B	Mihic-Probst D
3.23A,B	Kaliki S
3.24	Mihic-Probst D
3.25	Mihic-Probst D
3.26	Verdijk RM
3.27A,B	Verdijk RM
3.28	Verdijk RM
3.29	Verdijk RM
3.30A,B	Debnam JM
3.31A–D	Salomao DR
3.32	Grossniklaus HE
3.33A,B	Milman T
3.34A	Eagle RC Jr
3.34B	Milman T
3.35A	Jennifer Tan, Ophthalmology Department, Royal Hallamshire Hospital, Sheffield
3.35B	Tetzlaff M
3.36A	Zanna Currie, Ophthalmology Department, Royal Hallamshire Hospital, Sheffield
3.36B,C	Mudhar HS
3.37A,B	Mudhar HS
3.38	Grossniklaus HE
3.39A	Sangüeza OP
3.39B,C	Mudhar HS
3.40	Zanna Currie, Ophthalmology Department, Royal Hallamshire Hospital, Sheffield
3.41A,B	Mudhar HS
3.42	Mudhar HS
3.43A,B	Mudhar HS
3.44A,B	Mudhar HS
3.45	Jennifer Tan, Ophthalmology Department, Royal Hallamshire Hospital Sheffield
3.46	Mudhar HS
3.47A,B	Mudhar HS
3.48A–C	Ferreira TA
3.49	Adel Alsuhaibani, Department of Ophthalmology, College of Medicine, King Saud University, Riyadh
3.50A	Mudhar HS
3.50B	Alkatan H
3.51	Zanna Currie, Ophthalmology Department, Royal Hallamshire Hospital, Sheffield
3.52	Mudhar HS
3.53A,B	Mudhar HS
3.54	Mudhar HS
3.55A,B	Esmaeli B
3.56A–C	Mudhar HS
3.57A,B	Mudhar HS
3.58	Esmaeli B
3.59A–C	Mudhar HS
3.59D	Zembowicz A
3.60	Eberhart CG
3.61	Ludovic Benichou, Service de chirurgie maxillo-faciale et stomatologie, Hôpital Paris Saint-Joseph, Paris; and Goldman-Lévy G
3.62A,B	Roberts F
3.62C	Mudhar HS
3.63A–C	Mudhar HS
3.64	Debnam JM
3.65	Esmaeli B
3.66A–D	Eberhart CG
3.67	Jennifer Tan, Ophthalmology Department, Royal Hallamshire Hospital, Sheffield
3.68A	Agni M
3.68B	Robert E. LeBlanc, Department of Pathology and Laboratory Medicine, Dartmouth Geisel School of Medicine, Hanover NH
3.69	Robert E. LeBlanc, Department of Pathology and Laboratory Medicine, Dartmouth Geisel School of Medicine, Hanover NH
3.70	Robert E. LeBlanc, Department of Pathology and Laboratory Medicine, Dartmouth Geisel School of Medicine, Hanover NH
3.71	Jennifer Tan, Ophthalmology Department, Royal Hallamshire Hospital, Sheffield
3.72A–C	Zembowicz A
3.73	Mudhar HS
3.74	Jennifer Tan, Ophthalmology Department, Royal Hallamshire Hospital, Sheffield
3.75A–E	Mudhar HS
3.76	Grossniklaus HE
3.77	Mihic-Probst D
3.78A,B	Mihic-Probst D
3.79	Mudhar HS
3.80	Mudhar HS
3.81A,B	Moulin A
3.82A,B	Moulin A
3.83	Mudhar HS
3.84	Barnhill RL; Cassoux N
3.85	Mudhar HS
3.86	Mihic-Probst D
3.87A–C	Mihic-Probst D
4.01	Grossniklaus HE
4.02A,B	Grossniklaus HE
4.03	Auw-Haedrich C and Eye Center Freiburg
4.04	Eagle RC Jr
4.05A,B	Mudhar HS
4.06	Sagoo MS
4.07A,B	Eagle RC Jr
4.08	Vishnevskia Dai V
4.09	Vishnevskia Dai V
4.10A,B	Mudhar HS
4.11A,B	Grossniklaus HE
4.12	Grossniklaus HE
4.13A,B	Grossniklaus HE
4.14	Verdijk RM
4.15	Verdijk RM
4.16A,B	Sachin M. Salvi, Ocular Oncology, Orbits and Oculoplastics, Sheffield Ocular Oncology Service, Royal Hallamshire Hospital, Sheffield
4.17A–C	Mudhar HS
4.18A,B	Mudhar HS
4.19A–D	Damato BE
4.20A–C	Beenakker JWM
4.21A,B	Damato BE
4.22A,B	Madigan MC
4.23	Alkatan H
4.24	Salomao DR
4.25A,B	Salomao DR
4.26	Mudhar HS
4.27	Laver NM
4.28	Kivelä T
4.29	Kivelä T
4.30A,B	Sachin M. Salvi, Ocular Oncology, Orbits and Oculoplastics, Sheffield Ocular Oncology Service, Royal Hallamshire Hospital, Sheffield
4.31A,B	Mudhar HS
4.32A–C	Mudhar HS
4.33	Grossniklaus HE
4.34A	Grossniklaus HE
4.34B–D	Eagle RC Jr
4.35A,B	Grossniklaus HE
4.36	Grossniklaus HE
4.37A	Cassoux N
4.37B	Grossniklaus HE
4.37C	Beenakker JWM
4.38A	White VA
4.38B–D	Eagle RC Jr
4.39A,B	Grossniklaus HE
4.39C	Salomao DR
4.40A,B	Grossniklaus HE
5.01	Grossniklaus HE
5.02	Grossniklaus HE
5.03A–D	Grossniklaus HE
5.04A,B	Grossniklaus HE, Eberhart CG, Kivelä TT, editors. WHO classification of tumours of the eye. Lyon (France): International Agency for Research on Cancer; 2018. (WHO classification of tumours series, 4th ed.; vol. 12). https://publications.iarc.who.int/561; and Reprinted, with permission, from: Hudson LE, Mendoza PR, Yan J, Grossniklaus HE. Reactive retinal astrocytic tumor (focal nodular gliosis): a case report. Ocul Oncol Pathol. 2017;3(1):1–7. PMID:28275595. Copyright © 2017 Karger Publishers, Basel (Switzerland).
5.05A,B	Eberhart CG
5.06A–C	Grossniklaus HE
5.07	Eagle RC Jr
5.08A,B	Eagle RC Jr
5.09	Eagle RC Jr
5.10A,B	Chevez-Barrios P
5.11A–E	Eagle RC Jr
5.12	Eagle RC Jr
5.13A–I	Eagle RC Jr
5.14A–D	Chevez-Barrios P
5.15A–C	Chevez-Barrios P
5.16A–C	Chevez-Barrios P
5.17A,B	Grossniklaus HE
5.18	Carol L. Shields, Ocular Oncology Service, Wills Eye

	Hospital, Philadelphia PA
5.19A,B	Carol L. Shields, Ocular Oncology Service, Wills Eye Hospital, Philadelphia PA
5.20A	Grossniklaus HE, Eberhart CG, Kivelä TT, editors. WHO classification of tumours of the eye. Lyon (France): International Agency for Research on Cancer; 2018. (WHO classification of tumours series, 4th ed.; vol. 12). https://publications.iarc.who.int/561.
5.20B	Eagle RC Jr
5.21A,B	Eagle RC Jr
5.22	Eagle RC Jr
5.23A	Kivelä T
5.23B,C	Eagle RC Jr
5.24A	Heinrich Heimann, NHS Liverpool Ocular Oncology Service, Royal Liverpool University Hospital, Liverpool
5.24B,C	Eagle RC Jr
5.25A–E	Eagle RC Jr
5.26	Roberts F
5.27A	Roberts F
5.27B	Kivelä T
5.28	Roberts F
5.29A,B	Roberts F
5.30	Grossniklaus HE, Eberhart CG, Kivelä TT, editors. WHO classification of tumours of the eye. Lyon (France): International Agency for Research on Cancer; 2018. (WHO classification of tumours series, 4th ed.; vol. 12). https://publications.iarc.who.int/561.
5.31A,B	Moulin A
5.32A–D	Mudhar HS
5.33A	Mudhar HS
5.33B	Rao N
5.34A–D	Mudhar HS
5.35A,B	Laver NM
5.36	Eagle RC Jr
5.37	Eagle RC Jr
5.38A,B	Rodríguez Reyes AA
5.39	Eagle RC Jr
5.40	Eagle RC Jr
5.41A,B	Eagle RC Jr
5.42A–C	Eagle RC Jr
6.01	Grossniklaus HE, Eberhart CG, Kivelä TT, editors. WHO classification of tumours of the eye. Lyon (France): International Agency for Research on Cancer; 2018. (WHO classification of tumours series, 4th ed.; vol. 12). https://publications.iarc.who.int/561.
6.02	Cummings TJ
6.03A–C	Cummings TJ
6.04A,C	Cummings TJ
6.04B,D	Rodriguez FJ
6.05A–C	Rodriguez FJ
6.06	Adapted, with permission from Elsevier, from: Corrêa ZM, Augsburger JJ, Spaulding AG. Medulloepithelioma of the optic disc. Hum Pathol. 2011;42(12):2047–51. PMID:21676432.
6.07	Eberhart CG
6.08	Eberhart CG
6.09	Pekmezci M
6.10A	Cummings TJ
6.10B	Verdijk RM
6.10C	Rodriguez FJ
6.11A,B	Cummings TJ
7.01	Debnam JM
7.02A,B	Debnam JM
7.03	Mittal R
7.04	Mittal R
7.05	Salomao DR
7.06A–C	Esmaeli B
7.07A–D	Salomao DR
7.08A–D	Salomao DR
7.09	Iacob CE
7.10A–C	Iacob CE
7.11A,C	Grossniklaus HE
7.11B	Iacob CE
7.12A,B	Bret Wehrli, Schulich School of Medicine and Dentistry, Western University, London ON
7.13A,B	Bret Wehrli, Schulich School of Medicine and Dentistry, Western University, London ON
7.14A–C	Debnam JM
7.15A–C	Salomao DR
7.16A,B	Esmaeli B
7.17A–C	Chan ASY
7.18A,B	Chan ASY
7.19	Chan ASY
7.20A–C	Pekmezci M
7.21A,B	Pekmezci M
7.22A,B	White VA
7.23	Mudhar HS
7.24A	White VA
7.24B	Mudhar HS
7.25A–D	Milman T
7.26	Milman T
7.27	Adapted, with permission from Elsevier, from: Alkatan HM, Al-Harkan DH, Al-Mutlaq M, et al. Epithelial lacrimal gland tumors: a comprehensive clinicopathologic review of 26 lesions with radiologic correlation. Saudi J Ophthalmol. 2014 Jan;28(1):49–57. PMID:24526859.
7.28A,B	Debnam JM
7.28C	Alkatan H
7.29A,B	Mudhar HS
7.29C	Alkatan H
7.30A,B	White VA
7.30C	Reprinted, with permission, from: Wiwatwongwana D, Berean KW, Dolman PJ, et al. Unusual carcinomas of the lacrimal gland: epithelial-myoepithelial carcinoma and myoepithelial carcinoma. Arch Ophthalmol. 2009 Aug;127(8):1054–6. PMID:19667347.
7.31A,B	Reprinted, with permission, from: Wiwatwongwana D, Berean KW, Dolman PJ, et al. Unusual carcinomas of the lacrimal gland: epithelial-myoepithelial carcinoma and myoepithelial carcinoma. Arch Ophthalmol. 2009 Aug;127(8):1054–6. PMID:19667347.
7.32A,B	Reprinted, with permission, from: Rosenbaum PS, Mahadevia PS, Goodman LA, et al. Acinic cell carcinoma of the lacrimal gland. Arch Ophthalmol. 1995 Jun;113(6):781–5. PMID:7540387.
7.33	Reprinted, with permission, from: Rosenbaum PS, Mahadevia PS, Goodman LA, et al. Acinic cell carcinoma of the lacrimal gland. Arch Ophthalmol. 1995 Jun;113(6):781–5. PMID:7540387.
7.34A,B	Debnam JM
7.35A–C	Milman T
8.01	International Agency for Research on Cancer (IARC)
8.02	Grossniklaus HE, Eberhart CG, Kivelä TT, editors. WHO classification of tumours of the eye. Lyon (France): International Agency for Research on Cancer; 2018. (WHO classification of tumours series, 4th ed.; vol. 12). https://publications.iarc.who.int/561.
8.03A–C	Grossniklaus HE, Eberhart CG, Kivelä TT, editors. WHO classification of tumours of the eye. Lyon (France): International Agency for Research on Cancer; 2018. (WHO classification of tumours series, 4th ed.; vol. 12). https://publications.iarc.who.int/561.
8.04A,B	Mittal R
8.05	Heegaard S
8.06	Heegaard S
8.07A,B	Heegaard S
8.08A,B	Mudhar HS
8.09A,B	Mudhar HS
8.10A	Stagner AM
8.10B,C	Heegaard S
8.11	Heegaard S
8.12	Heegaard S
8.13	Heegaard S
8.14A–C	Farmer J
8.15A,B	Debnam JM
8.16	Heegaard S
8.17	Heegaard S
8.18A–C	Heegaard S
8.19A–C	Eberhart CG
9.01A–C	Debnam JM
9.02A,B	Adel Alsuhaibani, Department of Ophthalmology, College of Medicine, King Saud University, Riyadh
9.03	Alkatan H

9.04A–C	Alkatan H
9.05A	Alkatan H
9.05B	Maktabi A
9.06	Alkatan H
9.07A,B	Kaliki S
9.08	Kaliki S
9.09	Kaliki S
9.10A–C	Flucke U
9.11A,B	Kaliki S
9.11C	Colmenero I
9.12A–C	Colmenero I
9.12D	Mudhar HS
9.13A,B	Adapted, with permission, from: Nassiri N, Rootman J, Rootman DB, et al. Orbital lymphaticovenous malformations: current and future treatments. Surv Ophthalmol. 2015 Sep-Oct;60(5):383–405. PMID:26077629.
9.14	Kaliki S
9.15A–C	Debnam JM
9.16	Kaliki S
9.17A,B	Flucke U
9.18	Rootman DB
9.19A–C	Rootman DB
9.20	Flucke U
9.21	Debnam JM
9.22A,B	Cummings TJ
9.23A,B	Proia AD
9.24A,B	Proia AD
9.25A,B	Proia AD
9.26A–C	Mishra DK
9.27A,B	Mishra DK
9.28A,B	Mishra DK
9.29A,B	Proia AD
9.29C	Mishra DK
9.30A,B	Sachin M. Salvi, Ocular Oncology, Orbits and Oculoplastics, Sheffield Ocular Oncology Service, Royal Hallamshire Hospital, Sheffield
9.31	Mudhar HS
9.32A–D	Mudhar HS
9.33A,B	Mudhar HS
10.01	WHO Classification of Tumours Editorial Board. Haematolymphoid tumours. Lyon (France): International Agency for Research on Cancer; 2024. (WHO classification of tumours series, 5th ed.; vol. 11). https://publications.iarc.who.int/637; and Adapted, with permission, from: Vegh P, Fletcher J, Dixon D, et al. Mononuclear phagocyte system; first published: 2017 May 15. In: Encyclopedia of Life Sciences (eLS) [Internet]. Chichester (UK): John Wiley & Sons, Ltd. Available from: https://onlinelibrary.wiley.com/doi/10.1002/9780470015902.a0001217.pub2
10.02	Debnam JM
10.03	Salomao DR
10.04A–D	Salomao DR
10.05A,B	Debnam JM
10.06A,D	Salomao DR
10.06B,C	Verdijk RM
10.07	Salomao DR
10.08A,B	Reprinted, with permission from Springer, from: Damato BE. Extraocular lesions. In: Clinical atlas of ocular oncology. Cham (Switzerland): Springer; 2022. doi:10.1007/978-3-030-90127-1_1.
10.09A,B	Coupland SE
10.10A,B	Coupland SE
10.11	Chan ASY
10.12	Chan ASY
10.13A–C	Coupland SE
10.14	Ferry JA
10.15A,B	Debnam JM
10.16A–E	Ferry JA
10.17	Mulay K
10.18A,B	Debnam JM
10.19A–C	Ferry JA
10.20A–C	Ferry JA
10.21A–D	Debnam JM
10.22A,B	Coupland SE
10.23A,B	Coupland SE
10.24	Verdijk RM
10.25A	Chevez-Barrios P
10.25B	Verdijk RM
10.26A–C	Verdijk RM
10.27	Verdijk RM
10.28	Verdijk RM
10.29A–D	Verdijk RM
10.30A,B	Mudhar HS
10.31A–C	Mudhar HS
10.32	Milman T
10.33	Kempf W
10.34A–C	Milman T
10.35A–C	Milman T
10.36	Christian van Oterendorp, University Eye Hospital Göttingen, Göttingen
10.37	Christian van Oterendorp, University Eye Hospital Göttingen, Göttingen
10.38	Verdijk RM
10.39A–D	Verdijk RM
10.40A,B	Mittal R
10.41	Alkatan H
10.42A	Alkatan H
10.42B	Grossniklaus HE
10.43	Maktabi A
10.44A,B	Alkatan H
10.45A	Alkatan H
10.45B	Maktabi A
10.46A,B	Grossniklaus HE
10.47A,B	Antonio Augusto Cruz, Department of Ophthalmology, Ribeirão Preto Medical School, University of São Paulo, São Paulo
10.48A,B	Debnam JM
10.49	Alkatan H
10.50A	Fernando Chahud, Department of Pathology, Ribeirão Preto Medical School, University of São Paulo, São Paulo
10.50B	Maktabi A
10.50C	Alkatan H
10.51A	With permission from the Mayo Foundation for Medical Education and Research. All rights reserved.
10.51B	Dion Paridaens, Rotterdam Eye Hospital, Erasmus University Medical Center, Rotterdam
10.52A	With permission from the Mayo Foundation for Medical Education and Research. All rights reserved.
10.52B	Salomao DR
10.53	Salomao DR
10.54A–C	Salomao DR
10.55A,B	Cor van den Bos, Department of Hemato-oncology, Princess Máxima Center for Pediatric Oncology, Utrecht
10.55C,D	Debnam JM
10.56	McKelvie PA
10.57A–C	McKelvie PA
10.58	Salomao DR
10.59A,B	Mudhar HS
10.60A	Laver NM
10.60B,C	Debnam JM
10.61A,B	Mudhar HS
10.62A,B	Mudhar HS
10.63	Mudhar HS
11.01	Milman T
11.02	Sachin M. Salvi, Ocular Oncology, Orbits and Oculoplastics, Sheffield Ocular Oncology Service, Royal Hallamshire Hospital, Sheffield
11.03A,B	Mudhar HS
11.04A	Sachin M. Salvi, Ocular Oncology, Orbits and Oculoplastics, Sheffield Ocular Oncology Service, Royal Hallamshire Hospital, Sheffield
11.04B,C	Mudhar HS
11.05	Mudhar HS
11.06A,B	Mudhar HS
11.07A–C	Mudhar HS
11.08	Milman T
11.09A,B	Milman T
11.10A,B	Stagner AM
11.11	Yasser H. Al-Faky, Department of Ophthalmology, College of Medicine, King Saud University, Riyadh
11.12A,B	Debnam JM
11.13A,B	Alkatan H
11.14	Alkatan H
11.15	Yamamoto H
11.16A,B	Yamamoto H
11.17	Yamamoto H
11.18	Kashyap S
11.19	Kashyap S
11.20	Kashyap S
11.21	Kashyap S
11.22A,B	Grossniklaus HE
11.23	Grossniklaus HE
11.24A,B	Grossniklaus HE
11.25	Adapted, with permission from Wolters Kluwer Health, from: Kang JY, Kim HJ, Wojno TH, et al. Atypical lipomatous tumor/well-differentiated liposarcoma of the orbit: three cases and review of the literature. Ophthalmic Plast Reconstr Surg. 2021;37(3S):S134–S140. PMID:32991496.

11.26A	Adapted, with permission from Wolters Kluwer Health, from: Kang JY, Kim HJ, Wojno TH, et al. Atypical lipomatous tumor/well-differentiated liposarcoma of the orbit: three cases and review of the literature. Ophthalmic Plast Reconstr Surg. 2021;37(3S):S134–S140. PMID:32991496.
11.26B	Grossniklaus HE
11.27A,B	Milman T
11.28A,B	Roberts F
11.29	Roberts F
11.30	Grossniklaus HE
11.31	Roberts F
11.32	Debnam JM
11.33	Milman T
11.34	Bahrami A
11.35	Bahrami A
11.36A	Bahrami A
11.36B	Milman T
11.37	Milman T
11.38A,B	Subramanian K
11.39A,B	Subramanian K
11.40	Paul Rundle, Sheffield Ocular Oncology Service, Royal Hallamshire Hospital, Sheffield
11.41A,B	Mudhar HS
11.42A–C	Mudhar HS
11.43	Mishra DK
11.44A–C	Mishra DK
11.45	Rodriguez FJ
11.46	Mudhar HS
11.47A–D	Rodriguez FJ
11.48A,B	Eagle RC Jr
11.49	Rodriguez FJ
11.50	Stemmer-Rachamimov AO
11.51	Cummings TJ
11.52A,B	Verdijk RM
11.53	Verdijk RM
11.54A	Eagle RC Jr
11.54B,C	Stemmer-Rachamimov AO
11.55	Verdijk RM
11.56A–D	Verdijk RM
11.57	Verdijk RM
11.58	Grossniklaus HE
11.59	Verdijk RM
11.60	Verdijk RM
11.61A,B	Verdijk RM
11.62A,B,D	Perry A
11.62C	Nielsen GP
11.63	Nielsen GP
11.64	Milman T
11.65A–C	Milman T
11.66A,B	Milman T
11.67	Milman T
11.68	Milman T
11.69	Mudhar HS
11.70A,B	Mudhar HS
11.71	Mudhar HS
11.72A,B	Mudhar HS
11.73	Proia AD
11.74A–C	Proia AD
11.75	El-Naggar AK, Chan JKC, Grandis JR, Takata T, Slootweg PJ, editors. WHO classification of head and neck tumours. Lyon (France): International Agency for Research on Cancer; 2017. (WHO classification of tumours series, 4th ed.; vol. 9). https://publications.iarc.who.int/548.
11.76A,B	Grossniklaus HE
11.77A–C	Flucke U
11.78	Dickson BC
11.79	Dickson BC
11.80	Dickson BC
11.81	Dickson BC
11.82A,B	Ng T
11.83A,B	Subramanian K
11.84	Sandhya Sundaram, Department of Pathology, Sri Ramachandra Medical College, Sri Ramachandra Institute of Higher Education and Research, Chennai, Tamil Nadu
11.85A,B	Subramanian K
11.86	Oca Y
11.87A,B	Oca Y
11.88	Milman T
11.89A,C	Suurmeijer AJH
11.89B	Milman T
11.90	Suurmeijer AJH
11.91	Suurmeijer AJH
11.92	Milman T
11.93	Adapted, with permission, from: Mulay K, Chougule SS, Honavar SG. Orbital alveolar soft part sarcoma. Ophthalmology. 2016 Jul;123(7):1420. PMID:27342327
11.94A	Adapted, with permission, from Mulay K, Chougule SS, Honavar SG. Orbital alveolar soft part sarcoma. Ophthalmology. 2016 Jul;123(7):1420. PMID:27342327
11.94B	Mulay K
11.95A,B	Mulay K
11.95C	Jambhekar NA
11.96	Rogozhin DV
11.97	Mudhar HS
11.98	Paul O'Donnell, Royal National Orthopaedic Hospital, Brockley Hill, Stanmore, Middlesex
11.99A,B	Amary F
11.100	Rodríguez-Reyes AA
11.101	Fanburg-Smith JC
11.102A–C	Saumya Jakati, Ophthalmic Pathology Laboratory and Prof Brien Holden Eye Research Centre, LV Prasad Eye Institute (LVPEI), Kallam Anji Reddy Campus, Hyderabad
11.103	Fanburg-Smith JC
11.104A–D	Fanburg-Smith JC
11.105A,B	Bertin F
11.106	Mudhar HS
11.107	Righi A
11.108	Righi A
11.109	Flucke U
11.100A,B	Flucke U
11.111	Righi A
11.112A,B	Agaram NP
11.113	Agaram NP
11.114A,B	Agaram NP
11.115A,B	Proia AD
11.116A–C	Proia AD
11.117A,B	Debnam JM
11.118	de Álava E
12.01	Esmaeli B
12.02	Esmaeli B
12.03	Debnam JM
12.04A–C	Verdijk RM
12.05A–C	Verdijk RM
12.06	Sachin M Salvi, Ocular Oncology, Orbits and Oculoplastics, Sheffield Ocular Oncology Service, Royal Hallamshire Hospital, Sheffield
12.07A–C	Mudhar HS
12.08	Mudhar HS
12.09A,B	Mudhar HS
12.10A–C	Mudhar HS
13.01A–C	Cassoux N
13.02A,B	Abdel-Rahman MH
13.03A–C	de la Fouchardière A
13.04A,B	Milman T
13.05A,B	Mudhar HS
13.06A,B	Alkatan H
13.07	Rodriguez FJ
13.08A	Strianese D; and WHO Classification of Tumours Editorial Board. Head and neck tumours. Lyon (France): International Agency for Research on Cancer; 2024. (WHO classification of tumours series, 5th ed.; vol. 9). https://publications.iarc.who.int/629.
13.08B,C	Rodriguez FJ
13.09A,B	Midena E
13.10	Midena E
13.11	Stagner AM
13.12	Stagner AM
13.13A,B	Milman T
13.14A,B	Milman T
13.15A–C	Milman T

Tables

2.01	Mudhar HS
2.02	Mudhar HS
2.03	Eberhart CG; Folberg R; Milman T; Zembowicz A
3.01	WHO Classification of Tumours Editorial Board. Skin tumours. Lyon (France): International Agency for Research on Cancer; 2025. (WHO classification of tumours series, 5th ed.; vol. 12). https://publications.iarc.who.int/650.
3.02	de la Fouchardière A; Gerami P
4.01	Mudhar HS
5.01	Chevez-Barrios P
6.01	Louis DN, Ohgaki H, Wiestler OD, et al., editors. WHO classification of tumours of the central nervous system. Lyon (France): International Agency for Research on Cancer; 2016. (WHO classification of tumours series, 4th rev. ed.; vol. 1). https://publications.iarc.who.int/543;

	and Adapted from: Collins VP, Jones DT, Giannini C. Pilocytic astrocytoma: pathology, molecular mechanisms and markers. Acta Neuropathol. 2015 Jun;129(6):775–88. PMID:25792358
9.01	Milman T
9.02	Alkatan H
10.01	Coupland SE
10.02	WHO Classification of Tumours Editorial Board. Head and neck tumours. Lyon (France): International Agency for Research on Cancer; 2024. (WHO classification of tumours series, 5th ed.; vol. 9). https://publications.iarc.who.int/629.
10.03	WHO Classification of Tumours Editorial Board. Haematolymphoid tumours. Lyon (France): International Agency for Research on Cancer; 2024. (WHO classification of tumours series, 5th ed.; vol. 11). https://publications.iarc.who.int/637.
10.04	WHO Classification of Tumours Editorial Board. Haematolymphoid tumours. Lyon (France): International Agency for Research on Cancer; 2024. (WHO classification of tumours series, 5th ed.; vol. 11). https://publications.iarc.who.int/637.
10.05	Coupland SE
11.01	Milman T
11.02	Milman T
11.03	Milman T
11.04	Milman T
11.05	Milman T
11.06	Mudhar HS
11.07	Demicco EG
12.01	Verdijk RM
12.02	Mudhar HS
13.01	Hodge JC
13.02	Santagata S; Abdel-Rahman MH
13.03	Reprinted from: Louis DN, Ohgaki H, Wiestler OD, et al., editors. WHO classification of tumours of the central nervous system. Lyon (France): International Agency for Research on Cancer; 2016. (WHO classification of tumours series, 4th rev. ed.; vol. 1). https://publications.iarc.who.int/543.
13.04	Francis JH

Boxes

3.01	Messina JL
11.01	WHO Classification of Tumours Editorial Board. Central nervous system tumours. Lyon (France): International Agency for Research on Cancer; 2022. (WHO classification of tumours series, 5th ed.; vol. 6). https://publications.iarc.who.int/601.
13.01	WHO Classification of Tumours Editorial Board. Central nervous system tumours. Lyon (France): International Agency for Research on Cancer; 2022. (WHO classification of tumours series, 5th ed.; vol. 6). https://publications.iarc.who.int/601.

Images on the cover

Top left	Fig. 3.29: Verdijk RM
Middle left	Fig. 3.31A: Salomao DR
Bottom left	Fig. 3.31B: Salomao DR
Top centre	Fig. 7.16A: Esmaeli B
Middle centre	Fig. 3.59D: Zembowicz A
Bottom centre	Fig. 3.60: Eberhart CG
Top right	Fig. 11.02: Sachin M. Salvi, Ocular Oncology, Orbits and Oculoplastics, Sheffield Ocular Oncology Service, Royal Hallamshire Hospital, Sheffield
Middle right	Fig. 11.66A: Milman T
Bottom right	Fig. 11.66B: Milman T

Images on the chapter title pages

Chapter 1	Fig. 3.46: Mudhar HS
Chapter 2	Fig. 2.41D: Zembowicz A
Chapter 3	Fig. 3.10B: Verdijk RM
Chapter 4	Fig. 4.17B: Mudhar HS
Chapter 5	Fig. 5.06C: Grossniklaus HE
Chapter 6	Fig. 6.04B: Rodriguez FJ
Chapter 7	Fig. 7.17A: Chan ASY
Chapter 8	Fig. 8.10A: Stagner AM
Chapter 9	Fig. 9.24A: Proia AD
Chapter 10	Fig. 10.03: Salomao DR
Chapter 11	Fig. 11.47D: Rodriguez FJ
Chapter 12	Fig. 12.05A: Verdijk RM
Chapter 13	Fig. 13.03A: de la Fouchardière A

References

1. Ababtain RM, Alsharif HM, Alkatan HM, et al. Primary Mucinous Adenocarcinoma of the Eyelid: A Case with Initial Clinical Misdiagnosis Requiring Surgical Re-Excision of the Tumor. Int J Surg Case Rep. 2021 Aug;85:106185. PMID:34252644

2. Abbas HA, Reville PK, Geppner A, et al. Clinical and Molecular Characterization of Myeloid Sarcoma Without Medullary Leukemia. Leuk Lymphoma. 2021 Dec;62(14):3402–10. PMID:34380367

3. Abbas O, Mahalingam M. Cutaneous Sebaceous Neoplasms as Markers of Muir-Torre Syndrome: A Diagnostic Algorithm. J Cutan Pathol. 2009 Jun;36(6):613–9. PMID:19515040

4. Abbott DW, Simons K, Giorgadze T. Choroidal Melanoma Diagnosed by Aspiration Cytology: A Case Report with Cyto-Histologic Correlation and Review of the Literature. Ann Diagn Pathol. 2019 Oct;42:39–41. PMID:31306857

5. Abbott JJ, Oliveira AM, Nascimento AG. The Prognostic Significance of Fibrosarcomatous Transformation in Dermatofibrosarcoma Protuberans. Am J Surg Pathol. 2006 Apr;30(4):436–43. PMID:16625088

6. Abdalla MI, Hosni F. Osteoclastoma of the Orbit. Case Report. Br J Ophthalmol. 1966 Feb;50(2):95–8. PMID:4952464

7. Abdelbaki MS, Abu-Arja MH, Davidson TB, et al. Pineoblastoma in Children Less Than Six Years of Age: The Head Start I, II, and III Experience. Pediatr Blood Cancer. 2020 Jun;67(6):e28252. PMID:32187454

8. Abdelhakim AH, Dunbar KE, Godfrey KJ, et al. Unique Histopathologic Features of the Eyelid Dermatofibroma. Orbit. 2019 Aug;38(4):274–8. PMID:30183445

9. Abdellatief A, Mason CM, Ytterberg SR, et al. Choroidal Involvement in Erdheim-Chester Disease. Ophthalmic Surg Lasers Imaging Retina. 2015 Jun;46(6):674–6. PMID:26114850

10. Abdel-Rahman MH, Pilarski R, Cebulla CM, et al. Germline BAP1 Mutation Predisposes to Uveal Melanoma, Lung Adenocarcinoma, Meningioma, and Other Cancers. J Med Genet. 2011 Dec;48(12):856–9. PMID:21941004

11. AbdelRazek M, Stone JH. Neurologic Features of Immunoglobulin G4-Related Disease. Rheum Dis Clin North Am. 2017 Nov;43(4):621–31. PMID:29061247

12. Abdolrahimzadeh S, Plateroti AM, Recupero SM, et al. An Update on the Ophthalmologic Features in the Phakomatoses. J Ophthalmol. 2016;2016:3043026. PMID:27493794

13. Abdolrahimzadeh S, Pugi DM, de Paula A, et al. Ocular Manifestations in Phakomatosis Pigmentovascularis: Current Concepts on Pathogenesis, Diagnosis, and Management. Surv Ophthalmol. 2021 May-Jun;66(3):482–92. PMID:33058925

14. Abdulkader M, Kuhar M, Hattab E, et al. GATA3 Positivity in Endocrine Mucin-Producing Sweat Gland Carcinoma and Invasive Mucinous Carcinoma of the Eyelid: Report of 2 Cases. Am J Dermatopathol. 2016 Oct;38(10):789–91. PMID:27533071

15. Abeck D, Tetsch L, Lüftl M, et al. Extragenital Cutaneous Warts - Clinical Presentation, Diagnosis and Treatment. J Dtsch Dermatol Ges. 2019 Jun;17(6):613–34. PMID:31241843

16. Abesamis-Cubillan E, El-Shabrawi-Caelen L, LeBoit PE. Merkel Cells and Sclerosing Epithelial Neoplasms. Am J Dermatopathol. 2000 Aug;22(4):311–5. PMID:10949455

17. Abla O, Jacobsen E, Picarsic J, et al. Consensus Recommendations for the Diagnosis and Clinical Management of Rosai-Dorfman-Destombes Disease. Blood. 2018 Jun 28;131(26):2877–90. PMID:29720485

18. Abouzeid H, Balmer A, Moulin AP, et al. Phenotypic Variability of Retinocytomas: Preregression and Postregression Growth Patterns. Br J Ophthalmol. 2012 Jun;96(6):884–9. PMID:22328814

19. Abouzeid H, Schorderet DF, Balmer A, et al. Germline Mutations in Retinoma Patients: Relevance to Low-Penetrance and Low-Expressivity Molecular Basis. Mol Vis. 2009;15:771–7. PMID:19390654

20. Abramson DH. Cell Free DNA (CfDNA) in the Blood of Retinoblastoma Patients The Robert M. Ellsworth Lecture. Ophthalmic Genet. 2022 Dec;43(6):731–5. PMID:35382685

21. Abramson DH, Dunkel IJ, Brodie SE, et al. A Phase I/II Study of Direct Intraarterial (Ophthalmic Artery) Chemotherapy with Melphalan for Intraocular Retinoblastoma Initial Results. Ophthalmology. 2008 Aug;115(8):1398–404, 1404.E1. PMID:18342944

22. Abramson DH, Fallon J, Biran N, et al. Lacrimal Sac Adenocarcinoma Managed with Androgen Deprivation. Am J Ophthalmol Case Rep. 2020 Jul 24;19:100607. PMID:32760849

23. Abramson DH, Frank CM, Susman M, et al. Presenting Signs of Retinoblastoma. J Pediatr. 1998 Mar;132(3 Pt 1):505–8. PMID:9544909

24. AbuHilal M, Walsh S, Shear N. Associated Hematolymphoid Malignancies in Patients With Lymphomatoid Papulosis: A Canadian Retrospective Study. J Cutan Med Surg. 2017 Nov/Dec;21(6):507–12. PMID:28614957

25. Adam P, Baumann R, Schmidt J, et al. The BCL2 E17 and SP66 Antibodies Discriminate 2 Immunophenotypically and Genetically Distinct Subgroups of Conventionally BCL2-"Negative" Grade 1/2 Follicular Lymphomas. Hum Pathol. 2013 Sep;44(9):1817–26. PMID:23642737

26. Adamski WZ, Maciejewski J, Adamska K, et al. The Prevalence of Various Eyelid Skin Lesions in a Single-Centre Observation Study. Postepy Dermatol Alergol. 2021 Oct;38(5):804–7. PMID:34849127

27. Addison DJ, Font RL. Glioneuroma of Iris and Ciliary Body. Arch Ophthalmol. 1984 Mar;102(3):419–21. PMID:6703991

28. Adefusika JA, Pimentel JD, Chavan RN, et al. Primary Mucinous Carcinoma of the Skin: The Mayo Clinic Experience Over the Past 2 Decades. Dermatol Surg. 2015 Feb;41(2):201–8. PMID:25627628

29. Adekunle AN, Mendoza PR, Wojno TH, et al. Pleomorphic Adenoma With Prominent Clear Cell Myoepithelioma Component of the Lacrimal Gland. Ophthalmic Plast Reconstr Surg. 2016 Jan-Feb;32(1):e18–21. PMID:25603534

30. Adetunji MO, McGeehan B, Lee V, et al. Primary Orbital Melanoma: A Report of a Case and Comprehensive Review of the Literature. Orbit. 2021 Dec;40(6):461–9. PMID:32900269

31. Adler BL, Krausz AE, Minuti A, et al. Epidemiology and Treatment of Angiolymphoid Hyperplasia with Eosinophilia (ALHE): A Systematic Review. J Am Acad Dermatol. 2016 Mar;74(3):506–12.E11. PMID:26685720

32. Afghani T, Khan FA, Mansoor H. Conjunctival Leiomyoma; a Rare Tumor of the Ocular Surface. J Ophthalmic Vis Res. 2016 Oct-Dec;11(4):433–5. PMID:27994813

33. Afrogheh AH, Jakobiec FA, Hammon R, et al. Evaluation for High-Risk HPV in Squamous Cell Carcinomas and Precursor Lesions Arising in the Conjunctiva and Lacrimal Sac. Am J Surg Pathol. 2016 Apr;40(4):519–28. PMID:26735858

34. Agaimy A, Bieg M, Michal M, et al. Recurrent Somatic PDGFRB Mutations in Sporadic Infantile/Solitary Adult Myofibromas But Not in Angioleiomyomas and Myopericytomas. Am J Surg Pathol. 2017 Feb;41(2):195–203. PMID:27776010

35. Agaimy A, Bishop JA. SWI/SNF-Deficient Head and Neck Neoplasms: An Overview. Semin Diagn Pathol. 2021 May;38(3):175–82. PMID:33663878

36. Agaimy A, Michal M, Stoehr R, et al. Recurrent Novel HMGA2-NCOR2 Fusions Characterize a Subset of Keratin-Positive Giant Cell-Rich Soft Tissue Tumors. Mod Pathol. 2021 Aug;34(8):1507–20. PMID:33742141

37. Agaram NP, Huang SC, Tap WD, et al. Clinicopathologic and Survival Correlates of Embryonal Rhabdomyosarcoma Driven by RAS/RAF Mutations. Genes Chromosomes Cancer. 2022 Mar;61(3):131–7. PMID:34755412

38. Agaram NP, Prakash S, Antonescu CR. Deep-Seated Plexiform Schwannoma: A Pathologic Study of 16 Cases and Comparative Analysis with the Superficial Variety. Am J Surg Pathol. 2005 Aug;29(8):1042–8. PMID:16006798

39. Agaram NP, Sung YS, Zhang L, et al. Dichotomy of Genetic Abnormalities in PEComas With Therapeutic Implications. Am J Surg Pathol. 2015 Jun;39(6):813–25. PMID:25651471

40. Agaram NP, Zhang L, Jungbluth AA, et al. A Molecular Reappraisal of Glomus Tumors and Related Pericytic Neoplasms With Emphasis on NOTCH-Gene Fusions. Am J Surg Pathol. 2020 Nov;44(11):1556–62. PMID:32604167

40A. Agelli M, Clegg LX. Epidemiology of Primary Merkel Cell Carcinoma in the United States. J Am Acad Dermatol. 2003 Nov;49(5):832–41. Erratum in: J Am Acad Dermatol. 2004 May;50(5):733. PMID:14576661.

41. Aggarwal E, Mulay K, Honavar SG. Orbital Extra-Medullary Granulocytic Sarcoma: Clinicopathologic Correlation with Immunohistochemical Features. Surv Ophthalmol. 2014 Mar-Apr;59(2):232–5. PMID:24556444

42. Agiannidis C, Pana ZD, Molyva D, et al. Metachronous Occurrence of Colorectal Cancer in a Muir-Torre Syndrome Patient Presenting with Recurrent Sebaceous Adenoma of the Eyelid: Case Report and Updated Review of the Literature. J Cutan Med Surg. 2012 Nov-Dec;16(6):394–9. PMID:23149194

43. Agni M, Raven ML, Bowen RC, et al. An Update on Endocrine Mucin-Producing Sweat Gland Carcinoma: Clinicopathologic Study of 63 Cases and Comparative Analysis. Am J Surg Pathol. 2020 Aug;44(8):1005–16. PMID:32452870

44. Agnihotri S, Jalali S, Wilson MR, et al. The Genomic Landscape of Schwannoma. Nat Genet. 2016 Nov;48(11):1339–48. PMID:27723760

45. Agrawal R, Dey P, Lal A. Fine-Needle Aspiration Cytology of Orbital and Eyelid Lesions. Diagn Cytopathol. 2013 Nov;41(11):1000–11. PMID:23457033

46. Aguilera NS, Kapadia SB, Nalesnik MA, et al. Extramedullary Plasmacytoma of the Head and Neck: Use of Paraffin Sections to Assess Clonality with In Situ Hybridization, Growth Fraction, and the Presence of Epstein-Barr Virus. Mod Pathol. 1995 Jun;8(5):503–8. PMID:7675768

47. Ahmad M, Chen HC, Chang JR, et al. Tarsal Epithelial Cysts: Prevalence, Case Series, and Synthesis of Existing Literature. Ophthalmic Plast Reconstr Surg. 2021 May-Jun 01;37(3):255–61. PMID:32826823

48. Ahmad SM, Esmaeli B. Metastatic Tumors of the Orbit and Ocular Adnexa. Curr Opin Ophthalmol. 2007 Sep;18(5):405–13. PMID:17700235

49. Ahmad SM, Esmaeli B, Williams M, et al. American Joint Committee on Cancer Classification Predicts Outcome of Patients with Lacrimal Gland Adenoid Cystic Carcinoma. Ophthalmology. 2009 Jun;116(6):1210–5. PMID:19395039

50. Ahmad Z, Khurshid A, Qureshi A. Primary Orbital Yolk Sac Tumour in a 14-Year-Old Girl. BMJ Case Rep. 2009;2009:Bcr04.2009.1821. PMID:22096462

51. Ahmed AH, Foster CS, Shields CL. Association of Disease Location and Treatment With Survival in Diffuse Large B-Cell Lymphoma of the Eye and Ocular Adnexal Region. JAMA Ophthalmol. 2017 Oct 1;135(10):1062–8. PMID:28880986

52. Ahmed OM, Ma AK, Ahmed TM, et al. Epidemiology, Outcomes, and Prognostic Factors of Orbital Lymphoma in the United States. Orbit. 2020 Dec;39(6):397–402. PMID:31894703

53. Ahmed RA, Eltanamly RM. Orbital Epidermoid Cysts: A Diagnosis to Consider. J Ophthalmol. 2014;2014:508425. PMID:25276416

54. Ahn D, Lee GJ, Sohn JH, et al. Fine-Needle Aspiration Cytology Versus Core-Needle Biopsy for the Diagnosis of Extracranial Head and Neck Schwannoma. Head Neck. 2018 Dec;40(12):2695–700. PMID:30457183

55. Ahn IE, Underbayev C, Albitar A, et al. Clonal Evolution Leading to Ibrutinib Resistance in Chronic Lymphocytic Leukemia. Blood. 2017 Mar 16;129(11):1469–79. PMID:28049639

56. Ahn S, Kim Y, Oh YL. Fine Needle Aspiration Cytology of Benign Salivary Gland Tumors with Myoepithelial Cell Participation: An Institutional Experience of 575 Cases. Acta Cytol. 2013;57(6):567–74. PMID:24107383

57. Ahn SS, Song JJ, Park YB, et al. Malignancies in Korean Patients with Immunoglobulin G4-Related Disease. Int J Rheum Dis. 2017 Aug;20(8):1028–35. PMID:28544157

58. Ait Ouakrim D, Dashti SG, Chau R, et al. Aspirin, Ibuprofen, and the Risk of Colorectal Cancer in Lynch Syndrome. J Natl Cancer Inst. 2015 Jun 24;107(9):djv170. PMID:26109217

59. Aiyub S, Chan W, Szetu J, et al. Congenital Orbital Teratoma. Indian J Ophthalmol. 2013 Dec;61(12):767–9. PMID:23619505

60. AJCC Ophthalmic Oncology Task Force. International Validation of the American Joint Committee on Cancer's 7th Edition Classification of Uveal Melanoma. JAMA Ophthalmol. 2015 Apr;133(4):376–83. PMID:25555246
61. Akda F, Hafezi F, Heule-Dieleman HA, et al. [Orbital Metastases of Breast Cancer. Radiologic Features]. Ophthalmologe. 2010 Aug;107(8):728–32. German. PMID:20393728
62. Akhtar S, Oza KK, Khan SA, et al. Muir-Torre Syndrome: Case Report of a Patient with Concurrent Jejunal and Ureteral Cancer and a Review of the Literature. J Am Acad Dermatol. 1999 Nov;41(5 Pt 1):681–6. PMID:10534628
63. Akpek EK, Polcharoen W, Ferry JA, et al. Conjunctival Lymphoma Masquerading as Chronic Conjunctivitis. Ophthalmology. 1999 Apr;106(4):757–60. PMID:10201599
64. Akuzawa Y, Tsukasaki K, Saeki T, et al. A Case Series of Adult T-Cell Leukemia-Lymphoma, Associated with Human T-Cell Leukemia Virus Type-1, at a Single Center in a Non-Viral-Endemic Metropolitan Area. J Clin Exp Hematop. 2019;59(3):108–11. PMID:31564712
65. Al Harby L, Sagoo MS, O'Day R, et al. Distinguishing Choroidal Nevi from Melanomas Using the MOLES Algorithm: Evaluation in an Ocular Nevus Clinic. Ocul Oncol Pathol. 2021 Sep;7(4):294–302. PMID:34604203
66. AlAkeely AG, Alkatan HM, Alsuhaibani AH, et al. Benign Reactive Lymphoid Hyperplasia of the Conjunctiva in Childhood. Br J Ophthalmol. 2017 Jul;101(7):933–9. PMID:27899370
67. Alam MS, Chandran VA, KrishnaKumar S. Primary Apocrine Adenocarcinoma of the Lacrimal Sac: An Extremely Rare Variant of Lacrimal Sac Neoplasm. Orbit. 2022 Apr;41(2):241–4. PMID:32964761
68. Alam MS, Mukherjee B, Krishnakumar S, et al. Malignant Perivascular Epithelioid Cell Tumor of the Orbit: Report of a Case and Review of Literature. Indian J Ophthalmol. 2017 Sep;65(9):889–91. PMID:28905842
69. Alam MS, Subramanian N, Desai AS, et al. Mesenchymal Chondrosarcoma of the Orbit: A Case Report with 5 Years of Follow-Up. Orbit. 2018 Feb;37(1):73–5. PMID:28812954
70. Albergo JI, Gaston CL, Laitinen M, et al. Ewing's Sarcoma: Only Patients with 100% of Necrosis After Chemotherapy Should Be Classified as Having a Good Response. Bone Joint J. 2016 Aug;98-B(8):1138–44. PMID:27482030
71. Albert DM, Rubenstein RA, Scheie HG. Tumor Metastasis to the Eye. I. Incidence in 213 Adult Patients with Generalized Malignancy. Am J Ophthalmol. 1967 Apr;63(4):723–6. PMID:6022244
72. Albores-Saavedra J, Batich K, Chable-Montero F, et al. Merkel Cell Carcinoma Demographics, Morphology, and Survival Based on 3870 Cases: A Population Based Study. J Cutan Pathol. 2010 Jan;37(1):20–7. PMID:19638070
73. Aldossary MM, Alkatan HM, Maktabi AM. Epibulbar Complex and Osseous Choristoma: Clinicopathological Study with Interesting Associations. Ann Med Surg (Lond). 2018 Oct 31;36:135–41. PMID:30510760
74. Alefounder PR, Ferguson SJ. The Location of Dissimilatory Nitrite Reductase and the Control of Dissimilatory Nitrate Reductase by Oxygen in Paracoccus Denitrificans. Biochem J. 1980 Oct 15;192(1):231–40. PMID:7197918
75. Alemayehu AM, Yibekal BT, Fekadu SA. Prevalence of Vernal Keratoconjunctivitis and its Associated Factors Among Children in Gambella Town, Southwest Ethiopia, June 2018. PLoS One. 2019 Apr 18;14(4):e0215528. PMID:30998721
76. Alenda C, Aranda FI, Payá A, et al. Mesectodermal Leiomyoma of Ciliary Body. Int J Surg Pathol. 2002 Oct;10(4):309–12. PMID:12490985
77. AlHammad F, Edward DP, Alkatan HM, et al. Eyelid Sebaceous Gland Carcinoma: An Assessment of the T Classification of the American Joint Committee of Cancer TNM Staging System 8th Versus 7th Edition. Eur J Ophthalmol. 2021 Jul;31(4):2055–63. PMID:32567368
78. al-Hazzaa SA, Specht CS, McLean IW, et al. Subcutaneous Neuroglial Choristoma: An Immunohistopathological Case Study. Br J Ophthalmol. 1993 Dec;77(12):817–8. PMID:8110681
79. Ali MJ, Bothra N, Naik MN. Transitional Cell Carcinoma of Lacrimal Sac. Ophthalmic Plast Reconstr Surg. 2018 May/Jun;34(3):e106. PMID:28582372
80. Ali MJ, Honavar SG, Naik MN, et al. Malherbe's Calcifying Epithelioma (Pilomatrixoma): An Uncommon Periocular Tumor. Int J Trichology. 2011 Jan;3(1):31–3. PMID:21769234
81. Ali MJ, Honavar SG, Naik MN, et al. Primary Adenoid Cystic Carcinoma: An Extremely Rare Eyelid Tumor. Ophthalmic Plast Reconstr Surg. 2012 Mar-Apr;28(2):e35–6. PMID:21629138
82. Ali MJ, Honavar SG, Vemuganti GK. Ciliary Body Medulloepithelioma in an Adult. Surv Ophthalmol. 2013 May-Jun;58(3):266–72. PMID:23218809
83. Ali MJ, Kamal S, Vemuganti GK, et al. Glial Heterotopia or Ectopic Brain Masquerading as a Dacyrocystocele. Ophthalmic Plast Reconstr Surg. 2015 Mar-Apr;31(2):e26–8. PMID:24492734
84. Ali N, Child CS, Michaelides M, et al. Recurrence of a Rare Skin Tumour: Superficial Angiomyxoma in the Eyelid. Can J Ophthalmol. 2011 Apr;46(2):205–6. PMID:21708097
85. Al-Ibraheemi A, Inwards CY, Zreik RT, et al. Histologic Spectrum of Giant Cell Tumor (GCT) of Bone in Patients 18 Years of Age and Below: A Study of 63 Patients. Am J Surg Pathol. 2016 Dec;40(12):1702–12. PMID:27526293
86. Al-Ibraheemi A, Martinez A, Weiss SW, et al. Fibrous Hamartoma of Infancy: A Clinicopathologic Study of 145 Cases, Including 2 with Sarcomatous Features. Mod Pathol. 2017 Apr;30(4):474–85. PMID:28059097
87. Alipour F, Khaheshi S, Soleimanzadeh M, et al. Contact Lens-Related Complications: A Review. J Ophthalmic Vis Res. 2017 Apr-Jun;12(2):193–204. PMID:28540012
88. Ali-Ridha A, Brownstein S, O'Connor M, et al. Benign Solitary Fibrous Histiocytoma of Xanthomatous Subtype of the Perilimbal Conjunctiva and Adjacent Sclera in a Youth. Ocul Oncol Pathol. 2018 Nov;4(6):341–4. PMID:30574484
89. Al-Jamal RT, Cassoux N, Desjardins L, et al. The Pediatric Choroidal and Ciliary Body Melanoma Study: A Survey by the European Ophthalmic Oncology Group. Ophthalmology. 2016 Apr;123(4):898–907. PMID:26854035
90. Al-Jamal RT, Mäkitie T, Kivelä T. Nucleolar Diameter and Microvascular Factors as Independent Predictors of Mortality from Malignant Melanoma of the Choroid and Ciliary Body. Invest Ophthalmol Vis Sci. 2003 Jun;44(6):2381–9. PMID:12766034
91. Aljerian K, Fathaddin A, Almajed N, et al. Angiolipoma of the Orbit. Ophthalmic Plast Reconstr Surg. 2019 May/Jun;35(3):e81–2. PMID:30908468
92. Alkatan H, Al-Shedoukhy AA, Chaudhry IA, et al. Orbital Alveolar Soft Part Sarcoma: Histopathologic Report of Two Cases. Saudi J Ophthalmol. 2010 Apr;24(2):57–61. PMID:23960876
93. Alkatan HM, Al Otaibi M, Maktabi AMY, et al. Clinical, Radiological and Histopathological Characteristics of Surgically Removed Orbital Hematic Cysts: A Case Series. Saudi J Ophthalmol. 2018 Jan-Mar;32(1):45–51. PMID:29755271
94. Alkatan HM, Al-Arfaj KM, Maktabi A. Conjunctival Nevi: Clinical and Histopathologic Features in a Saudi Population. Ann Saudi Med. 2010 Jul-Aug;30(4):306–12. PMID:20622349
95. Alkatan HM, Al-Dahmash SA, Aljaedi H. A Case of Ciliary Body Mesectodermal Leiomyoma with Rapid Growth and Loss of Vision Necessitating Enucleation. Ann Med Surg (Lond). 2020 Nov 27;60:651–3. PMID:33304581
96. Alkatan HM, Al-Harkan DH, Al-Mutlaq M, et al. Epithelial Lacrimal Gland Tumors: A Comprehensive Clinicopathologic Review of 26 Lesions with Radiologic Correlation. Saudi J Ophthalmol. 2014 Jan;28(1):49–57. PMID:24526859
97. Alkatan HM, Alhothali W, Alnuhayer O, et al. Pilomatrixoma in a Child Mimicking a Ruptured Epidermal Cyst Clinically and Histopathologically: Case Report. Int J Surg Case Rep. 2021 Jul;84:106068. PMID:34119944
98. Alkatan HM, Al-Kofide A, Al-Hussain H. Yolk Sac Tumor: Histopathologic Report of 2 Cases. Can J Ophthalmol. 2008 Feb;43(1):125–6. PMID:18219360
99. Alkatan HM, Al Marek F, Elkhamary S. Demographics of Pediatric Orbital Lesions: A Tertiary Eye Center Experience in Saudi Arabia. J Epidemiol Glob Health. 2019 Mar;9(1):3–10. PMID:30932383
100. Alkatan HM, Al-Motlak MA, Al-Shedoukhy AA. Metastatic Squamous Spindle Cell Carcinoma of the Conjunctiva. Saudi J Ophthalmol. 2010 Oct;24(4):155–8. PMID:23960894
101. Alkatan HM, AlObaidan OS, Kfoury H, et al. Orbital Immature Teratoma: A Rare Entity with Diagnostic Challenges. Saudi J Ophthalmol. 2018 Jan-Mar;32(1):75–8. PMID:29755277
102. Alkatan HM, Al Qahtani AA, Maktabi AM. Intraocular Adenocarcinoma: Histopathological Report of Two Cases with Different Origin. Can J Ophthalmol. 2016 Apr;51(2):e67–70. PMID:27085283
103. Alkatan HM, Alsalamah AK, Almizel A, et al. Orbital Solitary Fibrous Tumors: A Multi-Centered Histopathological and Immunohistochemical Analysis with Radiological Description. Ann Saudi Med. 2020 May-Jun;40(3):227–33. PMID:32493043
104. Alkatan HM, Alyousef NA, Alshabib NS, et al. A Comprehensive Review of Biopsy Techniques for Oculoplastic and Orbital Surgeons from Ophthalmic Pathologists' Perspective. Saudi J Ophthalmol. 2021 Nov 17;35(3):174–8. PMID:35601859
105. Alkatan HM, Alzahem TA, Maktabi AMY. Ophthalmic Histiocytic Lesions: A Baseline Demographic and Clinicopathological Study of 28 Cases from Two Eye Centers. Int Ophthalmol. 2022 Apr;42(4):1221–32. PMID:34727265
106. Alkatan HM, Bedaiwi KM, Al-Faky YH, et al. Demographics and Histopathological Characteristics of Enucleated Microphthalmic Globes. Sci Rep. 2022 Mar 28;12(1):5283. PMID:35347187
107. Alkatan HM, Chaudhry I, Alayoubi A. Mature Teratoma Presenting as Orbital Cellulitis in a 5-Month-Old Baby. Ann Saudi Med. 2013 Nov-Dec;33(6):623–6. PMID:24413870
108. Alkatan HM, Chaudhry I, Al-Qahtani A. Epithelioid Sarcoma of the Orbit. Ann Saudi Med. 2011 Mar-Apr;31(2):187–9. PMID:21242638
109. Alkatan HM, Eberhart CG, Alshomar KM, et al. Primary Mesenchymal Chondrosarcoma of the Orbit: Histopathological Report of 3 Pediatric Cases. Saudi J Ophthalmol. 2018 Jan-Mar;32(1):69–74. PMID:29755276
110. Alkhadar H, Macluskey M, White S, et al. Nerve Growth Factor-Induced Migration in Oral and Salivary Gland Tumour Cells Utilises the PI3K/Akt Signalling Pathway: Is There a Link to Perineural Invasion? J Oral Pathol Med. 2020 Mar;49(3):227–34. PMID:31782565
111. Allen CE, Merad M, McClain KL. Langerhans-Cell Histiocytosis. N Engl J Med. 2018 Aug 30;379(9):856–68. PMID:30157397
112. Allen CE, Parsons DW. Biological and Clinical Significance of Somatic Mutations in Langerhans Cell Histiocytosis and Related Histiocytic Neoplastic Disorders. Hematology Am Soc Hematol Educ Program. 2015;2015:559–64. PMID:26637772
113. Allen PW, Dymock RB, MacCormac LB. Superficial Angiomyxomas with and Without Epithelial Components. Report of 30 Tumors in 28 Patients. Am J Surg Pathol. 1988 Jul;12(7):519–30. PMID:3389450
114. Allingham RR, Seo B, Rampersaud E, et al. A Duplication in Chromosome 4q35 is Associated with Hereditary Benign Intraepithelial Dyskeratosis. Am J Hum Genet. 2001 Feb;68(2):491–4. PMID:11170897
115. Almasri M, Amer M, Ghanej J, et al. Druggable Molecular Pathways in Chronic Lymphocytic Leukemia. Life (Basel). 2022 Feb 14;12(2):283. PMID:35207569
116. Al-Mujaini A, Wali U, Ganesh A, et al. Ocular Adnexal Reactive Lymphoid Hyperplasia in Children. Middle East Afr J Ophthalmol. 2012 Oct;19(4):406–9. PMID:23248544
117. Alniemi ST, Griepentrog GJ, Diehl N, et al. Incidence and Clinical Characteristics of Periocular Infantile Hemangiomas. Arch Ophthalmol. 2012 Jul;130(7):889–93. PMID:22776927
118. Al-Rohil RN, Meyer D, Slodkowska EA, et al. Pigmented Eyelid Cysts Revisited: Apocrine Retention Cyst Chromhidrosis. Am J Dermatopathol. 2014 Apr;36(4):318–26. PMID:24247572
119. AlRubaian A, Alkatan HM, Al-Faky YH, et al. Clinical Features Differentiating Intratarsal Keratinous Cyst from Chalazion. Int Ophthalmol. 2020 Aug;40(8):2041–5. PMID:32367161
120. Alsalamah AK, Maktabi AM, Alkatan HM. Adult Orbital Lesions in Saudi Arabia: A Multi-Centered Demographic Study with Clinicopathological Correlation. J Epidemiol Glob Health. 2020 Dec;10(4):359–66. PMID:32959608
121. Al-Sawaf O, Zhang C, Lu T, et al. Minimal Residual Disease Dynamics After Venetoclax-Obinutuzumab Treatment: Extended Off-Treatment Follow-Up From the Randomized CLL14 Study. J Clin Oncol. 2021 Dec 20;39(36):4049–60. PMID:34709929
122. AlSemari MA, Perrotta M, Russo C, et al. Orbital Myeloid Sarcoma (Chloroma): Report of 2 Cases and Literature Review. Am J Ophthalmol Case Rep. 2020 Jul 11;19:100806. PMID:32775766
123. Alshomar KM, Altariqi SM, Alrikabi AC, et al. Primary Extramedullary Plasmacytoma of the Eyelid Conjunctiva - A Case Report and Review of the Literature. Ann Med Surg (Lond). 2020 May 7;55:1–4. PMID:32435472
124. Alston RD, Tatevossian RG, McNally RJ, et al. Incidence and Survival of Childhood Langerhans Cell Histiocytosis in Northwest England from 1954 to 1998. Pediatr Blood Cancer. 2007 May;48(5):555–60. PMID:16652350
125. Alsulaiman HM, Fatani DR, Al Sheikh O, et al. Krause's Accessory Lacrimal Gland Dacryops - Case Report and Literature Review. Orbit. 2020 Dec;39(6):441–5. PMID:31914837
126. Altan-Yaycioglu R, Canan H, Sizmaz S, et al. Nasolacrimal Duct Obstruction: Clinicopathologic Analysis of 205 Cases. Orbit. 2010 Oct;29(5):254–8. PMID:20704489
127. Alturkistany W, Althaqib R, Alsulaiman N, et al. Lacrimal Gland Lesions Biopsied in a Tertiary Eye Center in Saudi Arabia: A Clinical, Radiological, Surgical, and Histological Review. Clin Ophthalmol. 2022 Jan 25;16:191–200.

PMID:35115759
128. Alves A, Constantinidou A, Thway K, et al. The Evolving Management of Epithelioid Sarcoma. Eur J Cancer Care (Engl). 2021 Nov;30(6):e13489. PMID:34278633
129. Alyahya GA, Stenman G, Persson F, et al. Pleomorphic Adenoma Arising in an Accessory Lacrimal Gland of Wolfring. Ophthalmology. 2006 May;113(5):879–82. PMID:16530838
130. Alzahem TA, Cruz AA, Maktabi AMY, et al. Ophthalmic Rosai-Dorfman Disease: A Multi-Centre Comprehensive Study. BMC Ophthalmol. 2021 Nov 23;21(1):404. PMID:34814862
131. Al-Zaid T, Ditelberg JS, Prieto VG, et al. Trichilemmomas Show Loss of PTEN in Cowden Syndrome But Only Rarely in Sporadic Tumors. J Cutan Pathol. 2012 May;39(5):493–9. PMID:22486434
132. Amary F, Berisha F, Ye H, et al. H3F3A (Histone 3.3) G34W Immunohistochemistry: A Reliable Marker Defining Benign and Malignant Giant Cell Tumor of Bone. Am J Surg Pathol. 2017 Aug;41(8):1059–68. PMID:28505000
133. Amary F, Markert E, Berisha F, et al. FOS Expression in Osteoid Osteoma and Osteoblastoma: A Valuable Ancillary Diagnostic Tool. Am J Surg Pathol. 2019 Dec;43(12):1661–7. PMID:31490237
134. Amary F, Perez-Casanova L, Ye H, et al. Synovial Chondromatosis and Soft Tissue Chondroma: Extraosseous Cartilaginous Tumor Defined by FN1 Gene Rearrangement. Mod Pathol. 2019 Dec;32(12):1762–71. PMID:31273315
135. Amary MF, Bacsi K, Maggiani F, et al. IDH1 and IDH2 Mutations Are Frequent Events in Central Chondrosarcoma and Central and Periosteal Chondromas But Not in Other Mesenchymal Tumours. J Pathol. 2011 Jul;224(3):334–43. PMID:21598255
136. Amary MF, Berisha F, Bernardi FdelC, et al. Detection of SS18-SSX Fusion Transcripts in Formalin-Fixed Paraffin-Embedded Neoplasms: Analysis of Conventional RT-PCR, QRT-PCR and Dual Color FISH as Diagnostic Tools for Synovial Sarcoma. Mod Pathol. 2007 Apr;20(4):482–96. PMID:17334349
137. Ambrosio MR, De Falco G, Gozzetti A, et al. Plasmablastic Transformation of a Pre-Existing Plasmacytoma: A Possible Role for Reactivation of Epstein Barr Virus Infection. Haematologica. 2014 Nov;99(11):e235–7. PMID:25193957
138. Amemiya T, Hayashida H, Dake Y. Metastatic Orbital Tumors in Japan: A Review of the Literature. Ophthalmic Epidemiol. 2002 Feb;9(1):35–47. PMID:11815894
139. Amin MB, Edge SB, Greene FL, et al., editors. AJCC Cancer Staging Manual. 8th ed. New York (NY): Springer; 2017.
140. Amin S, AlJboor M, Toro MD, et al. Management and Outcomes of Unilateral Group D Tumors in Retinoblastoma. Clin Ophthalmol. 2021 Jan 7;15:65–72. PMID:33447011
140A. Amin SM, Haugh AM, Lee CY, et al. A Comparison of Morphologic and Molecular Features of BRAF, ALK, and NTRK1 Fusion Spitzoid Neoplasms. Am J Surg Pathol. 2017 Apr;41(4):491–98. PMID:27776007
141. Ammerman JM, Lonser RR, Dambrosia J, et al. Long-Term Natural History of Hemangioblastomas in Patients with von Hippel-Lindau Disease: Implications for Treatment. J Neurosurg. 2006 Aug;105(2):248–55. PMID:17219830
142. Amram AL, Rico G, Kim JW, et al. Vitreous Seeds in Retinoblastoma: Clinicopathologic Classification and Correlation. Ophthalmology. 2017 Oct;124(10):1540–7. PMID:28528011
143. Amstutz CA, Michel S, Thiel MA. Follicular Conjunctivitis Caused by a Mantle Cell Lymphoma. Klin Monbl Augenheilkd. 2004 May;221(5):398–400. PMID:15162290
144. An S, Kim K, Moon S, et al. Indoor Tanning and the Risk of Overall and Early-Onset Melanoma and Non-Melanoma Skin Cancer: Systematic Review and Meta-Analysis. Cancers (Basel). 2021 Nov 25;13(23):5940. PMID:34885049
145. Anastassiou G, Heiligenhaus A, Bechrakis N, et al. Prognostic Value of Clinical and Histopathological Parameters in Conjunctival Melanomas: A Retrospective Study. Br J Ophthalmol. 2002 Feb;86(2):163–7. PMID:11815341
146. Ancona-Lezama D, Dalvin LA, Shields CL. Modern Treatment of Retinoblastoma: A 2020 Review. Indian J Ophthalmol. 2020 Nov;68(11):2356–65. PMID:33120616
147. Ancona-Lezama D, Garza-Garza LA, Ruiz-Lozano RE, et al. Diffuse Infiltrative Retinoblastoma with Retinal Detachment in "Cinnamon-Roll" Configuration: A Case Report. J AAPOS. 2021 Feb;25(1):59–62. PMID:33348043
148. Anderson KK, Lessner AM, Hood I, et al. Invasive Transitional Cell Carcinoma of the Lacrimal Sac Arising in an Inverted Papilloma. Arch Ophthalmol. 1994 Mar;112(3):306–7. PMID:8129653
149. Andrea T, Giulio G, Giuliana L, et al. Primary Dedifferentiated Liposarcoma of the Orbit, a Rare Entity: Case Report and Review of Literature. Saudi J Ophthalmol. 2019 Jul-Sep;33(3):312–5. PMID:31686978
150. Andreasen S, Esmaeli B, Holstein SL, et al. An Update on Tumors of the Lacrimal Gland. Asia Pac J Ophthalmol (Phila). 2017 Mar-Apr;6(2):159–72. PMID:28399336
151. Andreasen S, Grauslund M, Heegaard S. Lacrimal Gland Ductal Carcinomas: Clinical, Morphological and Genetic Characterization and Implications for Targeted Treatment. Acta Ophthalmol. 2017 May;95(3):299–306. PMID:27808478
152. Andreasen S, Heegaard S, Grauslund M, et al. The Interleukin-6/Janus Kinase/STAT3 Pathway in Pleomorphic Adenoma and Carcinoma Ex Pleomorphic Adenoma of the Lacrimal Gland. Acta Ophthalmol. 2016 Dec;94(8):798–804. PMID:27286739
153. Andreasen S, von Holstein SL, Homøe P, et al. Recurrent Rearrangements of the PLAG1 and HMGA2 Genes in Lacrimal Gland Pleomorphic Adenoma and Carcinoma Ex Pleomorphic Adenoma. Acta Ophthalmol. 2018 Nov;96(7):e768–71. PMID:29437290
154. Andreoli MT, Aakalu V, Setabutr P. Epidemiological Trends in Malignant Lacrimal Gland Tumors. Otolaryngol Head Neck Surg. 2015 Feb;152(2):279–83. PMID:25385802
155. Andrew NH, Coupland SE, Pirbhai A, et al. Lymphoid Hyperplasia of the Orbit and Ocular Adnexa: A Clinical Pathologic Review. Surv Ophthalmol. 2016 Nov-Dec;61(6):778–90. PMID:27127077
156. Andrew NH, Sladden N, Kearney DJ, et al. An Analysis of IgG4-Related Disease (IgG4-RD) Among Idiopathic Orbital Inflammations and Benign Lymphoid Hyperplasias Using Two Consensus-Based Diagnostic Criteria for IgG4-RD. Br J Ophthalmol. 2015 Mar;99(3):376–81. PMID:25185258
157. Anesi A, Negrello S, Lucchetti D, et al. Clinical Management of Acinic Cell Carcinoma of the Lacrimal Gland. Case Rep Oncol. 2019 Oct 16;12(3):777–90. PMID:31762749
158. Angi M, Damato B, Kalirai H, et al. Immunohistochemical Assessment of Mitotic Count in Uveal Melanoma. Acta Ophthalmol. 2011 Mar;89(2):e155–60. PMID:19900200
159. Angi M, Kalirai H, Taktak A, et al. Prognostic Biopsy of Choroidal Melanoma: An Optimised Surgical and Laboratory Approach. Br J Ophthalmol. 2017 Aug;101(8):1143–6. PMID:28596284
160. Anguria P, Kitinya J, Ntuli S, et al. The Role of Heredity in Pterygium Development. Int J Ophthalmol. 2014 Jun 18;7(3):563–73. PMID:24967209
161. Anjum S, Modaboyina S, Sen S, et al. Epithelial-Myoepithelial Carcinoma of the Lacrimal Gland: Case Report of Youngest Patient. Ophthalmic Plast Reconstr Surg. 2020 Nov/Dec;36(6):e141–4. PMID:32332692
162. Anjum S, Sen S, Pushker N, et al. Prognostic Impact of Notch1 Receptor and Clinicopathological High-Risk Predictors in Lacrimal Gland Adenoid Cystic Carcinoma. Acta Ophthalmol. 2021 Dec;99(8):e1467–73. PMID:33675181
163. Anninga JK, Gelderblom H, Fiocco M, et al. Chemotherapeutic Adjuvant Treatment for Osteosarcoma: Where Do We Stand? Eur J Cancer. 2011 Nov;47(16):2431–45. PMID:21703851
164. Ansai S, Koseki S, Hozumi Y, et al. An Immunohistochemical Study of Lysozyme, CD-15 (Leu M1), and Gross Cystic Disease Fluid Protein-15 in Various Skin Tumors. Assessment of the Specificity and Sensitivity of Markers of Apocrine Differentiation. Am J Dermatopathol. 1995 Jun;17(3):249–55. PMID:8599433
165. Ansai S, Watanabe S, Aso K. A Case of Tubular Apocrine Adenoma with Syringocystadenoma Papilliferum. J Cutan Pathol. 1989 Aug;16(4):230–6. PMID:2551940
166. Ansai SI. Topics in Histopathology of Sweat Gland and Sebaceous Neoplasms. J Dermatol. 2017 Mar;44(3):315–26. PMID:28256768
167. Ansari AN, Bobos M, Shih S, et al. Renal Cell Carcinoma Antigen Expression in Primary Cutaneous Endocrine Mucinous Carcinomas: A Case Series of 14 Patients and Review of the Literature. Am J Dermatopathol. 2019 Aug;41(8):571–7. PMID:31335409
168. Antonescu CR, Chen HW, Zhang L, et al. ZFP36-FOSB Fusion Defines a Subset of Epithelioid Hemangioma with Atypical Features. Genes Chromosomes Cancer. 2014 Nov;53(11):951–9. PMID:25043949
169. Antonescu CR, Huang SC, Sung YS, et al. Novel GATA6-FOXO1 Fusions in a Subset of Epithelioid Hemangioma. Mod Pathol. 2021 May;34(5):934–41. PMID:33318580
170. Antonescu CR, Le Loarer F, Mosquera JM, et al. Novel YAP1-TFE3 Fusion Defines a Distinct Subset of Epithelioid Hemangioendothelioma. Genes Chromosomes Cancer. 2013 Aug;52(8):775–84. PMID:23737213
171. Antonescu CR, Sung YS, Zhang L, et al. Recurrent SRF-RELA Fusions Define a Novel Subset of Cellular Myofibroma/Myopericytoma: A Potential Diagnostic Pitfall With Sarcomas With Myogenic Differentiation. Am J Surg Pathol. 2017 May;41(5):677–84. PMID:28248815
172. Anzeljc AJ, Oliveira AM, Grossniklaus HE, et al. Nodular Fasciitis of the Orbit: A Case Report Confirmed by Molecular Cytogenetic Analysis. Ophthalmic Plast Reconstr Surg. 2017 May/Jun;33(3S Suppl 1):S152–5. PMID:26882059
173. Aozasa K, Zaki MA. Epidemiology and Pathogenesis of Nasal NK/T-Cell Lymphoma: A Mini-Review. ScientificWorldJournal. 2011 Feb 14;11:422–8. PMID:21336457
174. Apple DJ, Craythorn JM, Reidy JJ, et al. Malignant Transformation of an Optic Nerve Melanocytoma. Can J Ophthalmol. 1984 Dec;19(7):320–5. PMID:6525581
175. Arai A, Takase H, Yoshimori M, et al. Gene Expression Profiling of Primary Vitreoretinal Lymphoma. Cancer Sci. 2020 Apr;111(4):1417–21. PMID:32056332
176. Arat YO, Font RL, Chaudhry IA, et al. Leiomyoma of the Orbit and Periocular Region: A Clinicopathologic Study of Four Cases. Ophthalmic Plast Reconstr Surg. 2005 Jan;21(1):16–22. PMID:15677948
177. Araujo I, Coupland SE. Primary Vitreoretinal Lymphoma – A Review. Asia Pac J Ophthalmol (Phila). 2017 May-Jun;6(3):283–9. PMID:28558176
178. Arbajian E, Magnusson L, Brosjö O, et al. A Benign Vascular Tumor with a New Fusion Gene: EWSR1-NFATC1 in Hemangioma of the Bone. Am J Surg Pathol. 2013 Apr;37(4):613–6. PMID:23480395
179. Arber DA, Weiss LM, Albújar PF, et al. Nasal Lymphomas in Peru. High Incidence of T-Cell Immunophenotype and Epstein-Barr Virus Infection. Am J Surg Pathol. 1993 Apr;17(4):392–9. PMID:8388175
180. Arentsen JJ, Green WR. Melanoma of the Iris: Report of 72 Cases Treated Surgically. Ophthalmic Surg. 1975 Summer;6(2):23–37. PMID:1153157
181. Arepalli S, Kaliki S, Shields CL. Choroidal Metastases: Origin, Features, and Therapy. Indian J Ophthalmol. 2015 Feb;63(2):122–7. PMID:25827542
182. Arepalli S, Kaliki S, Shields JA, et al. Growth of Congenital Hypertrophy of the Retinal Pigment Epithelium Over 22 Years. J Pediatr Ophthalmol Strabismus. 2012 Dec 18;49 Online:e73–5. PMID:23244302
183. Arepalli S, Pellegrini M, Ferenczy SR, et al. Combined Hamartoma of the Retina and Retinal Pigment Epithelium: Findings on Enhanced Depth Imaging Optical Coherence Tomography in Eight Eyes. Retina. 2014 Nov;34(11):2202–7. PMID:25102194
184. Argani P, Antonescu CR, Illei PB, et al. Primary Renal Neoplasms with the ASPL-TFE3 Gene Fusion of Alveolar Soft Part Sarcoma: A Distinctive Tumor Entity Previously Included Among Renal Cell Carcinomas of Children and Adolescents. Am J Pathol. 2001 Jul;159(1):179–92. PMID:11438465
185. Argani P, Aulmann S, Illei PB, et al. A Distinctive Subset of PEComas Harbors TFE3 Gene Fusions. Am J Surg Pathol. 2010 Oct;34(10):1395–406. PMID:20871214
186. Argani P, Lal P, Hutchinson B, et al. Aberrant Nuclear Immunoreactivity for TFE3 in Neoplasms with TFE3 Gene Fusions: A Sensitive and Specific Immunohistochemical Assay. Am J Surg Pathol. 2003 Jun;27(6):750–61. PMID:12766578
187. Argani P, Zhang L, Sung YS, et al. Novel SS18-NEDD4 Gene Fusion in a Primary Renal Synovial Sarcoma. Genes Chromosomes Cancer. 2020 Mar;59(3):203–8. PMID:31595587
188. Argani P, Zhong M, Reuter VE, et al. TFE3-Fusion Variant Analysis Defines Specific Clinicopathologic Associations Among Xp11 Translocation Cancers. Am J Surg Pathol. 2016 Jun;40(6):723–37. PMID:26975036
189. Argenyi ZB. Immunohistochemical Characterization of Palisaded, Encapsulated Neuroma. J Cutan Pathol. 1990 Dec;17(6):329–35. PMID:1705947
190. Argenyi ZB, Cooper PH, Santa Cruz D. Plexiform and Other Unusual Variants of Palisaded Encapsulated Neuroma. J Cutan Pathol. 1993 Feb;20(1):34–9. PMID:8468415
191. Argyris PP, Pambuccian SE, Cayci Z, et al. Lacrimal Gland Adenoid Cystic Carcinoma with High-Grade Transformation to Myoepithelial Carcinoma: Report of a Case and Review of Literature. Head Neck Pathol. 2013 Mar;7(1):85–92. PMID:22829347
192. Aricò M, Girschikofsky M, Généreau T, et al. Langerhans Cell Histiocytosis in Adults. Report from the International Registry of the Histiocyte Society. Eur J Cancer. 2003 Nov;39(16):2341–8. PMID:14556926

193. Armijos PO, Uhlenhake E, Milman T. Secretory Carcinoma of the Eyelid Arising in an Adnexal Gland. Ophthalmology. 2022 Oct;129(10):1218. PMID:35753863
194. Arnold A, Imada EL, Zhang ML, et al. Differential Gene Methylation and Expression of HOX Transcription Factor Family in Orbitofacial Neurofibroma. Acta Neuropathol Commun. 2020 May 4;8(1):62. PMID:32366326
195. Arnold MA, Anderson JR, Gastier-Foster JM, et al. Histology, Fusion Status, and Outcome in Alveolar Rhabdomyosarcoma With Low-Risk Clinical Features: A Report From the Children's Oncology Group. Pediatr Blood Cancer. 2016 Apr;63(4):634–9. PMID:26756883
196. Aronow ME, Nakagawa JA, Gupta A, et al. Tuberous Sclerosis Complex: Genotype/Phenotype Correlation of Retinal Findings. Ophthalmology. 2012 Sep;119(9):1917–23. PMID:22608477
197. Arora A, Nanda A, Lamba S. Cyto-Histopathological Correlation of Skin Adnexal Tumors: A Short Series. J Cytol. 2018 Oct-Dec;35(4):204–7. PMID:30498290
198. Arora R, Monga S, Mehta DK, et al. Malignant Fibrous Histiocytoma of the Conjunctiva. Clin Exp Ophthalmol. 2006 Apr;34(3):275–8. PMID:16671910
199. Asano J, Watanabe T, Oguchi T, et al. Association Between Immunoglobulin G4-Related Disease and Malignancy Within 12 Years After Diagnosis: An Analysis After Longterm Followup. J Rheumatol. 2015 Nov;42(11):2135–42. PMID:26472416
200. Asensio-Sánchez VM. Presumed Solitary Circumscribed Retinal Astrocytic Proliferation: A Lesion that Can Regress. Int Med Case Rep J. 2019 Apr 5;12:85–8. PMID:31118830
201. Ashok Kumar P, Paulraj S, Mirchia K, et al. Ductal Adenocarcinoma Ex Pleomorphic Adenoma of the Lacrimal Gland: A Rare and Morbid Malignancy. Case Rep Oncol Med. 2020 Feb 3;2020:1790106. PMID:32089922
202. Ashton N. Primary Tumours of the Iris. Br J Ophthalmol. 1964 Dec;48(12):650–68. PMID:14249186
203. Ashur-Fabian O, Blumenthal DT, Bakon M, et al. Long-Term Response in High-Grade Optic Glioma Treated with Medically Induced Hypothyroidism and Carboplatin: A Case Report and Review of the Literature. Anticancer Drugs. 2013 Mar;24(3):315–23. PMID:23348245
204. Asnaghi L, Alkatan H, Mahale A, et al. Identification of Multiple DNA Copy Number Alterations Including Frequent 8p11.22 Amplification in Conjunctival Squamous Cell Carcinoma. Invest Ophthalmol Vis Sci. 2014 Dec 9;55(12):8604–13. PMID:25491297
205. Asproudis I, Kanari M, Ntountas I, et al. Successful Treatment with Rituximab of IgG4-Related Disease Coexisting with Adult-Onset Asthma and Periocular Xanthogranuloma. Rheumatol Int. 2020 Apr;40(4):671–7. PMID:31392499
206. Asthagiri AR, Parry DM, Butman JA, et al. Neurofibromatosis Type 2. Lancet. 2009 Jun 6;373(9679):1974–86. PMID:19476995
207. Augsburger JJ. Fine Needle Aspiration Biopsy of Suspected Metastatic Cancers to the Posterior Uvea. Trans Am Ophthalmol Soc. 1988;86:499–560. PMID:2979028
208. Augsburger JJ, Corrêa ZM, Trichopoulos N, et al. Size Overlap Between Benign Melanocytic Choroidal Nevi and Choroidal Malignant Melanomas. Invest Ophthalmol Vis Sci. 2008 Jul;49(7):2823–8. PMID:18408179
209. Augsburger JJ, Henson GL, Hershberger VS, et al. Topographical Distribution of Typical Unifocal Congenital Hypertrophy of Retinal Pigment Epithelium. Graefes Arch Clin Exp Ophthalmol. 2006 Nov;244(11):1412–4. PMID:16568286
210. Aukema SM, Hoster E, Rosenwald A, et al. Expression of TP53 is Associated with the Outcome of MCL Independent of MIPI and Ki-67 in Trials of the European MCL Network. Blood. 2018 Jan 25;131(4):417–20. PMID:29196411
211. Aung PP, Batrani M, Mirzabeigi M, et al. Extraocular Sebaceous Carcinoma In Situ: Report of Three Cases and Review of the Literature. J Cutan Pathol. 2014 Jul;41(7):592–6. PMID:24666211
212. Aurias A, Rimbaut C, Buffe D, et al. Translocation Involving Chromosome 22 in Ewing's Sarcoma. A Cytogenetic Study of Four Fresh Tumors. Cancer Genet Cytogenet. 1984 May;12(1):21–5. PMID:6713357
213. Auw-Hädrich C, Bredow L, Reinhard T. [Conjunctival Degenerative Lesions and Tumours]. Klin Monbl Augenheilkd. 2013 Apr;230(4):445–63. German. PMID:23629804
214. Auw-Haedrich C, Danielewicz KD, Mendoza PR, et al. Conjunctival Stromal Tumor: Expansion of Findings in a Newly Described Entity. Ophthalmology. 2016 May;123(5):1166–7. PMID:26778331
215. Auw-Haedrich C, Sundmacher R, Freudenberg N, et al. Expression of P63 in Conjunctival Intraepithelial Neoplasia and Squamous Cell Carcinoma. Graefes Arch Clin Exp Ophthalmol. 2006 Jan;244(1):96–103. PMID:16021499
216. Avedschmidt SE, Stagner AM, Eagle RC Jr, et al. The Targetable Epigenetic Tumor Protein EZH2 is Enriched in Intraocular Medulloepithelioma. Invest Ophthalmol Vis Sci. 2016 Nov 1;57(14):6242–6. PMID:27842164
217. Awdry P. Lymphangiectasia Haemorrhagica Conjunctivae. Br J Ophthalmol. 1969 Apr;53(4):274–8. PMID:5781037
218. Aytekin MN, Öztürk R, Amer K, et al. Epidemiology, Incidence, and Survival of Synovial Sarcoma Subtypes: SEER Database Analysis. J Orthop Surg (Hong Kong). 2020 Jan-Apr;28(2):2309499020936009. PMID:32618221
219. Azari AA, Arabi A. Conjunctivitis: A Systematic Review. J Ophthalmic Vis Res. 2020 Aug 6;15(3):372–95. PMID:32864068
220. Azari AA, Kanavi MR, Lucarelli M, et al. Angiolymphoid Hyperplasia with Eosinophilia of the Orbit and Ocular Adnexa: Report of 5 Cases. JAMA Ophthalmol. 2014 May;132(5):633–6. PMID:24676051
221. Azzopardi JG, Laurini R. Inverted Follicular Keratosis. J Clin Pathol. 1975 Jun;28(6):465–71. PMID:1141446
222. Baab S, Le PH, Kinzer EE. Allergic Conjunctivitis. In: StatPearls. Treasure Island (FL): StatPearls Publishing; 2022. PMID:28846256.
223. Babu N, Dey P. Medulloepithelioma of Ciliary Body Diagnosed by Fine Needle Aspiration Cytology. Cytopathology. 2003 Apr;14(2):93–4. PMID:12713484
224. Babu NA, Rajesh E, Krupaa J, et al. Genodermatoses. J Pharm Bioallied Sci. 2015 Apr;7(Suppl 1):S203–6. PMID:26015711
225. Bachur CD, Comi AM. Sturge-Weber Syndrome. Curr Treat Options Neurol. 2013 Oct;15(5):607–17. PMID:23907585
226. Badami A, Bianciotto CG, Shields CL, et al. Combined Hamartoma of the Retina and Retinal Pigment Epithelium in a Child with Branchial Cleft Cysts. J Pediatr Ophthalmol Strabismus. 2012 Mar 13;49 Online:e9–11. PMID:22420620
227. Bagger M, Andersen MT, Andersen KK, et al. The Prognostic Effect of American Joint Committee on Cancer Staging and Genetic Status in Patients with Choroidal and Ciliary Body Melanoma. Invest Ophthalmol Vis Sci. 2014 Dec 23;56(1):438–44. PMID:25537201
228. Bagheri A, Abbaszadeh M, Torbati P, et al. Mesenchymal Chondrosarcoma of the Orbit Attached to the Optic Nerve. J Craniofac Surg. 2018 Sep;29(6):e591–4. PMID:29863559
229. Bahmad HF, Stoyanov K, Mendez T, et al. Keratoacanthoma Versus Squamous-Cell Carcinoma: Histopathological Features and Molecular Markers. Dermatopathology (Basel). 2024 Oct 8;11(4):272–85. PMID:39449378
230. Bahrami A, Dalton JD, Krane JF, et al. A Subset of Cutaneous and Soft Tissue Mixed Tumors Are Genetically Linked to Their Salivary Gland Counterpart. Genes Chromosomes Cancer. 2012 Feb;51(2):140–8. PMID:22038920
231. Bairey O, Kremer I, Rakowsky E, et al. Orbital and Adnexal Involvement in Systemic Non-Hodgkin's Lymphoma. Cancer. 1994 May 1;73(9):2395–9. PMID:8168043
232. Bajaj MS, Mehta M, Kashyap S, et al. Clinical and Pathologic Profile of Angiomyxomas of the Orbit. Ophthalmic Plast Reconstr Surg. 2011 Mar-Apr;27(2):76–80. PMID:20562663
233. Bajaj MS, Pushker N, Chaturvedi A, et al. Orbital Space-Occupying Lesions in Indian Children. J Pediatr Ophthalmol Strabismus. 2007 Mar-Apr;44(2):106–11. PMID:17410962
234. Bajric J, Griepentrog GJ, Mohney BG. Pediatric Periocular Dermoid Cysts: Incidence, Clinical Characteristics, and Surgical Outcomes. Ophthalmic Epidemiol. 2019 Apr;26(2):117–20. PMID:30260262
235. Bakalian S, Marshall JC, Logan P, et al. Molecular Pathways Mediating Liver Metastasis in Patients with Uveal Melanoma. Clin Cancer Res. 2008 Feb 15;14(4):951–6. PMID:18281525
236. Baker MS, Yin VT, Ivan D, et al. Epidemiology and Prognosis of Primary Periocular Sweat Gland Carcinomas. Ophthalmic Plast Reconstr Surg. 2017 Mar/Apr;33(2):101–5. PMID:26974419
237. Bakhti S, Terkmani F, Tighilt N, et al. Glial Heterotopia of the Orbit: A Rare Cause of Proptosis. Childs Nerv Syst. 2016 Nov;32(11):2239–41. PMID:27179534
238. Bakst R, Powers A, Yahalom J. Diagnostic and Therapeutic Considerations for Extramedullary Leukemia. Curr Oncol Rep. 2020 Jun 24;22(7):75. PMID:32577912
239. Balachandran C, Millar MJ, Murali R, et al. Malignant Optic Glioma Presenting as an Acute Anterior Optic Neuropathy. Retin Cases Brief Rep. 2009 Spring;3(2):156–60. PMID:25391062
240. Baliakas P, Jeromin S, Iskas M, et al. Cytogenetic Complexity in Chronic Lymphocytic Leukemia: Definitions, Associations, and Clinical Impact. Blood. 2019 Mar 14;133(11):1205–16. PMID:30602617
241. Balikov DA, Hu K, Liu CJ, et al. Comparative Molecular Analysis of Primary Central Nervous System Lymphomas and Matched Vitreoretinal Lymphomas by Vitreous Liquid Biopsy. Int J Mol Sci. 2021 Sep 16;22(18):9992. PMID:34576156
242. Ballard TN, Elner VM, Briceño CA. Lower Eyelid Lesion. JAMA Ophthalmol. 2015 Aug;133(8):955–6. PMID:26270402
243. Ballester LY, Cantu MD, Lim KPH, et al. The Use of BRAF V600E Mutation-Specific Immunohistochemistry in Pediatric Langerhans Cell Histiocytosis. Hematol Oncol. 2018 Feb;36(1):307–15. PMID:28219109
244. Balmer A, Munier F, Gailloud C. Retinoma. Case Studies. Ophthalmic Paediatr Genet. 1991 Sep;12(3):131–7. PMID:1754160
245. Bamps S, Oyen T, Legius E, et al. Multiple Granular Cell Tumors in a Child with Noonan Syndrome. Eur J Pediatr Surg. 2013 Jun;23(3):257–9. PMID:22915371
246. Ban M, Sugie S, Kamiya H, et al. Microcystic Adnexal Carcinoma with Lymph Node Metastasis. Dermatology. 2003;207(4):395–7. PMID:14657634
247. Bandyopadhyay A, Gangopadhyay M, Chakraborty S. Juvenile Xanthogranuloma-Diagnostic Challenge on Fine-Needle Aspiration Cytology. J Cytol. 2011 Oct;28(4):217–8. PMID:22090701
248. Banerjee P, Koka K, Alam MS, et al. The Spectrum and Clinicopathological Correlation of Eyelid Lesions: Twenty Years' Experience at a Tertiary Eye Care Center in South India. Indian J Ophthalmol. 2022 Jan;70(1):43–50. PMID:34937206
249. Bannister M, Lawson G. Papillary-Cystic Variant of Acinic Cell Carcinoma in the Lacrimal Gland. Case Rep Ophthalmol Med. 2014;2014:285485. PMID:24959368
250. Bansal S, Khan AL, Hsuan J. Lacrimal Sac Mucus-Secreting Adenocarcinoma. Orbit. 2008;27(3):199–201. PMID:18569829
251. Bao Y, Li J, Zhu Y. Mammary Analog Secretory Carcinoma With ETV6 Rearrangement Arising in the Conjunctiva and Eyelid. Am J Dermatopathol. 2018 Jul;40(7):531–5. PMID:29251639
252. Baranov E, Hornick JL. Soft Tissue Special Issue: Fibroblastic and Myofibroblastic Neoplasms of the Head and Neck. Head Neck Pathol. 2020 Mar;14(1):43–58. PMID:31950474
253. Baranov E, McBride MJ, Bellizzi AM, et al. A Novel SS18-SSX Fusion-Specific Antibody for the Diagnosis of Synovial Sarcoma. Am J Surg Pathol. 2020 Jul;44(7):922–33. PMID:32141887
254. Barbaro NM, Rosenblum ML, Maitland CG, et al. Malignant Optic Glioma Presenting Radiologically as a "Cystic" Suprasellar Mass: Case Report and Review of the Literature. Neurosurgery. 1982 Dec;11(6):787–9. PMID:6298650
255. Baredes S, Ludwin DB, Troublefield YL, et al. Adenocarcinoma Ex-Pleomorphic Adenoma of the Lacrimal Sac and Nasolacrimal Duct: A Case Report. Laryngoscope. 2003 Jun;113(6):940–2. PMID:12782801
256. Barker D, Wright E, Nguyen K, et al. Gene for von Recklinghausen Neurofibromatosis is in the Pericentromeric Region of Chromosome 17. Science. 1987 May 29;236(4805):1100–2. PMID:3107130
257. Barker-Griffith AE, McDonald PR, Green WR. Malignant Melanoma Arising in a Choroidal Magnacellular Nevus (Melanocytoma). Can J Ophthalmol. 1976 Apr;11(2):140–6. PMID:1078332
258. Barker-Griffith AE, Streeten BW, Charles NC. Moll Gland Neoplasms of the Eyelid: A Clinical and Pathological Spectrum in 5 Cases. Arch Ophthalmol. 2006 Nov;124(11):1645–9. PMID:17102015
259. Barnes AC, Goldman DR, Laver NV, et al. Congenital Simple Hamartoma of the Retinal Pigment Epithelium: Clinical, Optical Coherence Tomography, and Histopathological Correlation. Eye (Lond). 2014 Jun;28(6):765–6. PMID:24603418
260. Barnhill RL. The Spitzoid Lesion: Rethinking Spitz Tumors, Atypical Variants, 'Spitzoid Melanoma' and Risk Assessment. Mod Pathol. 2006 Feb;19(Suppl 2):S21–33. PMID:16446713
261. Barnhill RL, Lemaitre S, Lévy-Gabrielle C, et al. Satellite in Transit Metastases in Rapidly Fatal Conjunctival Melanoma: Implications for Angiotropism and Extravascular Migratory Metastasis (Description of a Murine Model for Conjunctival Melanoma). Pathology. 2016 Feb;48(2):166–76. PMID:27020389
262. Barr CC, Zimmerman LE, Curtin VT, et al. Bilateral Diffuse Melanocytic Uveal Tumors Associated with Systemic Malignant Neoplasms. A Recently Recognized Syndrome. Arch Ophthalmol. 1982 Feb;100(2):249–55. PMID:7065942

263. Barr FG, Galili N, Holick J, et al. Rearrangement of the PAX3 Paired Box Gene in the Paediatric Solid Tumour Alveolar Rhabdomyosarcoma. Nat Genet. 1993 Feb;3(2):113–7. PMID:8098985

264. Barrantes PC, Zhou P, MacDonald SM, et al. Granular Cell Tumor of the Orbit: Review of the Literature and a Proposed Treatment Modality. Ophthalmic Plast Reconstr Surg. 2022 Mar-Apr 01;38(2):122–31. PMID:34406152

265. Barreira Rodríguez JR, Cabal Díaz V, Costa García A, et al. Voltammetric Assay of Heroin in Illicit Dosage Forms. Analyst. 1990 Feb;115(2):209–12. PMID:2321771

266. Barresi V, Vitarelli E, Branca G, et al. Expression of Brachyury in Hemangioblastoma: Potential Use in Differential Diagnosis. Am J Surg Pathol. 2012 Jul;36(7):1052–7. PMID:22446946

267. Barrott JJ, Illum BE, Jin H, et al. Paracrine Osteoprotegerin and β-Catenin Stabilization Support Synovial Sarcomagenesis in Periosteal Cells. J Clin Invest. 2018 Jan 2;128(1):207–18. PMID:29202462

268. Barry JS, Reddy MA. The Association of an Epibulbar Dermoid and Duane Syndrome in a Patient with a SALL1 Mutation (Townes-Brocks Syndrome). Ophthalmic Genet. 2008 Dec;29(4):177–80. PMID:19005989

269. Barsegian A, Ahmad A, Shinder R. Leiomyoma of the Palpebral Conjunctiva. Ophthalmology. 2017 Jan;124(1):65. PMID:27993264

270. Bartoletti-Stella A, Salfi NC, Ceccarelli C, et al. Mitochondrial DNA Mutations in Oncocytic Adnexal Lacrimal Glands of the Conjunctiva. Arch Ophthalmol. 2011 May;129(5):664–6. PMID:21555623

271. Bartuma H, Nord KH, Macchia G, et al. Gene Expression and Single Nucleotide Polymorphism Array Analyses of Spindle Cell Lipomas and Conventional Lipomas with 13q14 Deletion. Genes Chromosomes Cancer. 2011 Aug;50(8):619–32. PMID:21563233

272. Baselga E. Sturge-Weber Syndrome. Semin Cutan Med Surg. 2004 Jun;23(2):87–98. PMID:15295918

273. Bashir S, Tariq M, Aslam HM, et al. Orbital Dermatofibrosarcoma Protuberans with Intracranial Extension Preceded by Recurrent Leiomyoma of the Orbit: A Case Report. J Med Case Rep. 2015 Apr 29;9:96. PMID:25924890

274. Bastian BC. The Molecular Pathology of Melanoma: An Integrated Taxonomy of Melanocytic Neoplasia. Annu Rev Pathol. 2014;9:239–71. PMID:24460190

275. Bata BM, Salvi SM, Mudhar HS. Conjunctival Invasive Squamous Carcinoma Arising from a Dysplastic Inverted Papilloma, Both Positive for HPV16. Can J Ophthalmol. 2021 Dec;56(6):e180–2. PMID:33901465

276. Baum JL, Feingold M. Ocular Aspects of Goldenhar's Syndrome. Am J Ophthalmol. 1973 Feb;75(2):250–7. PMID:4697181

277. Baumann F, Flores E, Napolitano A, et al. Mesothelioma Patients with Germline BAP1 Mutations Have 7-Fold Improved Long-Term Survival. Carcinogenesis. 2015 Jan;36(1):76–81. PMID:25380601

278. Baumhoer D, Amary F, Flanagan AM. An Update of Molecular Pathology of Bone Tumors. Lessons Learned from Investigating Samples by Next Generation Sequencing. Genes Chromosomes Cancer. 2019 Feb;58(2):88–99. PMID:30582658

279. Baumhoer D, Berthold R, Isfort I, et al. Recurrent CTNNB1 Mutations in Craniofacial Osteomas. Mod Pathol. 2022 Apr;35(4):489–94. PMID:34725446

280. Bautista MJ, Perumal B, Jones DM, et al. Proliferative Fasciitis of the Orbit. Ophthalmic Plast Reconstr Surg. 2017 May/Jun;33(3S Suppl 1):S151–2. PMID:26226235

281. Becerra EM, Saornil MA, Blanco G, et al. Cavitary Choroidal Melanoma. Can J Ophthalmol. 2005 Oct;40(5):619–22. PMID:16391628

282. Bechrakis NE, Lee WR. Dedifferentiation Potential of Iris Melanomas. Fortschr Ophthalmol. 1991;88(6):651–6. PMID:1794785

283. Becker JC, Houben R, Ugurel S, et al. MC Polyomavirus is Frequently Present in Merkel Cell Carcinoma of European Patients. J Invest Dermatol. 2009 Jan;129(1):248–50. PMID:18633441

284. Beekman R, Amador V, Campo E. SOX11, a Key Oncogenic Factor in Mantle Cell Lymphoma. Curr Opin Hematol. 2018 Jul;25(4):299–306. PMID:29738333

285. Begna KH, Kittur J, Yui J, et al. De Novo Isolated Myeloid Sarcoma: Comparative Analysis of Survival in 19 Consecutive Cases. Br J Haematol. 2021 Nov;195(3):413–6. PMID:34346084

286. Behbahani S, Pinto JO, Wassef D, et al. Analysis of Head and Neck Primary Cutaneous Mucinous Carcinoma: An Indolent Tumor of the Eccrine Sweat Glands. J Craniofac Surg. 2021 May 1;32(3):e244–7. PMID:32890173

287. Behera M, Chatterjee S. A Case of Syringocystadenoma Papilliferum of Eyelid with Literature Review. Indian J Ophthalmol. 2015 Jun;63(6):550–1. PMID:26265653

288. Behjati S, Tarpey PS, Haase K, et al. Recurrent Mutation of IGF Signalling Genes and Distinct Patterns of Genomic Rearrangement in Osteosarcoma. Nat Commun. 2017 Jun 23;8:15936. PMID:28643781

289. Behjati S, Tarpey PS, Presneau N, et al. Distinct H3F3A and H3F3B Driver Mutations Define Chondroblastoma and Giant Cell Tumor of Bone. Nat Genet. 2013 Dec;45(12):1479–82. PMID:24162739

290. Behjati S, Tarpey PS, Sheldon H, et al. Recurrent PTPRB and PLCG1 Mutations in Angiosarcoma. Nat Genet. 2014 Apr;46(4):376–9. PMID:24633157

291. Bejjanki KM, Mishra DK, Kaliki S. Periocular Lobular Capillary Hemangioma in Adults: A Clinicopathological Study. Middle East Afr J Ophthalmol. 2019 Sep 30;26(3):138–40. PMID:31619900

292. Bekkenk MW, Geelen FA, van Voorst Vader PC, et al. Primary and Secondary Cutaneous CD30(+) Lymphoproliferative Disorders: A Report from the Dutch Cutaneous Lymphoma Group on the Long-Term Follow-Up Data of 219 Patients and Guidelines for Diagnosis and Treatment. Blood. 2000 Jun 15;95(12):3653–61. PMID:10845893

293. Belhouachi N, Xochelli A, Boudjoghra M, et al. Primary Vitreoretinal Lymphomas Display a Remarkably Restricted Immunoglobulin Gene Repertoire. Blood Adv. 2020 Apr 14;4(7):1357–66. PMID:32267931

294. Bell D, Sniegowski MC, Wani K, et al. Mutational Landscape of Lacrimal Gland Carcinomas and Implications for Treatment. Head Neck. 2016 Apr;38(Suppl 1):e724–9. PMID:25899808

295. Bell WR, Singh K, Rajan Kd A, et al. Expression of P16 and P53 in Intraepithelial Periocular Sebaceous Carcinoma. Ocul Oncol Pathol. 2015 Dec;2(2):71–5. PMID:27171611

296. Bellerive C, Berry JL, Polski A, et al. Conjunctival Squamous Neoplasia: Staging and Initial Treatment. Cornea. 2018 Oct;37(10):1287–91. PMID:29863543

297. Ben Rejeb S, Charfi L, Sahraoui G, et al. Cyclin D1: Potential Utility as Marker for Langerhans Cell Histiocytosis. J Immunoassay Immunochem. 2021 Jul 4;42(4):370–9. PMID:33444078

298. Benali K, Benmessaoud H, Aarab J, et al. Lacrimal Gland Adenoid Cystic Carcinoma: Report of an Unusual Case with Literature Review. Radiat Oncol J. 2021 Jun;39(2):152–8. PMID:34619831

299. Benner MF, Jansen PM, Meijer CJ, et al. Diagnostic and Prognostic Evaluation of Phenotypic Markers TRAF1, MUM1, BCL2 and CD15 in Cutaneous CD30-Positive Lymphoproliferative Disorders. Br J Dermatol. 2009 Jul;161(1):121–7. PMID:19416236

300. Benner MF, Willemze R. Applicability and Prognostic Value of the New TNM Classification System in 135 Patients with Primary Cutaneous Anaplastic Large Cell Lymphoma. Arch Dermatol. 2009 Dec;145(12):1399–404. PMID:20026848

301. Bennett JA, Braga AC, Pinto A, et al. Uterine PEComas: A Morphologic, Immunohistochemical, and Molecular Analysis of 32 Tumors. Am J Surg Pathol. 2018 Oct;42(10):1370–83. PMID:30001237

302. Bennett SL, Basko-Plluska JL, Shea CR, et al. Role of Wnt Signaling in Dermatofibroma Induction Phenomenon. J Cutan Pathol. 2021 Feb;48(2):217–20. PMID:32767564

303. Benton S, Zhao J, Zhang B, et al. Impact of Next-Generation Sequencing on Interobserver Agreement and Diagnosis of Spitzoid Neoplasms. Am J Surg Pathol. 2021 Dec 1;45(12):1597–605. PMID:34757982

304. Berenbom A, Milman T, Finger PT. FIT Biopsy for Conjunctival Squamous Cell Carcinoma with Extensive Intraocular Invasion. Graefes Arch Clin Exp Ophthalmol. 2008 Mar;246(3):467–9. PMID:17972091

305. Berg JC, Scheithauer BW, Spinner RJ, et al. Plexiform Schwannoma: A Clinicopathologic Overview with Emphasis on the Head and Neck Region. Hum Pathol. 2008 May;39(5):633–40. PMID:18439936

306. Bergeron S, Ito H, Dossous YE, et al. Histopathological Variability and Concomitant Lesions in Pterygium in a Large Case Series. J Ophthalmol. 2021 Mar 19;2021:6623794. PMID:33828861

307. Berk DR, Culican SM, Bayliss SJ. Scleral Hemangioma: Case Report and Response to Propranolol. Pediatr Dermatol. 2013 May-Jun;30(3):e16–7. PMID:22486338

308. Berman A, Winkelmann RK. Involuting Common Warts. Clinical and Histopathologic Findings. J Am Acad Dermatol. 1980 Oct;3(4):356–62. PMID:7430456

309. Berman EL, Shields CL, Sagoo MS, et al. Multifocal Blue Nevus of the Conjunctiva. Surv Ophthalmol. 2008 Jan-Feb;53(1):41–9. PMID:18191656

310. Bernardini FP, Croxatto JO, Nozza P, et al. Primary Diffuse Leptomeningeal Gliomatosis in Children: A Clinical Pathologic Correlation. Ophthalmic Plast Reconstr Surg. 2013 Mar-Apr;29(2):93–7. PMID:23247038

311. Bernardini FP, de Conciliis C, Schneider S, et al. Solitary Fibrous Tumor of the Orbit: Is it Rare? Report of a Case Series and Review of the Literature. Ophthalmology. 2003 Jul;110(7):1442–8. PMID:12867407

312. Bernardini FP, Devoto MH, Croxatto JO. Epithelial Tumors of the Lacrimal Gland: An Update. Curr Opin Ophthalmol. 2008 Sep;19(5):409–13. PMID:18772674

313. Bernardini FP, Orcioni GF, Croxatto JO. Oncocytic Carcinoma of the Lacrimal Gland in a Patient with Neurofibromatosis. Ophthalmic Plast Reconstr Surg. 2010 Nov-Dec;26(6):486–8. PMID:20700068

314. Bernard-Pierrot I, Brams A, Dunois-Lardé C, et al. Oncogenic Properties of the Mutated Forms of Fibroblast Growth Factor Receptor 3b. Carcinogenesis. 2006 Apr;27(4):740–7. PMID:16338952

315. Bernstein KE, Lattes R. Nodular (Pseudosarcomatous) Fasciitis, a Nonrecurrent Lesion: Clinicopathologic Study of 134 Cases. Cancer. 1982 Apr 15;49(8):1668–78. PMID:6279273

316. Berres ML, Lim KP, Peters T, et al. BRAF-V600E Expression in Precursor Versus Differentiated Dendritic Cells Defines Clinically Distinct LCH Risk Groups. J Exp Med. 2014 Apr 7;211(4):669–83. PMID:24638167

317. Berry JL, Bechtold M, Shah S, et al. Not All Seeds Are Created Equal: Seed Classification Is Predictive of Outcomes in Retinoblastoma. Ophthalmology. 2017 Dec;124(12):1817–25. PMID:28655537

318. Berry M, Mankin H, Gebhardt M, et al. Osteoblastoma: A 30-Year Study of 99 Cases. J Surg Oncol. 2008 Sep 1;98(3):179–83. PMID:18561153

319. Bertagnoli R, Cook DL, Goldman GD. Bilateral Primary Mucinous Carcinoma of the Eyelid Treated with Mohs Surgery. Dermatol Surg. 1999 Jul;25(7):566–8. PMID:10469115

320. Bertoni F, Bacchini P, Capanna R, et al. Solid Variant of Aneurysmal Bone Cyst. Cancer. 1993 Feb 1;71(3):729–34. PMID:8431852

321. Bertschinger D, Oberic A, Moulin A, et al. Malignant Transformation of a 'Benign' Lacrimal Gland Tumor. Klin Monbl Augenheilkd. 2010 Apr;227(4):321–3. PMID:20408086

322. Betharia SM, Arora R, Kishore K, et al. Leiomyoma of the Orbit. Indian J Ophthalmol. 1991 Jan-Mar;39(1):35–7. PMID:1894345

323. Betz CS, Leunig A, Janda P, et al. [Adenocarcinoma in the Tear Sack After Endonasal Dacryocystorhinostomy]. HNO. 2005 Mar;53(3):257–62. German. PMID:15060713

324. Beutler BD, Cohen PR. Molluscum Contagiosum of the Eyelid: Case Report in a Man Receiving Methotrexate and Literature Review of Molluscum Contagiosum in Patients Who Are Immunosuppressed Secondary to Methotrexate or HIV Infection. Dermatol Online J. 2016 Mar 16;22(3):13030/Qt8vz669cj. PMID:27136625

325. Beutner KR, Becker TM, Stone KM. Epidemiology of Human Papillomavirus Infections. Dermatol Clin. 1991 Apr;9(2):211–8. PMID:1647901

326. Beykin G, Pe'er J, Amir G, et al. Paediatric and Adolescent Elevated Conjunctival Lesions in the Plical Area: Lymphoma or Reactive Lymphoid Hyperplasia? Br J Ophthalmol. 2014 May;98(5):645–50. PMID:24162623

327. Bhaijee F, Brown AS. Muir-Torre Syndrome. Arch Pathol Lab Med. 2014 Dec;138(12):1685–9. PMID:25427047

328. Bhatia A, Hatzoglou V, Ulaner G, et al. Neurologic and Oncologic Features of Erdheim-Chester Disease: A 30-Patient Series. Neuro Oncol. 2020 Jul 7;22(7):979–92. PMID:31950179

329. Bhatnagar R, Kalra VK. Intraoperative Induced Miosis in Posterior Chamber I.O.L. Implantation. Indian J Ophthalmol. 1987;35(5-6):242–5. PMID:3508781

330. Bhawan J, Silva C, Taungjaruwinai WM. Inconsistent Immunohistochemical Expression of Lymphatic and Blood Endothelial Cell Markers in Cutaneous Lymphangiomas. J Cutan Pathol. 2013 Sep;40(9):801–6. PMID:23782346

331. Bhushan G, Raina UK, Gupta A, et al. Inverted Mucoepidermoid Papilloma of Conjunctiva in a Child. J AAPOS. 2015 Jun;19(3):266–7. PMID:25813286

332. Bi YW, Chen RJ, Li XP. [Clinical and Pathological Analysis of Primary Lacrimal Sac Tumors]. Zhonghua Yan Ke Za Zhi. 2007 Jun;43(6):499–504. Chinese. PMID:17897525

333. Bianciotto C, Demirci H, Shields CL, et al. Metastatic Tumors to the Eyelid: Report of 20 Cases and Review of the Literature. Arch Ophthalmol. 2009 Aug;127(8):999–1005. PMID:19667336

334. Bihr S, Ohashi R, Moore AL, et al. Expression and Mutation Patterns of PBRM1,

BAP1 and SETD2 Mirror Specific Evolutionary Subtypes in Clear Cell Renal Cell Carcinoma. Neoplasia. 2019 Feb;21(2):247–56. PMID:30660076
335. Billecke L, Murga Penas EM, May AM, et al. Cytogenetics of Extramedullary Manifestations in Multiple Myeloma. Br J Haematol. 2013 Apr;161(1):87–94. PMID:23368088
336. Binderup ML, Bisgaard ML, Harbud V, et al. Von Hippel-Lindau Disease (VHL). National Clinical Guideline for Diagnosis and Surveillance in Denmark. 3rd Edition. Dan Med J. 2013 Dec;60(12):b4763. PMID:24355456
337. Binderup MLM, Stendell AS, Galanakis M, et al. Retinal Hemangioblastoma: Prevalence, Incidence and Frequency of Underlying von Hippel-Lindau Disease. Br J Ophthalmol. 2018 Jul;102(7):942–7. PMID:28972023
338. Bink K, Haralambieva E, Kremer M, et al. Primary Extramedullary Plasmacytoma: Similarities with and Differences from Multiple Myeloma Revealed by Interphase Cytogenetics. Haematologica. 2008 Apr;93(4):623–6. PMID:18326524
339. Binotti W, Hamrah P. COVID-19-Related Conjunctivitis Review: Clinical Features and Management. Ocul Immunol Inflamm. 2023 May;31(4):778–84. PMID:35394858
340. Bisceglia M, Muscarella LA, Galliani CA, et al. Extraneuraxial Hemangioblastoma: Clinicopathologic Features and Review of the Literature. Adv Anat Pathol. 2018 May;25(3):197–215. PMID:29189208
341. Bishop JA. OSPs and ESPs and ISPs, Oh My! An Update on Sinonasal (Schneiderian) Papillomas. Head Neck Pathol. 2017 Sep;11(3):269–77. PMID:28321771
342. Bishop JA, Guo TW, Smith DF, et al. Human Papillomavirus-Related Carcinomas of the Sinonasal Tract. Am J Surg Pathol. 2013 Feb;37(2):185–92. PMID:23095507
343. Bishop JA, Rooper LM, Sangoi AR, et al. The Myoepithelial Cells of Salivary Intercalated Duct-Type Intraductal Carcinoma Are Neoplastic: A Study Using Combined Whole-Slide Imaging, Immunofluorescence, and RET Fluorescence In Situ Hybridization. Am J Surg Pathol. 2021 Apr 1;45(4):507–15. PMID:33086236
344. Bishop JA, Westra WH. MYB Translocation Status in Salivary Gland Epithelial-Myoepithelial Carcinoma: Evaluation of Classic, Variant, and Hybrid Forms. Am J Surg Pathol. 2018 Mar;42(3):319–25. PMID:29135517
345. Bishop JA, Yonescu R, Batista DA, et al. Cytopathologic Features of Mammary Analogue Secretory Carcinoma. Cancer Cytopathol. 2013 May;121(5):228–33. PMID:23042752
346. Biswas J, Bhushan B, Jayakumar N, et al. Teratoid Malignant Medulloepithelioma of the Optic Nerve: Report of a Case and Review of the Literature. Orbit. 1999 Sep;18(3):191–6. PMID:12045984
347. Biswas J, Kabra S, Krishnakumar S, et al. Clinical and Histopathological Characteristics of Uveal Melanoma in Asian Indians. A Study of 103 Patients. Indian J Ophthalmol. 2004 Mar;52(1):41–4. PMID:15132378
348. Bjorkengren AG, Resnick D, Haghighi P, et al. Intraosseous Glomus Tumor: Report of a Case and Review of the Literature. AJR Am J Roentgenol. 1986 Oct;147(4):739–41. PMID:3019113
349. Blackburn PR, Davila JI, Jackson RA, et al. RNA Sequencing Identifies a Novel USP9X-USP6 Promoter Swap Gene Fusion in a Primary Aneurysmal Bone Cyst. Genes Chromosomes Cancer. 2019 Aug;58(8):589–94. PMID:30767316
350. Blakeley JO, Bakker A, Barker A, et al. The Path Forward: 2015 International Children's Tumor Foundation Conference on Neurofibromatosis Type 1, Type 2, and Schwannomatosis. Am J Med Genet A. 2017 Jun;173(6):1714–21. PMID:28436162
351. Blakeley JO, Plotkin SR. Therapeutic Advances for the Tumors Associated with Neurofibromatosis Type 1, Type 2, and Schwannomatosis. Neuro Oncol. 2016 May;18(5):624–38. PMID:26851632
352. Blasi MA, Maceroni M, Musarra T, et al. Adenocarcinoma NOS Arising from Accessory Lacrimal Glands: A Case Report and a Review of the Literature. Eur J Ophthalmol. 2022 Jul;32(4):nP71–7. PMID:33663254
353. Bledsoe JR, Wallace ZS, Deshpande V, et al. Atypical IgG4+ Plasmacytic Proliferations and Lymphomas: Characterization of 11 Cases. Am J Clin Pathol. 2017 Sep 1;148(3):215–35. PMID:28821195
354. Bledsoe JR, Wallace ZS, Stone JH, et al. Lymphomas in IgG4-Related Disease: Clinicopathologic Features in a Western Population. Virchows Arch. 2018 May;472(5):839–52. PMID:29285637
355. Bleeker JS, Quevedo JF, Folpe AL. "Malignant" Perivascular Epithelioid Cell Neoplasm: Risk Stratification and Treatment Strategies. Sarcoma. 2012;2012:541626. PMID:22619565
356. Blesinger H, Kaulfuß S, Aung T, et al. PIK3CA Mutations Are Specifically Localized to Lymphatic Endothelial Cells of Lymphatic Malformations. PLoS One. 2018 Jul 9;13(7):e0200343. PMID:29985963
357. Blessing NW, Bermudez-Magner JA, Fernandez MP, et al. Solitary Fibrous Tumor of the Orbit: A Case Series With Clinicopathologic Correlation and Evaluation of STAT6 as a Diagnostic Marker. Ophthalmic Plast Reconstr Surg. 2020 Mar/Apr;36(2):164–71. PMID:31876648
358. Blicker JA, Rootman J, White VA. Cellular Blue Nevus of the Conjunctiva. Ophthalmology. 1992 Nov;99(11):1714–7. PMID:1454347
359. Bloch RS, Gartner S. The Incidence of Ocular Metastatic Carcinoma. Arch Ophthalmol. 1971 Jun;85(6):673–5. PMID:5562786
360. Blodi FC. Leiomyoma of the Ciliary Body. Am J Ophthalmol. 1950 Jun;33(6):939–42. PMID:15419251
361. Blodi FC, Reuling FH, Sornson ET. Pseudomelanocytoma at the Optic Nervehead: An Adenoma of the Retinal Pigment Epithelium. Arch Ophthalmol. 1965 Mar;73:353–5. PMID:14246189
362. Blombery P, Anderson MA, Gong JN, et al. Acquisition of the Recurrent Gly101Val Mutation in BCL2 Confers Resistance to Venetoclax in Patients with Progressive Chronic Lymphocytic Leukemia. Cancer Discov. 2019 Mar;9(3):342–53. PMID:30514704
363. Boehlke CS, Frueh BR, Flint A, et al. Malignant Fibrous Histiocytoma of the Lateral Conjunctiva and Anterior Orbit. Ophthalmic Plast Reconstr Surg. 2007 Jul-Aug;23(4):338–40. PMID:17667121
364. Bogusiak K, Puch A, Arkuszewski P. Goldenhar Syndrome: Current Perspectives. World J Pediatr. 2017 Oct;13(5):405–15. PMID:28623555
365. Böhringer D, Birnbaum F, Reinhard T. [Cyclosporin A Eyedrops for Keratitis Nummularis After Adenovirus Keratoconjunctivitis]. Ophthalmologe. 2008 Jun;105(6):592–4. German. PMID:18365204
366. Boldrey EE, Schwartz A. Enlargement of Congenital Hypertrophy of the Retinal Pigment Epithelium. Am J Ophthalmol. 1982 Jul;94(1):64–6. PMID:7091284
367. Boley S, Sloan JL, Pemov A, et al. A Quantitative Assessment of the Burden and Distribution of Lisch Nodules in Adults with Neurofibromatosis Type 1. Invest Ophthalmol Vis Sci. 2009 Nov;50(11):5035–43. PMID:19516012
368. Bolzoni A, Pianta L, Farina D, et al. Benign Myoepithelioma of the Lacrimal Gland: Report of a Case. Eur Arch Otorhinolaryngol. 2005 Mar;262(3):186–8. PMID:15138773
369. Bonavolontà G, Tranfa F, de Conciliis C, et al. Dermoid Cysts: 16-Year Survey. Ophthalmic Plast Reconstr Surg. 1995 Sep;11(3):187–92. PMID:8541260
370. Bonder D, Fischer MJ, Levine MR. Squamous Cell Carcinoma of the Lacrimal Sac. Ophthalmology. 1983 Sep;90(9):1133–5. PMID:6646653
371. Bonetti F, Martignoni G, Colato C, et al. Abdominopelvic Sarcoma of Perivascular Epithelioid Cells. Report of Four Cases in Young Women, One with Tuberous Sclerosis. Mod Pathol. 2001 Jun;14(6):563–8. PMID:11406657
372. Boniuk M, Zimmerman LE. Epibulbar Osteoma (Episcleral Osseous Choristoma). Am J Ophthalmol. 1962 Feb;53:290–6. PMID:13871021
373. Boniuk M, Zimmerman LE. Pilomatrixoma (Benign Calcifying Epithelioma) of the Eyelids and Eyebrow. Arch Ophthalmol. 1963 Sep;70:399–406. PMID:14048805
374. Bonnet LA, Conway RM, Lim LA. Congenital Hypertrophy of the Retinal Pigment Epithelium (CHRPE) as a Screening Marker for Familial Adenomatous Polyposis (FAP): Systematic Literature Review and Screening Recommendations. Clin Ophthalmol. 2022 Mar 15;16:765–74. PMID:35321042
375. Bonnet P, Chasset F, Moguelet P, et al. Erdheim-Chester Disease Associated with Chronic Myelomonocytic Leukemia Harboring the Same Clonal Mutation. Haematologica. 2019 Nov;104(11):e530–3. PMID:31221777
376. Bonometti A, Berti E; for Associazione Italiana Ricerca Istiocitosi ONLUS. Reticulohistiocytoses: A Revision of the Full Spectrum. J Eur Acad Dermatol Venereol. 2020 Aug;34(8):1684–94. PMID:31955466
377. Bonometti A; for Associazione Italiana Ricerca Istiocitosi AIRI ONLUS. The Triptych of Mixed Histiocytosis: A Systematic Review of 105 Cases and Proposed Clinical Classification. Leuk Lymphoma. 2021 Jan;62(1):32–44. PMID:32969291
378. Bonzheim I, Giese S, Deuter C, et al. High Frequency of MYD88 Mutations in Vitreoretinal B-Cell Lymphoma: A Valuable Tool to Improve Diagnostic Yield of Vitreous Aspirates. Blood. 2015 Jul 2;126(1):76–9. PMID:25900979
379. Bonzheim I, Sander P, Salmerón-Villalobos J, et al. The Molecular Hallmarks of Primary and Secondary Vitreoretinal Lymphoma. Blood Adv. 2022 Mar 8;6(5):1598–607. PMID:34448823
380. Booman M, Douwes J, Glas AM, et al. Mechanisms and Effects of Loss of Human Leukocyte Antigen Class II Expression in Immune-Privileged Site-Associated B-Cell Lymphoma. Clin Cancer Res. 2006 May 1;12(9):2698–705. PMID:16675561
381. Boon LM, Mulliken JB, Enjolras O, et al. Glomuvenous Malformation (Glomangioma) and Venous Malformation: Distinct Clinicopathologic and Genetic Entities. Arch Dermatol. 2004 Aug;140(8):971–6. PMID:15313813
382. Borbolla-Pertierra AM, Morales-Baños DR, Martínez-Nava LR, et al. Orbital Liposarcoma. Arch Soc Esp Oftalmol. 2017 Feb;92(2):86–92. PMID:27236610
383. Borges T, Silva S. IgG4-Related Disease: How to Place it in the Spectrum of Immune-Mediated and Rheumatologic Disorders? Mod Rheumatol. 2020 Jul;30(4):609–16. PMID:31852351
384. Borit A, Richardson EP Jr. The Biological and Clinical Behaviour of Pilocytic Astrocytomas of the Optic Pathways. Brain. 1982 Mar;105(Pt 1):161–87. PMID:7066671
385. Bor-Shavit E, Hammel N, Nahum Y, et al. Visual Disability Rates in a Ten-Year Cohort of Patients with Anterior Visual Pathway Meningiomas. Disabil Rehabil. 2015;37(11):958–62. PMID:25133857
386. Bortz JG, Zhang PJL, Eagle RC Jr, et al. Secretory Carcinoma of the Lacrimal Gland: A Rare Case Report. Ophthalmic Plast Reconstr Surg. 2018 Sep/Oct;34(5):e154–7. PMID:30059394
387. Bosch MM, Wichmann WW, Boltshauser E, et al. Optic Nerve Sheath Meningiomas in Patients with Neurofibromatosis Type 2. Arch Ophthalmol. 2006 Mar;124(3):379–85. PMID:16534058
388. Boscolo E, Coma S, Luks VL, et al. AKT Hyper-Phosphorylation Associated with PI3K Mutations in Lymphatic Endothelial Cells from a Patient with Lymphatic Malformation. Angiogenesis. 2015 Apr;18(2):151–62. PMID:25424831
389. Bott M, Brevet M, Taylor BS, et al. The Nuclear Deubiquitinase BAP1 is Commonly Inactivated by Somatic Mutations and 3p21.1 Losses in Malignant Pleural Mesothelioma. Nat Genet. 2011 Jun 5;43(7):668–72. PMID:21642991
390. Boudhas A, Allaoui M, El Asri F, et al. Inflammatory Myofibroblastic Tumor of the Lacrimal Gland: Case Report of an Exceptional Location. BMC Clin Pathol. 2017 Aug 17;17:12. PMID:28824333
391. Boulland ML, Wechsler J, Bagot M, et al. Primary CD30-Positive Cutaneous T-Cell Lymphomas and Lymphomatoid Papulosis Frequently Express Cytotoxic Proteins. Histopathology. 2000 Feb;36(2):136–44. PMID:10672058
392. Bourlon C, Lipton JH, Deotare U, et al. Extramedullary Disease at Diagnosis of AML Does Not Influence Outcome of Patients Undergoing Allogeneic Hematopoietic Cell Transplant in CR1. Eur J Haematol. 2017 Sep;99(3):234–9. PMID:28556258
393. Boussemart L, Routier E, Mateus C, et al. Prospective Study of Cutaneous Side-Effects Associated with the BRAF Inhibitor Vemurafenib: A Study of 42 Patients. Ann Oncol. 2013 Jun;24(6):1691–7. PMID:23406731
394. Bouzas EA, Mastorakos G, Chrousos GP, et al. Lisch Nodules in Cushing's Disease. Arch Ophthalmol. 1993 Apr;111(4):439–40. PMID:8470969
395. Bowen JH, Christensen FH, Klintworth GK, et al. A Clinicopathologic Study of a Cartilaginous Hamartoma of the Orbit: A Rare Cause of Proptosis. Ophthalmology. 1981 Dec;88(12):1356–60. PMID:7322488
396. Bowman CB, Guber D, Brown CH 3rd, et al. Cutaneous Malignant Melanoma with Diffuse Intraocular Metastases. Arch Ophthalmol. 1994 Sep;112(9):1213–6. PMID:8085965
397. Boyd LC, O'Brien KJ, Ozkaya N, et al. Neurological Manifestations of Erdheim-Chester Disease. Ann Clin Transl Neurol. 2020 Apr;7(4):497–506. PMID:32227455
398. Boye E, Yu Y, Paranya G, et al. Clonality and Altered Behavior of Endothelial Cells from Hemangiomas. J Clin Invest. 2001 Mar;107(6):745–52. PMID:11254674
399. Bradfield Y, Burkat CN, Albert DM, et al. Capillary Hemangioma Presenting as a Scleral Vascular Lesion in a Child. Ophthalmic Plast Reconstr Surg. 2019 Sep/Oct;35(5):e115–6. PMID:31503170
400. Brandwein-Gensler M, Hille J, Wang BY, et al. Low-Grade Salivary Duct Carcinoma: Description of 16 Cases. Am J Surg Pathol. 2004 Aug;28(8):1040–4. PMID:15252310
401. Brannan PA, Cetinkaya A, Kim AS, et al. Solitary Orbital Plasmacytoma Associated with Chronic Hepatitis C: A Case Report. Orbit. 2009;28(1):71–3. PMID:19229750
402. Brannan PA, Kersten RC, Schneider S, et al. A Case of Primary Adenocarcinoma of the

Lacrimal Sac. Orbit. 2005 Dec;24(4):291–3. PMID:16354642
403. Brannan SO, Cheung D, Trotter S, et al. A Conjunctival Leiomyoma. Am J Ophthalmol. 2003 Oct;136(4):749–50. PMID:14516824
404. Branstetter DG, Nelson SD, Manivel JC, et al. Denosumab Induces Tumor Reduction and Bone Formation in Patients with Giant-Cell Tumor of Bone. Clin Cancer Res. 2012 Aug 15;18(16):4415–24. PMID:22711702
405. Brazzo BG, Saffra N. Dermatofibrosarcoma Protuberans of the Brow and Eyelid. Ophthalmic Plast Reconstr Surg. 2004 Jul;20(4):332–4. PMID:15266155
406. Bredow L, Martin G, Reinhard T, et al. Recurrent Conjunctival Papilloma Progressing into Squamous Cell Carcinoma with Change of HPV-Finding During the Course. Br J Ophthalmol. 2009 Nov;93(11):1437, 1451. PMID:19692355
407. Brems H, Beert E, de Ravel T, et al. Mechanisms in the Pathogenesis of Malignant Tumours in Neurofibromatosis Type 1. Lancet Oncol. 2009 May;10(5):508–15. PMID:19410195
408. Brems H, Park C, Maertens O, et al. Glomus Tumors in Neurofibromatosis Type 1: Genetic, Functional, and Clinical Evidence of a Novel Association. Cancer Res. 2009 Sep 15;69(18):7393–401. PMID:19738042
409. Brent AJ, Mota PM, Nebojsa A, et al. Squamous Cell Carcinoma Arising from Syringocystadenoma Papilliferum of the Eyelid. Can J Ophthalmol. 2017 Dec;52(6):e235–7. PMID:29217053
410. Bresler SC, Simon C, Shields CL, et al. Conjunctival Melanocytic Lesions. Arch Pathol Lab Med. 2022 May 1;146(5):632–46. PMID:34424954
411. Bresters D, Zwaan CM, Veerman AJ, et al. A Three-Year-Old Girl with a Yolk Sac Tumor in the Orbit/Maxillary Sinus. Med Pediatr Oncol. 2003 Jan;40(1):70–1. PMID:12426694
412. Brice SL, Jester JD, Friednash M, et al. Examination of Cutaneous T-Cell Lymphoma for Human Herpesviruses by Using the Polymerase Chain Reaction. J Cutan Pathol. 1993 Aug;20(4):304–7. PMID:8227605
413. Bridge JA, Bhatia PS, Anderson JR, et al. Biologic and Clinical Significance of Cytogenetic and Molecular Cytogenetic Abnormalities in Benign and Malignant Cartilaginous Lesions. Cancer Genet Cytogenet. 1993 Sep;69(2):79–90. PMID:8402563
414. Brierley JD, Gospodarowicz MK, Wittekind C, editors. TNM Classification of Malignant Tumours. 8th ed. Oxford (UK): Wiley-Blackwell; 2017.
415. Bright CJ, Hawkins MM, Winter DL, et al. Risk of Soft-Tissue Sarcoma Among 69 460 Five-Year Survivors of Childhood Cancer in Europe. J Natl Cancer Inst. 2018 Jun 1;110(6):649–60. PMID:29165710
416. Broaddus E, Topham A, Singh AD. Incidence of Retinoblastoma in the USA: 1975-2004. Br J Ophthalmol. 2009 Jan;93(1):21–3. PMID:18621794
417. Broekaert SM, Flux K, Kyrpychova L, et al. Squared-Off Nuclei and "Appliqué" Pattern as a Histopathological Clue to Periocular Sebaceous Carcinoma: A Clinicopathological Study of 50 Neoplasms From 46 Patients. Am J Dermatopathol. 2017 Apr;39(4):275–8. PMID:28323778
418. Bronkhorst IH, Ly LV, Jordanova ES, et al. Detection of M2-Macrophages in Uveal Melanoma and Relation with Survival. Invest Ophthalmol Vis Sci. 2011 Feb 3;52(2):643–50. PMID:20811059
419. Bronkhorst IH, Vu TH, Jordanova ES, et al. Different Subsets of Tumor-Infiltrating Lymphocytes Correlate with Macrophage Influx and Monosomy 3 in Uveal Melanoma. Invest Ophthalmol Vis Sci. 2012 Aug 9;53(9):5370–8. PMID:22743317
420. Brookes JL, Bentley C, Verma S, et al. Microcystic Adnexal Carcinoma Masquerading as a Chalazion. Br J Ophthalmol. 1998 Feb;82(2):196–7. PMID:9613389
421. Broughton WL, Zimmerman LE. A Clinicopathologic Study of 56 Cases of Intraocular Medulloepitheliomas. Am J Ophthalmol 1978 Mar;85(3):407–18. PMID:655220
422. Brouillard P, Boon LM, Mulliken JB, et al. Mutations in a Novel Factor, Glomulin, Are Responsible for Glomuvenous Malformations ("Glomangiomas"). Am J Hum Genet. 2002 Apr;70(4):866–74. PMID:11845407
423. Brouwer NJ, Gezgin G, Wierenga AFA, et al. Tumour Angiogenesis in Uveal Melanoma Is Related to Genetic Evolution. Cancers (Basel). 2019 Jul 13;11(7):979. PMID:31337000
424. Brouwer NJ, Marinkovic M, Bleeker JC, et al. Anterior Segment OCTA of Melanocytic Lesions of the Conjunctiva and Iris. Am J Ophthalmol. 2021 Feb;222:137–47. PMID:32926848
425. Brouwer NJ, Marinkovic M, Luyten GPM, et al. Lack of Tumour Pigmentation in Conjunctival Melanoma is Associated with Light Iris Colour and Worse Prognosis. Br J Ophthalmol. 2019 Mar;103(3):332–7. PMID:29777046
426. Brouwer NJ, Marinkovic M, van Duinen SG, et al. Treatment of Conjunctival Melanoma in a Dutch Referral Centre. Br J Ophthalmol. 2018 Sep;102(9):1277–82. PMID:29122819
427. Brouwer NJ, Verdijk RM, Heegaard S, et al. Conjunctival Melanoma: New Insights in Tumour Genetics and Immunology, Leading to New Therapeutic Options. Prog Retin Eye Res. 2022 Jan;86:100971. PMID:34015548
428. Brown HA, Sawyer DM, Woo T. Intraepidermal Merkel Cell Carcinoma with No Dermal Involvement. Am J Dermatopathol. 2000 Feb;22(1):65–9. PMID:10698220
429. Brownstein MH, Shapiro L. Trichilemmoma. Analysis of 40 New Cases. Arch Dermatol. 1973 Jun;107(6):866–9. PMID:4711118
430. Brownstein S, Little JM. Ocular Neurofibromatosis. Ophthalmology. 1983 Dec;90(12):1595–9. PMID:6429597
431. Bruce-Brand C, Schneider JW, Schubert P. Rosai-Dorfman Disease: An Overview. J Clin Pathol. 2020 Nov;73(11):697–705. PMID:32591351
432. Bruder E, Alaggio R, Kozakewich HP, et al. Vascular and Perivascular Lesions of Skin and Soft Tissues in Children and Adolescents. Pediatr Dev Pathol. 2012;15(1 Suppl):26–61. PMID:22420724
432A. Bruford EA, Antonescu CR, Carroll AJ, et al. HUGO Gene Nomenclature Committee (HGNC) Recommendations for the Designation of Gene Fusions. Leukemia. 2021 Nov;35(11):3040–3. PMID:34615987.
433. Bruggink SC, Eekhof JA, Egberts PF, et al. Natural Course of Cutaneous Warts Among Primary Schoolchildren: A Prospective Cohort Study. Ann Fam Med. 2013 Sep-Oct;11(5):437–41. PMID:24019275
434. Bryar P, Sun R, Ebroon D. Nasolacrimal Duct Obstruction Secondary to Dermatofibrosarcoma Protuberans. Ophthalmology. 2004 Jul;111(7):1398–400. PMID:15234144
435. Bubien V, Bonnet F, Brouste V, et al. High Cumulative Risks of Cancer in Patients with PTEN Hamartoma Tumour Syndrome. J Med Genet. 2013 Apr;50(4):255–63. PMID:23335809
436. Bueno R, Stawiski EW, Goldstein LD, et al. Comprehensive Genomic Analysis of Malignant Pleural Mesothelioma Identifies Recurrent Mutations, Gene Fusions and Splicing Alterations. Nat Genet. 2016 Apr;48(4):407–16. PMID:26928227
437. Buettner H. Congenital Hypertrophy of the Retinal Pigment Epithelium. Am J Ophthalmol. 1975 Feb;79(2):177–89. PMID:1115190
438. Bui M, Frank SJ, Nasser QJ, et al. Multidisciplinary Management of Primary Adenoid Cystic Carcinoma of the Eyelid with Perineural Invasion. Ophthalmic Plast Reconstr Surg. 2013 Nov-Dec;29(6):e143–6. PMID:23446295
439. Bui T, Young JW, Frausto RF, et al. Hereditary Benign Intraepithelial Dyskeratosis: Report of a Case and Re-Examination of the Evidence for Locus Heterogeneity. Ophthalmic Genet. 2016;37(1):76–80. PMID:24555743
440. Bulbul A. Lacrimal Gland Adenocarcinoma Responding to Checkpoint Inhibition and Androgen Deprivation. Oxf Med Case Reports. 2018 Aug 25;2018(9):omy066. PMID:30159157
441. Bullen R, Snow SN, Larson PO, et al. Multiple Agminated Spitz Nevi: Report of Two Cases and Review of the Literature. Pediatr Dermatol. 1995 Jun;12(2):156–8. PMID:7659643
442. Bullock JD, Goldberg SH, Rakes SM. Orbital Tumors in Children. Ophthalmic Plast Reconstr Surg. 1989;5(1):13–6. PMID:2487190
443. Bunod R, Adams D, Cauquil C, et al. Conjunctival Lymphangiectasia as a Biomarker of Severe Systemic Disease in Ser-77Tyr Hereditary Transthyretin Amyloidosis. Br J Ophthalmol. 2020 Oct;104(10):1363–7. PMID:31949094
444. Burg G, Kempf W, Kazakov DV, et al. Pyogenic Lymphoma of the Skin: A Peculiar Variant of Primary Cutaneous Neutrophil-Rich CD30+ Anaplastic Large-Cell Lymphoma. Clinicopathological Study of Four Cases and Review of the Literature. Br J Dermatol. 2003 Mar;148(3):580–6. PMID:12653754
445. Burgdorf WH, Pitha J, Fahmy A. Muir-Torre Syndrome. Histologic Spectrum of Sebaceous Proliferations. Am J Dermatopathol. 1986 Jun;8(3):202–8. PMID:3728878
446. Burger JA, Barr PM, Robak T, et al. Long-Term Efficacy and Safety of First-Line Ibrutinib Treatment for Patients with CLL/SLL: 5 Years of Follow-Up from the Phase 3 RESONATE-2 Study. Leukemia. 2020 Mar;34(3):787–98. PMID:31628428
447. Burk RO, Völcker HE, Daus W, et al. [Mesectodermal Leiomyoma of the Ciliary Body–Clinical Aspects, Surgery and Immunohistochemistry]. Fortschr Ophthalmol. 1989;86(6):631–5. German. PMID:2696714
448. Burkat CN, Van Buren JJ, Lucarelli MJ. Characteristics of Orbital Multiple Myeloma: A Case Report and Literature Review. Surv Ophthalmol. 2009 Nov-Dec;54(6):697–704. PMID:19709708
449. Burr JM, Mitry E, Rachet B, et al. Survival from Uveal Melanoma in England and Wales 1986 to 2001. Ophthalmic Epidemiol. 2007 Jan-Feb;14(1):3–8. PMID:17365812
450. Burris CK, Rodriguez ME, Raven ML. Melanomalytic Glaucoma. Ophthalmology. 2015 Dec;122(12):2422. PMID:26592671
451. Bursztyn LL, Hyrcza MD, Allen LH, et al. Low-Grade Intraductal Carcinoma of the Lacrimal Gland. Orbit. 2014 Apr;33(2):135–8. PMID:24195727
452. Busam KJ, Fang Y, Jhanwar SC, et al. Distinction of Conjunctival Melanocytic Nevi from Melanomas by Fluorescence In Situ Hybridization. J Cutan Pathol. 2010 Feb;37(2):196–203. PMID:20100177
453 Cabaret O, Perron E, Bressac-de Paillerets B, et al. Occurrence of BAP1 Germline Mutations in Cutaneous Melanocytic Tumors with Loss of BAP1-Expression: A Pilot Study. Genes Chromosomes Cancer. 2017 Sep;56(9):691–4. PMID:28560743
454. Cacciamani A, Scarinci F, Parravano M, et al. Choroidal Thickness Changes with Photodynamic Therapy for a Diffuse Choroidal Hemangioma in Sturge–Weber Syndrome. Int Ophthalmol. 2014 Oct;34(5):1131–5. PMID:24658736
455. Cadet J, Douki T. Formation of UV-Induced DNA Damage Contributing to Skin Cancer Development. Photochem Photobiol Sci. 2018 Dec 5;17(12):1816–41. PMID:29405222
456. Caers J, Paiva B, Zamagni E, et al. Diagnosis, Treatment and Response Assessment in Solitary Plasmacytoma: Updated Recommendations from a European Expert Panel. J Hematol Oncol. 2018 Jan 16;11(1):10. PMID:29338789
457. Cai R, Zhang C, Chen R, et al. Clinicopathological Features of a Suspected Case of Hereditary Benign Intraepithelial Dyskeratosis with Bilateral Corneas Involved: A Case Report and Mini Review. Cornea. 2011 Dec;30(12):1481–4. PMID:21993456
458. Cai Y, Shi Z, Bai Y. Review of Rosai-Dorfman Disease: New Insights into the Pathogenesis of This Rare Disorder. Acta Haematol 2017;138(1):14–23. PMID:28614806
459. Cajucom-Uy H, Tong L, Wong TY, et al. The Prevalence of and Risk Factors for Pterygium in an Urban Malay Population: The Singapore Malay Eye Study (SiMES). Br J Ophthalmol. 2010 Aug;94(8):977–81. PMID:19965830
460. Calandriello L, Grimaldi G, Petrone G, et al. Cavernous Venous Malformation (Cavernous Hemangioma) of the Orbit: Current Concepts and a Review of the Literature. Surv Ophthalmol. 2017 Jul-Aug;62(4):393–403. PMID:28131871
461. Calle CA, Castillo G, Eagle RC, et al. Oncocytoma of the Lacrimal Gland: Case Report and Review of the Literature. Orbit. 2006 Sep;25(3):243–7. PMID:16987774
462. Calonje E, Fletcher CD. Myoid Differentiation in Dermatofibrosarcoma Protuberans and its Fibrosarcomatous Variant: Clinicopathologic Analysis of 5 Cases. J Cutan Pathol. 1996 Feb;23(1):30–6. PMID:8720984
463. Caltabiano R, Magro G, Polizzi A, et al. A Mosaic Pattern of INI1/SMARCB1 Protein Expression Distinguishes Schwannomatosis and NF2-Associated Peripheral Schwannomas from Solitary Peripheral Schwannomas and NF2-Associated Vestibular Schwannomas. Childs Nerv Syst. 2017 Jun;33(6):933–40. PMID:28365909
464. Cambiaghi S, Restano L, Caputo R. Juvenile Xanthogranuloma Associated with Neurofibromatosis 1: 14 Patients Without Evidence of Hematologic Malignancies. Pediatr Dermatol. 2004 Mar-Apr;21(2):97–101. PMID:15078345
465. Campbell RJ, Min KW, Bolling JP. Skeinoid Fibers in Mesectodermal Leiomyoma of the Ciliary Body. Ultrastruct Pathol. 1997 Nov-Dec;21(6):559–67. PMID:9355238
466. Campo E, Cymbalista F, Ghia P, et al. TP53 Aberrations in Chronic Lymphocytic Leukemia: An Overview of the Clinical Implications of Improved Diagnostics. Haematologica. 2018 Dec;103(12):1956–68. PMID:30442727
467. Campochiaro C, Ramirez GA, Bozzolo EP, et al. IgG4-Related Disease in Italy: Clinical Features and Outcomes of a Large Cohort of Patients. Scand J Rheumatol. 2016;45(2):135–45. PMID:26398142
468. Cancer Genome Atlas Network. Genomic Classification of Cutaneous Melanoma. Cell. 2015 Jun 18;161(7):1681–96. PMID:26091043
469. Cancer Genome Atlas Research Network. Comprehensive and Integrated Genomic Characterization of Adult Soft Tissue Sarcomas. Cell. 2017 Nov 2;171(4):950–965.E28. PMID:29100075
470. Canelas MM, Cardoso JC, Andrade PF et al. Fibrous Histiocytomas: Histopathologic Review of 95 Cases. An Bras Dermatol. 2010

Mar-Apr;85(2):211–5. PMID:20520936
471. Cani AK, Soliman M, Hovelson DH, et al. Comprehensive Genomic Profiling of Orbital and Ocular Adnexal Lymphomas Identifies Frequent Alterations in MYD88 and Chromatin Modifiers: New Routes to Targeted Therapies. Mod Pathol. 2016 Jul;29(7):685–97. PMID:27102345
472. Cani AK, Toral MA, Balikov DA, et al. Molecular Characterization of a Rare Case of Bilateral Vitreoretinal T Cell Lymphoma Through Vitreous Liquid Biopsy. Int J Mol Sci. 2021 Jun 5;22(11):6099. PMID:34198843
473. Cantley LC. The Phosphoinositide 3-Kinase Pathway. Science. 2002 May 31;296(5573):1655–7. PMID:12040186
474. Canturk S, Qaddoumi I, Khetan V, et al. Survival of Retinoblastoma in Less-Developed Countries Impact of Socioeconomic and Health-Related Indicators. Br J Ophthalmol. 2010 Nov;94(11):1432–6. PMID:20733021
475. Cao J, Brouwer NJ, Richards KE, et al. PD-L1/PD-1 Expression and Tumor-Infiltrating Lymphocytes in Conjunctival Melanoma. Oncotarget. 2017 May 20;8(33):54722–34. PMID:28903377
476. Cao J, Heijkants RC, Jochemsen AG, et al. Targeting of the MAPK and AKT Pathways in Conjunctival Melanoma Shows Potential Synergy. Oncotarget. 2016 Jul 22;8(35):58021–36. PMID:28938534
477. Capó H, Palmer E, Nicholson DH. Congenital Cysts of the Iris Stroma. Am J Ophthalmol. 1993 Aug 15;116(2):228–32. PMID:8352310
478. Capper D, Jones DTW, Sill M, et al. DNA Methylation-Based Classification of Central Nervous System Tumours. Nature. 2018 Mar 22;555(7697):469–74. PMID:29539639
479. Carbone M, Ferris LK, Baumann F, et al. BAP1 Cancer Syndrome: Malignant Mesothelioma, Uveal and Cutaneous Melanoma, and MBAITs. J Transl Med. 2012 Aug 30;10:179. PMID:22935333
480. Carbone M, Flores EG, Emi M, et al. Combined Genetic and Genealogic Studies Uncover a Large BAP1 Cancer Syndrome Kindred Tracing Back Nine Generations to a Common Ancestor from the 1700s. PLoS Genet. 2015 Dec 18;11(12):e1005633. PMID:26683624
481. Cardoso JC, Calonje E. Cutaneous Manifestations of Human Papillomaviruses: A Review. Acta Dermatovenerol Alp Pannonica Adriat. 2011 Sep;20(3):145–54. PMID:22131115
482. Carney EM, Banerjee P, Ellis CL, et al. PAX2(-)/PAX8(-)/Inhibin A(+) Immunoprofile in Hemangioblastoma: A Helpful Combination in the Differential Diagnosis with Metastatic Clear Cell Renal Cell Carcinoma to the Central Nervous System. Am J Surg Pathol. 2011 Feb;35(2):262–7. PMID:21263247
483. Carr RA, Mesiano D, Heffron C, et al. Aberrant P16, P53 and Ki-67 Immunohistochemistry Staining Patterns Can Distinguish Solitary Keratoacanthoma from Cutaneous Squamous Cell Carcinoma. Pathology. 2023 Oct;55(6):772–84. PMID:37573161
484. Carrau RL, Stillman E, Canaan RE. Mucoepidermoid Carcinoma of the Conjunctiva. Ophthalmic Plast Reconstr Surg. 1994 Sep;10(3):163–8. PMID:7947443
485. Carreira H, Coutinho F, Carrilho C, et al. HIV and HPV Infections and Ocular Surface Squamous Neoplasia: Systematic Review and Meta-Analysis. Br J Cancer. 2013 Oct 1;109(7):1981–8. PMID:24030075
486. Carreño E, Saornil MA, Garcia-Alvarez C, et al. Prevalence of Ocular and Oculodermal Melanocytosis in Spanish Population with Uveal Melanoma. Eye (Lond). 2012 Jan;26(1):159–62. PMID:22020174
487. Carroll GS, Haik BG, Fleming JC, et al. Peripheral Nerve Tumors of the Orbit. Radiol Clin North Am. 1999 Jan;37(1):195–202, Xi–Xii. PMID:10026738
488. Carruth BP, Meyer DR. Angiolipoma of the Orbit: A Rare Tumor in an Unusual Location. Ophthalmic Plast Reconstr Surg. 2015 Nov-Dec;31(6):e142–5. PMID:24927028
489. Carruthers MN, Khosroshahi A, Augustin T, et al. The Diagnostic Utility of Serum IgG4 Concentrations in IgG4-Related Disease. Ann Rheum Dis. 2015 Jan;74(1):14–8. PMID:24651618
490. Carvalho RM, Taleb A, Carvalho GL, et al. [Conjunctival Fibrous Histiocytoma Simulating Atipical Pterygium in the Amazon Region: Case Report]. Arq Bras Oftalmol. 2010 Nov-Dec;73(6):534–6. Portuguese. PMID:21271031
491. Castillejo Becerra CM, Dalvin LA, Jevremovic D, et al. Clinical Characteristics and Outcomes of Ocular Adnexal Mantle Cell Lymphoma. Orbit. 2022 Feb;41(1):97–104. PMID:35100932
492. Castori M, Morrone A, Kanitakis J, et al. Genetic Skin Diseases Predisposing to Basal Cell Carcinoma. Eur J Dermatol. 2012 May-Jun;22(3):299–309. PMID:22391625
493. Castrén E, Salminen P, Vikkula M, et al. Inheritance Patterns of Infantile Hemangioma. Pediatrics. 2016 Nov;138(5):e20161623. PMID:27940781
494. Castro EC, Blazquez C, Boyd J, et al. Clinicopathologic Features of Histiocytic Lesions Following ALL, with a Review of the Literature. Pediatr Dev Pathol. 2010 May-Jun;13(3):225–37. PMID:19642834
495. Cates JMM. Modeling Continuous Prognostic Factors in Survival Analysis: Implications for Tumor Staging and Assessing Chemotherapy Effect in Osteosarcoma. Am J Surg Pathol. 2018 Apr;42(4):485–91. PMID:29200101
496. Cavazza S, Laffi GL, Lodi L, et al. Orbital Dermoid Cyst of Childhood: Clinical Pathologic Findings, Classification and Management. Int Ophthalmol. 2011 Apr;31(2):93–7. PMID:21267629
497. Cavazza S, Laffi GL, Lodi L, et al. Primary Cutaneous Adenoid Cystic Carcinoma of the Upper Lid: A Case Report and Literature Review. Int Ophthalmol. 2012 Feb;32(1):31–5. PMID:22228272
498. Cavicchio A, Freitag SK, Rabinovich A, et al. Eyelid Abscess Arising from an Epidermal Inclusion Cyst. Ophthalmic Surg Lasers Imaging. 2010 Jul 29;41 Online:1–3. PMID:21158377
499. Cawthon RM, Weiss R, Xu GF, et al. A Major Segment of the Neurofibromatosis Type 1 Gene: CDNA Sequence, Genomic Structure, and Point Mutations. Cell. 1990 Jul 13;62(1):193–201. PMID:2114220
500. Cellier L, Jacquemus J, Youssef-Provençal N, et al. Tri-Phenotypic Naevus: A Case Report. Pathology. 2018 Oct;50(6):691–3. PMID:30122258
501. Centers for Disease Control and Prevention (CDC). Notes from the Field: Acute Hemorrhagic Conjunctivitis Outbreaks Caused by Coxsackievirus A24v --- Uganda and Southern Sudan, 2010. MMWR Morb Mortal Wkly Rep. 2010 Aug 20;59(32):1024. PMID:20724969
502. Ceppi F, Abla O. Juvenile Xanthogranuloma and Related Non-LCH Disorders. In: Abla O, Janka G, editors. Histiocytic Disorders. Cham (Switzerland): Springer International Publishing; 2018. pp. 293–311.
503. Chacko JG, Lam BL, Adusumilli J, et al. Multicentric Malignant Glioma of Adulthood Masquerading as Optic Neuritis. Br J Ophthalmol. 2010 Jun;94(6):782–3, 812. PMID:18977790
504. Chadha V, Awan MA, Gonzalez P, et al. Orbital Venous-Lymphatic Malformation. Eye (Lond). 2009 Dec;23(12):2265–6. PMID:19218988
505. Chahud F, Young RH, Remulla JF, et al. Bilateral Diffuse Uveal Melanocytic Proliferation Associated with Extraocular Cancers: Review of a Process Particularly Associated with Gynecologic Cancers. Am J Surg Pathol. 2001 Feb;25(2):212–8. PMID:11176070
506. Chai P, Luo Y, Zhou C, et al. Clinical Characteristics and Mutation Spectrum of NF1 in 12 Chinese Families with Orbital/Periorbital Plexiform Neurofibromatosis Type 1. BMC Med Genet. 2019 Sep 18;20(1):158. PMID:31533651
507. Chakrabarti I, Mondal S, Goswami BK. Pigmented Malignant Teratoid Medulloepithelioma of Ciliary Body - An Extremely Rare Intraocular Tumor in Adult. Saudi J Ophthalmol. 2014 Jul;28(3):247–9. PMID:25278807
508. Chakraborty R, Abdel-Wahab O, Durham BH. MAP-Kinase-Driven Hematopoietic Neoplasms: A Decade of Progress in the Molecular Age. Cold Spring Harb Perspect Med. 2021 May 3;11(5):a034892. PMID:32601132
509. Chakraborty R, Hampton OA, Abhyankar H, et al. Activating MAPK1 (ERK2) Mutation in an Aggressive Case of Disseminated Juvenile Xanthogranuloma. Oncotarget. 2017 Jul 11;8(28):46065–70. PMID:28512266
510. Chakraborty R, Hampton OA, Shen X, et al. Mutually Exclusive Recurrent Somatic Mutations in MAP2K1 and BRAF Support a Central Role for ERK Activation in LCH Pathogenesis. Blood. 2014 Nov 6;124(19):3007–15. PMID:25202140
511. Chakrapani A, Warrick A, Nelson D, et al. BRAF and KRAS Mutations in Sporadic Glomus Tumors. Am J Dermatopathol. 2012 Jul;34(5):533–5. PMID:22317887
512. Chalkia AK, Spandidos DA, Detorakis ET. Viral Involvement in the Pathogenesis and Clinical Features of Ophthalmic Pterygium (Review). Int J Mol Med. 2013 Sep;32(3):539–43. PMID:23856952
513. Chamberlain BK, McClain CM, Gonzalez RS, et al. Alveolar Soft Part Sarcoma and Granular Cell Tumor: An Immunohistochemical Comparison Study. Hum Pathol. 2014 May;45(5):1039–44. PMID:24746209
514. Champion R, Daicker BC. Congenital Hypertrophy of the Pigment Epithelium: Light Microscopic and Ultrastructural Findings in Young Children. Retina. 1989;9(1):44–8. PMID:2717803
515. Chan CC, Collins AB, Chew EY. Molecular Pathology of Eyes with von Hippel-Lindau (VHL) Disease: A Review. Retina. 2007 Jan;27(1):1–7. PMID:17218907
516. Chan CC, Vortmeyer AO, Chew EY, et al. VHL Gene Deletion and Enhanced VEGF Gene Expression Detected in the Stromal Cells of Retinal Angioma. Arch Ophthalmol. 1999 May;117(5):625–30. PMID:10326959
517. Chan EH, Kapadia M, Cheung NC. Asymptomatic Follicular Conjunctivitis in an Elderly Man. JAMA Ophthalmol. 2019 Apr 1;137(4):451–2. PMID:30653223
518. Chan JK, Sin VC, Wong KF, et al. Nonnasal Lymphoma Expressing the Natural Killer Cell Marker CD56: A Clinicopathologic Study of 49 Cases of an Uncommon Aggressive Neoplasm. Blood. 1997 Jun 15;89(12):4501–13. PMID:9192774
519. Chan JK, Yip TT, Tsang WY, et al. Detection of Epstein-Barr Viral RNA in Malignant Lymphomas of the Upper Aerodigestive Tract. Am J Surg Pathol. 1994 Sep;18(9):938–46. PMID:8067515
520. Chan MP, Plouffe KR, Liu CJ, et al. Next-Generation Sequencing Implicates Oncogenic Roles for P53 and JAK/STAT Signaling in Microcystic Adnexal Carcinomas. Mod Pathol. 2020 Jun;33(6):1092–103. PMID:31857679
521. Chan WM, Liu DT, Lam LY, et al. Primary Epithelial-Myoepithelial Carcinoma of the Lacrimal Gland. Arch Ophthalmol. 2004 Nov;122(11):1714–7. PMID:15534138
522. Chang M, Lee Y, Baek S, et al. Orbital Glomus Tumor in an Asian Patient. BMC Ophthalmol. 2012 Dec 5;12:62. PMID:23216695
523. Chang MW, Frieden IJ, Good W. The Risk Intraocular Juvenile Xanthogranuloma: Survey of Current Practices and Assessment of Risk. J Am Acad Dermatol. 1996 Mar;34(3):445–9. PMID:8609257
524. Chang SH, Worley LA, Onken MD, et al. Prognostic Biomarkers in Uveal Melanoma: Evidence for a Stem Cell-Like Phenotype Associated with Metastasis. Melanoma Res. 2008 Jun;18(3):191–200. PMID:18477893
525. Chang Y, Wei WB, Shi JT, et al. Clinical and Histopathological Features of Adenomas of the Ciliary Pigment Epithelium. Acta Ophthalmol. 2016 Nov;94(7):e637–43. PMID:27130243
526. Chanudet E, Ye H, Ferry J, et al. A20 Deletion is Associated with Copy Number Gain at the TNFA/B/C Locus and Occurs Preferentially in Translocation-Negative MALT Lymphoma of the Ocular Adnexa and Salivary Glands. J Pathol. 2009 Feb;217(3):420–30. PMID:19006194
527. Chaput F, Amer R, Baglivo E, et al. Intraocular T-Cell Lymphoma: Clinical Presentation, Diagnosis, Treatment, and Outcome. Ocul Immunol Inflamm. 2017 Oct;25(5):639–48. PMID:27002464
528. Chapuy B, Stewart C, Dunford AJ, et al. Molecular Subtypes of Diffuse Large B Cell Lymphoma Are Associated with Distinct Pathogenic Mechanisms and Outcomes. Nat Med. 2018 May;24(5):679–90. PMID:29713087
529. Char DH, Cole TB, Miller TR. False Negative Orbital Fine Needle Biopsy. Orbit. 2012 Jun;31(3):194–6. PMID:22551376
530. Char DH, Crawford JB, Kroll S. Iris Melanomas. Diagnostic Problems. Ophthalmology. 1996 Feb;103(2):251–5. PMID:8594510
531. Char DH, Kemlitz AE, Miller T, et al. Iris Ring Melanoma: Fine Needle Biopsy. Br J Ophthalmol. 2006 Apr;90(4):420–2. PMID:16547317
532. Char DH, Miller T, Crawford JB. Uveal Tumour Resection. Br J Ophthalmol. 2001 Oct;85(10):1213–9. PMID:11567967
533. Char DH, Miller TR, Crawford JB. Cytopathologic Diagnosis of Benign Lesions Simulating Choroidal Melanomas. Am J Ophthalmol. 1991 Jul 15;112(1):70–5. PMID:1882925
534. Char DH, Miller TR, Crawford JB. Cytopathologic Diagnosis of Benign Lesions Simulating Choroidal Melanomas. Trans Am Ophthalmol Soc. 1991;89:235–44. PMID:1808809
535. Char DH, Stone RD, Crawford JB, et al. Diffuse Melanoma of the Choroid. Br J Ophthalmol. 1980 Mar;64(3):178–80. PMID:6966937
536. Charles NC, Fox DM, Avendaño JA, et al. Conjunctival Neurilemoma. Report of 3 Cases. Arch Ophthalmol. 1997 Apr;115(4):547–9. PMID:9109769
537. Charles NC, Kim ET. Ossifying Pilomatrixoma of the Eyelid. Ophthalmic Plast Reconstr Surg. 2020 Nov/Dec;36(6):e147–9. PMID:32304502
538. Charles NC, Ostriker GE. Epibulbar Conjunctival Fibroma. Ophthalmic Plast Reconstr Surg. 2007 May-Jun;23(3):249–50. PMID:17519675
539. Charles NC, Patel P. Solid Variant of a Proliferative Apocrine Hidrocystoma. Ophthalmic Plast Reconstr Surg. 2019 May/Jun;35(3):e72–4. PMID:30893188
540. Charles NC, Stagner AM, Raju LV, et al. Conjunctival Exophytic Schneiderian-Type Papillomas: A Rare Occurrence. Ophthalmic Plast

Reconstr Surg. 2021 Sep-Oct 01;37(5):e179–81. PMID:34284422

541. Charles SJ, Moore AT, Yates JR, et al. Lisch Nodules in Neurofibromatosis Type 2. Case Report. Arch Ophthalmol. 1989 Nov;107(11):1571–2. PMID:2510706

542. Chase DR, Enzinger FM. Epithelioid Sarcoma. Diagnosis, Prognostic Indicators, and Treatment. Am J Surg Pathol. 1985 Apr;9(4):241–63. PMID:4014539

543. Chasset F, Barete S, Charlotte F, et al. Cutaneous Manifestations of Erdheim-Chester Disease (ECD): Clinical, Pathological, and Molecular Features in a Monocentric Series of 40 Patients. J Am Acad Dermatol. 2016 Mar;74(3):513–20. PMID:26785805

544. Chau C, van Doorn R, van Poppelen NM, et al. Families with BAP1-Tumor Predisposition Syndrome in The Netherlands: Path to Identification and a Proposal for Genetic Screening Guidelines. Cancers (Basel). 2019 Aug 4;11(8):1114. PMID:31382694

545. Chaudhari PB, Pathy S, Deo SSV, et al. Alveolar Soft Part Sarcoma of Orbit: A Rare Diagnosis. J Egypt Natl Canc Inst. 2017 Sep;29(3):167–70. PMID:28844593

546. Chaudhry IA, Morales J, Shamsi FA, et al. Orbitofacial Neurofibromatosis: Clinical Characteristics and Treatment Outcome. Eye (Lond). 2012 Apr;26(4):583–92. PMID:22193879

547. Chaugule SS, Putambekar A, Gavade S, et al. Primary Orbital Leiomyosarcoma in an Adult Male. Ophthalmic Plast Reconstr Surg. 2019 Mar/Apr;35(2):e27–9. PMID:30601462

548. Chauhan S, Sen S, Sharma A, et al. Human Papillomavirus: A Predictor of Better Survival in Ocular Surface Squamous Neoplasia Patients. Br J Ophthalmol. 2012 Dec;96(12):1517–21. PMID:22942158

549. Chaussade A, Millot G, Wells C, et al. Correlation Between RB1germline Mutations and Second Primary Malignancies in Hereditary Retinoblastoma Patients Treated with External Beam Radiotherapy. Eur J Med Genet. 2019 Mar;62(3):217–23. PMID:30031154

550. Chavez M, Mafee MF, Castillo B, et al. Medulloepithelioma of the Optic Nerve. J Pediatr Ophthalmol Strabismus. 2004 Jan-Feb;41(1):48–52. PMID:14974835

551. Chawda SJ, Moseley IF. Computed Tomography of Orbital Dermoids: A 20-Year Review. Clin Radiol. 1999 Dec;54(12):821–5. PMID:10619299

552. Chawla B, Kashyap S, Sen S, et al. Clinicopathologic Review of Epithelial Tumors of the Lacrimal Gland. Ophthalmic Plast Reconstr Surg. 2013 Nov-Dec;29(6):440–5. PMID:24145905

553. Chawla B, Khurana S, Kashyap S. Giant Cell Reparative Granuloma of the Orbit. Ophthalmic Plast Reconstr Surg. 2013 Jul-Aug;29(4):e94–5. PMID:23511994

554. Chawla S, Blay JY, Rutkowski P, et al. Denosumab in Patients with Giant-Cell Tumour of Bone: A Multicentre, Open-Label, Phase 2 Study. Lancet Oncol. 2019 Dec;20(12):1719–29. PMID:31704134

555. Chebib I, Hornicek FJ, Nielsen GP, et al. Cytomorphologic Features that Distinguish Schwannoma from Other Low-Grade Spindle Cell Lesions. Cancer Cytopathol. 2015 Mar;123(3):171–9. PMID:25641870

556. Chellapandian D, Hines MR, Zhang R, et al. A Multicenter Study of Patients with Multisystem Langerhans Cell Histiocytosis Who Develop Secondary Hemophagocytic Lymphohistiocytosis. Cancer. 2019 Mar 15;125(6):963–71. PMID:30521100

557. Chen BJ, Mariño-Enríquez A, Fletcher CD, et al. Loss of Retinoblastoma Protein Expression in Spindle Cell/Pleomorphic Lipomas and Cytogenetically Related Tumors: An Immunohistochemical Study with Diagnostic Implications. Am J Surg Pathol. 2012 Aug;36(8):1119–28. PMID:22790852

558. Chen HC, Brownstein S, Tang T et al. Pilomatrixoma of the Ocular Adnexa: Report of 3 Cases with Variations in the Histopathological Findings. Can J Ophthalmol. 2019 Aug;54(4):413–6. PMID:31358136

559. Chen J, Yanuck RR 3rd, Abbondanzo SL, et al. C-Kit (CD117) Reactivity in Extramedullary Myeloid Tumor/Granulocytic Sarcoma. Arch Pathol Lab Med. 2001 Nov;125(11):1448–52. PMID:11698000

560. Chen JJ, Costello F, Kardon RH. Sex Disparities in Neuro-Ophthalmologic Disorders. Curr Eye Res. 2015 Feb;40(2):247–65. PMID:24911098

561. Chen KT. Intraductal Carcinoma of the Minor Salivary Gland. J Laryngol Otol. 1983 Feb;97(2):189–91. PMID:6298331

562. Chen L, Liu M, Zhang Z, et al. Ocular Manifestations of a Hospitalised Patient with Confirmed 2019 Novel Coronavirus Disease. Br J Ophthalmol. 2020 Jun;104(6):748–51. PMID:32265202

563. Chen TY, Keeney MG, Chintakuntlawar AV, et al. Adenoid Cystic Carcinoma of the Lacrimal Gland is Frequently Characterized by MYB Rearrangement. Eye (Lond). 2017 May;31(5):720–5. PMID:28085142

564. Chen W, Hornick JL, Fletcher CDM. NKX3.1 Immunoreactivity is Not Identified in Mesenchymal Chondrosarcoma: A 25-Case Cohort Study. Histopathology. 2021 Jan;78(2):334–7. PMID:32779239

565. Chen W, Jaffe R, Zhang L, et al. Langerhans Cell Sarcoma Arising from Chronic Lymphocytic Lymphoma/Small Lymphocytic Leukemia: Lineage Analysis and BRAF V600E Mutation Study. N Am J Med Sci. 2013 Jun;5(6):386–91. PMID:23923114

566. Chen X, Maniotis AJ, Majumdar D, et al. Uveal Melanoma Cell Staining for CD34 and Assessment of Tumor Vascularity. Invest Ophthalmol Vis Sci. 2002 Aug;43(8):2533–9. PMID:12147581

567. Chen X, Wu Q, Depeille P, et al. RasGRP3 Mediates MAPK Pathway Activation in GNAQ Mutant Uveal Melanoma. Cancer Cell. 2017 May 8;31(5):685–696.E6. PMID:28486107

568. Chen Y, Lin W, Yang H, et al. Aberrant Expansion and Function of Follicular Helper T Cell Subsets in IgG4-Related Disease. Arthritis Rheumatol. 2018 Nov;70(11):1853–65. PMID:29781221

569. Chen YF, Zhang WD, Wu MW, et al. Inflammatory Myofibroblastic Tumor of the Head and Neck. Med Oncol. 2011 Dec;28(Suppl 1):s349–53. PMID:21042957

570. Chen YW, Guo T, Shen L, et al. Receptor-Type Tyrosine-Protein Phosphatase κ Directly Targets STAT3 Activation for Tumor Suppression in Nasal NK/T-Cell Lymphoma. Blood. 2015 Mar 5;125(10):1589–600. PMID:25612622

571. Chen Z, Ni W, Li JL, et al. The CRTC1-MAML2 Fusion is the Major Oncogenic Driver in Mucoepidermoid Carcinoma. JCI Insight. 2021 Apr 8;6(7):e139497. PMID:33830080

572. Cheng F, Yu F, Wang X, et al. A Pedigree Analysis and Clonal Correlations of the Coexistence of B-Cell Lymphoma and Histiocytic/Dendritic Cell Tumor. Int J Surg Pathol. 2021 Dec;29(8):906–14. PMID:33939500

573. Cheng TW, Yu NY, Seetharam M, et al. Radiotherapy for Malignant Melanoma of the Lacrimal Sac. Rare Tumors. 2020 Nov 11;12:2036361320971943. PMID:33240474

574. Cheson BD, Fisher RI, Barrington SF, et al. Recommendations for Initial Evaluation, Staging, and Response Assessment of Hodgkin and Non-Hodgkin Lymphoma: The Lugano Classification. J Clin Oncol. 2014 Sep 20;32(27):3059–68. PMID:25113753

575. Cheuk W, Miliauskas JR, Chan JK. Intraductal Carcinoma of the Oral Cavity: A Case Report and a Reappraisal of the Concept of Pure Ductal Carcinoma In Situ in Salivary Duct Carcinoma. Am J Surg Pathol. 2004 Feb;28(2):266–70. PMID:15043319

576. Cheuk W, Tam FK, Chan AN, et al. Idiopathic Cervical Fibrosis–a New Member of IgG4-Related Sclerosing Diseases: Report of 4 Cases, 1 Complicated by Composite Lymphoma. Am J Surg Pathol. 2010 Nov;34(11):1678–85. PMID:20871392

577. Cheuk W, Yuen HK, Chan AC, et al. Ocular Adnexal Lymphoma Associated with IgG4+ Chronic Sclerosing Dacryoadenitis: A Previously Undescribed Complication of IgG4-Related Sclerosing Disease. Am J Surg Pathol. 2008 Aug;32(8):1159–67. PMID:18580683

578. Cheuk W, Yuen HK, Chan JK. Chronic Sclerosing Dacryoadenitis: Part of the Spectrum of IgG4-Related Sclerosing Disease? Am J Surg Pathol. 2007 Apr;31(4):643–5. PMID:17414116

579. Cheuk W, Yuen HK, Chu SY, et al. Lymphadenopathy of IgG4-Related Sclerosing Disease. Am J Surg Pathol. 2008 May;32(5):671–81. PMID:18344866

580. Cheung M, Testa JR. BAP1, a Tumor Suppressor Gene Driving Malignant Mesothelioma. Transl Lung Cancer Res. 2017 Jun;6(3):270–8. PMID:28713672

581. Cheung YH, Gayden T, Campeau PM, et al. A Recurrent PDGFRB Mutation Causes Familial Infantile Myofibromatosis. Am J Hum Genet. 2013 Jun 6;92(6):996–1000. PMID:23731537

582. Chévez-Barrios P, Eagle RC Jr, Krailo M, et al. Study of Unilateral Retinoblastoma With and Without Histopathologic High-Risk Features and the Role of Adjuvant Chemotherapy: A Children's Oncology Group Study. J Clin Oncol. 2019 Nov 1;37(31):2883–91. PMID:31539297

583. Chew EY. Ocular Manifestations of von Hippel-Lindau Disease: Clinical and Genetic Investigations. Trans Am Ophthalmol Soc. 2005;103:495–511. PMID:17057815

584. Chheda P, Ramamurthy S, Raval V, et al. Oculodermal Melanocytosis in Asian Indian Patients: Prevalence, Clinical Presentation, and Association with Choroidal Melanoma. Indian J Ophthalmol. 2025 Jan 1;73(Suppl 1):S88–94. PMID:39723871

585. Chidambaram B, Santosh V, Balasubramaniam V. Medulloepithelioma of the Optic Nerve with Intradural Extension–Report of Two Cases and a Review of the Literature. Childs Nerv Syst. 2000 Jun;16(6):329–33. PMID:10933227

586. Childress MA, Himmelberg SM, Chen H, et al. ALK Fusion Partners Impact Response to ALK Inhibition: Differential Effects on Sensitivity, Cellular Phenotypes, and Biochemical Properties. Mol Cancer Res. 2018 Nov;16(11):1724–36. PMID:30002191

587. Chiller K, Passaro D, Scheuller M, et al. Microcystic Adnexal Carcinoma: Forty-Eight Cases, Their Treatment, and Their Outcome. Arch Dermatol. 2000 Nov;136(11):1355–9. PMID:11074698

588. Chilton J, Caughron MR, Kepes JJ. Ganglioglioma of the Optic Chiasm: Case Report and Review of the Literature. Neurosurgery. 1990 Jun;26(6):1042–5. PMID:2194139

589. Chin B, Sassoon J, Farhat N, et al. Reactive Lymphoid Hyperplasia of the Eyelid. Ophthalmic Plast Reconstr Surg. 2020 Mar/Apr;36(2):e55. PMID:31261162

590. Chmielecki J, Crago AM, Rosenberg M, et al. Whole-Exome Sequencing Identifies a Recurrent NAB2-STAT6 Fusion in Solitary Fibrous Tumors. Nat Genet. 2013 Feb;45(2):131–2. PMID:23313954

591. Choi CJ, Jakobiec FA, Zakka FR, et al. Conjunctival Squamous Cell Neoplasia Associated With Ocular Cicatricial Pemphigoid. Ophthalmic Plast Reconstr Surg. 2017 Nov/Dec;33(6):e157–60. PMID:28509683

592. Choi CJ, Tran AQ, Anagnostopoulos AG, et al. A Single-Institution Review of Lacrimal Gland Biopsies Between 1962 and 2017. Orbit. 2023 Apr;42(2):148–56. PMID:35298320

593. Choi EK, Chévez-Barrios P. Inflamed Conjunctival Nevi: Histopathological Criteria. Arch Pathol Lab Med. 2014 Sep;138(9):1242–6. PMID:25171709

594. Choi G, Lee U, Won NH. Fibrous Histiocytoma of the Lacrimal Sac. Head Neck. 1997 Jan;19(1):72–5. PMID:9030950

595. Choi JS, Bae YC, Lee JW, et al. Dermoid Cysts: Epidemiology and Diagnostic Approach Based on Clinical Experiences. Arch Plast Surg. 2018 Nov 45(6) 512–6. PMID:30463230

596. Choi K, Kennedy M, Kazarov A, et al. A Common Precursor for Hematopoietic and Endothelial Cells. Development. 1998 Feb;125(4):725–32. PMID:9435292

597. Choi M, Jeon YK, Sun CH, et al. RTK-RAS Pathway Mutation is Enriched in Myeloid Sarcoma. Blood Cancer J. 2018 May 23;8(5):43. PMID:29789584

598. Choi MB, Salomão DR, Smith WM, et al. Ophthalmic Findings of Rosai-Dorfman Disease. Am J Ophthalmol. 2018 Apr;188:164–72. PMID:29428455

599. Choi SH, Hwang JM, Kim N. Orbital Fibrous Hamartoma of Infancy. J AAPOS. 2016 Feb;20(1):68–9. PMID:26917076

600. Choi YK, Yang JH, Ahn SY, et al. Retroperitoneal Fibrosis in the Era of Immunoglobulin G4-Related Disease. Kidney Res Clin Pract. 2019 Mar 31;38(1):42–8. PMID:30754935

601. Chong DY, Demirci H, Ronan SM, et al. Orbital Rhabdomyosarcoma in Li-Fraumeni Syndrome. Arch Ophthalmol. 2007 Apr;125(4):566–9. PMID:17420382

602. Choong PF, Pritchard DJ, Rock MG, et al. Low Grade Central Osteogenic Sarcoma. A Long-Term Followup of 20 Patients. Clin Orthop Relat Res. 1996 Jan; (322):198–206. PMID:8542697

603. Chorost MS, Yakopson V, Chou E. Posttraumatic Encapsulated Orbital Lipoma. Mil Med. 2020 Sep 18;185(9-10):e1876–9. PMID:32426822

604. Chott A, Vonderheid EC, Olbricht S, et al. The Dominant T Cell Clone is Present in Multiple Regressing Skin Lesions and Associated T Cell Lymphomas of Patients with Lymphomatoid Papulosis. J Invest Dermatol. 1996 Apr;106(4):696–700. PMID:8618007

605. Chou AJ, Geller DS, Gorlick R. Therapy for Osteosarcoma: Where Do We Go from Here? Paediatr Drugs. 2008;10(5):315–27. PMID:18754698

606. Chougule A, Bal A, Das A, et al. A Comparative Study of Inflammatory Myofibroblastic Tumors and Tumefactive IgG4-Related Inflammatory Lesions: The Relevance of IgG4 Plasma Cells. Appl Immunohistochem Mol Morphol. 2016 Nov/Dec;24(10):721–8. PMID:26469330

607. Chowdhury Z, Raphael V, Khonglah Y, et al. Mélange of Lymphoepithelial Lesions of Salivary Glands from a Tertiary Care Center of North East India: Diagnostic Conundrums. J Lab Physicians. 2021 Jul 12;13(4):338–45. PMID:34975253

608. Chowdhury Z, Sharma JD, Kakoti LM, et al. Experience with Orbital Tumors from a Tertiary Cancer Centre of North East India: A Pathology Perspective. J Lab Physicians. 2020 Dec;12(3):171–7. PMID:33268934

609. Chowdhury Z, Varshney J, Singh A, et al. Nodal Langerhans Cell Neoplasm: Detailing the Diagnostic Quandaries. Autops Case Rep. 2021 Dec 10;11:e2021344. PMID:35004363
610. Chowsilpa S, An D, Maleki Z. Adenoid Cystic Carcinoma Cytology: Salivary Gland and Nonsalivary Gland. Diagn Cytopathol. 2020 Dec;48(12):1282–9. PMID:32809258
611. Chowsilpa S, Chaiyasate S, Wannasai K, et al. Localised Nasopharyngeal Amyloidosis: The Importance of Postoperative Follow-Up. BMJ Case Rep. 2018 Feb 14;2018:Bcr2017222067. PMID:29444790
612. Christensen WN, Smith RR. Schneiderian Papillomas: A Clinicopathologic Study of 67 Cases. Hum Pathol. 1986 Apr;17(4):393–400. PMID:3957337
613. Chronopoulos A, Kilic E, Joussen AM, et al. Small Incision Iris Tumour Biopsy Using a Cavernous Sampling Forceps. Br J Ophthalmol. 2014 Nov;98(11):1539–42. PMID:24964795
614. Chudasama P, Mughal SS, Sanders MA, et al. Integrative Genomic and Transcriptomic Analysis of Leiomyosarcoma. Nat Commun. 2018 Jan 10;9(1):144. PMID:29321523
615. Chung EB, Enzinger FM. Infantile Myofibromatosis. Cancer. 1981 Oct 15;48(8):1807–18. PMID:7284977
616. Chung EB, Enzinger FM. Proliferative Fasciitis. Cancer. 1975 Oct;36(4):1450–8. PMID:1058047
617. Chung EM, Murphey MD, Specht CS, et al. From the Archives of the AFIP. Pediatric Orbit Tumors and Tumorlike Lesions: Osseous Lesions of the Orbit. Radiographics. 2008 Jul-Aug;28(4):1193–214. PMID:18635637
618. Chung YM, Lin YC, Huang DF, et al. Conjunctival Biopsy in Sarcoidosis. J Chin Med Assoc. 2006 Oct;69(10):472–7. PMID:17098671
619. Cialdini AP, Sahel JA, Jalkh AE, et al. Malignant Transformation of an Iris Melanocytoma. A Case Report. Graefes Arch Clin Exp Ophthalmol. 1989;227(4):348–54. PMID:2777104
620. Cimino L, Chan CC, Shen D, et al. Ocular Involvement in Nasal Natural Killer T-Cell Lymphoma. Int Ophthalmol. 2009 Aug;29(4):275–9. PMID:18438613
621. Cina SJ, Radentz SS, Smialek JE. A Case of Familial Angiolipomatosis with Lisch Nodules. Arch Pathol Lab Med. 1999 Oct;123(10):946–8. PMID:10506451
622. Cinotti E, Singer A, Labeille B, et al. Handheld In Vivo Reflectance Confocal Microscopy for the Diagnosis of Eyelid Margin and Conjunctival Tumors. JAMA Ophthalmol. 2017 Aug 1;135(8):845–51. PMID:28654937
623. Cipriani NA, Lusardi JJ, McElherne J, et al. Mucoepidermoid Carcinoma: A Comparison of Histologic Grading Systems and Relationship to MAML2 Rearrangement and Prognosis. Am J Surg Pathol. 2019 Jul;43(7):885–97. PMID:31021855
624. Cisarova K, Folcher M, El Zaoui I, et al. Genomic and Transcriptomic Landscape of Conjunctival Melanoma. PLoS Genet. 2020 Dec 31;16(12):e1009201. PMID:33383577
625. Cives M, Mannavola F, Lospalluti L, et al. Non-Melanoma Skin Cancers: Biological and Clinical Features. Int J Mol Sci. 2020 Jul 29;21(15):5394. PMID:32751327
626. Clark WH Jr, Elder DE, Guerry D 4th, et al. A Study of Tumor Progression: The Precursor Lesions of Superficial Spreading and Nodular Melanoma. Hum Pathol. 1984 Dec;15(12):1147–65. PMID:6500548
627. Clark WH Jr, Elder DE, Van Horn M. The Biologic Forms of Malignant Melanoma. Hum Pathol. 1986 May;17(5):443–50. PMID:3699806
628. Clark WH Jr, From L, Bernardino EA, et al. The Histogenesis and Biologic Behavior of Primary Human Malignant Melanomas of the Skin. Cancer Res. 1969 Mar;29(3):705–27. PMID:5773814
629. Clay MR, Martinez AP, Weiss SW, et al. MDM2 Amplification in Problematic Lipomatous Tumors: Analysis of FISH Testing Criteria. Am J Surg Pathol. 2015 Oct;39(10):1433–9. PMID:26146760
630. Clearkin KP, Enzinger FM. Intravascular Papillary Endothelial Hyperplasia. Arch Pathol Lab Med. 1976 Aug;100(8):441–4. PMID:947306
631. Clement CI, Genge J, O'Donnell BA, et al. Orbital and Periorbital Microcystic Adnexal Carcinoma. Ophthalmic Plast Reconstr Surg. 2005 Mar;21(2):97–102. PMID:15778661
632. Cleven AH, Höcker S, Briaire-de Bruijn I, et al. Mutation Analysis of H3F3A and H3F3B as a Diagnostic Tool for Giant Cell Tumor of Bone and Chondroblastoma. Am J Surg Pathol. 2015 Nov;39(11):1576–83. PMID:26457357
633. Coban DT, Erol MK, Suren D, et al. Primary Cutaneous Adenoid Cystic Carcinoma of the Eyelid and Literature Review. Arq Bras Oftalmol. 2015 Sep-Oct;78(5):323–5. PMID:26466235
634. Coban-Karatas M, Bal N, Altan-Yaycioglu R, et al. Spindle Cell Carcinoma of the Conjunctiva: A Rare Entity. Indian J Ophthalmol. 2016 May;64(5):402–4. PMID:27380985
635. Cobb MW. Human Papillomavirus Infection. J Am Acad Dermatol. 1990 Apr;22(4):547–66. PMID:2156916
636. Coca-Pelaz A, Rodrigo JP, Triantafyllou A, et al. Salivary Mucoepidermoid Carcinoma Revisited. Eur Arch Otorhinolaryngol. 2015 Apr;272(4):799–819. PMID:24771140
637. Coffin CM, Hornick JL, Fletcher CD. Inflammatory Myofibroblastic Tumor: Comparison of Clinicopathologic, Histologic, and Immunohistochemical Features Including ALK Expression in Atypical and Aggressive Cases. Am J Surg Pathol. 2007 Apr;31(4):509–20. PMID:17414097
638. Coffin CM, Watterson J, Priest JR, et al. Extrapulmonary Inflammatory Myofibroblastic Tumor (Inflammatory Pseudotumor). A Clinicopathologic and Immunohistochemical Study of 84 Cases. Am J Surg Pathol. 1995 Aug;19(8):859–72. PMID:7611533
639. Coggshall K, Tello TL, North JP, et al. Merkel Cell Carcinoma: An Update and Review: Pathogenesis, Diagnosis, and Staging. J Am Acad Dermatol. 2018 Mar;78(3):433–42. PMID:29229574
640. Cohen Aubart F, Emile JF, Carrat F, et al. Targeted Therapies in 54 Patients with Erdheim-Chester Disease, Including Follow-Up After Interruption (the LOVE Study). Blood. 2017 Sep 14;130(11):1377–80. PMID:28667012
641. Cohen Aubart F, Roos-Weil D, Armand M, et al. High Frequency of Clonal Hematopoiesis in Erdheim-Chester Disease. Blood. 2021 Jan 28;137(4):485–92. PMID:33067622
642. Cohen LM, Goldberg RA, Rootman DB. Recurrence of Distensible Orbital Venous-Dominant Venolymphatic Malformations After Sclerotherapy Versus Embolization With Excision. Ophthalmic Plast Reconstr Surg. 2022 May-Jun 01;38(3):283–8. PMID:34798656
643. Cohen MM Jr. The New Bone Biology: Pathologic, Molecular, and Clinical Correlates. Am J Med Genet A. 2006 Dec 1;140(23):2646–706. PMID:17103447
644. Cohen PR. Verruca Vulgaris Occurring on a Tattoo: Case Report and Review of Tattoo-Associated Human Papillomavirus Infections. Cureus. 2021 Aug 30;13(8):e17575. PMID:34646630
645. Cohen VM, Shields CL, Furuta M, et al. Vitreous Seeding from Retinal Astrocytoma in Three Cases. Retina. 2008 Jun;28(6):884–8. PMID:18536607
646. Cohen-Aubart F, Emile JF, Carrat F, et al. Phenotypes and Survival in Erdheim-Chester Disease: Results from a 165-Patient Cohort. Am J Hematol. 2018 May;93(5):e114–7. PMID:29396850
647. Cohn AD, Quiram PA, Drenser KA, et al. Surgical Outcomes of Epiretinal Membranes Associated with Combined Hamartoma of the Retina and Retinal Pigment Epithelium. Retina. 2009 Jun;29(6):825–30. PMID:19276871
648. Colarossi C, Milazzo M, Paglierani M, et al. A Juvenile Case of Conjunctival Atypical Nevus. Diagn Pathol. 2013 Apr 22;8:64. PMID:23607499
649. Collaborative Ocular Melanoma Study Group. Assessment of Metastatic Disease Status at Death in 435 Patients with Large Choroidal Melanoma in the Collaborative Ocular Melanoma Study (COMS): COMS Report No. 15. Arch Ophthalmol. 2001 May;119(5):670–6. PMID:11346394
650. Collgros H, Rodriguez-Lomba E, Regio Pereira A, et al. Lentiginous Melanoma (Lentigo Maligna and Lentigo Maligna Melanoma) in Australia: Clinicopathological Characteristics, Management and Recurrence Rates After 10-Year Follow-Up at a Tertiary Centre. J Eur Acad Dermatol Venereol. 2021 Jun;35(6):1315–22. PMID:33502077
651. Collins R, Lafford G, Meghji S, et al. Adult Nasal Chondromesenchymal Hamartoma: A Rare and Benign Tumour with Aggressive Malignant Transformation. BMJ Case Rep. 2021 Jul 28;14(7):e240643. PMID:34321260
652. Collins VP, Jones DT, Giannini C. Pilocytic Astrocytoma: Pathology, Molecular Mechanisms and Markers. Acta Neuropathol. 2015 Jun;129(6):775–88. PMID:25792358
653. Colman SD, Williams CA, Wallace MR. Benign Neurofibromas in Type 1 Neurofibromatosis (NF1) Show Somatic Deletions of the NF1 Gene. Nat Genet. 1995 Sep;11(1):90–2. PMID:7550323
654. Colombo F, Holbach LM, Naumann GO. Chronic Inflammation in Dermoid Cysts: A Clinicopathologic Study of 115 Patients. Orbit. 2000 Jun;19(2):97–107. PMID:12045954
655. Colombo F, Holbach LM, Naumann GO. Conjunctival Cyst and Conjunctival Dermoid of the Orbit. Orbit. 2000 Mar;19(1):13–9. PMID:12045960
656. Comfere NI, Gonzalez Santiago TM, Peters MS, et al. Cutaneous Extramedullary Plasmacytoma: Clinical, Prognostic, and Interphase Cytogenetic Analysis. Am J Dermatopathol. 2013 May;35(3):357–63. PMID:23000906
657. Comi AM. Presentation, Diagnosis, Pathophysiology, and Treatment of the Neurological Features of Sturge-Weber Syndrome. Neurologist. 2011 Jul;17(4):179–84. PMID:21712663
658. Compton CJ, Clark JD, Thompson MP, et al. Nodular Fasciitis of the Orbit. Ophthalmic Plast Reconstr Surg. 2016 Nov/Dec;32(6):e154–6. PMID:25393905
659. Conboy E, Dhamija R, Wang M, et al. Paraspinal Neurofibromas and Hypertrophic Neuropathy in Noonan Syndrome with Multiple Lentigines. J Med Genet. 2016 Feb;53(2):123–6. PMID:26337637
660. Concha Del Río LE, Duarte González GA, Mayorquín Ruiz M, et al. Characterization of Cyclitic Membranes by Ultrabiomicroscopy in Patients with Pars Planitis. J Ophthalmic Inflamm Infect. 2020 Jan 27;10(1):7. PMID:31997032
661. Condoluci A, Terzi Di Bergamo L, Langerbeins P, et al. International Prognostic Score for Asymptomatic Early-Stage Chronic Lymphocytic Leukemia. Blood. 2020 May 21;135(21):1859–69. PMID:32267500
662. Cooling RJ, Wright JE. Arachnoid Hyperplasia in Optic Nerve Glioma: Confusion with Orbital Meningioma. Br J Ophthalmol. 1979 Sep;63(9):596–9. PMID:486377
663. Copson B, McKelvie PA, Khong JJ. Massive Retinal Gliosis with Episcleral Extension. Clin Exp Ophthalmol. 2017 Dec;45(9):923–4. PMID:28516476
664. Cordel N, Tressières B, D'Incan M, et al. Frequency and Risk Factors for Associated Lymphomas in Patients With Lymphomatoid Papulosis. Oncologist. 2016 Jan;21(1):76–83. PMID:26668250
665. Corio RL, Sciubba JJ, Brannon RB, et al. Epithelial-Myoepithelial Carcinoma of Intercalated Duct Origin. A Clinicopathologic and Ultrastructural Assessment of Sixteen Cases. Oral Surg Oral Med Oral Pathol. 1982 Mar;53(3):280–7. PMID:6950345
666. Coroneo M. Ultraviolet Radiation and the Anterior Eye. Eye Contact Lens. 2011 Jul;37(4):214–24. PMID:21670690
667. Coroneo MT. Pterygium as an Early Indicator of Ultraviolet Insolation: A Hypothesis. Br J Ophthalmol. 1993 Nov;77(11):734–9. PMID:8280691
668. Correa R, Salpea P, Stratakis CA. Carney Complex: An Update. Eur J Endocrinol. 2015 Oct;173(4):m85–97. PMID:26130139
669. Corrêa ZM, Augsburger JJ. Independent Prognostic Significance of Gene Expression Profile Class and Largest Basal Diameter of Posterior Uveal Melanomas. Am J Ophthalmol. 2016 Feb;162:20–27.E1. PMID:26596399
670. Corrêa ZM, Augsburger JJ, Spaulding AG. Medulloepithelioma of the Optic Disc. Hum Pathol. 2011 Dec;42(12):2047–51. PMID:21676432
671. Corson TW, Gallie BL. One Hit, Two Hits, Three Hits, More? Genomic Changes in the Development of Retinoblastoma. Genes Chromosomes Cancer. 2007 Jul;46(7):617–34. PMID:17437278
672. Cortes Barrantes P, Jakobiec FA, Dryja TP. A Review of the Role of Cytogenetics in the Diagnosis of Orbital Rhabdomyosarcoma. Semin Ophthalmol. 2019;34(4):243–51. PMID:31146616
673. Costa S, Byrne M, Pissaloux D, et al. Melanomas Associated With Blue Nevi or Mimicking Cellular Blue Nevi: Clinical, Pathologic, and Molecular Study of 11 Cases Displaying a High Frequency of GNA11 Mutations, BAP1 Expression Loss, and a Predilection for the Scalp. Am J Surg Pathol. 2016 Mar;40(3):368–77. PMID:26645730
674. Costea CF, Turliuc MD, Dimitriu G, et al. Inflammatory Juvenile Compound Conjunctival Nevi. A Clinicopathological Study and Literature Review. Rom J Morphol Embryol. 2017;58(3):739–47. PMID:29250649
675. Coupland S, Heegaard S. Can Conjunctival Lymphoma Be a Clinical Diagnosis? Br J Ophthalmol. 2014 May;98(5):574–5. PMID:24307715
676. Coupland SE, Anastassiou G, Bornfeld N, et al. Primary Intraocular Lymphoma of T-Cell Type: Report of a Case and Review of the Literature. Graefes Arch Clin Exp Ophthalmol. 2005 Mar;243(3):189–97. PMID:15806372
677. Coupland SE, Damato B. Understanding Intraocular Lymphomas. Clin Exp Ophthalmol. 2008 Aug;36(6):564–78. PMID:18954321
678. Coupland SE, Foss HD, Assaf C, et al. T-Cell and T/Natural Killer-Cell Lymphomas Involving Ocular and Ocular Adnexal Tissues: A Clinicopathologic, Immunohistochemical, and Molecular Study of Seven Cases. Ophthalmology. 1999 Nov;106(11):2109–20. PMID:10571346
679. Coupland SE, Foss HD, Hidayat AA, et al.

Extranodal Marginal Zone B Cell Lymphomas of the Uvea: An Analysis of 13 Cases. J Pathol. 2002 Jul;197(3):333–40. PMID:12115879
680. Coupland SE, Heimann H, Bechrakis NE. Primary Intraocular Lymphoma: A Review of the Clinical, Histopathological and Molecular Biological Features. Graefes Arch Clin Exp Ophthalmol. 2004 Nov;242(11):901–13. PMID:15565454
681. Coupland SE, Hellmich M, Auw-Haedrich C, et al. Prognostic Value of Cell-Cycle Markers in Ocular Adnexal Lymphoma: An Assessment of 230 Cases. Graefes Arch Clin Exp Ophthalmol. 2004 Feb;242(2):130–45. PMID:14685876
682. Coupland SE, Hummel M, Müller HH, et al. Molecular Analysis of Immunoglobulin Genes in Primary Intraocular Lymphoma. Invest Ophthalmol Vis Sci. 2005 Oct;46(10):3507–14. PMID:16186327
683. Coupland SE, Joussen A, Anastassiou G, et al. Diagnosis of a Primary Uveal Extranodal Marginal Zone B-Cell Lymphoma by Chorioretinal Biopsy: Case Report. Graefes Arch Clin Exp Ophthalmol. 2005 May;243(5):482–6. PMID:15586289
684. Coupland SE, Krause L, Delecluse HJ, et al. Lymphoproliferative Lesions of the Ocular Adnexa. Analysis of 112 Cases. Ophthalmology. 1998 Aug;105(8):1430–41. PMID:9709754
685. Coupland SE, Lake SL, Zeschnigk M, et al. Molecular Pathology of Uveal Melanoma. Eye (Lond). 2013 Feb;27(2):230–42. PMID:23222563
686. Coupland SE, Loddenkemper C, Smith JR, et al. Expression of Immunoglobulin Transcription Factors in Primary Intraocular Lymphoma and Primary Central Nervous System Lymphoma. Invest Ophthalmol Vis Sci. 2005 Nov;46(11):3957–64. PMID:16249468
687. Cozzolino I, Varone V, Picardi M, et al. CD10, BCL6, and MUM1 Expression in Diffuse Large B-Cell Lymphoma on FNA Samples. Cancer Cytopathol. 2016 Feb;124(2):135–43. PMID:26414904
688. Crawford JB, Howes EL Jr, Char DH. Combined Nevi of the Conjunctiva. Arch Ophthalmol. 1999 Sep;117(9):1121–7. PMID:10496382
689. Crawford JB, Howes EL Jr, Char DH. Combined Nevi of the Conjunctiva. Trans Am Ophthalmol Soc. 1999;97:170–83. PMID:10703123
690. Creager HM, Kumar A, Zeng H, et al. Infection and Replication of Influenza Virus at the Ocular Surface. J Virol. 2018 Mar 14;92(7):e02192-17. PMID:29321303
691. Cree IA, Foss AJ, Luthert PJ. Undefined High-Power Fields. Lancet. 1996 Jan 27;347(8996):273–4. PMID:8551926
691A. Cree IA, Tan PH, Travis WD, et al. Counting Mitoses: SI(ze) Matters! Mod Pathol. 2021 Sep;34(9):1651–7. PMID:34079071.
692. Croci GA, Hoster E, Beà S, et al. Reproducibility of Histologic Prognostic Parameters for Mantle Cell Lymphoma: Cytology, Ki67, P53 and SOX11. Virchows Arch. 2020 Aug;477(2):259–67. PMID:31975037
693. Cruz NFSD, Cruz SFSD, Ishigai DH, et al. Conjunctival Tattoo: Report on an Emerging Body Modification Trend. Arq Bras Oftalmol. 2017 Nov-Dec;80(6):399–400. PMID:29267580
694. Cubie HA. Diseases Associated with Human Papillomavirus Infection. Virology. 2013 Oct;445(1-2):21–34. PMID:23932731
695. Cummings TJ, Dodd LG, Eedes CR, et al. Hereditary Benign Intraepithelial Dyskeratosis: An Evaluation of Diagnostic Cytology. Arch Pathol Lab Med. 2008 Aug;132(8):1325–8. PMID:18684035
696. Curran AE, Allen CM, Beck FM, et al. Distinctive Pattern of Glial Fibrillary Acidic Protein Immunoreactivity Useful in Distinguishing Fragmented Pleomorphic Adenoma, Canalicular Adenoma and Polymorphous Low Grade Adenocarcinoma of Minor Salivary Glands. Head Neck Pathol. 2007 Sep;1(1):27–32. PMID:20614277
697. Cu-Unjieng AB, Shields CL, Shields JA, et al. Iris Melanoma in Ocular Melanocytosis. Cornea. 1995 Mar;14(2):206–9. PMID:7743806
698. Da Costa CE, Annels NE, Faaij CM, et al. Presence of Osteoclast-Like Multinucleated Giant Cells in the Bone and Nonostotic Lesions of Langerhans Cell Histiocytosis. J Exp Med. 2005 Mar 7;201(5):687–93. PMID:15753204
699. Da Silva AD, Silva CA, de Camargo Moraes P, et al. Recurrent Oral Pyogenic Granuloma in Port-Wine Stain. J Craniofac Surg. 2011 Nov;22(6):2356–8. PMID:22134277
700. Da Silva LCM, Da Silva Platner F, Da Silva Fonseca L, et al. Ocular Manifestations of Chikungunya Infection: A Systematic Review. Pathogens. 2022 Mar 29;11(4):412. PMID:35456087
701. D'Adamo DR. Appraising the Current Role of Chemotherapy for the Treatment of Sarcoma. Semin Oncol. 2011 Oct;38(Suppl 3):S19–29. PMID:22055968
702. Dadone-Montaudié B, Alberti L, Duc A, et al. Alternative PDGFD Rearrangements in Dermatofibrosarcomas Protuberans Without PDGFB Fusions. Mod Pathol. 2018 Nov;31(11):1683–93. PMID:29955147
703. Dagklis A, Ponzoni M, Govi S, et al. Immunoglobulin Gene Repertoire in Ocular Adnexal Lymphomas: Hints on the Nature of the Antigenic Stimulation. Leukemia. 2012 Apr;26(4):814–21. PMID:22024723
704. Dahlén A, Debiec-Rychter M, Pedeutour F, et al. Clustering of Deletions on Chromosome 13 in Benign and Low-Malignant Lipomatous Tumors. Int J Cancer. 2003 Feb 20;103(5):616–23. PMID:12494468
705. Dahlén A, Mertens F, Rydholm A, et al. Fusion, Disruption, and Expression of HMGA2 in Bone and Soft Tissue Chondromas. Mod Pathol. 2003 Nov;16(11):1132–40. PMID:14614053
706. Dal Cin P, Kozakewich HP, Goumnerova L, et al. Variant Translocations Involving 16q22 and 17p13 in Solid Variant and Extraosseous Forms of Aneurysmal Bone Cyst. Genes Chromosomes Cancer. 2000 Jun;28(2):233–4. PMID:10825009
707. D'Ali L, Tulisso A, Mariuzzi L. Primary Mesenchymal Chondrosarcoma of the Orbit in a Young Female: Imaging and Histopathological Features. J Surg Case Rep. 2020 Mar 28;2020(3):rjaa037. PMID:32257101
708. Dalia S, Sagatys E, Sokol L, et al. Rosai-Dorfman Disease: Tumor Biology, Clinical Features, Pathology, and Treatment. Cancer Control. 2014 Oct;21(4):322–7. PMID:25310213
709. Dallachy R. Ectopic Lacrimal Glandular Tissue Within the Eyeball. Br J Ophthalmol. 1961 Dec;45(12):808–15. PMID:18170741
710. Dalland JC, Meyer R, Ketterling RP, et al. Myeloid Sarcoma With CBFB-MYH11 Fusion (Inv(16) or T(16;16)) Prevails in the Abdomen. Am J Clin Pathol. 2020 Feb 8;153(3):333–41. PMID:31671434
711. Dalvin LA, Lim LS, Chang M, et al. Circumscribed Choroidal Hemangioma: Clinical Features and Outcomes by Age Category in 458 Cases. Saudi J Ophthalmol. 2019 Jul-Sep;33(3):219–28. PMID:31686962
712. Dalvin LA, Yu MD, Ancona-Lezama DA, et al. Retinal Haemangioblastoma Associated with Peripheral Non-Perfusion: Widefield Fluorescein Angiography Analysis of 41 Cases. Br J Ophthalmol. 2020 Feb;104(2):167–72. PMID:31097435
713. Damato B, Bever GJ, Kim DJ, et al. An Audit of Retinal Lymphoma Treatment at the University of California San Francisco. Eye (Lond). 2020 Mar;34(3):515–22. PMID:31358925
714. Damato B, Coupland SE. Conjunctival Melanoma and Melanosis: A Reappraisal of Terminology, Classification and Staging. Clin Exp Ophthalmol. 2008 Nov;36(8):786–95. PMID:19128387
715. Damato B, Coupland SE. Management of Conjunctival Melanoma. Expert Rev Anticancer Ther. 2009 Sep;9(9):1227–39. PMID:19761427
716. Damato B, Eleuteri A, Hussain R, et al. Parsimonious Models for Predicting Mortality from Choroidal Melanoma. Invest Ophthalmol Vis Sci. 2020 Apr 9;61(4):35. PMID:32334433
717. Damato BE. Can the MOLES Acronym and Scoring System Improve the Management of Patients with Melanocytic Choroidal Tumours? Eye (Lond). 2023 Apr;37(5):830–6. PMID:35764877
718. Damato BE, Coupland SE. Differences in Uveal Melanomas Between Men and Women from the British Isles. Eye (Lond). 2012 Feb;26(2):292–9. PMID:22079972
719. Damle RN, Wasil T, Fais F, et al. Ig V Gene Mutation Status and CD38 Expression as Novel Prognostic Indicators in Chronic Lymphocytic Leukemia. Blood. 1999 Sep 15;94(6):1840–7. PMID:10477712
720. Daniel CS, Beaconsfield M, Rose GE, et al. Pleomorphic Lipoma of the Orbit: A Case Series and Review of Literature. Ophthalmology. 2003 Jan;110(1):101–5. PMID:12511353
721. Daniel L, Rao S, Muthusamy R, et al. Mucoepidermoid Carcinoma Ex Pleomorphic Adenoma of the Lacrimal Gland: A Rare Presentation. Indian J Ophthalmol. 2014 Jun;62(6):743–6. PMID:25005213
722. Darwich R, Ghazawi FM, Le M, et al. Epidemiology of Invasive Ocular Surface Squamous Neoplasia in Canada During 1992-2010. Br J Ophthalmol. 2020 Oct;104(10):1368–72. PMID:31949098
723. Dasgupta T, Wilson LD, Yu JB. A Retrospective Review of 1349 Cases of Sebaceous Carcinoma. Cancer. 2009 Jan 1;115(1):158–65. PMID:18988294
724. Dave TV, Mishra D, Mittal R, et al. Accidentally Diagnosed Transitional Cell Papilloma of the Lacrimal Sac. Saudi J Ophthalmol. 2017 Jul-Sep;31(3):177–9. PMID:28860918
725. Davies HR, Broad KD, Onadim Z, et al. Whole-Genome Sequencing of Retinoblastoma Reveals the Diversity of Rearrangements Disrupting RB1 and Uncovers a Treatment-Related Mutational Signature. Cancers (Basel). 2021 Feb 11;13(4):754. PMID:33670346
726. Davis JL, Viciana AL, Ruiz P. Diagnosis of Intraocular Lymphoma by Flow Cytometry. Am J Ophthalmol. 1997 Sep;124(3):362–72. PMID:9439362
727. Davis RC, Broadwater G, Foo WC, et al. Evaluation of Pelvic Washing Specimens in Patients with Endometrial Cancer: Cytomorphological Features, Diagnostic Agreement, and Pathologist Experience. Cancer Cytopathol. 2021 Jul;129(7):517–25. PMID:33481348
728. Davis RJ, D'Cruz CM, Lovell MA, et al. Fusion of PAX7 to FKHR by the Variant T(1;13)(P36;Q14) Translocation in Alveolar Rhabdomyosarcoma. Cancer Res. 1994 Jun 1;54(11):2869–72. PMID:8187070
729. Davis TH, Morton CC, Miller-Cassman R, et al. Hodgkin's Disease, Lymphomatoid Papulosis, and Cutaneous T-Cell Lymphoma Derived from a Common T-Cell Clone. N Engl J Med. 1992 Apr 23;326(17):1115–22. PMID:1532439
730. Day AM, McCulloch CE, Hammill AM, et al. Physical and Family History Variables Associated With Neurological and Cognitive Development in Sturge-Weber Syndrome. Pediatr Neurol. 2019 Jul;96:30–6. PMID:30853154
731. de Alba MA, Villegas VM, Gold AS, et al. Clinical Findings and Genetic Expression Profiling of Three Pigmented Lesions of the Optic Nerve. Case Rep Ophthalmol Med. 2015;2015:590659. PMID:25984377
732. de Barros GF, Hakim JR, Passos JP, et al. Orbital Alveolar Soft Part Sarcoma: Case Report and Literature Review. Can J Ophthalmol. 2019 Dec;54(6):e292–4. PMID:31836117
733. de Boer CJ, Schuuring E, Dreef E, et al. Cyclin D1 Protein Analysis in the Diagnosis of Mantle Cell Lymphoma. Blood. 1995 Oct 1;86(7):2715–23. PMID:7670110
734. de Boer CJ, van Krieken JH, Kluin-Nelemans HC, et al. Cyclin D1 Messenger RNA Overexpression as a Marker for Mantle Cell Lymphoma. Oncogene. 1995 May 4;10(9):1833–40. PMID:7753558
735. De Giorgi V, Trane L, Pieretti G, et al. Treatment of Periocular Advanced Basal Cell Carcinoma with Hedgehog Pathway Inhibitors: A Single-Center Study and a New Dedicated Therapeutic Protocol. Dermatol Reports 2021 Aug 5;13(3):9240. PMID:35003569
736. de Graaf P, Göricke S, Rodjan F, et al. Guidelines for Imaging Retinoblastoma: Imaging Principles and MRI Standardization. Pediatr Radiol. 2012 Jan;42(1):2–14. PMID:21850471
737. De Gregorio A, Cerini A, Scala A, et al. Floppy Eyelid, an Under-Diagnosed Syndrome: A Review of Demographics, Pathogenesis, and Treatment. Ther Adv Ophthalmol. 2021 Dec 5;13:25158414211059247. PMID:35187400
738. De Groot V, Verhelst E, Hogendoorn PCW, et al. Conjunctival Leiomyosarcoma, a Rare Neoplasm Always Originating at the Limbus? Report of a New Case and Review of 11 Published Cases. Ocul Oncol Pathol. 2019 Aug;5(5):333–9. PMID:31559244
739. de Jong MC, de Graaf P, Noij DP, et al. Diagnostic Performance of Magnetic Resonance Imaging and Computed Tomography for Advanced Retinoblastoma: A Systematic Review and Meta-Analysis. Ophthalmology. 2014 May;121(5):1109–18. PMID:24589388
740. de Jong MC, Kors WA, de Graaf P, et al. The Incidence of Trilateral Retinoblastoma: A Systematic Review and Meta-Analysis. Am J Ophthalmol. 2015 Dec;160(6):1116–1126.E5. PMID:26374932
741. de Jong MC, Kors WA, Moll AC, et al. Screening for Pineal Trilateral Retinoblastoma Revisited: A Meta-Analysis. Ophthalmology. 2020 May;127(5):601–7. PMID:32061409
742. de Jong S, Itinteang T, Withers AH, et al. Does Hypoxia Play a Role in Infantile Hemangioma? Arch Dermatol Res. 2016 May;308(4):219–27. PMID:26940670
743. de Koning MN, Quint KD, Bruggink SC, et al. High Prevalence of Cutaneous Warts in Elementary School Children and the Ubiquitous Presence of Wart-Associated Human Papillomavirus on Clinically Normal Skin. Br J Dermatol. 2015 Jan;172(1):196–201. PMID:24976535
743A. de La Fouchardière A, Tee MK, Peternel S, et al. Fusion Partners of NTRK3 Affect Subcellular Localization of the Fusion Kinase and Cytomorphology of Melanocytes. Mod Pathol. 2021 Apr;34(4):735–47. PMID:32968185
743B. de La Fouchardiere A, Tirode F, Castillo C, et al. Attempting to Solve the Pigmented Epithelioid Melanocytoma (PEM) Conundrum: PRKAR1A Inactivation Can Occur in Different Genetic Backgrounds (Common, Blue, and Spitz Subgroups) With Variation in Their Clinicopathologic Characteristics. Am J Surg Pathol. 2022 Aug;46(8):1106–15. PMID:35319525
744. de La Garza Bravo MM, Patel KP, Loghavi S, et al. Shared Clonality in Distinctive Lesions of Lymphomatoid Papulosis and Mycosis Fungoides Occurring in the Same Patients Suggests a Common Origin. Hum Pathol. 2015 Apr;46(4):558–69. PMID:25666664
745. De La Torre AJ, Luat AF, Juhász C, et

al. A Multidisciplinary Consensus for Clinical Care and Research Needs for Sturge-Weber Syndrome. Pediatr Neurol. 2018 Jul;84:11–20. PMID:29803545
746. De Potter P, Stanescu D, Caspers-Velu L, et al. Photo Essay: Combined Hamartoma of the Retina and Retinal Pigment Epithelium in Gorlin Syndrome. Arch Ophthalmol. 2000 Jul;118(7):1004–5. PMID:10900122
747. De Raedt T, Beert E, Pasmant E, et al. PRC2 Loss Amplifies Ras-Driven Transcription and Confers Sensitivity to BRD4-Based Therapies. Nature. 2014 Oct 9;514(7521):247–51. PMID:25119042
748. De Rosa G, Zeppa P, Tranfa F, et al. Acinic Cell Carcinoma Arising in a Lacrimal Gland. First Case Report. Cancer. 1986 May 15;57(10):1988–91. PMID:3955504
749. de Souza A, El-Azhary RA, Camilleri MJ, et al. In Search of Prognostic Indicators for Lymphomatoid Papulosis: A Retrospective Study of 123 Patients. J Am Acad Dermatol. 2012 Jun;66(6):928–37. PMID:21982062
750. DeBarge LR, Chan CC, Greenberg SC, et al. Chorioretinal, Iris, and Ciliary Body Infiltration by Juvenile Xanthogranuloma Masquerading as Uveitis. Surv Ophthalmol. 1994 Jul-Aug;39(1):65–71. PMID:7974193
751. Decatur CL, Ong E, Garg N, et al. Driver Mutations in Uveal Melanoma: Associations With Gene Expression Profile and Patient Outcomes. JAMA Ophthalmol. 2016 Jul 1;134(7):728–33. PMID:27123562
752. Decock C, Stefaan R, Vandenbroecke C, et al. Diagnosis and Treatment of a Superficial Upper Eyelid Arteriovenous Malformation. Orbit. 2008;27(4):301–3. PMID:18716969
753. DeCoteau JF, Butmarc JR, Kinney MC, et al. The T(2;5) Chromosomal Translocation is Not a Common Feature of Primary Cutaneous CD30+ Lymphoproliferative Disorders: Comparison with Anaplastic Large-Cell Lymphoma of Nodal Origin. Blood. 1996 Apr 15;87(8):3437–41. PMID:8605362
754. de Feraudy S, Fletcher CD. Intradermal Nodular Fasciitis: A Rare Lesion Analyzed in a Series of 24 Cases. Am J Surg Pathol. 2010 Sep;34(9):1377–81. PMID:20716998
755. Dehainault C, Garancher A, Castéra L, et al. The Survival Gene MED4 Explains Low Penetrance Retinoblastoma in Patients with Large RB1 Deletion. Hum Mol Genet. 2014 Oct 1;23(19):5243–50. PMID:24858910
756. Dehner LP. Juvenile Xanthogranulomas in the First Two Decades of Life: A Clinicopathologic Study of 174 Cases with Cutaneous and Extracutaneous Manifestations. Am J Surg Pathol. 2003 May;27(5):579–93. PMID:12717244
757. Dei Tos AP, Seregard S, Calonje E, et al. Giant Cell Angiofibroma. A Distinctive Orbital Tumor in Adults. Am J Surg Pathol. 1995 Nov;19(11):1286–93. PMID:7573691
758. Del Valle Estopinal M, Middleton LP, Esmaeli B, et al. Primary Signet Ring Cell/Histiocytoid Carcinoma of the Eyelid: Clinicopathologic Analysis with Evaluation of the E-Cadherin/β-Catenin Complex and Associated Genetic Alterations. Case Rep Pathol. 2021 Nov 11;2021:6628150. PMID:34804623
759. Delestre F, Blanche P, Bouayed E, et al. Ophthalmic Involvement of Chronic Lymphocytic Leukemia: A Systematic Review of 123 Cases. Surv Ophthalmol. 2021 Jan-Feb;66(1):124–31. PMID:32407752
760. Deliganis AV, Geyer JR, Berger MS. Prognostic Significance of Type 1 Neurofibromatosis (von Recklinghausen Disease) in Childhood Optic Glioma. Neurosurgery. 1996 Jun;38(6):1114–8. PMID:8727140
761. de Melo AC, Santos Thuler LC. Trends in the Incidence and Morbidity of Merkel Cell Carcinoma in Brazil. Future Oncol. 2021 Aug;17(22):2857–65. PMID:33960199
762. Demicco EG, Harms PW, Patel RM, et al. Extensive Survey of STAT6 Expression in a Large Series of Mesenchymal Tumors. Am J Clin Pathol. 2015 May;143(5):672–82. PMID:25873501
763. Demicco EG, Park MS, Araujo DM, et al. Solitary Fibrous Tumor: A Clinicopathological Study of 110 Cases and Proposed Risk Assessment Model. Mod Pathol. 2012 Sep;25(9):1298–306. PMID:22575866
764. Demicco EG, Wagner MJ, Maki RG, et al. Risk Assessment in Solitary Fibrous Tumors: Validation and Refinement of a Risk Stratification Model. Mod Pathol. 2017 Oct;30(10):1433–42. PMID:28731041
765. Demirci H, Demirci FY, Ciftci S, et al. Integrative Exome and Transcriptome Analysis of Conjunctival Melanoma and Its Potential Application for Personalized Therapy. JAMA Ophthalmol. 2019 Dec 1;137(12):1444–8. PMID:31647501
766. Demirci H, Mashayekhi A, Shields CL, et al. Iris Melanocytoma: Clinical Features and Natural Course in 47 Cases. Am J Ophthalmol. 2005 Mar;139(3):468–75. PMID:15767055
767. Demirci H, McCormick SA, Finger PT. Topical Mitomycin Chemotherapy for Conjunctival Malignant Melanoma and Primary Acquired Melanosis with Atypia: Clinical Experience with Histopathologic Observations. Arch Ophthalmol. 2000 Jul;118(7):885–91. PMID:10900099
768. Demirci H, Shields CL, Eagle RC Jr, et al. Giant Cell Angiofibroma, a Variant of Solitary Fibrous Tumor, of the Orbit in a 16-Year-Old Girl. Ophthalmic Plast Reconstr Surg. 2009 Sep-Oct;25(5):402–4. PMID:19966660
769. Demirci H, Shields CL, Shields JA. Bilateral Optic Disk Melanocytoma in a 10-Month-Old Infant. Am J Ophthalmol. 2003 Jul;136(1):190–2. PMID:12834694
770. Demirci H, Shields CL, Shields JA. New Ophthalmic Manifestations of Branchio-Oculo-Facial Syndrome. Am J Ophthalmol. 2005 Feb;139(2):362–4. PMID:15734008
771. Demirci H, Shields CL, Shields JA, et al. Diffuse Iris Melanoma: A Report of 25 Cases. Ophthalmology. 2002 Aug;109(8):1553–60. PMID:12153810
772. Demirci H, Shields CL, Shields JA, et al. Malignant Melanoma Arising from Unusual Conjunctival Blue Nevus. Arch Ophthalmol. 2000 Nov;118(11):1581–4. PMID:11074819
773. Demirci H, Shields CL, Shields JA, et al. Orbital Tumors in the Older Adult Population. Ophthalmology. 2002 Feb;109(2):243–8. PMID:11825802
774. Demirci H, Shields CL, Shields JA, et al. Ring Melanoma of the Anterior Chamber Angle: A Report of Fourteen Cases. Am J Ophthalmol. 2001 Sep;132(3):336–42. PMID:11530045
775. Demirci H, Shields CL, Shields JA, et al. Ring Melanoma of the Ciliary Body: Report on Twenty-Three Patients. Retina. 2002 Dec;22(6):698–706. PMID:12476094
776. Deprez M, Uffer S. Clinicopathological Features of Eyelid Skin Tumors. A Retrospective Study of 5504 Cases and Review of Literature. Am J Dermatopathol. 2009 May;31(3):256–62. PMID:19384066
777. Dermarkarian CR, Patel KR, Fuller MY, et al. Inflammatory Myofibroblastic Tumor of the Orbit in an 8-Month Old. Ophthalmic Plast Reconstr Surg. 2020 May/Jun;36(3):e65–8. PMID:31880682
778. Dermawan JK, Azzato EM, Billings SD, et al. YAP1-TFE3-Fused Hemangioendothelioma: A Multi-Institutional Clinicopathologic Study of 24 Genetically-Confirmed Cases. Mod Pathol. 2021 Dec;34(12):2211–21. PMID:34381186
779. Derzko-Dzulynsky L. IgG4-Related Disease in the Eye and Ocular Adnexa. Curr Opin Ophthalmol. 2017 Nov;28(6):617–22. PMID:28858963
780. De Salvo G, Krebs I, Binder S. High-Definition Optical Coherence Tomography in a Case of Congenital Hypertrophy of the Retinal Pigment Epithelium. Ophthalmic Surg Lasers Imaging. 2010 Nov-Dec;41(Suppl):S93–5. PMID:21117611
781. Deshpande V, Zen Y, Chan JK, et al. Consensus Statement on the Pathology of IgG4-Related Disease. Mod Pathol. 2012 Sep;25(9):1181–92. PMID:22596100
782. Detiger SE, Hötte GJ, Verdijk RM, et al. Adult Orbital Xanthogranuloma: Long-Term Follow-Up of Treated Cases. Eye (Lond). 2023 Aug;37(12):2475–81. PMID:36526862
783. Detiger SE, Karim AF, Verdijk RM, et al. The Treatment Outcomes in IgG4-Related Orbital Disease: A Systematic Review of the Literature. Acta Ophthalmol. 2019 Aug;97(5):451–9. PMID:30734497
784. Detiger SE, Karim F, Monserez D, et al. IgG4-Related Disease of Skull Base: Case Series of 3 Patients with Headache. World Neurosurg. 2020 Feb;134:536–9. PMID:31669684
785. Dey A, Seshasayee D, Noubade R, et al. Loss of the Tumor Suppressor BAP1 Causes Myeloid Transformation. Science. 2012 Sep 21;337(6101):1541–6. PMID:22878500
786. Dharmasena A, Lee PW, Irion LC, et al. Non-Keratinising Undifferentiated Nasopharyngeal-Type Carcinoma of the Lacrimal Sac. Int J Ophthalmol. 2016 Aug 18;9(8):1238–42. PMID:27588283
787. Dhermy P, Dugelay-Magnaud J. [Juvenile Melanoma of the Eyelid (Sophie Spitz Melanoma)]. Bull Soc Ophtalmol Fr. 1964 May-Jun;64:503–12. French. PMID:14300797
788. Dhupper M, Biswas J, Gopal L, et al. Clinicopathological Correlation of Choroidal Melanoma in Indian Population: A Study of 113 Cases. Oman J Ophthalmol. 2012 Jan;5(1):42–5. PMID:22557876
789. Di Cesare S, Marshall JC, Fernandes BF, et al. In Vitro Characterization and Inhibition of the CXCR4/CXCL12 Chemokine Axis in Human Uveal Melanoma Cell Lines. Cancer Cell Int. 2007 Nov 14;7:17. PMID:18001467
790. Di Cesare S, Marshall JC, Logan P, et al. Expression and Migratory Analysis of 5 Human Uveal Melanoma Cell Lines for CXCL12, CXCL8, CXCL1, and HGF. J Carcinog. 2007 Jan 29;6:2. PMID:17261188
791. Di Girolamo N, Atik A, McCluskey PJ, et al. Matrix Metalloproteinases and Their Inhibitors in Squamous Cell Carcinoma of the Conjunctiva. Ocul Surf. 2013 Jul;11(3):193–205. PMID:23838020
792. Diamond EL, Durham BH, Haroche J, et al. Diverse and Targetable Kinase Alterations Drive Histiocytic Neoplasms. Cancer Discov. 2016 Feb;6(2):154–65. PMID:26566875
793. Diamond EL, Durham BH, Ulaner GA, et al. Efficacy of MEK Inhibition in Patients with Histiocytic Neoplasms. Nature. 2019 Mar;567(7749):521–4. PMID:30867592
794. Dianzani C, Conforti C, Giuffrida R, et al. Current Therapies for Actinic Keratosis. Int J Dermatol. 2020 Jun;59(6):677–84. PMID:32012240
795. Díaz-Flores L, Gutiérrez R, Madrid JF, et al. Intravascular Papillary Endothelial Hyperplasia (IPEH). Evidence Supporting a Piecemeal Mode of Angiogenesis from Vein Endothelium, with Vein Wall Neovascularization and Papillary Formation. Histol Histopathol. 2016 Nov;31(11):1271–9. PMID:27323848
796. Diaz-Perez JA, Barajas-Gamboa JS. Complex Choristoma of the Lacrimal Caruncle: A Case Report of an Unusual Congenital Tumor with Clinical and Histopathological Classification. Int Ophthalmol. 2012 Feb;32(1):37–9. PMID:22213061
797. Dickens TA, Franchina M, Gajdatsy A, et al. Primary Orbital Melanoma Arising in an Atypical Diffuse (Plaque-Like) Blue Naevus/Melanocytosis: A Case Report and Review of Literature. BMC Ophthalmol. 2021 Dec 9;21(1):425. PMID:34886849
798. Dickson BC, Hornick JL, Fletcher CDM, et al. Dermatofibrosarcoma Protuberans with a Novel COL6A3-PDGFD Fusion Gene and Apparent Predilection for Breast. Genes Chromosomes Cancer. 2018 Sep;57(9):437–45. PMID:30014607
799. Di Girolamo N. Association of Human Papilloma Virus with Pterygia and Ocular-Surface Squamous Neoplasia. Eye (Lond). 2012 Feb;26(2):202–11. PMID:22134594
800. Dimaras H, Corson TW, Cobrinik D, et al. Retinoblastoma. Nat Rev Dis Primers. 2015 Aug 27;1:15021. PMID:27189421
801. Dimaras H, Khetan V, Halliday W, et al. Loss of RB1 Induces Non-Proliferative Retinoma: Increasing Genomic Instability Correlates with Progression to Retinoblastoma. Hum Mol Genet. 2008 May 15;17(10):1363–72. PMID:18211953
802. Dimaras H, Khetan V, Halliday W, et al. Retinoma Underlying Retinoblastoma Revealed After Tumor Response to 1 Cycle of Chemotherapy. Arch Ophthalmol. 2009 Aug;127(8):1066–8. PMID:19667353
803. Dinakaran S, Rundle PA, Parsons MA, et al. Adenoma of Ciliary Pigment Epithelium: A Case Series. Br J Ophthalmol. 2003 Apr;87(4):504–5. PMID:12642323
804. Dithmar S, Völcker HE, Grossniklaus HE. Multifocal Intraocular Malignant Melanoma: Report of Two Cases and Review of the Literature. Ophthalmology. 1999 Jul;106(7):1345–8. PMID:10406619
805. Dithmar SA, Rusciano DA, Armstrong CA, et al. Depletion of NK Cell Activity Results in Growth of Hepatic Micrometastases in a Murine Ocular Melanoma Model. Curr Eye Res. 1999 Nov;19(5):426–31. PMID:10520219
806. Ditta LC, Zhang J, Bibars W, et al. Cutaneous Angiomyolipoma of the Eyelid in a 2-Year-Old With Tuberous Sclerosis Complex. J Neuroophthalmol. 2021 Mar 1;41(1):e69–70. PMID:31609834
807. Divisato G, Formicola D, Esposito T, et al. ZNF687 Mutations in Severe Paget Disease of Bone Associated with Giant Cell Tumor. Am J Hum Genet. 2016 Feb 4;98(2):275–86. PMID:26849110
808. Dogru M, Matsuo H, Inoue M, et al. Management of Eyelid Sebaceous Carcinomas. Ophthalmologica. 1997;211(1):40–3. PMID:8958530
809. Dogrusöz M, Bagger M, van Duinen SG, et al. The Prognostic Value of AJCC Staging in Uveal Melanoma Is Enhanced by Adding Chromosome 3 and 8q Status. Invest Ophthalmol Vis Sci. 2017 Feb 1;58(2):833–42. PMID:28159971
810. Döhner H, Stilgenbauer S, Benner A, et al. Genomic Aberrations and Survival in Chronic Lymphocytic Leukemia. N Engl J Med. 2000 Dec 28;343(26):1910–6. PMID:11136261
811. Dommering CJ, Mol BM, Moll AC, et al. RB1 Mutation Spectrum in a Comprehensive Nationwide Cohort of Retinoblastoma Patients. J Med Genet. 2014 Jun;51(6):366–74. PMID:24688104
812. Dompmartin A, van Der Vleuten CJM, Dekeuleneer V, et al. GNA11-Mutated Sturge-Weber Syndrome Has Distinct Neurological and Dermatological Features. Eur J Neurol. 2022 Oct;29(10):3061–70. PMID:35715928
813. Dompmartin A, Vikkula M, Boon LM. Venous Malformation: Update on

Aetiopathogenesis, Diagnosis and Management. Phlebology. 2010 Oct;25(5):224–35. PMID:20870869

814. Donadieu J, Larabi IA, Tardieu M, et al. Vemurafenib for Refractory Multisystem Langerhans Cell Histiocytosis in Children: An International Observational Study. J Clin Oncol. 2019 Nov 1;37(31):2857–65. PMID:31513482

815. Donegan P, Law J, Schauwecker SM, et al. Use of an Ultrasonic Aspirator in Removal of an Orbital Rim Hemangioma. Ophthalmic Plast Reconstr Surg. 2021 May-Jun 01;37(3):e117–20. PMID:33481536

816. Dornbos D 3rd, Kim HJ, Butman JA, et al. Review of the Neurological Implications of von Hippel-Lindau Disease. JAMA Neurol. 2018 May 1;75(5):620–7. PMID:29379961

817. Dorsey CS, Montgomery H. Blue Nevus and its Distinction from Mongolian Spot and the Nevus of Ota. J Invest Dermatol. 1954 Mar;22(3):225–36. PMID:13130904

818. Dos Santos NR, de Bruijn DR, van Kessel AG. Molecular Mechanisms Underlying Human Synovial Sarcoma Development. Genes Chromosomes Cancer. 2001 Jan;30(1):1–14. PMID:11107170

819. Dottermusch M, Sumisławski P, Krevet J, et al. Co-Activation of Sonic Hedgehog and Wnt Signaling in Murine Retinal Precursor Cells Drives Ocular Lesions with Features of Intraocular Medulloepithelioma. Oncogenesis. 2021 Nov 16;10(11):78. PMID:34785636

820. Doyle LA, Fletcher CD. Peripheral Hemangioblastoma: Clinicopathologic Characterization in a Series of 22 Cases. Am J Surg Pathol. 2014 Jan;38(1):119–27. PMID:24145646

821. Doyle LA, Hornick JL, Fletcher CD. PEComa of the Gastrointestinal Tract: Clinicopathologic Study of 35 Cases with Evaluation of Prognostic Parameters. Am J Surg Pathol. 2013 Dec;37(12):1769–82. PMID:24061520

822. Doyle LA, Vivero M, Fletcher CD, et al. Nuclear Expression of STAT6 Distinguishes Solitary Fibrous Tumor from Histologic Mimics. Mod Pathol. 2014 Mar;27(3):390–5. PMID:24030747

823. Dreux N, Marty M, Chibon F, et al. Value and Limitation of Immunohistochemical Expression of HMGA2 in Mesenchymal Tumors: About a Series of 1052 Cases. Mod Pathol. 2010 Dec;23(12):1657–66. PMID:20834238

824. Drier A, Haroche J, Savatovsky J, et al. Cerebral, Facial, and Orbital Involvement in Erdheim-Chester Disease: CT and MR Imaging Findings. Radiology. 2010 May;255(2):586–94. PMID:20413768

825. Drilon A. TRK Inhibitors in TRK Fusion-Positive Cancers. Ann Oncol. 2019 Nov;30 Suppl 8:Viii23-Viii30. PMID:32223935

826. Drilon A, Li G, Dogan S, et al. What Hides Behind the MASC: Clinical Response and Acquired Resistance to Entrectinib After ETV6-NTRK3 Identification in a Mammary Analogue Secretory Carcinoma (MASC). Ann Oncol. 2016 May;27(5):920–6. PMID:26884591

827. Driskill JH, Zheng Y, Wu BK, et al. WWTR1(TAZ)-CAMTA1 Reprograms Endothelial Cells to Drive Epithelioid Hemangioendothelioma. Genes Dev. 2021 Apr 1;35(7-8):495–511. PMID:33766984

828. Drolet BA, Frieden IJ. Characteristics of Infantile Hemangiomas as Clues to Pathogenesis: Does Hypoxia Connect the Dots? Arch Dermatol. 2010 Nov;146(11):1295–9. PMID:21079070

829. Drummond SR, Kemp EG. Retinal Astrocytoma Managed by Brachytherapy. Ophthalmology. 2009 Mar;116(3):597–597.E1. PMID:19264224

830. Dryden SC, Marsili S, Meador AG, et al. Intravascular Papillary Endothelial Hyperplasia of the Orbit: A Case of Masson's Tumor. Cureus. 2019 Dec 1;11(12):e6266. PMID:31903303

831. Dryja TP, Zakov ZN, Albert DM. Adenocarcinoma Arising from the Epithelium of the Iris and Ciliary Body. Int Ophthalmol Clin. 1980 Summer;20(2):177–90. PMID:6995386

832. Du J, Wang J, Cui Y, et al. Clinicopathologic Study of Endolymphatic Sac Tumor (ELST) and Differential Diagnosis of Papillary Tumors Located at the Cerebellopontine Angle. Neuropathology. 2015 Oct;35(5):410–20. PMID:25944396

833. Du MQ. MALT Lymphoma : Recent Advances in Aetiology and Molecular Genetics. J Clin Exp Hematop. 2007 Nov;47(2):31–42. PMID:18040143

834. Du MQ. MALT Lymphoma: A Paradigm of NF-κB Dysregulation. Semin Cancer Biol. 2016 Aug;39:49–60. PMID:27452667

835. Duarte AF, Alpuim Costa D, Caçador N, et al. Adenoid Cystic Carcinoma of the Palpebral Lobe of the Lacrimal Gland - Case Report and Literature Review. Orbit. 2022 Oct;41(5):605–10. PMID:33749533

836. Dubb M, Michelow P. Cytologic Features of Chondroid Syringoma in Fine Needle Aspiration Biopsies: A Report of 3 Cases. Acta Cytol. 2010 Mar-Apr;54(2):183–6. PMID:20391975

837. Dubbink HJ, Bakels H, Post E, et al. TERT Promoter Mutations and BRAF Mutations Are Rare in Sporadic, and TERT Promoter Mutations Are Absent in NF1-Related Malignant Peripheral Nerve Sheath Tumors. J Neurooncol. 2014 Nov;120(2):267–72. PMID:25035100

838. Dubovy SR, Clark BJ. Palisaded Encapsulated Neuroma (Solitary Circumscribed Neuroma of Skin) of the Eyelid: Report of Two Cases and Review of the Literature. Br J Ophthalmol. 2001 Aug;85(8):949–51. PMID:11466253

839. Ducatman BS, Scheithauer BW, Piepgras DG, et al. Malignant Peripheral Nerve Sheath Tumors. A Clinicopathologic Study of 120 Cases. Cancer. 1986 May 15;57(10):2006–21. PMID:3082508

840. Duffy MT, Harris M, Hornblass A. Infantile Myofibromatosis of Orbital Bone. A Case Report with Computed Tomography, Magnetic Resonance Imaging, and Histologic Findings. Ophthalmology. 1997 Sep;104(9):1471–4. PMID:9307643

841. Duffy MT, Harrison W, Sassoon J, et al. Sclerosing Sweat Duct Carcinoma of the Eyelid Margin: Unusual Presentation of a Rare Tumor. Ophthalmology. 1999 Apr;106(4):751–6. PMID:10201598

842. Dujardin F, Binh MB, Bouvier C, et al. MDM2 and CDK4 Immunohistochemistry is a Valuable Tool in the Differential Diagnosis of Low-Grade Osteosarcomas and Other Primary Fibro-Osseous Lesions of the Bone. Mod Pathol. 2011 May;24(5):624–37. PMID:21336260

843. Duncan J, Chen Y, Fuchs D, et al. Follicular Lymphoma Presenting Solely as Chronic Follicular Conjunctivitis. Cornea. 2016 Mar;35(3):395–8. PMID:26606298

844. Duncan JL, Golabi M, Fredrick DR, et al. Complex Limbal Choristomas in Linear Nevus Sebaceous Syndrome. Ophthalmology. 1998 Aug;105(8):1459–65. PMID:9709758

845. Dupré A, Carrère S, Bonafé JL, et al. [Eruptive Generalized Syringomas, Milium and Atrophoderma Vermiculata. Nicolau and Balus' Syndrome (Author's Transl)]. French. Dermatologica. 1981;162(4):281–6. PMID:7262384

846. Dupree WB, Langloss JM, Weiss SW. Pigmented Dermatofibrosarcoma Protuberans (Bednar Tumor). A Pathologic, Ultrastructural, and Immunohistochemical Study. Am J Surg Pathol. 1985 Sep;9(9):630–9. PMID:3901787

847. Durham BH. Molecular Characterization of the Histiocytoses: Neoplasia of Dendritic Cells and Macrophages. Semin Cell Dev Biol. 2019 Feb;86:62–76. PMID:29526544

848. Durham BH, Lopez Rodrigo E, Picarsic J, et al. Activating Mutations in CSF1R and Additional Receptor Tyrosine Kinases in Histiocytic Neoplasms. Nat Med. 2019 Dec;25(12):1839–42. PMID:31768065

849. Durham BH, Roos-Weil D, Baillou C, et al. Functional Evidence for Derivation of Systemic Histiocytic Neoplasms from Hematopoietic Stem/Progenitor Cells. Blood. 2017 Jul 13;130(2):176–80. PMID:28566492

850. Durieux E, Descotes F, Nguyen AM, et al. Somatic DICER1 Gene Mutation in Sporadic Intraocular Medulloepithelioma Without Pleuropulmonary Blastoma Syndrome. Hum Pathol. 2015 May;46(5):783–7. PMID:25791583

851. Dutton JJ. Optic Nerve Gliomas and Meningiomas. Neurol Clin. 1991 Feb;9(1):163–77. PMID:2011108

852. Dutton JJ. Optic Nerve Sheath Meningiomas. Surv Ophthalmol. 1992 Nov-Dec;37(3):167–83. PMID:1475751

853. Dyall-Smith D, Trowell H, Dyall-Smith ML. Benign Human Papillomavirus Infection in Renal Transplant Recipients. Int J Dermatol. 1991 Nov;30(11):785–9. PMID:1661712

854. Dymerska M, Kirkorian AY, Offermann EA, et al. Size of Facial Port-Wine Birthmark May Predict Neurologic Outcome in Sturge-Weber Syndrome. J Pediatr. 2017 Sep;188:205–209.E1. PMID:28711177

855. Eade E, Tumuluri K, Do H, et al. Visual Outcomes and Late Complications in Paediatric Orbital Rhabdomyosarcoma. Clin Exp Ophthalmol. 2017 Mar;45(2):168–73. PMID:27473389

856. Eagle RC Jr. High-Risk Features and Tumor Differentiation in Retinoblastoma: A Retrospective Histopathologic Study. Arch Pathol Lab Med. 2009 Aug;133(8):1203–9. PMID:19653710

857. Eagle RC Jr, Shields JA, Donoso L, et al. Malignant Transformation of Spontaneously Regressed Retinoblastoma, Retinoma/Retinocytoma Variant. Ophthalmology. 1989 Sep;96(9):1389–95. PMID:2780006

858. Eagle RC. Eye Pathology: An Atlas and Text. 3rd ed. Philadelphia (PA): Wolters Kluwer; 2017. pp. 200–1.

859. Ebbelaar CF, Schrader AMR, van Dijk M, et al. Towards Diagnostic Criteria for Malignant Deep Penetrating Melanocytic Tumors Using Single Nucleotide Polymorphism Array and Next-Generation Sequencing. Mod Pathol. 2022 Aug;35(8):1110–20. PMID:35184152

860. Ebbo M, Patient M, Grados A, et al. Ophthalmic Manifestations in IgG4-Related Disease: Clinical Presentation and Response to Treatment in a French Case-Series. Medicine (Baltimore). 2017 Mar;96(10):e6205. PMID:28272212

861. Ebrahimi-Fakhari D, Mann LL, Poryo M, et al. Incidence of Tuberous Sclerosis and Age at First Diagnosis: New Data and Emerging Trends from a National, Prospective Surveillance Study. Orphanet J Rare Dis. 2018 Jul 17;13(1):117. PMID:30016967

862. Edelstein C, Shields CL, Shields JA, et al. Presumed Adenocarcinoma of the Retinal Pigment Epithelium in a Blind Eye with a Staphyloma. Arch Ophthalmol. 1998 Apr;116(4):525–8. PMID:9565054

863. Edward DP, Alkatan H, Rafiq Q, et al. MicroRNA Profiling in Intraocular Medulloepitheliomas. PLoS One. 2015 Mar 25;10(3):e0121706. PMID:25807141

864. Efebera Y, Blanchard E, Allam C, et al. Complete Response to Thalidomide and Dexamethasone in a Patient with Necrobiotic Xanthogranuloma Associated with Monoclonal Gammopathy: A Case Report and Review of the Literature. Clin Lymphoma Myeloma Leuk. 2011 Jun;11(3):298–302. PMID:21658660

865. Egan KM, Seddon JM, Glynn RJ, et al. Epidemiologic Aspects of Uveal Melanoma. Surv Ophthalmol. 1988 Jan-Feb;32(4):239–51. PMID:3279559

866. Eggers H, Jakobiec FA, Jones IS. Tumors of the Optic Nerve. Doc Ophthalmol. 1976 Apr 28;41(1):43–128. PMID:7736[illegible]7

867. Ehara Y, Yoshida Y, Kataoka S, et al. Rhabdomyomatous Mesenchymal Hamartoma: A New Proposed Clinical Classification of Adult Onset Acquired Type. Acta Derm Venereol. 2022 Jan 5;102:Adv00627. PMID:34904686

868. Eiger-Moscovich M, Eagle RC Jr, Lally SE, et al. Conjunctival Melanocytic Nevi With Granular Cell Change. Arch Pathol Lab Med. 2020 Apr;144(4):457–65. PMID:31469587

869. Eiger-Moscovich M, Eagle RC, Milman T. β-Catenin and Periodic Acid-Schiff Distinguish Granular Cell Nevus From Deep Penetrating Nevus. Arch Pathol Lab Med. 2021 Dec 1;145(12):1475–6. PMID:34818422

870. Eiger-Moscovich M, Eagle RC Jr, Shields CL, et al. Muir-Torre Syndrome Associated Periocular Sebaceous Neoplasms: Screening Patterns in the Literature and in Clinical Practice. Ocul Oncol Pathol. 2020 Aug;6(4):226–37. PMID:33005611

871. Eiger-Moscovich M, Reich E, Tauber G, et al. Efficacy of Vismodegib for the Treatment of Orbital and Advanced Periocular Basal Cell Carcinoma. Am J Ophthalmol. 2019 Nov;207:62–70. PMID:31077664

872. Eiger-Moscovich M, Zhang PJL, Lally SE, et al. Tubular Apocrine Adenoma of the Eyelid - A Case Report and Literature Review. Saudi J Ophthalmol. 2019 Jul-Sep;33(3):304–7. PMID:31686976

873. Eisen DB, Asgari MM, Bennett DD, et al. Guidelines of Care for the Management of Actinic Keratosis. J Am Acad Dermatol. 2021 Oct;85(4):e209–33. PMID:33820677

874. Eissa SS, Clay MR, Santiago T, et al. Dasatinib Induces a Dramatic Response in a Child with Refractory Juvenile Xanthogranuloma with a Novel MRC1-PDGFRB Fusion. Blood Adv. 2020 Jul 14;4(13):2991–5. PMID:32609843

875. Ekin MA, Ugurlu SK, Cakalagaoglu F. Unusual Intraconal Localization of Orbital Giant Cell Angiofibroma. Indian J Ophthalmol. 2018 Jan;66(1):160–3. PMID:29283151

876. El Beaino M, Roszik J, Livingston JA, et al. Mesenchymal Chondrosarcoma: A Review with Emphasis on its Fusion-Driven Biology. Curr Oncol Rep. 2018 Mar 26;20(5):37. PMID:29582189

877. El Zaoui I, Bucher M, Rimoldi D, et al. Conjunctival Melanoma Targeted Therapy: MAPK and PI3K/MTOR Pathways Inhibition. Invest Ophthalmol Vis Sci. 2019 Jun 3;60(7):2764–72. PMID:31247083

878. Eldaly H, Eldaly Z. Melanocytoma of the Optic Nerve Head, Thirty-Month Follow-Up. Semin Ophthalmol. 2015;30(5-6):464–9. PMID:24506313

879. Eldesouky MA, Elbakary MA. Orbital Dermoid Cyst: Classification and its Impact on Surgical Management. Semin Ophthalmol. 2018;33(2):170–4. PMID:27599687

880. Elenitoba-Johnson KS, Zarate-Osorno A, Meneses A, et al. Cytotoxic Granular Protein Expression, Epstein-Barr Virus Strain Type and Latent Membrane Protein-1 Oncogene Deletions in Nasal T-Lymphocyte/Natural Killer Cell Lymphomas from Mexico. Mod Pathol. 1998 Aug;11(8):754–61. PMID:9720504

881. Eletr ZM, Wilkinson KD. An Emerging Model for BAP1's Role in Regulating Cell Cycle Progression. Cell Biochem Biophys. 2011 Jun;60(1-2):3–11. PMID:21484256

882. El-Hadad C, Koka K, Dong W, et al. Multidisciplinary Management of Orbital Metastasis and Survival Outcomes. Ophthalmic Plast Reconstr Surg. 2021 Nov-Dec 01;37(6):541–5. PMID:33587417

883. Eliassi-Rad B, Albert DM, Green WR. Frequency of Ocular Metastases in Patients Dying of Cancer in Eye Bank Populations. Br J Ophthalmol. 1996 Feb;80(2):125–8. PMID:8814741

884. El-Jabbour JN, Bennett MH, Burke MM, et al. Proliferative Myositis. An Immunohistochemical and Ultrastructural Study. Am J Surg Pathol. 1991 Jul;15(7):654–9. PMID:2058761

885. Elkhamary SM, Cruz AAV, Zotin MC, et al. Involvement of Multiple Trigeminal Nerve Branches in IgG4-Related Orbital Disease. Ophthalmic Plast Reconstr Surg. 2021 Mar-Apr 01;37(2):176–8. PMID:32501880

886. Eller AW, Bernardino VB Jr. Blue Nevi of the Conjunctiva. Ophthalmology. 1983 Dec;90(12):1469–71. PMID:6677846

887. El-Rifai W, Sarlomo-Rikala M, Knuutila S, et al. DNA Copy Number Changes in Development and Progression in Leiomyosarcomas of Soft Tissues. Am J Pathol. 1998 Sep;153(3):985–90. PMID:9736047

888. Elsas FJ, Green WR. Epibulbar Tumors in Childhood. Am J Ophthalmol. 1975 Jun;79(6):1001–7. PMID:166560

889. El-Sawy T, Frank SJ, Hanna E, et al. Multidisciplinary Management of Lacrimal Sac/Nasolacrimal Duct Carcinomas. Ophthalmic Plast Reconstr Surg. 2013 Nov-Dec;29(6):454–7. PMID:24195987

890. El-Sawy T, Sabichi AL, Myers JN, et al. Epidermal Growth Factor Receptor Inhibitors for Treatment of Orbital Squamous Cell Carcinoma. Arch Ophthalmol. 2012 Dec;130(12):1608–11. PMID:23229707

891. El Shabrawi-Caelen L, Kerl H, Cerroni L. Lymphomatoid Papulosis: Reappraisal of Clinicopathologic Presentation and Classification into Subtypes A, B, and C. Arch Dermatol. 2004 Apr;140(4):441–7. PMID:15096372

892. Elsner RA, Shlomchik MJ. Germinal Center and Extrafollicular B Cell Responses in Vaccination, Immunity, and Autoimmunity. Immunity. 2020 Dec 15;53(6):1136–50. PMID:33326765

893. Ely A, Evans J, Sundstrom JM, et al. Orbital Involvement in Extranodal Natural Killer T Cell Lymphoma: An Atypical Case Presentation and Review of the Literature. Orbit. 2012 Aug;31(4):267–9. PMID:22681504

894. Emerick GT, Shields CL, Shields JA, et al. Chewing-Induced Visual Impairment from a Dumbbell Dermoid Cyst. Ophthalmic Plast Reconstr Surg. 1997 Mar;13(1):57–61. PMID:9076785

895. Emile JF, Abla O, Fraitag S, et al. Revised Classification of Histiocytoses and Neoplasms of the Macrophage-Dendritic Cell Lineages. Blood. 2016 Jun 2;127(22):2672–81. PMID:26966089

896. Emile JF, Cohen-Aubart F, Collin M, et al. Histiocytosis. Lancet. 2021 Jul 10;398(10295):157–70. PMID:33901419

897. Emmanuel B, Ruder E, Lin SW, et al. Incidence of Squamous-Cell Carcinoma of the Conjunctiva and Other Eye Cancers in the NIH-AARP Diet and Health Study. Ecancermedicalscience. 2012;6:254. PMID:22654961

898. Engel A, Eichner R, Aebi U. Polymorphism of Reconstituted Human Epidermal Keratin Filaments: Determination of Their Mass-Per-Length and Width by Scanning Transmission Electron Microscopy (STEM). J Ultrastruct Res. 1985 Mar;90(3):323–35. PMID:2416949

899. Ennishi D, Jiang A, Boyle M, et al. Double-Hit Gene Expression Signature Defines a Distinct Subgroup of Germinal Center B-Cell-Like Diffuse Large B-Cell Lymphoma. J Clin Oncol. 2019 Jan 20;37(3):190–201. PMID:30523716

900. Enzinger FM. Fibrous Hamartoma of Infancy. Cancer. 1965 Feb;18:241–8. PMID:14254080

901. Erickson BP, Henry C, Alabiad CR. Recurrent Dermatofibrosarcoma Protuberans Masquerading as a Lacrimal Sac Neoplasm: A Case Report and Review. Ophthalmic Plast Reconstr Surg. 2015 Sep-Oct;31(5):e135–8. PMID:24988500

902. Erickson BP, Modi YS, Ko MJ, et al. Transitional Cell-Type Papillary Carcinoma of the Lacrimal Sac Manifesting as a Medial Canthal Skin Lesion. Orbit. 2014 Oct;33(5):378–81. PMID:24911210

903. Erie JC, Campbell RJ, Liesegang TJ. Conjunctival and Corneal Intraepithelial and Invasive Neoplasia. Ophthalmology. 1986 Feb;93(2):176–83. PMID:3951824

904. Errani C, Zhang L, Panicek DM, et al. Epithelioid Hemangioma of Bone and Soft Tissue: A Reappraisal of a Controversial Entity. Clin Orthop Relat Res. 2012 May;470(5):1498–506. PMID:21948309

905. Errani C, Zhang L, Sung YS, et al. A Novel WWTR1-CAMTA1 Gene Fusion is a Consistent Abnormality in Epithelioid Hemangioendothelioma of Different Anatomic Sites. Genes Chromosomes Cancer. 2011 Aug;50(8):644–53. PMID:21584898

906. Erşahin Y, Yünten N. Bilateral Optic Nerve Glioma. Pediatr Neurosurg. 1999 Sep;31(3):168. PMID:10708361

907. Eshraghi B, Jahanbani-Ardakani HR, Abtahi SM, et al. Ophthalmologic Aspects of Dermatofibrosarcoma Protuberans: A Systematic Review in the Context of a Rare Case of Primary Orbital Involvement. J Fr Ophtalmol. 2019 Oct;42(8):913–24. PMID:30981544

908. Eskelin S, Kivelä T. Mode of Presentation and Time to Treatment of Uveal Melanoma in Finland. Br J Ophthalmol. 2002 Mar;86(3):333–8. PMID:11864894

909. Eskelin S, Tommila P, Palosaari T, et al. Photodynamic Therapy with Verteporfin to Induce Regression of Aggressive Retinal Astrocytomas. Acta Ophthalmol. 2008 Nov;86(7):794–9. PMID:18759802

910. Esmaeli B, Naderi A, Hidaji L, et al. Merkel Cell Carcinoma of the Eyelid with a Positive Sentinel Node. Arch Ophthalmol. 2002 May;120(5):646–8. PMID:12003618

911. Esmaeli B, Roberts D, Ross M, et al. Histologic Features of Conjunctival Melanoma Predictive of Metastasis and Death (an American Ophthalmological Thesis). Trans Am Ophthalmol Soc. 2012 Dec;110:64–73. PMID:23818735

912. Esmaeli B, Rubin ML, Xu S, et al. Greater Tumor Thickness, Ulceration, and Positive Sentinel Lymph Node Are Associated With Worse Prognosis in Patients With Conjunctival Melanoma: Implications for Future AJCC Classifications. Am J Surg Pathol. 2019 Dec;43(12):1701–10. PMID:31425167

913. Esmaeli B, Wang X, Youssef A, et al. Patterns of Regional and Distant Metastasis in Patients with Conjunctival Melanoma: Experience at a Cancer Center Over Four Decades. Ophthalmology. 2001 Nov;108(11):2101–5. PMID:11713086

914. Esmaili DD, Mukai S, Jakobiec FA, et al. Ocular Melanocytoma. Int Ophthalmol Clin. 2009 Winter;49(1):165–75. PMID:19125075

915. Esmaili N, Harris GJ. Langerhans Cell Histiocytosis of the Orbit: Spectrum of Disease and Risk of Central Nervous System Sequelae in Unifocal Cases. Ophthalmic Plast Reconstr Surg. 2016 Jan-Feb;32(1):28–34. PMID:25689784

916. Esteban F, González-Pérez JM, Benaixa JP, et al. Malignant Melanomas of the Nasolacrimal Duct. J Laryngol Otol. 2007 Mar;121(3):285–8. PMID:17123453

917. Evangelista MT, North JP. Comparative Analysis of Cytokeratin 15, TDAG51, Cytokeratin 20 and Androgen Receptor in Sclerosing Adnexal Neoplasms and Variants of Basal Cell Carcinoma. J Cutan Pathol. 2015 Nov;42(11):824–31. PMID:26016446

918. Evangelista MT, North JP. MYB, CD117 and SOX-10 Expression in Cutaneous Adnexal Tumors. J Cutan Pathol. 2017 May;44(5):444–50. PMID:28098399

919. Evans DG. Neurofibromatosis Type 2. Handb Clin Neurol. 2015;132:87–96. PMID:26564072

920. Evans DG, Bowers N, Burkitt-Wright E, et al. Comprehensive RNA Analysis of the NF1 Gene in Classically Affected NF1 Affected Individuals Meeting NIH Criteria Has High Sensitivity and Mutation Negative Testing is Reassuring in Isolated Cases With Pigmentary Features Only. EBioMedicine. 2016 May;7:212–20. PMID:27322474

921. Evans DG, O'Hara C, Wilding A, et al. Mortality in Neurofibromatosis 1: In North West England: An Assessment of Actuarial Survival in a Region of the UK Since 1989. Eur J Hum Genet. 2011 Nov;19(11):1187–91. PMID:21694737

922. Everett JN, Raymond VM, Dandapani M, et al. Screening for Germline Mismatch Repair Mutations Following Diagnosis of Sebaceous Neoplasm. JAMA Dermatol. 2014 Dec;150(12):1315–21. PMID:25006859

923. Eweiss AZ, Lund VJ, Jay A, et al. Transitional Cell Tumours of the Lacrimal Drainage Apparatus. Rhinology. 2013 Dec;51(4):349–54. PMID:24260768

924. Exner JH, Dahod S, Pochi PE. Pyogenic Granuloma-Like Acne Lesions During Isotretinoin Therapy. Arch Dermatol. 1983 Oct;119(10):808–11. PMID:6225396

925. Faaij CM, Willemze AJ, Révész T, et al. Chemokine/Chemokine Receptor Interactions in Extramedullary Leukaemia of the Skin in Childhood AML: Differential Roles for CCR2, CCR5, CXCR4 and CXCR7. Pediatr Blood Cancer. 2010 Aug;55(2):344–8. PMID:20582977

926. Faber W, Kock E, Landau I, et al. [Para-Trochlear Chondroma of the Orbit]. Klin Monbl Augenheilkd. 1992 Feb;200(2):138–9. German. PMID:1578865

927. Fabian ID, Stacey AW, Foster A, et al. Travel Burden and Clinical Presentation of Retinoblastoma: Analysis of 1024 Patients from 43 African Countries and 518 Patients from 40 European Countries. Br J Ophthalmol. 2021 Oct;105(10):1435–43. PMID:32933936

928. Famà R, Bomben R, Rasi S, et al. Ibrutinib-Naïve Chronic Lymphocytic Leukemia Lacks Bruton Tyrosine Kinase Mutations Associated with Treatment Resistance. Blood. 2014 Dec 11;124(25):3831–3. PMID:25498455

929. Fanburg-Smith JC, Auerbach A, Marwaha JS, et al. Immunoprofile of Mesenchymal Chondrosarcoma: Aberrant Desmin and EMA Expression, Retention of INI1, and Negative Estrogen Receptor in 22 Female-Predominant Central Nervous System and Musculoskeletal Cases. Ann Diagn Pathol. 2010 Feb;14(1):8–14. PMID:20123451

930. Fanburg-Smith JC, Auerbach A, Marwaha JS, et al. Reappraisal of Mesenchymal Chondrosarcoma: Novel Morphologic Observations of the Hyaline Cartilage and Endochondral Ossification and Beta-Catenin, Sox9, and Osteocalcin Immunostaining of 22 Cases. Hum Pathol. 2010 May;41(5):653–62. PMID:20138330

931. Fanburg-Smith JC, Meis-Kindblom JM, Fante R, et al. Malignant Granular Cell Tumor of Soft Tissue: Diagnostic Criteria and Clinicopathologic Correlation. Am J Surg Pathol. 1998 Jul;22(7):779–94. PMID:9669341

932. Fanburg-Smith JC, Miettinen M, Folpe AL, et al. Lingual Alveolar Soft Part Sarcoma; 14 Cases: Novel Clinical and Morphological Observations. Histopathology. 2004 Nov;45(5):526–37. PMID:15500657

933. Fang H, Reichard KK, Rabe KG, et al. IGH Translocations in Chronic Lymphocytic Leukemia: Clinicopathologic Features and Clinical Outcomes. Am J Hematol. 2019 Mar;94(3):338–45. PMID:30575108

934. Farah SE, Konrad H, Huang DT, et al. Ectopic Orbital Meningioma: A Case Report and Review. Ophthalmic Plast Reconstr Surg. 1999 Nov;15(6):463–6. PMID:10588262

935. Farah-Klibi F, Ferchichi L, Zaïri I, et al. Lipomatous Hemangiopericytoma (Adipocytic Variant of Solitary Fibrous Tumor) of the Orbit. A Case Report with Review of the Literature. Pathologica. 2006 Dec;98(6):645–8. PMID:17285842

936. Fardeau C, Lee CP, Merle-Béral H, et al. Retinal Fluorescein, Indocyanine Green Angiography, and Optic Coherence Tomography in Non-Hodgkin Primary Intraocular Lymphoma. Am J Ophthalmol. 2009 May;147(5):886–94, 894.E1. PMID:19243734

937. Farley MN, Schmidt LS, Mester JL, et al. A Novel Germline Mutation in BAP1 Predisposes to Familial Clear-Cell Renal Cell Carcinoma. Mol Cancer Res. 2013 Sep;11(9):1061–71. PMID:23709298

938. Farmer JP, Lamba M, Lamba WR, et al. Lymphoproliferative Lesions of the Lacrimal Gland: Clinicopathological, Immunohistochemical and Molecular Genetic Analysis. Can J Ophthalmol. 2005 Apr;40(2):151–60. PMID:16049528

939. Farrahi F, Egbert BM, Swetter SM. Histologic Similarities Between Lentigo Maligna and Dysplastic Nevus: Importance of Clinicopathologic Distinction. J Cutan Pathol. 2005 Jul;32(6):405–12. PMID:15953373

940. Fasina O, Adeoye A, Akang E. Orbital Intravascular Papillary Endothelial Hyperplasia in a Nigerian Child: A Case Report and Review of the Literature. J Med Case Rep. 2012 Sep 13;6:300. PMID:22974134

941. Fatima A, Matalia HP, Vemuganti GK, et al. Pseudoepitheliomatous Hyperplasia Mimicking Ocular Surface Squamous Neoplasia Following Cultivated Limbal Epithelium Transplantation. Clin Exp Ophthalmol. 2006 Dec;34(9):889–91. PMID:17181623

942. Fazal MI, Patel BC. Blepharoconjunctivitis. In: StatPearls. Treasure Island (FL): StatPearls Publishing; 2022. PMID:32644328

943. Feely MM, Gonzalo DH, Corbera M, et al. IgG4-Related Cholecystitis Presenting as Biliary Malignancy: Report of Three Cases. J Gastrointest Surg. 2014 Sep;18(9):1710–5. PMID:24944152

944. Fehr A, Werenicz S, Trocchi P, et al. Mucoepidermoid Carcinoma of the Salivary Glands Revisited with Special Reference to Histologic Grading and CRTC1/3-MAML2 Genotyping. Virchows Arch. 2021 Nov;479(5):975–85. PMID:34231055

945. Fei P, Liu X, Sun Y, et al. Acinic Cell Carcinoma in the Lacrimal Gland–a Case Report and Pathologic Study. Chin Med Sci J. 1991 Jun;6(2):110–2. PMID:1804375

946. Feijó ED, Alencastro Landim G, de Melo Dias M, et al. Giant Bilateral Cysts of the Accessory Lacrimal Glands of Wolfring in a Child. Ophthalmic Plast Reconstr Surg. 2020 Jan/Feb;36(1):e4–6. PMID:31593037

947. Feinfield RE, Hesse RJ, Scharfenberg JC. Orbital Angiolipoma. Arch Ophthalmol. 1988 Aug;106(8):1093–5. PMID:3401137

948. Fend F, Ferreri AJ, Coupland SE. How We Diagnose and Treat Vitreoretinal Lymphoma.

Br J Haematol. 2016 Jun;173(5):680–92. PMID:27133587
949. Fereydooni A, Dardik A, Nassiri N. Molecular Changes Associated with Vascular Malformations. J Vasc Surg. 2019 Jul;70(1):314–326.E1. PMID:30922748
950. Fernandes BF, Castiglione E, Belfort RN, et al. Orbital Leiomyoma: Histopathologic and Immunohistochemical Findings of a Rare Tumor. Ophthalmic Plast Reconstr Surg. 2009 Jan-Feb;25(1):59–61. PMID:19273932
951. Fernandes BF, Odashiro AN, Saraiva VS, et al. Immunohistochemical Expression of Melan-A and Tyrosinase in Uveal Melanoma. J Carcinog. 2007 Apr 20;6:6. PMID:17445277
952. Fernandez C, Figarella-Branger D, Girard N, et al. Pilocytic Astrocytomas in Children: Prognostic Factors–a Retrospective Study of 80 Cases. Neurosurgery. 2003 Sep;53(3):544–53. PMID:12943571
953. Fernández-Figueras MT, Malvehy J, Tschandl P, et al. Position Paper on a Simplified Histopathological Classification of Basal Cell Carcinoma: Results of the European Consensus Project. J Eur Acad Dermatol Venereol. 2022 Mar;36(3):351–9. PMID:34931722
954. Fernandez-Flores A, Cassarino DS. Endocrine Mucin-Producing Sweat Gland Carcinoma: A Study of Three Cases and CK8, CK18 and CD5/6 Immunoexpression. J Cutan Pathol. 2015 Aug;42(8):578–86. PMID:25925290
955. Ferreira I, Wiedemeyer K, Demetter P, et al. Update on the Pathology, Genetics and Somatic Landscape of Sebaceous Tumours. Histopathology. 2020 Apr;76(5):640–9. PMID:31821583
956. Ferreira TA, Jaarsma-Coes MG, Marinkovic M, et al. MR Imaging Characteristics of Uveal Melanoma with Histopathological Validation. Neuroradiology. 2022 Jan;64(1):171–84. PMID:34718831
957. Ferreira TA, Pinheiro CF, Saraiva P, et al. MR and CT Imaging of the Normal Eyelid and its Application in Eyelid Tumors. Cancers (Basel). 2020 Mar 12;12(3):658. PMID:32178233
958. Ferreri AJ, Guidoboni M, Ponzoni M, et al. Evidence for an Association Between Chlamydia Psittaci and Ocular Adnexal Lymphomas. J Natl Cancer Inst. 2004 Apr 21;96(8):586–94. PMID:15100336
959. Ferreri AJ, Ponzoni M, Guidoboni M, et al. Bacteria-Eradicating Therapy with Doxycycline in Ocular Adnexal MALT Lymphoma: A Multicenter Prospective Trial. J Natl Cancer Inst. 2006 Oct 4;98(19):1375–82. PMID:17018784
960. Ferreri AJ, Ponzoni M, Guidoboni M, et al. Regression of Ocular Adnexal Lymphoma After Chlamydia Psittaci-Eradicating Antibiotic Therapy. J Clin Oncol. 2005 Aug 1;23(22):5067–73. PMID:15968003
961. Ferri E, Minotto C, Ianniello F, et al. Maxillo-Ethmoidal Chloroma in Acute Myeloid Leukaemia: Case Report. Acta Otorhinolaryngol Ital. 2005 Jun;25(3):195–9. PMID:16450777
962. Ferry AP. Granular Cell Tumor (Myoblastoma) of the Palpebral Conjunctiva Causing Pseudoepitheliomatous Hyperplasia of the Conjunctival Epithelium. Am J Ophthalmol. 1981 Feb;91(2):234–8. PMID:6258438
963. Ferry AP, Font RL. Carcinoma Metastatic to the Eye and Orbit II. A Clinicopathological Study of 26 Patients with Carcinoma Metastatic to the Anterior Segment of the Eye. Arch Ophthalmol. 1975 Jul;93(7):472–82. PMID:166633
964. Ferry AP, Font RL. Carcinoma Metastatic to the Eye and Orbit. I. A Clinicopathologic Study of 227 Cases. Arch Ophthalmol. 1974 Oct;92(4):276–86. PMID:4412321
965. Ferry JA, Fung CY, Lucarelli MJ, et al. Ocular Adnexal Lymphoma: Long-Term Outcome, Patterns of Failure and Prognostic Factors in 174 Patients. J Hematopathol. 2021;14:41–52. doi:10.1007/S12308-020-00424-6.
966. Ferry JA, Fung CY, Zukerberg L, et al. Lymphoma of the Ocular Adnexa: A Study of 353 Cases. Am J Surg Pathol. 2007 Feb;31(2):170–84. PMID:17255761
967. Fetsch JF, Sesterhenn IA, Miettinen M, et al. Epithelioid Hemangioma of the Penis: A Clinicopathologic and Immunohistochemical Analysis of 19 Cases, with Special Reference to Exuberant Examples Often Confused with Epithelioid Hemangioendothelioma and Epithelioid Angiosarcoma. Am J Surg Pathol. 2004 Apr;28(4):523–33. PMID:15087672
968. Feu-Basilio S, Matas J, Dotti-Boada M, et al. Orbital TFE3-Rearranged Perivascular Epithelioid Cell Tumor: A Case Report and Review of the Literature. Am J Dermatopathol. 2021 Dec 1;43(12):e263–6. PMID:34291749
969. Field MG, Decatur CL, Kurtenbach S, et al. PRAME as an Independent Biomarker for Metastasis in Uveal Melanoma. Clin Cancer Res. 2016 Mar 1;22(5):1234–42. PMID:26933176
970. Field MG, Durante MA, Decatur CL, et al. Epigenetic Reprogramming and Aberrant Expression of PRAME Are Associated with Increased Metastatic Risk in Class 1 and Class 2 Uveal Melanomas. Oncotarget. 2016 Sep 13;7(37):59209–19. PMID:27486988
971. Figueira E, Rajak S, McKelvie P, et al. Primary Orbital Melanoma: A Case Series and Literature Review. Orbit. 2018 Oct;37(5):352–7. PMID:29388848
972. Figueira EC, Danks J, Watanabe A, et al. Apocrine Adenocarcinoma of the Eyelid: Case Series and Review. Ophthalmic Plast Reconstr Surg. 2013 Nov-Dec;29(6):417–23. PMID:24217473
973. Finger PT, Latkany P, Kurli M, et al. The Finger Iridectomy Technique: Small Incision Biopsy of Anterior Segment Tumours. Br J Ophthalmol. 2005 Aug;89(8):946–9. PMID:16024840
974. Firestone BK, Arias JD, Shields CL, et al. Bilateral Combined Hamartomas of the Retina and Retinal Pigment Epithelium as the Presenting Feature of Neurofibromatosis Type 2 (Wishart Type). J Pediatr Ophthalmol Strabismus. 2014;51. PMID:25922868
975. Firsova MV, Mendeleeva LP, Kovrigina AM, et al. Plasmacytoma in Patients with Multiple Myeloma: Morphology and Immunohistochemistry. BMC Cancer. 2020 Apr 22;20(1):346. PMID:32321465
976. Fischer K, Al-Sawaf O, Bahlo J, et al. Venetoclax and Obinutuzumab in Patients with CLL and Coexisting Conditions. N Engl J Med. 2019 Jun 6;380(23):2225–36. PMID:31166681
977. Fischer K, Bahlo J, Fink AM, et al. Long-Term Remissions After FCR Chemoimmunotherapy in Previously Untreated Patients with CLL: Updated Results of the CLL8 Trial. Blood. 2016 Jan 14;127(2):208–15. PMID:26486789
978. Fishman MA, Baram TZ. Megalencephaly Due to Impaired Cerebral Venous Return in a Sturge-Weber Variant Syndrome. J Child Neurol. 1986 Apr;1(2):115–8. PMID:3598114
979. Fittall MW, Lyskjaer I, Ellery P, et al. Drivers Underpinning the Malignant Transformation of Giant Cell Tumour of Bone. J Pathol. 2020 Dec;252(4):433–40. PMID:32866294
980. Fittall MW, Mifsud W, Pillay N, et al. Recurrent Rearrangements of FOS and FOSB Define Osteoblastoma. Nat Commun. 2018 Jun 1;9(1):2150. PMID:29858576
981. Fitzpatrick TB. The Validity and Practicality of Sun-Reactive Skin Types I Through VI. Arch Dermatol. 1988 Jun;124(6):869–71. PMID:3377516
982. Flamme I, Krieg M, Plate KH. Up-Regulation of Vascular Endothelial Growth Factor in Stromal Cells of Hemangioblastomas is Correlated with Up-Regulation of the Transcription Factor HRF/HIF-2alpha. Am J Pathol. 1998 Jul;153(1):25–9. PMID:9665461
983. Fletcher CD. Solitary Circumscribed Neuroma of the Skin (So-Called Palisaded, Encapsulated Neuroma). A Clinicopathologic and Immunohistochemical Study. Am J Surg Pathol. 1989 Jul;13(7):574–80. PMID:2660609
984. Fletcher CD, Davies SE. Benign Plexiform (Multinodular) Schwannoma: A Rare Tumour Unassociated with Neurofibromatosis. Histopathology. 1986 Sep;10(9):971–80. PMID:3096870
985. Flieder A, Koerner FC, Pilch BZ, et al. Endocrine Mucin-Producing Sweat Gland Carcinoma: A Cutaneous Neoplasm Analogous to Solid Papillary Carcinoma of Breast. Am J Surg Pathol. 1997 Dec;21(12):1501–6. PMID:9414195
986. Flores Pimentel M, Heath A, Wan MJ, et al. Prevalence of Choroidal Abnormalities and Lisch Nodules in Children Meeting Clinical and Molecular Diagnosis of Neurofibromatosis Type 1. Transl Vis Sci Technol. 2022 Feb 1;11(2):10. PMID:35119474
987. Flucke U, Karanian M, Broek RWT, et al. Soft Tissue Special Issue: Perivascular and Vascular Tumors of the Head and Neck. Head Neck Pathol. 2020 Mar;14(1):21–32. PMID:31950476
988. Flucke U, Palmedo G, Blankenhorn N, et al. EWSR1 Gene Rearrangement Occurs in a Subset of Cutaneous Myoepithelial Tumors: A Study of 18 Cases. Mod Pathol. 2011 Nov;24(11):1444–50. PMID:21725291
989. Flucke U, van Noesel MM, Siozopoulou V, et al. EWSR1-The Most Common Rearranged Gene in Soft Tissue Lesions, Which Also Occurs in Different Bone Lesions: An Updated Review. Diagnostics (Basel). 2021 Jun 15;11(6):1093. PMID:34203801
990. Flucke U, Vogels RJ, de Saint Aubain Somerhausen N, et al. Epithelioid Hemangioendothelioma: Clinicopathologic, Immunhistochemical, and Molecular Genetic Analysis of 39 Cases. Diagn Pathol. 2014 Jul 1;9:131. PMID:24986479
991. Flux K, Kutzner H, Rütten A, et al. Infundibulocystic Structures and Prominent Squamous Metaplasia in Sebaceoma-A Rare Feature. A Clinicopathologic Study of 10 Cases. Am J Dermatopathol. 2016 Sep;38(9):678–82. PMID:26760686
992. Folberg R, Hendrix MJ, Maniotis AJ. Vasculogenic Mimicry and Tumor Angiogenesis. Am J Pathol. 2000 Feb;156(2):361–81. PMID:10666364
993. Folberg R, Jakobiec FA, Bernardino VB, et al. Benign Conjunctival Melanocytic Lesions. Clinicopathologic Features. Ophthalmology. 1989 Apr;96(4):436–61. PMID:2657539
994. Folberg R, McLean IW, Zimmerman LE. Primary Acquired Melanosis of the Conjunctiva. Hum Pathol. 1985 Feb;16(2):129–35. PMID:3972395
995. Folberg R, Rummelt V, Parys-Van Ginderdeuren R, et al. The Prognostic Value of Tumor Blood Vessel Morphology in Primary Uveal Melanoma. Ophthalmology. 1993 Sep;100(9):1389–98. PMID:8371929
996. Foley KM, Woodruff JM, Ellis FT, et al. Radiation-Induced Malignant and Atypical Peripheral Nerve Sheath Tumors. Ann Neurol. 1980 Apr;7(4):311–8. PMID:7377756
997. Folpe AL, Deyrup AT. Alveolar Soft-Part Sarcoma: A Review and Update. J Clin Pathol. 2006 Nov;59(11):1127–32. PMID:17071801
998. Folpe AL, Fanburg-Smith JC, Miettinen M, et al. Atypical and Malignant Glomus Tumors: Analysis of 52 Cases, with a Proposal for the Reclassification of Glomus Tumors. Am J Surg Pathol. 2001 Jan;25(1):1–12. PMID:11145243
999. Folpe AL, Kwiatkowski DJ. Perivascular Epithelioid Cell Neoplasms: Pathology and Pathogenesis. Hum Pathol. 2010 Jan;41(1):1–15. PMID:19604538
1000. Folpe AL, McKenney JK, Bridge JA, et al. Sclerosing Rhabdomyosarcoma in Adults: Report of Four Cases of a Hyalinizing, Matrix-Rich Variant of Rhabdomyosarcoma that May Be Confused with Osteosarcoma, Chondrosarcoma, or Angiosarcoma. Am J Surg Pathol. 2002 Sep;26(9):1175–83. PMID:12218574
1001. Folpe AL, Mentzel T, Lehr HA, et al. Perivascular Epithelioid Cell Neoplasms of Soft Tissue and Gynecologic Origin: A Clinicopathologic Study of 26 Cases and Review of the Literature. Am J Surg Pathol. 2005 Dec;29(12):1558–75. PMID:16327428
1002. Fonseca RA, Dantas MA, Kaga T, et al. Combined Hamartoma of the Retina and Retinal Pigment Epithelium Associated with Juvenile Nasopharyngeal Angiofibroma. Am J Ophthalmol. 2001 Jul;132(1):131–2. PMID:11438076
1003. Font RL, Chaqués-Alepuz V. [Giant Optic Disk Melanocytoma Complicated with Massive Intraocular Seeding]. Arch Soc Esp Oftalmol. 2011 May;86(5):158–61. Spanish. PMID:21624657
1004. Font RL, Del Valle M, Avedaño J, et al. Primary Adenoid Cystic Carcinoma of the Conjunctiva Arising from the Accessory Lacrimal Glands: A Clinicopathologic Study of Three Cases. Cornea. 2008 May;27(4):494–7. PMID:18434856
1005. Font RL, Hidayat AA. Fibrous Histiocytoma of the Orbit. A Clinicopathologic Study of 150 Cases. Hum Pathol. 1982 Mar;13(3):199–209. PMID:6281162
1006. Font RL, Jurco S 3rd, Brechner RJ. Postradiation Leiomyosarcoma of the Orbit Complicating Bilateral Retinoblastoma. Arch Ophthalmol. 1983 Oct;101(10):1557–61. PMID:6626009
1007. Font RL, Moura RA, Shetlar DJ, et al. Combined Hamartoma of Sensory Retina and Retinal Pigment Epithelium. Retina. 1989;9(4):302–11. PMID:2627919
1008. Font RL, Wheeler TM Boniuk M. Intravascular Papillary Endothelial Hyperplasia of the Orbit and Ocular Adnexa. A Report of Five Cases. Arch Ophthalmol. 1983 Nov;101(11):1731–6. PMID:6635471
1009. Font RL, Zimmerman LE. Nodular Fasciitis of the Eye and Adnexa. A Report of Ten Cases. Arch Ophthalmol. 1966 Apr;75(4):475–81. PMID:5905201
1010. Font RL, Zimmerman LE, Fine BS. Adenoma of the Retinal Pigment Epithelium: Histochemical and Electron Microscopic Observations. Am J Ophthalmol. 1972 Apr;73(4):544–54. PMID:4111985
1011. Forbat E, Al-Niaimi F, Ali FR. Molluscum Contagiosum: Review and Update on Management. Pediatr Dermatol. 2017 Sep;34(5):504–15. PMID:28884917
1012. Forbis R Jr, Helwig EB. Pilomatrixoma (Calcifying Epithelioma). Arch Dermatol. 1961 Apr;83:606–18. PMID:13700704
1013. Ford J, Thakar S, Thuro B, et al. Prognostic Value of the Staging System for Eyelid Tumors in the 7th Edition of the American Joint Committee on Cancer Staging Manual. Ophthalmic Plast Reconstr Surg. 2017 Sep/Oct;33(5):317–24. PMID:28350693
1014. Ford J, Thuro BA, Thakar S, et al. Immune Checkpoint Inhibitors for Treatment of Metastatic Melanoma of the Orbit and Ocular Adnexa. Ophthalmic Plast Reconstr Surg. 2017 Jul/Aug;33(4):e82–5. PMID:27662198
1015. Ford JR, Rubin ML, Frank SJ, et al. Prognostic Factors for Local Recurrence and Survival and Impact of Local Treatments

on Survival in Lacrimal Gland Carcinoma. Br J Ophthalmol. 2021 Jun;105(6):768–74. PMID:32680839
1016. Forshew T, Tatevossian RG, Lawson AR, et al. Activation of the ERK/MAPK Pathway: A Signature Genetic Defect in Posterior Fossa Pilocytic Astrocytomas. J Pathol. 2009 Jun;218(2):172–81. PMID:19373855
1017. Foss AJ, Alexander RA, Hungerford JL, et al. Reassessment of the PAS Patterns in Uveal Melanoma. Br J Ophthalmol. 1997 Mar;81(3):240–6. PMID:9135390
1018. Foss AJ, Alexander RA, Jefferies LW, et al. Microvessel Count Predicts Survival in Uveal Melanoma. Cancer Res. 1996 Jul 1;56(13):2900–3. PMID:8674036
1019. Fotouhi A, Hashemi H, Khabazkhoob M, et al. Prevalence and Risk Factors of Pterygium and Pinguecula: The Tehran Eye Study. Eye (Lond). 2009 May;23(5):1125–9. PMID:18600244
1020. Foucar E, Rosai J, Dorfman R. Sinus Histiocytosis with Massive Lymphadenopathy (Rosai-Dorfman Disease): Review of the Entity. Semin Diagn Pathol. 1990 Feb;7(1):19–73. PMID:2180012
1021. Foucar E, Rosai J, Dorfman RF. The Ophthalmologic Manifestations of Sinus Histiocytosis with Massive Lymphadenopathy. Am J Ophthalmol. 1979 Mar;87(3):354–67. PMID:434097
1022. Fox CP, Civallero M, Ko YH, et al. Survival Outcomes of Patients with Extranodal Natural-Killer T-Cell Lymphoma: A Prospective Cohort Study from the International T-Cell Project. Lancet Haematol. 2020 Apr;7(4):e284–94. PMID:32105608
1023. França JA, Gayden T, Bareke E, et al. Whole-Exome Sequencing Reveals Novel Vacuolar ATPase Genes' Variants and Variants in Genes Involved in Lysosomal Biology and Autophagosomal Formation in Oral Granular Cell Tumors. J Oral Pathol Med. 2021 Apr;50(4):410–7. PMID:33289181
1024. Francis JH, Berry D, Abramson DH, et al. Intravitreous Cutaneous Metastatic Melanoma in the Era of Checkpoint Inhibition: Unmasking and Masquerading. Ophthalmology. 2020 Feb;127(2):240–8. PMID:31708274
1025. Francis JH, Grossniklaus HE, Habib LA, et al. BRAF, NRAS, and GNAQ Mutations in Conjunctival Melanocytic Nevi. Invest Ophthalmol Vis Sci. 2018 Jan 1;59(1):117–21. PMID:29332123
1026. Francis JH, Marr BP, Abramson DH. Classification of Vitreous Seeds in Retinoblastoma: Correlations with Patient, Tumor, and Treatment Characteristics. Ophthalmology. 2016 Jul;123(7):1601–5. PMID:27030103
1027. Francis JH, Wiesner T, Milman T, et al. Investigation of Somatic GNAQ, GNA11, BAP1 and SF3B1 Mutations in Ophthalmic Melanocytomas. Ocul Oncol Pathol. 2016 Apr;2(3):171–7. PMID:27239460
1028. Franz DN, Belousova E, Sparagana S, et al. Long-Term Use of Everolimus in Patients with Tuberous Sclerosis Complex: Final Results from the EXIST-1 Study. PLoS One. 2016 Jun 28;11(6):e0158476. PMID:27351628
1029. Fraunfelder FW. Liquid Nitrogen Cryotherapy for Conjunctival Lymphangiectasia: A Case Series. Trans Am Ophthalmol Soc. 2009 Dec;107:229–32. PMID:20126499
1030. Frayer WC. Reactivity of the Retinal Pigment Epithelium: An Experimental and Histopathologic Study. Trans Am Ophthalmol Soc. 1966;64:586–643. PMID:5965122
1031. Freedman MI, Folk JC. Metastatic Tumors to the Eye and Orbit. Patient Survival and Clinical Characteristics. Arch Ophthalmol. 1987 Sep;105(9):1215–9. PMID:3307718
1032. Freeman C, Berg JW, Cutler SJ. Occurrence and Prognosis of Extranodal Lymphomas. Cancer. 1972 Jan;29(1):252–60. PMID:5007387
1033. Freitag SK, Aakalu VK, Tao JP, et al. Sentinel Lymph Node Biopsy for Eyelid and Conjunctival Malignancy: A Report by the American Academy of Ophthalmology. Ophthalmology. 2020 Dec;127(12):1757–65. PMID:32698034
1034. Freyer DR, Kennedy R, Bostrom BC, et al. Juvenile Xanthogranuloma: Forms of Systemic Disease and Their Clinical Implications. J Pediatr. 1996 Aug;129(2):227–37. PMID:8765620
1035. Fried I, Tabori U, Tihan T, et al. Optic Pathway Gliomas: A Review. CNS Oncol. 2013 Mar;2(2):143–59. PMID:25057976
1036. Friedberg JW, Byrtek M, Link BK, et al. Effectiveness of First-Line Management Strategies for Stage I Follicular Lymphoma: Analysis of the National LymphoCare Study. J Clin Oncol. 2012 Sep 20;30(27):3368–75. PMID:22915662
1037. Friedman BJ, Sahu J, Solomides CC, et al. Contiguous Verrucous Proliferations in Syringocystadenoma Papilliferum: A Retrospective Analysis with Additional Evaluation Via Mutation-Specific BRAFV600E Immunohistochemistry. J Cutan Pathol. 2018 Mar;45(3):212–6. PMID:29206289
1038. Friedman HD, Sanderson SO, Stein CK, et al. Extramedullary Granulopoiesis Mimicking Recurrent Lymphoma After Prolonged Administration of Human Recombinant Granulocyte Colony-Stimulating Factor. Ann Hematol. 1998 Jul-Aug;77(1-2):79–83. PMID:9760159
1039. Friedman JM. Neurofibromatosis 1. In: Adam MP, Feldman J, Mirzaa GM, et al., editors. GeneReviews. Seattle (WA): University of Washington, Seattle; 1993-2025. PMID:20301288.
1040. Friedman PM, Friedman RH, Jiang SB, et al. Microcystic Adnexal Carcinoma: Collaborative Series Review and Update. J Am Acad Dermatol. 1999 Aug;41(2 Pt 1):225–31. PMID:10426893
1041. Frierson HF, Cooper PH. Myxoid Variant of Dermatofibrosarcoma Protuberans. Am J Surg Pathol. 1983 Jul;7(5):445–50. PMID:6614310
1041A. Fritz A, Percy C, Jack A, et al., editors. International Classification of Diseases for Oncology (ICD-O). 3rd ed. 1st Rev. Geneva (Switzerland): World Health Organization; 2013.
1042. Froehlich M, Cook J, Bruner E, et al. Endocrine Mucin-Producing Sweat Gland Carcinoma of the Eyelid With Locoregional Metastasis to the Parotid Gland. Dermatol Surg. 2020 Aug;46(8):1116–8. PMID:31977506
1043. Froehlich MH, Conti KR, Norris II, et al. Endocrine Mucin-Producing Sweat Gland Carcinoma: A Systematic Review and Meta-Analysis. J Dermatolog Treat. 2022 Jun;33(4):2182–91. PMID:34057875
1044. Frouin E, Vignon-Pennamen MD, Balme B, et al. Anatomoclinical Study of 30 Cases of Sclerosing Sweat Duct Carcinomas (Microcystic Adnexal Carcinoma, Syringomatous Carcinoma and Squamoid Eccrine Ductal Carcinoma). J Eur Acad Dermatol Venereol. 2015 Oct;29(10):1978–94. PMID:25873411
1045. Fu K, Weisenburger DD, Greiner TC, et al. Cyclin D1-Negative Mantle Cell Lymphoma: A Clinicopathologic Study Based on Gene Expression Profiling. Blood. 2005 Dec 15;106(13):4315–21. PMID:16123218
1046. Fujii M, Kiura K, Kamei H, et al. [Antiemetic Effects of Combinations of Metoclopramide, Droperidol and Dexamethasone for the Prevention of Cisplatin-Induced Gastro-Intestinal Toxicity: A Randomized Crossover Trial]. Gan To Kagaku Ryoho. 1987 Jul;14(7):2257–61. Japanese. PMID:3300561
1047. Fukuda H, Tsuchida D, Koda K, et al. Inhibition of Sympathetic Pathways Restores Postoperative Ileus in the Upper and Lower Gastrointestinal Tract. J Gastroenterol Hepatol. 2007 Aug;22(8):1293–9. PMID:17688668
1048. Fukuda T, Igarashi T, Hiraki H, et al. Abnormal Pigmentation of Schwannoma Attributed to Excess Production of Neuromelanin-Like Pigment. Pathol Int. 2000 Mar;50(3):230–7. PMID:10792787
1049. Fukunaga M. Expression of D2-40 in Lymphatic Endothelium of Normal Tissues and in Vascular Tumours. Histopathology. 2005 Apr;46(4):396–402. PMID:15810951
1050. Fung AT, Pellegrini M, Shields CL. Congenital Hypertrophy of the Retinal Pigment Epithelium: Enhanced-Depth Imaging Optical Coherence Tomography in 18 Cases. Ophthalmology. 2014 Jan;121(1):251–6. PMID:24126031
1051. Furdova A, Kapitanova K, Kollarova A, et al. Periocular Basal Cell Carcinoma - Clinical Perspectives. Oncol Rev. 2020 Apr 30;14(1):420. PMID:32395200
1052. Furusato E, Cameron JD, Newsom RW, et al. Ocular Perivascular Epithelioid Cell Tumor: Report of 2 Cases with Distinct Clinical Presentations. Hum Pathol. 2010 May;41(5):768–72. PMID:20236689
1053. Furusato E, Valenzuela IA, Fanburg-Smith JC, et al. Orbital Solitary Fibrous Tumor: Encompassing Terminology for Hemangiopericytoma, Giant Cell Angiofibroma, and Fibrous Histiocytoma of the Orbit: Reappraisal of 41 Cases. Hum Pathol. 2011 Jan;42(1):120–8. PMID:21056898
1054. Fuster C, Martín-Garcia D, Balagué O, et al. Cryptic Insertions of the Immunoglobulin Light Chain Enhancer Region Near CCND1 in T(11;14)-Negative Mantle Cell Lymphoma. Haematologica. 2020 Aug;105(8):e408–11. PMID:31753927
1055. Gabillot-Carré M, Weill F, Mamelle G, et al. Microcystic Adnexal Carcinoma: Report of Seven Cases Including One with Lung Metastasis. Dermatology. 2006;212(3):221–8. PMID:16549917
1056. Gadner H, Minkov M, Grois N, et al. Therapy Prolongation Improves Outcome in Multisystem Langerhans Cell Histiocytosis. Blood. 2013 Jun 20;121(25):5006–14. PMID:23589673
1057. Gahankari MD, Jehangir R, Bhatti SS. Melanocytoma of the Optic Disc. J Postgrad Med. 1992 Jul-Sep;38(3):135–6. PMID:1303415
1058. Galati L, Combes JD, Gupta P, et al. Detection of a Large Spectrum of Viral Infections in Conjunctival Premalignant and Malignant Lesions. Int J Cancer. 2020 Nov 15;147(10):2862–70. PMID:32525572
1059. Galgano MA, Goulart CR, Iwenofu H, et al. Osteoblastomas of the Spine: A Comprehensive Review. Neurosurg Focus. 2016 Aug;41(2):e4. PMID:27476846
1060. Galili N, Davis RJ, Fredericks WJ, et al. Fusion of a Fork Head Domain Gene to PAX3 in the Solid Tumour Alveolar Rhabdomyosarcoma. Nat Genet. 1993 Nov;5(3):230–5. PMID:8275086
1061. Galindo-Ferreiro A, Alkatan HM, ElKhamary SM, et al. Recurrent Orbital Inflammation Mimicking Orbital Cellulitis Associated With Orbitopalpebral Venous Lymphatic Malformation. Ophthalmic Plast Reconstr Surg. 2017 Sep/Oct;33(5):e112–4. PMID:27879620
1062. Galindo-Ferreiro A, Elkhamary SM, Aldossari S, et al. Sensitivity of Computed Tomography for the Assessment of Spontaneous Dermoid Cyst Localized Rupture with Granulomatous Reaction. Semin Ophthalmol. 2018;33(5):629–33. PMID:28991502
1063. Gallagher MJ, Giannoudis A, Herrington CS, et al. Human Papillomavirus in Pterygium. Br J Ophthalmol. 2001 Jul;85(7):782–4. PMID:11423447
1064. Gallie BL, Ellsworth RM, Abramson DH, et al. Retinoma: Spontaneous Regression of Retinoblastoma or Benign Manifestation of the Mutation? Br J Cancer. 1982 Apr;45(4):513–21. PMID:7073943
1065. Gan L, Luo X, Fei Y, et al. Ophthalmic Involvement Disparities in Clinical Characteristics of IgG4-Related Disease: A Retrospective Study of 573 Patients. BMC Ophthalmol. 2021 Dec 27;21(1):447. PMID:34961492
1066. Gandhi NG, Lin LK, O'Hara M. Sildenafil for Pediatric Orbital Lymphangioma. JAMA Ophthalmol. 2013 Sep;131(9):1228–30. PMID:23828510
1067. Gandini S, Sera F, Cattaruzza MS, et al. Meta-Analysis of Risk Factors for Cutaneous Melanoma: I. Common and Atypical Naevi. Eur J Cancer. 2005 Jan;41(1):28–44. PMID:15617989
1068. Gange WS, Holland SM, De Alba F. IgG4-Related Ophthalmic Disease Presenting as Choroidal and Orbital Lesions. Retin Cases Brief Rep. 2019 Summer;13(3):283–6. PMID:28346259
1069. Gao S, Zhou Y, Jin X, et al. Primary Vitreoretinal Natural Killer/T-Cell Lymphoma with Breast Involvement: A Case Report and Review of the Literature. Surv Ophthalmol. 2019 Mar-Apr;64(2):225–32. PMID:30321569
1070. Gao Y, Chen G, Chow C, et al. Ocular PEComas Are Frequently Melanotic and TFE3-Translocated: Report of Two Cases Including the First Description of PRCC-TFE3 Fusion in PEComa. Virchows Arch. 2021 May;478(5):1025–31. PMID:32676967
1071. Garbutcheon-Singh KB, Curchin DJ, McCormack CJ, et al. Trends in the Incidence of Merkel Cell Carcinoma in Victoria, Australia, Between 1986 and 2016. Australas J Dermatol. 2020 Feb;61(1):e34–8. PMID:32040877
1072. Garces S, Khoury JD, Kanagal-Shamanna R, et al. Chronic Lymphocytic Leukemia with Proliferation Centers in Bone Marrow is Associated with Younger Age at Initial Presentation, Complex Karyotype, and TP53 Disruption. Hum Pathol. 2018 Dec;82:215–31. PMID:30086334
1073. Garces S, Medeiros LJ, Patel KP, et al. Mutually Exclusive Recurrent KRAS and MAP2K1 Mutations in Rosai-Dorfman Disease. Mod Pathol. 2017 Oct;30(10):1367–77. PMID:28664935
1074. Gardrat S, Houy A, Brooks K, et al. Definition of Biologically Distinct Groups of Conjunctival Melanomas According to Etiological Factors and Implications for Precision Medicine. Cancers (Basel). 2021 Jul 30;13(15):3836. PMID:34359736
1075. Garneski KM, Warcola AH, Feng Q, et al. Merkel Cell Polyomavirus is More Frequently Present in North American Than Australian Merkel Cell Carcinoma Tumors. J Invest Dermatol. 2009 Jan;129(1):246–8. PMID:18650846
1076. Garoon RB, Medina CA, Scelfo C, et al. Retinocytoma with Vitreous Seeding: New Insights from Enhanced Depth Imaging Optical Coherence Tomography and High-Resolution Posterior Segment Ultrasonography. Retin Cases Brief Rep. 2021 Jan 1;15(1):68–70. PMID:29470300
1076A. Garrity JA, Henderson JW, Cameron JD. Chapter 13: Metastatic Carcinomas. In: Henderson's Orbital Tumors. 4th ed. New York (NY): Raven Press; 2007. pp. 313–26.
1077. Garvayo M, Cossu G, Broome M, et al. Pediatric Cranial Osteoblastoma: Technical

1214. Gupta S, Verma R, Sen R, et al. Solitary Fibrous Tumor of the Orbit. Asian J Neurosurg. 2016 Jan-Mar;11(1):78. PMID:26889300

1215. Guseva NV, Jaber O, Tanas MR, et al. Anchored Multiplex PCR for Targeted Next-Generation Sequencing Reveals Recurrent and Novel USP6 Fusions and Upregulation of USP6 Expression in Aneurysmal Bone Cyst. Genes Chromosomes Cancer. 2017 Apr;56(4):266–77. PMID:27910166

1216. Guthoff R, Guthoff T, Mueller-Hermelink HK, et al. Perivascular Epithelioid Cell Tumor of the Orbit. Arch Ophthalmol. 2008 Jul;126(7):1009–11. PMID:18625958

1217. Gutmann DH, Donahoe J, Brown T, et al. Loss of Neurofibromatosis 1 (NF1) Gene Expression in NF1-Associated Pilocytic Astrocytomas. Neuropathol Appl Neurobiol. 2000 Aug;26(4):361–7. PMID:10931370

1218. Gutmann DH, Ferner RE, Listernick RH, et al. Neurofibromatosis Type 1. Nat Rev Dis Primers. 2017 Feb 23;3:17004. PMID:28230061

1218A. Gutmann DH, McLellan MD, Hussain I, et al. Somatic Neurofibromatosis Type 1 (NF1) Inactivation Characterizes NF1-Associated Pilocytic Astrocytoma. Genome Res. 2013 Mar;23(3):431–9. PMID:23222849

1219. Guy JR, Rao NA. Graphite Foreign Body of the Conjunctiva Simulating Melanoma. Cornea. 1985-1986-1986;4(4):263–5. PMID:3836032

1220. Guyot-Goubin A, Donadieu J, Barkaoui M, et al. Descriptive Epidemiology of Childhood Langerhans Cell Histiocytosis in France, 2000-2004. Pediatr Blood Cancer. 2008 Jul;51(1):71–5. PMID:18260117

1221. Hada M, Meel R, Kashyap S, et al. Eyelid Pilomatrixoma Masquerading as Chalazion. Can J Ophthalmol. 2017 Apr;52(2):e62–4. PMID:28457306

1222. Hadden PW, Damato BE, McKay IC. Bilateral Uveal Melanoma: A Series of Four Cases. Eye (Lond). 2003 Jul;17(5):613–6. PMID:12855969

1223. Hadi R, Xu H, Barber BR, et al. A Case of Endocrine Mucin-Producing Sweat Gland Carcinoma with Distant Metastasis. J Cutan Pathol. 2021 Jul;48(7):937–42. PMID:33660318

1224. Hadjistilianou T, Mastrangelo D, Gragnoli A, et al. Letter to the Editor: Neurofibromatosis Type 1 (NF 1) Associated with Embryonal Rhabdomyosarcoma of the Orbit. Med Pediatr Oncol. 2002 Jun;38(6):449. PMID:11984810

1225. Hafeez F, Krakowski AC, Lian CG, et al. Sporadic Superficial Angiomyxomas Demonstrate Loss of PRKAR1A Expression. Histopathology. 2022 May;80(6):1001–3. PMID:34532875

1226. Hafner C, Di Martino E, Pitt E, et al. FGFR3 Mutation Affects Cell Growth, Apoptosis and Attachment in Keratinocytes. Exp Cell Res. 2010 Jul 15;316(12):2008–16. PMID:20420824

1227. Hafner C, Landthaler M, Mentzel T, et al. FGFR3 and PIK3CA Mutations in Stucco Keratosis and Dermatosis Papulosa Nigra. Br J Dermatol. 2010 Mar;162(3):508–12. PMID:19845664

1228. Hafner C, van Oers JM, Hartmann A, et al. High Frequency of FGFR3 Mutations in Adenoid Seborrheic Keratoses. J Invest Dermatol. 2006 Nov;126(11):2404–7. PMID:16778799

1229. Haisley-Royster CA, Allingham RR, Klintworth GK, et al. Hereditary Benign Intraepithelial Dyskeratosis: Report of Two Cases with Prominent Oral Lesions. J Am Acad Dermatol. 2001 Oct;45(4):634–6. PMID:11568764

1230. Hakimi AA, Ostrovnaya I, Reva B, et al. Adverse Outcomes in Clear Cell Renal Cell Carcinoma with Mutations of 3p21 Epigenetic Regulators BAP1 and SETD2: A Report by MSKCC and the KIRC TCGA Research Network. Clin Cancer Res. 2013 Jun 15;19(12):3259–67. PMID:23620406

1231. Hale PN, Allen RA, Straatsma BR. Benign Melanomas (Nevi) of the Choroid and Ciliary Body. Arch Ophthalmol. 1965 Oct;74(4):532–8. PMID:5838370

1232. Hallek M. Chronic Lymphocytic Leukemia: 2020 Update on Diagnosis, Risk Stratification and Treatment. Am J Hematol. 2019 Nov;94(11):1266–87. PMID:31364186

1233. Haller F, Bieg M, Will R, et al. Enhancer Hijacking Activates Oncogenic Transcription Factor NR4A3 in Acinic Cell Carcinomas of the Salivary Glands. Nat Commun. 2019 Jan 21;10(1):368. PMID:30664630

1234. Haller F, Skálová A, Ihrler S, et al. Nuclear NR4A3 Immunostaining Is a Specific and Sensitive Novel Marker for Acinic Cell Carcinoma of the Salivary Glands. Am J Surg Pathol. 2019 Sep;43(9):1264–72. PMID:31094928

1235. Hamam R, Bhat P, Foster CS. Conjunctival/Corneal Intraepithelial Neoplasia. Int Ophthalmol Clin. 2009 Winter;49(1):63–70. PMID:19125065

1236. Hamblin TJ, Davis Z, Gardiner A, et al. Unmutated Ig V(H) Genes Are Associated with a More Aggressive Form of Chronic Lymphocytic Leukemia. Blood. 1999 Sep 15;94(6):1848–54. PMID:10477713

1237. Hamburg A. Medulloepithelioma Arising from the Posterior Pole. Ophthalmologica. 1980;181(3-4):152–9. PMID:7231881

1238. Hämmerl L, Ferlay J, Borok M, et al. The Burden of Squamous Cell Carcinoma of the Conjunctiva in Africa. Cancer Epidemiol. 2019 Aug;61:150–3. PMID:31255960

1239. Han K, Ha HJ, Kong JS, et al. Importance of Individual Ghost Cells in Fine-Needle Aspiration Cytology Diagnosis of Pilomatricoma. J Pathol Transl Med. 2018 Jan;52(1):45–50. PMID:29370510

1240. Han LM, Khanafshar E, Afshar AR, et al. The Diagnostic Utility of Next-Generation Sequencing on FNA Biopsies of Melanocytic Uveal Lesions. Cancer Cytopathol. 2020 Jul;128(7):499–505. PMID:32196967

1241. Han R, Jiang Y, Bian A, et al. Extranodal Natural Killer/T-Cell Lymphoma Nasal Type with Extensive Ocular Tissue Involvement: A Case Report. Diagn Pathol. 2021 Nov 11;16(1):104. PMID:34763717

1242. Han SB, Jeon HS, Kim M, et al. Quantification of Astigmatism Induced by Pterygium Using Automated Image Analysis. Cornea. 2016 Mar;35(3):370–6. PMID:26684048

1243. Hanbazazh M, Barrantes PC, DeVience E, et al. Overlapping Immunohistochemical Features of Adenocarcinoma of the Nonpigmented Ciliary Body Epithelium and Renal Cell Carcinoma. Am J Ophthalmol. 2021 Jun;226:191–200. PMID:33529584

1244. Handa U, Chhabra S, Mohan H. Epidermal Inclusion Cyst: Cytomorphological Features and Differential Diagnosis. Diagn Cytopathol. 2008 Dec;36(12):861–3. PMID:18855902

1245. Handorf CR, Kulkarni A, Grenert JP, et al. A Multicenter Study Directly Comparing the Diagnostic Accuracy of Gene Expression Profiling and Immunohistochemistry for Primary Site Identification in Metastatic Tumors. Am J Surg Pathol. 2013 Jul;37(7):1067–75. PMID:23648464

1246. Hankinson TC, Ogden AT, Canoll P, et al. Intraorbital and Intracranial Soft-Tissue Glomus Tumor in an 8-Year-Old Child. Case Report. J Neurosurg Pediatr. 2008 May;1(5):389–91. PMID:18447675

1247. Hans CP, Weisenburger DD, Greiner TC, et al. Confirmation of the Molecular Classification of Diffuse Large B-Cell Lymphoma by Immunohistochemistry Using a Tissue Microarray. Blood. 2004 Jan 1;103(1):275–82. PMID:14504078

1248. Hao J, Yang MB, Liu H, et al. Distribution of Propranolol in Periocular Tissues: A Comparison of Topical and Systemic Administration. J Ocul Pharmacol Ther. 2011 Oct;27(5):453–9. PMID:21810027

1249. Harbour JW, Brantley MA Jr, Hollingsworth H, et al. Association Between Posterior Uveal Melanoma and Iris Freckles, Iris Naevi, and Choroidal Naevi. Br J Ophthalmol. 2004 Jan;88(1):36–8. PMID:14693769

1250. Harbour JW, Onken MD, Roberson ED, et al. Frequent Mutation of BAP1 in Metastasizing Uveal Melanomas. Science. 2010 Dec 3;330(6009):1410–3. PMID:21051595

1251. Harbour JW, Roberson ED, Anbunathan H, et al. Recurrent Mutations at Codon 625 of the Splicing Factor SF3B1 in Uveal Melanoma. Nat Genet. 2013 Feb;45(2):133–5. PMID:23313955

1252. Harbour JW, Wilson D, Finger PT, et al. Gene Expressing Profiling of Iris Melanomas. Ophthalmology. 2013 Jan;120(1):213, 213.E1–3. PMID:23283188

1253. Hardy AW, Dwivedi RC, Masterson L, et al. Inverted Papilloma of Lacrimal Sac Invading into the Orbit: Case Report and Review of Literature. J Cancer Res Ther. 2015 Jan-Mar;11(1):238–40. PMID:25879369

1254. Harkins A, Bassig-Santos C, Cirone M. Frontal Arteriovenous Malformation Presenting as Painful Unilateral Conjunctiva Injection. Clin Pract Cases Emerg Med. 2022 Feb;6(1):96–8. PMID:35226863

1255. Harms KL, Healy MA, Nghiem P, et al. Analysis of Prognostic Factors from 9387 Merkel Cell Carcinoma Cases Forms the Basis for the New 8th Edition AJCC Staging System. Ann Surg Oncol. 2016 Oct;23(11):3564–71. PMID:27198511

1256. Haroche J, Abla O. Uncommon Histiocytic Disorders: Rosai-Dorfman, Juvenile Xanthogranuloma, and Erdheim-Chester Disease. Hematology Am Soc Hematol Educ Program. 2015;2015:571–8. PMID:26637774

1257. Haroche J, Charlotte F, Arnaud L, et al. High Prevalence of BRAF V600E Mutations in Erdheim-Chester Disease But Not in Other Non-Langerhans Cell Histiocytoses. Blood. 2012 Sep 27;120(13):2700–3. PMID:22879539

1258. Haroche J, Cohen-Aubart F, Amoura Z. Erdheim-Chester Disease. Blood. 2020 Apr 16;135(16):1311–8. PMID:32107533

1259. Haroche J, Cohen-Aubart F, Emile JF, et al. Reproducible and Sustained Efficacy of Targeted Therapy with Vemurafenib in Patients with BRAF(V600E)-Mutated Erdheim-Chester Disease. J Clin Oncol. 2015 Feb 10;33(5):411–8. PMID:25422482

1260. Harold Lee HB, Garrity JA, Cameron JD, et al. Primary Optic Nerve Sheath Meningioma in Children. Surv Ophthalmol. 2008 Nov-Dec;53(6):543–58. PMID:19026318

1261. Harooni H, Schoenfield LR, Singh AD. Current Appraisal of Conjunctival Melanocytic Tumors: Classification and Treatment. Future Oncol. 2011 Mar;7(3):435–46. PMID:21417906

1262. Harper PS. Calcifying Epithelioma of Malherbe. Association with Myotonic Muscular Dystrophy. Arch Dermatol. 1972 Jul;106(1):41–4. PMID:5039107

1263. Harris BF, Harris JP, Ducey TJ, et al. Phakomatous Choristoma of the Orbit With Involvement of the Inferior Oblique Muscle. Ophthalmic Plast Reconstr Surg. 2019 Jan/Feb;35(1):e10–9. PMID:30407999

1264. Harris JL, Gumucio CC, Ohanion MB. Adenocarcinoma of the Ciliary Epithelium. Arch Ophthalmol. 1968 Aug;80(2):217–9. PMID:5661889

1265. Harrison A, Loftus S, Pambuccian S. Orbital Chondroma. Ophthalmic Plast Reconstr Surg. 2006 Nov-Dec;22(6):484–5. PMID:17117112

1266. Harrison W, Pittman P, Cummings T. Optic Nerve Choristoma. Saudi J Ophthalmol. 2018 Jan-Mar;32(1):90–1. PMID:29755281

1267. Harrison W, Pittman P, Cummings T. Pleomorphic Adenoma of the Lacrimal Gland: A Review with Updates on Malignant Transformation and Molecular Genetics. Saudi J Ophthalmol. 2018 Jan-Mar;32(1):13–6. PMID:29755265

1268. Harvey NT, Tabone T, Erber W, et al. Circumscribed Sebaceous Neoplasms: A Morphological, Immunohistochemical and Molecular Analysis. Pathology. 2016 Aug;48(5):454–62. PMID:27311873

1269. Hasegawa SL, Mentzel T, Fletcher CD. Schwannomas of the Sinonasal Tract and Nasopharynx. Mod Pathol. 1997 Aug;10(8):777–84. PMID:9267819

1270. Hasegawa T, Matsuno Y, Shimoda T, et al. Proximal-Type Epithelioid Sarcoma: A Clinicopathologic Study of 20 Cases. Mod Pathol. 2001 Jul;14(7):655–63. PMID:11454997

1271. Hashemian H, Mahbod M, Amoli FA, et al. Histopathology of Conjunctivochalasis Compared to Normal Conjunctiva. J Ophthalmic Vis Res. 2016 Oct-Dec;11(4):345–9. PMID:27994801

1272. Hashimoto H, Daimaru Y, Enjoji M. Intravascular Papillary Endothelial Hyperplasia. A Clinicopathologic Study of 91 Cases. Am J Dermatopathol. 1983 Dec;5(6):539–46. PMID:6666836

1273. Hashimoto K, Sasajima Y, Ando M, et al. Immunohistochemical Profile for Unknown Primary Adenocarcinoma. PLoS One. 2012;7(1):e31181. PMID:22299055

1274. Hassane S, Fouad E, Said I, et al. Orbital Metastatic Angiosarcoma. Korean J Ophthalmol. 2010 Dec;24(6):364–6. PMID:21165236

1275. Hassenstein A, Bialasiewicz AA, von Domarus D, et al. Tapioca Melanomas of the Iris: Immunohistology and Report on Two Cases. Graefes Arch Clin Exp Ophthalmol. 1999 May;237(5):424–8. PMID:10333110

1276. Hasson A, Farias MM, Nicklas C, et al. Periorbital Syringoma Treated with Radiofrequency and Carbon Dioxide (CO2) Laser in 5 Patients. J Drugs Dermatol. 2012 Jul;11(7):879–80. PMID:22777235

1277. Hauben EI, Weeden S, Pringle J, et al. Does the Histological Subtype of High-Grade Central Osteosarcoma Influence the Response to Treatment with Chemotherapy and Does it Affect Overall Survival? A Study on 570 Patients of Two Consecutive Trials of the European Osteosarcoma Intergroup. Eur J Cancer. 2002 Jun;38(9):1218–25. PMID:12044509

1278. Haugh AM, Njauw CN, Bubley JA, et al. Genotypic and Phenotypic Features of BAP1 Cancer Syndrome: A Report of 8 New Families and Review of Cases in the Literature. JAMA Dermatol. 2017 Oct 1;153(10):999–1006. PMID:28793149

1279. Haupt R, Minkov M, Astigarraga I, et al. Langerhans Cell Histiocytosis (LCH): Guidelines for Diagnosis, Clinical Work-Up, and Treatment for Patients Till the Age of 18 Years. Pediatr Blood Cancer. 2013 Feb;60(2):175–84. PMID:23109216

1280. Haupt R, Nanduri V, Calevo MG, et al. Permanent Consequences in Langerhans Cell Histiocytosis Patients: A Pilot Study from the Histiocyte Society-Late Effects Study Group. Pediatr Blood Cancer. 2004 May;42(5):438–44. PMID:15049016

1281. Håvik AL, Bruland O, Myrseth E, et al. Genetic Landscape of Sporadic Vestibular Schwannoma. J Neurosurg. 2018 Mar;128(3):911–22. PMID:28409725

1282. Hayani KM, Zelger BG, Kind P, et al.

Seborrheic Keratosis With Sebaceous Differentiation, a Series of 8 Cases and Critical Review of the Literature. Am J Dermatopathol. 2021 Nov 1;43(11):801–10. PMID:33958512
1283. Hayashi N, Borodic G, Karesh JW, et al. Giant Cell Angiofibroma of the Orbit and Eyelid. Ophthalmology. 1999 Jun;106(6):1223–9. PMID:10366097
1284. Hayashi N, Komatsu T, Komatsu T, et al. Juvenile Xanthogranuloma Presenting with Unilateral Prominent Nodule of the Eyelid: Report of a Case and Clinicopathological Findings. Jpn J Ophthalmol. 2004 Sep-Oct;48(5):435–9. PMID:15486764
1285. Hayden A, Wilson DJ, Rosenbaum JT. Management of Orbital Xanthogranuloma with Methotrexate. Br J Ophthalmol. 2007 Apr;91(4):434–6. PMID:17135338
1286. Hayek S, Adam C, Adams D, et al. Conjunctival Lymphangiectasia: A Novel Ocular Manifestation of Hereditary Transthyretin Amyloidosis. Amyloid. 2019 Jun;26(2):94–5. PMID:31074309
1287. Hayward DM, Yoo D, Lee JM, et al. Myoepithelioma of the Orbital Apex and Middle Cranial Fossa: Case Report and Review of the Literature. Neuroophthalmology. 2014 Jan 28;38(1):14–20. PMID:27928268
1288. Hazim AZ, Ruan GJ, Ravindran A, et al. Efficacy of BRAF-Inhibitor Therapy in BRAFV600E -Mutated Adult Langerhans Cell Histiocytosis. Oncologist. 2020 Dec;25(12):1001–4. PMID:32985015
1289. He CY, Dong GH, Yang DM, et al. Inflammatory Myofibroblastic Tumors of the Nasal Cavity and Paranasal Sinus: A Clinicopathologic Study of 25 Cases and Review of the Literature. Eur Arch Otorhinolaryngol. 2015 Apr;272(4):789–97. PMID:24756612
1290. He S, Huang Y, Dong S, et al. MiR-199a-3p/5p Participated in TGF-β and EGF Induced EMT by Targeting DUSP5/MAP3K11 in Pterygium. J Transl Med. 2020 Sep 1;18(1):332. PMID:32867783
1291. He X, Pang Z, Zhang X, et al. Consistent Amplification of FRS2 and MDM2 in Low-Grade Osteosarcoma: A Genetic Study of 22 Cases With Clinicopathologic Analysis. Am J Surg Pathol. 2018 Sep;42(9):1143–55. PMID:30001240
1292. Heald B, Mester J, Rybicki L, et al. Frequent Gastrointestinal Polyps and Colorectal Adenocarcinomas in a Prospective Series of PTEN Mutation Carriers. Gastroenterology. 2010 Dec;139(6):1927–33. PMID:20600018
1293. Heaps RS, Miller NR, Albert DM, et al. Primary Adenocarcinoma of the Lacrimal Gland. A Retrospective Study. Ophthalmology. 1993 Dec;100(12):1856–60. PMID:8259287
1294. Heath P. Tumors of the Iris: Classification and Clinical Follow-Up. Trans Am Ophthalmol Soc. 1964;62:51–85. PMID:14269906
1295. Heathcote JG. Transitional Neoplasms of the Naso-Lacrimal System: A Review of the Histopathology and Histogenesis. Saudi J Ophthalmol. 2012 Apr;26(2):125–31. PMID:23960982
1296. Heegaard S, Grossniklaus H, editors. Eye Pathology: An Illustrated Guide. Heidelberg (Germany): Springer; 2014.
1297. Heegaard S, Jensen OA, Prause JU. Immunohistochemical Diagnosis of Malignant Melanoma of the Conjunctiva and Uvea: Comparison of the Novel Antibody Against Melan-A with S100 Protein and HMB-45. Melanoma Res. 2000 Aug;10(4):350–4. PMID:10985669
1298. Heegaard S, Larsen JN, Fledelius HC, et al. Neoplasia Versus Hyperplasia of the Retinal Pigment Epithelium. A Comparison of Two Cases. Acta Ophthalmol Scand. 2001 Dec;79(6):626–33. PMID:11782230
1299. Heegaard S, Prause JU. Leiomyoma of the Caruncle. Acta Ophthalmol Scand. 1998 Dec;76(6):731–3. PMID:9881563
1300. Heerema MG, Suurmeijer AJ. Sox10 Immunohistochemistry Allows the Pathologist to Differentiate Between Prototypical Granular Cell Tumors and Other Granular Cell Lesions. Histopathology. 2012 Nov;61(5):997–9. PMID:22804786
1301. Heeringa JJ, Karim AF, van Laar JAM, et al. Expansion of Blood IgG4+ B, TH2, and Regulatory T Cells in Patients with IgG4-Related Disease. J Allergy Clin Immunol. 2018 May;141(5):1831–1843.E10. PMID:28830675
1302. Hegde P, Venugopal M, Ramesh S, et al. An Eye-Opening Case of Periorbital Oedema: A Clinicodiagnostic Dilemma. Clin Exp Dermatol. 2022 Apr;47(4):780–2. PMID:34923671
1303. Hei Y, Kang L, Yang X, et al. Orbital Alveolar Soft Part Sarcoma: A Report of 8 Cases and Review of the Literature. Oncol Lett. 2018 Jan;15(1):304–14. PMID:29285193
1304. Heidari P, Verdijk RM, van Den Bosch WA, et al. Biopsy-Proven Recurrence of Unilateral IgG4-Related Orbital Inflammation After 20 Years. Orbit. 2014 Oct;33(5):388–91. PMID:24911364
1305. Heidenreich B, Denisova E, Rachakonda S, et al. Genetic Alterations in Seborrheic Keratoses. Oncotarget. 2017 May 30;8(22):36639–49. PMID:28410231
1306. Heindl LM, Jünemann AG, Kruse FE, et al. Tumors of the Lacrimal Drainage System. Orbit. 2010 Oct;29(5):298–306. PMID:20958177
1307. Heindl LM, Naumann GO, Kruse FE, et al. Aggressive Metastasising Adenocarcinoma of the Retinal Pigment Epithelium with Trisomy 21. Br J Ophthalmol. 2008 Mar;92(3):389–91. PMID:18303161
1308. Helgager J, Lidov HG, Mahadevan NR, et al. A Novel GIT2-BRAF Fusion in Pilocytic Astrocytoma. Diagn Pathol. 2017 Nov 15;12(1):82. PMID:29141672
1309. Helm K, Findeis-Hosey J. Immunohistochemistry of Pigmented Actinic Keratoses, Actinic Keratoses, Melanomas In Situ and Solar Lentigines with Melan-A. J Cutan Pathol. 2008 Oct;35(10):931–4. PMID:18494818
1310. Helmi HA, Alkatan HM, Al-Essa RS, et al. Choroidal Hemangioma in Sturge Weber Syndrome: Case Series with Confirmed Tissue Diagnosis. Int J Surg Case Rep. 2021 Dec;89:106626. PMID:34847393
1311. Helmi HA, Alsarhani W, Alkatan HM, et al. Sebaceous Gland Carcinoma with Misleading Clinical Appearance: A Case Report of an Eyelid Lesion. Am J Case Rep. 2020 Aug 13;21:e925134. PMID:32788569
1312. Hendrix MJ, Seftor EA, Seftor RE, et al. Biologic Determinants of Uveal Melanoma Metastatic Phenotype: Role of Intermediate Filaments as Predictive Markers. Lab Invest. 1998 Feb;78(2):153–63. PMID:9484713
1313. Hendrix MJ, Seftor EA, Seftor RE, et al. Regulation of Uveal Melanoma Interconverted Phenotype by Hepatocyte Growth Factor/Scatter Factor (HGF/SF). Am J Pathol. 1998 Apr;152(4):855–63. PMID:9546344
1314. Henner MS, Shapiro PE, Ritter JH, et al. Solitary Syringoma. Report of Five Cases and Clinicopathologic Comparison with Microcystic Adnexal Carcinoma of the Skin. Am J Dermatopathol. 1995 Oct;17(5):465–70. PMID:8599451
1315. Hennessy MP, Collins F, Coroneo MT. The Distinction Between Multiple Retinal Pigment Epithelial Hamartomata (MRPEH) in Familial Adenomatous Polyposis (FAP) and Congenital Hypertrophy of the Retinal Pigment Epithelium (CHRPE). Aust N Z J Ophthalmol. 1993 Nov;21(4):275–6. PMID:8148147
1316. Henning B, Stieger P, Kamarachev J, et al. Pyogenic Granuloma in Patients Treated with Selective BRAF Inhibitors: Another Manifestation of Paradoxical Pathway Activation. Melanoma Res. 2016 Jun;26(3):304–7. PMID:27116335
1317. Heran MK, Rootman J, Sangha BS, et al. Dynamic Arterial and Valsalva-Augmented Venous Phase Multidetector CT for Orbital Vascular Lesions: A Pictorial Review*. Ophthalmic Plast Reconstr Surg. 2014 Mar-Apr;30(2):180–5. PMID:24614549
1318. Herbert HM, Sun MT, Selva D, et al. Merkel Cell Carcinoma of the Eyelid: Management and Prognosis. JAMA Ophthalmol. 2014 Feb;132(2):197–204. PMID:24287584
1319. Hered RW, Hiles DA. Epibulbar Osseous Choristoma and Ectopic Lacrimal Gland Underlying a Dermolipoma. J Pediatr Ophthalmol Strabismus. 1987 Sep-Oct;24(5):255–8. PMID:3681614
1320. Héritier S, Barkaoui MA, Miron J, et al. Incidence and Risk Factors for Clinical Neurodegenerative Langerhans Cell Histiocytosis: A Longitudinal Cohort Study. Br J Haematol. 2018 Nov;183(4):608–17. PMID:30421536
1321. Héritier S, Emile JF, Barkaoui MA, et al. BRAF Mutation Correlates With High-Risk Langerhans Cell Histiocytosis and Increased Resistance to First-Line Therapy. J Clin Oncol. 2016 Sep 1;34(25):3023–30. PMID:27382093
1322. Hernandez-Martin A, Baselga E, Drolet BA, et al. Juvenile Xanthogranuloma. J Am Acad Dermatol. 1997 Mar;36(3 Pt 1):355–67. PMID:9091465
1323. Hernández-Núñez A, Nájera Botello L, Romero Maté A, et al. Retrospective Study of Pilomatricoma: 261 Tumors in 239 Patients. Actas Dermosifiliogr. 2014 Sep;105(7):699–705. PMID:24838222
1324. Herrera A, Ortega C, Reyes G, et al. Primary Orbital Mesenchymal Chondrosarcoma: Case Report and Review of the Literature. Case Rep Med. 2012;2012:292147. PMID:22761622
1325. Herrera-Goepfert R. Postradiation Synovial Sarcoma of the Common Bile Duct: A Previously Unreported Anatomic Site. Int J Surg Pathol. 2018 Aug;26(5):469–74. PMID:29336183
1326. Herschorn BJ, Jakobiec FA, Hornblass A, et al. Epibulbar Subconjunctival Fibroma. A Tumor Possibly Arising from Tenon's Capsule. Ophthalmology. 1983 Dec;90(12):1490–4. PMID:6677850
1327. Herschorn BJ, Jakobiec FA, Hornblass A, et al. Mucoepidermoid Carcinoma of the Palpebral Mucocutaneous Junction. A Clinical, Light Microscopic and Electron Microscopic Study of an Unusual Tubular Variant. Ophthalmology. 1983 Dec;90(12):1437–46. PMID:6677843
1328. Hervier B, Haroche J, Arnaud L, et al. Association of Both Langerhans Cell Histiocytosis and Erdheim-Chester Disease Linked to the BRAFV600E Mutation. Blood. 2014 Aug 14;124(7):1119–26. PMID:24894769
1329. Herwig MC, Wells JR, Grossniklaus HE. Conjunctival Stromal Tumor: Report of 4 Cases. Ophthalmology. 2012 Apr;119(4):682–7. PMID:22200094
1330. Herwig-Carl MC, Loeffler KU, Grossniklaus HE. Melanocytoma of the Conjunctiva: Clinicopathologic Features of Three Cases. Ocul Oncol Pathol. 2019 Jun;5(4):290–7. PMID:31367593
1331. Hesse RJ, Scharfenberg JC, Ratz JL, et al. Eyelid Microcystic Adnexal Carcinoma. Arch Ophthalmol. 1995 Apr;113(4):494–6. PMID:7710401
1332. Hidayat AA, Flint A, Marentette L, et al. Myxomas and Angiomyxomas of the Orbit: A Clinicopathologic Study of 6 Cases. Ophthalmology. 2007 May;114(5):1012–9. PMID:17467533
1333. Hidayat AA, Font RL. Trichilemmoma of Eyelid and Eyebrow. A Clinicopathologic Study of 31 Cases. Arch Ophthalmol. 1980 May;98(5):844–7. PMID:6990903
1334. Hiddemann W, Kneba M, Dreyling M, et al. Frontline Therapy with Rituximab Added to the Combination of Cyclophosphamide, Doxorubicin, Vincristine, and Prednisone (CHOP) Significantly Improves the Outcome for Patients with Advanced-Stage Follicular Lymphoma Compared with Therapy with CHOP Alone: Results of a Prospective Randomized Study of the German Low-Grade Lymphoma Study Group. Blood. 2005 Dec 1;106(12):3725–32. PMID:16123223
1335. Hiemcke-Jiwa LS, Ten Dam-van Loon NH, Leguit RJ, et al. Potential Diagnosis of Vitreoretinal Lymphoma by Detection of MYD88 Mutation in Aqueous Humor With Ultrasensitive Droplet Digital Polymerase Chain Reaction. JAMA Ophthalmol. 2018 Oct 1;136(10):1098–104. PMID:30027272
1336. Higuchi K, Urano M, Takahashi RH, et al. Cytological Features of Mammary Analogue Secretory Carcinoma of Salivary Gland: Fine-Needle Aspiration of Seven Cases. Diagn Cytopathol. 2014 Oct;42(10):846–55. PMID:24585770
1337. Hilal T, DiCaudo DJ, Connolly SM, et al. Necrobiotic Xanthogranuloma: A 30-Year Single-Center Experience. Ann Hematol. 2018 Aug;97(8):1471–9. PMID:29568990
1338. Hildebrand GD, Timms C, Thompson DA, et al. Juvenile Xanthogranuloma with Presumed Involvement of the Optic Disc and Retina. Arch Ophthalmol. 2004 Oct;122(10):1551–5. PMID:15477475
1339. Hill JC, Maske R. Pathogenesis of Pterygium. Eye (Lond). 1989;3(Pt 2):218–26. PMID:2695353
1340. Hilliard NJ, Wakefield DN, Krahl D, et al. P16 Expression in Conventional and Desmoplastic Trichilemmomas. Am J Dermatopathol. 2009 Jun;31(4):342–9. PMID:19461237
1341. Hindsø TG, Esmaeli B, Holm F, et al. International Multicentre Retrospective Cohort Study of Ocular Adnexal Marginal Zone B-Cell Lymphoma. Br J Ophthalmol. 2020 Mar;104(3):357–62. PMID:31177189
1342. Hirano K, Tada M, Sasahira N, et al. Incidence of Malignancies in Patients with IgG4-Related Disease. Intern Med. 2014;53(3):171–6. PMID:24492683
1343. Hiscott P, Seitz B, Naumann GO. Epithelioid Cell Spitz Nevus of the Eyelid. Am J Ophthalmol. 1998 Nov;126(5):735–7. PMID:9822246
1344. Ho CY, Bornhorst M, Almira-Suarez MI, et al. Clinicopathologic Features of Diencephalic Neuronal and Glioneuronal Tumors. J Neuropathol Exp Neurol. 2020 Jan 1;79(1):67–73. PMID:31793986
1345. Ho CY, Mosier S, Safneck J, et al. Genetic Profiling by Single-Nucleotide Polymorphism-Based Array Analysis Defines Three Distinct Subtypes of Orbital Meningioma. Brain Pathol. 2015 Mar;25(2):193–201. PMID:24773246
1346. Ho SF, Brown L, Bamford M, et al. 5 Years Review of Periocular Basal Cell Carcinoma and Proposed Follow-Up Protocol. Eye (Lond). 2013 Jan;27(1):78–83. PMID:23154501
1347. Hoang MP, Amirkhan RH. Inhibin Alpha Distinguishes Hemangioblastoma from Clear Cell Renal Cell Carcinoma. Am J Surg Pathol. 2003 Aug;27(8):1152–6. PMID:12883249
1348. Hoang MP, Dresser KA, Kapur P, et al. Microcystic Adnexal Carcinoma: An Immunohistochemical Reappraisal. Mod Pathol. 2008 Feb;21(2):178–85. PMID:18065959
1349. Hoang VT, Trinh CT, Nguyen CH, et al. Overview of Epidermoid Cyst. Eur J Radiol Open. 2019 Sep 5;6:291–301. PMID:31516916
1350. Hodge JC, Pearce KE, Wang X, et al.

Molecular Cytogenetic Analysis for TFE3 Rearrangement in Xp11.2 Renal Cell Carcinoma and Alveolar Soft Part Sarcoma: Validation and Clinical Experience with 75 Cases. Mod Pathol. 2014 Jan;27(1):113–27. PMID:23828314
1351. Holling M, Wildförster U, Verheggen R, et al. Myopericytoma: A Series of 5 Cases Affecting the Nervous System. World Neurosurg. 2015 Nov;84(5):1493.E5–8. PMID:25931311
1352. Hollowell KL, Agle SC, Zervos EE et al. Cutaneous Apocrine Adenocarcinoma: Defining Epidemiology, Outcomes, and Optimal Therapy for a Rare Neoplasm. J Surg Oncol. 2012 Mar 15;105(4):415–9. PMID:21913192
1353. Holm F, Mikkelsen LH, Kamper P, et al. Ocular Adnexal Lymphoma in Denmark: A Nationwide Study of 387 Cases from 1980 to 2017. Br J Ophthalmol. 2021 Jul;105(7):914–20. PMID:32732342
1354. Honavar SG, Manjandavida FP. Tumors of the Ocular Surface: A Review. Indian J Ophthalmol. 2015 Mar;63(3):187–203. PMID:25971163
1355. Honavar SG, Shields CL, Maus M, et al. Primary Intraepithelial Sebaceous Gland Carcinoma of the Palpebral Conjunctiva. Arch Ophthalmol. 2001 May;119(5):764–7. PMID:11346408
1356. Honavar SG, Shields CL, Singh AD, et al. Two Discrete Choroidal Melanomas in an Eye with Ocular Melanocytosis. Surv Ophthalmol. 2002 Jan-Feb;47(1):36–41. PMID:11801268
1357. Honda Y, Nakamizo S, Dainichi T, et al. Adult-Onset Asthma and Periocular Xanthogranuloma Associated with IgG4-Related Disease with Infiltration of Regulatory T Cells. J Eur Acad Dermatol Venereol. 2017 Feb;31(2):e124–5. PMID:27519554
1358. Hongo H, Miyawaki S, Teranishi Y, et al. Somatic GJA4 Gain-of-Function Mutation in Orbital Cavernous Venous Malformations. Angiogenesis. 2023 Feb;26(1):37–52. PMID:35902510
1359. Hongo T, Yamamoto H, Jiromaru R, et al. Clinicopathologic Significance of EGFR Mutation and HPV Infection in Sinonasal Squamous Cell Carcinoma. Am J Surg Pathol. 2021 Jan;45(1):108–18. PMID:32868526
1360. Hongo T, Yamamoto H, Tanabe M, et al. High-Risk HPV-Related Squamous Cell Carcinoma in the Conjunctiva and Lacrimal Sac: Clinicopathologic Characteristics and Diagnostic Utility of P16 and Rb Immunohistochemistry. Am J Surg Pathol. 2022 Jul 1;46(7):977–87. PMID:34985043
1361. Honma K, Tsuzuki S, Nakagawa M, et al. TNFAIP3/A20 Functions as a Novel Tumor Suppressor Gene in Several Subtypes of Non-Hodgkin Lymphomas. Blood. 2009 Sep 17;114(12):2467–75. PMID:19608751
1362. Hoppenreijs VP, Reuser TT, Mooy CM, et al. Syringomatous Carcinoma of the Eyelid and Orbit: A Clinical and Histopathological Challenge. Br J Ophthalmol. 1997 Aug;81(8):668–72. PMID:9349155
1363. Horn H, Ziepert M, Becher C, et al. MYC Status in Concert with BCL2 and BCL6 Expression Predicts Outcome in Diffuse Large B-Cell Lymphoma. Blood. 2013 Mar 21;121(12):2253–63. PMID:23335369
1364. Hornblass A, Jakobiec FA, Bosniak S, et al. The Diagnosis and Management of Epithelial Tumors of the Lacrimal Sac. Ophthalmology. 1980 Jun;87(6):476–90. PMID:7413136
1365. Hornick JL, Dal Cin P, Fletcher CD. Loss of INI1 Expression is Characteristic of Both Conventional and Proximal-Type Epithelioid Sarcoma. Am J Surg Pathol. 2009 Apr;33(4):542–50. PMID:19033866
1366. Hornick JL, Fletcher CD. Sclerosing PEComa: Clinicopathologic Analysis of a Distinctive Variant with a Predilection for the Retroperitoneum. Am J Surg Pathol. 2008 Apr;32(4):493–501. PMID:18223480
1367. Hornick JL, Sholl LM, Dal Cin P, et al. Expression of ROS1 Predicts ROS1 Gene Rearrangement in Inflammatory Myofibroblastic Tumors. Mod Pathol. 2015 May;28(5):732–9. PMID:25612511
1368. Hoshida Y, Li T, Dong Z, et al. Lymphoproliferative Disorders in Renal Transplant Patients in Japan. Int J Cancer. 2001 Mar 15;91(6):869–75. PMID:11275994
1369. Hosten N, Bornfeld N, Wassmuth R, et al. Uveal Melanoma: Detection of Extraocular Growth with MR Imaging and US. Radiology. 1997 Jan;202(1):61–7. PMID:8988193
1370. Hoster E, Dreyling M, Klapper W, et al. A New Prognostic Index (MIPI) for Patients with Advanced-Stage Mantle Cell Lymphoma. Blood. 2008 Jan 15;111(2):558–65. PMID:17962512
1371. Hoster E, Klapper W, Hermine O, et al. Confirmation of the Mantle-Cell Lymphoma International Prognostic Index in Randomized Trials of the European Mantle-Cell Lymphoma Network. J Clin Oncol. 2014 May 1;32(13):1338–46. PMID:24687837
1372. Hoster E, Rosenwald A, Berger F, et al. Prognostic Value of Ki-67 Index, Cytology, and Growth Pattern in Mantle-Cell Lymphoma: Results From Randomized Trials of the European Mantle Cell Lymphoma Network. J Clin Oncol. 2016 Apr 20;34(12):1386–94. PMID:26926679
1373. Hou LC, Murphy MA, Tung GA. Primary Orbital Leiomyosarcoma: A Case Report with MRI Findings. Am J Ophthalmol. 2003 Mar;135(3):408–10. PMID:12614772
1374. Houston SK, Bourne TD, Lopes MB, et al. Bilateral Massive Retinal Gliosis Associated with Retinopathy of Prematurity. Arch Pathol Lab Med. 2009 Aug;133(8):1242–5. PMID:19653718
1375. Houtzagers LE, Wierenga APA, Ruys AAM, et al. Iris Colour and the Risk of Developing Uveal Melanoma. Int J Mol Sci. 2020 Sep 28;21(19):7172. PMID:32998469
1376. Howard JE, Dwivedi RC, Masterson L, et al. Langerhans Cell Sarcoma: A Systematic Review. Cancer Treat Rev. 2015 Apr;41(4):320–31. PMID:25805533
1377. Howrey RP, Lipham WJ, Schultz WH, et al. Sebaceous Gland Carcinoma: A Subtle Second Malignancy Following Radiation Therapy in Patients with Bilateral Retinoblastoma. Cancer. 1998 Aug 15;83(4):767–71. PMID:9708943
1378. Hristodulopulos V, Medel R. Intramuscular Lipoma of Superior Rectus Muscle. Ophthalmic Plast Reconstr Surg. 2016 May-Jun;32(3):e52–5. PMID:25029341
1379. Hsieh SC, Shen CY, Liao HT, et al. The Cellular and Molecular Bases of Allergy, Inflammation and Tissue Fibrosis in Patients with IgG4-Related Disease. Int J Mol Sci. 2020 Jul 18;21(14):5082. PMID:32708432
1380. Hsu A, Frank SJ, Ballo MT, et al. Postoperative Adjuvant External-Beam Radiation Therapy for Cancers of the Eyelid and Conjunctiva. Ophthalmic Plast Reconstr Surg. 2008 Nov-Dec;24(6):444–9. PMID:19033839
1381. Hsu CR, Chen YY, Yao M, et al. Orbital and Ocular Adnexal Lymphoma: A Review of Epidemiology and Prognostic Factors in Taiwan. Eye (Lond). 2021 Jul;35(7):1946–53. PMID:32994547
1382. Hsueh C, Hsueh S, Gonzalez-Crussi F, et al. Nasal Chondromesenchymal Hamartoma in Children: Report of 2 Cases with Review of the Literature. Arch Pathol Lab Med. 2001 Mar;125(3):400–3. PMID:11231491
1383. Hu DN, McCormick SA, Yu GP. Latitude and Uveal Melanoma. Ophthalmology. 2008 Apr;115(4):757. PMID:18387420
1384. Hu DN, Yu G, McCormick SA, et al. Population-Based Incidence of Conjunctival Melanoma in Various Races and Ethnic Groups and Comparison with Other Melanomas. Am J Ophthalmol. 2008 Mar;145(3):418–23. PMID:18191091
1385. Hu DN, Yu GP, McCormick SA, et al. Population-Based Incidence of Uveal Melanoma in Various Races and Ethnic Groups. Am J Ophthalmol. 2005 Oct;140(4):612–7. PMID:16226513
1386. Huang FW, Hodis E, Xu MJ, et al. Highly Recurrent TERT Promoter Mutations in Human Melanoma. Science. 2013 Feb 22;339(6122):957–9. PMID:23348506
1387. Huang JT, Liang MG. Vascular Malformations. Pediatr Clin North Am. 2010 Oct;57(5):1091–110. PMID:20888460
1388. Huang KL, Mashl RJ, Wu Y, et al. Pathogenic Germline Variants in 10,389 Adult Cancers. Cell. 2018 Apr 5;173(2):355–370.E14. PMID:29625052
1389. Huang S, Juniat V, Satchi K, et al. Bilateral Lacrimal Gland Disease: Clinical Features and Outcomes. Eye (Lond). 2022 Nov;36(11):2163–71. PMID:34725471
1390. Huang SC, Alaggio R, Sung YS, et al. Frequent HRAS Mutations in Malignant Ectomesenchymoma: Overlapping Genetic Abnormalities With Embryonal Rhabdomyosarcoma. Am J Surg Pathol. 2016 Jul;40(7):876–85. PMID:26872011
1391. Huang SC, Zhang L, Sung YS, et al. Frequent FOS Gene Rearrangements in Epithelioid Hemangioma: A Molecular Study of 58 Cases With Morphologic Reappraisal. Am J Surg Pathol. 2015 Oct;39(10):1313–21. PMID:26135557
1392. Huang Y, de Reyniès A, de Leval L, et al. Gene Expression Profiling Identifies Emerging Oncogenic Pathways Operating in Extranodal NK/T-Cell Lymphoma, Nasal Type. Blood. 2010 Feb 11;115(6):1226–37. PMID:19965620
1393. Huang YM, Huang YY, Yang HY, et al. Conjunctival Papilloma: Clinical Features, Outcome, and Factors Related to Recurrence. Taiwan J Ophthalmol. 2018 Jan-Mar;8(1):15–8. PMID:29675344
1394. Huang YY, Liang WY, Tsai CC, et al. Comparison of the Clinical Characteristics and Outcome of Benign and Malignant Eyelid Tumors: An Analysis of 4521 Eyelid Tumors in a Tertiary Medical Center. Biomed Res Int. 2015;2015:453091. PMID:26634208
1395. Hudson LE, Mendoza P, Hudson WH, et al. Distinct Gene Expression Profiles Define Anaplastic Grade in Retinoblastoma. Am J Pathol. 2018 Oct;188(10):2328–38. PMID:30036517
1396. Hudson LE, Mendoza PR, Yan J, et al. Reactive Retinal Astrocytic Tumor (Focal Nodular Gliosis): A Case Report. Ocul Oncol Pathol. 2017 Jan;3(1):1–7. PMID:28275595
1397. Huggett MT, Culver EL, Kumar M, et al. Type 1 Autoimmune Pancreatitis and IgG4-Related Sclerosing Cholangitis is Associated with Extrapancreatic Organ Failure, Malignancy, and Mortality in a Prospective UK Cohort. Am J Gastroenterol. 2014 Oct;109(10):1675–83. PMID:25155229
1398. Huggins AB, Carrasco JR, Evans JJ, et al. Solitary Extramedullary Plasmacytoma of the Orbital Apex and Dura Masquerading as Idiopathic Inflammation. Ophthalmic Plast Reconstr Surg. 2017 May/Jun;33(3S Suppl 1):S92–4. PMID:26226234
1399. Huggins AB, Stefanyszyn MA, Nyquist G, et al. Basaloid Adenocarcinoma of the Lacrimal Sac: A Rare Entity and Approach to Management. Orbit. 2017 Dec;36(6):441–4. PMID:28837389
1400. Hughes E, Fogarty H, Fortune A, et al. Ocular Presentation of Natural Killer/T-Cell Lymphoma in a Caucasian Man. BMJ Case Rep. 2016 Apr 26;2016:Bcr2016215089. PMID:27118749
1401. Hui JI, Buchser NM, Dubovy SR. Primary Eyelid Leiomyoma. Ophthalmic Plast Reconstr Surg. 2011 Jul-Aug;27(4):e102–3. PMID:20966798
1402. Hung CC, Lin SY, Lee CN, et al. Low Penetrance of Retinoblastoma for P.V654L Mutation of the RB1 Gene. BMC Med Genet. 2011 May 26;12:76. PMID:21615945
1403. Hung CH, Lo CY. Immunoglobulin G4-Related Orbital Disease with Bilateral Optic Perineuritis and Maxillary Nerves Involvement: A Case Report. Ophthalmol Ther. 2020 Dec;9(4):1089–99. PMID:33068257
1404. Hung YP. Vascular Tumors of Bone: Updates and Diagnostic Pitfall. Surg Pathol Clin. 2021 Dec;14(4):645–63. PMID:34742485
1405. Hung YP, Fletcher CD, Hornick JL. FOSB is a Useful Diagnostic Marker for Pseudomyogenic Hemangioendothelioma. Am J Surg Pathol. 2017 May;41(5):596–606. PMID:28009608
1406. Hung YP, Fletcher CDM. Myopericytomatosis: Clinicopathologic Analysis of 11 Cases With Molecular Identification of Recurrent PDGFRB Alterations in Myopericytomatosis and Myopericytoma. Am J Surg Pathol. 2017 Aug;41(8):1034–44. PMID:28505006
1407. Hunt SJ, Kilzer B, Santa Cruz DJ. Desmoplastic Trichilemmoma: Histologic Variant Resembling Invasive Carcinoma. J Cutan Pathol. 1990 Feb;17(1):45–52. PMID:2319039
1408. Huntington AC, Langloss JM, Hidayat AA. Spindle Cell Carcinoma of the Conjunctiva. An Immunohistochemical and Ultrastructural Study of Six Cases. Ophthalmology. 1990 Jun;97(6):711–7. PMID:1695722
1409. Husain M, Nguyen GK. Alveolar Soft Part Sarcoma. Report of a Case Diagnosed by Needle Aspiration Cytology and Electron Microscopy. Acta Cytol. 1995 Sep-Oct;39(5):951–4. PMID:7571976
1410. Hussain RN, Kalirai H, Groenewald C, et al. Prognostic Biopsy of Choroidal Melanoma After Proton Beam Radiation Therapy. Ophthalmology. 2016 Oct;123(10):2264–5. PMID:27324683
1411. Hussaini HM, Angel CM, Speight PM, et al. A Double-Clear Variant of Epithelial-Myoepithelial Carcinoma of the Parotid Gland. Head Neck Pathol. 2012 Dec;6(4):471–5. PMID:22427262
1412. Hyrcza MD, Andreasen S, Melchior LC, et al. Primary Secretory Carcinoma of the Lacrimal Gland: Report of a New Entity. Am J Ophthalmol. 2018 Sep;193:178–83. PMID:29963997
1413. Hyrcza MD, Gilbert RW, Yu E, et al. Mucoepidermoid Carcinoma Ex-Inverted Papilloma. Diagn Histopathol. 2015 May 1;21(5):212–5.
1414. IARC Working Group on the Evaluation of Carcinogenic Risks to Humans. Human Papillomaviruses. IARC Monogr Eval Carcinog Risks Hum. 2007;90:1–670. Available from: https://publications.iarc.fr/108. PMID:18354839
1415. Idos G, Valle L. Lynch Syndrome. In: Adam MP, Everman DB, Mirzaa GM, et al., editors. GeneReviews. Seattle (WA): University of Washington, Seattle; 1993–2025. PMID:20301390
1416. Ikediobi NI, Iyengar V, Hwang L, et al. Infantile Myofibromatosis: Support for Autosomal Dominant Inheritance. J Am Acad Dermatol. 2003 Aug;49(2 Suppl Case Reports):S148–50. PMID:12894106
1417. Im S, Cho U, Choi HJ, et al. Palisading and Verocay Body Prominent Orbital Leiomyosarcoma, Masquerading as a Schwannoma.

Int J Surg Pathol. 2019 Jun;27(4):409–10. PMID:30326763
1418. Imaizumi M, Nakatsuka K. Oncocytoma of the Peripunctum. Int Ophthalmol. 2005 Jun;26(3):111–3. PMID:17091220
1419. Inamori O, Fukuoka H, Nagamine M, et al. Mesectodermal Leiomyoma of the Ciliary Body: A Unique Variant of Leiomyoma with Myogenic and Neurogenic Histological Features. Int J Surg Pathol. 2022 Feb;30(1):114–9. PMID:34424080
1420. Inayama Y, Hanashi M, Yazawa T, et al. Massive Gliosis of the Retina: Report of a Case Investigated by Immunohistochemistry and Clonality Assays. Hum Pathol. 2005 Jun;36(6):702–5. PMID:16021579
1421. Infante-Cossio P, Infante-Cossio M, Herce-Lopez J, et al. Supraorbital Leiomyoma. Ophthalmic Plast Reconstr Surg. 2018 Mar/Apr;34(2):e71. PMID:28151824
1422. Inoue D, Chew GL, Liu B, et al. Spliceosomal Disruption of the Non-Canonical BAF Complex in Cancer. Nature. 2019 Oct;574(7778):432–6. PMID:31597964
1423. Inoue D, Yoshida K, Yoneda N, et al. IgG4-Related Disease: Dataset of 235 Consecutive Patients. Medicine (Baltimore). 2015 Apr;94(15):e680. PMID:25881845
1424. Inoue R, Saishin Y, Shima C, et al. A Case of Iris Melanocytoma Transformed to Malignant Melanoma. Jpn J Ophthalmol. 2009 May;53(3):271–3. PMID:19484449
1424A. International Association of Cancer Registries (IACR) [Internet]. Lyon (France): International Agency for Research on Cancer; 2021. International Classification of Diseases for Oncology (ICD-O) – ICD-O-3.2; Updated 2021 Jan 25. Available from: http://www.iacr.com.fr/index.php?option=com_content&view=-category&layout=blog&id=100&itemid=577.
1425. International CLL-IPI Working Group. An International Prognostic Index for Patients with Chronic Lymphocytic Leukaemia (CLL-IPI): A Meta-Analysis of Individual Patient Data. Lancet Oncol. 2016 Jun;17(6):779–90. PMID:27185642
1426. Ioannidis AS, Rai P, Mulholland B. Conjunctival Lymphoid Hyperplasia Presenting with Bilateral Panuveitis. Am J Ophthalmol. 2005 Mar;139(3):566–8. PMID:15767083
1427. Iordanous Y, Belrose JC, Cadieux DC, et al. P63 Positive Mucoepidermoid Tumor of the Lacrimal Sac with Associated Papilloma. Orbit. 2015;34(4):220–2. PMID:26121166
1428. Iovino C, Casini G, Peiretti E. Bilateral Noncalcified Astrocytic Hamartomas in Retinitis Pigmentosa: Multimodal Imaging Evaluation Over 8 Years of Follow-Up. Eur J Ophthalmol. 2019 Sep;29(5):nP18–21. PMID:30280590
1429. Iqbal J, Kucuk C, Deleeuw RJ, et al. Genomic Analyses Reveal Global Functional Alterations that Promote Tumor Growth and Novel Tumor Suppressor Genes in Natural Killer-Cell Malignancies. Leukemia. 2009 Jun;23(6):1139–51. PMID:19194464
1430. Isaacs H Jr. Fetal and Neonatal Histiocytoses. Pediatr Blood Cancer. 2006 Aug;47(2):123–9. PMID:16416419
1431. Isaacson PG, Du MQ. MALT Lymphoma: From Morphology to Molecules. Nat Rev Cancer. 2004 Aug;4(8):644–53. PMID:15286744
1432. Isager P, Østerlind A, Engholm G, et al. Uveal and Conjunctival Malignant Melanoma in Denmark, 1943-97: Incidence and Validation Study. Ophthalmic Epidemiol. 2005 Aug;12(4):223–32. PMID:16033743
1433. Ishida M, Iwai M, Yoshida K, et al. Primary Ductal Adenocarcinoma of the Lacrimal Sac: The First Reported Case. Int J Clin Exp Pathol. 2013 Aug 15;6(9):1929–34. PMID:24040460
1434. Ishida Y, Takahashi Y, Takahashi E, et al. Solitary Circumscribed Neuroma of the Palpebral Conjunctiva: A Rare Location. Cont Lens Anterior Eye. 2016 Dec;39(6):471–3. PMID:27522960
1435. Ishikawa MK, Arps DP, Chow C, et al. Histopathological Features of Molluscum Contagiosum Other Than Molluscum Bodies. Histopathology. 2015 Dec;67(6):836–42. PMID:25891863
1436. International Society for the Study of Vascular Anomalies [Internet]. Milwaukee (WI): International Society for the Study of Vascular Anomalies; 2018 [Cited 2022 Apr 18]. ISSVA Classification of Vascular Anomalies. Available from: https://www.issva.org/classification.
1437. Italiano A, Di Mauro I, Rapp J, et al. Clinical Effect of Molecular Methods in Sarcoma Diagnosis (GENSARC): A Prospective, Multicentre, Observational Study. Lancet Oncol. 2016 Apr;17(4):532–8. PMID:26970672
1438. Ito Y, Ishibashi K, Masaki A, et al. Mammary Analogue Secretory Carcinoma of Salivary Glands: A Clinicopathologic and Molecular Study Including 2 Cases Harboring ETV6-X Fusion. Am J Surg Pathol. 2015 May;39(5):602–10. PMID:25651470
1439. Iwata J, Fletcher CD. Lipidized Fibrous Histiocytoma: Clinicopathologic Analysis of 22 Cases. Am J Dermatopathol. 2000 Apr;22(2):126–34. PMID:10770432
1440. Iyengar P, Deangelis DD, Greenberg M, et al. Perivascular Epithelioid Cell Tumor of the Orbit: A Case Report and Review of the Literature. Pediatr Dev Pathol. 2005 Jan-Feb;8(1):98–104. PMID:15803216
1441. Jabarin B, Solomon A, Amer R. Interleukin-17 and its Correlation with Vascular Endothelial Growth Factor Expression in Ocular Surface Pathologies: A Histologic Study. Eur J Ophthalmol. 2016 Jun 10;26(4):283–6. PMID:26615952
1442. Jabbarpoor Bonyadi MH, Ownagh V, Rahimy E, et al. Giraffe or Leopard Spot Chorioretinopathy as an Outstanding Finding: Case Report and Literature Review. Int Ophthalmol. 2019 Jun;39(6):1405–12. PMID:29948498
1443. Jaber OI, Kirby PA. Alveolar Soft Part Sarcoma. Arch Pathol Lab Med. 2015 Nov;139(11):1459–62. PMID:26516944
1444. Jacobs JL, Merriam JC, Chadburn A, et al. Mesenchymal Chondrosarcoma of the Orbit. Report of Three New Cases and Review of the Literature. Cancer. 1994 Jan 15;73(2):399–405. PMID:8293407
1445. Jacobsen E, Shanmugam V, Jagannathan J. Rosai-Dorfman Disease with Activating KRAS Mutation - Response to Cobimetinib. N Engl J Med. 2017 Dec 14;377(24):2398–9. PMID:29236635
1446. Jacoby LB, MacCollin M, Barone R, et al. Frequency and Distribution of NF2 Mutations in Schwannomas. Genes Chromosomes Cancer. 1996 Sep;17(1):45–55. PMID:8889506
1447. Jadusingh IH. Fine Needle Aspiration Cytology of Fibrous Hamartoma of Infancy. Acta Cytol. 1997 Jul-Aug;41(4 Suppl):1391–3. PMID:9990282
1448. Jagan L, Zoroquiain P, Bravo-Filho V, et al. Sebaceous Adenomas of the Eyelid and Muir-Torre Syndrome. Br J Ophthalmol. 2015 Jul;99(7):909–13. PMID:25595178
1449. Jager MJ, Brouwer NJ, Esmaeli B. The Cancer Genome Atlas Project: An Integrated Molecular View of Uveal Melanoma. Ophthalmology. 2018 Aug;125(8):1139–42. PMID:30032793
1450. Jager MJ, Shields CL, Cebulla CM, et al. Uveal Melanoma. Nat Rev Dis Primers. 2020 Apr 9;6(1):24. PMID:32273508
1451. Jaggi GP, Mironov A, Huber AR, et al. Optic Nerve Compartment Syndrome in a Patient with Optic Nerve Sheath Meningioma. Eur J Ophthalmol. 2007 May-Jun;17(3):454–8. PMID:17534836
1452. Jain A, Goyal P, Nigam PK, et al. Xanthelasma Palpebrarum-Clinical and Biochemical Profile in a Tertiary Care Hospital of Delhi. Indian J Clin Biochem. 2007 Sep;22(2):151–3. PMID:23105704
1453. Jain D, Ebrahimi KB, Miller NR, et al. Intraorbital Meningiomas: A Pathologic Review Using Current World Health Organization Criteria. Arch Pathol Lab Med. 2010 May;134(5):766–70. PMID:20441509
1454. Jain P, Finger PT, Damato B, et al. Multicenter, International Assessment of the Eighth Edition of the American Joint Committee on Cancer Cancer Staging Manual for Conjunctival Melanoma. JAMA Ophthalmol. 2019 Aug 1;137(8):905–11. PMID:31169891
1455. Jain P, Surrey LF, Straka J, et al. BRAF Fusions in Pediatric Histiocytic Neoplasms Define Distinct Therapeutic Responsiveness to RAF Paradox Breakers. Pediatr Blood Cancer. 2021 Jun;68(6):e28933. PMID:33565241
1456. Jain SU, Khazaei S, Marchione DM, et al. Histone H3.3 G34 Mutations Promote Aberrant PRC2 Activity and Drive Tumor Progression. Proc Natl Acad Sci U S A. 2020 Nov 3;117(44):27354–64. PMID:33067396
1457. Jakobiec FA. Conjunctival Primary Acquired Melanosis: Is It Time for a New Terminology? Am J Ophthalmol. 2016 Feb;162:3–19.E1. PMID:26556007
1458. Jakobiec FA. Ocular Adnexal Lymphoid Tumors: Progress in Need of Clarification. Am J Ophthalmol. 2008 Jun;145(6):941–50. PMID:18405875
1459. Jakobiec FA, Barrantes PC, Ma L, et al. Epibulbar Proliferative Fasciitis, a Variant of Nodular Fasciitis: A Differential Diagnosis of Conditions With Focal or Diffuse Myxoid Stromas. Ophthalmic Plast Reconstr Surg. 2021 Sep-Oct 01;37(5):399–407. PMID:33481533
1460. Jakobiec FA, Bhat P, Colby KA. Immunohistochemical Studies of Conjunctival Nevi and Melanomas. Arch Ophthalmol. 2010 Feb;128(2):174–83. PMID:20142539
1461. Jakobiec FA, Bonanno PA, Sigelman J. Conjunctival Adnexal Cysts and Dermoids. Arch Ophthalmol. 1978 Aug;96(8):1404–9. PMID:678180
1462. Jakobiec FA, Brodie SE, Haik B, et al. Giant Cell Astrocytoma of the Retina. A Tumor of Possible Mueller Cell Origin. Ophthalmology. 1983 Dec;90(12):1565–76. PMID:6677857
1463. Jakobiec FA, Colby K, Bajart AM, et al. Immunohistochemical Studies of Atypical Conjunctival Melanocytic Nevi. Arch Ophthalmol. 2009 Aug;127(8):970–80. PMID:19667333
1464. Jakobiec FA, Cortes Barrantes P, Aronow ME. Relationship Between Conjunctival Intraepithelial Dendritic Melanocytes and Nevocytes. Ocul Oncol Pathol. 2020 Aug;6(4):251–8. PMID:33005614
1465. Jakobiec FA, Folberg R, Iwamoto T. Clinicopathologic Characteristics of Premalignant and Malignant Melanocytic Lesions of the Conjunctiva. Ophthalmology. 1989 Feb;96(2):147–66. PMID:2649838
1466. Jakobiec FA, Font RL, Tso MO, et al. Mesectodermal Leiomyoma of the Ciliary Body: A Tumor of Presumed Neural Crest Origin. Cancer. 1977 May;39(5):2102–13. PMID:870167
1467. Jakobiec FA, Hanbazazh M, Cortes Barrantes P, et al. Adult Primary Capillary Hemangioma of the Sclera: A Previously Undescribed Entity With a Review of Epibulbar Vascular Lesions. Ophthalmic Plast Reconstr Surg. 2020 Jul/Aug;36(4):327–33. PMID:31895731
1468. Jakobiec FA, Howard GM, Rosen M, et al. Leiomyoma and Leiomyosarcoma of the Orbit. Am J Ophthalmol. 1975 Dec;80(6):1028–42. PMID:1200096
1469. Jakobiec FA, Jones IS, Tannenbaum M. Leiomyoma. An Unusual Tumour of the Orbit. Br J Ophthalmol. 1973 Nov;57(11):825–31. PMID:4361898
1470. Jakobiec FA, Kool M, Stagner AM, et al. Intraocular Medulloepitheliomas and Embryonal Tumors With Multilayered Rosettes of the Brain: Comparative Roles of LIN28A and C19MC. Am J Ophthalmol. 2015 Jun;159(6):1065–1074.E1. PMID:25748578
1471. Jakobiec FA, Mehta M, Iwamoto M, et al. Intratarsal Keratinous Cysts of the Meibomian Gland: Distinctive Clinicopathologic and Immunohistochemical Features in 6 Cases. Am J Ophthalmol. 2010 Jan;149(1):82–94. PMID:19875094
1472. Jakobiec FA, Mendoza PR, Colby KA. Clinicopathologic and Immunohistochemical Studies of Conjunctival Large Cell Acanthoma, Epidermoid Dysplasia, and Squamous Papilloma. Am J Ophthalmol. 2013 Oct;156(4):830–46. PMID:23786782
1473. Jakobiec FA, Nguyen J, Bhat P, et al. MDM2-Positive Atypical Lipomatous Neoplasm/Well-Differentiated Liposarcoma Versus Spindle Cell Lipoma of the Orbit. Ophthalmic Plast Reconstr Surg. 2010 Nov-Dec;26(6):413–5. PMID:20639786
1474. Jakobiec FA, Rai R, Yoon MK. Fibrous Histiocytoma of the Tarsus: Clinical and Immunohistochemical Observations with a Differential Diagnosis. Cornea. 2014 May;33(5):536–9. PMID:24608257
1475. Jakobiec FA, Rashid A, Lewis K. Massive Retinal Gliosis in Neurofibromatosis Type 1. JAMA Ophthalmol. 2015 Jan;133(1):100–2. PMID:25317586
1476. Jakobiec FA, Rose MF, Trief D, et al. Immunohistochemical Investigations of Adult Intraocular Medulloepitheliomas. Clin Exp Ophthalmol. 2015 May-Jun;43(4):379–85. PMID:25251824
1477. Jakobiec FA, Sacks E, Lisman RL, et al. Epibulbar Fibroma of the Conjunctival Substantia Propria. Arch Ophthalmol. 1988 May;106(5):661–4. PMID:3358733
1478. Jakobiec FA, Silbert G. Are Most Iris "Melanomas" Really Nevi? A Clinicopathologic Study of 189 Lesions. Arch Ophthalmol. 1981 Dec;99(12):2117–32. PMID:7305709
1479. Jakobiec FA, Stacy RC, Thakker MM. Blue Nevus of the Tarsus as the Predominant Component of a Combined Nevus of the Eyelid. Ophthalmic Plast Reconstr Surg. 2011 Jul-Aug;27(4):e94–6. PMID:20940655
1480. Jakobiec FA, Stagner AM, Colby KA. Pigmented Caruncular Apocrine Hidrocystoma With Oncocytic Features. Ophthalmic Plast Reconstr Surg. 2017 May/Jun;33(3S Suppl 1):S42–5. PMID:25794031
1481. Jakobiec FA, Stagner AM, Eagle RC Jr, et al. Unusual Pleomorphic Adenoma of the Lacrimal Gland: Immunohistochemical Demonstration of PLAG1 and HMGA2 Oncoproteins. Surv Ophthalmol. 2017 Mar-Apr;62(2):219–26. PMID:27567603
1482. Jakobiec FA, Stagner AM, Katowitz WR, et al. A Microanatomic Abnormality of the Lacrimal Gland Associated with Goldenhar Syndrome. Surv Ophthalmol. 2016 Sep-Oct;61(5):654–63. PMID:26892494
1483. Jakobiec FA, Stagner AM, Rubin PAD. Lymphoepithelial Carcinoma of the Nasolacrimal Duct: Clinical, Radiologic, and Immunopathologic Features. Ophthalmic Plast Reconstr Surg. 2017 May/Jun;33(3S Suppl 1):S18–21. PMID:25902392
1484. Jakobiec FA, Thanos A, Stagner AM, et al. So-Called Massive Retinal Gliosis: A Critical Review and Reappraisal. Surv Ophthalmol. 2016 May-Jun;61(3):339–56. PMID:26703887
1485. Jakobiec FA, Trief D, Rashid A, et al. New Insights into the Development of Infantile

Intraocular Medulloepithelioma. Am J Ophthalmol. 2014 Dec;158(6):1275–1296.E1. PMID:25174896

1486. Jakobiec FA, Werdich XQ, Chodosh J, et al. An Analysis of Conjunctival and Periocular Venous Malformations: Clinicopathologic and Immunohistochemical Features with a Comparison of Racemose and Cirsoid Lesions. Surv Ophthalmol. 2014 Mar-Apr;59(2):236–44. PMID:24355066

1487. Jakobiec FA, Zakka FR. A Reappraisal of Eyelic Eccrine and Apocrine Hidrocystomas: Microanatomic and Immunohistochemical Studies of 40 Lesions. Am J Ophthalmol. 2011 Feb;151(2):358–74.E2. PMID:21168812

1488. Jakobiec FA, Zakka FR, Hatton MP. Eyelid Basal Cell Carcinoma Developing in an Epidermoid Cyst: A Previously Unreported Event. Ophthalmic Plast Reconstr Surg. 2010 Nov-Dec;26(6):491–4. PMID:20736874

1489. Jakobiec FA, Zakka FR, Perry LP. The Cytologic Composition of Dacryops: An Immunohistochemical Investigation of 15 Lesions Compared to the Normal Lacrimal Gland. Am J Ophthalmol. 2013 Feb;155(2):380–396.E1. PMID:23114708

1490. Jakobiec FA, Zimmerman LE, Spencer WH, et al. Metastatic Colloid Carcinoma Versus Primary Carcinoma of the Ciliary Epithelium. Ophthalmology. 1987 Nov;94(11):1469–80. PMID:2825094

1491. Jakobiec FA, Zuckerman BD, Berlin AJ, et al. Unusual Melanocytic Nevi of the Conjunctiva. Am J Ophthalmol. 1985 Jul 15;100(1):100–13. PMID:4014368

1492. James CR, Lyness R, Wright JE. Respiratory Epithelium Lined Cysts Presenting in the Orbit Without Associated Mucocele Formation. Br J Ophthalmol. 1986 May;70(5):387–90. PMID:3964639

1493. Jamshidi F, Bashashati A, Shumansky K, et al. The Genomic Landscape of Epithelioid Sarcoma Cell Lines and Tumours. J Pathol. 2016 Jan;238(1):63–73. PMID:26365879

1494. Jamshidian-Tehrani M, Eshraghi B, Zarei M, et al. Successful Total Resection of an Orbital Epithelioid Hemangioendothelioma with the Aid of Endovascular Embolization. Ocul Oncol Pathol. 2019 Jan;5(1):50–3. PMID:30675477

1495. Janakiram TN, Sagar S, Sharma SB, et al. Primary Mucoepidermoid Carcinoma of the Lacrimal Sac -a Case Report and Literature Review. Klin Onkol. 2016;29(4):291–4. PMID:27534787

1496. Janatpour KA, Choo PH, Lloyd WC 3rd. Primary Orbital Peripheral T-Cell Lymphoma: Histologic, Immunophenotypic, and Genotypic Features. Arch Ophthalmol. 2007 Sep;125(9):1289–92. PMID:17846377

1497. Jang J, Kie JH, Lee SY, et al. Acinic Cell Carcinoma of the Lacrimal Gland with Intracranial Extension: A Case Report. Ophthalmic Plast Reconstr Surg. 2001 Nov;17(6):454–7. PMID:11766029

1498. Jang JH, Chang SD, Choe MS. A Case of Recurrent Schneiderian Papilloma of the Lacrimal Sac Invading the Nasal Cavity. Korean J Ophthalmol. 2009 Jun;23(2):100–3. PMID:19568358

1499. Jansen JC, Van Calster J, Pulido JS, et al. Early Diagnosis and Successful Treatment of Paraneoplastic Melanocytic Proliferation. Br J Ophthalmol. 2015 Jul;99(7):943–8. PMID:25908835

1500. Jansen RW, de Bloeme CM, Brisse HJ, et al. MR Imaging Features to Differentiate Retinoblastoma from Coats' Disease and Persistent Fetal Vasculature. Cancers (Basel). 2020 Nov 30;12(12):3592. PMID:33266342

1501. Janssen D, Harms D. Juvenile Xanthogranuloma in Childhood and Adolescence: A Clinicopathologic Study of 129 Patients from the Kiel Pediatric Tumor Registry. Am J Surg Pathol. 2005 Jan;29(1):21–8. PMID:15613853

1501A. Janzarik WG, Kratz CP, Loges NT, et al. Further Evidence for a Somatic KRAS Mutation in a Pilocytic Astrocytoma. Neuropediatrics. 2007 Apr;38(2):61–3. PMID:17712732

1502. Jastrzebski A, Brownstein S, Jordan DR, et al. Histochemical Analysis and Immunohistochemical Profile of Mucoepidermoid Carcinoma of the Conjunctiva. Saudi J Ophthalmol. 2012 Apr;26(2):205–10. PMID:23960993

1503. Jastrzebski A, Brownstein S, Manusow J, et al. Isolated Conjunctival Lymphangioma. Can J Ophthalmol. 2011 Aug;46(4):369–70. PMID:21816261

1504. Jauregui HO, Klintworth GK. Pigmented Squamous Cell Carcinoma of Cornea and Conjunctiva: A Light Microscopic, Histochemical, and Ultrastructural Study. Cancer. 1976 Aug;38(2):778–88. PMID:974995

1505. Jawad MU, Extein J, Min ES, et al. Prognostic Factors for Survival in Patients with Epithelioid Sarcoma: 441 Cases from the SEER Database. Clin Orthop Relat Res. 2009 Nov;467(11):2939–48. PMID:19224301

1506. Jaworski A, Wolffsohn JS, Napper GA. Detection, Aetiology and Management of Conjunctival Intraepithelial Neoplasia. Ophthalmic Physiol Opt. 2000 Sep;20(5):371–80. PMID:11045245

1507. Jayaprakasam A, O'Donovan D, Rene C. Infraorbital Nerve Enlargement Due to IgG4-Related Disease. Eye (Lond). 2014 May;28(5):628–9. PMID:24577252

1508. Jayaraman SS, Rayhan DJ, Hazany S, et al. Mutational Landscape of Basal Cell Carcinomas by Whole-Exome Sequencing. J Invest Dermatol. 2014 Jan;134(1):213–20. PMID:23774526

1509. Jebastin Thangaiah J, Hanley K, Noman L, et al. Cytologic Features and Immunohistochemical Findings of Epithelioid Hemangioendothelioma (EHE) in Effusion: A Case Series. Diagn Cytopathol. 2021 Jan;49(1):e24–30. PMID:32797671

1510. Jedrych JJ, Duraisamy S, Karunamurthy A. Aneurysmal Fibrous Histiocytomas with Recurrent Rearrangement of the PRKCD Gene and LAMTOR1-PRKCD Fusions. J Cutan Pathol. 2018 Dec;45(12):966–8. PMID:30094855

1511. Jensen DE, Proctor M, Marquis ST, et al. BAP1: A Novel Ubiquitin Hydrolase Which Binds to the BRCA1 RING Finger and Enhances BRCA1-Mediated Cell Growth Suppression. Oncogene. 1998 Mar 5;16(9):1097–112. PMID:9528852

1512. Jensen OA. Glomus Tumor (Glomangioma) of Eyelid. Arch Ophthalmol. 1965 Apr;73:511–3. PMID:14270138

1513. Jensen OA. Metastatic Tumours of the Eye and Orbit. A Histopathological Analysis of a Danish Series. Acta Pathol Microbiol Scand Suppl. 1970;212(Suppl 212:201+). PMID:5267091

1514. Jeon S, Paik JS, Yang SW. A Case of Microcystic Adnexal Carcinoma. Jpn J Ophthalmol. 2010 Jan;54(1):104–5. PMID:20151289

1515. Jeon YK, Cheon JE, Kim SK, et al. Clinicopathological Features and Global Genomic Copy Number Alterations of Pilomyxoid Astrocytoma in the Hypothalamus/Optic Pathway: Comparative Analysis with Pilocytic Astrocytoma Using Array-Based Comparative Genomic Hybridization. Mod Pathol. 2008 Nov;21(11):1345–56. PMID:18622384

1516. Jepson CN, Wetzig PC. Pure Chondroma of the Trochlea. A Case Report. Surv Ophthalmol. 1966 Dec;11(6):656–9. PMID:5981161

1517. Jessup CJ, Redston M, Tilton E, et al. Importance of Universal Mismatch Repair Protein Immunohistochemistry in Patients with Sebaceous Neoplasia as an Initial Screening Tool for Muir-Torre Syndrome. Hum Pathol. 2016 Mar;49:1–9. PMID:26826402

1518. Jett K, Friedman JM. Clinical and Genetic Aspects of Neurofibromatosis 1. Genet Med. 2010 Jan;12(1):1–11. PMID:20027112

1519. Jia S, Zhu T, Shi H, et al. American Joint Committee on Cancer Tumor Staging System Predicts the Outcome and Metastasis Pattern in Conjunctival Melanoma. Ophthalmology. 2022 Jul;129(7):771–80. PMID:35245602

1520. Jiang L, Gu ZH, Yan ZX, et al. Exome Sequencing Identifies Somatic Mutations of DDX3X in Natural Killer/T-Cell Lymphoma. Nat Genet. 2015 Sep;47(9):1061–6. PMID:26192917

1521. Jiménez I, Laé M, Tanguy ML, et al. Craniofacial Second Primary Tumors in Patients with Germline Retinoblastoma Previously Treated with External Beam Radiotherapy: A Retrospective Institutional Analysis. Pediatr Blood Cancer. 2020 Apr;67(4):e28158. PMID:31904159

1522. Jing H, Weiwen C, Meihong C, et al. Glomus Tumour of the Iris: A Case Report. Eur J Ophthalmol. 2022 Jan;32(1):NP203–7. PMID:32962404

1523. Jo VY, Fletcher CD. Epithelioid Malignant Peripheral Nerve Sheath Tumor: Clinicopathologic Analysis of 63 Cases. Am J Surg Pathol. 2015 May;39(5):673–82. PMID:25602794

1524. Joag MG, Gupta A, Galor A, et al. Conjunctival Intraepithelial Neoplasia with Mucoepidermoid Differentiation: A Case Report of a Subtle Lesion. Ocul Oncol Pathol. 2015 Jun;1(4):278–82. PMID:27171853

1525. Johansson P, Aoude LG, Wadt K, et al. Deep Sequencing of Uveal Melanoma Identifies a Recurrent Mutation in PLCB4. Oncotarget. 2016 Jan 26;7(4):4624–31. PMID:26683228

1526. Johansson PA, Brooks K, Newell F, et al. Whole Genome Landscapes of Uveal Melanoma Show an Ultraviolet Radiation Signature in Iris Tumours. Nat Commun. 2020 May 15;11(1):2408. PMID:32415113

1527. John AM, Schwartz RA. Muir-Torre Syndrome (MTS): An Update and Approach to Diagnosis and Management. J Am Acad Dermatol. 2016 Mar;74(3):558–66. PMID:26892655

1528. Johnson MW, Eberhart CG, Perry A, et al. Spectrum of Pilomyxoid Astrocytomas: Intermediate Pilomyxoid Tumors. Am J Surg Pathol. 2010 Dec;34(12):1783–91. PMID:21107083

1529. Johnson NA, Slack GW, Savage KJ, et al. Concurrent Expression of MYC and BCL2 in Diffuse Large B-Cell Lymphoma Treated with Rituximab Plus Cyclophosphamide, Doxorubicin, Vincristine, and Prednisone. J Clin Oncol. 2012 Oct 1;30(28):3452–9. PMID:22851565

1530. Johnson TE, Alabiad C, Wei L, et al. Extensive Juvenile Xanthogranuloma Involving the Orbit, Sinuses, Brain, and Subtemporal Fossa in a Newborn. Ophthalmic Plast Reconstr Surg. 2010 Mar-Apr;26(2):133–4. PMID:20305521

1531. Jokinen CH, Ragsdale BD, Argenyi ZB. Expanding the Clinicopathologic Spectrum of Palisaded Encapsulated Neuroma. J Cutan Pathol. 2010 Jan;37(1):43–8. PMID:19614730

1532. Jolly SS, Brownstein S, Jordan DR. Leiomyoma of the Anterior Orbit and Eyelid. Can J Ophthalmol. 1995 Dec;30(7):366–70. PMID:8963938

1533. Jolson AS, Jolson SC. Suture Barb Giant Papillary Conjunctivitis. Ophthalmic Surg. 1984 Feb;15(2):139–40. PMID:6709289

1534. Jonas RA, Ung L, Rajaiya J, et al. Mystery Eye: Human Adenovirus and the Enigma of Epidemic Keratoconjunctivitis. Prog Retin Eye Res. 2020 May;76:100826. PMID:31891773

1535. Jones AC, Prihoda TJ, Kacher JE, et al. Osteoblastoma of the Maxilla and Mandible: A Report of 24 Cases, Review of the Literature, and Discussion of its Relationship to Osteoid Osteoma of the Jaws. Oral Surg Oral Med Oral Pathol Oral Radiol Endod. 2006 Nov;102(5):639–50. PMID:17052641

1536. Jones D, Woyach JA, Zhao W, et al. PLCG2 C2 Domain Mutations Co-Occur with BTK and PLCG2 Resistance Mutations in Chronic Lymphocytic Leukemia Undergoing Ibrutinib Treatment. Leukemia. 2017 Jul;31(7):1645–7. PMID:28366935

1537. Jones DT, Hutter B, Jäger N, et al. Recurrent Somatic Alterations of FGFR1 and NTRK2 in Pilocytic Astrocytoma. Nat Genet. 2013 Aug;45(8):927–32. PMID:23817572

1537A. Jones DT, Kocialkowski S, Liu L, et al. Oncogenic RAF1 Rearrangement and a Novel BRAF Mutation as Alternatives to KIAA1549:BRAF Fusion in Activating the MAPK Pathway in Pilocytic Astrocytoma. Oncogene. 2009 May;28(20):2119–23. PMID:19363522

1538. Jones DT, Kocialkowski S, Liu L, et al. Tandem Duplication Producing a Novel Oncogenic BRAF Fusion Gene Defines the Majority of Pilocytic Astrocytomas. Cancer Res. 2008 Nov 1;68(21):8673–7. PMID:18974108

1539. Jones KB, Barrott JJ, Xie M, et al. The Impact of Chromosomal Translocation Locus and Fusion Oncogene Coding Sequence in Synovial Sarcomagenesis. Oncogene. 2016 Sep 22;35(38):5021–32. PMID:26947017

1540. Jones N, Gibb A, Irion L, et al. Gamma-Delta T-Cell Lymphoma of Skin, Eye and Brain Presenting with Visual Loss. BMJ Case Rep. 2017 Jun;2017

1541. Jong R, Kandel R, Fornasier V, et al. Alveolar Soft Part Sarcoma: Review of Nine Cases Including Two Cases with Unusual Histology. Histopathology. 1998 Jan;32(1):63–8. PMID:9522219

1542. Jordan M, Carmignac V, Sorlin A, et al. Reverse Phenotyping in Patients with Skin Capillary Malformations and Mosaic GNAQ or GNA11 Mutations Defines a Clinical Spectrum with Genotype-Phenotype Correlation. J Invest Dermatol. 2020 May;140(5):1106–1110.E2. PMID:31726051

1543. Jordanova ES, Riemersma SA, Philippo K, et al. Beta2-Microglobulin Aberrations in Diffuse Large B-Cell Lymphoma of the Testis and the Central Nervous System. Int J Cancer. 2003 Jan 20;103(3):393–8. PMID:12471623

1544. Jordanova ES, Riemersma SA, Philippo K, et al. Hemizygous Deletions in the HLA Region Account for Loss of Heterozygosity in the Majority of Diffuse Large B-Cell Lymphomas of the Testis and the Central Nervous System. Genes Chromosomes Cancer. 2002 Sep;35(1):38–48. PMID:12203788

1544A. Jørgensen M, Heegaard S. A Review of Nasal, Paranasal, and Skull Base Tumors Invading the Orbit. Surv Ophthalmol. 2018 May-Jun;63(3):389–405. PMID:28739401

1545. Jouary T, Kubica E, Dalle S, et al. Sentinel Node Status and Immunosuppression: Recurrence Factors in Localized Merkel Cell Carcinoma. Acta Derm Venereol. 2015 Sep;95(7):835–40. PMID:25784178

1546. Jouenne F, Chevret S, Bugnet E, et al. Genetic Landscape of Adult Langerhans Cell Histiocytosis with Lung Involvement. Eur Respir J. 2020 Feb 27;55(2):1901190. PMID:31806714

1547. Jouhi S, Al-Jamal RT, Täll M, et al. Presumed Incipient Choroidal Melanoma: Proposed Diagnostic Criteria and Management. Br J Ophthalmol. 2023 Mar;107(3):412–7. PMID:34666992

1548. Julian CG, Bowers PW. A Clinical Review of 209 Pilomatricomas. J Am Acad Dermatol. 1998 Aug;39(2 Pt 1):191–5. PMID:9704827

1549. Jünemann A, Holbach LM. [Epithelial Giant Inclusion Cyst 50 Years After Enucleation

Without Orbital Implant]. Klin Monbl Augenheilkd. 1998 Feb;212(2):127–8. German. PMID:9577816
1550. Jung A, Bechthold S, Pfluger T, et al. Orbital Rhabdomyosarcoma in Noonan Syndrome. J Pediatr Hematol Oncol. 2003 Apr;25(4):330–2. PMID:12679651
1551. Jung CS, Hubbard GB 3rd, Grossniklaus HE. Giant Cell Astrocytoma of the Retina in a 1-Month-Old Infant. J Pediatr Ophthalmol Strabismus. 2009 Nov 2. PMID:19873950
1552. Jung EH, Avila SA, Gordon AA, et al. Phakomatous Choristomas: A Case Report and Review of Literature. Ophthalmic Plast Reconstr Surg. 2022 Jul-Aug 01;38(4):330–5. PMID:34750316
1553. Jung JH, Shin DH, Cho KS, et al. Nasolacrimal Duct Obstruction Caused by Oncocytic Carcinoma. Korean J Ophthalmol. 2013 Apr;27(2):126–9. PMID:23543280
1554. Jung JY, Kim JH, Kim ST, et al. MR Features of Intraocular Ectopic Lacrimal Tissue. AJNR Am J Neuroradiol. 2006 Nov-Dec;27(10):2196–8. PMID:17110692
1555. Jung SK, Lim J, Yang SW, et al. Nationwide Trends in the Incidence of Orbital Lymphoma from 1999 to 2016 in South Korea. Br J Ophthalmol. 2021 Oct;105(10):1341–5. PMID:32863278
1556. Jung SK, Paik JS, Park GS, et al. Refractory Follicular Conjunctival Lesions: Overlook as Just Inflammation or Not? Br J Ophthalmol. 2019 Nov;103(11):1660–5. PMID:30709807
1557. Jung SM, Lin HC, Chu PH, et al. Expression of Cell Cycle-Regulatory Proteins, MIB-1, P16, P53, and P63, in Squamous Cell Carcinoma of Conjunctiva: Not Associated with Human Papillomavirus Infection. Virchows Arch. 2006 Mar;448(3):301–5. PMID:16328355
1558. Jurczyk M, Peevey JF, Vande Haar MA, et al. Pitfalls of Fine-Needle Aspiration Cytology of Parotid Membranous Basal Cell Adenoma-A Review of Pitfalls in FNA Cytology of Salivary Gland Neoplasms with Basaloid Cell Features. Diagn Cytopathol. 2015 May;43(5):432–7. PMID:25431027
1559. Kabra RS, Patel SB, Shanbhag SS. Orbital Chondroma: A Rare Mesenchymal Tumor of Orbit. Indian J Ophthalmol. 2015 Jun;63(6):551–4. PMID:26265654
1560. Kadaba P, Arepalli S, Shields JA, et al. Combined Hamartoma of the Retina and Retinal Pigment Epithelium in Branchio-Otic Syndrome. J AAPOS. 2014 Apr;18(2):201–3. PMID:24698626
1561. Kadariya Y, Cheung M, Xu J, et al. Bap1 Is a Bona Fide Tumor Suppressor: Genetic Evidence from Mouse Models Carrying Heterozygous Germline Bap1 Mutations. Cancer Res. 2016 May 1;76(9):2836–44. PMID:26896281
1562. Kadin ME, Hamilton RG, Vonderheid EC. Evidence Linking Atopy and Staphylococcal Superantigens to the Pathogenesis of Lymphomatoid Papulosis, a Recurrent CD30+ Cutaneous Lymphoproliferative Disorder. PLoS One. 2020 Feb 12;15(2):e0228751. PMID:32049976
1563. Kadin ME, Vonderheid EC, Weiss LM. Absence of Epstein-Barr Viral RNA in Lymphomatoid Papulosis. J Pathol. 1993 Jun;170(2):145–8. PMID:8393923
1564. Kadoch C, Crabtree GR. Reversible Disruption of MSWI/SNF (BAF) Complexes by the SS18-SSX Oncogenic Fusion in Synovial Sarcoma. Cell. 2013 Mar 28;153(1):71–85. PMID:23540691
1565. Kager L, Zoubek A, Pötschger U, et al. Primary Metastatic Osteosarcoma: Presentation and Outcome of Patients Treated on Neoadjuvant Cooperative Osteosarcoma Study Group Protocols. J Clin Oncol. 2003 May 15;21(10):2011–8. PMID:12743156
1566. Kai K, Minesaki A, Suzuki K, et al. Difficulty in the Cytodiagnosis of Mammary Analogue Secretory Carcinoma: Survey of 109 Cytologists with a Case Originating from a Minor Salivary Gland. Acta Cytol. 2017;61(6):469–76. PMID:28738326
1567. Kajino Y, Yamaguchi A, Hashimoto N, et al. Beta-Catenin Gene Mutation in Human Hair Follicle-Related Tumors. Pathol Int. 2001 Jul;51(7):543–8. PMID:11472567
1568. Kalapesi FB, Garrott HM, Moldovan C, et al. IgG4 Orbital Inflammation in a 5-Year-Old Child Presenting as an Orbital Mass. Orbit. 2013 Apr;32(2):137–40. PMID:23480695
1569. Kale SM, Patil SB, Khare N, et al. Clinicopathological Analysis of Eyelid Malignancies - A Review of 85 Cases. Indian J Plast Surg. 2012 Jan;45(1):22–8. PMID:22754148
1570. Kaliki S, Arepalli S, Shields CL, et al. Conjunctival Papilloma: Features and Outcomes Based on Age at Initial Examination. JAMA Ophthalmol. 2013 May;131(5):585–93. PMID:23538642
1571. Kaliki S, Bothra N, Bejjanki KM, et al. Malignant Eyelid Tumors in India: A Study of 536 Asian Indian Patients. Ocul Oncol Pathol. 2019 Apr;5(3):210–9. PMID:31049330
1572. Kaliki S, Eagle RC, Grossniklaus HE, et al. Inadvertent Implantation of Aqueous Tube Shunts in Glaucomatous Eyes with Unrecognized Intraocular Neoplasms: Report of 5 Cases. JAMA Ophthalmol. 2013 Jul;131(7):925–8. PMID:23699787
1573. Kaliki S, Ji X, Zou Y, et al. Lag Time Between Onset of First Symptom and Treatment of Retinoblastoma: An International Collaborative Study of 692 Patients from 10 Countries. Cancers (Basel). 2021 Apr 19;13(8):1956. PMID:33921566
1574. Kaliki S, Maniar A, Patel A, et al. Clinical Presentation and Outcome of Retinoblastoma Based on Age at Presentation: A Review of 1450 Children. Int Ophthalmol. 2020 Jan;40(1):99–107. PMID:31444587
1575. Kaliki S, Palkonda VAR. Second Primary Tumors in Retinoblastoma Survivors: A Study of 7 Asian Indian Patients. Int Ophthalmol. 2020 Dec;40(12):3303–8. PMID:32737729
1576. Kaliki S, Rathi SG, Palkonda VAR. Primary Orbital Ewing Sarcoma Family of Tumors: A Study of 12 Cases. Eye (Lond). 2018 Mar;32(3):615–21. PMID:29219959
1577. Kaliki S, Shields CL, Eagle RC Jr, et al. Ciliary Body Medulloepithelioma: Analysis of 41 Cases. Ophthalmology. 2013 Dec;120(12):2552–9. PMID:23796765
1578. Kaliki S, Shields CL, Shah SU, et al. Postenucleation Adjuvant Chemotherapy with Vincristine, Etoposide, and Carboplatin for the Treatment of High-Risk Retinoblastoma. Arch Ophthalmol. 2011 Nov;129(11):1422–7. PMID:22084213
1579. Kaliki S, Shields CL, Shields JA. Uveal Melanoma: Estimating Prognosis. Indian J Ophthalmol. 2015 Feb;63(2):93–102. PMID:25827538
1580. Kaliki S, Vempuluru VS, Ghose N, et al. Ocular Surface Squamous Neoplasia in India: A Study of 438 Patients. Int Ophthalmol. 2022 Jun;42(6):1915–26. PMID:35094225
1581. Kaliki S, Vempuluru VS, Priya Y, et al. Risk Factors for Recurrent Retinoblastoma After Intravenous Chemotherapy. Int Ophthalmol. 2021 Jun;41(6):2033–9. PMID:33611762
1582. Kalina PH, Bartley GB, Campbell RJ, et al. Isolated Neurofibromas of the Conjunctiva. Am J Ophthalmol. 1991 Jun 15;111(6):694–8. PMID:2039037
1583. Kalirai H, Dodson A, Faqir S, et al. Lack of BAP1 Protein Expression in Uveal Melanoma is Associated with Increased Metastatic Risk and Has Utility in Routine Prognostic Testing. Br J Cancer. 2014 Sep 23;111(7):1373–80. PMID:25058347
1584. Kalisa P, Van Zieleghem B, Roux P, et al. Orbital Lymphangioma: Clinical Features and Management. Bull Soc Belge Ophtalmol. 2001;(282):59–68. PMID:12455141
1585. Kam AW, Galvin J, Cherepanoff S, et al. Primary Choroidal Lymphoma Diagnosed with 27-Gauge Pars Plana Vitrectomy Choroidal Biopsy. Case Rep Ophthalmol. 2019 Jul 23;10(2):213–20. PMID:31692619
1586. Kamal S, Kaliki S, Sreedhar A, et al. Primary Orbital Yolk Sac Tumor: Report of a Case and Review of Literature. Int Ophthalmol. 2016 Jun;36(3):435–44. PMID:26481249
1587. Kamalpour L, Brindise RT, Nodzenski M, et al. Primary Cutaneous Mucinous Carcinoma: A Systematic Review and Meta-Analysis of Outcomes After Surgery. JAMA Dermatol. 2014 Apr;150(4):380–4. PMID:24452370
1588. Kamekura R, Takahashi H, Ichimiya S. New Insights into IgG4-Related Disease: Emerging New CD4+ T-Cell Subsets. Curr Opin Rheumatol. 2019 Jan;31(1):9–15. PMID:30422824
1589. Kamisawa T, Nakazawa T, Tazuma S, et al. Clinical Practice Guidelines for IgG4-Related Sclerosing Cholangitis. J Hepatobiliary Pancreat Sci. 2019 Jan;26(1):9–42. PMID:30575336
1590. Kamoshima Y, Sawamura Y, Imai T, et al. Giant Cell Tumor of the Frontal Bone in a Girl: Case Report. Neurol Med Chir (Tokyo). 2011;51(11):798–800. PMID:22123486
1591. Kanakis M, Petrou P, Lourida G, et al. Erdheim-Chester Disease: A Comprehensive Review from the Ophthalmologic Perspective. Surv Ophthalmol. 2022 Mar-Apr;67(2):388–410. PMID:34081930
1592. Kanemitsu N, Isobe Y, Masuda A, et al. Expression of Epstein-Barr Virus-Encoded Proteins in Extranodal NK/T-Cell Lymphoma, Nasal Type (ENKL): Differences in Biologic and Clinical Behaviors of LMP1-Positive and -Negative ENKL. Clin Cancer Res. 2012 Apr 15;18(8):2164–72. PMID:22371452
1593. Kang JY, Kim HJ, Wojno TH, et al. Atypical Lipomatous Tumor/Well-Differentiated Liposarcoma of the Orbit: Three Cases and Review of the Literature. Ophthalmic Plast Reconstr Surg. 2021 May-Jun 01;37 3S:S134–40. PMID:32991496
1594. Kang Y, Pekmezci M, Folpe AL, et al. Diagnostic Utility of SOX10 to Distinguish Malignant Peripheral Nerve Sheath Tumor from Synovial Sarcoma, Including Intraneural Synovial Sarcoma. Mod Pathol. 2014 Jan;27(1):55–61. PMID:23929265
1595. Kantelip B, Nores JM, Boccard R, et al. [A Case of Fibrous Histiocytoma of the Conjunctiva]. Presse Med. 1988 May 7;17(17):859–61. French. PMID:2838836
1596. Kanthan GL, Jayamohan J, Yip D, et al. Management of Metastatic Carcinoma of the Uveal Tract: An Evidence-Based Analysis. Clin Exp Ophthalmol. 2007 Aug;35(6):553–65. PMID:17760639
1597. Kao AA, Galor A, Karp CL, et al. Clinicopathologic Correlation of Ocular Surface Squamous Neoplasms at Bascom Palmer Eye Institute: 2001 to 2010. Ophthalmology. 2012 Sep;119(9):1773–6. PMID:22771047
1598. Kao SC, Yeh LK, Tsai CC, et al. Ectopic Lacrimal Gland Cyst of the Orbit. Zhonghua Yi Xue Za Zhi (Taipei). 2000 Apr;63(4):334–8. PMID:10820914
1599. Karai LJ, Kadin ME, Hsi ED, et al. Chromosomal Rearrangements of 6p25.3 Define a New Subtype of Lymphomatoid Papulosis. Am J Surg Pathol. 2013 Aug;37(8):1173–81. PMID:23648461
1600. Karamchandani JR, Nielsen TO, van de Rijn M, et al. Sox10 and S100 in the Diagnosis of Soft-Tissue Neoplasms. Appl Immunohistochem Mol Morphol. 2012 Oct;20(5):445–50. PMID:22495377
1601. Karamzadeh Dashti N, Bahrami A, Lee SJ, et al. BRAF V600E Mutations Occur in a Subset of Glomus Tumors, and Are Associated With Malignant Histologic Characteristics. Am J Surg Pathol. 2017 Nov;41(11):1532–41. PMID:28834810
1602. Karanian M, Kelsey A, Paindavoine S, et al. SRF Fusions Other Than With RELA Expand the Molecular Definition of SRF-fused Perivascular Tumors. Am J Surg Pathol. 2020 Dec;44(12):1725–35. PMID:33021523
1603. Karanian M, Pérot G, Coindre JM, et al. Fluorescence In Situ Hybridization Analysis is a Helpful Test for the Diagnosis of Dermatofibrosarcoma Protuberans. Mod Pathol. 2015 Feb;28(2):230–7. PMID:25081750
1604. Karcioglu ZA, Fleming JC, Haik BG. A Prospective Comparison of Fine-Needle Aspiration Cytopathology and Histopathology in the Diagnosis of Orbital Mass Lesions. Br J Ophthalmol. 2010 Jan;94(1):128–30. PMID:19628495
1605. Karcioglu ZA, Hadjistilianou D, Rozans M, et al. Orbital Rhabdomyosarcoma. Cancer Control. 2004 Sep-Oct;11(5):328–33. PMID:15377992
1606. Karcioglu ZA, Mullaney PB. Diagnosis and Management of Iris Juvenile Xanthogranuloma. J Pediatr Ophthalmol Strabismus. 1997 Jan-Feb;34(1):44–51. PMID:9027680
1607. Karczewski KJ, Francioli LC, Tiao G, et al. The Mutational Constraint Spectrum Quantified from Variation in 141,456 Humans. Nature. 2020 May;581(7809):434–43. PMID:32461654
1608. Karim AF, Verdijk RM, Nagtegaal AP, et al. To Distinguish IgG4-Related Disease from Seronegative Granulomatosis with Polyangiitis. Rheumatology (Oxford). 2017 Dec 1;56(12):2245–7. PMID:28968906
1609. Karim F, Clahsen-van Groningen M, van Laar JA. AA Amyloidosis and IgG4-Related Disease. N Engl J Med. 2017 Feb 9;376(6):599–600. PMID:28177871
1610. Karim F, de Hoog J, Paridaens D, et al. IgG4-Related Disease as an Emerging Cause of Scleritis. Acta Ophthalmol. 2017 Dec;95(8):e795–6. PMID:28229544
1611. Karim F, Loeffen J, Bramer W, et al. IgG4-Related Disease: A Systematic Review of This Unrecognized Disease in Pediatrics. Pediatr Rheumatol Online J. 2016 Mar 25;14(1):18. PMID:27012661
1612. Karlin JN, Ahankoob N, Rootman DB. Multiple Arterial Vascular Anomalies in the Periorbital, Paranasal, and Intracranial Spaces Treated With Systemic Bevacizumab. J Craniofac Surg. 2021 Nov-Dec 01;32(8):e768–71. PMID:34224454
1613. Karlsson M, Boeryd B, Carstensen J, et al. Correlations of Ki-67 and PCNA to DNA Ploidy, S-Phase Fraction and Survival in Uveal Melanoma. Eur J Cancer. 1996 Feb;32A(2):357–62. PMID:8664054
1614. Karp CL, Mercado C, Venkateswaran N, et al. Use of High-Resolution Optical Coherence Tomography in the Surgical Management of Ocular Surface Squamous Neoplasia: A Pilot Study. Am J Ophthalmol. 2019 Oct;206:17–31. PMID:31163136
1615. Karpinets TV, Mitani Y, Liu B, et al. Whole-Genome Sequencing of Common Salivary Gland Carcinomas: Subtype-Restricted and Shared Genetic Alterations. Clin Cancer Res. 2021 Jul 15;27(14):3960–9. PMID:34011559
1616. Karube K, Nakagawa M, Tsuzuki S, et al. Identification of FOXO3 and PRDM1 as Tumor-Suppressor Gene Candidates in NK-Cell Neoplasms by Genomic and Functional

Analyses. Blood. 2011 Sep 22;118(12):3195–204. PMID:21690554
1617. Kase S, Ishida S. Adenosquamous Carcinoma Arising in Bulbar Conjunctiva. Ophthalmic Plast Reconstr Surg. 2019 Sep/Oct;35(5):e109–10. PMID:31356465
1618. Kase S, Yoshikawa H, Nakajima Y, et al. Adenosquamous Carcinoma of the Conjunctiva: A Case Report. Oncol Lett. 2014 Jun;7(6):1941–3. PMID:24932264
1619. Kashima TG, Nishiyama T, Shimazu K, et al. Periostin, a Novel Marker of Intramembranous Ossification, is Expressed in Fibrous Dysplasia and in C-Fos-Overexpressing Bone Lesions. Hum Pathol. 2009 Feb;40(2):226–37. PMID:18799196
1620. Kashofer K, Gornicec M, Lind K, et al. Detection of Prognostically Relevant Mutations and Translocations in Myeloid Sarcoma by Next Generation Sequencing. Leuk Lymphoma. 2018 Feb;59(2):501–4. PMID:28633614
1621. Kasprzak JM, Xu YG. Diagnosis and Management of Lentigo Maligna: A Review. Drugs Context. 2015 May 29;4:212281. PMID:26082796
1622. Katabi N, Xu B, Jungbluth AA, et al. PLAG1 Immunohistochemistry is a Sensitive Marker for Pleomorphic Adenoma: A Comparative Study with PLAG1 Genetic Abnormalities. Histopathology. 2018 Jan;72(2):285–93. PMID:28796899
1623. Katircioglu YA, Altiparmak UE, Akmansu H, et al. Squamous Cell Carcinoma of the Lacrimal Sac. Orbit. 2003 Sep;22(3):151–3. PMID:12868021
1624. Kato H, Mizuno N, Nakagawa K, et al. Microcystic Adnexal Carcinoma: A Light Microscopic, Immunohistochemical and Ultrastructural Study. J Cutan Pathol. 1990 Apr;17(2):87–95. PMID:2187025
1625. Kato K, Takeuchi M, Yonekawa Y, et al. Management of Inflamed Conjunctival Nevus with Topical Antiallergic Medications: Case Series. Clin Ophthalmol. 2021 Feb 12;15:559–64. PMID:33603334
1626. Kaur A, Kishore P, Agrawal A, et al. Mesenchymal Chondrosarcoma of the Orbit: A Report of Two Cases and Review of the Literature. Orbit. 2008;27(1):63–7. PMID:18307151
1627. Kaur H, Cameron JD, Mohney BG. Severe Astigmatic Amblyopia Secondary to Subcutaneous Juvenile Xanthogranuloma of the Eyelid. J AAPOS. 2006 Jun;10(3):277–8. PMID:16814185
1628. Kaur K, Gurnani B. Vernal Keratoconjunctivitis. In: StatPearls. Treasure Island (FL): StatPearls Publishing; 2022. PMID:35015458
1629. Kaur V, Swami A, Alapat D, et al. Clinical Characteristics, Molecular Profile and Outcomes of Myeloid Sarcoma: A Single Institution Experience Over 13 Years. Hematology. 2018 Jan;23(1):17–24. PMID:28574302
1630. Kausar A, Zafar SN, Altaf S, et al. Ophthalmic Manifestations of Linear Nevus Sebaceous/Organoid Nevus Syndrome. J Coll Physicians Surg Pak. 2015 Mar;25(3):220–2. PMID:25772967
1631. Kaw YT, Cuesta RA. Nodular Fasciitis of the Orbit Diagnosed by Fine Needle Aspiration Cytology. A Case Report. Acta Cytol. 1993 Nov-Dec;37(6):957–60. PMID:8249520
1632. Kaya EA, Broadbent TJ, Thomas CJ, et al. Primary Epithelioid Sarcoma of Orbit: A Case Report and Review of the Literature. Case Rep Oncol Med. 2018 Dec 17;2018:3989716. PMID:30652038
1633. Kazakov DV, Bisceglia M, Spagnolo DV, et al. Apocrine Mixed Tumors of the Skin with Architectural and/or Cytologic Atypia: A Retrospective Clinicopathologic Study of 18 Cases. Am J Surg Pathol. 2007 Jul;31(7):1094–102. PMID:17592277
1634. Kazakov DV, Bouda J Jr, Kacerovska D, et al. Vulvar Syringomas with Deep Extension: A Potential Histopathologic Mimic of Microcystic Adnexal Carcinoma. Int J Gynecol Pathol. 2011 Jan;30(1):92–4. PMID:21131826
1635. Kazakov DV, Kacerovska D, Hantschke M, et al. Cutaneous Mixed Tumor, Eccrine Variant: A Clinicopathologic and Immunohistochemical Study of 50 Cases, with Emphasis on Unusual Histopathologic Features. Am J Dermatopathol. 2011 Aug;33(6):557–68. PMID:21697702
1636. Kazakov DV, Kacerovska D, Michal M. Microcystic Adnexal Carcinoma with Multiple Areas of Follicular Differentiation Toward Germinative Cells and Specific Follicular Stroma (Trichoblastomatous Areas). Am J Dermatopathol. 2011 Jun;33(4):e47–9. PMID:21252639
1637. Kazakov DV, Kutzner H, Rütten A, et al. Carcinoid-Like Pattern in Sebaceous Neoplasms: Another Distinctive, Previously Unrecognized Pattern in Extraocular Sebaceous Carcinoma and Sebaceoma. Am J Dermatopathol. 2005 Jun;27(3):195–203. PMID:15900121
1638. Kazakov DV, Kutzner H, Spagnolo DV, et al. What is Extraocular Cutaneous Sebaceous Carcinoma In Situ? Am J Dermatopathol. 2010 Dec;32(8):857–8. PMID:20966738
1639. Kazakov DV, Suster S, LeBoit PE, et al. Mucinous Carcinoma of the Skin, Primary and Secondary: A Clinicopathologic Study of 63 Cases with Emphasis on the Morphologic Spectrum of Primary Cutaneous Forms: Homologies with Mucinous Lesions in the Breast. Am J Surg Pathol. 2005 Jun;29(6):764–82. PMID:15897743
1640. Keelawat S, Tirakunwichcha S, Saonanon P, et al. Cytokeratin-Negative Undifferentiated (Lymphoepithelial) Carcinoma of the Lacrimal Sac. Ophthalmic Plast Reconstr Surg. 2017 Jan/Feb;33(1):e16–8. PMID:25719371
1641. Kehrer-Sawatzki H, Cooper DN. Classification of NF1 Microdeletions and its Importance for Establishing Genotype/Phenotype Correlations in Patients with NF1 Microdeletions. Hum Genet. 2021 Dec;140(12):1635–49. PMID:34535841
1642. Kehrer-Sawatzki H, Farschtschi S, Mautner VF, et al. The Molecular Pathogenesis of Schwannomatosis, a Paradigm for the Co-Involvement of Multiple Tumour Suppressor Genes in Tumorigenesis. Hum Genet. 2017 Feb;136(2):129–48. PMID:27921248
1643. Kelishadi M, Kelishadi M, Moradi A, et al. Human Adenoviruses Role in Ophthalmic Pterygium Formation. Jundishapur J Microbiol. 2015 Apr 18;8(4):e16871. PMID:26034543
1644. Kellermann N, Maier M, Feucht N. [Vitreous Metastasis of Malignant Cutaneous Melanoma During Treatment with Ipilimumab]. Ophthalmologe. 2017 Feb;114(2):163–6. German. PMID:27260623
1645. Kemp PS, Allen RC, Longmuir SQ. Cryptic Respiratory Epithelial Cyst of the Lateral Orbit in a 3 Year Old with Strabismus and Amblyopia. J Pediatr Ophthalmol Strabismus. 2014 Mar 4;51 Online:e19–21. PMID:25314310
1646. Kempf W. CD30+ Lymphoproliferative Disorders: Histopathology, Differential Diagnosis, New Variants, and Simulators. J Cutan Pathol. 2006 Feb;33(Suppl 1):58–70. PMID:16412214
1647. Kempf W, Kadin ME, Dvorak AM, et al. Endogenous Retroviral Elements, But Not Exogenous Retroviruses, Are Detected in CD30-Positive Lymphoproliferative Disorders of the Skin. Carcinogenesis. 2003 Feb;24(2):301–6. PMID:12584181
1648. Kempf W, Kadin ME, Kutzner H, et al. Lymphomatoid Papulosis and Human Herpesviruses–A PCR-Based Evaluation for the Presence of Human Herpesvirus 6, 7 and 8 Related Herpesviruses. J Cutan Pathol. 2001 Jan;28(1):29–33. PMID:11168749
1649. Kempf W, Kazakov DV, Schärer L, et al. Angioinvasive Lymphomatoid Papulosis: A New Variant Simulating Aggressive Lymphomas. Am J Surg Pathol. 2013 Jan;37(1):1–13. PMID:23026936
1650. Kempf W, Kerl K, Mitteldorf C. Cutaneous CD30-Positive T-Cell Lymphoproliferative Disorders-Clinical and Histopathologic Features, Differential Diagnosis, and Treatment. Semin Cutan Med Surg. 2018 Mar;37(1):24–9. PMID:29719017
1651. Kempf W, Pfaltz K, Vermeer MH, et al. EORTC, ISCL, and USCLC Consensus Recommendations for the Treatment of Primary Cutaneous CD30-Positive Lymphoproliferative Disorders: Lymphomatoid Papulosis and Primary Cutaneous Anaplastic Large-Cell Lymphoma. Blood. 2011 Oct 13;118(15):4024–35. PMID:21841159
1652. Kemps PG, Hebeda KM, Pals ST, et al. Spectrum of Histiocytic Neoplasms Associated with Diverse Haematological Malignancies Bearing the Same Oncogenic Mutation. J Pathol Clin Res. 2021 Jan;7(1):10–26. PMID:32852896
1653. Kemps PG, Picarsic J, Durham BH, et al. ALK-Positive Histiocytosis: A New Clinicopathologic Spectrum Highlighting Neurologic Involvement and Responses to ALK Inhibition. Blood. 2022 Jan 13;139(2):256–80. PMID:34727172
1654. Kemps PG, Zondag TCE, Arnardóttir HB, et al. Clinicogenomic Associations in Childhood Langerhans Cell Histiocytosis: An International Cohort Study. Blood Adv. 2023 Feb 28;7(4):664–79. PMID:36083130
1655. Kenawy N, Coupland SE, Austin M, et al. Conjunctival Leiomyosarcoma. Clin Exp Ophthalmol. 2012 Apr;40(3):328–30. PMID:21718409
1656. Kenawy N, Kalirai H, Sacco JJ, et al. Conjunctival Melanoma Copy Number Alterations and Correlation with Mutation Status, Tumor Features, and Clinical Outcome. Pigment Cell Melanoma Res. 2019 Jul;32(4):564–75. PMID:30672666
1657. Kenawy N, Lake SL, Coupland SE, et al. Conjunctival Melanoma and Melanocytic Intra-Epithelial Neoplasia. Eye (Lond). 2013 Feb;27(2):142–52. PMID:23222568
1658. Kenny SE, Tye CB, Johnson DA, et al. Giant Papillary Conjunctivitis: A Review. Ocul Surf. 2020 Jul;18(3):396–402. PMID:32339665
1659. Keren S, Hildebrand D, Wilson S, et al. The Management of Periorbital Nodular Fasciitis Using Intra-Lesional Triamcinolone: A Case Report and Review of the Literature. Orbit. 2021 Aug;40(4):333–7. PMID:32646258
1660. Kerjaschki D. The Lymphatic Vasculature Revisited. J Clin Invest. 2014 Mar;124(3):874–7. PMID:24590271
1661. Kerr DA, Thompson LDR, Tafe LJ, et al. Clinicopathologic and Genomic Characterization of Inflammatory Myofibroblastic Tumors of the Head and Neck: Highlighting a Novel Fusion and Potential Diagnostic Pitfall. Am J Surg Pathol. 2021 Dec 1;45(12):1707–19. PMID:34001695
1662. Kersten RC, Tse DT, Anderson R. Iris Melanoma. Nevus or Malignancy? Surv Ophthalmol. 1985 May-Jun;29(6):423–33. PMID:4012597
1663. Kerstetter J, Wang J. Adult Orbital Xanthogranulomatous Disease: A Review with Emphasis on Etiology, Systemic Associations, Diagnostic Tools, and Treatment. Dermatol Clin. 2015 Jul;33(3):457–63. PMID:26143425
1664. Kervarrec T, Collin C, Larousserie F, et al. H3F3 Mutation Status of Giant Cell Tumors of the Bone, Chondroblastomas and Their Mimics: A Combined High Resolution Melting and Pyrosequencing Approach. Mod Pathol. 2017 Mar;30(3):393–406. PMID:28059095
1664A. Kervarrec T, Pissaloux D, Tirode F, et al. Morphologic Features in a Series of 352 Spitz Melanocytic Proliferations Help Predict Their Oncogenic Drivers. Virchows Arch. 2022 Feb;480(2):369–82. PMID:34761304
1665. Kestelyn P, van Liefferinge T, Goes F, et al. A Rare Case of Chronic Papillary Conjunctivitis Diagnosed After Several Years of Evolution. Clinical and Pathological Findings. Bull Soc Belge Ophtalmol. 1993;248:61–6. PMID:8044334
1666. Ketteler P, Hülsenbeck I, Frank M, et al. The Impact of RB1 Genotype on Incidence of Second Tumours in Heritable Retinoblastoma. Eur J Cancer. 2020 Jul;133:47–55. PMID:32434110
1667. Khafaga Y, Hassounah M, Kandil A, et al. Optic Gliomas: A Retrospective Analysis of 50 Cases. Int J Radiat Oncol Biol Phys. 2003 Jul 1;56(3):807–12. PMID:12788189
1668. Khalil MK. Balloon Cell Malignant Melanoma of the Choroid: Ultrastructural Studies. Br J Ophthalmol. 1983 Sep;67(9):579–84. PMID:6882713
1669. Khan S, Finger PT, Yu GP, et al. Clinical and Pathologic Characteristics of Biopsy-Proven Iris Melanoma: A Multicenter International Study. Arch Ophthalmol. 2012 Jan;130(1):57–64. PMID:21911649
1670. Khan SK, Yadav PS, Elliott G, et al. Induced GnasR201H Expression from the Endogenous Gnas Locus Causes Fibrous Dysplasia by Up-Regulating Wnt/β-Catenin Signaling. Proc Natl Acad Sci U S A. 2018 Jan 16;115(3):e418–27. PMID:29158412
1671. Khanam S, Agarwal A, Goel R, et al. Immunoglobulin G4-Related Disease Masquerading as Metastatic Malignant Melanoma of the Choroid. BMJ Case Rep. 2021 Apr 1;14(4):e241605. PMID:33795286
1672. Khanlari M, Chapman JR. Follicular Lymphoma: Updates for Pathologists. J Pathol Transl Med. 2022 Jan;56(1):1–15. PMID:34942689
1673. Khazaei S, De Jay N, Deshmukh S, et al. H3.3 G34W Promotes Growth and Impedes Differentiation of Osteoblast-Like Mesenchymal Progenitors in Giant Cell Tumor of Bone. Cancer Discov. 2020 Dec;10(12):1968–87. PMID:32967858
1674. Kheirkhah A, Mahbod M, Farzbod F, et al. Repeated Applications of Impression Cytology to Increase Sensitivity for Diagnosis of Conjunctival Intraepithelial Neoplasia. Br J Ophthalmol. 2012 Feb;96(2):229–33. PMID:21498806
1675. Khoja L, Atenafu EG, Suciu S, et al. Meta-Analysis in Metastatic Uveal Melanoma to Determine Progression Free and Overall Survival Benchmarks: An International Rare Cancers Initiative (IRCI) Ocular Melanoma Study. Ann Oncol. 2019 Aug 1;30(8):1370–80. PMID:31150059
1676. Khong JJ, Hardy TG, McNab AA. Prevalence of Oculo-Auriculo-Vertebral Spectrum in Dermolipoma. Ophthalmology. 2013 Aug;120(8):1529–32. PMID:23683920
1677. Khosroshahi A, Wallace ZS, Crowe JL, et al. International Consensus Guidance Statement on the Management and Treatment of IgG4-Related Disease. Arthritis Rheumatol. 2015 Jul;67(7):1688–99. PMID:25809420
1678. Khoury JD, Cher W. Myeloid Diseases in the Lung and Pleura. Semin Diagn Pathol. 2020 Nov;37(6):296–302. PMID:32591154
1679. Kiernan M, Fabian ID, Smith V, et al. Strabismus as a Presenting Sign in Retinoblastoma. J Pediatr Ophthalmol Strabismus. 2021 Sep-Oct;58(5):324–30. PMID:34592118
1680. Kiire CA, Stewart RMK, Srinivasan S, et al. A Prospective Study of the Incidence,

Associations and Outcomes of Ocular Surface Squamous Neoplasia in the United Kingdom. Eye (Lond). 2019 Feb;33(2):283–94. PMID:30593587
1681. Kilkenny M, Merlin K, Young R, et al. The Prevalence of Common Skin Conditions in Australian School Students: 1. Common, Plane and Plantar Viral Warts. Br J Dermatol. 1998 May;138(5):840–5. PMID:9666831
1682. Kim BH, Henderson BA. Intraocular Choristoma. Semin Ophthalmol. 2005 Oct-Dec;20(4):223–9. PMID:16352493
1682A. Kim D, Compres EV, Zhang B, et al. A Series of RET Fusion Spitz Neoplasms With Plaque-Like Silhouette and Dyscohesive Nesting of Epithelioid Melanocytes. Am J Dermatopathol. 2021 Apr;43(4):243–51. PMID:33742998
1683. Kim DH, Kim MY, Park YM, et al. Agminated Lobular Capillary Hemangiomas Presumably Associated with an Acquired Arteriovenous Malformation. J Dermatol. 2006 Sep;33(9):646–8. PMID:16958814
1684. Kim HJ, Kim HJ, Kim YD, et al. Solitary Fibrous Tumor of the Orbit: CT and MR Imaging Findings. AJNR Am J Neuroradiol. 2008 May;29(5):857–62. PMID:18272558
1685. Kim HJ, McCormick SA, Nath S, et al. Melanocytic Nevi of the Tarsal Conjunctiva: Clinicopathologic Case Series with Review of Literature. Ophthalmic Plast Reconstr Surg. 2010 Nov-Dec;26(6):438–42. PMID:20683369
1686. Kim HJ, Shields CL, Eagle RC Jr, et al. Fibrous Histiocytoma of the Conjunctiva. Am J Ophthalmol. 2006 Dec;142(6):1036–43. PMID:17157587
1687. Kim J, Steeples LR, Jones NP. Ocular Involvement in the Histiocytoses: A Literature Review with an Illustrative Case Series. Ocul Immunol Inflamm. 2022 Apr 3;30(3):600–14. PMID:34637661
1688. Kim JM, Hall LB, Elia M, et al. Acute Presentation of Mesectodermal Leiomyoma of the Ciliary Body. Ocul Oncol Pathol. 2017 Nov;3(4):304–9. PMID:29344486
1689. Kim JS, Proia AD, Liss J, et al. Multiple Cranial Neuropathies as the Initial Presentation of Primary Ductal Adenocarcinoma of the Lacrimal Gland. Ophthalmic Plast Reconstr Surg. 2022 May-Jun 01;38(3):e75–7. PMID:35030152
1690. Kim JY, Park Y. Treatment of Retinoblastoma: The Role of External Beam Radiotherapy. Yonsei Med J. 2015 Nov;56(6):1478–91. PMID:26446627
1691. Kim ME, Polski A, Xu L, et al. Comprehensive Somatic Copy Number Analysis Using Aqueous Humor Liquid Biopsy for Retinoblastoma. Cancers (Basel). 2021 Jul 3;13(13):3340. PMID:34283049
1692. Kim MH, Sa HS, Woo K, et al. Fibrolipoma of the Orbit. Ophthalmic Plast Reconstr Surg. 2011 Jan-Feb;27(1):e16–8. PMID:20700070
1693. Kim N, Yang HK, Kim JH, et al. IgG4-Related Ophthalmic Disease Involving Extraocular Muscles: Case Series. BMC Ophthalmol. 2018 Jul 3;18(1):162. PMID:29970061
1694. Kim S, Jun JH, Kim J, et al. HIF-1α and VEGF Expression Correlates with Thrombus Remodeling in Cases of Intravascular Papillary Endothelial Hyperplasia. Int J Clin Exp Pathol. 2013 Nov 15;6(12):2912–8. PMID:24294378
1695. Kim SE, Kim JH, Yang SW. Dedifferentiated Transformation in Metastatic Liposarcoma of Orbit and Brain. Orbit. 2020 Dec;39(6):437–40. PMID:31910682
1696. Kim SJ, Lee SU, Kang MS, et al. IgG4-Related Disease Presenting as Recurrent Scleritis Combined with Optic Neuropathy. BMC Ophthalmol. 2021 Jan 5;21(1):5. PMID:33402162
1697. Kim SJ, Yoon DH, Jaccard A, et al. A Prognostic Index for Natural Killer Cell Lymphoma After Non-Anthracycline-Based Treatment: A Multicentre, Retrospective Analysis. Lancet Oncol. 2016 Mar;17(3):389–400. PMID:26873565
1698. Kim SW, Choi MK, Han HS, et al. A Case of Pulmonary Langerhans Cell Sarcoma Simultaneously Diagnosed with Cutaneous Langerhans Cell Histiocytosis Studied by Whole-Exome Sequencing. Acta Haematol. 2017;138(1):24–30. PMID:28614815
1699. Kim UR, Shah AD, Shanti R, et al. Primary Adenoid Cystic Carcinoma of the Eyelid. Ophthalmic Plast Reconstr Surg. 2010 Mar-Apr;26(2):134–6. PMID:20305522
1700. Kim YD, Goldberg RA. Orbital Fat Prolapse and Dermolipoma: Two Distinct Entities. Korean J Ophthalmol. 1994 Jun;8(1):42–3. PMID:7933633
1701. Kim YH, Willemze R, Pimpinelli N, et al. TNM Classification System for Primary Cutaneous Lymphomas Other Than Mycosis Fungoides and Sezary Syndrome: A Proposal of the International Society for Cutaneous Lymphomas (ISCL) and the Cutaneous Lymphoma Task Force of the European Organization of Research and Treatment of Cancer (EORTC). Blood. 2007 Jul 15;110(2):479–84. PMID:17339420
1702. Kim YR, Han KH. Familial Hypercholesterolemia and the Atherosclerotic Disease. Korean Circ J. 2013 Jun;43(6):363–7. PMID:23882283
1703. Kimura K, Usui Y, Goto H; Japanese Intraocular Lymphoma Study Group. Clinical features and diagnostic significance of the intraocular fluid of 217 patients with intraocular lymphoma. Jpn J Ophthalmol. 2012 Jul;56(4):383–9. PMID:22661396
1704. Kincaid MC, Green WR, Hoover RE, et al. Iododerma of the Conjunctiva and Skin. Ophthalmology. 1981 Dec;88(12):1216–20. PMID:7322470
1705. Kinch K, Roberts F. Primary Orbital Sarcoma in Adults: A Case Series with Emphasis on Post-Irradiation Sarcoma. Orbit. 2024 Jun;43(3):417–28. PMID:36622318
1706. King R, Hayzen BA, Page RN, et al. Recurrent Nevus Phenomenon: A Clinicopathologic Study of 357 Cases and Histologic Comparison with Melanoma with Regression. Mod Pathol. 2009 May;22(5):611–7. PMID:19270643
1707. King-Smith PE, Mauger TF, Begley CG, et al. Optical Analysis and Reappraisal of the Peripheral Light Focusing Theory of Nasal Pterygia Formation. Invest Ophthalmol Vis Sci. 2020 Feb 7;61(2):42. PMID:32106293
1708. Kiratli H, Ağın A, Önder S. Ciliary Body Mesectodermal Leiomyoma Diagnosed by Fine Needle Aspiration Biopsy. Ocul Oncol Pathol. 2017 Sep;3(3):199–203. PMID:29071270
1709. Kiratli H, Deniz Y, Büyükeren B, et al. Mesenchymal Chondrosarcoma of the Lacrimal Gland. Ophthalmic Plast Reconstr Surg. 2018 May/Jun;34(3):e77–9. PMID:29342030
1710. Kiratli H, Erkan Balci K, Güler G. Primary Orbital Endodermal Sinus Tumor (Yolk Sac Tumor). J AAPOS. 2008 Dec;12(6):623–5. PMID:18835732
1711. Kiratli H, Kiliç M, Tarlan B, et al. Adult Orbital Xanthogranulomas: Clinical Features and Management. Eur J Ophthalmol. 2015 Jul-Aug;25(4):288–92. PMID:25612656
1712. Kiratli H, Koç I. Malignant Transformation of Retinocytoma Treated with Intra-Arterial Chemotherapy. Can J Ophthalmol. 2016 Jun;51(3):e105–7. PMID:27316281
1713. Kiratli H, Koç İ, Özkayar Ö, et al. Sequential Development of Dermatofibrosarcoma Protuberans in the Forehead and Eyelid. Can J Ophthalmol. 2017 Dec;52(6):e228–30. PMID:29217050
1714. Kiratli H, Sekeroğlu MA, Tezel GG. Orbital Heterotopic Glial Tissue Presenting as Exotropia. Orbit. 2008;27(3):165–8. PMID:18569821
1715. Kiratli H, Shields CL, Shields JA, et al. Metastatic Tumours to the Conjunctiva: Report of 10 Cases. Br J Ophthalmol. 1996 Jan;80(1):5–8. PMID:8664233
1716. Kiratli H, Tarlan B, Ruacan S. Epitheloid Hemangioendothelioma of the Palpebral Lobe of the Lacrimal Gland. Orbit. 2013 Apr;32(2):120–3. PMID:23514025
1717. Kirchner J, Hatzoglou V, Buthorn JB, et al. 18F-FDG PET/CT Versus Anatomic Imaging for Evaluating Disease Extent and Clinical Trial Eligibility in Erdheim-Chester Disease: Results from 50 Patients in a Registry Study. Eur J Nucl Med Mol Imaging. 2021 Apr;48(4):1154–65. PMID:33057928
1718. Kirkegaard MK, Minderman M, Sjö LD, et al. Prevalence and Prognostic Value of MYD88 and CD79B Mutations in Ocular Adnexal Large B-Cell Lymphoma: A Reclassification of Ocular Adnexal Large B-Cell Lymphoma. Br J Ophthalmol. 2023 Apr;107(4):576–81. PMID:34706861
1719. Kirkegaard MM, Coupland SE, Prause JU, et al. Malignant Lymphoma of the Conjunctiva. Surv Ophthalmol. 2015 Sep-Oct;60(5):444–58. PMID:26003619
1720. Kiryakoza LC, Diaz JD, Priluck J, et al. A Case of Bilateral Diffuse Uveal Melanocytic Proliferation in the Setting of Urothelial Carcinoma of the Ureter: A Failed Response to Plasmapheresis. Ophthalmic Surg Lasers Imaging Retina. 2022 Jun;53(6):350–3. PMID:35724372
1721. Kisser U, Heichel J, Glien A. Rare Diseases of the Orbit. Laryngorhinootologie. 2021 Apr;100 S 01:S1–79. PMID:34352903
1722. Kivelä T, Simpson ER, Grossniklaus HE, Jager MJ, Singh AD, Caminal JM, et al. Uveal Melanoma. In: Amin MB, Edge SB, Greene FL, et al., editors. AJCC cancer staging manual. 8th ed. New York: Springer; 2017. pp. 805–17.
1723. Kivelä T. Incidence, Prevalence and Epidemiology of Ocular Melanoma. In: Murray TG, Boldt HC, editors. Ocular Melanoma: Advances in Diagnostic and Therapeutic Strategies. London (UK): Future Medicine; 2014. pp. 20–38.
1724. Kivelä T. The Epidemiological Challenge of the Most Frequent Eye Cancer: Retinoblastoma, an Issue of Birth and Death. Br J Ophthalmol. 2009 Sep;93(9):1129–31. PMID:19704035
1725. Kivelä T, Eskelin S. Transformation of Nevus to Melanoma. Ophthalmology. 2006 May;113(5):887–8.e1. PMID:16650691
1726. Kivelä T, Kauniskangas L, Miettinen P, et al. Glioneuroma Associated with Colobomatous Dysplasia of the Anterior Uvea and Retina. A Case Simulating Medulloepithelioma. Ophthalmology. 1989 Dec;96(12):1799–808. PMID:2622623
1727. Kivelä T, Summanen P. Retinoinvasive Malignant Melanoma of the Uvea. Br J Ophthalmol. 1997 Aug;81(8):691–7. PMID:9349160
1728. Kivelä T, Tarkkanen A. Orbital Germ Cell Tumors Revisited: A Clinicopathological Approach to Classification. Surv Ophthalmol. 1994 May-Jun;38(6):541–54. PMID:8066543
1729. Kivelä T, Tarkkanen A. Recurrent Medulloepithelioma of the Ciliary Body. Immunohistochemical Characteristics. Ophthalmology. 1988 Nov;95(11):1565–75. PMID:3211466
1730. Kivelä TT. The First Description of the Complete Natural History of Uveal Melanoma by Two Scottish Surgeons, Allan Burns and James Wardrop. Acta Ophthalmol. 2018 Mar;96(2):203–14. PMID:28834323
1731. Kivelä TT, Piperno-Neumann S, Desjardins L, et al. Validation of a Prognostic Staging for Metastatic Uveal Melanoma: A Collaborative Study of the European Ophthalmic Oncology Group. Am J Ophthalmol. 2016 Aug;168:217–26. PMID:27296487
1732. Klaber R. Morbus Recklinghausen with Glomoid Tumours. Proc R Soc Med. 1938 Feb;31(4):347. PMID:19991403
1733. Klapper W, Hoster E, Determann O, et al. Ki-67 as a Prognostic Marker in Mantle Cell Lymphoma-Consensus Guidelines of the Pathology Panel of the European MCL Network. J Hematop. 2009 Jul;2(2):103–11. PMID:19669190
1734. Klein A, Barak A, Habot-Wilner Z, et al. The Appearance of Congenital Hypertrophy of Retinal Pigment Epithelium by High-Resolution Optical Coherence Tomography. Retina. 2011 Sep;31(8):1740–1. PMID:21817965
1735. Kleinerman RA, Schonfeld SJ, Sigel BS, et al. Bone and Soft-Tissue Sarcoma Risk in Long-Term Survivors of Hereditary Retinoblastoma Treated With Radiation. J Clin Oncol. 2019 Dec 10;37(35):3436–45. PMID:31622129
1736. Kleinerman RA, Tucker MA, Tarone RE, et al. Risk of New Cancers After Radiotherapy in Long-Term Survivors of Retinoblastoma: An Extended Follow-Up. J Clin Oncol. 2005 Apr 1;23(10):2272–9. PMID:15800318
1737. Klemp K, Kiilgaard JF, Heegaard S, et al. Bilateral Diffuse Uveal Melanocytic Proliferation: Case Report and Literature Review. Acta Ophthalmol. 2017 Aug;95(5):439–45. PMID:28636126
1738. Klijanienko J, El-Naggar AK, Servois V, et al. Mucoepidermoid Carcinoma Ex Pleomorphic Adenoma: Nonspecific Preoperative Cytologic Findings in Six Cases. Cancer. 1998 Aug 25;84(4):231–4. PMID:9723598
1739. Klijanienko J, El-Naggar AK, Vielh P. Fine-Needle Sampling Findings in 26 Carcinoma Ex Pleomorphic Adenomas: Diagnostic Pitfalls and Clinical Considerations. Diagn Cytopathol. 1999 Sep;21(3):163–6. PMID:10450099
1740. Klijanienko J, Vielh P. Fine-Needle Sampling of Salivary Gland Lesions. IV. Review of 50 Cases of Mucoepidermoid Carcinoma with Histologic Correlation. Diagn Cytopathol. 1997 Aug;17(2):92–8. PMID:9258615
1741. Klijanienko J, Vielh P. Fine-Needle Sampling of Salivary Gland Lesions. VII. Cytology and Histology Correlation of Five Cases of Epithelial-Myoepithelial Carcinoma. Diagn Cytopathol. 1998 Dec;19(6):405–9. PMID:9839128
1742. Knapp AN, Samara WA, Shields CL, et al. Conjunctival Fibrous Histiocytoma in an 8-Year-Old Boy. J AAPOS. 2016 Aug;20(4):368–70. PMID:27282913
1743. Knežević M, Stojković M, Jovanović M, et al. A 7-Year Prospective Study of Routine Histopathological Evaluation of the Lacrimal Sac Wall Incisional Biopsy Specimens Obtained During External Dacryocystorhinostomy in Adults and a Review of the Literature. Med Oncol. 2012 Mar;29(1):396–400. PMID:21264538
1744. Kniggendorf VF, Neto ET, Maia EM, et al. Bilateral Diffuse Uveal Melanocytic Proliferation Associated with Renal Cancer: The Importance of Indocyanine Green Angiography and Early Diagnosis. Retin Cases Brief Rep. 2018 Summer;12(3):166–71. PMID:27861254
1745. Knight J, Ratnasingham K. Metastasising Pleomorphic Adenoma: Systematic Review. Int J Surg. 2015 Jul;19:137–45. PMID:25958295
1746. Knop N, Knop E. Regulation of the Inflammatory Component in Chronic Dry Eye Disease by the Eye-Associated Lymphoid Tissue (EALT). Dev Ophthalmol. 2010;45:23–39. PMID:20502024
1747. Knowles DM, Jakobiec FA, McNally L, et al. Lymphoid Hyperplasia and Malignant Lymphoma Occurring in the Ocular Adnexa (Orbit, Conjunctiva, and Eyelids): A Prospective Multiparametric Analysis of 108 Cases During 1977 to 1987. Hum Pathol. 1990 Sep;21(9):959–73. PMID:2394438

1748. Knudsen MKH, Rasmussen PK, Coupland SE, et al. Clinicopathological Features of Ocular Adnexal Mantle-Cell Lymphoma in an International Multicenter Cohort. JAMA Ophthalmol. 2017 Dec 1;135(12):1367–74. PMID:29121219
1749. Knutsen T, Gobu V, Knaus R, et al. The Interactive Online SKY/M-FISH & CGH Database and the Entrez Cancer Chromosomes Search Database: Linkage of Chromosomal Aberrations with the Genome Sequence. Genes Chromosomes Cancer. 2005 Sep;44(1):52–64. PMID:15934046
1750. Kobayashi N, Oda T, Takizawa M, et al. Integrin α7 and Extracellular Matrix Laminin 211 Interaction Promotes Proliferation of Acute Myeloid Leukemia Cells and Is Associated with Granulocytic Sarcoma. Cancers (Basel). 2020 Feb;12(2):363. PMID:32033262
1751. Koch KR, Ortmann M, Heindl LM. Conjunctival Mucoepidermoid Carcinoma. Ophthalmology. 2016 Mar;123(3):616. PMID:26902565
1752. Kodama T, Tane N, Ohira A, et al. Sclerosing Sweat Duct Carcinoma of the Eyelid. Jpn J Ophthalmol. 2004 Jan-Feb;48(1):7–11. PMID:14767643
1753. Kodet R, Newton WA Jr, Hamoudi AB, et al. Childhood Rhabdomyosarcoma with Anaplastic (Pleomorphic) Features. A Report of the Intergroup Rhabdomyosarcoma Study. Am J Surg Pathol. 1993 May;17(5):443–53. PMID:8470759
1754. Kodet R, Newton WA Jr, Hamoudi AB, et al. Orbital Rhabdomyosarcomas and Related Tumors in Childhood: Relationship of Morphology to Prognosis–an Intergroup Rhabdomyosarcoma Study. Med Pediatr Oncol. 1997 Jul;29(1):51–60. PMID:9142207
1755. Koelsche C, Hovestadt V, Jones DT, et al. Melanotic Tumors of the Nervous System Are Characterized by Distinct Mutational, Chromosomal and Epigenomic Profiles. Brain Pathol. 2015 Mar;25(2):202–8. PMID:25399693
1756. Koelsche C, Schrimpf D, Stichel D, et al. Sarcoma Classification by DNA Methylation Profiling. Nat Commun. 2021 Jan 21;12(1):498. PMID:33479225
1757. Koelsche C, Schweizer L, Renner M, et al. Nuclear Relocation of STAT6 Reliably Predicts NAB2-STAT6 Fusion for the Diagnosis of Solitary Fibrous Tumour. Histopathology. 2014 Nov;65(5):613–22. PMID:24702701
1758. Kohashi K, Oda Y, Yamamoto H, et al. Reduced Expression of SMARCB1/INI1 Protein in Synovial Sarcoma. Mod Pathol. 2010 Jul;23(7):981–90. PMID:20305614
1759. Kohn R, Nofsinger K, Freedman SI. Rapid Recurrence of Papillary Squamous Cell Carcinoma of the Canaliculus. Am J Ophthalmol. 1981 Sep;92(3):363–7. PMID:7294095
1760. Kolesnikov IS, Lytkin MI, Tishchenko MI, et al. [Integral Rheography of the Body as a Method of Evaluation of the Circulatory System in Surgical Diseases]. Vestn Khir Im I I Grek. 1981 Jan;126(1):9–15. Russian. PMID:7222429
1761. Koletsa T, Karayannopoulou G, Dereklis D, et al. Mesectodermal Leiomyoma of the Ciliary Body: Report of a Case and Review of the Literature. Pathol Res Pract. 2009;205(2):125–30. PMID:18930601
1762. Komotar RJ, Burger PC, Carson BS, et al. Pilocytic and Pilomyxoid Hypothalamic/Chiasmatic Astrocytomas. Neurosurgery. 2004 Jan;54(1):72–9. PMID:14683543
1763. Kong YY, Kong JC, Shi DR, et al. Cutaneous Rosai-Dorfman Disease: A Clinical and Histopathologic Study of 25 Cases in China. Am J Surg Pathol. 2007 Mar;31(3):341–50. PMID:17325475
1764. Konstantinidis L, Damato B. Intraocular Metastases–A Review. Asia Pac J Ophthalmol (Phila). 2017 Mar-Apr;6(2):208–14. PMID:28399345
1765. Konstantinova AM, Michal M, Kacerovska D, et al. Hidradenoma Papilliferum: A Clinicopathologic Study of 264 Tumors From 261 Patients, With Emphasis on Mammary-Type Alterations. Am J Dermatopathol. 2016 Aug;38(8):598–607. PMID:26863059
1766. Kontos G, Borooah S, Khan A, et al. The Epidemiology, Clinical Characteristics, Histopathology and Management of Juvenile- and Adult-Onset Corneoscleral Limbus Xanthogranuloma. Graefes Arch Clin Exp Ophthalmol. 2016 Mar;254(3):413–20. PMID:26794218
1767. Koo GC, Tan SY, Tang T, et al. Janus Kinase 3-Activating Mutations Identified in Natural Killer/T-Cell Lymphoma. Cancer Discov. 2012 Jul;2(7):591–7. PMID:22705984
1768. Kooi IE, Mol BM, Massink MP, et al. A Meta-Analysis of Retinoblastoma Copy Numbers Refines the List of Possible Driver Genes Involved in Tumor Progression. PLoS One. 2016 Apr 26;11(4):e0153323. PMID:27115612
1769. Kooi IE, Mol BM, Massink MP, et al. Somatic Genomic Alterations in Retinoblastoma Beyond RB1 Are Rare and Limited to Copy Number Changes. Sci Rep. 2016 Apr 29;6:25264. PMID:27126562
1770. Koopmans AE, Ober K, Dubbink HJ, et al. Prevalence and Implications of TERT Promoter Mutation in Uveal and Conjunctival Melanoma and in Benign and Premalignant Conjunctival Melanocytic Lesions. Invest Ophthalmol Vis Sci. 2014 Aug 26;55(9):6024–30. PMID:25159205
1771. Koopmans AE, Verdijk RM, Brouwer RW, et al. Clinical Significance of Immunohistochemistry for Detection of BAP1 Mutations in Uveal Melanoma. Mod Pathol. 2014 Oct;27(10):1321–30. PMID:24633195
1772. Kopsidas K, Mudhar H, Sisley K, et al. Aggressive Ciliary Body Adenocarcinoma with Bilateral Lung Metastases: Histological, Molecular, Genetic and Clinical Aspects. Ocul Oncol Pathol. 2019 Feb;5(2):79–84. PMID:30976584
1773. Korshunov A, Jakobiec FA, Eberhart CG et al. Comparative Integrated Molecular Analysis of Intraocular Medulloepitheliomas and Central Nervous System Embryonal Tumors with Multilayered Rosettes Confirms that They Are Distinct Nosologic Entities. Neuropathology. 2015 Dec;35(6):538–44. PMID:26183384
1774. Korswagen LA, Moll AC, Imhof SM, et al. A Second Primary Tumor in a Patient with Retinoma. Ophthalmic Genet. 2004 Mar;25(1):45–8. PMID:15255114
1775. Koshy J, Schnadig V, Nawgiri R. Is Fine Needle Aspiration Cytology a Useful Diagnostic Tool for Granular Cell Tumors? A Cytohistological Review with Emphasis on Pitfalls. Cytojournal. 2014 Oct 21;11:28. PMID:25379050
1776. Kossard S, Xenias SJ, Palestine RF, et al. Inflammatory Changes in Verruca Vulgaris. J Cutan Pathol. 1980 Aug 7(4):217–21. PMID:7430479
1777. Koubaa Mahjoub W, Jouini R, Khanchel F, et al. Neuroblastoma-Like Schwannoma with Giant Rosette: A Potential Diagnostic Pitfall for Hyalinizing Spindle Cell Tumor. J Cutan Pathol. 2019 Mar;46(3):234–7. PMID:30582192
1778. Koutlas IG, Scheithauer BW. Palisaded Encapsulated ("Solitary Circumscribed") Neuroma of the Oral Cavity: A Review of 55 Cases. Head Neck Pathol. 2010 Mar;4(1):15–26. PMID:20237984
1779. Kramer GD, Arepalli S, Shields CL, et al. Ciliary Body Medulloepithelioma Association with Pleuropulmonary Blastoma in a Familial Tumor Predisposition Syndrome. J Pediatr Ophthalmol Strabismus. 2014 Jul 16;51 Online:e48–50. PMID:25032694
1780. Kransdorf MJ, Sweet DE. Aneurysmal Bone Cyst: Concept, Controversy, Clinical Presentation, and Imaging. AJR Am J Roentgenol. 1995 Mar;164(3):573–80. PMID:7863874
1781. Krantz BA, Dave N, Komatsubara KM, et al. Uveal Melanoma: Epidemiology, Etiology, and Treatment of Primary Disease. Clin Ophthalmol. 2017 Jan 31;11:279–89. PMID:28203054
1782. Krauss T, Ferrara AM, Links TP, et al. Preventive Medicine of von Hippel-Lindau Disease-Associated Pancreatic Neuroendocrine Tumors. Endocr Relat Cancer. 2018 Sep;25(9):783–93. PMID:29748190
1783. Krauthammer M, Kong Y, Bacchiocchi A, et al. Exome Sequencing Identifies Recurrent Mutations in NF1 and RASopathy Genes in Sun-Exposed Melanomas. Nat Genet. 2015 Sep;47(9):996–1002. PMID:26214590
1784. Krema H, Simpson ER, Pavlin CJ, et al. Management of Ciliary Body Melanoma with Iodine-125 Plaque Brachytherapy. Can J Ophthalmol. 2009 Aug;44(4):395–400. PMID:19606159
1785. Kremer I, Sandbank J, Weinberger D, et al. Pigmented Epithelial Tumours of the Conjunctiva. Br J Ophthalmol. 1992 May;76(5):294–6. PMID:1390513
1786. Kremer M, Ott G, Nathrath M, et al. Primary Extramedullary Plasmacytoma and Multiple Myeloma: Phenotypic Differences Revealed by Immunohistochemical Analysis. J Pathol. 2005 Jan;205(1):92–101. PMID:15586381
1787. Kretzmer H, Biran A, Purroy N, et al. Preneoplastic Alterations Define CLL DNA Methylome and Persist through Disease Progression and Therapy. Blood Cancer Discov. 2021 Jan;2(1):54–69. PMID:33604581
1788. Krieg M, Marti HH, Plate KH. Coexpression of Erythropoietin and Vascular Endothelial Growth Factor in Nervous System Tumors Associated with von Hippel-Lindau Tumor Suppressor Gene Loss of Function. Blood. 1998 Nov 1;92(9):3388–93. PMID:9787178
1789. Krishna M. Diagnosis of Metastatic Neoplasms: An Immunohistochemical Approach. Arch Pathol Lab Med. 2010 Feb;134(2):207–15. PMID:20121608
1790. Krishna Y, Coupland SE. Lacrimal Sac Tumors–A Review. Asia Pac J Ophthalmol (Phila). 2017 Mar-Apr;6(2):173–8. PMID:28399337
1791. Krishna Y, Kalirai H, Thornton S, et al. Genetic Findings in Treatment-Naïve and Proton-Beam-Radiated Iris Melanomas. Br J Ophthalmol. 2016 Jul;100(7):1012–6. PMID:27098748
1792. Krishnakumar S, Subramanian N, Mohan ER, et al. Solitary Fibrous Tumor of the Orbit: A Clinicopathologic Study of Six Cases with Review of the Literature. Surv Ophthalmol. 2003 Sep-Oct;48(5):544–54. PMID:14499820
1793. Krohn J, Frøystein T, Dahl O. Topographical Distribution of Choroidal Naevi in the Ocular Fundus. Eye (Lond). 2009 Aug;23(8):1685–90. PMID:19039331
1794. Krohn J, Frøystein T, Dahl O. Topography of Solitary Congenital Hypertrophy of the Retinal Pigment Epithelium in the Ocular Fundus. Acta Ophthalmol. 2009 Nov;87(8):921–2. PMID:19604161
1795. Krohn J, Rishi P, Frøystein T, et al. Circumscribed Choroidal Haemangioma: Clinical and Topographical Features. Br J Ophthalmol. 2019 Oct;103(10):1448–52. PMID:30602446
1796. Krohn J, Sundal KV, Frøystein T. Topography and Clinical Features of Iris Melanoma. BMC Ophthalmol. 2022 Jan 3;22(1):6. PMID:34980044
1797. Kronish JW, Sneed SR, Tse DT. Epidermal Cysts of the Eyelid. Arch Ophthalmol. 1988 Feb;106(2):270. PMID:3341987
1798. Krzystolik Z, Czerniak B, Woyke S. [Diagnosis of Intraocular Melanoma by Thin-Needle Aspiration Biopsy]. Klin Oczna. 1982 Sep;84(9):279–82. Polish. PMID:7162114
1799. Kubota T, Moritani S. High Incidence of Autoimmune Disease in Japanese Patients with Ocular Adnexal Reactive Lymphoid Hyperplasia. Am J Ophthalmol. 2007 Jul;144(1):148–9. PMID:17601445
1800. Kubota T, Moritani S, Ichihara S. Clinicopathologic and Immunohistochemical Features of Primary Ductal Adenocarcinoma of Lacrimal Gland: Five New Cases and Review of Literature. Graefes Arch Clin Exp Ophthalmol. 2013 Aug;251(8):2071–6. PMID:23613093
1801. Kujala E, Damato B, Coupland SE, et al. Staging of Ciliary Body and Choroidal Melanomas Based on Anatomic Extent. J Clin Oncol. 2013 Aug 1;31(22):2825–31. PMID:23816968
1802. Kujala E, Mäkitie T, Kivelä T. Very Long-Term Prognosis of Patients with Malignant Uveal Melanoma. Invest Ophthalmol Vis Sci. 2003 Nov;44(11):4651–9. PMID:14578381
1803. Kulkarni V, Rajshekhar V, Chandi SM. Orbital Apex Leiomyoma with Intracranial Extension. Surg Neurol. 2000 Oct;54(4):327–30. PMID:11136938
1804. Kumar S, Zafar SF, Raufi AM, et al. Apocrine Carcinoma of the Face in a 62-Year-Old Asian Man. Clin Pract. 2011 Jul 1;1(3):e50. PMID:24765311
1805. Kumar VA, Esmaeli B, Ahmed S, et al. Imaging Features of Malignant Lacrimal Sac and Nasolacrimal Duct Tumors. AJNR Am J Neuroradiol. 2016 Nov;37(11):2134–7. PMID:27418476
1806. Kumari N, Das S, Gandhi A, et al. Primary Orbital Yolk Sac Tumor Presenting as Fungating Mass. Orbit. Aug;42(4):459–62. PMID:35258404
1807. Kummer JA, Vermeer MH, Dukers D, et al. Most Primary Cutaneous CD30-Positive Lymphoproliferative Disorders Have a CD4-Positive Cytotoxic T-Cell Phenotype. J Invest Dermatol. 1997 Nov;109(5):636–40. PMID:9347791
1808. Kunieda J, Yamashita K, Togashi Y, et al. High Prevalence of TERT Aberrations in Myxoid Liposarcoma: TERT Reactivation May Play a Crucial Role in Tumorgenesis. Cancer Sci. 2022 Mar;113(3):1078–89. PMID:34971481
1809. Kunimoto K, Yamamoto Y, Jinnin M. ISSVA Classification of Vascular Anomalies and Molecular Biology. Int J Mol Sci. 2022 Feb 21;23(4):2358. PMID:35216474
1810. Kuo PK, Puliafito CA, Wang KM, et al. Uveal Melanoma in China. Int Ophthalmol Clin. 1982 Fall;22(3):57–71. PMID:7107133
1811. Kurisu Y, Shibayama Y, Tsuji M, et al. A Case of Primary Ductal Adenocarcinoma of the Lacrimal Gland: Histopathological and Immunohistochemical Study. Pathol Res Pract. 2005;201(1):49–53. PMID:15807311
1812. Kurli M, Finger PT. Melanocytic Conjunctival Tumors. Ophthalmol Clin North Am. 2005 Mar;18(1):15–24, Vii. PMID:15763188
1813. Kurli M, Finger PT, Manor T, et al. Finding Malignant Change in a Necrotic Choroidal Melanocytoma: A Clinical Challenge. Br J Ophthalmol. 2005 Jul;89(7):921–2. PMID:15965181
1814. Kurosawa A, Kurosawa H. Ovoid Bodies in Choroidal Neurofibromatosis. Arch Ophthalmol. 1982 Dec;100(12):1939–41. PMID:6816197
1815. Kurt AM, Unni KK, McLeod RA, et al. Low-Grade Intraosseous Osteosarcoma. Cancer. 1990 Mar 15;65(6):1418–28. PMID:2306687
1816. Kuruvilla R, Escaravage GK Jr, Finn AJ, et al. Infiltrative Subcutaneous Juvenile Xanthogranuloma of the Eyelid in a Neonate. Ophthalmic Plast Reconstr Surg. 2009 Jul-Aug;25(4):330–2. PMID:19617803
1817. Küry S, Ebstein F, Mollé A, et al. Rare

Germline Heterozygous Missense Variants in BRCA1-Associated Protein 1, BAP1, Cause a Syndromic Neurodevelopmental Disorder. Am J Hum Genet. 2022 Feb 3;109(2):361–72. PMID:35051358
1818. Kutlubay Z, Bairamov O, Sevim A, et al. Rosai-Dorfman Disease: A Case Report with Nodal and Cutaneous Involvement and Review of the Literature. Am J Dermatopathol. 2014 Apr;36(4):353–7. PMID:23863552
1819. Kuznetsov JN, Aguero TH, Owens DA, et al. BAP1 Regulates Epigenetic Switch from Pluripotency to Differentiation in Developmental Lineages Giving Rise to BAP1-Mutant Cancers. Sci Adv. 2019 Sep 18;5(9):eaax1738. PMID:31555735
1820. Kwong YL, Lam CC, Chan TM. Post-Transplantation Lymphoproliferative Disease of Natural Killer Cell Lineage: A Clinicopathological and Molecular Analysis. Br J Haematol. 2000 Jul;110(1):197–202. PMID:10930998
1821. Kyllo RL, Brady KL, Hurst EA. Sebaceous Carcinoma: Review of the Literature. Dermatol Surg. 2015 Jan;41(1):1–15. PMID:25521100
1822. La Rosa M, Lionetti E, Reibaldi M, et al. Allergic Conjunctivitis: A Comprehensive Review of the Literature. Ital J Pediatr. 2013 Mar 14;39:18. PMID:23497516
1823. Labauge P, Krivosic V, Denier C, et al. Frequency of Retinal Cavernomas in 60 Patients with Familial Cerebral Cavernomas: A Clinical and Genetic Study. Arch Ophthalmol. 2006 Jun;124(6):885–6. PMID:16769843
1824. Labrador Velandia S, García Lagarto E, Saornil MA, et al. Primary Conjunctival Follicular Lymphoma Mimicking Chronic Conjunctivitis. Arch Soc Esp Oftalmol. 2016 Feb;91(2):86–9. PMID:26560164
1825. Lacey B, Rootman J, Marotta TR. Distensible Venous Malformations of the Orbit: Clinical and Hemodynamic Features and a New Technique of Management. Ophthalmology. 1999 Jun;106(6):1197–209. PMID:10366093
1826. Lack EE, Worsham GF, Callihan MD, et al. Granular Cell Tumor: A Clinicopathologic Study of 110 Patients. J Surg Oncol. 1980;13(4):301–16. PMID:6246310
1827. LaCroce SJ, Wilson MN, Romanowski JE, et al. Moraxella Nonliquefaciens and M. Osloensis Are Important Moraxella Species That Cause Ocular Infections. Microorganisms. 2019 Jun 4;7(6):163. PMID:31167433
1828. Lacy SE, Barrans SL, Beer PA, et al. Targeted Sequencing in DLBCL, Molecular Subtypes, and Outcomes: A Haematological Malignancy Research Network Report. Blood. 2020 May 14;135(20):1759–71. PMID:32187361
1829. Ladanyi M, Antonescu CR, Drobnjak M, et al. The Precrystalline Cytoplasmic Granules of Alveolar Soft Part Sarcoma Contain Monocarboxylate Transporter 1 and CD147. Am J Pathol. 2002 Apr;160(4):1215–21. PMID:11943706
1830. Ladanyi M, Antonescu CR, Leung DH, et al. Impact of SYT-SSX Fusion Type on the Clinical Behavior of Synovial Sarcoma: A Multi-Institutional Retrospective Study of 243 Patients. Cancer Res. 2002 Jan 1;62(1):135–40. PMID:11782370
1831. Ladanyi M, Lui MY, Antonescu CR, et al. The Der(17)T(X;17)(P11;Q25) of Human Alveolar Soft Part Sarcoma Fuses the TFE3 Transcription Factor Gene to ASPL, a Novel Gene at 17q25. Oncogene. 2001 Jan 4;20(1):48–57. PMID:11244503
1832. Lafaut BA, Mietz H, Ortmann M, et al. Melanocytoma of the Choroid: Angiographic and Histopathologic Findings. Ophthalmic Surg Lasers. 2002 Mar-Apr;33(2):158–62. PMID:11942551
1833. Laharanne E, Oumouhou N, Bonnet F, et al. Genome-Wide Analysis of Cutaneous T-Cell Lymphomas Identifies Three Clinically Relevant Classes. J Invest Dermatol. 2010 Jun;130(6):1707–18. PMID:20130593
1834. Lahat G, Dhuka AR, Hallevi H, et al. Angiosarcoma: Clinical and Molecular Insights. Ann Surg. 2010 Jun;251(6):1098–106. PMID:20485141
1835. Lahlou G, Classe M, Wassef M, et al. Sinonasal Inflammatory Myofibroblastic Tumor with Anaplastic Lymphoma Kinase 1 Rearrangement: Case Study and Literature Review. Head Neck Pathol. 2017 Jun;11(2):131–8. PMID:27443585
1836. Lai CT, Tai MC, Liang CM, et al. Unusual Uveal Tract Tumor: Mesectodermal Leiomyoma of the Ciliary Body. Pathol Int. 2004 May;54(5):337–42. PMID:15086838
1837. Laird PW, Grossniklaus HE, Hubbard GB. Ciliary Body Medulloepithelioma Associated with Pleuropulmonary Blastoma. Br J Ophthalmol. 2013 Aug;97(8):1079, 1086–7. PMID:23613510
1838. Lakatos K, Sterlich K, Pötschger U, et al. Langerhans Cell Histiocytosis of the Orbit: Spectrum of Clinical and Imaging Findings. J Pediatr. 2021 Mar;230:174–181.E1. PMID:33157073
1839. Lakhey M, Thakur SK, Mishra A, et al. Pleomorphic Adenoma of Lacrimal Gland: Diagnosis Based on Fine Needle Aspiration Cytology. Indian J Pathol Microbiol. 2001 Jul;44(3):333–5. PMID:12024925
1840. Lal G, Leavitt JA, Lindor NM, et al. Unilateral Lisch Nodules in the Absence of Other Features of Neurofibromatosis 1. Am J Ophthalmol. 2003 Apr;135(4):567–8. PMID:12654389
1841. Lally DR, Eagle RC, Wasserman BN. Occult Intraorbital Conjunctival Inclusion Cyst Discovered Almost 70 Years After Strabismus Surgery. J Pediatr Ophthalmol Strabismus. 2013 Apr 2:50 Online:e15-7. PMID:23557018
1842. Lally SE, Milman T, Orloff M, et al. Mutational Landscape and Outcomes of Conjunctival Melanoma in 101 Patients. Ophthalmology. 2022 Jun;129(6):679–93. PMID:35085662
1843. Lam A, Shields CL, Manquez ME, et al. Progressive Resorption of a Presumed Spontaneously Regressed Retinoblastoma Over 20 Years. Retina. 2005 Feb-Mar;25(2):230–1. PMID:15689823
1844. Lam C, Ou JC, Billingsley EM. "PTCH"-Ing it Together: A Basal Cell Nevus Syndrome Review. Dermatol Surg. 2013 Nov;39(11):1557–72. PMID:23725561
1845. Lam DS, Chow LT, Gandhi SR, et al. Benign Fibrous Histiocytoma of the Choroid. Eye (Lond). 1998;12(Pt 2):208–11. PMID:9683939
1846. Lam K, Brownstein S, Jordan DR, et al. Dacryops: A Series of 5 Cases and a Proposed Pathogenesis. JAMA Ophthalmol. 2013 Jul;131(7):929–32. PMID:23846204
1847. Lam KY. Langerhans Cell Histiocytosis (Histiocytosis X). Postgrad Med J. 1997 Jul;73(861):391–4. PMID:9338021
1848. Lam SC, Yuen HKL. Medical and Sclerosing Agents in the Treatment of Orbital Lymphatic Malformations: What's New? Curr Opin Ophthalmol. 2019 Sep;30(5):380–5. PMID:31232717
1849. Lam SW, Cleton-Jansen AM, Cleven AHG, et al. Molecular Analysis of Gene Fusions in Bone and Soft Tissue Tumors by Anchored Multiplex PCR-Based Targeted Next-Generation Sequencing. J Mol Diagn. 2018 Sep;20(5):653–63. PMID:30139549
1850. Lam SW, Cleven AHG, Kroon HM, et al. Utility of FOS as Diagnostic Marker for Osteoid Osteoma and Osteoblastoma. Virchows Arch. 2020 Mar;476(3):455–63. PMID:31768625
1851. Landau DA, Sun C, Rosebrock D, et al. The Evolutionary Landscape of Chronic Lymphocytic Leukemia Treated with Ibrutinib Targeted Therapy. Nat Commun. 2017 Dec 19;8(1):2185. PMID:29259203
1852. Landry M, Winkelmann RK. An Unusual Tubular Apocrine Adenoma. Arch Dermatol. 1972 Jun;105(6):869–79. PMID:4113017
1853. Lang FF, Miller DC, Pisharody S, et al. High Frequency of P53 Protein Accumulation Without P53 Gene Mutation in Human Juvenile Pilocytic, Low Grade and Anaplastic Astrocytomas. Oncogene. 1994 Mar;9(3):949–54. PMID:8108140
1854. Lang PG Jr, McKelvey AC, Nicholson JH. Three-Dimensional Reconstruction of the Superficial Multicentric Basal Cell Carcinoma Using Serial Sections and a Computer. Am J Dermatopathol. 1987 Jun;9(3):198–203. PMID:3631446
1855. Langham ME, Kramer T. Decreased Choroidal Blood Flow Associated with Retinitis Pigmentosa. Eye (Lond). 1990;4(Pt 2):374–81. PMID:2379647
1856. Laplant J, Cockerham K. Primary Malignant Orbital Tumors. J Neurol Surg B Skull Base. 2021 Feb;82(1):81–90. PMID:33777620
1857. Larque AB, Hakim S, Ordi J, et al. High-Risk Human Papillomavirus is Transcriptionally Active in a Subset of Sinonasal Squamous Cell Carcinomas. Mod Pathol. 2014 Mar;27(3):343–51. PMID:24030745
1858. Larrea-Oyarbide N, Valmaseda-Castellón E, Berini-Aytés L, et al. Osteomas of the Craniofacial Region. Review of 106 Cases. J Oral Pathol Med. 2008 Jan;37(1):38–42. PMID:18154576
1859. Larsen AC, Dahl C, Dahmcke CM, et al. BRAF Mutations in Conjunctival Melanoma: Investigation of Incidence, Clinicopathological Features, Prognosis and Paired Premalignant Lesions. Acta Ophthalmol. 2016 Aug;94(5):463–70. PMID:27009410
1860. Larsen AC, Dahmcke CM, Dahl C, et al. A Retrospective Review of Conjunctival Melanoma Presentation, Treatment, and Outcome and an Investigation of Features Associated With BRAF Mutations. JAMA Ophthalmol. 2015 Nov;133(11):1295–303. PMID:26425792
1861. Larsson PA, Lidén S. Prevalence of Skin Diseases Among Adolescents 12–16 Years of Age. Acta Derm Venereol. 1980;60(5):415–23. PMID:6162313
1862. Laskin WB, Weiss SW, Bratthauer GL. Epithelioid Variant of Malignant Peripheral Nerve Sheath Tumor (Malignant Epithelioid Schwannoma). Am J Surg Pathol. 1991 Dec;15(12):1136–45. PMID:1746681
1863. Lassaletta L, Torres-Martín M, Peña-Granero C, et al. NF2 Genetic Alterations in Sporadic Vestibular Schwannomas: Clinical Implications. Otol Neurotol. 2013 Sep;34(7):1355–61. PMID:23921927
1864. Lassalle S, Maschi C, Caujolle JP, et al. Inverted Conjunctival Papilloma: A Certainly Underestimated High-Risk Lesion for Carcinomatous Transformation-a Case Report. Can J Ophthalmol. 2017 Feb;52(1):e30–1. PMID:28237169
1865. Lassalle S, Nahon-Esteve S, Frouin E, et al. PD-L1 Expression in 65 Conjunctival Melanomas and Its Association with Clinical Outcome. Int J Mol Sci. 2020 Nov 30;21(23):9147. PMID:33266349
1866. Lattier JM, Yang H, Crawford S, et al. Host Pigment Epithelium-Derived Factor (PEDF) Prevents Progression of Liver Metastasis in a Mouse Model of Uveal Melanoma. Clin Exp Metastasis. 2013 Dec;30(8):969–76. PMID:23793989
1867. Lau LL, Lung CK, Ahmad SS. A Benign Presentation of Primary Ductal Adenocarcinoma of Lacrimal Gland: A Rare Malignancy. Indian J Ophthalmol. 2015 Nov;63(11):856–8. PMID:26669339
1868. Laukkanen K, Saarinen M, Mallet F, et al. Cutaneous T-Cell Lymphoma (CTCL) Cell Line-Derived Extracellular Vesicles Contain HERV-W-Encoded Fusogenic Syncytin-1. J Invest Dermatol. 2020 Jul;140(7):1466–1469. E4. PMID:31883959
1869. Launbjerg K, Bache I, Galanakis M, et al. von Hippel-Lindau Development in Children and Adolescents. Am J Med Genet A. 2017 Sep;173(9):2381–94. PMID:28650583
1870. Laver NM, Hidayat AA, Croxatto JO. Pleomorphic Adenocarcinomas of the Ciliary Epithelium. Immunohistochemical and Ultrastructural Features of 12 Cases. Ophthalmology. 1999 Jan;106(1):103–10. PMID:9917789
1871. Lavric A, Tsimpida M, Hungerford JL, et al. Mesectodermal Leiomyoma of the Ciliary Body Presenting as Anterior Staphyoma. Retin Cases Brief Rep. 2017 Summer;11(3):266–8. PMID:27258538
1872. Lazar AJ, Lyle S, Calonje E. Sebaceous Neoplasia and Torre-Muir Syndrome. Curr Diagn Pathol. 2007 Aug;13(4):301–19. PMID:18670585
1873. Lazo de La Vega L, Bick N, Hu K, et al. Invasive Squamous Cell Carcinomas and Precursor Lesions on UV-Exposed Epithelia Demonstrate Concordant Genomic Complexity in Driver Genes. Mod Pathol. 2020 Nov;33(11):2280–94. PMID:32461624
1874. Lazovich D, Isaksson Vogel R, Weinstock MA, et al. Association Between Indoor Tanning and Melanoma in Younger Men and Women. JAMA Dermatol. 2016 Mar;152(3):268–75. PMID:26818409
1875. Le Guellec S, Decouvelaere AV, Filleron T, et al. Malignant Peripheral Nerve Sheath Tumor Is a Challenging Diagnosis: A Systematic Pathology Review, Immunohistochemistry, and Molecular Analysis in 160 Patients From the French Sarcoma Group Database. Am J Surg Pathol. 2016 Jul;40(7):896–908. PMID:27158754
1876. Le Guin CHD, Metz KA, Kreis SH, et al. GNAQ Q209R Mutations Are Highly Specific for Circumscribed Choroidal Hemangioma. Cancers (Basel). 2019 Jul 22;11(7):1031. PMID:31336681
1877. Leatherbarrow B, Nerad JA, Carter KD, et al. Phakomatous Choristoma of the Orbit: A Case Report. Br J Ophthalmol. 1992 Aug;76(8):507–8. PMID:1390539
1878. LeBlanc RE, Miller DM, Zegans ME. PRAME Immunohistochemistry is Useful in the Evaluation of Conjunctival Melanomas, Nevi, and Primary Acquired Melanosis. J Cutan Pathol. 2021 Dec;48(12):1442–8. PMID:34089198
1879. LeBoit PE, Sexton M. Microcystic Adnexal Carcinoma of the Skin. A Reappraisal of the Differentiation and Differential Diagnosis of an Underrecognized Neoplasm. J Am Acad Dermatol. 1993 Oct;29(4):609–18. PMID:7691906
1880. Ledesma-Gil G, Essilfie J, Onishi A, et al. Presumed Retinal Pericapillary Astrocytic Hamartoma: Multimodal Imaging Findings of a Novel Hamartomatous Lesion. Br J Ophthalmol. 2021 Dec;105(12):1711–5. PMID:32980819
1881. Lee A, Yuen HKL, Tham CCY, et al. Conjunctival Adenosquamous Carcinoma Lacks MAML2 Translocation: A Variant of Squamous Cell Carcinoma With Mucoepidermoid Differentiation and Aggressive Behavior? Int J Surg Pathol. 2020 Dec;28(8):893–8. PMID:32476556
1882. Lee CS, Bae JH, Jeon IH, et al. Melanocytoma of the Optic Disk in the Korean Population. Retina. 2010 Nov-Dec;30(10):1714–20. PMID:20829742

1883. Lee DH, Jung SH, Yoon TM, et al. Characteristics of Paranasal Sinus Osteoma and Treatment Outcomes. Acta Otolaryngol. 2015 Jun;135(6):602–7. PMID:25719573

1884. Lee DW, Kwak SH, Kim JH, et al. Sebaceous Carcinoma Arising from Sebaceoma. Arch Craniofac Surg. 2021 Apr;22(2):126–30. PMID:33957741

1885. Lee DW, Yang JH, Chang S, et al. Clinical and Pathological Characteristics of Extradigital and Digital Glomus Tumours: A Retrospective Comparative Study. J Eur Acad Dermatol Venereol. 2011 Dec;25(12):1392–7. PMID:21371130

1886. Lee GA, Hirst LW. Incidence of Ocular Surface Epithelial Dysplasia in Metropolitan Brisbane. A 10-Year Survey. Arch Ophthalmol. 1992 Apr;110(4):525–7. PMID:1562262

1887. Lee GA, Hirst LW. Ocular Surface Squamous Neoplasia. Surv Ophthalmol. 1995 May-Jun;39(6):429–50. PMID:7660300

1888. Lee GL, Witman PM, Mosser JL, et al. A Case Series of Giant Molluscum Contagiosum in an Immigrant African Pediatric Population. Pediatr Dermatol. 2021 Nov;38(Suppl 2):113–6. PMID:34409645

1889. Lee HE, Zhang L. Immunoglobulin G4-Related Hepatobiliary Disease. Semin Diagn Pathol. 2019 Nov;36(6):423–33. PMID:31358425

1890. Lee J, Kim B, Lee H, et al. Whole Exome Sequencing Identifies Mutational Signatures of Vitreoretinal Lymphoma. Haematologica. 2020 Sep 1;105(9):e458–60. PMID:33054063

1891. Lee JA, Bank WO, Gonzalez-Melendez M, et al. Giant Cell Tumor of the Skull. Radiographics. 1998 Sep-Oct;18(5):1295–302. PMID:9747621

1892. Lee JS, Ko GH, Kim HC, et al. Langerhans Cell Sarcoma Arising from Langerhans Cell Histiocytosis: A Case Report. J Korean Med Sci. 2006 Jun;21(3):577–80. PMID:16778410

1893. Lee JY, Chung H, Cho H, et al. Clinical Characteristics and Treatment Outcomes of Isolated Myeloid Sarcoma Without Bone Marrow Involvement: A Single-Institution Experience. Blood Res. 2017 Sep;52(3):184–92. PMID:29043233

1894. Lee LH, Krupski C, Clark J, et al. High-Risk LCH in Infants is Serially Transplantable in a Xenograft Model But Responds Durably to Targeted Therapy. Blood Adv. 2020 Feb 25;4(4):717–27. PMID:32092141

1895. Lee MJ, Lee MY, Choe JY, et al. Ultra-Low-Dose Radiation Treatment for Early-Stage Ocular Adnexal MALT Lymphoma. Eur J Ophthalmol. 2022 Sep;32(5):3092–6. PMID:34318737

1896. Lee S, Park HY, Kang SY, et al. Genetic Alterations of JAK/STAT Cascade and Histone Modification in Extranodal NK/T-Cell Lymphoma Nasal Type. Oncotarget. 2015 Jul 10;6(19):17764–76. PMID:25980440

1897. Lee SE, Lee EH, Park H, et al. The Diagnostic Utility of the GNAS Mutation in Patients with Fibrous Dysplasia: Meta-Analysis of 168 Sporadic Cases. Hum Pathol. 2012 Aug;43(8):1234–42. PMID:22245114

1898. Lee SW, Park SH, Kim IH, et al. Nonsurgical Treatment of an Incompletely Excised Primary Adenocarcinoma of Nonpigmented Ciliary Epithelium. Tumori. 2007 Sep-Oct;93(5):514–7. PMID:18038890

1899. Lee V, Azari AA, Nehls S, et al. Leiomyoma of the Lower Eyelid. JAMA Ophthalmol. 2013 Aug;131(8):1085. PMID:23929515

1900. Lee V, Cree IA, Hungerford JL. Ring Melanoma–a Rare Cause of Refractory Glaucoma. Br J Ophthalmol. 1999 Feb;83(2):194–8. PMID:10396198

1901. Lee W, Teckie S, Wiesner T, et al. PRC2 is Recurrently Inactivated Through EED or SUZ12 Loss in Malignant Peripheral Nerve Sheath Tumors. Nat Genet. 2014 Nov;46(11):1227–32. PMID:25240281

1902. Lee YJ, Lee C, Kim MK, et al. Conjunctival Pigmented Lesion: Clinicopathological Analysis of 85 Cases in Korean Population. Sci Rep. 2019 Dec 3;9(1):18204. PMID:31796811

1903. Leeksma AC, Baliakas P, Moysiadis T et al. Genomic Arrays Identify High-Risk Chronic Lymphocytic Leukemia with Genomic Complexity: A Multi-Center Study. Haematologica. 2021 Jan 1;106(1):87–97. PMID:31974198

1904. Legius E, Marchuk DA, Collins FS, et al. Somatic Deletion of the Neurofibromatosis Type 1 Gene in a Neurofibrosarcoma Supports a Tumour Suppressor Gene Hypothesis. Nat Genet. 1993 Feb;3(2):122–6. PMID:8499945

1905. Legius E, Messiaen L, Wolkenstein P, et al. Revised Diagnostic Criteria for Neurofibromatosis Type 1 and Legius Syndrome: An International Consensus Recommendation. Genet Med. 2021 Aug;23(8):1506–13. PMID:34012067

1906. Lehman LJ, Hohberger GG, Buettner H, et al. Necrotic Melanocytoma of the Choroid in a 2-Year-Old Child. J Pediatr Ophthalmol Strabismus. 1997 Jan-Feb;34(1):40–3. PMID:9027679

1907. Lehrich BM, Goshtasbi K, Abiri A, et al. Treatment Modalities and Overall Survival Outcomes for Sinonasal Extranodal Natural Killer/T-Cell Lymphoma. Leuk Lymphoma. 2021 Mar;62(3):727–30. PMID:33054461

1908. Leibovitch I, Huilgol SC, Richards S, et al. Periocular Microcystic Adnexal Carcinoma: Management and Outcome with Mohs' Micrographic Surgery. Ophthalmologica. 2006;220(2):109–13. PMID:16491033

1909. Leibovitch I, Huilgol SC, Selva D, et al. Basal Cell Carcinoma Treated with Mohs Surgery in Australia III. Perineural Invasion. J Am Acad Dermatol. 2005 Sep;53(3):458–63. PMID:16112353

1910. Leibovitch I, McNab A, Sullivan T, et al. Orbital Invasion by Periocular Basal Cell Carcinoma. Ophthalmology. 2005 Apr;112(4):717–23. PMID:15808267

1911. Leidenix M, Mamalis N, Goodart R, et al. Malignant Transformation of a Necrotic Melanocytoma of the Choroid in an Amblyopic Eye. Ann Ophthalmol. 1994 Mar-Apr;26(2):42–6. PMID:8010703

1912. Leithner A, Windhager R, Lang S, et al. Aneurysmal Bone Cyst. A Population Based Epidemiologic Study and Literature Review. Clin Orthop Relat Res. 1999 Jun; (363):176–9. PMID:10379320

1913. Lemaître S, Lecler A, Lévy-Gabriel C, et al. Evisceration and Ocular Tumors: What Are the Consequences? J Fr Ophtalmol. 2017 Feb;40(2):93–101. PMID:28126270

1914. Lemke AJ, Hosten N, Bornfeld N, et al. Uveal Melanoma: Correlation of Histopathologic and Radiologic Findings by Using Thin-Section MR Imaging with a Surface Coil. Radiology. 1999 Mar;210(3):775–83. PMID:10207481

1915. Lenci LT, Shams P, Shriver EM, et al. Dermoid Cysts: Clinical Predictors of Complex Lesions and Surgical Complications. J AAPOS. 2017 Feb;21(1):44–7. PMID:28089745

1916. Lentzsch AM, Siggel R, Spital C, et al. Long-Time Follow-Up of Asymmetric Bilateral Diffuse Uveal Melanocytic Proliferation (BDUMP) in a Patient with Metastasized Urothelial Carcinoma. Retin Cases Brief Rep. 2023 Mar;17(2):105–10. PMID:33492075

1917. Leonardo D, Shields CL, Shields JA, et al. Recurrent Giant Orbital Dermoid of Infancy. J Pediatr Ophthalmol Strabismus. 1994 Jan-Feb;31(1):50–2. PMID:8195964

1918. Leporati P, Landek-Salgado MA, Lupi I, et al. IgG4-Related Hypophysitis: A New Addition to the Hypophysitis Spectrum. J Clin Endocrinol Metab. 2011 Jul;96(7):1971–80. PMID:21593109

1919. Leung KCP, Ko TCS. Orbital Hybrid Peripheral Nerve Sheath Tumors. Taiwan J Ophthalmol. 2020 Jul 27;10(3):181–3. PMID:33110748

1920. Levasseur SD, Wittenberg LA, White VA. Vitreoretinal Lymphoma: A 20-Year Review of Incidence, Clinical and Cytologic Features, Treatment, and Outcomes. JAMA Ophthalmol. 2013 Jan;131(1):50–5. PMID:23307208

1921. Levin LA, Jakobiec FA. Optic Nerve Tumors of Childhood: A Decision-Analytical Approach to Their Diagnosis. Int Ophthalmol Clin. 1992 Winter;32(1):223–40. PMID:1537660

1922. Levi-Schaffer F, Micera A, Zamir E, et al. Nerve Growth Factor and Eosinophils in Inflamed Juvenile Conjunctival Nevus. Invest Ophthalmol Vis Sci. 2002 Jun;43(6):1850–6. PMID:12036989

1923. Levy J, Ilsar M, Deckel Y, et al. Eyelid Pilomatrixoma: A Description of 16 Cases and a Review of the Literature. Surv Ophthalmol. 2008 Sep-Oct;53(5):526–35. PMID:18929763

1924. Levy J, Ilsar M, Deckel Y, et al. Lesions of the Caruncle: A Description of 42 Cases and a Review of the Literature. Eye (Lond). 2009 May;23(5):1004–18. PMID:18927596

1925. Lezcano C, Ho J, Seethala RR. Sox10 and DOG1 Expression in Primary Adnexal Tumors of the Skin. Am J Dermatopathol. 2017 Dec;39(12):896–902. PMID:28394798

1926. Lezcano C, Jungbluth AA, Nehal KS, et al. PRAME Expression in Melanocytic Tumors. Am J Surg Pathol. 2018 Nov;42(11):1456–65. PMID:30045064

1927. Li BK, Vasiljevic A, Dufour C, et al. Pineoblastoma Segregates into Molecular Sub-Groups with Distinct Clinico-Pathologic Features: A Rare Brain Tumor Consortium Registry Study. Acta Neuropathol. 2020 Feb;139(2):223–41. PMID:31820118

1928. Li E, Distefano A, Sinard J, et al. Epithelial-Myoepithelial Carcinoma Presenting as a Pseudo Veno-Lymphatic Malformation. Ophthalmic Plast Reconstr Surg. 2018 Sep/Oct;34(5):e157–60. PMID:30080758

1929. Li E, Silbert J, Sinard J. Pleomorphic Lipoma of the Bulbar Conjunctiva. BMJ Case Rep. 2018 Dec 13;11(1):e226548. PMID:30567236

1930. Li HC, Roux JJ, Pranikoff T, et al. Deep Juvenile Xanthogranuloma Presenting as a Chest Wall Mass: A Case Report. Acta Cytol. 2008 Sep-Oct;52(5):607–11. PMID:18833826

1931. Li HH, Zhou G, Fu XB, et al. Antigen Expression of Human Eccrine Sweat Glands. J Cutan Pathol. 2009 Mar;36(3):318–24. PMID:19032382

1932. Li J, Perry A, James CD, et al. Cancer-Related Gene Expression Profiles in NF1-Associated Pilocytic Astrocytomas. Neurology. 2001 Apr 10;56(7):885–90. PMID:11294925

1933. Li JY, Gaillard F, Moreau A, et al. Detection of Translocation T(11;14)(Q13;Q32) in Mantle Cell Lymphoma by Fluorescence In Situ Hybridization. Am J Pathol. 1999 May;154(5):1449–52. PMID:10329598

1934. Li S, Xu J, You MJ. The Pathologic Diagnosis of Mantle Cell Lymphoma. Histol Histopathol. 2021 Oct;36(10):1037–51. PMID:34114641

1935. Li W, Chen Y, Sun ZP, et al. Clinicopathological Characteristics of Immunoglobulin G4-Related Sialadenitis. Arthritis Res Ther. 2015 Jul 21;17(1):186. PMID:26194097

1936. Li W, Gragoudas ES, Egan KM. Metastatic Melanoma Death Rates by Anatomic Site After Proton Beam Irradiation for Uveal Melanoma. Arch Ophthalmol. 2000 Aug;118(8):1066–70. PMID:10922199

1937. Li WL, Buckley J, Sanchez-Lara PA, et al. A Rapid and Sensitive Next-Generation Sequencing Method to Detect RB1 Mutations Improves Care for Retinoblastoma Patients and Their Families. J Mol Diagn. 2016 Jul;18(4):480–93. PMID:27155049

1938. Li Y, Gao H, Li Z, et al. Clinical Characteristics of 76 Patients with IgG4-Related Hypophysitis: A Systematic Literature Review. Int J Endocrinol. 2019 Dec 18;2019:5382640. PMID:31929792

1939. Li Y, Yang QX, Tian XT, et al. Malignant Transformation of Nasal Chondromesenchymal Hamartoma in Adult: A Case Report and Review of the Literature. Histol Histopathol. 2013 Mar;28(3):337–44. PMID:23348387

1940. Liau JY, Tsai JH, Huang WC, et al. BRAF and KRAS Mutations in Tubular Apocrine Adenoma and Papillary Eccrine Adenoma of the Skin. Hum Pathol. 2018 Mar;73:59–65. PMID:29241739

1941. Lieb WE, Shields JA, Eagle RC Jr, et al. Cystic Adenoma of the Pigmented Ciliary Epithelium. Clinical, Pathologic, and Immunohistopathologic Findings. Ophthalmology. 1990 Nov;97(11):1489–93. PMID:1701528

1942. Liersch J, Carlson JA, Schaller J. Histopathological and Clinical Findings in Cutaneous Manifestation of Erdheim-Chester Disease and Langerhans Cell Histiocytosis Overlap Syndrome Associated With the BRAFV600E Mutation. Am J Dermatopathol. 2017 Jul;39(7):493–503. PMID:27898473

1943. Liesegang TJ. Pigmented Conjunctival and Scleral Lesions. Mayo Clin Proc. 1994 Feb;69(2):151–61. PMID:8309267

1944. Ligon AH, Moore SD, Parisi MA, et al. Constitutional Rearrangement of the Architectural Factor HMGA2: A Novel Human Phenotype Including Overgrowth and Lipomas. Am J Hum Genet. 2005 Feb;76(2):340–8. PMID:15593017

1945. Lim KPH, Milne P, Poidinger M, et al. Circulating CD1c+ Myeloid Dendritic Cells Are Potential Precursors to LCH Lesion CD1a+CD207+ Cells. Blood Adv. 2020 Jan 14;4(1):87–99. PMID:31899802

1946. Lim YH, Bacchiocchi A, Qiu J, et al. GNA14 Somatic Mutation Causes Congenital and Sporadic Vascular Tumors by MAPK Activation. Am J Hum Genet. 2016 Aug 4;99(2):443–50. PMID:27476652

1947. Lin CY, Tsai CC, Kao HC, et al. HMB-45 Negative Angiomyolipoma of the Orbit: A Case Report and Review of the Literature. BMC Ophthalmol. 2016 Jan 11;16:8. PMID:26754205

1948. Lin HC, Chu PH, Jung SM, et al. MUC5AC in Juvenile Conjunctival Nevus. Jpn J Ophthalmol. 2012 Mar;56(2):107–12. PMID:22139382

1949. Lin IC, Wu CT, Liao SL, et al. Primary Orbital Leiomyosarcoma. Ophthalmic Plast Reconstr Surg. 2005 Nov;21(6):451–3. PMID:16304526

1950. Lin PH, Kitaguchi Y, Mupas-Uy J, et al. Rescue Technique for Complete Removal of an Accidentally Ruptured Orbital Dumbbell Deep Dermoid Cyst: A Case Report. Am J Ophthalmol Case Rep. 2018 Feb 1;10:55–8. PMID:29780914

1951. Lin SY, Liao SL, Hong JB, et al. TERT Promoter Mutations in Periocular Carcinomas: Implications of Ultraviolet Light in Pathogenesis. Br J Ophthalmol. 2016 Feb;100(2):274–7. PMID:26472403

1952. Lin W, Lu S, Chen H, et al. Clinical Characteristics of Immunoglobulin G4-Related Disease: A Prospective Study of 118 Chinese Patients. Rheumatology (Oxford). 2015 Nov;54(11):1982–90. PMID:26106212

1953. Lincoff NS, Chung C, Balos L, et al. Combing the Globe for Terrorism. J Neuroophthalmol. 2012 Mar;32(1):82–5. PMID:22330854

1954. Lindau M, Bote R. [Hard Odontomas]. Stomatol DDR. 1987 Jun;37(6):356–62. German. PMID:3483101
1955. Lindegaard J, Heegaard S, Toft PB, et al. Malignant Transformation of a Medulloepithelioma of the Optic Nerve. Orbit. 2010 Jun;29(3):161–4. PMID:20497085
1956. Lindegaard J, Isager P, Prause JU, et al. Optic Nerve Invasion of Uveal Melanoma. APMIS. 2007 Jan;115(1):1–16. PMID:17223846
1957. Lindegaard J, Isager P, Prause JU, et al. Optic Nerve Invasion of Uveal Melanoma: Clinical Characteristics and Metastatic Pattern. Invest Ophthalmol Vis Sci. 2006 Aug;47(8):3268–75. PMID:16877391
1958. Linder JS, Harris GJ, Segura AD. Periorbital Infantile Myofibromatosis. Arch Ophthalmol. 1996 Feb;114(2):219–22. PMID:8573030
1959. Linn Murphree A. Intraocular Retinoblastoma: The Case for a New Group Classification. Ophthalmol Clin North Am. 2005 Mar;18(1):41–53, Viii. PMID:15763190
1960. Listernick R, Charrow J, Greenwald M, et al. Natural History of Optic Pathway Tumors in Children with Neurofibromatosis Type 1: A Longitudinal Study. J Pediatr. 1994 Jul;125(1):63–6. PMID:8021787
1961. Listernick R, Charrow J, Gutmann DH. Intracranial Gliomas in Neurofibromatosis Type 1. Am J Med Genet. 1999 Mar 26;89(1):38–44. PMID:10469435
1962. Listernick R, Darling C, Greenwald M, et al. Optic Pathway Tumors in Children: The Effect of Neurofibromatosis Type 1 on Clinical Manifestations and Natural History. J Pediatr. 1995 Nov;127(5):718–22. PMID:7472822
1963. Listernick R, Louis DN, Packer RJ, et al. Optic Pathway Gliomas in Children with Neurofibromatosis 1: Consensus Statement from the NF1 Optic Pathway Glioma Task Force. Ann Neurol. 1997 Feb;41(2):143–9. PMID:9029062
1964. Liu GY, Song H, Xu XL. Multiple Palisaded Encapsulated Neuromas in Siblings: A Case Report and Review of the Published Work. J Dermatol. 2016 May;43(5):560–3. PMID:26460241
1965. Liu H, Perugino CA, Ghebremichael M, et al. Disease Severity Linked to Increase in Autoantibody Diversity in IgG4-Related Disease. Arthritis Rheumatol. 2020 Apr;72(4):687–93. PMID:31612628
1966. Liu HL, Hoppe RT, Kohler S, et al. CD30+ Cutaneous Lymphoproliferative Disorders: The Stanford Experience in Lymphomatoid Papulosis and Primary Cutaneous Anaplastic Large Cell Lymphoma. J Am Acad Dermatol. 2003 Dec;49(6):1049–58. PMID:14639383
1967. Liu J, Ottaviani D, Sefta M, et al. A High-Risk Retinoblastoma Subtype with Stemness Features, Dedifferentiated Cone States and Neuronal/Ganglion Cell Gene Expression. Nat Commun. 2021 Sep 22;12(1):5578. PMID:34552068
1968. Liu L, Wu J, Geng J, et al. Geographical Prevalence and Risk Factors for Pterygium: A Systematic Review and Meta-Analysis. BMJ Open. 2013 Nov 19;3(11):e003787. PMID:24253031
1969. Liu M, Qin W, Yin Z. An Unusual Case of Primary Mesenchymal Chondrosarcoma in Orbit with Intracranial Extension. Clin Imaging. 2010 Sep-Oct;34(5):379–81. PMID:20813303
1970. Liu Q, Liu DY, Yang ZQ. Characteristics of Human Infection with Avian Influenza Viruses and Development of New Antiviral Agents. Acta Pharmacol Sin. 2013 Oct;34(10):1257–69. PMID:24096642
1971. Liu R, Wang N, Zhang H, et al. Clinical analysis of 109 cases of lacrimal gland pleomorphic adenoma. Int J Ophthalmol. 2021 Dec 18;14(12):1852–7. PMID:34926199
1972. Liu TYA, Ediriwickrema LS, Vizcaino MA, et al. Optic Nerve Infiltration and Vitreous Seeding by a Cerebral Glioblastoma. JAMA Ophthalmol. 2017 Apr 1;135(4):400–1. PMID:28208187
1973. Liu W, Yang Y, Qi S, et al. Treatment, Survival, and Prognosis of Advanced-Stage Natural Killer/T-Cell Lymphoma: An Analysis From the China Lymphoma Collaborative Group. Front Oncol. 2021 Feb 19;10:583050. PMID:33718104
1974. Liu Y, Su M, Yang Y, et al. Prognostic Factors Associated With Decreased Survival in Patients With Acinic Cell Carcinoma of the Parotid Gland. J Oral Maxillofac Surg. 2017 Feb;75(2):416–22. PMID:27474461
1975. Liu Y, Zheng Q, Wang C, et al. Granular Cell Tumors Overexpress TFE3 Without Gene Rearrangement: Evaluation of Immunohistochemistry and Break-Apart FISH in 45 Cases. Oncol Lett. 2019 Dec;18(6):6355–60. PMID:31788112
1976. Liu Z, Karp CL, Galor A, et al. Role of Optical Coherence Tomography Angiography in the Characterization of Vascular Network Patterns of Ocular Surface Squamous Neoplasia. Ocul Surf. 2020 Oct;18(4):926–35. PMID:32344147
1977. Liyanage SE, Saleh GM, Rose GE, et al. Delayed Diagnosis of Microcystic Adnexal Carcinoma in Progressive Eyelid Distortion. Arch Ophthalmol. 2010 Jan;128(1):132–5. PMID:20065232
1978. Liyanage SE, Watson GM, Wearne MJ. Late Ocular Manifestation of a Childhood Venous-Lymphatic Malformation. Eye (Lond). 2008 Sep;22(9):1194–5. PMID:18034192
1979. Liy-Wong C, Mohammed J, Carleton A, et al. The Relationship Between Neurofibromatosis Type 1, Juvenile Xanthogranuloma, and Malignancy: A Retrospective Case-Control Study. J Am Acad Dermatol. 2017 Jun;76(6):1084–7. PMID:28189268
1980. Llamas-Velasco M, Kempf W, Cota C, et al. Multiple Eruptive Epithelioid Hemangiomas: A Subset of Cutaneous Cellular Epithelioid Hemangioma With Expression of FOS-B. Am J Surg Pathol. 2019 Jan;43(1):26–34. PMID:29266025
1981. Llavero-Valero P, Garrido-Hermosilla AM, Díaz-Ruiz MC, et al. Giant Cell Tumour of Frontal Bone in a Patient with Bilateral Retinoblastoma. Arch Soc Esp Oftalmol (Engl Ed). 2019 Apr;94(4):200–3. PMID:30449636
1982. Lloyd WC 3rd, Eagle RC Jr, Shields JA, et al. Congenital Hypertrophy of the Retinal Pigment Epithelium. Electron Microscopic and Morphometric Observations. Ophthalmology. 1990 Aug;97(8):1052–60. PMID:2402417
1983. Lo C, Patel P, Charles NC. Langerhans Cell Histiocytosis Presenting as a Nodulo-Ulcerative Eyelid Lesion. Ophthalmic Plast Reconstr Surg. 2017 May/Jun;33(3S Suppl 1):S51–2. PMID:26359698
1984. Lochhead J, Benjamin L. Lymphangiectasia Haemorrhagica Conjunctivae. Eye (Lond). 1998;12(Pt 4):627–9. PMID:9850253
1985. Loeffler KU, Kivelä T, Borgmann H, et al. Malignant Tumor of the Retinal Pigment Epithelium with Extraocular Extension in a Phthisical Eye. Graefes Arch Clin Exp Ophthalmol. 1996 Aug;234(Suppl 1):S70–5. PMID:8871153
1986. Loghavi S, Khoury JD, Medeiros LJ. Epstein-Barr Virus-Positive Plasmacytoma in Immunocompetent Patients. Histopathology. 2015 Aug;67(2):225–34. PMID:25556356
1987. Logié A, Dunois-Lardé C, Rosty C, et al. Activating Mutations of the Tyrosine Kinase Receptor FGFR3 Are Associated with Benign Skin Tumors in Mice and Humans. Hum Mol Genet. 2005 May 1;14(9):1153–60. PMID:15772091
1988. Loh SH, Oh YJ, Lew BL, et al. Primary Cutaneous Apocrine Carcinoma. Ann Dermatol. 2016 Oct;28(5):669–70. PMID:27746659
1989. Lohmann DR, Gallie BL. Retinoblastoma. 2000 Jul 18 [Updated 2023 Sep 21]. In: Adam MP, Feldman J, Mirzaa GM, et al., editors. GeneReviews. Seattle (WA): University of Washington, Seattle; 1993-2025. PMID:20301625
1990. Löhr JM, Beuers U, Vujasinovic M, et al. European Guideline on IgG4-Related Digestive Disease - UEG and SGF Evidence-Based Recommendations. United European Gastroenterol J. 2020 Jul;8(6):637–66. PMID:32552502
1991. Lois N, Shields CL, Shields JA, et al. Primary Iris Stromal Cysts. A Report of 17 Cases. Ophthalmology. 1998 Jul;105(7):1317–22. PMID:9663240
1992. London J, Martin A, Soussan M, et al. Adult Onset Asthma and Periocular Xanthogranuloma (AAPOX), a Rare Entity With a Strong Link to IgG4-Related Disease: An Observational Case Report Study. Medicine (Baltimore). 2015 Oct;94(43):e1916. PMID:26512617
1993. Lopes M, Duffau H, Fleuridas G. Primary Spheno-Orbital Angiosarcoma: Case Report and Review of the Literature. Neurosurgery. 1999 Feb;44(2):405–7. PMID:9932897
1994. Lopez DR, Forcucci JA, O'Connor H, et al. PReferentially Expressed Antigen in MElanoma (PRAME) Expression in BRCA1-Associated Protein (BAP1)-Inactivated Melanocytic Tumors and Deep Penetrating Nevi: A Pilot Study. J Cutan Pathol. 2021 Apr;48(4):597–600. PMID:33094849
1995. Lopez-Nunez O, John I, Panasiti RN, et al. Infantile Inflammatory Myofibroblastic Tumors: Clinicopathological and Molecular Characterization of 12 Cases. Mod Pathol. 2020 Apr;33(4):576–90. PMID:31690781
1996. Lorillon G, Mourah S, Vercellino L, et al. Sustained Response to Salvage Therapy for Dabrafenib-Resistant Metastatic Langerhans Cell Sarcoma. Ann Oncol. 2016 Dec;27(12):2305–7. PMID:27502715
1997. LoRusso FJ, Boniuk M, Font RL. Melanocytoma (Magnocellular Nevus) of the Ciliary Body: Report of 10 Cases and Review of the Literature. Ophthalmology. 2000 Apr;107(4):795–800. PMID:10768345
1998. Louis DN, Perry A, Wesseling P, et al. The 2021 WHO Classification of Tumors of the Central Nervous System: A Summary. Neuro Oncol. 2021 Aug 2;23(8):1231–51. PMID:34185076
1999. Low JR, Bian Ng S, Sundar G. Undifferentiated Carcinoma of the Lacrimal Sac: Case Report and Review of Literature. Orbit. 2011 Dec;30(6):293–6. PMID:21957907
2000. Lu WY, Goldman M, Young B, et al. Optic Nerve Ganglioglioma. Case Report. J Neurosurg. 1993 Jun;78(6):979–82. PMID:8487083
2001. Lubo I, Fermin I, Massarelli O, et al. Perivascular Epithelioid Cell Tumour with Intraorbital Location: Report of a Case and Review of the Literature. Case Rep Pathol. 2016;2016:1936421. PMID:26925281
2002. Lubs ML, Bauer MS, Formas ME, et al. Lisch Nodules in Neurofibromatosis Type 1. N Engl J Med. 1991 May 2;324(18):1264–6. PMID:1901624
2003. Lucas DR, Unni KK, McLeod RA, et al. Osteoblastoma: Clinicopathologic Study of 306 Cases. Hum Pathol. 1994 Feb;25(2):117–34. PMID:8119712
2004. Lucas F, Larkin K, Gregory CT, et al. Novel BCL2 Mutations in Venetoclax-Resistant, Ibrutinib-Resistant CLL Patients with BTK/PLCG2 Mutations. Blood. 2020 Jun 11;135(24):2192–5. PMID:32232486
2005. Lucci LM, Anderson RL, Harrie RP, et al. Solitary Fibrous Tumor of the Orbit in a Child. Ophthalmic Plast Reconstr Surg. 2001 Sep;17(5):369–73. PMID:11642494
2006. Lue JK, O'Connor OA, Bertoni F. Targeting Pathogenic Mechanisms in Marginal Zone Lymphoma: From Concepts and Beyond. Ann Lymphoma. 2020 Sep 30;4:7. PMID:34667996
2007. Luengo-Alonso G, Mellado-Romero M, Shemesh S, et al. Denosumab Treatment for Giant-Cell Tumor of Bone: A Systematic Review of the Literature. Arch Orthop Trauma Surg. 2019 Oct;139(10):1339–49. PMID:30877429
2008. Lundgren L, Kindblom LG, Willems J, et al. Proliferative Myositis and Fasciitis. A Light and Electron Microscopic, Cytologic, DNA-Cytometric and Immunohistochemical Study. APMIS. 1992 May;100(5):437–48. PMID:1586481
2009. Luthra CL, Doxanas MT, Green WR. Lesions of the Caruncle: A Clinicohistopathologic Study. Surv Ophthalmol. 1978 Nov-Dec;23(3):183–95. PMID:216128
2010. Luthra R, Nemesure BB, Wu SY, et al. Frequency and Risk Factors for Pterygium in the Barbados Eye Study. Arch Ophthalmol. 2001 Dec;119(12):1827–32. PMID:11735795
2011. Lutsik P, Baude A, Mancarella D, et al. Globally Altered Epigenetic Landscape and Delayed Osteogenic Differentiation in H3.3-G34W-Mutant Giant Cell Tumor of Bone. Nat Commun. 2020 Oct 27;11(1):5414. PMID:33110075
2012. Lv M, Dong ZJ, Tong YX, et al. Retrospective Analysis of Clinicopathological Characteristics of Lacrimal Gland Pleomorphic Adenoma and Mechanism of Tumorigenesis by the Imbalance Between Apoptosis and Proliferation. Med Sci Monit. 2021 Mar 19;27:e929152. PMID:33737504
2013. Lynch TM, Gutmann DH. Neurofibromatosis 1. Neurol Clin. 2002 Aug;20(3):841–65. PMID:12432832
2014. Lyon DB, Tang TT, Kidder TM. Epithelioid Hemangioendothelioma of the Orbital Bones. Ophthalmology. 1992 Dec;99(12):1773–8. PMID:1480392
2015. Lyons LJ, Vrcek I, Somogyi M, et al. Natural Killer/T-Cell Lymphoma Invading the Orbit and Globe. Proc (Bayl Univ Med Cent). 2017 Oct;30(4):447–9. PMID:28966461
2016. Ma K, Xu L, Jie Y, et al. Prevalence of and Factors Associated with Pterygium in Adult Chinese: The Beijing Eye Study. Cornea. 2007 Dec;26(10):1184–6. PMID:18043173
2017. Maat W, Ly LV, Jordanova ES, et al. Monosomy of Chromosome 3 and an Inflammatory Phenotype Occur Together in Uveal Melanoma. Invest Ophthalmol Vis Sci. 2008 Feb;49(2):505–10. PMID:18234992
2018. Macagno N, Sohier P, Kervarrec T, et al. Recent Advances on Immunohistochemistry and Molecular Biology for the Diagnosis of Adnexal Sweat Gland Tumors. Cancers (Basel). 2022 Jan 18;14(3):476. PMID:35158743
2019. MacCarthy A, Birch JM, Draper GJ, et al. Retinoblastoma in Great Britain 1963-2002. Br J Ophthalmol. 2009 Jan;93(1):33–7. PMID:18838413
2020. Machado I, Cruz J, Lavernia J, et al. Solitary, Multiple, Benign, Atypical, or Malignant: The "Granular Cell Tumor" Puzzle. Virchows Arch. 2016 May;468(5):527–38. PMID:26637199
2021. Machado I, Yoshida A, Morales MGN, et al. Review with Novel Markers Facilitates Precise Categorization of 41 Cases of Diagnostically Challenging, "Undifferentiated Small Round Cell Tumors". A Clinicopathologic, Immunophenotypic and Molecular Analysis. Ann Diagn Pathol. 2018 Jun;34:1–12. PMID:29661713
2022. Machein MR, Plate KH. VEGF in Brain Tumors. J Neurooncol. 2000 Oct-Nov;50(1-2):109–20. PMID:11245271

2023. Mackie IA, Seal DV. The Questionably Dry Eye. Br J Ophthalmol. 1981 Jan;65(1):2–9. PMID:7448154
2024. Madreperla SA, Green WR, Daniel R, et al. Human Papillomavirus in Primary Epithelial Tumors of the Lacrimal Sac. Ophthalmology. 1993 Apr;100(4):569–73. PMID:8386822
2025. Maeda M, Morimoto A, Shioda Y, et al. Long-Term Outcomes of Children with Extracutaneous Juvenile Xanthogranulomas in Japan. Pediatr Blood Cancer. 2020 Jul;67(7):e28381. PMID:32383820
2026. Maegawa J, Yasumura K, Iwai T, et al. Malignant Melanoma of the Lacrimal Sac: A Case Report. Int J Dermatol. 2014 Feb;53(2):243–5. PMID:24261959
2027. Maeng M, Petrakos P, Zhou M, et al. Bi-Institutional Retrospective Study on the Demographics and Basic Clinical Presentation of Hidrocystomas. Orbit. 2017 Dec;36(6):433–5. PMID:28722532
2028. Magan T, Rapuano CJ, Ayres BD, et al. Actinic Granuloma of the Conjunctiva: Case Series and Review of the Literature. Am J Ophthalmol. 2021 Sep;229:120–6. PMID:33895150
2029. Magrini E, Pragliola A, Farnedi A, et al. Cytogenetic Analysis of Myoepithelial Cell Carcinoma of Salivary Gland. Virchows Arch. 2004 Jan;444(1):82–6. PMID:14994730
2030. Mahale A, Alkatan H, Alwadani S, et al. Altered Gene Expression in Conjunctival Squamous Cell Carcinoma. Mod Pathol. 2016 May;29(5):452–60. PMID:26916071
2031. Mahalingam M. MSH6, Past and Present and Muir-Torre Syndrome-Connecting the Dots. Am J Dermatopathol. 2017 Apr;39(4):239–49. PMID:28323777
2032. Mahdjoubi A, Cassoux N, Levy-Gabriel C, et al. Adult Ocular Medulloepithelioma Diagnosed by Transscleral Fine Needle Aspiration: A Case Report. Diagn Cytopathol. 2017 Jun;45(6):561–4. PMID:28217870
2033. Mahesh L, Krishnakumar S, Subramanian N, et al. Malignant Teratoma of the Orbit: A Clinicopathological Study of a Case. Orbit. 2003 Dec;22(4):305–9. PMID:14685907
2034. Mairot K, Sahakian N, Salgues B, et al. Somatostatin Receptor PET/CT Scan as a Helpful Diagnostic Tool for Optic Nerve Sheath Meningioma. J Fr Ophtalmol. 2021 Dec;44(10):e619–21. PMID:34229893
2035. Majewski S, Jablonska S. Human Papillomavirus-Associated Tumors of the Skin and Mucosa. J Am Acad Dermatol. 1997 May;36(5 Pt 1):659–85. PMID:9146528
2036. Majumdar K, Saran R, Tyagi I, et al. Cytodiagnosis of Alveolar Soft Part Sarcoma: Report of Two Cases with Special Emphasis on the First Orbital Lesion Diagnosed by Aspiration Cytology. J Cytol. 2013 Jan;30(1):58–61. PMID:23661945
2037. Mak ST. Eyelid Tumours and Pseudotumours in Hong Kong. Hong Kong Med J. 2013 Jun;19(3):277. PMID:23732436
2038. Makhlouf HR, Ishak KG, Shekar R, et al. Melanoma Markers in Angiomyolipoma of the Liver and Kidney: A Comparative Study. Arch Pathol Lab Med. 2002 Jan;126(1):49–55. PMID:11800647
2039. Makino K, Nakajima K, Tsutsumi S, et al. Mucoepidermoid Carcinoma of the Lacrimal Gland in a Patient with the CRTC1-MAML2 Fusion Gene. Radiol Case Rep. 2021 Oct 2;16(12):3643–6. PMID:34630791
2040. Mäkitie T, Summanen P, Tarkkanen A, et al. Microvascular Density in Predicting Survival of Patients with Choroidal and Ciliary Body Melanoma. Invest Ophthalmol Vis Sci. 1999 Oct;40(11):2471–80. PMID:10509639
2041. Mäkitie T, Summanen P, Tarkkanen A, et al. Microvascular Loops and Networks as Prognostic Indicators in Choroidal and Ciliary Body Melanomas. J Natl Cancer Inst. 1999 Feb 17;91(4):359–67. PMID:10050870
2042. Mäkitie T, Summanen P, Tarkkanen A, et al. Tumor-Infiltrating Macrophages (CD68(+) Cells) and Prognosis in Malignant Uveal Melanoma. Invest Ophthalmol Vis Sci. 2001 Jun;42(7):1414–21. PMID:11381040
2043. Maklad AM, Bayoumi Y, Tunio M, et al. Steroid-Resistant Extranodal Rosai-Dorfman Disease of Cheek Mass and Ptosis Treated with Radiation Therapy. Case Rep Hematol. 2013;2013:428297. PMID:23738161
2044. Maktabi AM, Almater AI, Alkatan HM. Periocular Intravascular Papillary Endothelial Hyperplasia: A Retrospective Study. Eur J Ophthalmol. 2022 Jul;32(4):1934–41. PMID:34615394
2045. Malempati S, Hawkins DS. Rhabdomyosarcoma: Review of the Children's Oncology Group (COG) Soft-Tissue Sarcoma Committee Experience and Rationale for Current COG Studies. Pediatr Blood Cancer. 2012 Jul 15;59(1):5–10. PMID:22378628
2046. Malhas AM, Sumathi VP, James SL, et al. Low-Grade Central Osteosarcoma: A Difficult Condition to Diagnose. Sarcoma. 2012;2012:764796. PMID:22851905
2047. Malick H, Kumari R, Lokovitis V, et al. Squamous Carcinoma Ex Pleomorphic Adenoma of the Lacrimal Gland. Orbit. 2022 Apr;41(2):260–3. PMID:33172316
2048. Malinowska I, Kwiatkowski DJ, Weiss S, et al. Perivascular Epithelioid Cell Tumors (PEComas) Harboring TFE3 Gene Rearrangements Lack the TSC2 Alterations Characteristic of Conventional PEComas: Further Evidence for a Biological Distinction. Am J Surg Pathol. 2012 May;36(5):783–4. PMID:22456611
2049. Mallipatna A, Gallie BL, Chévez-Barrios P, et al. Retinoblastoma. In: Amin MB, Edge S, Greene F, et al., editors. AJCC Cancer Staging Manual. 8th ed. New York (NY): Springer; 2017.
2051. Malta PG, Vilani DSRA, de Miranda CF, et al. Goldenhar Syndrome: The Importance of an Ophthalmological Approach. Rom J Ophthalmol. 2020 Oct-Dec;64(4):444–8. PMID:33367184
2052. Maly A, Epstein D, Meir K, et al. Histological Criteria for Grading of Atypia in Melanocytic Conjunctival Lesions. Pathology. 2008 Dec;40(7):676–81. PMID:18985522
2053. Mamaï O, Boussofara L, Denguezli M, et al. Multiple Self-Healing Palmoplantar Carcinoma: A Familial Predisposition to Skin Cancer with Primary Palmoplantar and Conjunctival Lesions. J Invest Dermatol. 2015 Jan;135(1):304–8. PMID:25050600
2054. Mancera N, Smalley KSM, Margo CE. Melanoma of the Eyelid and Periocular Skin: Histopathologic Classification and Molecular Pathology. Surv Ophthalmol. 2019 May-Jun;64(3):272–88. PMID:30578807
2055. Mandahl N, Fletcher CD, Dal Cin P, et al. Comparative Cytogenetic Study of Spindle Cell and Pleomorphic Leiomyosarcomas of Soft Tissues: A Report from the CHAMP Study Group. Cancer Genet Cytogenet. 2000 Jan 1;116(1):66–73. PMID:10616536
2056. Mandeville JT, Roh JH, Woog JJ, et al. Cutaneous Benign Mixed Tumor (Chondroid Syringoma) of the Eyelid: Clinical Presentation and Management. Ophthalmic Plast Reconstr Surg. 2004 Mar;20(2):110–6. PMID:15083078
2057. Mannami T, Yoshino T, Oshima K, et al. Clinical, Histopathological, and Immunogenetic Analysis of Ocular Adnexal Lymphoproliferative Disorders: Characterization of Malt Lymphoma and Reactive Lymphoid Hyperplasia. Mod Pathol. 2001 Jul;14(7):641–9. PMID:11454995
2058. Mansour AM, Barber JC, Reinecke RD, et al. Ocular Choristomas. Surv Ophthalmol. 1989 Mar-Apr;33(5):339–58. PMID:2655139
2059. Mansour AM, Hidayat AA. Metastatic Eyelid Disease. Ophthalmology. 1987 Jun;94(6):667–70. PMID:3627715
2060. Mansour AM, Wang F, Henkind P, et al. Ocular Findings in the Facioauriculovertebral Sequence (Goldenhar-Gorlin Syndrome). Am J Ophthalmol. 1985 Oct 15;100(4):555–9. PMID:4050929
2061. Mantelli F, Bruscolini A, La Cava M, et al. Ocular Manifestations of Sturge-Weber Syndrome: Pathogenesis, Diagnosis, and Management. Clin Ophthalmol. 2016 May 13;10:871–8. PMID:27257371
2062. Manz HJ, Rosen DA, Macklin RD, et al. Neuroectodermal Tumor of Anterior Lip of the Optic Cup. Glioneuroma Transitional to Teratoid Medullo-Epithelioma. Arch Ophthalmol. 1973 May;89(5):382–6. PMID:4697214
2063. Marafioti T, Copie-Bergman C, Calaminici M, et al. Another Look at Follicular Lymphoma: Immunophenotypic and Molecular Analyses Identify Distinct Follicular Lymphoma Subgroups. Histopathology. 2013 May;62(6):860–75. PMID:23509938
2064. Marback EF, Costa AL, Nossa LM, et al. Eyelid Skin Adenoid Cystic Carcinoma: A Clinicopathological Study of One Case Simulating Sebaceous Gland Carcinoma. Br J Ophthalmol. 2003 Jan;87(1):118–9. PMID:12488275
2065. Marchese C, Montera M, Torrini M, et al. Granular Cell Tumor in a PHTS Patient with a Novel Germline PTEN Mutation. Am J Med Genet A. 2003 Jul 15;120A(2):286–8. PMID:12833416
2066. Marginean FE, Lesnik M, Gauthier A, et al. The Accurate Cytological Diagnosis of Salivary Carcinoma Ex Pleomorphic Adenoma May Be Hampered by Myoepithelial Differentiation. Cytopathology. 2021 Jul;32(4):527–30. PMID:33528074
2067. Margo C, Hidayat A, Kopelman J, et al. Retinocytoma. A Benign Variant of Retinoblastoma. Arch Ophthalmol. 1983 Oct;101(10):1519–31. PMID:6626001
2068. Margo CE, Bombardier T. The Diagnostic Value of Fungal Autofluorescence. Surv Ophthalmol. 1985 Mar-Apr;29(5):374–6. PMID:3992475
2069. Margo CE, Brooks HL Jr. Adenocarcinoma of the Ciliary Epithelium in a 12-Year-Old Black Child. J Pediatr Ophthalmol Strabismus. 1991 Jul-Aug;28(4):232–5. PMID:1919972
2070. Margo CE, Folberg R, Zimmerman LE, et al. Endodermal Sinus Tumor (Yolk Sac Tumor) of the Orbit. Ophthalmology. 1983 Dec;90(12):1426–32. PMID:6677841
2071. Margo CE, Groden LR. Intraepithelial Neoplasia of the Conjunctiva with Mucoepidermoid Differentiation. Am J Ophthalmol. 1989 Nov 15;108(5):600–1. PMID:2817062
2072. Margo CE, Grossniklaus HE. Pseudoadenomatous Hyperplasia of the Conjunctiva. Ophthalmology. 2001 Jan;108(1):135–8. PMID:11150278
2073. Margo CE, Lessner A, Stern GA. Intraepithelial Sebaceous Carcinoma of the Conjunctiva and Skin of the Eyelid. Ophthalmology. 1992 Feb;99(2):227–31. PMID:1553212
2074. Margo CE, Lowery RL, Kerschmann RL. Lack of P53 Protein Immunoreactivity in Bilateral Diffuse Uveal Melanocytic Proliferation. Retina. 1997;17(5):434–6. PMID:9355192
2075. Margo CE, Mulla Z, Billiris K. Incidence of Surgically Treated Uveal Melanoma by Race and Ethnicity. Ophthalmology. 1998 Jun;105(6):1087–90. PMID:9627661
2076. Margo CE, Mulla ZD; Analysis of the Florida Cancer Registry. Malignant Tumors of the Orbit. Ophthalmology. 1998 Jan;105(1):185–90. PMID:9442797
2077. Margo CE, Pavan PR, Gendelman D, et al. Bilateral Melanocytic Uveal Tumors Associated with Systemic Non-Ocular Malignancy. Malignant Melanomas or Benign Paraneoplastic Syndrome? Retina. 1987 Fall;7(3):137–41. PMID:3423428
2078. Margo CE, White AA. Ocular Surface Squamous Neoplasia: Terminology that is Conceptually Friendly But Clinically Perilous. Eye (Lond). 2014 May;28(5):507–9. PMID:24807632
2079. Margolis S, Aleksic S, Charles N, et al. Retinal and Optic Nerve Findings in Goldenhar-Gorlin Syndrome. Ophthalmology. 1984 Nov;91(11):1327–33. PMID:6514297
2080. María Moral R, Monteagudo C, Muriel J, et al. Fluorescent In Situ Hybridization (FISH): A Useful Diagnostic Tool for Childhood Conjunctival Melanoma. Eur J Ophthalmol. 2022 Nov;32(6):NP13–9. PMID:34240653
2081. Mariani P, Dureau S, Savignoni A, et al. Development of a Prognostic Nomogram for Liver Metastasis of Uveal Melanoma Patients Selected by Liver MRI. Cancers (Basel). 2019 Jun 21;11(6):863. PMID:31234340
2082. Maric I, Pittaluga S, Dale JK, et al. Histologic Features of Sinus Histiocytosis with Massive Lymphadenopathy in Patients with Autoimmune Lymphoproliferative Syndrome. Am J Surg Pathol. 2005 Jul;29(7):903–11. PMID:15958855
2083. Marie PJ, de Pollak C, Chanson P, et al. Increased Proliferation of Osteoblastic Cells Expressing the Activating Gs Alpha Mutation in Monostotic and Polyostotic Fibrous Dysplasia. Am J Pathol. 1997 Mar;150(3):1059–69. PMID:9060842
2084. Maritati F, Peyronel F, Vaglio A. IgG4-Related Disease: A Clinical Perspective. Rheumatology (Oxford). 2020 May 1;59(Suppl 3):iii123–31. PMID:32348524
2085. Marshall AF, White DR, Shockley WW. Pleomorphic Adenoma in the Palpebral Lobe of the Lacrimal Gland. Otolaryngol Head Neck Surg. 2005 Jan;132(1):141–3. PMID:15632926
2086. Martel A, Lassalle S, Picard-Gauci A, et al. New Targeted Therapies and Immunotherapies for Locally Advanced Periocular Malignant Tumours: Towards a New 'Eye-Sparing' Paradigm? Cancers (Basel). 2021 Jun 5;13(11):2822. PMID:34198863
2087. Martelli G, Giardini R. Pilomatrix Carcinoma: A Case Report and Review of the Literature. Eur J Surg Oncol. 1994 Dec;20(6):703–4. PMID:7995429
2088. Marthin JK, Lindegaard J, Prause JU, et al. Lesions of the Lacrimal Drainage System: A Clinicopathological Study of 643 Biopsy Specimens of the Lacrimal Drainage System in Denmark 1910-1999. Acta Ophthalmol Scand. 2005 Feb;83(1):94–9. PMID:15715565
2089. Martignetti JA, Tian L, Li D, et al. Mutations in PDGFRB Cause Autosomal-Dominant Infantile Myofibromatosis. Am J Hum Genet. 2013 Jun 6;92(6):1001–7. PMID:23731542
2090. Martignoni G, Gobbo S, Camparo P, et al. Differential Expression of Cathepsin K in Neoplasms Harboring TFE3 Gene Fusions. Mod Pathol. 2011 Oct;24(10):1313–9. PMID:21602817
2091. Martin M, Maßhöfer L, Temming P, et al. Exome Sequencing Identifies Recurrent Somatic Mutations in EIF1AX and SF3B1 in Uveal Melanoma with Disomy 3. Nat Genet. 2013 Aug;45(8):933–6. PMID:23793026
2092. Martin PS, Rodgers CD, Fantin A, et al. Conjunctival Myxoid Stroma Tumor of the Palpebral Conjunctiva: A Case Report. Am J Ophthalmol Case Rep. 2022 Feb 18;26:101427. PMID:35243164
2093. Martinez V, Sissons HA. Aneurysmal Bone Cyst. A Review of 123 Cases Including Primary Lesions and Those Secondary to Other Bone Pathology. Cancer. 1988 Jun

1;61(11):2291–304. PMID:2835141
2094. Martinez-Lopez A, Curiel-Olmo S, Mollejo M, et al. MYD88 (L265P) Somatic Mutation in Marginal Zone B-Cell Lymphoma. Am J Surg Pathol. 2015 May;39(5):644–51. PMID:25723115
2095. Martín-Garcia D, Navarro A, Valdés-Mas R, et al. CCND2 and CCND3 Hijack Immunoglobulin Light-Chain Enhancers in Cyclin D1- Mantle Cell Lymphoma. Blood. 2019 Feb 28;133(9):940–51. PMID:30538135
2096. Maruyama K, Kunikata H, Sugita S, et al. First Case of Primary Intraocular Natural Killer T-Cell Lymphoma. BMC Ophthalmol. 2015 Nov 19;15:169. PMID:26585973
2097. Masamune A, Kikuta K, Hamada S, et al. Nationwide Epidemiological Survey of Autoimmune Pancreatitis in Japan in 2016. J Gastroenterol. 2020 Apr;55(4):462–70. PMID:31872350
2098. Mashayekhi A, Kaliki S, Walker B, et al. Metastasis from Uveal Melanoma Associated with Congenital Ocular Melanocytosis: A Matched Study. Ophthalmology. 2013 Jul;120(7):1465–8. PMID:23522968
2099. Mashayekhi A, Shukla SY, Shields JA, et al. Choroidal Lymphoma: Clinical Features and Association with Systemic Lymphoma. Ophthalmology. 2014 Jan;121(1):342–51. PMID:23978622
2100. Mashayekhi A, Siu S, Shields CL, et al. Slow Enlargement of Choroidal Nevi: A Long-Term Follow-Up Study. Ophthalmology. 2011 Feb;118(2):382–8. PMID:20801518
2101. Masoomian B, Lally SE, Shields JA, et al. Ophthalmic Manifestations of Rosai-Dorfman Disease in Five Patients. J Curr Ophthalmol. 2020 Jul 4;32(3):238–43. PMID:32775797
2102. Massi D, Carli P, Franchi A, et al. Naevus-Associated Melanomas: Cause or Chance? Melanoma Res. 1999 Feb;9(1):85–91. PMID:10338338
2103. Massone C, Cerroni L. Phenotypic Variability in Primary Cutaneous Anaplastic Large T-Cell Lymphoma: A Study on 35 Patients. Am J Dermatopathol. 2014 Feb;36(2):153–7. PMID:24394302
2104. Massone C, El-Shabrawi-Caelen L, Kerl H, et al. The Morphologic Spectrum of Primary Cutaneous Anaplastic Large T-Cell Lymphoma: A Histopathologic Study on 66 Biopsy Specimens from 47 Patients with Report of Rare Variants. J Cutan Pathol. 2008 Jan;35(1):46–53. PMID:18095994
2105. Massop DJ, Frederick PA, Li HJ, et al. Epibulbar Nodular Fasciitis. Case Rep Ophthalmol. 2016 May 10;7(1):262–7. PMID:27462253
2106. Massoth LR, Hung YP, Ferry JA, et al. Histiocytic and Dendritic Cell Sarcomas of Hematopoietic Origin Share Targetable Genomic Alterations Distinct from Follicular Dendritic Cell Sarcoma. Oncologist. 2021 Jul;26(7):e1263–72. PMID:33904632
2107. Mastorakos P, Hays MA, Caruso JP, et al. Transtentorial Dissemination of Optic Nerve Glioblastoma: Case Report. J Neurosurg. 2018 Feb;128(2):406–13. PMID:28298017
2108. Mastrangelo D, De Francesco S, Di Leonardo A, et al. Does the Evidence Matter in Medicine? The Retinoblastoma Paradigm. Int J Cancer. 2007 Dec 1;121(11):2501–5. PMID:17657745
2109. Mataftsi A, Zografos L, Balmer A, et al. Chiasmatic Infiltration Secondary to Late Malignant Transformation of Retinoma. Ophthalmic Genet. 2012 Sep;33(3):155–8. PMID:21526971
2110. Matatall KA, Agapova OA, Onken MD, et al. BAP1 Deficiency Causes Loss of Melanocytic Cell Identity in Uveal Melanoma. BMC Cancer. 2013 Aug 5;13:371. PMID:23915344
2111. Mathew JG, Bowman AS, Saab J, et al. Next-Generation Sequencing Analysis Suggests Varied Multistep Mutational Pathogenesis for Endocrine Mucin-Producing Sweat Gland Carcinoma with Comments on INSM1 and MUC2 Suggesting a Conjunctival Origin. J Am Acad Dermatol. 2022 May;86(5):1072–9. PMID:33515627
2112. Mathis T, Jardel P, Loria O, et al. New Concepts in the Diagnosis and Management of Choroidal Metastases. Prog Retin Eye Res. 2019 Jan;68:144–76. PMID:30240895
2113. Mathur R, Seah LL, Lim W, et al. High-Flow Hemangioblastoma of the Orbit. Ophthalmic Plast Reconstr Surg. 2008 Jan-Feb;24(1):67–9. PMID:18209654
2114. Matsui S, Yamamoto H, Minamoto S, et al. Proposed Diagnostic Criteria for IgG4-Related Respiratory Disease. Respir Investig. 2016 Mar;54(2):130–2. PMID:26879484
2115. Matsuo T, Tanaka T, Ichimura K, et al. Intraocular Relapse with Hypopyon and Retinal Infiltrates After Chemotherapy and Peripheral Blood Stem Cell Transplantation for Extranodal NK/T-Cell Lymphoma. J Clin Exp Hematop. 2015;55(3):157–61. PMID:26763364
2116. Matsuo T, Tanaka T, Yamasaki O. Lacrimal Sac Malignant Melanoma in 15 Japanese Patients: Case Report and Literature Review. J Investig Med High Impact Case Rep. 2019 Jan-Dec;7:2324709619888052. PMID:31747798
2117. Matter MS, Bihl M, Juskevicius D, et al. Is Rosai-Dorfman Disease a Reactve Process? Detection of a MAP2K1 L115V Mutation in a Case of Rosai-Dorfman Disease. Virchows Arch. 2017 Oct;471(4):545–7. PMID:28597077
2118. Matthews BJ, Mudhar HS, Rennie IG. Trans-Corneal Fine Cannula Aspiration: Rycroft Cannula Aspiration Technique for Sampling Iris Tumours. Br J Ophthalmol. 2012 Mar;96(3):329–31. PMID:21856690
2119. Maudgil A, Wagner BE, Rundle P, et al. Ocular Surface Foreign Bodies: Novel Findings Mimicking Ocular Malignant Melanoma. Eye (Lond). 2014 Nov;28(11):1370–4. PMID:25104745
2120. Mauriello JA Jr, Abdelsalam A, McLean IW. Adenoid Squamous Carcinoma of the Conjunctiva–a Clinicopathological Study of 14 Cases. Br J Ophthalmol. 1997 Nov;81(11):1001–5. PMID:9505827
2121. Mauriello JA Jr, Napolitano J, McLean I. Actinic Keratosis and Dysplasia of the Conjunctiva: A Clinicopathological Study of 45 Cases. Can J Ophthalmol. 1995 Oct;30(6):312–6. PMID:8574978
2122. Maurus K, Appenzeller S, Roth S, et al. Recurrent Oncogenic JAK and STAT Alterations in Cutaneous CD30-Positive Lymphoproliferative Disorders. J Invest Dermatol. 2020 Oct;140(10):2023–2031.E1. PMID:32147503
2123. Mauzo SH, Ferrarotto R, Bell D, et al. Molecular Characteristics and Potential Therapeutic Targets in Merkel Cell Carcinoma. J Clin Pathol. 2016 May;69(5):382–90. PMID:26818033
2124. Mavrikakis I, White VA, Heran M, et al. Orbital Mesenchymal Hamartoma with Rhabdomyomatous Features. Br J Ophthalmol. 2007 May;91(5):692–3. PMID:17446511
2125. Máximo V, Rios E, Sobrinho-Simões M. Oncocytic Lesions of the Thyroid, Kidney, Salivary Glands, Adrenal Cortex, and Parathyroid Glands. Int J Surg Pathol. 2014 Feb;22(1):33–6. PMID:24406625
2126. Mazloumi M, Dalvin LA, Abtahi SH, et al. Photodynamic Therapy in Ocular Oncology. J Ophthalmic Vis Res. 2020 Oct 25;15(4):547–58. PMID:33133446
2127. McCartney A. Intraocular Metastasis. Br J Ophthalmol. 1993 Mar;77(3):133. PMID:8457500
2128. McCarty CA, Fu CL, Taylor HR. Epidemiology of Pterygium in Victoria, Australia. Br J Ophthalmol. 2000 Mar;84(3):289–92. PMID:10684840
2129. McCarville MB, Muzzafar S, Kao SC, et al. Imaging Features of Alveolar Soft-Part Sarcoma: A Report from Children's Oncology Group Study ARST0332. AJR Am J Roentgenol. 2014 Dec;203(6):1345–52. PMID:25415714
2130. McClain KL, Bigenwald C, Collin M, et al. Histiocytic Disorders. Nat Rev Dis Primers. 2021 Oct 7;7(1):73. PMID:34620874
2131. McClain KL, Natkunam Y, Swerdlow SH. Atypical Cellular Disorders. Hematology Am Soc Hematol Educ Program. 2004:283–96. PMID:15561688
2132. McClellan SF, Ainbinder DJ. Orbital Rosai-Dorfman Disease: A Literature Review. Orbit. 2013 Oct;32(5):341–6. PMID:23895540
2133. McClintic EA, Ting A, Yeatts RP. Oral Propranolol as an Alternative Therapy for Orbital Angiolymphoid Hyperplasia With Eosinophilia. Ophthalmic Plast Reconstr Surg. 2016 Nov/Dec;32(6):e139–40. PMID:26954109
2134. McCulley JP, Moore MB, Matoba AY. Mucus Fishing Syndrome. Ophthalmology. 1985 Sep;92(9):1262–5. PMID:4058886
2135. McDermott EM, Weiss AP. Glomus Tumors. J Hand Surg Am. 2006 Oct;31(8):1397–400. PMID:17027805
2136. McDermott MB, Ponder TB, Dehner LP. Nasal Chondromesenchymal Hamartoma: An Upper Respiratory Tract Analogue of the Chest Wall Mesenchymal Hamartoma. Am J Surg Pathol. 1998 Apr;22(4):425–33. PMID:9537469
2137. McEachren TM, Brownstein S, Jordan DR, et al. Epithelioid Hemangioma of the Orbit. Ophthalmology. 2000 Apr;107(4):806–10. PMID:10768347
2138. McEvoy J, Nagahawatte P, Finkelstein D, et al. RB1 Gene Inactivation by Chromothripsis in Human Retinoblastoma. Oncotarget. 2014 Jan 30;5(2):438–50. PMID:24509483
2139. McGrath LA, Bacon JF, Rundle P, et al. A Case of a Cavitary Iris Melanoma with Aqueous Cytological Modulation. Ocul Oncol Pathol. 2019 Apr;5(3):171–5. PMID:31049323
2140. McKay KM, Sambrano BL, Fox PS, et al. Thickness of Superficial Basal Cell Carcinoma (SBCC) Predicts Imiquimod Efficacy: A Proposal for a Thickness-Based Definition of SBCC. Br J Dermatol. 2013 Sep;169(3):549–54. PMID:23627639
2141. McKelvie PA. Ocular Adnexal Lymphomas: A Review. Adv Anat Pathol. 2010 Jul;17(4):251–61. PMID:20574170
2142. McKelvie PA, Daniell M, McNab A, et al. Squamous Cell Carcinoma of the Conjunctiva: A Series of 26 Cases. Br J Ophthalmol. 2002 Feb;86(2):168–73. PMID:11815342
2143. McKenzie CA, Chen AC, Choy B, et al. Classification of High Risk Basal Cell Carcinoma Subtypes: Experience of the ONTRAC Study with Proposed Definitions and Guidelines for Pathological Reporting. Pathology. 2016 Aug;48(5):395–7. PMID:27311865
2144. McKey K, Zhang PJL, Shields CL, et al. Orbital Atypical Lipomatous Tumor/Well-Differentiated Liposarcoma Masquerading as Pleomorphic Lipoma: A Diagnostic Challenge. Ophthalmic Plast Reconstr Surg. 2019 May/Jun;35(3):e76–80. PMID:30908464
2145. McLean IW, Foster WD, Zimmerman LE, et al. Modifications of Callender's Classification of Uveal Melanoma at the Armed Forces Institute of Pathology. Am J Ophthalmol. 1983 Oct;96(4):502–9. PMID:6624832
2146. McLean IW, Keefe KS, Burnier MN. Uveal Melanoma. Comparison of the Prognostic Value of Fibrovascular Loops, Mean of the Ten Largest Nucleoli, Cell Type, and Tumor Size. Ophthalmology. 1997 May;104(5):777–80. PMID:9160022
2147. McLean IW, Saraiva VS, Burnier MN Jr. Pathological and Prognostic Features of Uveal Melanomas. Can J Ophthalmol. 2004 Jun;39(4):343–50. PMID:15327098
2148. McMahon RT, Font RL, McLean IW. Phakomatous Choristoma of Eyelid: Electron Microscopical Confirmation of Lenticular Derivation. Arch Ophthalmol. 1976 Oct;94(10):1778–81. PMID:973823
2149. McNab AA. Orbital Myositis: A Comprehensive Review and Reclassification. Ophthalmic Plast Reconstr Surg. 2020 Mar/Apr;36(2):109–17. PMID:31261163
2150. McNab AA, Jones RS, Hardy TG. Spheno-Orbital Lesions-A Major Review of Non-meningioma Causes. Ophthalmic Plast Reconstr Surg. 2021 Nov-Dec 01;37(6):522–33. PMID:33782321
2151. McNab AA, McKelvie P. IgG4-Related Ophthalmic Disease. Part II: Clinical Aspects. Ophthalmic Plast Reconstr Surg. 2015 May-Jun;31(3):167–78. PMID:25564258
2152. McNab AA, Satchi K. Recurrent Lacrimal Gland Pleomorphic Adenoma: Clinical and Computed Tomography Features. Ophthalmology. 2011 Oct;118(10):2088–92. PMID:21684609
2153. Medawar PB. Immunity to Homologous Grafted Skin; the Fate of Skin Homografts Transplanted to the Brain, to Subcutaneous Tissue, and to the Anterior Chamber of the Eye. Br J Exp Pathol. 1948 Feb;29(1):58–69. PMID:18865105
2154. Mee JJ, McNab AA, McKelvie P. Respiratory Epithelial Orbital Cysts. Clin Exp Ophthalmol. 2002 Oct;30(5):356–60. PMID:12213161
2155. Mehrad M, Stelow EB, Bishop JA, et al. Transcriptionally Active HPV and Targetable EGFR Mutations in Sinonasal Inverted Papilloma: An Association Between Low-Risk HPV, Condylomatous Morphology, and Cancer Risk? Am J Surg Pathol. 2020 Mar;44(3):340–6. PMID:31743131
2156. Mehraein Y, Wagner M, Remberger K, et al. Parvovirus B19 Detected in Rosai-Dorfman Disease in Nodal and Extranodal Manifestations. J Clin Pathol. 2006 Dec;59(12):1320–6. PMID:17142576
2157. Mehta NS, Tenzel PA, Sharfi D, et al. Orbital Glial Heterotopia: A Report of 2 Cases and Review of the Literature. Ophthalmic Plast Reconstr Surg. 2020 Jan/Feb;36(1):2–6. PMID:31348112
2158. Mehta SH, Switzer JA, Biddinger P, et al. IgG4-Related Leptomeningitis: A Reversible Cause of Rapidly Progressive Cognitive Decline. Neurology. 2014 Feb 11;82(6):540–2. PMID:24384648
2159. Meisler DM, Eiferman RA, Ratliff NB, et al. Surgical Management of Conjunctival Lymphangiectasis by Conjunctival Resection. Am J Ophthalmol. 2003 Oct;136(4):735–6. PMID:14516817
2160. Meister P, Bückmann FW, Konrad E. Extent and Level of Fascial Involvement in 100 Cases with Nodular Fasciitis. Virchows Arch A Pathol Anat Histol. 1978 Oct 26;380(2):177–85. PMID:153036
2161. Melchers RC, Willemze R, Bekkenk MW, et al. Frequency and Prognosis of Associated Malignancies in 504 Patients with Lymphomatoid Papulosis. J Eur Acad Dermatol Venereol. 2020 Feb;34(2):260–6. PMID:31715046
2162. Meli GA, Meli L, Chiaramonte R, et al. Osteoblastoma of the Orbit. A Case Report and Review of the Literature. Neuroradiol J. 2008 Feb 18;21(1):71–6. PMID:24256752
2163. Melo JV, Catovsky D, Galton DA. The Relationship Between Chronic Lymphocytic Leukaemia and Prolymphocytic Leukaemia. II. Patterns of Evolution of 'Prolymphocytoid' Transformation. Br J Haematol. 1986 Sep;64(1):77–86. PMID:3463362

2164. Melton JL, Rasmussen JE. Clinical Manifestations of Human Papillomavirus Infection in Nongenital Sites. Dermatol Clin. 1991 Apr;9(2):219–33. PMID:1647902
2165. Mencía-Gutiérrez E, Gutiérrez-Díaz E, García-Suárez E, et al. Eyelid Pilomatricomas in Young Adults: A Report of 8 Cases. Cutis. 2002 Jan;69(1):23–6. PMID:11829174
2166. Méndez-Martínez S, Santiago Varela M, Blanco-Teijeiro MJ, et al. Diagnosis and Long-Term Monitoring of Adenomas of the Ciliary Body Epithelium by Ultrasound Biomicroscopy. Eur J Ophthalmol. 2021 Jul;31(4):2032–41. PMID:32830591
2167. Mendlick MR, Nelson M, Pickering D, et al. Translocation T(1;3)(P36.3;Q25) is a Nonrandom Aberration in Epithelioid Hemangioendothelioma. Am J Surg Pathol. 2001 May;25(5):684–7. PMID:11342784
2168. Mendoza PR, Grossniklaus HE. Sentinel Lymph Node Biopsy for Eyelid and Conjunctival Tumors: What is the Evidence? Int Ophthalmol Clin. 2015 Winter;55(1):123–36. PMID:25436498
2169. Mendoza PR, Grossniklaus HE. The Biology of Retinoblastoma. Prog Mol Biol Transl Sci. 2015;134:503–16. PMID:26310174
2170. Mendoza PR, Jakobiec FA, Krane JF. Immunohistochemical Features of Lacrimal Gland Epithelial Tumors. Am J Ophthalmol. 2013 Dec;156(6):1147–1158.E1. PMID:23972314
2171. Mennel S, Meyer CH, Peter S, et al. Current Treatment Modalities for Exudative Retinal Hamartomas Secondary to Tuberous Sclerosis: Review of the Literature. Acta Ophthalmo Scand. 2007 Mar;85(2):127–32. PMID:17305725
2172. Menon V, Deshmukh R, Mulay K. A Rare Masquerade of Chalazion: Adenoid Cystic Carcinoma. Indian J Ophthalmol. 2019 Aug;67(8):1371–3. PMID:31332148
2173. Mensink HW, Vaarwater J, de Keizer RJ, et al. Chromosomal Aberrations in Iris Melanomas. Br J Ophthalmol. 2011 Mar;95(3):424–8. PMID:20881029
2174. Menter T, Dirnhofer S, Tzankov A. LEF1: A Highly Specific Marker for the Diagnosis of Chronic Lymphocytic B Cell Leukaemia/Small Lymphocytic B Cell Lymphoma. J Clin Pathol. 2015 Jun;68(6):473–8. PMID:25713417
2175. Menter T, Gasser A, Juskevicius D, et al. Diagnostic Utility of the Germinal Center-Associated Markers GCET1, HGAL, and LMO2 in Hematolymphoid Neoplasms. Appl Immunohistochem Mo Morphol. 2015 Aug;23(7):491–8. PMID:25203428
2176. Menter T, Trivedi P, Ahmad R, et al. Diagnostic Utility of Lymphoid Enhancer Binding Factor 1 Immunohistochemistry in Small B-Cell Lymphomas. Am J Clin Pathol. 2017 Mar 1;147(3):292–300. PMID:28395058
2177. Mentzel T, Beham A, Katenkamp D, et al. Fibrosarcomatous ("High-Grade") Dermatofibrosarcoma Protuberans: Clinicopathologic and Immunohistochemical Study of a Series of 41 Cases with Emphasis on Prognostic Significance. Am J Surg Pathol. 1998 May;22(5):576–87. PMID:9591728
2178. Mentzel T, Dei Tos AP, Sapi Z, et al. Myopericytoma of Skin and Soft Tissues: Clinicopathologic and Immunohistochemical Study of 54 Cases. Am J Surg Pathol. 2006 Jan;30(1):104–13. PMID:16330949
2179. Mentzel T, Schildhaus HU, Palmedo G, et al. Postradiation Cutaneous Angiosarcoma After Treatment of Breast Carcinoma is Characterized by MYC Amplification in Contrast to Atypical Vascular Lesions After Radiotherapy and Control Cases: Clinicopathological, Immunohistochemical and Molecular Analysis of 66 Cases. Mod Pathol. 2012 Jan;25(1):75–85. PMID:21909081
2180. Menzies SW, Liyanarachchi S, Coates E, et al. Estimated Risk of Progression of Lentigo Maligna to Lentigo Maligna Melanoma. Melanoma Res. 2020 Apr;30(2):193–7. PMID:31095041
2181. Merani R, Khannah G, Mann S, et al. Orbital Leiomyoma: A Case Report with Clinical, Radiological and Pathological Correlation. Clin Exp Ophthalmol. 2005 Aug;33(4):408–11. PMID:16033356
2183. Merritt H, Pfeiffer ML, Richani K, et al. Erdheim-Chester Disease with Orbital Involvement: Case Report and Ophthalmic Literature Review. Orbit. 2016 Aug;35(4):221–6. PMID:27322549
2184. Merritt N, Garcia K, Rajendran D, et al. TAZ-CAMTA1 and YAP-TFE3 Alter the TAZ/YAP Transcriptome by Recruiting the ATAC Histone Acetyltransferase Complex. Elife. 2021 Apr 29;10(Apr):10. PMID:33913810
2185. Meshkani SE, Kooshan N, Moghadam AB, et al. Signaling Roadmap to Epithelial-Mesenchymal Transition in Pterygium, TWIST1 Centralized. J Cell Physiol. 2019 Aug;234(10):18146–55. PMID:30847945
2186. Messiaen LM, Callens T, Mortier G, et al. Exhaustive Mutation Analysis of the NF1 Gene Allows Identification of 95% of Mutations and Reveals a High Frequency of Unusual Splicing Defects. Hum Mutat. 2000;15(6):541–55. PMID:10862084
2187. Messmer E, Font RL, Laqua H, et al. Cavernous Hemangioma of the Retina. Immunohistochemical and Ultrastructural Observations. Arch Ophthalmol. 1984 Mar;102(3):413–8. PMID:6538410
2188. Messmer EP, Font RL, McCrary JA 3rd, et al. Epithelioid Angiosarcoma of the Orbit Presenting as Tolosa-Hunt Syndrome. A Clinicopathologic Case Report with Review of the Literature. Ophthalmology. 1983 Dec;90(12):1414–21. PMID:6687155
2189. Messner KS, Braniecki M. Palisaded Encapsulated Neuroma: An Entity to Consider in the Differential Diagnosis of the Eyelid Nodule. A Case Report. Ophthalmic Plast Reconstr Surg. 2011 Mar-Apr;27(2):e35–7. PMID:20683368
2190. Mester J, Eng C. Cowden Syndrome: Recognizing and Managing a Not-So-Rare Hereditary Cancer Syndrome. J Surg Oncol. 2015 Jan;111(1):125–30. PMID:25132236
2191. Meunier J, Lumbroso-Le Rouic L, Vincent-Salomon A, et al. Ophthalmologic and Intraocular Non-Hodgkin's Lymphoma: A Large Single Centre Study of Initial Characteristics, Natural History, and Prognostic Factors. Hematol Oncol. 2004 Dec;22(4):143–58. PMID:16134191
2192. Meyer CH, Becker R, Schmidt JC, et al. [When is Congenital Hypertrophy of the Retinal Pigment Epithelium (CHRPE) Associated with the Gardner's Syndrome? An Overview with Clinical Examples]. Klin Monbl Augenheilkd. 2002 Sep;219(9):644–8. German. PMID:12410463
2193. Meyerle CB, Dahr SS, Wetjen NM, et al. Clinical Course of Retrobulbar Hemangioblastomas in von Hippel-Lindau Disease. Ophthalmology. 2008 Aug;115(8):1382–9. PMID:18395800
2194. Meza-Romero R, Navarrete-Dechent C, Downey C. Molluscum Contagiosum: An Update and Review of New Perspectives in Etiology, Diagnosis, and Treatment. Clin Cosmet Investig Dermatol. 2019 May 30;12:373–81. PMID:31239742
2195. Michel JB, Nochy D, Choudat L, et al. Consequences of Renal Morphologic Damage Induced by Inhibition of Converting Enzyme in Rat Renovascular Hypertension. Lab Invest. 1987 Oct;57(4):402–11. PMID:2823006
2196. Michels RG, Knox DL, Erozan YS, et al. Intraocular Reticulum Cell Sarcoma. Diagnosis by Pars Plana Vitrectomy. Arch Ophthalmol. 1975 Dec;93(12):1331–5. PMID:1106372
2197. Miesbauerová M, Tommola S, Šteiner P, et al. Cytopathological Features of Secretory Carcinoma of Salivary Glands and Ancillary Techniques in its Diagnostics: Impact of New Milan System for Reporting Salivary Gland Cytopathology. APMIS. 2019 Jul;127(7):491–502. PMID:30942913
2198. Miettinen MM, Antonescu CR, Fletcher CDM, et al. Histopathologic Evaluation of Atypical Neurofibromatous Tumors and Their Transformation into Malignant Peripheral Nerve Sheath Tumor in Patients with Neurofibromatosis 1-a Consensus Overview. Hum Pathol. 2017 Sep;67:1–10. PMID:28551330
2199. Mihic-Probst D, Mnich CD, Oberholzer PA, et al. P16 Expression in Primary Malignant Melanoma is Associated with Prognosis and Lymph Node Status. Int J Cancer. 2006 May 1;118(9):2262–8. PMID:16331607
2200. Mikami M, Koizumi H, Ishii M, et al. The Identification of Monoclonality in Fibrous Dysplasia by Methylation-Specific Polymerase Chain Reaction for the Human Androgen Receptor Gene. Virchows Arch. 2004 Jan;444(1):56–60. PMID:14576938
2201. Mikkelsen LH, Andreasen S, Melchior LC, et al. Genomic and Immunohistochemical Characterisation of a Lacrimal Gland Oncocytoma and Review of Literature. Oncol Lett. 2017 Oct;14(4):4176–82. PMID:28943925
2202. Milbratz GH, Borges FP, Cintra MB, et al. Orbital Invasion by Squamous Cell Carcinoma Arising in Multiple Epidermoid Cysts. Ophthalmic Plast Reconstr Surg. 2012 Nov-Dec;28(6):e144–5. PMID:22460681
2203. Miles SL, Niles RM, Pittock S, et al. A Factor Found in the IgG Fraction of Serum of Patients with Paraneoplastic Bilateral Diffuse Uveal Melanocytic Proliferation Causes Proliferation of Cultured Human Melanocytes. Retina. 2012 Oct;32(9):1959–66. PMID:22791177
2204. Miliauskas JR, Orell SR. Fine-Needle Aspiration Cytological Findings in Five Cases of Epithelial-Myoepithelial Carcinoma of Salivary Glands. Diagn Cytopathol. 2003 Mar;28(3):163–7. PMID:12619100
2205. Miller CV, Wolf A, Klingenstein A, et al. Clinical Outcome of Advanced Squamous Cell Carcinoma of the Conjunctiva. Eye (Lond). 2014 Aug;28(8):962–7. PMID:24858526
2206. Miller NR. Primary Tumours of the Optic Nerve and its Sheath. Eye (Lond). 2004 Nov;18(11):1026–37. PMID:15534587
2207. Miller RS, Ball KL, Comi AM, et al. Growth Hormone Deficiency in Sturge-Weber Syndrome. Arch Dis Child. 2006 Apr;91(4):340–1. PMID:16551788
2208. Milman T, Eiger-Moscovich M, Henry RK, et al. Cyclin D1 Expression and Molecular Genetic Findings in Periocular Histiocytoses and Neoplasms of Macrophage-Dendritic Cell Lineage. Am J Ophthalmol. 2022 Oct;242:36–51. PMID:35594918
2209. Milman T, Eiger-Moscovich M, Henry RK, et al. Validation of the Newly Proposed World Health Organization Classification System for Conjunctival Melanocytic Intraepithelial Lesions: A Comparison with the C-MIN and PAM Classification Schemes. Am J Ophthalmol. 2021 Mar;223:60–74. PMID:33130046
2209A. Milman T, Grossniklaus HE, Eagle RC Jr, et al. Protocol for the Examination of Specimens from Patients with Retinoblastoma. Version: Retinoblastoma 4.1.0.0. Northfield (IL): College of American Pathologists; 2021 Jun. Available from: https://www.cap.org/protocols-and-guidelines/cancer-reporting-tools/cancer-protocol-templates.
2210. Milman T, Hu DN, McCormick SA, et al. Expression of Neurotrophin Receptors by Retinoinvasive Uveal Melanoma. Melanoma Res. 2012 Apr;22(2):164–8. PMID:22343487
2211. Milman T, Iacob C, Lauer S, et al. Adenocarcinoma, Not Otherwise Specified, Arising in Accessory Lacrimal Gland: A Diagnostic Challenge. Ocul Oncol Pathol. 2018 Sep;4(2):67–72. PMID:30320083
2212. Milman T, Iacob C, McCormick SA. Hybrid Cysts of the Eyelid with Follicular and Apocrine Differentiation: An Under-Recognized Entity? Ophthalmic Plast Reconstr Surg. 2008 Mar-Apr;24(2):122–5. PMID:18356717
2213. Milman T, Ida CM, Zhang PJL, et al. Gene Fusions in Ocular Adnexal Tumors. Am J Ophthalmol. 2021 Jan;221:211–25. PMID:32800827
2214. Milman T, Jakobiec FA, Lally SE, et al. Lacrimal Gland Hamartoma (Formerly Termed Dacryoadenoma). Am J Ophthalmol. 2020 Sep;217:189–97. PMID:32360334
2215. Milman T, McCormick SA. The Molecular Genetics of Eyelid Tumors: Recent Advances and Future Directions. Graefes Arch Clin Exp Ophthalmol. 2013 Feb;251(2):419–33. PMID:23275038
2216. Milman T, Mudhar HS, Eagle RC Jr. PAX8 Expression in the Crystalline Lens and Lens-Derived Lesions. Ophthalmol Sci. 2021 Apr 18;1(2):100024. PMID 36249298
2217. Milman T, Salomao DR, Ida CM, et al. Conjunctival Myxoid Lesions: Clinical-Pathologic Multiparametric Analysis, Including Molecular Genetics (An American Ophthalmological Society Thesis). Am J Ophthalmol. 2019 Sep;205:115–31. PMID:31078543
2218. Milman T, Shields CL, Brooks JSJ, et al. Primary Cutaneous Angiosarcoma of the Eyelid: A Diagnostic and Therapeutic Challenge. Ocul Oncol Pathol. 2018 Jun;4(4):230–5. PMID:30643767
2219. Milman T, Shields JA, Husson M, et al. Primary Ductal Adenocarcinoma of the Lacrimal Gland. Ophthalmology. 2005 Nov;112(11):2048–51. PMID:16271319
2220. Milman T, Zhang Q, Ang S, et al. Immunohistochemical Profiling of Conjunctival Melanocytic Intraepithelial Lesions, Including SOX10, HMB45, Ki67, and P16. Am J Ophthalmol. 2021 Feb;222:148–56. PMID:33002436
2221. Milne P, Bigley V, Bacon CM, et al. Hematopoietic Origin of Langerhans Cell Histiocytosis and Erdheim-Chester Disease in Adults. Blood. 2017 Jul 13;130(2):167–75. PMID:28512190
2222. Mir F, Alnajar H, Rohra P, et al. Metastatic Granular Cell Tumor to the Breast Diagnosed by Fine Needle Aspiration Cytology: A Case Report with Review of the Literature. Diagn Cytopathol. 2019 Mar;47(3):226–9. PMID:30589232
2223. Misago N, Mihara I, Ansai S, et al. Sebaceoma and Related Neoplasms with Sebaceous Differentiation: A Clinicopathologic Study of 30 Cases. Am J Dermatopathol. 2002 Aug;24(4):294–304. PMID:12142617
2224. Misago N, Toda S. Sebaceous Carcinoma Within Rippled/Carcinoid Pattern Sebaceoma. J Cutan Pathol. 2016 Jan;43(1):64–70. PMID:26268140
2225. Mishra A, Heathcote JG, LaRoche GR. Optic Nerve Choristoma Causing Vision Loss in an Adolescent. Can J Ophthalmol. 2017 Aug;52(4):e138–40. PMID:28774539
2226. Mishra DK, Jakati S, Bothra N, et al. Pleomorphic Lipoma of Conjunctiva - An Unusual Tumor at Unusual Site. Indian J Pathol Microbiol. 2020 Oct-Dec;63(4):654–5. PMID:33154330
2227. Mishra DK, Taneja S, Singh V, et al.

Histopathological Spectrum of Ocular Surface Squamous Neoplasia: A Retrospective Study of 776 Lesions. Indian J Pathol Microbiol. 2022 Jan-Mar;65(1):3–7. PMID:35074957
2228. Missotten GS, Gambrelle J, de Wolff-Rouendaal D, et al. Epistaxis or Epiphora as a Sign for Extension of a Conjunctival Melanoma. A Series of Six Patients with Nasolacrimal Recurrence. Br J Ophthalmol. 2010 Oct;94(10):1328–31. PMID:20584717
2229. Missotten GS, van Santbrink-Bakker H, de Keizer RJ. Dumbbell-Shaped Dermoid Cysts. Acta Ophthalmol. 2010 Mar;88(2):e11–2. PMID:19016659
2230. Mistry K, Levell NJ, Hollestein L, et al. Trends in Incidence, Treatment and Survival of Merkel Cell Carcinoma in England 2004-2018: A Cohort Study. Br J Dermatol. 2023 Feb 10;188(2):228–36. PMID:36763882
2231. Mittal R, Araujo I, Czanner G, et al. Perforin Expression in Eyelid Sebaceous Carcinomas: A Useful and Specific Immunomarker for the Differential Diagnosis of Eyelid Carcinomas. Acta Ophthalmol. 2016 Aug;94(5):e325–30. PMID:26843360
2232. Mittal R, Cherepanoff S, Thornton S, et al. Bilateral Diffuse Uveal Melanocytic Proliferation: Molecular Genetic Analysis of a Case and Review of the Literature. Ocul Oncol Pathol. 2015 Dec;2(2):94–9. PMID:27171825
2233. Mittal R, Ganguly A, Rath S, et al. IgG4-Related Orbital Inflammation Presenting as Bilateral Proptosis in a Child. Eye (Lond). 2014 Oct;28(10):1264–6. PMID:24993327
2234. Mittal R, Rath S, Vemuganti GK. Ocular Surface Squamous Neoplasia - Review of Etio-Pathogenesis and an Update on Clinico-Pathological Diagnosis. Saudi J Ophthalmol. 2013 Jul;27(3):177–86. PMID:24227983
2235. Mittal R, Tripathy D. Sebaceoma of the Eyelid: A Rare Entity. Can J Ophthalmol. 2014 Jun;49(3):e78–80. PMID:24862791
2236. Mittal S, Goswami C, Kanoria N, et al. Post-Irradiation Angiosarcoma of Bone. J Cancer Res Ther. 2007 Apr-Jun;3(2):96–9. PMID:17998731
2237. Mitter D, Ullmann R, Muradyan A, et al. Genotype-Phenotype Correlations in Patients with Retinoblastoma and Interstitial 13q Deletions. Eur J Hum Genet. 2011 Sep;19(9):947–58. PMID:21505449
2238. Miyazawa A, Inoue M, Hirakata A, et al. Expression of Inhibin Alpha by Stromal Cells of Retinal Angiomas Excised from a Patient with von Hippel-Lindau Disease. Jpn J Ophthalmol. 2009 Sep;53(5):501–5. PMID:19847606
2239. Mizushima I, Kasashima S, Fujinaga Y, et al. Clinical and Pathological Characteristics of IgG4-Related Periaortitis/Periarteritis and Retroperitoneal Fibrosis Diagnosed Based on Experts' Diagnosis. Ann Vasc Dis. 2019 Dec 25;12(4):460–72. PMID:31942203
2240. Mlakar J, Kocjan BJ, Hošnjak L, et al. Morphological Characteristics of Conjunctival Squamous Papillomas in Relation to Human Papillomavirus Infection. Br J Ophthalmol. 2015 Mar;99(3):431–6. PMID:25527693
2241. Mocan MC, Bozkurt B, Orhan D, et al. Juvenile Xanthogranuloma of the Corneal Limbus: Report of Two Cases and Review of the Literature. Cornea. 2008 Jul;27(6):739–42. PMID:18580271
2242. Mogaddam AS, Memar B, Aledavood A, et al. Isolated Orbital Endodermal Sinus Tumor. Ophthalmic Plast Reconstr Surg. 2007 Nov-Dec;23(6):477–9. PMID:18030121
2243. Mohadjer Y, Holds JB, Rootman J, et al. The Spectrum of Orbital Rosai-Dorfman Disease. Ophthalmic Plast Reconstr Surg. 2006 May-Jun;22(3):163–8. PMID:16714922
2244. Mohajeri A, Tayebwa J, Collin A, et al. Comprehensive Genetic Analysis Identifies a Pathognomonic NAB2/STAT6 Fusion Gene, Nonrandom Secondary Genomic Imbalances, and a Characteristic Gene Expression Profile in Solitary Fibrous Tumor. Genes Chromosomes Cancer. 2013 Oct;52(10):873–86. PMID:23761323
2245. Mohney BG, Robertson DM, Schomberg PJ, et al. Second Nonocular Tumors in Survivors of Heritable Retinoblastoma and Prior Radiation Therapy. Am J Ophthalmol. 1998 Aug;126(2):269–77. PMID:9727521
2246. Mojtahed A, Schrijver I, Ford JM, et al. A Two-Antibody Mismatch Repair Protein Immunohistochemistry Screening Approach for Colorectal Carcinomas, Skin Sebaceous Tumors, and Gynecologic Tract Carcinomas. Mod Pathol. 2011 Jul;24(7):1004–14. PMID:21499234
2247. Molho-Pessach V, Ramot Y, Camille F, et al. H Syndrome: The First 79 Patients. J Am Acad Dermatol. 2014 Jan;70(1):80–8. PMID:24172204
2248. Møller P, Seppälä T, Bernstein I, et al. Cancer Incidence and Survival in Lynch Syndrome Patients Receiving Colonoscopic and Gynaecological Surveillance: First Report from the Prospective Lynch Syndrome Database. Gut. 2017 Mar;66(3):464–72. PMID:26657901
2249. Møller P, Seppälä T, Bernstein I, et al. Incidence of and Survival After Subsequent Cancers in Carriers of Pathogenic MMR Variants with Previous Cancer: A Report from the Prospective Lynch Syndrome Database. Gut. 2017 Sep;66(9):1657–64. PMID:27261338
2250. Moloney TP, Trinh T, Farrah JJ. A Case of Conjunctival Mucoepidermoid Carcinoma in Australia. Clin Ophthalmol. 2014;8:11–4. PMID:24363552
2251. Molteni R, Biavasco R, Stefanoni D, et al. Oncogene-Induced Maladaptive Activation of Trained Immunity in the Pathogenesis and Treatment of Erdheim-Chester Disease. Blood. 2021 Oct 28;138(17):1554–69. PMID:34077954
2252. Mombaerts I, Ramberg I, Coupland SE, et al. Diagnosis of Orbital Mass Lesions: Clinical, Radiological, and Pathological Recommendations. Surv Ophthalmol. 2019 Nov-Dec;64(6):741–56. PMID:31276737
2253. Monroe AK, Burkholder BM, Butler NJ, et al. Sclerouveitis Associated with Rosai-Dorfman Disease in an HIV-Infected Patient. Ocul Immunol Inflamm. 2014 Jun;22(3):236–8. PMID:24564426
2254. Monroe EJ. Brief Description of ISSVA Classification for Radiologists. Tech Vasc Interv Radiol. 2019 Dec;22(4):100628. PMID:31864528
2255. Monsereenusorn C, Rodriguez-Galindo C. Clinical Characteristics and Treatment of Langerhans Cell Histiocytosis. Hematol Oncol Clin North Am. 2015 Oct;29(5):853–73. PMID:26461147
2256. Montalban A, Liétin B, Louvrier C, et al. Malignant Lacrimal Sac Tumors. Eur Ann Otorhinolaryngol Head Neck Dis. 2010 Nov;127(5):165–72. PMID:21036121
2257. Montes TL, Agra MV, Alonso MSM, et al. Conjunctival Leiomyosarcoma: A Case Report and Review of Literature. Indian J Ophthalmol. 2017 May;65(5):406–8. PMID:28573999
2258. Montes-Mojarro IA, Chen BJ, Ramirez-Ibarguen AF, et al. Mutational Profile and EBV Strains of Extranodal NK/T-Cell Lymphoma, Nasal Type in Latin America. Mod Pathol. 2020 May;33(5):781–91. PMID:31822801
2259. Montgomery EA, Dry SM. Pleomorphic Rhabdomyosarcoma. In: WHO Classification of Tumours Editorial Board. Soft Tissue and Bone Tumours. Lyon (France): International Agency for Research on Cancer; 2020. pp. 209–10. (WHO Classification of Tumours Series, 5th ed.; vol. 3). https://publications.iarc.who.int/588.
2260. Moody S, Escudero-Ibarz L, Wang M, et al. Significant Association Between TNFAIP3 Inactivation and Biased Immunoglobulin Heavy Chain Variable Region 4-34 Usage in Mucosa-Associated Lymphoid Tissue Lymphoma. J Pathol. 2017 Sep;243(1):3–8. PMID:28682481
2261. Moore RF, Zhang XR, Allison DB, et al. High-Risk Human Papillomavirus and ZEB1 in Ocular Adnexal Sebaceous Carcinoma. J Cutan Pathol. 2021 Aug;48(8):1027–33. PMID:33745190
2262. Mooy CM, Luyten GP, de Jong PT, et al. Immunohistochemical and Prognostic Analysis of Apoptosis and Proliferation in Uveal Melanoma. Am J Pathol. 1995 Oct;147(4):1097–104. PMID:7573354
2263. Mor JM, Rokohl AC, Koch KR, et al. Sentinel Lymph Node Biopsy in the Management of Conjunctival Melanoma: Current Insights. Clin Ophthalmol. 2019 Jul 23;13:1297–302. PMID:31440020
2264. Morales AT, Cignarella AG, Jabeen IS, et al. An Update on IgG4-Related Lung Disease. Eur J Intern Med. 2019 Aug;66:18–24. PMID:31227290
2265. Moran DJ, Hollows FC. Pterygium and Ultraviolet Radiation: A Positive Correlation. Br J Ophthalmol. 1984 May;68(5):343–6. PMID:6712914
2266. Moran JM, Phelps PO. Periocular Skin Cancer: Diagnosis and Management. Dis Mon. 2020 Oct;66(10):101046. PMID:32600650
2267. Moran S, Martínez-Cardús A, Sayols S, et al. Epigenetic Profiling to Classify Cancer of Unknown Primary: A Multicentre, Retrospective Analysis. Lancet Oncol. 2016 Oct;17(10):1386–95. PMID:27575023
2268. Morawala A, Bothra N, Dendukuri G, et al. Solitary Fibrous Tumors of the Lacrimal Drainage System With Variable Orbital and Sinonasal Extensions: Combined External and Endoscopic Surgical Approach. Ophthalmic Plast Reconstr Surg. 2020 Jul/Aug;36(4):403–9. PMID:31990895
2269. Morawala A, Bothra N, Mishra DK, et al. Poorly Differentiated Primary Adenocarcinoma of the Lacrimal Sac and the Nasolacrimal Duct. Orbit. 2020 Aug;39(4):289–92. PMID:31684800
2270. Morawala A, Mohamed A, Krishnamurthy A, et al. Sebaceous Gland Carcinoma: Analysis Based on the 8th Edition of American Joint Cancer Committee Classification. Eye (Lond). 2023 Mar;37(4):714–9. PMID:35347292
2271. Moret A, Tabareau-Delalande F, Joly A, et al. [Myoepithelial Carcinoma of the Lacrimal Gland]. Rev Stomatol Chir Maxillofac Chir Orale. 2014 Jun;115(3):172–7. French. PMID:24456911
2272. Morgan NV, Morris MR, Cangul H, et al. Mutations in SLC29A3, Encoding an Equilibrative Nucleoside Transporter ENT3, Cause a Familial Histiocytosis Syndrome (Faisalabad Histiocytosis) and Familial Rosai-Dorfman Disease. PLoS Genet. 2010 Feb 5;6(2):e1000833. PMID:20140240
2273. Morgan-Warren PJ, Madge SN. Lacrimal Duct Cyst (Dacryops) Following Ocular Chemical Injury. Orbit. 2012 Oct;31(5):335–7. PMID:22571599
2274. Mori H, Takahashi K. A Case of Adenocarcinoma of the Retinal Pigment Epithelium: An Immunohistochemical and Electron Microscopic Study. Ocul Oncol Pathol. 2017 Dec;4(1):38–43. PMID:29344497
2275. Mori T, Sukeda A, Sekine S, et al. SOX10 Expression as Well as BRAF and GNAQ/11 Mutations Distinguish Pigmented Ciliary Epithelium Neoplasms From Uveal Melanomas. Invest Ophthalmol Vis Sci. 2017 Oct 1;58(12):5445–51. PMID:29059311
2276. Morita M, Murase T, Okumura Y, et al. Clinicopathological Significance of EGFR Pathway Gene Mutations and CRTC1/3-MAML2 Fusions in Salivary Gland Mucoepidermoid Carcinoma. Histopathology. 2020 Jun;76(7):1013–22. PMID:32129900
2277. Moritz EN, Giacometti JN. Palisading Encapsulated Neuroma of the Eyelid. JAMA Ophthalmol. 2022 Feb 1;140(2):e214790. PMID:35175297
2278. Morotti RA, Nicol KK, Parham DM, et al. An Immunohistochemical Algorithm to Facilitate Diagnosis and Subtyping of Rhabdomyosarcoma: The Children's Oncology Group Experience. Am J Surg Pathol. 2006 Aug;30(8):962–8. PMID:16861966
2279. Morris WR, Fleming JC. Respiratory Choristomatous Cysts in the Temporal Orbit. Ophthalmic Plast Reconstr Surg. 2001 Nov;17(6):462–4. PMID:11766031
2280. Morrow NC, Tanas MR, Syed NA, et al. Solitary Adult Orbital Myofibroma: Report of a Case and Review of the Literature. Am J Ophthalmol Case Rep. 2020 Oct 9;20:100955. PMID:33089011
2281. Morschhauser F, Fowler NH, Feugier P, et al. Rituximab Plus Lenalidomide in Advanced Untreated Follicular Lymphoma. N Engl J Med. 2018 Sep 6;379(10):934–47. PMID:30184451
2282. Moser S, Borm J, Mihic-Probst D, et al. Metastatic Basal Cell Carcinoma: Report of a Case and Review of the Literature. Oral Surg Oral Med Oral Pathol Oral Radiol. 2014 Feb;117(2):e79–82. PMID:23313228
2283. Mosquera JM, Sboner A, Zhang L, et al. Novel MIR143-NOTCH Fusions in Benign and Malignant Glomus Tumors. Genes Chromosomes Cancer. 2013 Nov;52(11):1075–87. PMID:23999936
2284. Moss HB, Sines DT, Blatt J, et al. Epithelioid Hemangioma Responsive to Oral Propranolol. Ophthalmic Plast Reconstr Surg. 2012 Jul-Aug;28(4):e88–90. PMID:22186982
2285. Mossé YP, Voss SD, Lim MS, et al. Targeting ALK With Crizotinib in Pediatric Anaplastic Large Cell Lymphoma and Inflammatory Myofibroblastic Tumor: A Children's Oncology Group Study. J Clin Oncol. 2017 Oct 1;35(28):3215–21. PMID:28787259
2286. Mota CP, Silva Cunha JL, Magalhães MCSV, et al. Oral Juvenile Xanthogranuloma: A Clinicopathological, Immunohistochemical and BRAF V600E Study of Five New Cases, with Literature Review. Head Neck Pathol. 2022 Jun;16(2):407–15. PMID:34414559
2287. Mourah S, Lorillon G, Meignin V, et al. Dramatic Transient Improvement of Metastatic BRAF(V600E)-Mutated Langerhans Cell Sarcoma Under Treatment with Dabrafenib. Blood. 2015 Dec 10;126(24):2649–52. PMID:26468227
2288. Mouriaux F, Vincent S, Kherrouche Z, et al. Microphthalmia Transcription Factor Analysis in Posterior Uveal Melanomas. Exp Eye Res. 2003 Jun;76(6):653–61. PMID:12742347
2289. Movahedi M, Bishop DT, Macrae F, et al. Obesity, Aspirin, and Risk of Colorectal Cancer in Carriers of Hereditary Colorectal Cancer: A Prospective Investigation in the CAPP2 Study. J Clin Oncol. 2015 Nov 1;33(31):3591–7. PMID:26282643
2290. Movassaghian M, Brunner AM, Blonquist TM, et al. Presentation and Outcomes Among Patients with Isolated Myeloid Sarcoma: A Surveillance, Epidemiology, and End Results Database Analysis. Leuk Lymphoma. 2015 Jun;56(6):1698–703. PMID:25213180
2291. Moyer AB, Roberts J, Olsen RJ, et al. Human Papillomavirus-Driven Squamous Lesions: High-Risk Genotype Found in Conjunctival Papillomas, Dysplasia, and Carcinoma. Am J Dermatopathol. 2018

Jul;40(7):486–90. PMID:29533279
2292. Mudhar HS, Bata BM, Quhill H, et al. Uveal Melanoma and Paraneoplastic Perivascular Dermal Melanocytic Proliferation in the Setting of Bilateral Diffuse Uveal Melanocytic Proliferation: The Potential Role of the Hepatocyte Growth Factor/C-Met Axis in Their Pathogenesis. Ocul Oncol Pathol. 2021 Dec;7(6):418–27. PMID:35087819
2293. Mudhar HS, Doherty R, Salawu A, et al. Immunohistochemical and Molecular Pathology of Ocular Uveal Melanocytoma: Evidence for Somatic GNAQ Mutations. Br J Ophthalmol. 2013 Jul;97(7):924–8. PMID:23685997
2294. Mudhar HS, Doherty RE, Salvi SM, et al. Genetic Profiling of Primary Orbital Melanoma: An Analysis of 6 Cases with Clinicopathologic Correlation. Ophthalmology. 2019 Jul;126(7):1045–52. PMID:30605742
2295. Mudhar HS, Krishna Y, Cross S, et al. A Multicenter Study Validates the WHO 2022 Classification for Conjunctival Melanocytic Intraepithelial Lesions With Clinical and Prognostic Relevance. Lab Invest. 2024 Jan;104(1):100281. PMID:37924948
2296. Mudhar HS, McGrath LA, Chung AKK, et al. Ocular Surface Fibroma: Clinical, Histopathological, and Immunohistochemical Features of 10 Cases. Ocul Oncol Pathol. 2020 May;6(3):196–202. PMID:32509765
2297. Mudhar HS, Milman T, Eagle RC Jr, et al. Usefulness of PAX8 Immunohistochemistry in Adult Intraocular Tumor Diagnosis. Ophthalmology. 2021 May;128(5):765–78. PMID:33002562
2298. Mudhar HS, Milman T, Zhang PJL, et al. Conjunctival 'Mucoepidermoid Carcinoma' Revisited: A Revision of Terminology, Based on Morphologic, Immunohistochemical and Molecular Findings of 14 Cases, and the 2018 WHO Classification of Tumours of the Eye. Mod Pathol. 2020 Jul;33(7):1242–55. PMID:31932683
2299. Mudhar HS, Nurrudin M. Ossifying Cystic Odontogenic and Schneiderian Choristoma of the Orbit. Orbit. 2014 Feb;33(1):59–61. PMID:24171664
2300. Mudhar HS, Pavel M, Chung AKK, et al. Two Cases of STAT6-Positive, Primary Conjunctival Giant Cell-Rich Solitary Fibrous Tumour (Giant Cell Angiofibroma) with Some Unusual Histological Features. Ocul Oncol Pathol. 2020 Oct;6(5):328–32. PMID:33123525
2301. Mudhar HS, Salvi SS, Pissaloux D, et al. Single Time Frame Overview of the Genetic Changes in Conjunctival Melanoma from Intraepithelial Disease to Invasive Melanoma: A Study of 4 Exenteration Specimens Illustrating the Potential Role of Cyclin D1. Ocul Oncol Pathol. 2022 Feb;8(1):52–63. PMID:35356600
2302. Mudhar HS, Saunders E, Rundle P, et al. The In Vivo Modulatory Effects of an Anterior-Chamber Microenvironment on Uveal Melanoma. Br J Ophthalmol. 2009 Apr;93(4):535–40. PMID:19019926
2303. Mudhar HS, Scott I, Ul-Hassan A, et al. Bilateral Diffuse Uveal Melanocytic Hyperplasia: Molecular Characterization and Novel Association with Bilateral Renal Papillary Carcinoma. Histopathology. 2012 Oct;61(4):751–4. PMID:22803781
2304. Mudhar HS, Smith K, Talley P, et al. Fluorescence In Situ Hybridisation (FISH) in Histologically Challenging Conjunctival Melanocytic Lesions. Br J Ophthalmol. 2013 Jan;97(1):40–6. PMID:23137666
2305. Mueller AJ, Freeman WR, Schaller UC, et al. Complex Microcirculation Patterns Detected by Confocal Indocyanine Green Angiography Predict Time to Growth of Small Choroidal Melanocytic Tumors: MuSIC Report II. Ophthalmology. 2002 Dec;109(12):2207–14. PMID:12466160
2306. Mukherjee B, Kadaskar J, Priyadarshini O, et al. Angiolymphoid Hyperplasia with Eosinophilia of the Orbit and Adnexa. Ocul Oncol Pathol. 2015 Sep;2(1):40–7. PMID:27171790
2307. Mulay K, Aggarwal E, White VA. Periocular Sebaceous Gland Carcinoma: A Comprehensive Review. Saudi J Ophthalmol. 2013 Jul;27(3):159–65. PMID:24227981
2308. Mulay K, Ali MJ, Honavar SG, et al. Orbital Alveolar Soft-Part Sarcoma: Clinico-Pathological Profiles, Management and Outcomes. J Cancer Res Ther. 2014 Apr-Jun;10(2):294–8. PMID:25022380
2309. Mulay K, Puthyapurayil FM, Mohammad JA, et al. Adenoid Cystic Carcinoma of the Lacrimal Gland: Role of Nuclear Survivin (BIRC5) as a Prognostic Marker. Histopathology. 2013 May;62(6):840–6. PMID:23611357
2310. Mulay K, Rasmussen PK, Aggarwal E, et al. Accessory Lacrimal Gland Tumours of the Eye Region. Acta Ophthalmol. 2018 Nov;96(7):e772–5. PMID:29855174
2311. Mulay K, White VA, Shah SJ, et al. Sebaceous carcinoma: clinicopathologic features and diagnostic role of immunohistochemistry (Including Androgen Receptor). Can J Ophthalmol. 2014 Aug;49(4):326–32. PMID:25103648
2312. Mullaney J, Mooney D, O'Connor M, et al. Bilateral Ovarian Carcinoma with Bilateral Uveal Melanoma. Br J Ophthalmol. 1984 Apr;68(4):261–7. PMID:6704361
2313. Munch-Petersen HD, Rasmussen PK, Coupland SE, et al. Ocular Adnexal Diffuse Large B-Cell Lymphoma: A Multicenter International Study. JAMA Ophthalmol. 2015 Feb;133(2):165–73. PMID:25393033
2314. Mundra PA, Dhomen N, Rodrigues M, et al. Ultraviolet Radiation Drives Mutations in a Subset of Mucosal Melanomas. Nat Commun. 2021 Jan 11;12(1):259. PMID:33431815
2315. Munier FL. Classification and Management of Seeds in Retinoblastoma. Ellsworth Lecture Ghent August 24th 2013. Ophthalmic Genet. 2014 Dec;35(4):193–207. PMID:25321846
2316. Munier FL, Beck-Popovic M, Chantada GL, et al. Conservative Management of Retinoblastoma: Challenging Orthodoxy Without Compromising the State of Metastatic Grace. "Alive, with Good Vision and No Comorbidity". Prog Retin Eye Res. 2019 Nov;73:100764. PMID:31173880
2317. Munier FL, Gaillard MC, Balmer A, et al. Intravitreal Chemotherapy for Vitreous Disease in Retinoblastoma Revisited: From Prohibition to Conditional Indications. Br J Ophthalmol. 2012 Aug;96(8):1078–83. PMID:22694968
2318. Munier FL, Moulin A, Gaillard MC, et al. Intracameral Chemotherapy for Globe Salvage in Retinoblastoma with Secondary Anterior Chamber Invasion. Ophthalmology. 2018 Apr;125(4):615–7. PMID:29208450
2319. Murali R, Chandramohan R, Möller I, et al. Targeted Massively Parallel Sequencing of Angiosarcomas Reveals Frequent Activation of the Mitogen Activated Protein Kinase Pathway. Oncotarget. 2015 Nov 3;6(34):36041–52. PMID:26440310
2320. Murali R, McCarthy SW, Scolyer RA. Blue Nevi and Related Lesions: A Review Highlighting Atypical and Newly Described Variants, Distinguishing Features and Diagnostic Pitfalls. Adv Anat Pathol. 2009 Nov;16(6):365–82. PMID:19851128
2321. Murali R, Wiesner T, Scolyer RA. Tumours Associated with BAP1 Mutations. Pathology. 2013 Feb;45(2):116–26. PMID:23277170
2322. Murphy JT, Soeken T, Megison S, et al. Juvenile Xanthogranuloma: Diverse Presentations of Noncutaneous Disease. J Pediatr Hematol Oncol. 2014 Nov;36(8):641–5. PMID:24065046
2323. Muscarella LA, Bisceglia M, Galliani CA, et al. Extraneuraxial Hemangioblastoma: A Clinicopathologic Study of 10 Cases with Molecular Analysis of the VHL Gene. Pathol Res Pract. 2018 Aug;214(8):1156–65. PMID:29941223
2324. Mussavi M, Asadollahi K, Janbaz F, et al. The Evaluation of Red Reflex Sensitivity and Specificity Test Among Neonates in Different Conditions. Iran J Pediatr. 2014 Dec;24(6):697–702. PMID:26019774
2325. Mustapar N, Zawawi MSF, Tuan Sharif SE. The Value of H3K27me3 Immunohistochemistry in Differentiating Malignant Peripheral Nerve Sheath Tumour with Its Histologic Mimickers. Asian Pac J Cancer Prev. 2020 Mar 1;21(3):699–705. PMID:32212796
2326. Mwinula JH, Sagawa T, Tawara A, et al. Anterior Chamber Angle Vascularization in Sturge-Weber Syndrome. Report of a Case. Graefes Arch Clin Exp Ophthalmol. 1994 Jul;232(7):387–91. PMID:7523256
2327. Mynatt CJ, Feldman KA, Thompson LD. Orbital Infantile Myofibroma: A Case Report and Clinicopathologic Review of 24 Cases from the Literature. Head Neck Pathol. 2011 Sep;5(3):205–15. PMID:21512784
2328. Nabavizadeh SA, Santi M, Belasco JB, et al. Primary Atypical Optic Nerve Sheath Meningioma in a Child with Restricted Diffusion on Magnetic Resonance Imaging. J Neuroophthalmol. 2014 Jun;34(2):173–6. PMID:24705258
2329. Nacev BA, Jones KB, Intlekofer AM, et al. The Epigenomics of Sarcoma. Nat Rev Cancer. 2020 Oct;20(10):608–23. PMID:32782366
2330. Nadeu F, Martin-Garcia D, Clot G, et al. Genomic and Epigenomic Insights into the Origin, Pathogenesis, and Clinical Behavior of Mantle Cell Lymphoma Subtypes. Blood. 2020 Sep 17;136(12):1419–32. PMID:32584970
2331. Nadiarnykh O, McNeill-Badalova NA, Gaillard MC, et al. Optical Coherence Tomography (OCT) to Image Active and Inactive Retinoblastomas as Well as Retinomas. Acta Ophthalmol. 2020 Mar;98(2):158–65. PMID:31448879
2332. Nagafuchi S, Ishibashi H, Anzai K, et al. Budd-Chiari Syndrome and Epstein-Barr Virus (EBV) Associated Plasmacytoma in a Patient with Chronic Active EBV Infection. Clin Investig. 1994 Nov;72(11):883–6. PMID:7894217
2333. Nagao T. "Dedifferentiation" and High-Grade Transformation in Salivary Gland Carcinomas. Head Neck Pathol. 2013 Jul;7(Suppl 1):S37–47. PMID:23821210
2334. Nagarajan P, El-Hadad C, Gruschkus SK, et al. PD-L1/PD1 Expression, Composition of Tumor-Associated Immune Infiltrate, and HPV Status in Conjunctival Squamous Cell Carcinoma. Invest Ophthalmol Vis Sci. 2019 May 1;60(6):2388–98. PMID:31141610
2335. Nagatsuka H, Rivera RS, Gunduz M, et al. Microcystic Adnexal Carcinoma with Mandibular Bone Marrow Involvement: A Case Report with Immunohistochemistry. Am J Dermatopathol. 2006 Dec;28(6):518–22. PMID:17122497
2336. Nair AG, Gore SS, Ganvir AY, et al. Giant Perivascular Epithelioid Cell Tumor of the Orbit: A Clinicopathological Analysis and Review of the Literature. Ocul Oncol Pathol. 2018 Sep;4(5):272–9. PMID:30320097
2337. Nair AG, Kaliki S, Kamal S, et al. Conjunctival Leiomyosarcoma: A Report of Two Cases. Orbit. 2015;34(5):274–8. PMID:26214581
2338. Nair AG, Pathak RS, Iyer VR, et al. Optic Nerve Glioma: An Update. Int Ophthalmol. 2014 Aug;34(4):999–1005. PMID:24736941
2339. Nair PA, Singhal R. Xanthelasma Palpebrarum - a Brief Review. Clin Cosmet Investig Dermatol. 2018;11:1–5. PMID:29296091
2340. Nakaguro M, Nagao T. Epithelial-Myoepithelial Carcinoma. Surg Pathol Clin. 2021 Mar;14(1):97–109. PMID:33526226
2341. Nakaguro M, Tanigawa M, Hirai H, et al. The Diagnostic Utility of RAS Q61R Mutation-specific Immunohistochemistry in Epithelial-Myoepithelial Carcinoma. Am J Surg Pathol 2021 Jul 1;45(7):885–94. PMID:33481388
2342. Nakaguro M, Urano M, Suzuki H, et al. Low-Grade Intraductal Carcinoma of the Salivary Gland with Prominent Oncocytic Change: A Newly Described Variant. Histopathology. 2018 Aug;73(2):314–20. PMID:29574884
2343. Nakamine H, Yamakawa M, Yoshino T, et al. Langerhans Cell Histiocytosis and Langerhans Cell Sarcoma: Current Understanding and Differential Diagnosis. J Clin Exp Hematop. 2016;56(2):109–18. PMID:27980300
2344. Nakamura Y, Mashima Y, Kameyama K, et al. Detection of Human Papillomavirus Infection in Squamous Tumours of the Conjunctiva and Lacrimal Sac by Immunohistochemistry, In Situ Hybridisation, and Polymerase Chain Reaction. Br J Ophthalmol. 1997 Apr;81(4):308–13. PMID:9215061
2345. Nakano T, Yamamoto H, Hashimoto K, et al. HER2 and EGFR Gene Copy Number Alterations Are Predominant in High-Grade Salivary Mucoepidermoid Carcinoma Irrespective of MAML2 Fusion Status. Histopathology. 2013 Sep;63(3):378–92. PMID:23855785
2346. Nakashima Y, Tagawa H, Suzuki R, et al. Genome-Wide Array-Based Comparative Genomic Hybridization of Natural Killer Cell Lymphoma/Leukemia: Different Genomic Alteration Patterns of Aggressive NK-Cell Leukemia and Extranodal Nk/T-Cell Lymphoma, Nasal Type. Genes Chromosomes Cancer. 2005 Nov;44(3):247–55. PMID:16049916
2347. Nam SW, Woo KI, Kim YD. Characteristics of Primary Extranodal Marginal Zone B-Cell Lymphoma in Korea: Conjunctiva Versus Other Ocular Adnexa. Br J Ophthalmol. 2018 Apr;102(4):502–8. PMID:28814410
2348. Nann D, Schneckenburger P, Steinhilber J, et al. Pediatric Langerhans Cell Histiocytosis: The Impact of Mutational Profile on Clinical Progression and Late Sequelae. Ann Hematol. 2019 Jul;98(7):1617–26. PMID:30923995
2349. Narayan DS, Traber GL, Figueira E, et al. Natural History of Primary Paediatric Optic Nerve Sheath Meningioma: Case Series and Review. Br J Ophthalmol. 2018 Aug;102(8):1147–53. PMID:29146762
2350. Narchi H. Four Half-Siblings with Infantile Myofibromatosis: A Case for Autosomal-Recessive Inheritance. Clin Genet. 2001 Feb;59(2):134–5. PMID:11260217
2351. Nasany RA, Reiner AS, Francis JH, et al. Rosai-Dorfman-Destombes Disease of the Nervous System: A Systematic Literature Review. Orphanet J Rare Dis. 2022 Mar 2;17(1):92. PMID:35236371
2352. Nascimento AF, Fletcher CD. The Controversial Nosology of Benign Nerve Sheath Tumors: Neurofilament Protein Staining Demonstrates Intratumoral Axons in Many Sporadic Schwannomas. Am J Surg Pathol. 2007 Sep;31(9):1363–70. PMID:17721192
2353. Nasr AM, Blodi FC, Lindahl S, et al. Congenital Generalized Multicentric Myofibromatosis with Orbital Involvement. Am J Ophthalmol. 1986 Dec 15;102(6):779–87. PMID:3538883
2354. Nasser H, Ahmed Y, Szpunar SM, et al. Malignant Granular Cell Tumor: A Look into the Diagnostic Criteria. Patho Res Pract. 2011 Mar 15;207(3):164–8. PMID:21282016
2355. Nassiri N, Rootman J, Rootman DB, et al. Orbital Lymphaticovenous Malformations: Current and Future Treatments. Surv Ophthalmol. 2015 Sep-Oct;60(5):383–405. PMID:25077629
2356. Nasu M, Emi M, Pastorino S, et al. High Incidence of Somatic BAP1 Alterations in Sporadic Malignant Mesothelioma. J Thorac Oncol. 2015 Apr;10(4):565–76. PMID:25658628

2357. Nath K, Gogi R, Zaidi N, et al. Cystic Lesions of Conjunctiva (a Clinicopathogical Study). Indian J Ophthalmol. 1983 Jan;31(1):1–4. PMID:6629442
2358. Nath K, Shukla BR. Orbital Leiomyoma and its Origin. Br J Ophthalmol. 1963 Jun;47(6):369–71. PMID:14189707
2359. Naumann G, Yanoff M, Zimmerman LE. Histogenesis of Malignant Melanomas of the Uvea. I. Histopathologic Characteristics of Nevi of the Choroid and Ciliary Body. Arch Ophthalmol. 1966 Dec;76(6):784–96. PMID:5924936
2360. Nava-Castañeda Á, Kahuam-López N, De La Fuente Díez Y, et al. Primary Adenoid Cystic Carcinoma Arising from an Ectopic Lacrimal Gland Involving Both Nasal Orbits: A Rare Clinical Entity. Orbit. 2021 Dec;40(6):525–8. PMID:32912017
2361. Navarrete-Dechent C, Monnier J, Marghoob NG, et al. Bilateral Diffuse Uveal Melanocytic Proliferation with Multifocal Diffuse Integumentary Melanocytic Proliferation Paraneoplastic Syndrome: A Case Report. Australas J Dermatol. 2021 Aug;62(3):386–9. PMID:33974277
2362. Nayak B, Poddar C, Panigrahi MK, et al. Late Manifestation of Follicular Conjunctivitis in Ventilated Patient Following COVID-19 Positive Severe Pneumonia. Indian J Ophthalmol. 2020 Aug;68(8):1675–7. PMID:32709820
2363. Neerukonda VK, Carruth B, Estopinal MDV. Invasive Carcinoma Ex-Pleomorphic Adenoma of the Lacrimal Gland with a Cystadenocarcinoma Component: A Case Report and Review of the Literature. Case Rep Pathol. 2020 Aug 12;2020:6482837. PMID:32850170
2364. Nell RJ, Menger NV, Versluis M, et al. Involvement of Mutant and Wild-Type CYSLTR2 in the Development and Progression of Uveal Nevi and Melanoma. BMC Cancer. 2021 Feb 15;21(1):164. PMID:33588787
2365. Nellessen T, Aoki R, Kammerbauer C, et al. Relationship Between α-Genus Human Papillomavirus and Non-Genital Seborrheic Keratosis: Report of New Cases and Updated Review. J Cosmet Dermatol. 2023 Jan;22(1):306–10. PMID:35066969
2366. Nelson CC, Hertzberg BS, Klintworth GK. A Histopathologic Study of 716 Unselected Eyes in Patients with Cancer at the Time of Death. Am J Ophthalmol. 1983 Jun;95(6):788–93. PMID:6859188
2367. Nelson KD, McSoley JJ. Clinical Findings and Management of Conjunctival Intraepithelial Neoplasia. Optometry. 2011 Jan;82(1):15–21. PMID:21071282
2368. Nelson MA, Einspahr JG, Alberts DS, et al. Analysis of the P53 Gene in Human Precancerous Actinic Keratosis Lesions and Squamous Cell Cancers. Cancer Lett. 1994 Sep 30;85(1):23–9. PMID:7923098
2369. Nemer KM, Hurst EA. Confluent Verruca Vulgaris Arising Within Bilateral Eyebrow Tattoos: Successful Treatment With Ablative Laser and Topical 5% Imiquimod Cream. Dermatol Surg. 2019 Mar;45(3):473–5. PMID:29757860
2370. National Institutes of Health Consensus Development Conference. Neurofibromatosis. Conference Statement. Arch Neurol. 1988 May;45(5):575–8. PMID:3128965
2371. Nevares RL, Mulliken JB, Robb RM. Ocular Dermoids. Plast Reconstr Surg. 1988 Dec;82(6):959–64. PMID:3200959
2372. Newton C, Dutton JJ, Klintworth GK. A Respiratory Epithelial Choristomatous Cyst of the Orbit. Ophthalmology. 1985 Dec;92(12):1754–7. PMID:4088630
2373. Newton R, Ferlay J, Reeves G, et al. Effect of Ambient Solar Ultraviolet Radiation on Incidence of Squamous-Cell Carcinoma of the Eye. Lancet. 1996 May 25;347(9013):1450–1. PMID:8676629
2374. Newton R, Ziegler J, Ateenyi-Agaba C, et al. The Epidemiology of Conjunctival Squamous Cell Carcinoma in Uganda. Br J Cancer. 2002 Jul 29;87(3):301–8. PMID:12177799
2375. Newton-Bishop JA, Chang YM, Iles MM, et al. Melanocytic Nevi, Nevus Genes, and Melanoma Risk in a Large Case-Control Study in the United Kingdom. Cancer Epidemiol Biomarkers Prev. 2010 Aug;19(8):2043–54. PMID:20647408
2376. Ng A, Chiorazzi N. Potential Relevance of B-Cell Maturation Pathways in Defining the Cell(s) of Origin for Chronic Lymphocytic Leukemia. Hematol Oncol Clin North Am. 2021 Aug;35(4):665–85. PMID:34174979
2377. Ng SB, Chung TH, Kato S, et al. Epstein-Barr Virus-Associated Primary Nodal T/NK-Cell Lymphoma Shows a Distinct Molecular Signature and Copy Number Changes. Haematologica. 2018 Feb;103(2):278–87. PMID:29097495
2378. Nguyen HL, Boon LM, Vikkula M. Genetics of Vascular Anomalies. Semin Pediatr Surg. 2020 Oct;29(5):150967. PMID:33069286
2379. Ni C, D'Amico DJ, Fan CQ, et al. Tumors of the Lacrimal Sac: A Clinicopathological Analysis of 82 Cases. Int Ophthalmol Clin. 1982 Spring;22(1):121–40. PMID:6277817
2380. Ni C, Wagoner M, Kieval S, et al. Tumours of the Moll's Glands. Br J Ophthalmol. 1984 Jul;68(7):502–6. PMID:6329262
2381. Ni Z. [Histopathological Classification of 3,510 Cases with Eyelid Tumor]. Zhonghua Yan Ke Za Zhi. 1996 Nov;32(6):435–7. Chinese. PMID:9590811
2382. Nichols JC, Amato JE, Chung SM. Characteristics of Lisch Nodules in Patients with Neurofibromatosis Type 1. J Pediatr Ophthalmol Strabismus. 2003 Sep-Oct;40(5):293–6. PMID:14560838
2383. Nickoloff BJ, Fleischmann HE, Carmel J, et al. Microcystic Adnexal Carcinoma. Immunohistologic Observations Suggesting Dual (Pilar and Eccrine) Differentiation. Arch Dermatol. 1986 Mar;122(3):290–4. PMID:3513708
2384. Niffenegger JH, Soltero A, Niffenegger JS, et al. Prevalence of Hepatocyte Growth Factor and Autoantibodies to α-HGF as a New Etiology for Bilateral Diffuse Uveal Melanocytic Proliferation Masquerading as Neovascular Age-Related Macular Degeneration. J Clin Exp Ophthalmol. 2018;9(4):740. PMID:30370177
2385. Nijsten T, Curiel-Lewandrowski C, Kadin ME. Lymphomatoid Papulosis in Children: A Retrospective Cohort Study of 35 Cases. Arch Dermatol. 2004 Mar;140(3):306–12. PMID:15023774
2386. Nikiphorou E, Galloway J, Fragoulis GE. Overview of IgG4-Related Aortitis and Periaortitis. A Decade Since Their First Description. Autoimmun Rev. 2020 Dec;19(12):102694. PMID:33121641
2387. Nirankari VS, Karesh JW, Richards RD. Complications of Exposed Monofilament Sutures. Am J Ophthalmol. 1983 Apr;95(4):515–9. PMID:6837695
2388. Njauw CN, Kim I, Piris A, et al. Germline BAP1 Inactivation is Preferentially Associated with Metastatic Ocular Melanoma and Cutaneous-Ocular Melanoma Families. PLoS One. 2012;7(4):e35295. PMID:22545102
2389. Nolan GR, Hirst LW. Impression Cytology in the Diagnosis of Ocular Surface Squamous Neoplasia. Br J Ophthalmol. 2001 Jul;85(7):888. PMID:11423469
2390. Nolan GR, Hirst LW, Bancroft BJ. The Cytomorphology of Ocular Surface Squamous Neoplasia by Using Impression Cytology. Cancer. 2001 Feb 25;93(1):60–7. PMID:11241267
2391. Nolan GR, Hirst LW, Wright RG, et al. Application of Impression Cytology to the Diagnosis of Conjunctival Neoplasms. Diagn Cytopathol. 1994;11(3):246–9. PMID:7867466
2392. Nomura S, Suzuki R, Sugiyama S, et al. Optic Glioma with Characteristic Bilateral Optic Atrophy in a 3-Year-Old Girl. Pediatr Neurosurg. 1999 Oct;31(4):213–8. PMID:10705932
2393. Nomura T, Maki D, Matsumoto F, et al. A Rare Case of Coexisting Lacrimal Sac Adenocarcinoma and Transitional Cell Carcinoma. Ear Nose Throat J. 2018 Oct-Nov;97(10-11):e32–5. PMID:30481853
2394. Nonaka D, Chiriboga L, Rubin BP. Sox10: A Pan-Schwannian and Melanocytic Marker. Am J Surg Pathol. 2008 Sep;32(9):1291–8. PMID:18636017
2395. Nordstrom-O'Brien M, van Der Luijt RB, van Rooijen E, et al. Genetic Analysis of von Hippel-Lindau Disease. Hum Mutat. 2010 May;31(5):521–37. PMID:20151405
2396. Nork TM, Ghobrial MW, Peyman GA, et al. Massive Retinal Gliosis. A Reactive Proliferation of Müller Cells. Arch Ophthalmol. 1986 Sep;104(9):1383–9. PMID:3092790
2397. North JP. Molecular Genetics of Sebaceous Neoplasia. Surg Pathol Clin. 2021 Jun;14(2):273–84. PMID:34023105
2398. North JP, Golovato J, Vaske CJ, et al. Cell of Origin and Mutation Pattern Define Three Clinically Distinct Classes of Sebaceous Carcinoma. Nat Commun. 2018 May 14;9(1):1894. PMID:29760388
2399. North JP, McCalmont TH, Fehr A, et al. Detection of MYB Alterations and Other Immunohistochemical Markers in Primary Cutaneous Adenoid Cystic Carcinoma. Am J Surg Pathol. 2015 Oct;39(10):1347–56. PMID:26076064
2400. North JP, Solomon DA, Golovato J, et al. Loss of ZNF750 in Ocular and Cutaneous Sebaceous Carcinoma. J Cutan Pathol. 2019 Oct;46(10):736–41. PMID:31148199
2401. North PE. Pediatric Vascular Tumors and Malformations. Surg Pathol Clin. 2010 Sep;3(3):455–94. PMID:26839221
2402. North PE, Waner M, Mizeracki A, et al. A Unique Microvascular Phenotype Shared by Juvenile Hemangiomas and Human Placenta. Arch Dermatol. 2001 May;137(5):559–70. PMID:11346333
2403. North VS, Habib LA, Yoon MK. Merkel Cell Carcinoma of the Eyelid: A Review. Surv Ophthalmol. 2019 Sep-Oct;64(5):659–67. PMID:30871952
2404. Nusliha A, Dalpatadu U, Amarasinghe B, et al. Congenital Hypertrophy of Retinal Pigment Epithelium (CHRPE) in Patients with Familial Adenomatous Polyposis (FAP); a Polyposis Registry Experience. BMC Res Notes. 2014 Oct 18;7:734. PMID:25326340
2405. Oakes CC, Seifert M, Assenov Y, et al. DNA Methylation Dynamics During B Cell Maturation Underlie a Continuum of Disease Phenotypes in Chronic Lymphocytic Leukemia. Nat Genet. 2016 Mar;48(3):253–64. PMID:26780610
2406. O'Connell JX, Kattapuram SV, Mankin HJ, et al. Epithelioid Hemangioma of Bone. A Tumor Often Mistaken for Low-Grade Angiosarcoma or Malignant Hemangioendothelioma. Am J Surg Pathol. 1993 Jun;17(6):610–7. PMID:8333560
2407. Oda T, Kikuchi K, Togao O, et al. Alveolar Soft Part Sarcoma of the Orbit: A Case Report. Radiol Case Rep. 2021 Oct 2;16(12):3766–71. PMID:34630814
2408. Odashiro AN, Fernandes BF, Al-Kandari A, et al. Report of Two Cases of Ciliary Body Mesectodermal Leiomyoma: Unique Expression of Neural Markers. Ophthalmology. 2007 Jan;114(1):157–61. PMID:17070579
2409. Odashiro AN, Leite LV, Oliveira RS, et al. Primary Orbital Mesenchymal Chondrosarcoma: A Case Report and Literature Review. Int Ophthalmol. 2009 Jun;29(3):173–7. PMID:18188507
2410. Ognjanovic S, Olivier M, Bergemann TL, et al. Sarcomas in TP53 Germline Mutation Carriers: A Review of the IARC TP53 Database. Cancer. 2012 Mar 1;118(5):1387–96. PMID:21837677
2411. Ogun OA, Ogun GO, Brown BJ, et al. Congenital Orbital Teratoma: A Case Report and Challenges of its Management in a Resource Limited Setting. Pan Afr Med J. 2012;12:3. PMID:22826728
2412. Ogura K, Hosoda F, Nakamura H, et al. Highly Recurrent H3F3A Mutations with Additional Epigenetic Regulator Alterations in Giant Cell Tumor of Bone. Genes Chromosomes Cancer. 2017 Oct;56(10):711–8. PMID:28545165
2413. Oh JE, Ohta T, Satomi K, et al. Alterations in the NF2/LATS1/LATS2/YAP Pathway in Schwannomas. J Neuropathol Exp Neurol. 2015 Oct;74(10):952–9. PMID:26360373
2414. Oh JK, Dehghani A, Shinder R. Solitary Fibrous Tumor of the Conjunctiva. Orbit. 2020 Dec;39(6):458–9. PMID:31698970
2415. Ohar JA, Cheung M, Talarchek J, et al. Germline BAP1 Mutational Landscape of Asbestos-Exposed Malignant Mesothelioma Patients with Family History of Cancer. Cancer Res. 2016 Jan 15;76(2):206–15. PMID:26719535
2416. Ohguro H, Maruyama I, Nakazawa M. A Case of Pseudoadenomatous Hyperplasia of Ciliary Body Epithelium Successfully Treated by Local Resection. Tohoku J Exp Med. 2002 May;197(1):41–5. PMID:12180792
2417. Ohta N, Makihara S, Okano M, et al. Roles of IL-17, Th1, and Tc1 Cells in Patients with IgG4-Related Sclerosing Sialadenitis. Laryngoscope. 2012 Oct;122(10):2169–74. PMID:22786718
2418. Ohtsuka K, Hashimoto M, Suzuki Y. A Review of 244 Orbital Tumors in Japanese Patients During a 21-Year Period: Origins and Locations. Jpn J Ophthalmol. 2005 Jan-Feb;49(1):49–55. PMID:15692775
2419. Okano K, Ishida M, Sandoh K, et al. Cytological Features of Carcinoma Ex Pleomorphic Adenoma of the Salivary Glands: A Diagnostic Challenge. Diagn Cytopathol. 2020 Feb;48(2):149–53. PMID:31675185
2420. O'Keefe M, Fulcher T, Kelly P, et al. Medulloepithelioma of the Optic Nerve Head. Arch Ophthalmol. 1997 Oct;115(10):1325–7. PMID:9338683
2421. Okonkwo SN, Afghani T, Akbar M, et al. Bilateral Orbital Glial Heterotopia: A Rare Case Report. Oman J Ophthalmol. 2018 Sep-Dec;11(3):288–90. PMID:30505127
2422. Olenczak JB, Ford JR, Mericli AF, et al. Surgical and Ophthalmologic Outcomes of Reconstruction in Patients Treated With Eye-Sparing Surgery and Radiation Therapy for Tumors of the Lacrimal Drainage Apparatus. Ann Plast Surg. 2021 Mar 1;86(3):292–7. PMID:33555683
2423. Oliphant H, Rajak S, Selva D. Simple Lipoma of the Eyelid: A Rare Entity. Clin Exp Ophthalmol. 2017 May;45(4):412–3. PMID:27992661
2424. Oliveira AM, Hsi BL, Weremowicz S, et al. USP6 (Tre2) Fusion Oncogenes in Aneurysmal Bone Cyst. Cancer Res. 2004 Mar 15;64(6):1920–3. PMID:15026324
2425. Oliveira AM, Perez-Atayde AR, Dal Cin P, et al. Aneurysmal Bone Cyst Variant Translocations Upregulate USP6 Transcription by Promoter Swapping with the ZNF9, COL1A1, TRAP150, and OMD Genes. Oncogene. 2005 May 12;24(21):3419–26. PMID:15735689
2426. Oliveira AM, Perez-Atayde AR, Inwards CY, et al. USP6 and CDH11 Oncogenes Identify the Neoplastic Cell in Primary Aneurysmal Bone Cysts and Are Absent in So-Called Secondary

Aneurysmal Bone Cysts. Am J Pathol. 2004 Nov;165(5):1773–80. PMID:15509545
2427. Olsen GM, Nackers A, Drolet BA. Infantile and Congenital Hemangiomas. Semin Pediatr Surg. 2020 Oct;29(5):150969. PMID:33069287
2428. Olsen TG, Heegaard S. Orbital Lymphoma. Surv Ophthalmol. 2019 Jan-Feb;64(1):45–66. PMID:30144455
2429. Olsen TG, Helwig EB. Angiolymphoid Hyperplasia with Eosinophilia. A Clinicopathologic Study of 116 Patients. J Am Acad Dermatol. 1985 May;12(5 Pt 1):781–96. PMID:4008683
2430. Olsen TG, Holm F, Mikkelsen LH, et al. Orbital Lymphoma-An International Multicenter Retrospective Study. Am J Ophthalmol. 2019 Mar;199:44–57. PMID:30419193
2431. Olson NJ, Linos K. Dedifferentiated Solitary Fibrous Tumor: A Concise Review. Arch Pathol Lab Med. 2018 Jun;142(6):761–6. PMID:29848035
2432. O'Malley DP. Benign Extramedullary Myeloid Proliferations. Mod Pathol. 2007 Apr;20(4):405–15. PMID:17334344
2433. Omulecki W, Pruszczyński M, Borowski J. Ring Melanoma of the Iris and Ciliary Body. Br J Ophthalmol. 1985 Jul;69(7):514–8. PMID:4016045
2434. O'Neal KD, Butnor KJ, Perkinson KR, et al. Bilateral Diffuse Uveal Melanocytic Proliferation Associated with Pancreatic Carcinoma: A Case Report and Literature Review of This Paraneoplastic Syndrome. Surv Ophthalmol. 2003 Nov-Dec;48(6):613–25. PMID:14609707
2435. Ong HS, Ji T, Zhang CP, et al. Head and Neck Inflammatory Myofibroblastic Tumor (IMT): Evaluation of Clinicopathologic and Prognostic Features. Oral Oncol. 2012 Feb;48(2):141–8. PMID:22014665
2436. Ong LY, Mercer B, Campbell LJ, et al. Abnormal Cytogenetics in Orbital Lipoma. Ophthalmic Plast Reconstr Surg. 2009 May-Jun;25(3):243–5. PMID:19454946
2437. Ong SLM, Lam SW, van Den Akker BEWM, et al. Expanding the Spectrum of EWSR1-NFATC2-Rearranged Benign Tumors: A Common Genomic Abnormality in Vascular Malformation/Hemangioma and Simple Bone Cyst. Am J Surg Pathol. 2021 Dec 1;45(12):1669–81. PMID:34081036
2438. Onken MD, Li J, Cooper JA. Uveal Melanoma Cells Utilize a Novel Route for Transendothelial Migration. PLoS One. 2014 Dec 15;9(12):e115472. PMID:25506912
2439. Onken MD, Worley LA, Ehlers JP, et al. Gene Expression Profiling in Uveal Melanoma Reveals Two Molecular Classes and Predicts Metastatic Death. Cancer Res. 2004 Oct 15;64(20):7205–9. PMID:15492234
2440. Ordóñez NG. Granular Cell Tumor: A Review and Update. Adv Anat Pathol. 1999 Jul;6(4):186–203. PMID:10410172
2441. Orduña-Azcona J, Gili P, De Manuel-Triantafilo S, et al. Solitary Congenital Hypertrophy of the Retinal Pigment Epithelium Features by High-Definition Optical Coherence Tomography. Eur J Ophthalmol. 2014 Jul-Aug;24(4):566–9. PMID:24366775
2442. O'Reilly FM, Brat DJ, McAlpine BE, et al. Microphthalmia Transcription Factor Immunohistochemistry: A Useful Diagnostic Marker in the Diagnosis and Detection of Cutaneous Melanoma, Sentinel Lymph Node Metastases, and Extracutaneous Melanocytic Neoplasms. J Am Acad Dermatol. 2001 Sep;45(3):414–9. PMID:11511840
2443. O'Rourke MA, Cannon PS, Shaw JF, et al. Cutaneous Pleomorphic Adenoma of the Periocular Region - a Case Series. Orbit. 2022 Jun;41(3):361–4. PMID:33292052
2444. Orsey A, Paessler M, Lange BJ, et al. Central Nervous System Juvenile Xanthogranuloma with Malignant Transformation. Pediatr Blood Cancer. 2008 Apr;50(4):927–30. PMID:17520744
2445. Ortins-Pina A, Llamas-Velasco M, Turpin S, et al. FOSB Immunoreactivity in Endothelia of Epithelioid Hemangioma (Angiolymphoid Hyperplasia with Eosinophilia). J Cutan Pathol. 2018 Jun;45(6):395–402. PMID:29527734
2446. Ortiz MV, Dunkel IJ. Retinoblastoma. J Child Neurol. 2016 Feb;31(2):227–36. PMID:26023180
2447. Ortonne N, Wolkenstein P, Blakeley JO, et al. Cutaneous Neurofibromas: Current Clinical and Pathologic Issues. Neurology. 2018 Jul 10;91(2 Suppl 1):S5–13. PMID:29987130
2448. Ortube MC, Lazareff J, Vinters HV, et al. Orbital Ectopic Brain Tissue in Aicardi Syndrome. J Craniofac Surg. 2010 Sep;21(5):1551–3. PMID:20818257
2449. Osborn AJ, Dickie P, Neilson DE, et al. Activating PIK3CA Alleles and Lymphangiogenic Phenotype of Lymphatic Endothelial Cells Isolated from Lymphatic Malformations. Hum Mol Genet. 2015 Feb 15;24(4):926–38. PMID:25292196
2450. Østergaard J, Prause JU, Heegaard S. Oncocytic Lesions of the Ophthalmic Region: A Clinicopathological Study with Emphasis on Cytokeratin Expression. Acta Ophthalmol. 2011 May;89(3):263–7. PMID:19843013
2451. Ostler DA, Prieto VG, Reed JA, et al. Adipophilin Expression in Sebaceous Tumors and Other Cutaneous Lesions with Clear Cell Histology: An Immunohistochemical Study of 117 Cases. Mod Pathol. 2010 Apr;23(4):567–73. PMID:20118912
2452. Ostrom QT, Gittleman H, Truitt G, et al. CBTRUS Statistical Report: Primary Brain and Other Central Nervous System Tumors Diagnosed in the United States in 2011-2015. Neuro Oncol. 2018 Oct 1;20(Suppl_4):iv1–86. PMID:30445539
2453. Otsuka A, Levesque MP, Dummer R, et al. Hedgehog Signaling in Basal Cell Carcinoma. J Dermatol Sci. 2015 May;78(2):95–100. PMID:25766766
2454. Otsuka H, Kohashi K, Yoshimoto M, et al. Immunohistochemical Evaluation of H3K27 Trimethylation in Malignant Peripheral Nerve Sheath Tumors. Pathol Res Pract. 2018 Mar;214(3):417–25. PMID:29482987
2455. Otto J, Sorge I, Horn LC, et al. Magnetic Resonance Imaging of a Phakomatous Choristoma. Pediatr Radiol. 2015 Oct;45(11):1712–5. PMID:26070367
2456. Owen JL, Kibbi N, Worley B, et al. Sebaceous Carcinoma: Evidence-Based Clinical Practice Guidelines. Lancet Oncol. 2019 Dec;20(12):e699–714. PMID:31797796
2457. Oyama T, Takizawa J, Nakamura N, et al. Multifocal Mucosa-Associated Lymphoid Tissue Lymphoma Associated with IgG4-Related Disease: A Case Report. Jpn J Ophthalmol. 2011 May;55(3):304–6. PMID:21584726
2458. Oystreck DT, Morales J, Chauchry I, et al. Visual Loss in Orbitofacial Neurofibromatosis Type 1. Ophthalmology. 2012 Oct;119(10):2168–73. PMID:22709421
2459. Özcan G, Gündüz AK, Mirzayev I, et al. Presumed Retinal Metastasis from Lung Adenocarcinoma: A Case Report and Literature Review. Case Rep Ophthalmol Med. 2021 Jun 10;2021:6615284. PMID:34306783
2460. Ozkaya N, Rosenblum MK, Durham BH, et al. The Histopathology of Erdheim-Chester Disease: A Comprehensive Review of a Molecularly Characterized Cohort. Mod Pathol. 2018 Apr;31(4):581–97. PMID:29192649
2461. Paal E, Thompson LD, Heffess CS. A Clinicopathologic and Immunohistochemical Study of Ten Pancreatic Lymphangiomas and a Review of the Literature. Cancer. 1998 Jun 1;82(11):2150–8. PMID:9610694
2462. Paez-Escamilla M, Walter SD, Ramaiya KJ, et al. Diagnosis of Bilateral Retinocytoma in an Adolescent Patient Using Multimodal Imaging and Genetic Testing. Ophthalmic Surg Lasers Imaging Retina. 2018 Oct 1;49(10):812–4. PMID:30395669
2463. Pagano Boza C, Vigo R, Premoli JE, et al. A Case Report of a Primary Apocrine Adenocarcinoma of the Eyelid with Literature Review. Orbit. 2018 Oct;37(5):389–92. PMID:29313402
2464. Painter CA, Jain E, Tomson BN, et al. The Angiosarcoma Project: Enabling Genomic and Clinical Discoveries in a Rare Cancer Through Patient-Partnered Research. Nat Med. 2020 Feb;26(2):181–7. PMID:32042194
2465. Palakkamanil MM, Mahmood MN, Chan A. Diagnostic and Treatment Challenges of a Case of Primary Cutaneous Signet-Ring Cell/Histiocytoid Carcinoma of the Eyelid. BMC Ophthalmol. 2020 Oct 14;20(1):410. PMID:33054772
2466. Paliogiannis P, Palmieri G, Tanda F, et al. Perivascular Epithelioid Cell Tumors (PEComas) of the Orbit. J Pathol Transl Med. 2017 Jan;51(1):7–8. PMID:28063419
2467. Palioura S, Jakobiec FA, Zakka FR, et al. Pleomorphic Adenoma (Formerly Chondroid Syringoma) of the Eyelid Margin with a Pseudocystic Appearance. Surv Ophthalmol. 2013 Sep-Oct;58(5):486–91. PMID:23294914
2468. Palma J, Sasso DF, Dufort G, et al. Successful Treatment of Metastatic Retinoblastoma with High-Dose Chemotherapy and Autologous Stem Cell Rescue in South America. Bone Marrow Transplant. 2012 Apr;47(4):522–7. PMID:21602901
2469. Palomero J, Vegliante MC, Eguileor A, et al. SOX11 Defines Two Different Subtypes of Mantle Cell Lymphoma Through Transcriptional Regulation of BCL6. Leukemia. 2016 Jul;30(7):1596–9. PMID:26710884
2470. Pan CC, Chung MY, Ng KF, et al. Constant Allelic Alteration on Chromosome 16p (TSC2 Gene) in Perivascular Epithelioid Cell Tumour (PEComa): Genetic Evidence for the Relationship of PEComa with Angiomyolipoma. J Pathol. 2008 Feb;214(3):387–93. PMID:18085521
2471. Pan S, Li TJ. PTCH1 Mutations in Odontogenic Keratocysts: Are They Related to Epithelial Cell Proliferation? Oral Oncol. 2009 Oct;45(10):861–5. PMID:19362041
2472. Pan Y, Hysinger JD, Barron T, et al. NF1 Mutation Drives Neuronal Activity-Dependent Initiation of Optic Glioma. Nature. 2021 Jun;594(7862):277–82. PMID:34040258
2473. Panagopoulos I, Andersen K, Gorunova L, et al. Recurrent Fusion of the Genes for High-Mobility Group AT-Hook 2 (HMGA2) and Nuclear Receptor Co-Repressor 2 (NCOR2) in Osteoclastic Giant Cell-Rich Tumors of Bone. Cancer Genomics Proteomics. 2022 Mar-Apr;19(2):163–77. PMID:35181586
2474. Panagopoulos I, Gorunova L, Andersen K, et al. NDRG1-PLAG1 and TRPS1-PLAG1 Fusion Genes in Chondroid Syringoma. Cancer Genomics Proteomics. 2020 May-Jun;17(3):237–48. PMID:32345665
2475. Panagopoulos I, Gorunova L, Bjerkehagen B, et al. LAMTOR1-PRKCD and NUMA1-SFMBT1 Fusion Genes Identified by RNA Sequencing in Aneurysmal Benign Fibrous Histiocytoma with T(3;11)(P21;Q13). Cancer Genet. 2015 Nov;208(11):545–51. PMID:26432191
2476. Panarelli JF, Zoumalan CI, Mukkamala K, et al. Dedifferentiated Adenoid Cystic Carcinoma of the Lacrimal Gland. Ophthalmic Plast Reconstr Surg. 2011 Sep-Oct;27(5):e119–21. PMID:21283029
2477. Pande M, Lynch PM, Hopper JL, et al. Smoking and Colorectal Cancer in Lynch Syndrome: Results from the Colon Cancer Family Registry and the University of Texas M.D. Anderson Cancer Center. Clin Cancer Res. 2010 Feb 15;16(4):1331–9. PMID:20145170
2478. Panoutsakopoulos G, Pandis N, Kyriazoglou I, et al. Recurrent T(16;17)(Q22;P13) in Aneurysmal Bone Cysts. Genes Chromosomes Cancer. 1999 Nov;26(3):265–6. PMID:10502326
2479. Pantalon A, Ștefănache T, Danciu M, et al. Iris Juvenile Xanthogranuloma in an Infant - Spontaneous Hyphema and Secondary Glaucoma. Rom J Ophthalmol. 2017 Jul-Sep;61(3):229–36. PMID:29450403
2480. Papa BM, Prince HM, McNab AA, et al. IgG4-Related Ophthalmic Disease in Association with Adult-Onset Asthma and Periocular Xanthogranuloma: A Case Report. Orbit. 2023 Feb;42(1):98–103. PMID:34493168
2481. Papalas JA, Proia AD. Primary Mucinous Carcinoma of the Eyelid: A Clinicopathologic and Immunohistochemical Study of 4 Cases and an Update on Recurrence Rates. Arch Ophthalmol. 2010 Sep;128(9):1160–5. PMID:20837800
2482. Papale JJ, Akiwama K, Hirose T, et al. Adenocarcinoma of the Ciliary Body Pigment Epithelium in a Child. Arch Ophthalmol. 1984 Jan;102(1):100–3. PMID:6703952
2483. Papke DJ Jr, Hornick JL. What is New in Endothelial Neoplasia? Virchows Arch. 2020 Jan;476(1):17–28. PMID:31463731
2484. Papo M, Diamond EL, Cohen-Aubart F, et al. High Prevalence of Myeloid Neoplasms in Adults with Non-Langerhans Cell Histiocytosis. Blood. 2017 Aug 24;130(8):1007–13. PMID:28679734
2485. Paradela S, Castiñeiras I, Cuevas J, et al. Mucinous Carcinoma of the Skin: Evaluation of Lymphatic Invasion with D2-40. Am J Dermatopathol. 2008 Oct;30(5):504–8. PMID:18806507
2486. Pareja F, Brandes AH, Basili T, et al. Loss-of-Function Mutations in ATP6AP1 and ATP6AP2 in Granular Cell Tumors. Nat Commun. 2018 Aug 30;9(1):3533. PMID:30166553
2487. Paridaens AD, Deuble K, McCartney AC. Spontaneous Congenital Non-Pigmented Epithelial Cysts of the Iris Stroma. Br J Ophthalmol. 1992 Jan;76(1):39–42. PMID:1739690
2488. Paridaens AD, Minassian DC, McCartney AC, et al. Prognostic Factors in Primary Malignant Melanoma of the Conjunctiva: A Clinicopathological Study of 256 Cases. Br J Ophthalmol. 1994 Apr;78(4):252–9. PMID:8199108
2489. Park DY, Lee JH, Suh YL, et al. Metastatic Adenoid Cystic Carcinoma of the Eyelid. Ophthalmic Plast Reconstr Surg. 2012 Sep-Oct;28(5):e117–2. PMID:22366665
2490. Park IA, Sa HS, Chung YS, et al. Androgen Receptor-Positive Ductal Adenocarcinoma of the Nasolacrimal Duct: A Case Report. Am J Ophthalmol Case Rep. 2016 Nov 14;5:33–7. PMID:29503943
2491. Park JS, Ko DK. A Histopathologic Study of Epidermoid Cysts in Korea: Comparison Between Ruptured and Unruptured Epidermal Cyst. Int J Clin Exp Pathol. 2013;6(2):242–8. PMID:23330009
2492. Park JY, Cohen C, Lopez D, et al. EGFR Exon 20 Insertion/Duplication Mutations Characterize Fibrous Hamartoma of Infancy. Am J Surg Pathol. 2016 Dec;40(12):1713–8. PMID:27631514
2493. Park R, Centeno MG, Shinder R. Ocular Surface Leiomyoma in a Child After Strabismus Repair. Ophthalmology 2013 Dec;125(12):1958. PMID:30454719
2494. Park SH, Lee JH, Chae YS, et al. Recurrent Mesectodermal Leiomyoma of the Ciliary Body: A Case Report. J Korean Med Sci. 2003 Aug;18(4):614–7. PMID:12923346

2495. Parker RT, Ovens CA, Fraser CL, et al. Optic Nerve Sheath Meningiomas: Prevalence, Impact, and Management Strategies. Eye Brain. 2018 Oct 24;10:85–99. PMID:30498385
2496. Parkin B, Chew JB, White VA, et al. Lymphocytic Infiltration and Enlargement of the Lacrimal Glands: A New Subtype of Primary Sjögren's Syndrome? Ophthalmology. 2005 Nov;112(11):2040–7. PMID:16168486
2497. Parks SL, Glover AT. Benign Mixed Tumors Arising in the Palpebral Lobe of the Lacrimal Gland. Ophthalmology. 1990 Apr;97(4):526–30. PMID:2158030
2498. Parmar DN, Rose GE. Management of Lacrimal Sac Tumours. Eye (Lond). 2003 Jul;17(5):599–606. PMID:12855966
2499. Parmley VC, George DP, Fannin LA. Juvenile Xanthogranuloma of the Iris in an Adult. Arch Ophthalmol. 1998 Mar;116(3):377–9. PMID:9514494
2500. Parra O, Linos K, Yan S, et al. Comparative Performance of Insulinoma-Associated Protein 1 (INSM1) and Routine Immunohistochemical Markers of Neuroendocrine Differentiation in the Diagnosis of Endocrine Mucin-Producing Sweat Gland Carcinoma. J Cutan Pathol. 2021 Jan;48(1):41–6. PMID:32745280
2501. Parsons MA, Rennie IG, Rundle PA, et al. Congenital Hypertrophy of Retinal Pigment Epithelium: A Clinico-Pathological Case Report. Br J Ophthalmol. 2005 Jul;89(7):920–1. PMID:15965180
2502. Pascual-Castroviejo I, Díaz-Gonzalez C, García-Melian RM, et al. Sturge-Weber Syndrome: Study of 40 Patients. Pediatr Neurol. 1993 Jul-Aug;9(4):283–8. PMID:8216540
2503. Pasquale S, Strianese D, Mansueto G, et al. Epithelioid Myoepithelioma of Lacrimal Gland. Virchows Arch. 2005 Jan;446(1):97. PMID:15568156
2504. Pasqualucci L, Dalla-Favera R. The Genetic Landscape of Diffuse Large B-Cell Lymphoma. Semin Hematol. 2015 Apr;52(2):67–76. PMID:25805586
2505. Pastora-Salvador N, Abelairas-Gómez J, Peralta-Calvo J, et al. Atypical Clinical Presentation and Long-Term Survival in a Patient with Optic Nerve Medulloepithelioma: A Case Report. J Med Case Rep. 2012 May 9;6:123. PMID:22571440
2506. Pastoret C, Houot R, Llamas-Gutierrez F, et al. Detection of Clonal Heterogeneity and Targetable Mutations in Myeloid Sarcoma by High-Throughput Sequencing. Leuk Lymphoma. 2017 Apr;58(4):1008–12. PMID:27659839
2507. Pastorino S, Yoshikawa Y, Pass HI, et al. A Subset of Mesotheliomas With Improved Survival Occurring in Carriers of BAP1 and Other Germline Mutations. J Clin Oncol. 2018 Oct 30;36(35):JCO2018790352. PMID:30376426
2508. Patel NR, Chrisinger JSA, Demicco EG, et al. USP6 Activation in Nodular Fasciitis by Promoter-Swapping Gene Fusions. Mod Pathol. 2017 Nov;30(11):1577–88. PMID:28752842
2509. Patil S, Perry A, Maccollin M, et al. Immunohistochemical Analysis Supports a Role for INI1/SMARCB1 in Hereditary Forms of Schwannomas, But Not in Solitary, Sporadic Schwannomas. Brain Pathol. 2008 Oct;18(4):517–9. PMID:18422762
2509A. Pattwell SS, Konnick EQ, Liu YJ, et al. Neurotrophic Receptor Tyrosine Kinase 2 (NTRK2) Alterations in Low-Grade Gliomas: Report of a Novel Gene Fusion Partner in a Pilocytic Astrocytoma and Review of the Literature. Case Rep Pathol. 2020 Jan 30:2020:5903863. PMID:32082673
2510. Paul SK, Chou L, Shields CL. Cutaneous Melanoma Metastatic to Anterior Lens Capsule. JAMA Ophthalmol. 2018 Mar 8;136(3):e180095. PMID:29522164
2511. Paulli M, Berti E, Rosso R, et al. CD30/Ki-1-Positive Lymphoproliferative Disorders of the Skin–Clinicopathologic Correlation and Statistical Analysis of 86 Cases: A Multicentric Study from the European Organization for Research and Treatment of Cancer Cutaneous Lymphoma Project Group. J Clin Oncol. 1995 Jun;13(6):1343–54. PMID:7751878
2512. Paxton CN, O'Malley DP, Bellizzi AM, et al. Genetic Evaluation of Juvenile Xanthogranuloma: Genomic Abnormalities Are Uncommon in Solitary Lesions, Advanced Cases May Show More Complexity. Mod Pathol. 2017 Sep;30(9):1234–40. PMID:28752840
2513. Paysse EA, Coats D, Chévez-Barrios P. An Unusual Case of Leukocoria: Heterotopic Brain Arising from the Retina. Arch Ophthalmol. 2003 Jan;121(1):119–22. PMID:12523898
2514. Peck T, Gervasio KA, Zhang PJL, et al. Atypical Lipomatous Tumor/Well-Differentiated Liposarcoma with Myxoid Stroma in a Hereditary Retinoblastoma Survivor. Ocul Oncol Pathol. 2020 Mar;6(2):79–86. PMID:32258014
2515. Pecorella I, Ciocci L, Modesti M, et al. Adenoma of the Non-Pigmented Ciliary Epithelium: A Rare Intraocular Tumor with Unusual Immunohistochemical Findings. Pathol Res Pract. 2009;205(12):870–5. PMID:19346082
2516. Pecorella I, Cruciani F, Russo V. A Solitary Fibrous Tumour of the Eyelid. Med Princ Pract. 2014;23(2):170–3. PMID:24216606
2517. Pecorella I, Garner A. Ostensible Oncocytoma of Accessory Lacrimal Glands. Histopathology. 1997 Mar;30(3):264–70. PMID:9088957
2518. Pe'er J. Ocular Surface Squamous Neoplasia. Ophthalmol Clin North Am. 2005 Mar;18(1):1–13, Vii. PMID:15763187
2519. Pe'er J. Pathology of Eyelid Tumors. Indian J Ophthalmol. 2016 Mar;64(3):177–90. PMID:27146927
2520. Pe'er J, Blumenthal EZ, Frenkel S. Punch Biopsy of Iris Lesions: A Novel Technique for Obtaining Histology Samples. Br J Ophthalmol. 2007 May;91(5):660–2. PMID:17446506
2521. Pe'er J, Hidayat AA, Ilsar M, et al. Glandular Tumors of the Lacrimal Sac. Their Histopathologic Patterns and Possible Origins. Ophthalmology. 1996 Oct;103(10):1601–5. PMID:8874432
2522. Pe'er J, Levinger S, Ilsar M, et al. Malignant Fibrous Histiocytoma of the Conjunctiva. Br J Ophthalmol. 1990 Oct;74(10):624–8. PMID:1704795
2523. Pe'er JJ, Stefanyszyn M, Hidayat AA. Nonepithelial Tumors of the Lacrimal Sac. Am J Ophthalmol. 1994 Nov 15;118(5):650–8. PMID:7977578
2524. Pekmezci M, Cuevas-Ocampo AK, Perry A, et al. Significance of H3K27me3 Loss in the Diagnosis of Malignant Peripheral Nerve Sheath Tumors. Mod Pathol. 2017 Dec;30(12):1710–9. PMID:28776579
2525. Pekmezci M, Reuss DE, Hirbe AC, et al. Morphologic and Immunohistochemical Features of Malignant Peripheral Nerve Sheath Tumors and Cellular Schwannomas. Mod Pathol. 2015 Feb;28(2):187–200. PMID:25189642
2526. Pellegrini M, Preziosa C, Yaghy A, et al. Choroidal Lymphoma: Diagnostic Value of Combined Indocyanine Green Angiography and Optical Coherence Tomography. Ocul Immunol Inflamm. 2022 Jan 1-8. PMID:35050836
2527. Pellerano F, Gil G, Rosario A, et al. Survey of 138 Conjunctival Tumors in the Dominican Republic. Ophthalmic Epidemiol. 2020 Aug;27(4):278–82. PMID:32066308
2528. Pellerano F, Guillermo E, Garrido G, et al. Congenital Orbital Teratoma. Ocul Oncol Pathol. 2017 Jan;3(1):11–6. PMID:28275597
2529. Pelmus M, Guillou L, Hostein I, et al. Monophasic Fibrous and Poorly Differentiated Synovial Sarcoma: Immunohistochemical Reassessment of 60 T(X;18)(SYT-SSX)-Positive Cases. Am J Surg Pathol. 2002 Nov;26(11):1434–40. PMID:12409719
2530. Pemov A, Hansen NF, Sindiri S, et al. Low Mutation Burden and Frequent Loss of CDKN2A/B and SMARCA2, But Not PRC2, Define Premalignant Neurofibromatosis Type 1-Associated Atypical Neurofibromas. Neuro Oncol. 2019 Aug 5;21(8):981–92. PMID:30722027
2531. Penfield W, Editor. Cytology and Cellular Pathology of the Nervous System. 2nd ed. New York (NY): Hafner Publishing Company; 1965.
2532. Pereira PR, Odashiro AN, Rodrigues-Reyes AA, et al. Histopathological Review of Sebaceous Carcinoma of the Eyelid. J Cutan Pathol. 2005 Aug;32(7):496–501. PMID:16008694
2533. Pereira TDSF, de Amorim LSD, Pereira NB, et al. Oral Pyogenic Granulomas Show MAPK/ERK Signaling Pathway Activation, Which Occurs Independently of BRAF, KRAS, HRAS, NRAS, GNA11, and GNA14 Mutations. J Oral Pathol Med. 2019 Nov;48(10):906–10. PMID:31310691
2534. Pérez-Bañón MD, Moreno Moreno E, Won-Kim HR, et al. Childhood Proliferative Fasciitis of the Orbit Mimicking Sarcoma: A Case Report. Orbit. 2023 Feb;42(1):104–6. PMID:34470541
2535. Perra MT, Colombari R, Maxia C, et al. Finding of Conjunctival Melanocytic Pigmented Lesions Within Pterygium. Histopathology. 2006 Mar;48(4):387–93. PMID:16487360
2535A. Perron E, Pissaloux D, Charon Barra C, et al. Melanocytic Myxoid Spindle Cell Tumor With ALK Rearrangement (MMySTAR): Report of 4 Cases of a Nevus Variant With Potential Diagnostic Challenge. Am J Surg Pathol. 2018 May;42(5):595–603. PMID:29635259
2536. Perry A, Banerjee R, Lohse CM, et al. A Role for Chromosome 9p21 Deletions in the Malignant Progression of Meningiomas and the Prognosis of Anaplastic Meningiomas. Brain Pathol. 2002 Apr;12(2):183–90. PMID:11958372
2537. Perry HD, Font RL. Iris Nodules in von Recklinghausen's Neurofibromatosis. Electron Microscopic Confirmation of Their Melanocytic Origin. Arch Ophthalmol. 1982 Oct;100(10):1635–40. PMID:6814406
2538. Peshtani A, Kaliki S, Eagle RC, et al. Medulloepithelioma: A Triad of Clinical Features. Oman J Ophthalmol. 2014 May;7(2):93–5. PMID:25136238
2539. Peterson C, Moore R, Hicks JL, et al. NGS Analysis Confirms Common TP53 and RB1 Mutations, and Suggests MYC Amplification in Ocular Adnexal Sebaceous Carcinomas. Int J Mol Sci. 2021 Aug 6;22(16):8454. PMID:34445161
2540. Petrovic A, Obéric A, Moulin A, et al. Ocular Adnexal (Orbital) Solitary Fibrous Tumor: Nuclear STAT6 Expression and Literature Review. Graefes Arch Clin Exp Ophthalmol. 2015 Sep;253(9):1609–17. PMID:25761539
2541. Pfaff E, Aichmüller C, Sill M, et al. Molecular Subgrouping of Primary Pineal Parenchymal Tumors Reveals Distinct Subtypes Correlated with Clinical Parameters and Genetic Alterations. Acta Neuropathol. 2020 Feb;139(2):243–57. PMID:31768671
2542. Pfeifer FM, Bridge JA, Neff JR, et al. Cytogenetic Findings in Aneurysmal Bone Cysts. Genes Chromosomes Cancer. 1991 Nov;3(6):416–9. PMID:1777412
2543. Pfister S, Janzarik WG, Remke M, et al. BRAF Gene Duplication Constitutes a Mechanism of MAPK Pathway Activation in Low-Grade Astrocytomas. J Clin Invest. 2008 May;118(5):1739–49. PMID:18398503
2544. Phan IT, Courtney RJ, Marx DP, et al. Proptosis Caused by Rhabdomyomatous Mesenchymal Hamartomata Occurring in the Orbit. Ophthalmic Plast Reconstr Surg. 2016 May-Jun;32(3):e62–4. PMID:25105519
2545. Phulware RH, Guleria P, Iyer VK, et al. Cytological Diagnosis of Langerhans Cell Histiocytosis: A Series of 47 Cases. Cytopathology. 2019 Jul;30(4):413–8. PMID:31017324
2546. Picarsic J, Pysher T, Zhou H, et al. BRAF V600E Mutation in Juvenile Xanthogranuloma Family Neoplasms of the Central Nervous System (CNS-JXG): A Revised Diagnostic Algorithm to Include Pediatric Erdheim-Chester Disease. Acta Neuropathol Commun. 2019 Nov 4;7(1):168. PMID:31685033
2547. Pichi F, Dolz-Marco R, Francis JH, et al. Advanced OCT Analysis of Biopsy-Proven Vitreoretinal Lymphoma. Am J Ophthalmol. 2022 Jun;238:16–26. PMID:34843686
2548. Pichi F, Neri P, Agarwal A, et al. Vasoproliferative Tumors in Intermediate Uveitis. Retina. 2020 Sep;40(9):1765–73. PMID:31584561
2549. Pickering H, Chernet A, Sata E, et al. Genomics of Ocular Chlamydia Trachomatis After 5 Years of SAFE Interventions for Trachoma in Amhara, Ethiopia. J Infect Dis. 2022 Mar 15;225(6):994–1004. PMID:33034349
2550. Pilarski R, Burt R, Kohlman W, et al. Cowden Syndrome and the PTEN Hamartoma Tumor Syndrome: Systematic Review and Revised Diagnostic Criteria. J Natl Cancer Inst. 2013 Nov 6;105(21):1607–16. PMID:24136893
2551. Pilarski R, Byrne L, Carlo MI, et al. BAP1 Tumor Predisposition Syndrome. 2016 Oct 13 [Updated 2024 Dec 5]. In: Adam MP, Feldman J, Mirzaa GM, et al., editors. GeneReviews. Seattle (WA): University of Washington, Seattle; 1993–2025. PMID:27748099
2552. Pilarski R, Cebulla CM, Massengill JB, et al. Expanding the Clinical Phenotype of Hereditary BAP1 Cancer Predisposition Syndrome, Reporting Three New Cases. Genes Chromosomes Cancer. 2014 Feb;53(2):177–82. PMID:24243779
2553. Pilarski R, Stephens JA, Noss R, et al. Predicting PTEN Mutations: An Evaluation of Cowden Syndrome and Bannayan-Riley-Ruvalcaba Syndrome Clinical Features. J Med Genet. 2011 Aug;48(8):505–12. PMID:21659347
2554. Pileri SA, Ascani S, Cox MC, et al. Myeloid Sarcoma: Clinico-Pathologic, Phenotypic and Cytogenetic Analysis of 92 Adult Patients. Leukemia. 2007 Feb;21(2):340–50. PMID:17170724
2555. Pileri SA, Grogan TM, Harris NL, et al. Tumours of Histiocytes and Accessory Dendritic Cells: An Immunohistochemical Approach to Classification from the International Lymphoma Study Group Based on 61 Cases. Histopathology. 2002 Jul;41(1):1–29. PMID:12121233
2556. Pinkerton OD, Hokama Y, Shigemura LA. Immunologic Basis for the Pathogenesis of Pterygium. Am J Ophthalmol. 1984 Aug 15;98(2):225–8. PMID:6383051
2557. Pinnix CC, Dabaja BS, Milgrom SA, et al. Ultra-Low-Dose Radiotherapy for Definitive Management of Ocular Adnexal B-Cell Lymphoma. Head Neck. 2017 Jun;39(6):1095–100. PMID:28370694
2558. Pinnix CC, Dabaja BS, Milgrom SA, et al. Ultra-Low-Dose Radiotherapy for Definitive Management of Ocular Adnexal B-Cell Lymphoma. Head Neck. 2019 May;41(5):1546. PMID:30990235
2559. Pire A, Orbach D, Galmiche L, et al. Clinical, Pathologic, and Molecular Features of Inflammatory Myofibroblastic Tumors in Children and Adolescents. Pediatr Blood Cancer. 2022 May;69(5):e29460. PMID:34854544

2560. Pires A, Peng Y, Boussahmain C, et al. Cutaneous and Mammary Apocrine Carcinomas Have Different Immunoprofiles. Hum Pathol. 2014 Feb;45(2):320–6. PMID:24342430
2561. Piro P, Pappas HR, Erozan YS, et al. Diagnostic Vitrectomy in Metastatic Breast Carcinoma in the Vitreous. Retina. 1982;2(3):182–8. PMID:6294773
2562. Pirouzmanesh A, Reinisch JF, Gonzalez-Gomez I, et al. Pilomatrixoma: A Review of 346 Cases. Plast Reconstr Surg. 2003 Dec;112(7):1784–9. PMID:14663221
2563. Pitchamuthu H, Gonzalez P, Kyle P, et al. Fat-Forming Variant of Solitary Fibrous Tumour of the Orbit: The Entity Previously Known as Lipomatous Haemangiopericytoma. Eye (Lond). 2009 Jun;23(6):1479–81. PMID:18617906
2564. Pivetti-Pezzi P, Torce C, Colabelli-Gisoldi RA, et al. Relapsing Bilateral Uveitis and Papilledema in Sinus Histiocytosis with Massive Lymphadenopathy (Rosai-Dorfman Disease). Eur J Ophthalmol. 1995 Jan-Mar;5(1):59–62. PMID:7795403
2565. Płaszczyca A, Nilsson J, Magnusson L, et al. Fusions Involving Protein Kinase C and Membrane-Associated Proteins in Benign Fibrous Histiocytoma. Int J Biochem Cell Biol. 2014 Aug;53:475–81. PMID:24721208
2566. Platt S, Al Zahrani Y, Singh N, et al. Extranodal Marginal Zone Lymphoma of Ocular Adnexa: Outcomes Following Radiation Therapy. Ocul Oncol Pathol. 2017 Sep;3(3):181–7. PMID:29134184
2567. Plaza JA, Garrity JA, Dogan A, et al. Orbital Inflammation with IgG4-Positive Plasma Cells: Manifestation of IgG4 Systemic Disease. Arch Ophthalmol. 2011 Apr;129(4):421–8. PMID:21482868
2568. Plaza JA, Suster S. The Toker Tumor: Spectrum of Morphologic Features in Primary Neuroendocrine Carcinomas of the Skin (Merkel Cell Carcinoma). Ann Diagn Pathol. 2006 Dec;10(6):376–85. PMID:17126260
2569. Plemel DJA, Benson MD, Tong CM, et al. Nonosseous Periocular Manifestations of Langerhans Cell Histiocytosis: A Case Report and Systematic Review. Ophthalmic Plast Reconstr Surg. 2021 Sep-Oct 01;37(5):408–13. PMID:33315841
2570. Pofee SV, Pawar PS, Gaddewar NS, et al. Primary Yolk Sac Tumor of Orbit: Report of a Rare Case. Indian J Cancer. 2020 Jul-Sep;57(3):337–9. PMID:32594074
2571. Pokorny KS, Hyman BM, Jakobiec FA, et al. Epibulbar Choristomas Containing Lacrimal Tissue. Clinical Distinction from Dermoids and Histologic Evidence of an Origin from the Palpebral Lobe. Ophthalmology. 1987 Oct;94(10):1249–57. PMID:3684203
2572. Polito E, Pichierri P, Loffredo A, et al. Inflammatory Myofibroblastic Tumor of the Orbit. Ophthalmologica. 2007;221(5):353–5. PMID:17728559
2573. Pollard ZF, Calhoun J. Deep Orbital Dermoid with Draining Sinus. Am J Ophthalmol. 1975 Feb;79(2):310–3. PMID:1115198
2574. Pollock PM, Harper UL, Hansen KS, et al. High Frequency of BRAF Mutations in Nevi. Nat Genet. 2003 Jan;33(1):19–20. PMID:12447372
2575. Polubothu S, Al-Olabi L, Carmen Del Boente M, et al. GNA11 Mutation as a Cause of Sturge-Weber Syndrome: Expansion of the Phenotypic Spectrum of Gα/11 Mosaicism and the Associated Clinical Diagnoses. J Invest Dermatol. 2020 May;140(5):1110–3. PMID:31838126
2576. Pongpruttipan T, Sukpanichnant S, Assanasen T, et al. Extranodal NK/T-Cell Lymphoma, Nasal Type, Includes Cases of Natural Killer Cell and αβ, γδ, and αβ/γδ T-Cell Origin: A Comprehensive Clinicopathologic and Phenotypic Study. Am J Surg Pathol. 2012 Apr;36(4):481–99. PMID:22314189
2577. Ponti G, Losi L, Pedroni M, et al. Value of MLH1 and MSH2 Mutations in the Appearance of Muir-Torre Syndrome Phenotype in HNPCC Patients Presenting Sebaceous Gland Tumors or Keratoacanthomas. J Invest Dermatol. 2006 Oct;126(10):2302–7. PMID:16826164
2578. Ponzoni M, Ferreri AJ. Bacteria Associated with Marginal Zone Lymphomas. Best Pract Res Clin Haematol. 2017 Mar-Jun;30(1-2):32–40. PMID:28288714
2579. Poole Perry LJ, Jakobiec FA, Zakka FR, et al. Reactive Retinal Astrocytic Tumors (So-Called Vasoproliferative Tumors): Histopathologic, Immunohistochemical, and Genetic Studies of Four Cases. Am J Ophthalmol. 2013 Mar;155(3):593–608.E1. PMID:23219067
2580. Popova T, Hebert L, Jacquemin V, et al. Germline BAP1 Mutations Predispose to Renal Cell Carcinomas. Am J Hum Genet. 2013 Jun 6;92(6):974–80. PMID:23684012
2581. Porrini G, Giovannini A, Amato G, et al. Photodynamic Therapy of Circumscribed Choroidal Hemangioma. Ophthalmology. 2003 Apr;110(4):674–80. PMID:12689885
2582. Portell CA, Aronow ME, Rybicki LA, et al. Clinical Characteristics of 95 Patients with Ocular Adnexal and Uveal Lymphoma: Treatment Outcomes in Extranodal Marginal Zone Subtype. Clin Lymphoma Myeloma Leuk. 2014 Jun;14(3):203–10. PMID:24417911
2583. Porter N, Sandhu A, O'Connell TB, et al. Pleomorphic Adenoma of the Palpebral Lobe of the Lacrimal Gland. Otolaryngol Head Neck Surg. 2007 Feb;136(2):328–9. PMID:17275570
2584. Poulogiannis G, Frayling IM, Arends MJ. DNA Mismatch Repair Deficiency in Sporadic Colorectal Cancer and Lynch Syndrome. Histopathology. 2010 Jan;56(2):167–79. PMID:20102395
2585. Poveda J, Cassidy DP, Zhou Y, et al. Expression of Germinal Center Cell Markers by Extranodal Marginal Zone Lymphomas of MALT Type Within Colonized Follicles, a Diagnostic Pitfall with Follicular Lymphoma. Leuk Lymphoma. 2021 May;62(5):1116–22. PMID:33283568
2586. Powers DB, Fisher E, Erdmann D. Zygomatic Intraosseous Hemangioma: Case Report and Literature Review. Craniomaxillofac Trauma Reconstr. 2017 Mar;10(1):1–10. PMID:28210401
2587. Pradhan A, Tripathy D, Mittal R. Infantile Simple Dacryops: Clinicopathological Correlation and Immunocharacterization. J AAPOS. 2020 Feb;24(1):42–6. PMID:31821863
2588. Preechawai P, Della Roccad RC, Della Rocca D, et al. Transitional Cell Carcinoma of the Lacrimal Sac. J Med Assoc Thai. 2005 Nov;88(Suppl 9):S138–42. PMID:16681067
2589. Presneau N, Baumhoer D, Behjati S, et al. Diagnostic Value of H3F3A Mutations in Giant Cell Tumour of Bone Compared to Osteoclast-Rich Mimics. J Pathol Clin Res. 2015 Mar 16;1(2):113–23. PMID:27499898
2590. Preston DL, Ron E, Yonehara S, et al. Tumors of the Nervous System and Pituitary Gland Associated with Atomic Bomb Radiation Exposure. J Natl Cancer Inst. 2002 Oct 16;94(20):1555–63. PMID:12381708
2591. Price EA, Kolkiewicz K, Patel R, et al. Detection and Reporting of RB1 Promoter Hypermethylation in Diagnostic Screening. Ophthalmic Genet. 2018 Aug;39(4):526–31. PMID:29851531
2592. Price HN. Congenital Melanocytic Nevi: Update in Genetics and Management. Curr Opin Pediatr. 2016 Aug;28(4):476–82. PMID:27307047
2593. Price KM, Cummings TJ, Etter JR, et al. Ectopic Brain in the Orbit Presenting as Disc Edema in an Adult. Orbit. 2009;28(1):74–7. PMID:19229751
2594. Priest JR, Williams GM, Manera R, et al. Ciliary Body Medulloepithelioma: Four Cases Associated with Pleuropulmonary Blastoma–a Report from the International Pleuropulmonary Blastoma Registry. Br J Ophthalmol. 2011 Jul;95(7):1001–5. PMID:21156700
2595. Prieto-Granada CN, Wiesner T, Messina JL, et al. Loss of H3K27me3 Expression Is a Highly Sensitive Marker for Sporadic and Radiation-Induced MPNST. Am J Surg Pathol. 2016 Apr;40(4):479–89. PMID:26645727
2596. Prieto-Granada CN, Zhang L, Antonescu CR, et al. Primary Cutaneous Adenoid Cystic Carcinoma with MYB Aberrations: Report of Three Cases and Comprehensive Review of the Literature. J Cutan Pathol. 2017 Feb;44(2):201–9. PMID:27859477
2597. Pruksakorn V, Tirakunwichcha S, Assanasen T. Orbital Myeloid Sarcoma in Adult Mimicking Nasolacrimal Duct Obstruction: A Case Report. Am J Ophthalmol Case Rep. 2016 Aug 12;4:35–7. PMID:29503920
2598. Pugh TJ, Ballonoff A, Newman F, et al. Improved Survival in Patients with Early Stage Low-Grade Follicular Lymphoma Treated with Radiation: A Surveillance, Epidemiology, and End Results Database Analysis. Cancer. 2010 Aug 15;116(16):3843–51. PMID:20564102
2599. Pujari A, Ali MJ, Mulay K, et al. The Black Lacrimal Sac: A Clinicopathological Correlation of a Malignant Melanoma with Anterior Lacrimal Crest Infiltration. Int Ophthalmol. 2014 Feb;34(1):111–5. PMID:23456510
2600. Pujari A, Bajaj MS, Sen S, et al. Conjunctival Angiomyxoma-Rare But Needs Observation. Can J Ophthalmol. 2018 Apr;53(2):e60–2. PMID:29631843
2601. Pulido JS, Flotte TJ, Raja H, et al. Dermal and Conjunctival Melanocytic Proliferations in Diffuse Uveal Melanocytic Proliferation. Eye (Lond). 2013 Sep;27(9):1058–62. PMID:23788206
2602. Pulido JS, Johnston PB, Nowakowski GS, et al. The Diagnosis and Treatment of Primary Vitreoretinal Lymphoma: A Review. Int J Retina Vitreous. 2018 May 7;4:18. PMID:29760948
2603. Pulido JS, Salomao DR, Frederick LA, et al. MyD-88 L265P Mutations Are Present in Some Cases of Vitreoretinal Lymphoma. Retina. 2015 Apr;35(4):624–7. PMID:25768255
2604. Pulitzer MP, Amin BD, Busam KJ. Merkel Cell Carcinoma: Review. Adv Anat Pathol. 2009 May;16(3):135–44. PMID:19395876
2605. Punia RS, Nanda A, Mohan H, et al. Clinicopathological Study of Dermolipoma–a Report of Four Cases. Indian J Pathol Microbiol. 2006 Oct;49(4):605–7. PMID:17183873
2606. Pupić-Bakrač J, Pupić-Bakrač A, Bačić I, et al. Epidermoid and Dermoid Cysts of the Head and Neck. J Craniofac Surg. 2021 Jan-Feb 01;32(1):e25–7. PMID:32796308
2607. Purcell JJ Jr, Shields JA. Hypertrophy with Hyperpigmentation of the Retinal Pigment Epithelium. Arch Ophthalmol. 1975 Nov;93(11):1122–6. PMID:1191102
2608. Purohit BS, Vargas MI, Ailianou A, et al. Orbital Tumours and Tumour-Like Lesions: Exploring the Armamentarium of Multiparametric Imaging. Insights Imaging. 2016 Feb;7(1):43–68. PMID:26518678
2609. Pusateri A, Margo CE. Intraocular Astrocytoma and its Differential Diagnosis. Arch Pathol Lab Med. 2014 Sep;138(9):1250–4. PMID:25171711
2610. Pushker N, Meel R, Kumar A, et al. Orbital and Periorbital Dermoid/Epidermoid Cyst: A Series of 280 Cases and a Brief Review. Can J Ophthalmol. 2020 Apr;55(2):167–71. PMID:31712044
2611. Pushker N, Shrey D, Bajaj MS, et al. Malignant Non-Teratoid Medulloepithelioma of the Optic Nerve with Intraocular Extension. Clin Exp Ophthalmol. 2010 Oct;38(7):731–3. PMID:20497433
2612. Pushpa G, Karve PP, Subashini K, et al. Abrikossoff's Tumor: An Unusual Presentation. Indian J Dermatol. 2013 Sep;58(5):407. PMID:24082205
2613. Qannam A, Bello IO. Comparison of Histological Grading Methods in Mucoepidermoid Carcinoma of Minor Salivary Glands. Indian J Pathol Microbiol. 2016 Oct-Dec;59(4):457–62. PMID:27721274
2614. Qi W, Rosikiewicz W, Yin Z, et al. Genomic Profiling Identifies Genes and Pathways Dysregulated by HEY1-NCOA2 Fusion and Shines a Light on Mesenchymal Chondrosarcoma Tumorigenesis. J Pathol. 2022 Aug;257(5):579–92. PMID:35342947
2615. Qian Y, Zakov ZN, Schoenfield L, et al. Iris Melanoma Arising in Iris Nevus in Oculo(-Dermal) Melanocytosis. Surv Ophthalmol. 2008 Jul-Aug;53(4):411–5. PMID:18572057
2616. Qin V, Verdijk RM, Paridaens D. Epibulbar Osseous Choristoma: A Photo Essay Case Report. Int Ophthalmol. 2019 May;39(5):1137–9. PMID:29589231
2617. Qiu M, Shields CL. Choroidal Nevus in the United States Adult Population: Racial Disparities and Associated Factors in the National Health and Nutrition Examination Survey. Ophthalmology. 2015 Oct;122(10):2071–83. PMID:26255109
2618. Qualman S, Lynch J, Bridge J, et al. Prevalence and Clinical Impact of Anaplasia in Childhood Rhabdomyosarcoma : A Report from the Soft Tissue Sarcoma Committee of the Children's Oncology Group. Cancer. 2008 Dec 1;113(11):3242–7. PMID:18985676
2618A. Quan VL, Zhang B, Mohan LS, et al. Activating Structural Alterations in MAPK Genes Are Distinct Genetic Drivers in a Unique Subgroup Of Spitzoid Neoplasms. Am J Surg Pathol. 2019 Apr;43(4):538–48. PMID:30640733
2619. Quattrochi B, Russell-Goldman E. Utility of Insulinoma-Associated Protein 1 (INSM1) and Mucin 2 (MUC2) Immunohistochemistry in the Distinction of Endocrine Mucin-Producing Sweat Gland Carcinoma From Morphologic Mimics. Am J Dermatopathol. 2022 Feb 1;44(2):92–7. PMID:34086646
2620. Queisser A, Seront E, Boon LM, et al. Genetic Basis and Therapies for Vascular Anomalies. Circ Res. 2021 Jun 25;129(1):155–73. PMID:34166070
2621. Quhill H, Mudhar HS, Spiteri Cornish K, et al. Cutaneous Malignant Melanoma Metastasis to the Pseudophakic Lens Capsule with Associated Granulomatous Intraocular Inflammation. Ocul Oncol Pathol. 2020 Oct;6(5):339–43. PMID:33123527
2622. Quhill H, Rennie IG, Rundle PA, et al. Three Cases of Intraocular Mesectodermal Leiomyoma Expressing Progesterone and Androgen Receptors. Eye (Lond). 2013 May;27(5):669–72. PMID:23519275
2623. Quigg M, Rust RS, Miller JQ. Clinical Findings of the Phakomatoses: Sturge-Weber Syndrome. Neurology. 2006 Feb 28;66(4):e17–8. PMID:16505293
2624. Quinquenel A, Fornecker LM, Letestu R, et al. Prevalence of BTK and PLCG2 Mutations in a Real-Life CLL Cohort Still on Ibrutinib After 3 Years: A FILO Group Study. Blood. 2019 Aug 15;134(7):641–4. PMID:31243043
2625. Quintanilla-Martinez L, Franklin JL, Guerrero I, et al. Histological and Immunophenotypic Profile of Nasal NK/T Cell Lymphomas from Peru: High Prevalence of P53 Overexpression. Hum Pathol. 1999 Jul;30(7):849–55. PMID:10414505

2626. Quintanilla-Martinez L, Kremer M, Keller G, et al. P53 Mutations in Nasal Natural Killer/T-Cell Lymphoma from Mexico: Association with Large Cell Morphology and Advanced Disease. Am J Pathol. 2001 Dec;159(6):2095–105. PMID:11733360
2627. Qureshi HS, Salama ME, Chitale D, et al. Primary Cutaneous Mucinous Carcinoma: Presence of Myoepithelial Cells as a Clue to the Cutaneous Origin. Am J Dermatopathol. 2004 Oct;26(5):353–8. PMID:15365364
2628. Raches D, Hiscock M, Chapieski L. Behavioral and Academic Problems in Children with Sturge-Weber Syndrome: Differences Between Children with and Without Seizures. Epilepsy Behav. 2012 Nov;25(3):457–63. PMID:23000106
2629. Raderer M, Kiesewetter B, Ferreri AJ. Clinicopathologic Characteristics and Treatment of Marginal Zone Lymphoma of Mucosa-Associated Lymphoid Tissue (MALT Lymphoma). CA Cancer J Clin. 2016 Mar-Apr;66(2):153–71. PMID:26773441
2630. Rafizadeh SM, Ghadimi H, Nozarian Z. Phakomatous Choristoma of the Eyelid and Orbit: A Case Report. Pediatr Dev Pathol. 2020 Aug;23(4):296–300. PMID:31640459
2631. Ragge NK, Acheson J, Murphree AL. Iris Mammillations: Significance and Associations. Eye (Lond). 1996;10(Pt 1):86–91. PMID:8763309
2632. Raghavan SS, Clark M, Louie CY, et al. Molecular Profiling of a Primary Cutaneous Signet-Ring Cell/Histiocytoid Carcinoma of the Eyelid. J Cutan Pathol. 2020 Sep;47(9):860–4. PMID:32358805
2632A. Raghavan SS, Kapler ES, Dinges MM, et al. Eruptive Spitz Nevus, a Striking Example of Benign Metastasis. Sci Rep. 2020 Oct;10(1):16216. PMID:33004920
2633. Rahangdale SR, Castillo M, Shockley W. MR in Squamous Cell Carcinoma of the Lacrimal Sac. AJNR Am J Neuroradiol. 1995 Jun-Jul;16(6):1262–4. PMID:7677021
2634. Rahimy E, Coffee RE, McCannel TA. Bilateral Diffuse Uveal Melanocytic Proliferation as a Precursor to Multiple Systemic Malignancies. Semin Ophthalmol. 2015 May;30(3):206–9. PMID:24124896
2635. Rahman AM, Madge SN, Billing K, et al. Craniofacial Fibrous Dysplasia: Clinical Characteristics and Long-Term Outcomes. Eye (Lond). 2009 Dec;23(12):2175–81. PMID:19182771
2636. Rahman T, Bhattacharjee K, Sarma JD, et al. Primary Dermatofibrosarcoma Protuberans of Orbit–a Rare Entity. Orbit. 2013 Apr;32(2):127–9. PMID:23448305
2637. Rai K, Pilarski R, Boru G, et al. Germline BAP1 Alterations in Familial Uveal Melanoma. Genes Chromosomes Cancer. 2017 Feb;56(2):168–74. PMID:27718540
2638. Rai K, Pilarski R, Cebulla CM, et al. Comprehensive Review of BAP1 Tumor Predisposition Syndrome with Report of Two New Cases. Clin Genet. 2016 Mar;89(3):285–94. PMID:26096145
2639. Rajabi MT, Poursayed Lazarjani SZ, Mohammadi SS, et al. Giant Cell Tumor: Changing Behavior from Intraorbital to Intraosseous Mass. J Curr Ophthalmol. 2020 Dec 12;32(4):414–6. PMID:33553846
2640. Rajaii F, Aronow ME, Campbell AA, et al. A Case of Metastatic Giant Cell Tumor of Soft Tissue of the Orbit Associated With PALB2 Variant. JAMA Ophthalmol. 2020 Dec 1;138(12):1322–4. PMID:33090178
2641. Rajaii F, Ghafourian A, Eberhart CG. Intratarsal Keratinous Cyst - an Emerging Entity. Case Rep Ophthalmol. 2013 Oct 5;4(3):160–4. PMID:24403898
2642. Rajan Kd A, Burris C, Iliff N, et al. DNA Mismatch Repair Defects and Microsatellite Instability Status in Periocular Sebaceous Carcinoma. Am J Ophthalmol. 2014 Mar;157(3):640–7.E1, 2. PMID:24321472
2643. Rajkumar SV, Dimopoulos MA, Palumbo A, et al. International Myeloma Working Group Updated Criteria for the Diagnosis of Multiple Myeloma. Lancet Oncol. 2014 Nov;15(12):e538–48. PMID:25439696
2644. Rajyalakshmi R, Akhtar M, Swathi Y, et al. Cytological Diagnosis of Rosai-Dorfman Disease: A Study of Twelve Cases with Emphasis on Diagnostic Challenges. J Cytol. 2020 Jan-Mar;37(1):46–52. PMID:31942098
2645. Ramaesh K, Marshall JW, Wharton SB, et al. Intraocular Metastases of Cutaneous Malignant Melanoma: A Case Report and Review of the Literature. Eye (Lond). 1999 Apr;13(Pt 2):247–50. PMID:10450391
2646. Ramakrishnan R, Chaudhry IH, Ramdial P, et al. Primary Cutaneous Adenoid Cystic Carcinoma: A Clinicopathologic and Immunohistochemical Study of 27 Cases. Am J Surg Pathol. 2013 Oct;37(10):1603–11. PMID:24025525
2647. Ramaswamy PV, Storm CA, Filiano JJ, et al. Multiple Granular Cell Tumors in a Child with Noonan Syndrome. Pediatr Dermatol. 2010 Mar-Apr;27(2):209–11. PMID:20537083
2648. Ramberg I, Heegaard S. Human Papillomavirus Related Neoplasia of the Ocular Adnexa. Viruses. 2021 Aug 2;13(8):1522. PMID:34452388
2649. Ramberg I, Møller-Hansen M, Toft PB, et al. Human Papillomavirus Infection Plays a Role in Conjunctival Squamous Cell Carcinoma: A Systematic Review and Meta-Analysis of Observational Studies. Acta Ophthalmol. 2021 Aug;99(5):478–88. PMID:33191633
2650. Ramberg I, Sjö NC, Bonde JH, et al. Inverted Papilloma of the Conjunctiva. BMJ Open Ophthalmol. 2019 Feb 28;4(1):e000193. PMID:30997398
2651. Ramberg I, Toft PB, Georgsen JB, et al. Conjunctival Intraepithelial Neoplasia and Carcinoma: Distinct Clinical and Histological Features in Relation to Human Papilloma Virus Status. Br J Ophthalmol. 2021 Jun;105(6):878–83. PMID:31649051
2652. Ramberg I, Toft PB, Heegaard S. Carcinomas of the Lacrimal Drainage System. Surv Ophthalmol. 2020 Nov-Dec;65(6):691–707. PMID:32304675
2653. Ramberg I, Vieira FG, Toft PB, et al. Genomic Alterations in Human Papillomavirus-Positive and -Negative Conjunctival Squamous Cell Carcinomas. Invest Ophthalmol Vis Sci. 2021 Nov 1;62(14):11. PMID:34779821
2654. Ramberg I, Vieira FG, Toft PB, et al. Viral and Genomic Drivers of Squamous Cell Neoplasms Arising in the Lacrimal Drainage System. Cancers (Basel). 2022 May 23;14(10):2558. PMID:35626161
2655. Ramesh S, Duckwiler G, Goldberg RA, et al. Multimodality Management of Complex Periorbital Venolymphatic Malformations. Ophthalmic Plast Reconstr Surg. 2019 Jul/Aug;35(4):387–98. PMID:30601461
2656. Ramlee N, Ramli N, Tajudin LS. Pleomorphic Adenoma in the Palpebral Lobe of the Lacrimal Gland Misdiagnosed as Chalazion. Orbit. 2007 Jun;26(2):137–9. PMID:17613864
2657. Ramos A, Pozo CD, Chinchurreta A, et al. Adenoid Cystic Carcinoma of the Lacrimal Sac: Case Report. Arq Bras Oftalmol. 2016 Sep-Oct;79(5):333–5. PMID:27982216
2658. Ramos-Betancourt N, Field MG, Davila-Alquisiras JH, et al. Whole Exome Profiling and Mutational Analysis of Ocular Surface Squamous Neoplasia. Ocul Surf. 2020 Oct;18(4):627–32. PMID:32717381
2659. Randon M, Lévy-Gabriel C, Abbas R, et al. Results of External Beam Radiotherapy for Diffuse Choroidal Hemangiomas in Sturge-Weber Syndrome. Eye (Lond). 2018 Jun;32(6):1067–73. PMID:29403070
2660. Rantala ES, Hernberg M, Kivelä TT. Overall Survival After Treatment for Metastatic Uveal Melanoma: A Systematic Review and Meta-Analysis. Melanoma Res. 2019 Dec;29(6):561–8. PMID:30664106
2661. Rantala ES, Hernberg MM, Piperno-Neumann S, et al. Metastatic Uveal Melanoma: The Final Frontier. Prog Retin Eye Res. 2022 Sep;90:101041. PMID:34999237
2662. Rao NA, Font RL. Mucoepidermoid Carcinoma of the Conjunctiva: A Clinicopathologic Study of Five Cases. Cancer. 1976 Oct;38(4):1699–709. PMID:991088
2663. Rao NA, Hidayat AA, McLean IW, et al. Sebaceous Carcinomas of the Ocular Adnexa: A Clinicopathologic Study of 104 Cases, with Five-Year Follow-Up Data. Hum Pathol. 1982 Feb;13(2):113–22. PMID:7076199
2664. Rao Q, Shen Q, Xia QY, et al. PSF/SFPQ is a Very Common Gene Fusion Partner in TFE3 Rearrangement-Associated Perivascular Epithelioid Cell Tumors (PEComas) and Melanotic Xp11 Translocation Renal Cancers: Clinicopathologic, Immunohistochemical, and Molecular Characteristics Suggesting Classification as a Distinct Entity. Am J Surg Pathol. 2015 Sep;39(9):1181–96. PMID:26274027
2665. Rao R, Honavar SG, Mulay K. Primary Lacrimal Gland Teratoma in an Adult: A Clinicopathologic and Radiological Correlation. Indian J Ophthalmol. 2019 Jul;67(7):1238–40. PMID:31238481
2666. Raparia K, Chang CC, Chévez-Barrios P. Intraocular Lymphoma: Diagnostic Approach and Immunophenotypic Findings in Vitrectomy Specimens. Arch Pathol Lab Med. 2009 Aug;133(8):1233–7. PMID:19653716
2667. Rashid A, Jakobiec FA. Avoiding the Major Complication of Ophthalmic Pathology: Misdiagnosis. A Review of Three Common Diagnostic Challenges. Semin Ophthalmol. 2014 Sep-Nov;29(5-6):468–74. PMID:25325875
2668. Rashid T, Bagatell R, Pawel B, et al. More Than Meets the Eye? A Cautionary Tale of Malignant Ectomesenchymoma Treated as Low-Risk Orbital Rhabdomyosarcoma. J Pediatr Hematol Oncol. 2021 Aug 1;43(6):e854–8. PMID:32769567
2669. Rasmussen P, Sjö LD, Prause JU, et al. Mantle Cell Lymphoma in the Orbital and Adnexal Region. Br J Ophthalmol. 2009 Aug;93(8):1047–51. PMID:19429588
2670. Rasmussen PK, Coupland SE, Finger PT, et al. Ocular Adnexal Follicular Lymphoma: A Multicenter International Study. JAMA Ophthalmol. 2014 Jul;132(7):851–8. PMID:24763920
2671. Rasmussen PK, Ralfkiaer E, Prause JU, et al. Diffuse Large B-Cell Lymphoma of the Ocular Adnexal Region: A Nation-Based Study. Acta Ophthalmol. 2013 Mar;91(2):163–9. PMID:22551232
2672. Rasmussen PK, Ralfkiaer E, Prause JU, et al. Follicular Lymphoma of the Ocular Adnexal Region: A Nation-Based Study. Acta Ophthalmol. 2015 Mar;93(2):184–91. PMID:25125069
2673. Rasmussen SA, Yang Q, Friedman JM. Mortality in Neurofibromatosis 1: An Analysis Using U.S. Death Certificates. Am J Hum Genet. 2001 May;68(5):1110–8. PMID:11283797
2674. Rath S, Agarwal S, Charan Das P, et al. Orbital Myeloid Sarcoma in Adults Presenting with Exposure Keratopathy and Hearing Loss. Can J Ophthalmol. 2015 Oct;50(5):e78–81. PMID:26455987
2675. Rath S, Connors JM, Dolman PJ, et al. Comparison of American Joint Committee on Cancer TNM-Based Staging System (7th Edition) and Ann Arbor Classification for Predicting Outcome in Ocular Adnexal Lymphoma. Orbit. 2014 Feb;33(1):23–8. PMID:24180616
2676. Rath S, Honavar SG, Reddy VA, et al. Sebaceous Carcinoma of the Eyelid Metastasizing to the Lacrimal Sac After 5 Years. Orbit. 2009;28(5):309–12. PMID:19874127
2677. Raval V, Reddy R, Kaliki S, et al. Optic Nerve Head Melanocytoma: Optical Coherence Tomography/Angiography Features. Indian J Ophthalmol. 2021 Feb;69(2):332–6. PMID:33463586
2678. Ravindran A, Goyal G, Go RS, et al. Rosai-Dorfman Disease Displays a Unique Monocyte-Macrophage Phenotype Characterized by Expression of OCT2. Am J Surg Pathol. 2021 Jan;45(1):35–44. PMID:33177341
2679. Razanamahery J, Diamond EL, Cohen-Aubart F, et al. Erdheim-Chester Disease with Concomitant Rosai-Dorfman Like Lesions: A Distinct Entity Mainly Driven by MAP2K1. Haematologica. 2020 Jan;105(1):e5–8. PMID:31123032
2680. Razem B, Raiteb M, El Mrini S, et al. Orbital Myeloid Sarcoma Misdiagnosed for Subperiostal Hematoma: A Case Report. J Med Case Rep. 2021 Oct 8;15(1):501. PMID:34625114
2681. Read RW, Burnstine M, Rowland JM, et al. Rhabdomyomatous Mesenchymal Hamartoma of the Eyelid: Report of a Case and Literature Review. Ophthalmology. 2001 Apr;108(4):798–804. PMID:11297501
2682. Rech KL, He R. Challenges in the Histopathologic Diagnosis of Histiocytic Neoplasms. J Natl Compr Canc Netw. 2021 Nov;19(11):1305–11. PMID:34781270
2683. Rednam SP, Erez A, Druker H, et al. Von Hippel-Lindau and Hereditary Pheochromocytoma/Paraganglioma Syndromes: Clinical Features, Genetics, and Surveillance Recommendations in Childhood. Clin Cancer Res. 2017 Jun 15;23(12):e68–75. PMID:28620007
2684. Reed RJ. Fibrous Dysplasia of Bone. A Review of 25 Cases. Arch Pathol. 1963 May;75:480–95. PMID:13973557
2685. Reed RJ, Fine RM, Meltzer HD. Palisaded, Encapsulated Neuromas of the Skin. Arch Dermatol. 1972 Dec;106(6):865–70. PMID:4639250
2686. Reese A, Margo CE. Conjunctival Squamous Intraepithelial Neoplasia and its Differential Diagnosis. J Clin Pathol. 2022 May;75(5):354–8. PMID:33619216
2687. Regillo CD, Eagle RC Jr, Shields JA, et al. Histopathologic Findings in Congenital Grouped Pigmentation of the Retina. Ophthalmology. 1993 Mar;100(3):400–5. PMID:8460012
2688. Rehan S, Aye K. In Patients with a Positive Family History of Familial Adenomatous Polyposis Can the Condition Be Diagnosed from the Presence of Congenital Hypertrophy of the Retinal Pigment Epithelium Detected Via an Eye Examination: A Systematic Review. Clin Exp Ophthalmol. 2020 Jan;48(1):98–116. PMID:31525261
2688A. Reichgelt BA, Visser O. Epidemiology and Survival of Merkel Cell Carcinoma in the Netherlands. A Population-Based Study of 808 Cases in 1993-2007. Eur J Cancer. 2011 Mar;47(4):579–85. PMID: 21144740.
2689. Reiman A, Kikuchi H, Scocchia D, et al. Validation of an NGS Mutation Detection Panel for Melanoma. BMC Cancer. 2017 Feb 22;17(1):150. PMID:28228113
2690. Reimann JD, Fletcher CD. Myxoid Dermatofibrosarcoma Protuberans: A Rare Variant Analyzed in a Series of 23 Cases. Am J Surg Pathol. 2007 Sep;31(9):1371–7. PMID:17721193
2691. Reinecke RD, Kuwabara T. Corneal Deposits Secondary to Topical Epinephrine.

Arch Ophthalmol. 1963 Aug;70:170–2. PMID:14060094
2692. Reinhardt A, Stichel D, Schrimpf D, et al. Anaplastic Astrocytoma with Piloid Features, a Novel Molecular Class of IDH Wildtype Glioma with Recurrent MAPK Pathway, CDKN2A/B and ATRX Alterations. Acta Neuropathol. 2018 Aug;136(2):273–91. PMID:29564591
2693. Reis GF, Bloomer MM, Perry A, et a . Pilocytic Astrocytomas of the Optic Nerve and Their Relation to Pilocytic Astrocytomas Elsewhere in the Central Nervous System. Mod Pathol. 2013 Oct;26(10):1279–87. PMID:23702730
2694. Reisenauer JS, Mneimneh W, Jenkins S, et al. Comparison of Risk Stratification Models to Predict Recurrence and Survival in Pleuropulmonary Solitary Fibrous Tumor. J Thorac Oncol. 2018 Sep;13(9):1349–62. PMID:29935303
2695. Rekhi B, Ingle A, Agarwal M, et al. Alveolar Soft Part Sarcoma 'Revisited': Clinicopathological Review of 47 Cases from a Tertiary Cancer Referral Centre, Including Immunohistochemical Expression of TFE3 in 22 Cases and 21 Other Tumours. Pathology. 2012 Jan;44(1):11–7. PMID:22173238
2696. Remmer MH, Kaliki S, Eagle RC, et al. Giant Leiomyoma of the Ciliary Body. Oman J Ophthalmol. 2014 May;7(2):31–3. PMID:25136234
2697. Ren M, Zeng JH, Luo QL, et al. Primary Malignant Melanoma of Lacrimal Sac. Int J Ophthalmol. 2014 Dec 18;7(6):1069–70. PMID:25540768
2698. Renfro L, Grant-Kels JM, Brown SA. Multiple Agminate Spitz Nevi. Pediatr Dermatol. 1989 Jun;6(2):114–7. PMID:2748471
2699. Repo P, Järvinen RS, Jäntti JE, et al. Population-Based Analysis of BAP1 Germline Variations in Patients with Uveal Melanoma. Hum Mol Genet. 2019 Jul 15;28(14):2415–26. PMID:31058963
2700. Requena C, Requena L, Kutzner H, et al. Spitz Nevus: A Clinicopathological Study of 349 Cases. Am J Dermatopathol. 2009 Apr;31(2):107–16. PMID:19318795
2701. Requena L, Prieto VG, Requena C, et al. Primary Signet-Ring Cell/Histiocytoid Carcinoma of the Eyelid: A Clinicopathologic Study of 5 Cases and Review of the Literature. Am J Surg Pathol. 2011 Mar;35(3):378–91. PMID:21317710
2702. Requena L, Sangüeza O. Cutaneous Adnexal Neoplasms. Cham (Switzerland): Springer; 2017.
2703. Requena L, Sangüeza O. Cutaneous Adnexal Neoplasms. Cham (Switzerland): Springer; 2017. pp. 12–38.
2704. Reyes-Godinez N, Tamez-Tamez VE, Ruiz-Lozano RE, et al. Congenital Orbital Glial Heterotopia Associated with Clinicopathological Anophthalmia: A Case Report. Klin Monbl Augenheilkd. 2023 Sep;240(9):1103–6. PMID:35253133
2705. Ribeiro SF, Chahud F, Cruz AA. Oculomotor Disturbances Due to Granular Cell Tumor. Ophthalmic Plast Reconstr Surg. 2012 Jan-Feb;28(1):e23–7. PMID:21464781
2706. Ribeiro SF, Chahud F, Cruz AA. Orbital Hemangiopericytoma/Solitary Fibrous Tumor in Childhood. Ophthalmic Plast Reconstr Surg. 2012 May-Jun;28(3):e58–60. PMID:21743364
2706A. Richardson TE, Tang K, Vasudevaraja V, et al. GOPC-ROS1 Fusion Due to Microdeletion at 6q22 Is an Oncogenic Driver in a Subset of Pediatric Gliomas and Glioneuronal Tumors. J Neuropathol Exp Neurol. 2019 Dec;78(12):1089–99. PMID:31626289
2707. Richter S, Vandezande K, Chen N, et al. Sensitive and Efficient Detection of RB1 Gene Mutations Enhances Care for Families with Retinoblastoma. Am J Hum Genet. 2003 Feb;72(2):253–69. PMID:12541220
2708. Riddle ND, Bui MM. Fibrous Dysplasia. Arch Pathol Lab Med. 2013 Jan;137(1):134–8. PMID:23276185
2709. Riemersma SA, Jordanova ES, Schop RF, et al. Extensive Genetic Alterations of the HLA Region, Including Homozygous Deletions of HLA Class II Genes in B-Cell Lymphomas Arising in Immune-Privileged Sites. Blood. 2000 Nov 15;96(10):3569–77. PMID:11071656
2710. Riffle JE, Prosser AH, Lee JR, et al. Nodular Fasciitis of the Orbit: A Case Report and Brief Review of the Literature. Case Rep Ophthalmol Med. 2011;2011:235956. PMID:22611507
2711. Rigaud C, Barkaoui MA, Thomas C, et al. Langerhans Cell Histiocytosis: Therapeutic Strategy and Outcome in a 30-Year Nationwide Cohort of 1478 Patients Under 18 Years of Age. Br J Haematol. 2016 Sep;174(6):887–98. PMID:27273725
2712. Righi A, Sbaraglia M, Gambarotti M, et al. Primary Vascular Tumors of Bone: A Monoinstitutional Morphologic and Molecular Analysis of 427 Cases With Emphasis on Epithelioid Variants. Am J Surg Pathol. 2020 Sep;44(9):1192–203. PMID:32271190
2713. Rihani HT, Dalvin LA, Hodge DO, et al. Incidence of Sturge-Weber Syndrome and Associated Ocular Involvement in Olmsted County, Minnesota, United States. Ophthalmic Genet. 2020 Apr;41(2):108–24. PMID:32233696
2714. Riley FC. Metastatic Tumors of the Eyelids. Am J Ophthalmol. 1970 Feb;69(2):259–64. PMID:5414008
2715. Riminucci M, Fisher LW, Shenker A, et al. Fibrous Dysplasia of Bone in the McCune-Albright Syndrome: Abnormalities in Bone Formation. Am J Pathol. 1997 Dec;151(6):1587–600. PMID:9403710
2716. Rishi K, Font RL. Sebaceous Gland Tumors of the Eyelids and Conjunctiva in the Muir-Torre Syndrome: A Clinicopathologic Study of Five Cases and Literature Review. Ophthalmic Plast Reconstr Surg. 2004 Jan;20(1):31–6. PMID:14752307
2717. Rishi P, Hirawat RS, Verma A. Association of Bilateral, Multiple Presumed Retinal Astrocytic Proliferations with Combined Hamartoma of Retina and Retinal Pigment Epithelium in a 9-Year-Old Male Child with Neurofibromatosis Type 2. Indian J Ophthalmol. 2016 Nov;64(11):850–2. PMID:27958212
2718. Rismiller KP, Crowe DR, Knackstedt TJ. Prognostic Factors, Treatment, and Survival in Primary Cutaneous Mucinous Carcinoma: A SEER Database Analysis. Dermatol Surg. 2020 Sep;46(9):1141–7. PMID:31702595
2719. Rito M, Fonseca I. Carcinoma Ex-Pleomorphic Adenoma of the Salivary Glands Has a High Risk of Progression When the Tumor Invades More Than 2.5 Mm Beyond the Capsule of the Residual Pleomorphic Adenoma. Virchows Arch. 2016 Mar;468(3):297–303. PMID:26638158
2720. Ritter J, Bielack SS. Osteosarcoma. Ann Oncol. 2010 Oct;21(Suppl 7):vii320–5. PMID:20943636
2721. Ritter MR, Dorrell MI, Edmonds J, et al. Insulin-Like Growth Factor 2 and Potential Regulators of Hemangioma Growth and Involution Identified by Large-Scale Expression Analysis. Proc Natl Acad Sci U S A. 2002 May 28;99(11):7455–60. PMID:12032304
2722. Rivolta C, Royer-Bertrand B, Rimoldi D, et al. UV Light Signature in Conjunctival Melanoma; Not Only Skin Should Be Protected from Solar Radiation. J Hum Genet. 2016 Apr;61(4):361–2. PMID:26657935
2723. Roberts F, MacDuff EM. An Update on Mesenchymal Tumours of the Orbit with an Emphasis on the Value of Molecular/Cytogenetic Testing. Saudi J Ophthalmol. 2018 Jan-Mar;32(1):3–12. PMID:29755264
2724. Roberts ME, Riegert-Johnson DL, Thomas BC, et al. A Clinical Scoring System to Identify Patients with Sebaceous Neoplasms at Risk for the Muir-Torre Variant of Lynch Syndrome. Genet Med. 2014 Sep;16(9):711–6. PMID:24603434
2725. Roberts ME, Riegert-Johnson DL, Thomas BC, et al. Screening for Muir-Torre Syndrome Using Mismatch Repair Protein Immunohistochemistry of Sebaceous Neoplasms. J Genet Couns. 2013 Jun;22(3):393–405. PMID:23212176
2726. Robertson AG, Shih J, Yau C, et al. Integrative Analysis Identifies Four Molecular and Clinical Subsets in Uveal Melanoma. Cancer Cell. 2017 Aug 14;32(2):204–220.E15. PMID:28810145
2727. Robertson AG, Shih J, Yau C, et al. Integrative Analysis Identifies Four Molecular and Clinical Subsets in Uveal Melanoma. Cancer Cell. 2018 Jan 8;33(1):151. PMID:29316429
2728. Robertson DM, Campbell RJ, Salomão DR. Mushroom-Shaped Choroidal Melanocytoma Mimicking Malignant Melanoma. Arch Ophthalmol. 2002 Jan;120(1):82–5. PMID:11786063
2729. Robertson SJ, Elder JE, Bekhor PS. Infantile Hemangioma Affecting the Iris. Pediatr Dermatol. 2021 Nov;38(6):1579–80. PMID:34632621
2730. Robinson C, Collins MT, Boyce AM. Fibrous Dysplasia/McCune-Albright Syndrome: Clinical and Translational Perspectives. Curr Osteoporos Rep. 2016 Oct;14(5):178–86. PMID:27492469
2731. Robinson DR, Wu YM, Kalyana-Sundaram S, et al. Identification of Recurrent NAB2-STAT6 Gene Fusions in Solitary Fibrous Tumor by Integrative Sequencing. Nat Genet. 2013 Feb;45(2):180–5. PMID:23313952
2732. Robinson JW, Brownstein S, Jordan DR, et al. Conjunctival Mucoepidermoid Carcinoma in a Patient with Ocular Cicatricial Pemphigoid and a Review of the Literature. Surv Ophthalmol. 2006 Sep-Oct;51(5):513–9. PMID:16950250
2733. Robson A, Lazar AJ, Ben Nagi J, et al. Primary Cutaneous Apocrine Carcinoma: A Clinico-Pathologic Analysis of 24 Cases. Am J Surg Pathol. 2008 May;32(5):682–90. PMID:18347508
2734. Rodrigues EB, Shields CL, Eagle RC Jr, et al. Solitary Intraosseous Orbital Myofibroma in Four Cases. Ophthalmic Plast Reconstr Surg. 2006 Jul-Aug;22(4):292–5. PMID:16855503
2735. Rodrigues FW, Arruda JT, Silva RE, et al. TP53 Gene Expression, Codon 72 Polymorphism and Human Papillomavirus DNA Associated with Pterygium. Genet Mol Res. 2008;7(4):1251–8. PMID:19065760
2736. Rodrigues M, Hidayat A, Karesh J. Pleomorphic Adenocarcinoma of Ciliary Epithelium Simulating an Epibulbar Tumor. Am J Ophthalmol. 1988 Nov 15;106(5):595–600. PMID:2461084
2737. Rodriguez EF, Blakeley J, Langmead S, et al. Low-Grade Schwann Cell Neoplasms with Leptomeningeal Dissemination: Clinicopathologic and Autopsy Findings. Hum Pathol. 2017 Feb;60:121–8. PMID:27666764
2738. Rodriguez FJ, Brosnan-Cashman JA, Allen SJ, et al. Alternative Lengthening of Telomeres, ATRX Loss and H3-K27M Mutations in Histologically Defined Pilocytic Astrocytoma with Anaplasia. Brain Pathol. 2019 Jan;29(1):126–40. PMID:30192422
2739. Rodriguez FJ, Ligon AH, Horkayne-Szakaly I, et al. BRAF Duplications and MAPK Pathway Activation Are Frequent in Gliomas of the Optic Nerve Proper. J Neuropathol Exp Neurol. 2012 Sep;71(9):789–94. PMID:22892521
2740. Rodriguez FJ, Perry A, Gutmann DH, et al. Gliomas in Neurofibromatosis Type 1: A Clinicopathologic Study of 100 Patients. J Neuropathol Exp Neurol. 2008 Mar;67(3):240–9. PMID:18344915
2741. Rodriguez-Galindo C, Allen CE. Langerhans Cell Histiocytosis. Blood. 2020 Apr 16;135(16):1319–31. PMID:32106306
2742. Rodriguez-Galindo C, Wilson MW, Haik BG, et al. Treatment of Metastatic Retinoblastoma. Ophthalmology. 2003 Jun;110(6):1237–40. PMID:12799253
2743. Rodriguez-Sains RS. Pigmented Conjunctival Neoplasms. Orbit. 2002 Sep;21(3):231–8. PMID:12187419
2744. Roelofs KA, O'Day R, Harby LA, et al. The MOLES System for Planning Management of Melanocytic Choroidal Tumors: Is It Safe? Cancers (Basel). 2020 May 21;12(5):1311. PMID:32455720
2745. Rogers R, Zhou F, Grunes D, et al. Chondroid Syringoma of the Axilla: An Unusual Tumor Diagnosed by Fine Needle Aspiration. Diagn Cytopathol. 2016 Apr;44(4):342–6. PMID:26800260
2746. Rogers WO, Wirth DF. Kinetoplast DNA Minicircles: Regions of Extensive Sequence Divergence. Proc Natl Acad Sci U S A. 1987 Jan;84(2):565–9. PMID:3025880
2747. Roh MR, Eliades P, Gupta S, et al. Genetics of Melanocytic Nevi. Pigment Cell Melanoma Res. 2015 Nov;28(6):661–72. PMID:26300491
2748. Rohrbach JM, Steuhl KP, Pressler H, et al. Primary Extraskeletal Mesenchymal Chondrosarcoma of the Lid. Graefes Arch Clin Exp Ophthalmol. 1991;229(2):172–7. PMID:2044980
2749. Rohrbach JM, Steuhl KP, Thanos S. [Monoclonal Antibody HMB-45 in Diagnosis of Intra-Ocular Melanoma]. Klin Monbl Augenheilkd. 1991 Oct;199(4):274–7. German. PMID:1762354
2750. Röhrich M, Koelsche C, Schrimpf D, et al. Methylation-Based Classification of Benign and Malignant Peripheral Nerve Sheath Tumors. Acta Neuropathol. 2016 Jun;131(6):877–87. PMID:26857854
2751. Rohwedder A, Keminer O, Hendricks C, et al. Detection of HPV DNA in Trichilemmomas by Polymerase Chain Reaction. J Med Virol. 1997 Feb;51(2):119–25. PMID:9021542
2752. Rolston JD, Han SJ, Cotter JA, et al. Gangliogliomas of the Optic Pathway. J Clin Neurosci. 2014 Dec;21(12):2244–9. PMID:25043166
2753. Romanello DA, Imamguliyeva Z, Cavalieri S, et al. Multidisciplinary Management of Radiation-Induced Salivary Gland Carcinomas in the Modern Radiotherapy Era. Cancers (Basel). 2020 Dec 14;12(12):3769. PMID:33327563
2754. Ron E, Modan B, Boice JD Jr, et al. Tumors of the Brain and Nervous System After Radiotherapy in Childhood. N Engl J Med. 1988 Oct 20;319(16):1033–9. PMID:3173432
2755. Ronen S, Keiser E, Collins KM, et al. Langerhans Cell Sarcoma Involving Skin and Showing Epidermotropism: A Comprehensive Review. J Cutan Pathol. 2021 Apr;48(4):547–57. PMID:32644218
2756. Rones B, Zimmerman LE. The Prognosis of Primary Tumors of the Iris Treated by Iridectomy. AMA Arch Ophthalmol. 1958 Aug;60(2):193–205. PMID:13558786
2757. Ronquillo CC, Vegunta S, Ellis N, et al. Adenoid Cystic Carcinoma of the Eyelid Can Locally Recur and Mimic Basal Cell Carcinoma: Case Report and Review of the Literature. Ophthalmic Plast Reconstr Surg. 2020 Sep/Oct;36(5):e112–5. PMID:32118847

2758. Rooper LM, Karantanos T, Ning Y, et al. Salivary Secretory Carcinoma With a Novel ETV6-MET Fusion: Expanding the Molecular Spectrum of a Recently Described Entity. Am J Surg Pathol. 2018 Aug;42(8):1121–6. PMID:29683815
2759. Rooper LM, Lombardo KA, Oliai BR, et al. MYB RNA In Situ Hybridization Facilitates Sensitive and Specific Diagnosis of Adenoid Cystic Carcinoma Regardless of Translocation Status. Am J Surg Pathol. 2021 Apr 1;45(4):488–97. PMID:33165092
2760. Rootman DB, Diniz SB, Cohen LM. Clinical Assessment and Lesion-Specific Management of Orbital Vascular Malformations. J Neurol Surg B Skull Base. 2021 Feb;82(1):116–28. PMID:33777625
2761. Rootman DB, Heran MK, Rootman J, et al. Cavernous Venous Malformations of the Orbit (So-Called Cavernous Haemangioma): A Comprehensive Evaluation of Their Clinical, Imaging and Histologic Nature. Br J Ophthalmol. 2014 Jul;98(7):880–8. PMID:24627253
2762. Rootman DB, Rootman J, Gregory S, et al. Stereotactic Fractionated Radiotherapy for Cavernous Venous Malformations (Hemangioma) of the Orbit. Ophthalmic Plast Reconstr Surg. 2012 Mar-Apr;28(2):96–102. PMID:22410657
2763. Rootman J. Vascular Malformations of the Orbit: Hemodynamic Concepts. Orbit. 2003 Jun;22(2):103–20. PMID:12789590
2764. Rootman J, Hay E, Graeb D, et al. Orbital-Adnexal Lymphangiomas. A Spectrum of Hemodynamically Isolated Vascular Hamartomas. Ophthalmology. 1986 Dec;93(12):1558–70. PMID:3808616
2765. Rosales Santillan M, Tschen JA, Soparkar CN. Apocrine Adenocarcinoma of the Eyelid: Case Report and Literature Review on Management. Dermatol Online J. 2019 May 15;25(5):13030/Qt2p62h61q. PMID:31220897
2766. Rose AM, Cowen S, Jayasena CN, et al. Presentation, Treatment, and Prognosis of Secondary Melanoma Within the Orbit. Front Oncol. 2017 Jun 23;7:125. PMID:28690979
2767. Rose AM, Kabiru J, Rose GE. Alveolar Soft-Part Sarcoma of the Orbit. Afr J Paediatr Surg. 2011 Jan-Apr;8(1):82–4. PMID:21478594
2768. Rose AM, Luo R, Radia UK, et al. Detection of Mutations in SF3B1, EIF1AX and GNAQ in Primary Orbital Melanoma by Candidate Gene Analysis. BMC Cancer. 2018 Dec 17;18(1):1262. PMID:30558566
2769. Rose AM, Luthert PJ, Jayasena CN, et al. Primary Orbital Melanoma: Presentation, Treatment, and Long-Term Outcomes for 13 Patients. Front Oncol. 2017 Dec 18;7:316. PMID:29326884
2770. Rosenbaum PS, Mahadevia PS, Goodman LA, et al. Acinic Cell Carcinoma of the Lacrimal Gland. Arch Ophthalmol. 1995 Jun;113(6):781–5. PMID:7540387
2771. Rosenwald A, Wright G, Chan WC, et al. The Use of Molecular Profiling to Predict Survival After Chemotherapy for Diffuse Large-B-Cell Lymphoma. N Engl J Med. 2002 Jun 20;346(25):1937–47. PMID:12075054
2772. Rosner M, Zloto O. Periocular Molluscum Contagiosum: Six Different Clinical Presentations. Acta Ophthalmol. 2018 Aug;96(5):e600–5. PMID:29855150
2773. Rossi ED, Pantanowitz L, Hornick JL. Cytologic and Histological Features of Rare Nonepithelial and Nonlymphoid Tumors of the Thyroid. Cancer Cytopathol. 2021 Aug;129(8):583–602. PMID:33493367
2774. Rosso R, Colombo R, Ricevuti G. Neurilemmoma of the Ciliary Body: Report of a Case. Br J Ophthalmol. 1983 Sep;67(9):585–7. PMID:6882714
2775. Roth MJ, Medeiros LJ, Elenitoba-Johnson K, et al. Extramedullary Myeloid Cell Tumors. An Immunohistochemical Study of 29 Cases Using Routinely Fixed and Processed Paraffin-Embedded Tissue Sections. Arch Pathol Lab Med. 1995 Sep;119(9):790–8. PMID:7668936
2776. Rothová N, Houbová J. [Histiocytosis X]. Cesk Pediatr. 1968 Oct;23(10):890–3. Czech. PMID:5701259
2777. Rowley SA, O'Callaghan FJ, Osborne JP. Ophthalmic Manifestations of Tuberous Sclerosis: A Population Based Study. Br J Ophthalmol. 2001 Apr;85(4):420–3. PMID:11264130
2778. Roy P, Bullock MJ, Perez-Ordoñez B, et al. Epithelial-Myoepithelial Carcinoma with High Grade Transformation. Am J Surg Pathol. 2010 Sep;34(9):1258–65. PMID:20679885
2779. Royo C, Salaverria I, Hartmann EM, et al. The Complex Landscape of Genetic Alterations in Mantle Cell Lymphoma. Semin Cancer Biol. 2011 Nov;21(5):322–34. PMID:21945515
2780. Rubinstein LJ. Pathological Features of Optic Nerve and Chiasmatic Gliomas. Neurofibromatosis. 1988;1(3):152–8. PMID:3152462
2781. Ruhoy SM, Thomas D, Nuovo GJ. Multiple Inverted Follicular Keratoses as a Presenting Sign of Cowden's Syndrome: Case Report with Human Papillomavirus Studies. J Am Acad Dermatol. 2004 Sep;51(3):411–5. PMID:15337985
2782. Rujimethapass N, Manuskiatti W, Wanitphakdeedecha R, et al. Ocular Manifestations of Facial Port-Wine Stain, Nevus of Ota, and Phakomatosis Pigmentovascularis in Asian Patients. J Am Acad Dermatol. 2021 Nov;85(5):1194–200. PMID:32387657
2783. Rulon DB, Helwig EB. Cutaneous Sebaceous Neoplasms. Cancer. 1974 Jan;33(1):82–102. PMID:4129561
2784. Rummelt V, Folberg R, Rummelt C, et al. Microcirculation Architecture of Melanocytic Nevi and Malignant Melanomas of the Ciliary Body and Choroid. A Comparative Histopathologic and Ultrastructural Study. Ophthalmology. 1994 Apr;101(4):718–27. PMID:8152768
2785. Rummelt V, Folberg R, Woolson RF, et al. Relation Between the Microcirculation Architecture and the Aggressive Behavior of Ciliary Body Melanomas. Ophthalmology. 1995 May;102(5):844–51. PMID:7777286
2786. Ruocco E, Brunetti G, Del Vecchio M, et al. The Practical Use of Cytology for Diagnosis in Dermatology. J Eur Acad Dermatol Venereol. 2011 Feb;25(2):125–9. PMID:20553359
2787. Ruppenstein M, Straub BK, Ach T, et al. [Primary Intrastromal Iris Cysts]. Klin Monbl Augenheilkd. 2010 May;227(5):425–9. German. PMID:20490997
2788. Rusch A, Ziltener G, Nackaerts K, et al. Prevalence of BRCA-1 Associated Protein 1 Germline Mutation in Sporadic Malignant Pleural Mesothelioma Cases. Lung Cancer. 2015 Jan;87(1):77–9. PMID:25468148
2789. Rush A, Leone CR Jr. Ectopic Lacrimal Gland Cyst of the Orbit. Am J Ophthalmol. 1981 Aug;92(2):198–201. PMID:7270633
2790. Rush JA, Younge BR, Campbell RJ, et al. Optic Glioma. Long-Term Follow-Up of 85 Histopathologically Verified Cases. Ophthalmology. 1982 Nov;89(11):1213–9. PMID:6818504
2791. Rushlow D, Piovesan B, Zhang K, et al. Detection of Mosaic RB1 Mutations in Families with Retinoblastoma. Hum Mutat. 2009 May;30(5):842–51. PMID:19280657
2792. Rushlow DE, Mol BM, Kennett JY, et al. Characterisation of Retinoblastomas Without RB1 Mutations: Genomic, Gene Expression, and Clinical Studies. Lancet Oncol. 2013 Apr;14(4):327–34. PMID:23498719
2793. Russell-Goldman E, Dubuc A, Hanna J. Differential Expression of PLAG1 in Apocrine and Eccrine Cutaneous Mixed Tumors: Evidence for Distinct Molecular Pathogenesis. Am J Dermatopathol. 2020 Apr;42(4):251–7. PMID:30839344
2794. Ryan SJ, Font RL. Primary Epithelial Neoplasms of the Lacrimal Sac. Am J Ophthalmol. 1973 Jul;76(1):73–88. PMID:4352147
2794A. Ryall S, Zapotocky M, Fukuoka K, et al. Integrated Molecular and Clinical Analysis of 1,000 Pediatric Low-Grade Gliomas. Cancer Cell. 2020 Apr;37(4):569–83.E5. PMID:32289278
2795. Sa HS, Rubin ML, Ning J, et al. Association of T and N Categories of the American Joint Commission on Cancer, 8th Edition, With Metastasis and Survival in Patients With Orbital Sarcoma. JAMA Ophthalmol. 2020 Apr 1;138(4):374–81. PMID:32105303
2796. Sa HS, Tetzlaff MT, Esmaeli B. Predictors of Local Recurrence for Eyelid Sebaceous Carcinoma: Questionable Value of Routine Conjunctival Map Biopsies for Detection of Pagetoid Spread. Ophthalmic Plast Reconstr Surg. 2019 Sep/Oct;35(5):419–25. PMID:30865067
2797. Sabazade S, Herrspiegel C, Gill V, et al. No Differences in the Long-Term Prognosis of Iris and Choroidal Melanomas When Adjusting for Tumor Thickness and Diameter. BMC Cancer. 2021 Nov 24;21(1):1270. PMID:34819035
2798. Sabeti S, Ball KL, Burkhart C, et al. Consensus Statement for the Management and Treatment of Port-Wine Birthmarks in Sturge-Weber Syndrome. JAMA Dermatol. 2021 Jan 1;157(1):98–104. PMID:33175124
2799. Sabry AO, Patel BC. Papilloma. In: StatPearls. Treasure Island (FL): StatPearls Publishing; 2022. PMID:32809572
2800. Sadegh L, Chen PW, Brown JR, et al. NKT Cells Act Through Third Party Bone Marrow-Derived Cells to Suppress NK Cell Activity in the Liver and Exacerbate Hepatic Melanoma Metastases. Int J Cancer. 2015 Sep 1;137(5):1085–94. PMID:25683463
2801. Sadick M, Müller-Wille R, Wildgruber M, et al. Vascular Anomalies (Part I): Classification and Diagnostics of Vascular Anomalies. Rofo. 2018 Sep;190(9):825–35. PMID:29874693
2802. Sadun F, Hinton DR, Sadun AA. Rapid Growth of an Optic Nerve Ganglioglioma in a Patient with Neurofibromatosis 1. Ophthalmology. 1996 May;103(5):794–9. PMID:8637690
2803. Saeed MU, Chang BY, Anand S, et al. Diagnostic Surprise in an Evisceration Specimen. Orbit. 2007 Jun;26(2):129–31. PMID:17613862
2804. Saeed P, Rootman J, Nugent RA, et al. Optic Nerve Sheath Meningiomas. Ophthalmology. 2003 Oct;110(10):2019–30. PMID:14522782
2805. Saegusa M, Takano Y, Hashimura M, et al. HPV Type 16 in Conjunctival and Junctional Papilloma, Dysplasia, and Squamous Cell Carcinoma. J Clin Pathol. 1995 Dec;48(12):1106–10. PMID:8567996
2806. Saeki T, Kawano M, Nagasawa T, et al. Validation of the Diagnostic Criteria for IgG4-Related Kidney Disease (IgG4-RKD) 2011, and Proposal of a New 2020 Version. Clin Exp Nephrol. 2021 Feb;25(2):99–109. PMID:33398598
2807. Saffra N, Gorgani F, Panasci D, et al. Diplopia and Proptosis Due to Isolated Lateral Rectus Plasmacytoma in a Patient with Multiple Myeloma. BMJ Case Rep. 2019 Jul 8;12(7):e229178. PMID:31289159
2808. Safneck JR, Napier LB, Halliday WC. Malignant Astrocytoma of the Optic Nerve in a Child. Can J Neurol Sci. 1992 Nov;19(4):498–503. PMID:1330262
2809. Saggini A, Gulia A, Argenyi Z, et al. A Variant of Lymphomatoid Papulosis Simulating Primary Cutaneous Aggressive Epidermotropic CD8+ Cytotoxic T-Cell Lymphoma. Description of 9 Cases. Am J Surg Pathol. 2010 Aug;34(8):1168–75. PMID:20661014
2810. Sagoo MS, Mruthyunjaya P, Cree I, et al. Malignant Transformation of Iris Melanocytoma to Iris Ring Melanoma. Br J Ophthalmol. 2007 Nov;91(11):1571–2. PMID:17947283
2811. Sah RP, Chari ST. Serologic Issues in IgG4-Related Systemic Disease and Autoimmune Pancreatitis. Curr Opin Rheumatol. 2011 Jan;23(1):108–13. PMID:21124093
2812. Saha K, Leatherbarrow B. Orbital Lymphangiomas: A Review of Management Strategies. Curr Opin Ophthalmol. 2012 Sep;23(5):433–8. PMID:22828166
2813. Saharan N, Gupta N, Loordudasan L, et al. Fine Needle Aspiration Cytology from an Axillary Lymph Node: Finessing the Fine Distinctions. Diagn Cytopathol. 2021 Dec;49(12):1257–60. PMID:34708939
2814. Sahm F, Capper D, Preusser M, et al. BRAFV600E Mutant Protein is Expressed in Cells of Variable Maturation in Langerhans Cell Histiocytosis. Blood. 2012 Sep 20;120(12):e28–34. PMID:22859608
2815. Sahm F, Jakobiec FA, Meyer J, et al. Somatic Mutations of DICER1 and KMT2D Are Frequent in Intraocular Medulloepitheliomas. Genes Chromosomes Cancer. 2016 May;55(5):418–27. PMID:26841698
2816. Sahm F, Schrimpf D, Olar A, et al. TERT Promoter Mutations and Risk of Recurrence in Meningioma. J Natl Cancer Inst. 2015 Dec 13;108(5):djv377. PMID:26668184
2817. Sahm F, Schrimpf D, Stichel D, et al. DNA Methylation-Based Classification and Grading System for Meningioma: A Multicentre, Retrospective Analysis. Lancet Oncol. 2017 May;18(5):682–94. PMID:28314689
2818. Saiju R, Duwal S. Bilateral Retinoblastoma in Early Infancy. Nepal J Ophthalmol. 2013 Jan-Jun;5(1):124–8. PMID:23584660
2819. Sakai A, Tagami M, Kakehashi A, et al. Expression, Intracellular Localization, and Mutation of EGFR in Conjunctival Squamous Cell Carcinoma and the Association with Prognosis and Treatment. PLoS One. 2020 Aug 24;15(8):e0238120. PMID:32833992
2820. Sakaida H, Kobayashi M, Yuta A, et al. Squamous Cell Carcinoma of the Nasolacrimal Duct. Eur Arch Otorhinolaryngol. 2009 Mar;266(3):455–8. PMID:18488243
2821. Sakamoto A, Oda Y, Iwamoto Y, et al. A Comparative Study of Fibrous Dysplasia and Osteofibrous Dysplasia with Regard to Gsalpha Mutation at the Arg201 Codon: Polymerase Chain Reaction-Restriction Fragment Length Polymorphism Analysis of Paraffin-Embedded Tissues. J Mol Diagn. 2000 May;2(2):67–72. PMID:11272890
2822. Sakamoto K, Morimoto A, Shioda Y, et al. Central Diabetes Insipidus in Pediatric Patients with Langerhans Cell Histiocytosis: Results from the JLSG-96/02 Studies. Pediatr Blood Cancer. 2019 Jan;66(1):e27454. PMID:30207064
2823. Salam A, Barrett AW, Malhotra R, et al. Marsupialization for Lacrimal Ductular Cysts (Dacryops): A Case Series. Ophthalmic Plast Reconstr Surg. 2012 Jan-Feb;28(1):57–62. PMID:21956544
2824. Salamah MM, Hammoudi SM, Sadi AR. Infantile Myofibromatosis. J Pediatr Surg. 1988 Oct;23(10):975–7. PMID:3236168
2825. Salaverria I, Royo C, Carvajal-Cuenca A, et al. CCND2 Rearrangements Are the Most Frequent Genetic Events in Cyclin D1(-) Mantle Cell Lymphoma. Blood. 2013 Feb 21;121(8):1394–402. PMID:23255553
2826. Salib RJ, Afoakwah EO. De Novo Papillary Squamous Carcinoma of the Lacrimal Sac. Auris Nasus Larynx. 2003 May;30(2):205–8. PMID:12753996
2827. Salinas R, Puig M, Fry CL, et al.

Floppy Eyelid Syndrome: A Comprehensive Review. Ocul Surf. 2020 Jan;18(1):31–9. PMID:31593763
2828. Salinas-Souza C, De Andrea C, Bihl M, et al. GNAS Mutations Are Not Detected in Parosteal and Low-Grade Central Osteosarcomas. Mod Pathol. 2015 Oct;28(10):1336–42. PMID:26248895
2829. Salisbury JA, Szpak CA, Klintworth GK. Pigmented Squamous Cell Carcinoma of the Conjunctiva. A Clinicopathologic Ultrastructural Study. Ophthalmology. 1983 Dec;90(12):1477–81. PMID:6677848
2830. Salomão DR, Mathers WD, Sutphin JE, et al. Cytologic Changes in the Conjunctiva Mimicking Malignancy After Topical Mitomycin C Chemotherapy. Ophthalmology. 1999 Sep;106(9):1756–60. PMID:10485547
2831. Salomão DR, Pulido JS, Johnston PB, et al. Vitreoretinal Presentation of Secondary Large B-Cell Lymphoma in Patients with Systemic Lymphoma. JAMA Ophthalmol. 2013 Sep;131(9):1151–8. PMID:23744124
2832. Salotti JA, Nanduri V, Pearce MS, et al. Incidence and Clinical Features of Langerhans Cell Histiocytosis in the UK and Ireland. Arch Dis Child. 2009 May;94(5):376–80. PMID:19060008
2833. Salour H, Tavakoli M, Karimi S, et al. Granular Cell Tumor of the Orbit. J Ophthalmic Vis Res. 2013 Oct;8(4):376–9. PMID:24653826
2834. Salvador AH, Beabout JW, Dahlin DC. Mesenchymal Chondrosarcoma–Observations on 30 New Cases. Cancer. 1971 Sep;28(3):605–15. PMID:5096926
2835. Salzer-Kuntschik M, Delling G, Beron G, et al. Morphological Grades of Regression in Osteosarcoma After Polychemotherapy - Study COSS 80. J Cancer Res Clin Oncol. 1983;106 Suppl(Suppl 1):21–4. PMID:6577010
2836. Samara WA, Khoo CT, Say EA, et al. Juvenile Xanthogranuloma Involving the Eye and Ocular Adnexa: Tumor Control, Visual Outcomes, and Globe Salvage in 30 Patients. Ophthalmology. 2015 Oct;122(10):2130–8. PMID:26189188
2837. Sammour R, Lafaille P, Joncas V, et al. Adenoid Cystic Carcinoma of the Eyelid: A Rare Cutaneous Tumor Treated with Mohs Micrographic Surgery. Dermatol Surg. 2009 Jun;35(6):997–1000. PMID:19397655
2838. Sampieri K, Mencarelli MA, Epistolato MC, et al. Genomic Differences Between Retinoma and Retinoblastoma. Acta Oncol. 2008;47(8):1483–92. PMID:18785023
2839. Samson SI, Konty K, Lee WN, et al. Quantifying the Impact of Influenza Among Persons With Type 2 Diabetes Mellitus: A New Approach to Determine Medical and Physical Activity Impact. J Diabetes Sci Technol. 2021 Jan;15(1):44–52. PMID:31747789
2840. Samuelov L, Kinori M, Chamlin SL, et al. Risk of Intraocular and Other Extracutaneous Involvement in Patients with Cutaneous Juvenile Xanthogranuloma. Pediatr Dermatol. 2018 May;35(3):329–35. PMID:29488239
2841. Sanborn GE, Valenzuela RE, Green WR. Leiomyoma of the Orbit. Am J Ophthalmol. 1979 Mar;87(3):371–5. PMID:434098
2842. Sánchez-Vicente JL, Contreras-Díaz M, Rueda T, et al. Combined Hamartoma of the Retina and Retinal Pigment Epithelium in a Patient with Gorlin Syndrome: Spontaneous Partial Resolution of Traction Caused by Epiretinal Membrane. Case Rep Ophthalmol Med. 2016;2016:2312196. PMID:27595027
2843. Sandberg AA, Bridge JA. Updates on the Cytogenetics and Molecular Genetics of Bone and Soft Tissue Tumors. Dermatofibrosarcoma Protuberans and Giant Cell Fibroblastoma. Cancer Genet Cytogenet. 2003 Jan 1;140(1):1–12. PMID:12550751
2844. Sanders TE. Intraocular Juvenile Xanthogranuloma (Nevoxanthogranuloma): A Survey of 20 Cases. Trans Am Ophthalmol Soc. 1960;58:59–74. PMID:13746162
2845. Sane F, Sauter P, Fronval S, et al. [Fruit of the Emergence of an Enterovirus: Acute Haemorrhagic Conjunctivitis]. Ann Biol Clin (Paris). 2008 Sep-Oct;66(5):485–92. French. PMID:18957336
2846. Sanerkin NG, Mott MG, Roylance J. An Unusual Intraosseous Lesion with Fibroblastic, Osteoclastic, Osteoblastic, Aneurysmal and Fibromyxoid Elements. "Solid" Variant of Aneurysmal Bone Cyst. Cancer. 1983 Jun 15;51(12):2278–86. PMID:6850506
2847. Sangle NA, Schmidt RL, Patel JL, et al. Optimized Immunohistochemical Panel to Differentiate Myeloid Sarcoma from Blastic Plasmacytoid Dendritic Cell Neoplasm. Mod Pathol. 2014 Aug;27(8):1137–43. PMID:24390220
2848. Sant DW, Tao W, Field MG, et al. Whole Exome Sequencing of Lacrimal Gland Adenoid Cystic Carcinoma. Invest Ophthalmol Vis Sci. 2017 May 1;58(6):BIO240–6. PMID:28820917
2849. Saornil MA, Egan KM, Gragoudas ES, et al. Histopathology of Proton Beam-Irradiated Vs Enucleated Uveal Melanomas. Arch Ophthalmol. 1992 Aug;110(8):1112–8. PMID:1323252
2850. Sarangi J, Konkimalla A, Kaur K, et al. Endocrine Mucin Producing Sweat Gland Carcinoma with Metastasis to Parotid Gland: Not as Indolent as Perceived? Head Neck Pathol. 2022 Mar;16(1):331–7. PMID:34184156
2851. Sarfraz H, Gentille C, Ensor J, et al. Primary Cutaneous Anaplastic Large-Cell Lymphoma: A Review of the SEER Database from 2005 to 2016. Clin Exp Dermatol. 2021 Dec;46(8):1420–6. PMID:34081802
2852. Sarin V, Singh B, Prasher P. A Silent Nasal Mass with Ophthalmic Presentation. Orbit. 2010 Dec;29(6):367–9. PMID:21158582
2852A. Sarin KY, Sun BK, Bangs CD, et al. Activating HRAS Mutation in Agminated Spitz Nevi Arising in a Nevus Spilus. JAMA Dermatol. 2013 Sep;149(9):1077–81. PMID:23884457
2853. Saro F, Clua A, Esteva E, et al. Cytologic Diagnosis of Ocular Melanocytoma: A Case Report. Acta Cytol. 2008 Jan-Feb;52(1):87–90. PMID:18323281
2854. Sasco AJ, Jaquet A, Boidin E, et al. The Challenge of AIDS-Related Malignancies in Sub-Saharan Africa. PLoS One. 2010 Jan 11;5(1):e8621. PMID:20066157
2855. Sassani JW, Yanoff M. Inverted Follicular Keratosis. Am J Ophthalmol. 1979 Jun;87(6):810–3. PMID:453311
2856. Sastre X, Chantada GL, Doz F, et al. Proceedings of the Consensus Meetings from the International Retinoblastoma Staging Working Group on the Pathology Guidelines for the Examination of Enucleated Eyes and Evaluation of Prognostic Risk Factors in Retinoblastoma. Arch Pathol Lab Med. 2009 Aug;133(8):1199–202. PMID:19653709
2857. Sato H, Sato N, Gakiya M, et al. Neonatal Orbital Teratoma with Intracranial Extension–Case Report. Neurol Med Chir (Tokyo). 1985 Jan;25(1):50–4. PMID:2581161
2858. Saunders T, Margo CE. Intraocular Medulloepithelioma. Arch Pathol Lab Med. 2012 Feb;136(2):212–6. PMID:22288972
2859. Savar A, Ross MI, Prieto VG, et al. Sentinel Lymph Node Biopsy for Ocular Adnexal Melanoma: Experience in 30 Patients. Ophthalmology. 2009 Nov;116(11):2217–23. PMID:19766318
2860. Savino G, Midena G, Blasi MA, et al. Orbital and Eyelid B-Cell Lymphoma: A Multicenter Retrospective Study. Cancers (Basel). 2020 Sep 7;12(9):2538. PMID:32906630
2861. Say EA, Shields CL, Bianciotto C, et al. Oncocytic Lesions (Oncocytoma) of the Ocular Adnexa: Report of 15 Cases and Review of Literature. Ophthalmic Plast Reconstr Surg. 2012 Jan-Feb;28(1):14–21. PMID:21956543
2862. Sayed-Ahmed I, Murillo JC, Monsalve P, et al. Blue Nevi of the Ocular Surface: Clinical Characteristics, Pathologic Features, and Clinical Course. Ophthalmology. 2018 Aug;125(8):1189–98. PMID:29551421
2863. Schachat AP, Shields JA, Fine SL, et al. Combined Hamartomas of the Retina and Retinal Pigment Epithelium. Ophthalmology. 1984 Dec;91(12):1609–15. PMID:6521994
2864. Schachat AP, Wilkinson CP, Hinton DR, et al., editors. Ryan's Retina. 6th ed. Philadelphia (PA): Elsevier; 2018.
2865. Schaefer IM, Dong F, Garcia EP, et al. Recurrent SMARCB1 Inactivation in Epithelioid Malignant Peripheral Nerve Sheath Tumors. Am J Surg Pathol. 2019 Jun;43(6):835–43. PMID:30864974
2866. Schaefer IM, Fletcher CD, Hornick JL. Loss of H3K27 Trimethylation Distinguishes Malignant Peripheral Nerve Sheath Tumors from Histologic Mimics. Mod Pathol. 2016 Jan;29(1):4–13. PMID:26585554
2867. Schäfer T, Merkl J, Klemm E, et al. The Epidemiology of Nevi and Signs of Skin Aging in the Adult General Population: Results of the KORA-Survey 2000. J Invest Dermatol. 2006 Jul;126(7):1490–6. PMID:16645597
2868. Schalenbourg A, Coupland S, Kacperek A, et al. Iridocyclectomy for Neovascular Glaucoma Caused by Proton-Beam Radiotherapy of Pigmented Ciliary Adenocarcinoma. Graefes Arch Clin Exp Ophthalmol. 2008 Oct;246(10):1499–501. PMID:18581131
2869. Schaller J, Rohwedder A, Burgdorf WH, et al. Identification of Human Papillomavirus DNA in Cutaneous Lesions of Cowden Syndrome. Dermatology. 2003;207(2):134–40. PMID:12920361
2870. Schefler AC, Abramson DH. Retinoblastoma: What is New in 2007-2008. Curr Opin Ophthalmol. 2008 Nov;19(6):526–34. PMID:18854698
2871. Scheithauer BW, Silva AI, Ketterling RP, et al. Rosette-Forming Glioneuronal Tumor: Report of a Chiasmal-Optic Nerve Example in Neurofibromatosis Type 1: Special Pathology Report. Neurosurgery. 2009 Apr;64(4):e771–2. PMID:19349806
2872. Schepis C, Siragusa M, Palazzo R, et al. Perforating Milia-Like Idiopathic Calcinosis Cutis and Periorbital Syringomas in a Girl with Down Syndrome. Pediatr Dermatol. 1994 Sep;11(3):258–60. PMID:7971561
2873. Scherer D, Bermejo JL, Rudnai P, et al. MC1R Variants Associated Susceptibility to Basal Cell Carcinoma of Skin: Interaction with Host Factors and XRCC3 Polymorphism. Int J Cancer. 2008 Apr 15;122(8):1787–93. PMID:18067130
2874. Scheuermann JC, de Ayala Alonso AG, Oktaba K, et al. Histone H2A Deubiquitinase Activity of the Polycomb Repressive Complex PR-DUB. Nature. 2010 May 13;465(7295):243–7. PMID:20436459
2875. Schiefer TK, Parker WL, Anakwenze OA, et al. Extradigital Glomus Tumors: A 20-Year Experience. Mayo Clin Proc. 2006 Oct;81(10):1337–44. PMID:17036559
2875A. Schindler G, Capper D, Meyer J, et al. Analysis of BRAF V600E Mutation in 1,320 Nervous System Tumors Reveals High Mutation Frequencies in Pleomorphic Xanthoastrocytoma, Ganglioglioma and Extra-Cerebellar Pilocytic Astrocytoma. Acta Neuropathol. 2011 Mar;121(3):397–405. PMID:21274720
2876. Schittkowski MP, Wrede A. Dermatofibrosarcoma Protuberans with Primary Orbital Manifestation. Orbit. 2013 Apr;32(2):117–9. PMID:23514021
2877. Schlegel U. Primary CNS Lymphoma. Ther Adv Neurol Disord. 2009 Mar;2(2):93–104. PMID:21180644
2878. Schlesinger T, Appukuttan B, Hwang T, et al. Internal En Bloc Resection and Genetic Analysis of Retinal Capillary Hemangioblastoma. Arch Ophthalmol. 2007 Sep;125(9):1189–93. PMID:17846357
2879. Schlote T, Nagel G, Vecsei PV, et al. [Conjunctival Cysts of the Orbits: Clinical Aspects and Histology in 4 Patients]. Klin Monbl Augenheilkd. 1998 Aug;213(2):117–20. German. PMID:9782472
2880. Schmack I, Patel RM, Folpe AL, et al. Subconjunctival Herniated Orbital Fat: A Benign Adipocytic Lesion that May Mimic Pleomorphic Lipoma and Atypical Lipomatous Tumor. Am J Surg Pathol. 2007 Feb;31(2):193–8. PMID:17255763
2881. Scholz SL, Cosgarea I, Süßkind D, et al. NF1 Mutations in Conjunctival Melanoma. Br J Cancer. 2018 May;118(9):1243–7. PMID:29559732
2882. Scholz SL, Möller I, Reis H, et al. Frequent GNAQ, GNA11, and EIF1AX Mutations in Iris Melanoma. Invest Ophthalmol Vis Sci. 2017 Jul 1;58(9):3464–70. PMID:28700778
2883. Scholz SL, Murali R, Westekemper H, et al. Re: Van Poppelen et al.: Genetic Background of Iris Melanomas and Iris Melanocytic Tumors of Uncertain Malignant Potential (Ophthalmology. 2018;125:904-912). Ophthalmology. 2018 Nov;125(11):e78–9. PMID:30318043
2884. Scholz SL, Thomasen H, Reis H, et al. Frequent TERT Promoter Mutations in Ocular Surface Squamous Neoplasia. Invest Ophthalmol Vis Sci. 2015 Sep;56(10):5854–61. PMID:26348634
2885. Schoolmeester JK, Lastra RR. Granular Cell Tumors Overexpress TFE3 Without Corollary Gene Rearrangement. Hum Pathol. 2015 Aug;46(8):1242–3. PMID:26009539
2886. Schornack MM, Siemsen DW, Bradley EA, et al. Ocular Manifestations of Molluscum Contagiosum. Clin Exp Optom. 2006 Nov;89(6):390–3. PMID:17026608
2887. Schrader KA, Nelson TN, De Luca A, et al. Multiple Granular Cell Tumors Are an Associated Feature of LEOPARD Syndrome Caused by Mutation in PTPN11. Clin Genet. 2009 Feb;75(2):185–9. PMID:19054014
2888. Schwab C, Wackernagel W, Grinninger P, et al. A Unifying Concept of Uveal Pigment Cell Distribution and Dissemination Based on an Animal Model: Insights into Ocular Melanogenesis. Cells Tissues Organs. 2016;201(3):232–8. PMID:27002320
2889. Schwab C, Zalaudek I, Mayer C, et al. New Insights into Oculodermal Nevogenesis and Proposal for a New Iris Nevus Classification. Br J Ophthalmol. 2015 May;99(5):644–9. PMID:25359901
2890. Schwab JH, Antonescu CR, Athanasian EA, et al. A Comparison of Intramedullary and Juxtacortical Low-Grade Osteogenic Sarcoma. Clin Orthop Relat Res. 2008 Jun;466(6):1318–22. PMID:18425560
2891. Schwartz RA. Sign of Leser-Trélat. J Am Acad Dermatol. 1996 Jul;35(1):88–95. PMID:8682971
2892. Schwartz RA, Torre DP. The Muir-Torre Syndrome: A 25-Year Retrospect. J Am Acad Dermatol. 1995 Jul;33(1):90–104. PMID:7601953
2893. Schweizer L, Koelsche C, Sahm F, et al. Meningeal Hemangiopericytoma and Solitary Fibrous Tumors Carry the NAB2-STAT6 Fusion and Can Be Diagnosed by Nuclear Expression of STAT6 Protein. Acta Neuropathol. 2013 May;125(5):651–8. PMID:23575898
2894. Sciot R, Dorfman H, Brys P, et al. Cytogenetic-Morphologic Correlations in Aneurysmal

Bone Cyst, Giant Cell Tumor of Bone and Combined Lesions. A Report from the CHAMP Study Group. Mod Pathol. 2000 Nov;13(11):1206–10. PMID:11106078
2895. Scott CT, Holland GN, Glasgow BJ. Cavitation in Ciliary Body Melanoma. Am J Ophthalmol. 1997 Feb;123(2):269–71. PMID:9186143
2896. Scott DW, King RL, Staiger AM, et al. High-Grade B-Cell Lymphoma with MYC and BCL2 and/or BCL6 Rearrangements with Diffuse Large B-Cell Lymphoma Morphology. Blood. 2018 May 3;131(18):2060–4. PMID:29475959
2897. Searl SS, Krigstein HJ, Albert DM, et al. Invasive Squamous Cell Carcinoma with Intraocular Mucoepidermoid Features. Conjunctival Carcinoma with Intraocular Invasion and Diphasic Morphology. Arch Ophthalmol. 1982 Jan;100(1):109–11. PMID:7055460
2898. Seavey CN, Pobbati AV, Hallett A, et al. WWTR1(TAZ)-CAMTA1 Gene Fusion is Sufficient to Dysregulate YAP/TAZ Signaling and Drive Epithelioid Hemangioendothelioma Tumorigenesis. Genes Dev. 2021 Apr 1;35(7-8):512–27. PMID:33766982
2899. Seca M, Borges P, Reimão P, et al. Conjunctival Lymphangioma: A Case Report and Brief Review of the Literature. Case Rep Ophthalmol Med. 2012;2012:836573. PMID:22666617
2900. Seçkin D. Cutaneous Lymphoproliferative Disorders in Organ Transplant Recipients: Update 2014. G Ital Dermatol Venereol. 2014 Aug;149(4):401–8. PMID:25068227
2901. Seddon JM, Gragoudas ES, Glynn RJ, et al. Host Factors, UV Radiation, and Risk of Uveal Melanoma. A Case-Control Study. Arch Ophthalmol. 1990 Sep;108(9):1274–80. PMID:2400347
2902. See TRO, Stålhammar G, Tang T, et al. Primary Ductal Adenocarcinoma of the Lacrimal Gland: A Review and Report of Five Cases. Surv Ophthalmol. 2020 May-Jun;65(3):371–80. PMID:31837385
2903. Seely M, Jackson K, Meeker A, et al. Case Series of Patients With Hereditary Benign Intraepithelial Dyskeratosis. Cornea. 2022 Nov 1;41(11):1451–4. PMID:36219214
2904. Seethala RR, Barnes EL, Hunt JL. Epithelial-Myoepithelial Carcinoma: A Review of the Clinicopathologic Spectrum and Immunophenotypic Characteristics in 61 Tumors of the Salivary Glands and Upper Aerodigestive Tract. Am J Surg Pathol. 2007 Jan;31(1):44–57. PMID:17197918
2905. Seethala RR, Richmond JA, Hoschar AP, et al. New Variants of Epithelial-Myoepithelial Carcinoma: Oncocytic-Sebaceous and Apocrine. Arch Pathol Lab Med. 2009 Jun;133(6):950–9. PMID:19492889
2906. Segal A, Segal N, Gal A, et al. Mucinous Sweat Gland Adenocarcinoma of the Eyelid - Current Knowledge of a Rare Tumor. Orbit. 2010 Dec;29(6):334–40. PMID:21158574
2907. Sekimizu M, Yoshida A, Mitani S, et al. Frequent Mutations of Genes Encoding Vacuolar H+ -ATPase Components in Granular Cell Tumors. Genes Chromosomes Cancer. 2019 Jun;58(6):373–80. PMID:30597645
2908. Şekkeli MZ, Hoşal MB, Öcal E, et al. Conjunctival Pyogenic Granuloma During Pregnancy. Arq Bras Oftalmol. 2021 Sep 20;84(5):490–3. PMID:34550219
2909. Šekoranja D, Boštjančič E, Salapura V, et al. Primary Aneurysmal Bone Cyst with a Novel SPARC-USP6 Translocation Identified by Next-Generation Sequencing. Cancer Genet. 2018 Dec;228-229:12–6. PMID:30553465
2910. Šekoranja D, Hawlina G, Pižem J. PRAME Expression in Melanocytic Lesions of the Conjunctiva. Histopathology. 2021 Dec;79(6):989–96. PMID:34268800
2911. Šekoranja D, Vergot K, Hawlina G, et al. Combined Deep Penetrating Nevi of the Conjunctiva Are Relatively Common Lesions Characterised by BRAFV600E Mutation and Activation of the Beta Catenin Pathway: A Clinicopathological Analysis of 34 Lesions. Br J Ophthalmol. 2020 Jul;104(7):1016–21. PMID:31558492
2912. Sekundo W. [Pterygium]. Ophthalmologe. 2010 Jun;107(6):509–10. German. PMID:20544202
2913. Sellam A, Desjardins L, Barnhill R, et al. Fine Needle Aspiration Biopsy in Uveal Melanoma: Technique, Complications, and Outcomes. Am J Ophthalmol. 2016 Feb;162:28–34.E1. PMID:26556006
2914. Selmer J, Skov T, Spelman L, et al. Squamous Cell Carcinoma and Keratoacanthomas Are Biologically Distinct and Can Be Diagnosed by Light Microscopy: A Review. Histopathology. 2016 Oct;69(4):535–41. PMID:27323251
2914A. Selva D, White VA, O'Connell JX, et al. Primary Bone Tumors of the Orbit. Surv Ophthalmol. 2004 May-Jun;49(3):328–42. doi:10.1016/j.survophthal.2004.02.011. PMID:15110669
2915. Sen M, Honavar SG. Circumscribed Choroidal Hemangioma: An Overview of Clinical Manifestation, Diagnosis and Management. Indian J Ophthalmol. 2019 Dec;67(12):1965–73. PMID:31755430
2916. Sen M, Honavar SG, Sharma N, et al. COVID-19 and Eye: A Review of Ophthalmic Manifestations of COVID-19. Indian J Ophthalmol. 2021 Mar;69(3):488–509. PMID:33595463
2917. Sen S, Kashyap S, Betharia S. Primary Orbital Plasmacytoma: A Case Report. Orbit. 2003 Dec;22(4):317–9. PMID:14685909
2918. Sen S, Mahindrakar A, Betharia SM, et al. Pleomorphic Adenomas of the Lacrimal Gland: A Clinicopathological Analysis. Clin Exp Ophthalmol. 2004 Oct;32(5):523–5. PMID:15498065
2919. Sendele DD, Kenyon KR, Mobilia EF, et al. Superior Limbic Keratoconjunctivitis in Contact Lens Wearers. Ophthalmology. 1983 Jun;90(6):616–22. PMID:6888855
2920. Sendul SY, Atilgan CU, Kabukcuoglu F, et al. Anterior Orbital Leiomyoma Originating from the Supraorbital Neurovascular Bundle. SAGE Open Med Case Rep. 2017 Dec 11;5:X17740991. PMID:29276593
2921. Șerbănescu MS, Bungărdean RM, Georgiu C, et al. Nodular and Micronodular Basal Cell Carcinoma Subtypes Are Different Tumors Based on Their Morphological Architecture and Their Interaction with the Surrounding Stroma. Diagnostics (Basel). 2022 Jul 5;12(7):1636. PMID:35885545
2922. Seregard S. Apocrine Adenocarcinoma Arising in Moll Gland Cystadenoma. Ophthalmology. 1993 Nov;100(11):1716–9. PMID:8233400
2923. Seregard S. Phakomatous Choristoma May Be Located in the Eyelid or Orbit or Both. Acta Ophthalmol Scand. 1999 Jun;77(3):343–6. PMID:10406159
2924. Serin Ş, Bozkurt Oflaz A, Karabağlı P, et al. Eyelid Molluscum Contagiosum Lesions in Two Patients with Unilateral Chronic Conjunctivitis. Turk J Ophthalmol. 2017 Aug;47(4):226–30. PMID:28845328
2925. Serrano C, George S. Leiomyosarcoma. Hematol Oncol Clin North Am. 2013 Oct;27(5):957–74. PMID:24093170
2926. Sesenna E, Ferri A, Thai E, et al. Huge Orbital Teratoma with Intracranial Extension: A Case Report. J Pediatr Surg. 2010 May;45(5):e27–31. PMID:20438911
2927. Seykora J, Elder D. Dysplastic Nevi and Other Risk Markers for Melanoma. Semin Oncol. 1996 Dec;23(6):682–7. PMID:8970587
2928. Sha C, Barrans S, Cucco F, et al. Molecular High-Grade B-Cell Lymphoma: Defining a Poor-Risk Group That Requires Different Approaches to Therapy. J Clin Oncol. 2019 Jan 20;37(3):202–12. PMID:30523719
2929. Shabb N, Sneige N, Fanning CV, et al. Fine-Needle Aspiration Cytology of Alveolar Soft-Part Sarcoma. Diagn Cytopathol. 1991;7(3):293–8. PMID:1879268
2930. Shadan FF, Mascarello JT, Newbury RO, et al. Supernumerary Ring Chromosomes Derived from the Long Arm of Chromosome 12 as the Primary Cytogenetic Anomaly in a Rare Soft Tissue Chondroma. Cancer Genet Cytogenet. 2000 Apr 15;118(2):144–7. PMID:10748295
2931. Shafi F, Gonglore B, Sandramouli S, et al. Spindle Cell Lipoma of the Conjunctiva. Ophthalmic Plast Reconstr Surg. 2016 Mar-Apr;32(2):e28–30. PMID:24911538
2932. Shah CP, Weis E, Lajous M, et al. Intermittent and Chronic Ultraviolet Light Exposure and Uveal Melanoma: A Meta-Analysis. Ophthalmology. 2005 Sep;112(9):1599–607. PMID:16051363
2933. Shah NB, Chang WY, White VA, et al. Orbital Lipoma: 2 Cases and Review of Literature. Ophthalmic Plast Reconstr Surg. 2007 May-Jun;23(3):202–5. PMID:17519657
2934. Shah SS, Chandan VS, Wilbur DC, et al. Glial Fibrillary Acidic Protein and CD57 Immunolocalization in Cell Block Preparations is a Useful Adjunct in the Diagnosis of Pleomorphic Adenoma. Arch Pathol Lab Med. 2007 Sep;131(9):1373–7. PMID:17824792
2935. Shahraki T, Arabi A, Feizi S. Pterygium: An Update on Pathophysiology, Clinical Features, and Management. Ther Adv Ophthalmol. 2021 May 31;13:25158414211020152. PMID:34104871
2936. Shain AH, Bagger MM, Yu R, et al. The Genetic Evolution of Metastatic Uveal Melanoma. Nat Genet. 2019 Jul;51(7):1123–30. PMID:31253977
2937. Shain AH, Bastian BC. From Melanocytes to Melanomas. Nat Rev Cancer. 2016 Jun;16(6):345–58. PMID:27125352
2938. Shain AH, Garrido M, Botton T, et al. Exome Sequencing of Desmoplastic Melanoma Identifies Recurrent NFKBIE Promoter Mutations and Diverse Activating Mutations in the MAPK Pathway. Nat Genet. 2015 Oct;47(10):1194–9. PMID:26343386
2939. Shain AH, Yeh I, Kovalyshyn I, et al. The Genetic Evolution of Melanoma from Precursor Lesions. N Engl J Med. 2015 Nov 12;373(20):1926–36. PMID:26559571
2940. Shalin SC, Lyle S, Calonje E, et al. Sebaceous Neoplasia and the Muir-Torre Syndrome: Important Connections with Clinical Implications. Histopathology. 2010 Jan;56(1):133–47. PMID:20055911
2941. Shalini B, Akshi K, Namrata N, et al. Case of Chondroid Syringoma Mimicking a Nodular Hidradenoma: A Diagnostic Pitfall on Cytopathology. Diagn Cytopathol. 2018 Jan;46(1):59–62. PMID:28772003
2942. Shan Y, Xu Y, Lu Y, et al. Epidemiology and Survival Outcomes for Eyelid Primary Malignant Melanoma: An Analysis of 1397 Cases in the SEER Database. J Ophthalmol. 2020 Dec 8;2020:4858636. PMID:33520295
2943. Shankar GM, Abedalthagafi M, Vaubel RA, et al. Germline and Somatic BAP1 Mutations in High-Grade Rhabdoid Meningiomas. Neuro Oncol. 2017 Apr 1;19(4):535–45. PMID:28170043
2944. Shankar GM, Santagata S. BAP1 Mutations in High-Grade Meningioma: Implications for Patient Care. Neuro Oncol. 2017 Oct 19;19(11):1447–56. PMID:28482042
2945. Shanmugam V, Margolskee E, Kluk M, et al. Rosai-Dorfman Disease Harboring an Activating KRAS K117N Missense Mutation. Head Neck Pathol. 2016 Sep;10(3):394–9. PMID:26922062
2946. Shao H, Xi L, Raffeld M, et al. Clonally Related Histiocytic/Dendritic Cell Sarcoma and Chronic Lymphocytic Leukemia/Small Lymphocytic Lymphoma: A Study of Seven Cases. Mod Pathol. 2011 Nov;24(11):1421–32. PMID:21666687
2947. Shao JW, Yin JH, Xiang ST, et al. CT and MRI Findings in Relapsing Primary Malignant Melanoma of the Lacrimal Sac: A Case Report and Brief Literature Review. BMC Ophthalmol. 2020 May 14;20(1):191. PMID:32408870
2948. Shapey J, Sabin HI, Danesh-Meyer HV, et al. Diagnosis and Management of Optic Nerve Sheath Meningiomas. J Clin Neurosci. 2013 Aug;20(8):1045–56. PMID:23809100
2949. Shapira Y, Juniat V, Smith C, et al. Adult-Onset Xanthogranuloma With Frontal Nerve and Intracranial Involvement. Ophthalmic Plast Reconstr Surg. 2021 Sep-Oct 01;37(5):e167–70. PMID:33710041
2950. Sharara N, Holden JT, Wojno TH, et al. Ocular Adnexal Lymphoid Proliferations: Clinical, Histologic, Flow Cytometric, and Molecular Analysis of Forty-Three Cases. Ophthalmology. 2003 Jun;110(6):1245–54. PMID:12799255
2951. Sharara NA, Alexander RA, Luthert PJ, et al. Differential Immunoreactivity of Melanocytic Lesions of the Conjunctiva. Histopathology. 2001 Oct;39(4):426–31. PMID:11683945
2952. Sharma D, Neiweem A, Davis K, et al. Epithelial-Myoepithelial Carcinoma of the Lacrimal Sac and Literature Review of the Lacrimal System. Allergy Rhinol (Providence). 2020 Apr 20;11:2152656720920600. PMID:32341837
2953. Sharma D, Singh G, Kakkar N, et al. Orbital Dermatofibrosarcoma Protuberans with Frontal and Ethmoid Sinus Involvement: A Case Report and Brief Review of Literature. Indian J Ophthalmol. 2017 Sep;65(9):892–4. PMID:28905843
2954. Sharma MC, Mahapatra AK, Gaikwad S, et al. Pigmented Medulloepithelioma: Report of a Case and Review of the Literature. Childs Nerv Syst. 1998 Jan-Feb;14(1-2):74–8. PMID:9548346
2954A. Sharma MK, Zehnbauer BA, Watson MA, et al. RAS Pathway Activation and an Oncogenic RAS Mutation in Sporadic Pilocytic Astrocytoma. Neurology. 2005 Oct;65(8):1335–6. PMID:16247081
2955. Sharma P, Shields CL, Turaka K, et al. Ciliary Body Medulloepithelioma with Neoplastic Cyclitic Membrane Imaging with Fluorescein Angiography and Ultrasound Biomicroscopy. Graefes Arch Clin Exp Ophthalmol. 2011 Aug;249(8):1259–61. PMID:21505878
2956. Sharma S, Gupta N, Rajwanshi A, et al. Inflammatory Myofibroblastic Tumour: A Diagnostic Challenge on Fine Needle Aspiration Cytology. Cytopathology. 2016 Dec;27(6):512–6. PMID:27087029
2957. Sharma S, Kaur R, Bal A, et al. Primary Orbital Plasmacytoma: An Unusual Presentation in an Adolescent. Indian J Pathol Microbiol. 2018 Jan-Mar;61(1):158–9. PMID:29567915
2958. Shehri M, Bouhenni R, Ghazi NG, et al. Retinal Reactive Astrocytic Tumor: Gene Expression Profiling. JAMA Ophthalmol. 2014 Jun;132(6):773–5. PMID:24921169
2959. Shelsta HN, Jampol LM, Weinberg DV. Indolent Nonprogressive Multifocal Choroidal Lesions. Retina. 2012 Feb;32(2):289–92. PMID:21900853
2960. Shen AS, Peterhof E, Kind P, et al. Activating Mutations in the RAS/Mitogen-Activated Protein Kinase Signaling Pathway in Sporadic Trichoblastoma and Syringocystadenoma Papilliferum. Hum Pathol. 2015

Feb;46(2):272–6. PMID:25532942
2961. Shen J, Li H, Feng S, et al. Orbital Solitary Fibrous Tumor: A Clinicopathologic Study from a Chinese Tertiary Hospital with a Literature Review. Cancer Manag Res. 2018 May 9;10:1069–78. PMID:29780261
2962. Shern JF, Chen L, Chmielecki J, et al. Comprehensive Genomic Analysis of Rhabdomyosarcoma Reveals a Landscape of Alterations Affecting a Common Genetic Axis in Fusion-Positive and Fusion-Negative Tumors. Cancer Discov. 2014 Feb;4(2):216–31. PMID:24436047
2963. Shern JF, Yohe ME, Khan J. Pediatric Rhabdomyosarcoma. Crit Rev Oncog. 2015;20(3-4):227–43. PMID:26349418
2964. Shi Y, Jia R, Fan X. Ocular Basal Cell Carcinoma: A Brief Literature Review of Clinical Diagnosis and Treatment. Onco Targets Ther. 2017 May 8;10:2483–9. PMID:28507440
2965. Shia J. Immunohistochemistry Versus Microsatellite Instability Testing for Screening Colorectal Cancer Patients at Risk for Hereditary Nonpolyposis Colorectal Cancer Syndrome. Part I. The Utility of Immunohistochemistry. J Mol Diagn. 2008 Jul;10(4):293–300. PMID:18556767
2966. Shield PW, Crous H. Fine-Needle Aspiration Cytology of Merkel Cell Carcinoma-a Review of 69 Cases. Diagn Cytopathol. 2014 Nov;42(11):924–8. PMID:24678011
2967. Shields CL, Acaba-Berrocal LA, Selzer EB, et al. Uveal Metastasis Based on Patient Age in 1,111 Patients: Comparison of Clinical Features and Outcomes Per Age Category. Retina. 2020 Feb;40(2):204–13. PMID:31972789
2968. Shields CL, Alset AE, Boal NS, et al. Conjunctival Tumors in 5002 Cases. Comparative Analysis of Benign Versus Malignant Counterparts. The 2016 James D. Allen Lecture. Am J Ophthalmol. 2017 Jan;173:106–33. PMID:27725148
2969. Shields CL, Chien JL, Surakiatchanukul T, et al. Conjunctival Tumors: Review of Clinical Features, Risks, Biomarkers, and Outcomes–The 2017 J. Donald M. Gass Lecture. Asia Pac J Ophthalmol (Phila). 2017 Mar-Apr;6(2):109–20. PMID:28399347
2970. Shields CL, Dalvin LA, Ancona-Lezama D, et al. Choroidal Nevus Imaging Features in 3,806 Cases and Risk Factors for Transformation into Melanoma in 2,355 Cases: The 2020 Taylor R. Smith and Victor T. Curtin Lecture. Retina. 2019 Oct;39(10):1840–51. PMID:30608349
2971. Shields CL, Dalvin LA, Vichitvejpaisal P, et al. Prognostication of Uveal Melanoma is Simple and Highly Predictive Using The Cancer Genome Atlas (TCGA) Classification: A Review. Indian J Ophthalmol. 2019 Dec;67(12):1959–63. PMID:31755428
2972. Shields CL, Demirci H, Karatza E, et al. Clinical Survey of 1643 Melanocytic and Nonmelanocytic Conjunctival Tumors. Ophthalmology. 2004 Sep;111(9):1747–54. PMID:15350332
2973. Shields CL, Demirci H, Materin MA, et al. Clinical Factors in the Identification of Small Choroidal Melanoma. Can J Ophthalmol. 2004 Jun;39(4):351–7. PMID:15327099
2974. Shields CL, Douglass AM, Beggache M, et al. Intravitreous Chemotherapy for Active Vitreous Seeding from Retinoblastoma: Outcomes After 192 Consecutive Injections. The 2015 Howard Naquin Lecture. Retina. 2016 Jun;36(6):1184–90. PMID:26630319
2975. Shields CL, Eagle RC, Ip MS, et al. Two Discrete Uveal Melanomas in a Child with Ocular Melanocytosis. Retina. 2006 Jul-Aug;26(6):684–7. PMID:16829813
2976. Shields CL, Fasiuddin AF, Mashayekhi A, et al. Conjunctival Nevi: Clinical Features and Natural Course in 410 Consecutive Patients. Arch Ophthalmol. 2004 Feb;122(2):167–75. PMID:14769591
2977. Shields CL, Furuta M, Mashayekhi A, et al. Clinical Spectrum of Choroidal Nevi Based on Age at Presentation in 3422 Consecutive Eyes. Ophthalmology. 2008 Mar;115(3):546–552.E2. PMID:18067966
2978. Shields CL, Furuta M, Thangappan A, et al. Metastasis of Uveal Melanoma Millimeter-by-Millimeter in 8033 Consecutive Eyes. Arch Ophthalmol. 2009 Aug;127(8):989–98. PMID:19667335
2979. Shields CL, Ghassemi F, Tuncer S, et al. Clinical Spectrum of Diffuse Infiltrating Retinoblastoma in 34 Consecutive Eyes. Ophthalmology. 2008 Dec;115(12):2253–8. PMID:18962920
2980. Shields CL, Husson M, Shields JA, et al. Solitary Intraosseous Infantile Myofibroma of the Orbital Roof. Arch Ophthalmol. 1998 Nov;116(11):1528–30. PMID:9823360
2981. Shields CL, Kalafatis NE, Gad M, et al. Metastatic Tumours to the Eye. Review of Metastasis to the Iris, Ciliary Body, Choroid, Retina, Optic Disc, Vitreous, and/or Lens Capsule. Eye (Lond). 2023 Apr;37(5):809–14. PMID:35306540
2982. Shields CL, Kaliki S, Al-Dahmash S, et al. Retinal Vasoproliferative Tumors: Comparative Clinical Features of Primary Vs Secondary Tumors in 334 Cases. JAMA Ophthalmol. 2013 Mar;131(3):328–34. PMID:23494037
2983. Shields CL, Kaliki S, Arepalli S, et al. Uveal Melanoma in Children and Teenagers. Saudi J Ophthalmol. 2013 Jul;27(3):197–201. PMID:24227986
2984. Shields CL, Kaliki S, Crabtree GS, et al. Iris Metastasis from Systemic Cancer in 104 Patients: The 2014 Jerry A. Shields Lecture. Cornea. 2015 Jan;34(1):42–8. PMID:25343701
2985. Shields CL, Kaliki S, Furuta M, et al. Clinical Spectrum and Prognosis of Uveal Melanoma Based on Age at Presentation in 8,033 Cases. Retina. 2012 Jul;32(7):1363–72. PMID:22466491
2986. Shields CL, Kaliki S, Hutchinson A, et al. Iris Nevus Growth into Melanoma: Analysis of 1611 Consecutive Eyes: The ABCDEF Guide. Ophthalmology. 2013 Apr;120(4):766–72. PMID:23290981
2987. Shields CL, Kaliki S, Livesey M, et al. Association of Ocular and Oculodermal Melanocytosis with the Rate of Uveal Melanoma Metastasis: Analysis of 7872 Consecutive Eyes. JAMA Ophthalmol. 2013 Aug;131(8):993–1003. PMID:23681424
2988. Shields CL, Kaliki S, Shah SU, et al. Iris Melanoma: Features and Prognosis in 317 Children and Adults. J AAPOS. 2012 Feb;16(1):10–6. PMID:22370659
2989. Shields CL, Kancherla S, Patel J, et al. Clinical Survey of 3680 Iris Tumors Based on Patient Age at Presentation. Ophthalmology. 2012 Feb;119(2):407–14. PMID:22035581
2990. Shields CL, Kels JG, Shields JA. Melanoma of the Eye: Revealing Hidden Secrets, One at a Time. Clin Dermatol. 2015 Mar-Apr;33(2):183–96. PMID:25704938
2991. Shields CL, Lally SE, Leahey AM, et al. Targeted Retinoblastoma Management: When to Use Intravenous, Intra-Arterial, Periocular, and Intravitreal Chemotherapy. Curr Opin Ophthalmol. 2014 Sep;25(5):374–85. PMID:25014750
2992. Shields CL, Maktabi AM, Jahnle E, et al. Halo Nevus of the Choroid in 150 Patients: The 2010 Henry van Dyke Lecture. Arch Ophthalmol. 2010 Jul;128(7):859–64. PMID:20625046
2993. Shields CL, Manchandia A, Subbiah R, et al. Pigmented Squamous Cell Carcinoma In Situ of the Conjunctiva in 5 Cases. Ophthalmology. 2008 Oct;115(10):1673–8. PMID:18378314
2994. Shields CL, Manquez ME, Ehya H, et al. Fine-Needle Aspiration Biopsy of Iris Tumors in 100 Consecutive Cases: Technique and Complications. Ophthalmology. 2006 Nov;113(11):2080–6. PMID:17074566
2995. Shields CL, Markowitz JS, Belinsky I, et al. Conjunctival Melanoma: Outcomes Based on Tumor Origin in 382 Consecutive Cases. Ophthalmology. 2011 Feb;118(2):389–95.E1, 2. PMID:20723990
2996. Shields CL, Mashayekhi A, Au AK, et al. The International Classification of Retinoblastoma Predicts Chemoreduction Success. Ophthalmology. 2006 Dec;113(12):2276–80. PMID:16996605
2997. Shields CL, Mashayekhi A, Cater J, et al. Chemoreduction for Retinoblastoma: Analysis of Tumor Control and Risks for Recurrence in 457 Tumors. Trans Am Ophthalmol Soc. 2004;102:35–44. PMID:15747743
2998. Shields CL, Mashayekhi A, Ho T, et al. Solitary Congenital Hypertrophy of the Retinal Pigment Epithelium: Clinical Features and Frequency of Enlargement in 330 Patients. Ophthalmology. 2003 Oct;110(10):1968–76. PMID:14522773
2999. Shields CL, Materin MA, Walker C, et al. Photoreceptor Loss Overlying Congenital Hypertrophy of the Retinal Pigment Epithelium by Optical Coherence Tomography. Ophthalmology. 2006 Apr;113(4):661–5. PMID:16581426
3000. Shields CL, McMahon JF, Atalay HT, et al. Retinal Metastasis from Systemic Cancer in 8 Cases. JAMA Ophthalmol. 2014 Nov;132(11):1303–8. PMID:25033168
3001. Shields CL, Perez B, Benavides R, et al. Optical Coherence Tomography of Optic Disk Melanocytoma in 15 Cases. Retina. 2008 Mar;28(3):441–6. PMID:18327136
3002. Shields CL, Pirondini C, Bianciotto C, et al. Autofluorescence of Congenital Hypertrophy of the Retinal Pigment Epithelium. Retina. 2007 Oct;27(8):1097–100. PMID:18040252
3003. Shields CL, Qureshi A, Eagle RC Jr, et al. Epibulbar Osseous Choristoma in 8 Patients. Cornea. 2012 Jul;31(7):756–60. PMID:22516954
3004. Shields CL, Ramasubramanian A, Ganguly A, et al. Cytogenetic Testing of Iris Melanoma Using Fine Needle Aspiration Biopsy in 17 Patients. Retina. 2011 Mar;31(3):574–80. PMID:21336070
3005. Shields CL, Ramasubramanian A, Mellen PL, et al. Conjunctival Squamous Cell Carcinoma Arising in Immunosuppressed Patients (Organ Transplant, Human Immunodeficiency Virus Infection). Ophthalmology. 2011 Nov;118(11):2133–2137.E1. PMID:21762990
3006. Shields CL, Ramasubramanian A, Rosenwasser R, et al. Superselective Catheterization of the Ophthalmic Artery for Intraarterial Chemotherapy for Retinoblastoma. Retina. 2009 Sep;29(8):1207–9. PMID:19734768
3007. Shields CL, Say EAT, Fuller T, et al. Retinal Astrocytic Hamartoma Arises in Nerve Fiber Layer and Shows "Moth-Eaten" Optically Empty Spaces on Optical Coherence Tomography. Ophthalmology. 2016 Aug;123(8):1809–16. PMID:27157148
3008. Shields CL, Shields JA. Ocular Surface Squamous Neoplasia: From Blue Skies to Blue Dyes–We Still Need Our Ophthalmic Pathologists. JAMA Ophthalmol. 2015 Nov;133(11):1321–2. PMID:26378883
3009. Shields CL, Shields JA. Tumors of the Conjunctiva and Cornea. Indian J Ophthalmol. 2019 Dec;67(12):1930–48. PMID:31755426
3010. Shields CL, Shields JA. Tumors of the Conjunctiva and Cornea. Surv Ophthalmol. 2004 Jan-Feb;49(1):3–24. PMID:14711437
3011. Shields CL, Shields JA, Barrett J, et al. Vasoproliferative Tumors of the Ocular Fundus. Classification and Clinical Manifestations in 103 Patients. Arch Ophthalmol. 1995 May;113(5):615–23. PMID:7748132
3012. Shields CL, Shields JA, Buchanon HW. Solitary Orbital Involvement with Juvenile Xanthogranuloma. Arch Ophthalmol. 1990 Nov;108(11):1537–9. PMID:2123087
3013. Shields CL, Shields JA, De Potter P, et al. Diffuse Choroidal Melanoma. Clinical Features Predictive of Metastasis. Arch Ophthalmol. 1996 Aug;114(8):956–63. PMID:8694731
3014. Shields CL, Shields JA, De Potter P, et al. Plaque Radiotherapy in the Management of Retinoblastoma. Use as a Primary and Secondary Treatment. Ophthalmology. 1993 Feb;100(2):216–24. PMID:8437830
3015. Shields CL, Shields JA, Eagle RC Jr, et al. Progressive Enlargement of Acquired Retinal Astrocytoma in 2 Cases. Ophthalmology. 2004 Feb;111(2):363–8. PMID:15019391
3016. Shields CL, Shields JA, Gross NE, et al. Survey of 520 Eyes with Uveal Metastases. Ophthalmology. 1997 Aug;104(8):1265–76. PMID:9261313
3017. Shields CL, Shields JA, Honavar SG, et al. Clinical Spectrum of Primary Ophthalmic Rhabdomyosarcoma. Ophthalmology. 2001 Dec;108(12):2284–92. PMID:11733272
3018. Shields CL, Shields JA, Marr BP, et al. Congenital Simple Hamartoma of the Retinal Pigment Epithelium: A Study of Five Cases. Ophthalmology. 2003 May;110(5):1005–11. PMID:12750104
3019. Shields CL, Shields JA, Materin M, et al. Iris Melanoma: Risk Factors for Metastasis in 169 Consecutive Patients. Ophthalmology. 2001 Jan;108(1):172–8. PMID:11150284
3020. Shields CL, Shields JA, White D, et al. Types and Frequency of Lesions of the Caruncle. Am J Ophthalmol. 1986 Dec 15;102(6):771–8. PMID:3789057
3021. Shields CL, Sioufi K, Alset AE, et al. Clinical Features Differentiating Benign From Malignant Conjunctival Tumors in Children. JAMA Ophthalmol. 2017 Mar 1;135(3):215–24. PMID:28125759
3022. Shields CL, Srinivasan A, Lucio-Alvarez JA, et al. Retinocytoma/Retinoma: Comparative Analysis of Clinical Features in 78 Tumors and Rate of Transformation into Retinoblastoma Over 20 Years. J AAPOS. 2021 Jun;25(3):147.E1–8. PMID:34051357
3023. Shields CL, Thangappan A, Hartzell K, et al. Combined Hamartoma of the Retina and Retinal Pigment Epithelium in 77 Consecutive Patients Visual Outcome Based on Macular Versus Extramacular Tumor Location. Ophthalmology. 2008 Dec;115(12):2246–2252.E3. PMID:18995912
3024. Shields CL, Welch RJ, Malik K, et al. Uveal Metastasis: Clinical Features and Survival Outcome of 2214 Tumors in 1111 Patients Based on Primary Tumor Origin. Middle East Afr J Ophthalmol. 2018 Apr-Jun;25(2):81–90. PMID:30122853
3025. Shields JA, Bakewell B, Augsburger JJ, et al. Classification and Incidence of Space-Occupying Lesions of the Orbit. A Survey of 645 Biopsies. Arch Ophthalmol. 1984 Nov;102(11):1606–11. PMID:6497741
3026. Shields JA, Bakewell B, Augsburger JJ, et al. Space-Occupying Orbital Masses in Children. A Review of 250 Consecutive Biopsies. Ophthalmology. 1986 Mar;93(3):379–84. PMID:3703507
3027. Shields JA, Bianciotto CG, Kivela T, et al. Presumed Solitary Circumscribed Retinal Astrocytic Proliferation: The 2010 Jonathan W. Wirtschafter Lecture. Arch Ophthalmol. 2011

Sep;129(9):1189–94. PMID:21911666
3028. Shields JA, Demirci H, Marr BP, et al. Sebaceous Carcinoma of the Ocular Region: A Review. Surv Ophthalmol. 2005 Mar-Apr;50(2):103–22. PMID:15749305
3029. Shields JA, Demirci H, Mashayekhi A, et al. Melanocytoma of Optic Disc in 115 Cases: The 2004 Samuel Johnson Memorial Lecture, Part 1. Ophthalmology. 2004 Sep;111(9):1739–46. PMID:15350331
3030. Shields JA, Demirci H, Mashayekhi A, et al. Melanocytoma of the Optic Disk: A Review. Indian J Ophthalmol. 2019 Dec;67(12):1949–58. PMID:31755427
3031. Shields JA, Demirci H, Mashayekhi A, et al. Melanocytoma of the Optic Disk: A Review. Surv Ophthalmol. 2006 Mar-Apr;51(2):93–104. PMID:16500211
3032. Shields JA, Eagle RC Jr, Dutton J, et al. Adenocarcinoma of the Retinal Pigment Epithelium: Clinicopathologic Correlation with Paradoxical Immunohistochemical Findings. JAMA Ophthalmol. 2014 Oct;132(10):1249–52. PMID:24993572
3033. Shields JA, Eagle RC Jr, Ewing MQ, et al. Retinal Cavernous Hemangioma: Fifty-Two Years of Clinical Follow-Up with Clinicopathologic Correlation. Retina. 2014 Jun;34(6):1253–7. PMID:24849703
3034. Shields JA, Eagle RC Jr, Ferguson K, et al. Tumors of the Nonpigmented Epithelium of the Ciliary Body: The Lorenz E. Zimmerman Tribute Lecture. Retina. 2015 May;35(5):957–65. PMID:25545484
3035. Shields JA, Eagle RC Jr, Shields CL, et al. Acquired Neoplasms of the Nonpigmented Ciliary Epithelium (Adenoma and Adenocarcinoma). Ophthalmology. 1996 Dec;103(12):2007–16. PMID:9003334
3036. Shields JA, Eagle RC Jr, Shields CL, et al. Aggressive Retinal Astrocytomas in Four Patients with Tuberous Sclerosis Complex. Trans Am Ophthalmol Soc. 2004;102:139–47. PMID:15747752
3037. Shields JA, Eagle RC Jr, Shields CL, et al. Clinicopathologic Reports, Case Reports, and Small Case Series: Progressive Growth of Benign Adenoma of the Pigment Epithelium of the Ciliary Body. Arch Ophthalmol. 2001 Dec;119(12):1859–61. PMID:11735805
3038. Shields JA, Eagle RC Jr, Shields CL, et al. Congenital Neoplasms of the Nonpigmented Ciliary Epithelium (Medulloepithelioma). Ophthalmology. 1996 Dec;103(12):1998–2006. PMID:9003333
3039. Shields JA, Eagle RC Jr, Shields CL, et al. Malignant Transformation of Congenital Hypertrophy of the Retinal Pigment Epithelium. Ophthalmology. 2009 Nov;116(11):2213–6. PMID:19744732
3040. Shields JA, Eagle RC Jr, Shields CL, et al. Pigmented Adenoma of the Optic Nerve Head Simulating a Melanocytoma. Ophthalmology. 1992 Nov;99(11):1705–8. PMID:1454346
3041. Shields JA, Eagle RC Jr, Shields CL, et al. Pigmented Medulloepithelioma of the Ciliary Body. Arch Ophthalmol. 2002 Feb;120(2):207–10. PMID:11831926
3042. Shields JA, Kaden IH, Eagle RC Jr, et al. Orbital Dermoid Cysts: Clinicopathologic Correlations, Classification, and Management. The 1997 Josephine E. Schueler Lecture. Ophthalmic Plast Reconstr Surg. 1997 Dec;13(4):265–76. PMID:9430304
3043. Shields JA, Karan DS, Perry HD, et al. Epithelioid Cell Nevus of the Iris. Arch Ophthalmol. 1985 Feb;103(2):235–7. PMID:3977695
3044. Shields JA, Karcioglu ZA, Shields CL, et al. Orbital and Eyelid Involvement with Erdheim-Chester Disease. A Report of Two Cases. Arch Ophthalmol. 1991 Jun;109(6):850–4. PMID:2043074
3045. Shields JA, Marr BP, Shields CL, et al. Conjunctival Mascaroma Masquerading as Melanoma. Cornea. 2005 May;24(4):496–7. PMID:15829815
3046. Shields JA, Mashayekhi A, Kligman BE, et al. Vascular Tumors of the Conjunctiva in 140 Cases. Ophthalmology. 2011 Sep;118(9):1747–53. PMID:21788081
3047. Shields JA, Sanborn GE, Augsburger JJ. The Differential Diagnosis of Malignant Melanoma of the Iris. A Clinical Study of 200 Patients. Ophthalmology. 1983 Jun;90(6):716–20. PMID:6888862
3048. Shields JA, Shields CL. Cysts of the Iris Pigment Epithelium. What Is New and Interesting? The 2016 Jose Rizal International Medal Lecture. Asia Pac J Ophthalmol (Phila). 2017 Jan-Feb;6(1):64–9. PMID:28161919
3049. Shields JA, Shields CL. Glial Tumors of the Retina. The 2009 King Khaled Memorial Lecture. Saudi J Ophthalmol. 2009 Oct;23(3-4):197–201. PMID:23960860
3050. Shields JA, Shields CL. Malignant Transformation of Presumed Pleomorphic Adenoma of Lacrimal Gland After 60 Years. Arch Ophthalmol. 1987 Oct;105(10):1403–5. PMID:2821976
3051. Shields JA, Shields CL. Orbital Cysts of Childhood–Classification, Clinical Features, and Management. Surv Ophthalmol. 2004 May-Jun;49(3):281–99. PMID:15110666
3052. Shields JA, Shields CL. Rhabdomyosarcoma: Review for the Ophthalmologist. Surv Ophthalmol. 2003 Jan-Feb;48(1):39–57. PMID:12559326
3053. Shields JA, Shields CL. Tumors and Related Lesions of the Pigmented Epithelium. Asia Pac J Ophthalmol (Phila). 2017 Mar-Apr;6(2):215–23. PMID:28399346
3054. Shields JA, Shields CL, Christian C, et al. Orbital Nodular Fasciitis Simulating a Dermoid Cyst in an 8-Month-Old Child. Case Report and Review of the Literature. Ophthalmic Plast Reconstr Surg. 2001 Mar;17(2):144–8. PMID:11281591
3055. Shields JA, Shields CL, Davidson R, et al. Iris Melanoma Arising from Sector Congenital Ocular Melanocytosis in a Child. Cornea. 2009 Dec;28(10):1191–3. PMID:19770714
3056. Shields JA, Shields CL, Eagle RC Jr. Melanocytoma (Hyperpigmented Magnocellular Nevus) of the Uveal Tract: The 34th G. Victor Simpson Lecture. Retina. 2007 Jul-Aug;27(6):730–9. PMID:17621182
3057. Shields JA, Shields CL, Eagle RC Jr, et al. Adenocarcinoma Arising from Congenital Hypertrophy of Retinal Pigment Epithelium. Arch Ophthalmol. 2001 Apr;119(4):597–602. PMID:11296028
3058. Shields JA, Shields CL, Eagle RC Jr, et al. Malignant Melanoma Arising from a Large Uveal Melanocytoma in a Patient with Oculodermal Melanocytosis. Arch Ophthalmol. 2000 Jul;118(7):990–3. PMID:10900118
3059. Shields JA, Shields CL, Eagle RC Jr, et al. Observations on Seven Cases of Intraocular Leiomyoma. The 1993 Byron Demorest Lecture. Arch Ophthalmol. 1994 Apr;112(4):521–8. PMID:8155052
3060. Shields JA, Shields CL, Eagle RC Jr, et al. Ocular Manifestations of the Organoid Nevus Syndrome. Ophthalmology. 1997 Mar;104(3):549–57. PMID:9082288
3061. Shields JA, Shields CL, Eagle RC Jr, et al. Pigmented Conjunctival Squamous Cell Carcinoma Simulating a Conjunctival Melanoma. Am J Ophthalmol. 2001 Jul;132(1):104–6. PMID:11438062
3062. Shields JA, Shields CL, Eagle RC Jr, et al. Pilomatrixoma of the Eyelid. J Pediatr Ophthalmol Strabismus. 1995 Jul-Aug;32(4):260–1. PMID:7494166
3063. Shields JA, Shields CL, Ehya H, et al. Fine-Needle Aspiration Biopsy of Suspected Intraocular Tumors. The 1992 Urwick Lecture. Ophthalmology. 1993 Nov;100(11):1677–84. PMID:8233394
3064. Shields JA, Shields CL, Epstein JA, et al. Review: Primary Epithelial Malignancies of the Lacrimal Gland: The 2003 Ramon L. Font Lecture. Ophthalmic Plast Reconstr Surg. 2004 Jan;20(1):10–21. PMID:14752304
3065. Shields JA, Shields CL, Gündüz K, et al. Adenoma of the Ciliary Body Pigment Epithelium: The 1998 Albert Ruedemann, Sr, Memorial Lecture, Part 1. Arch Ophthalmol. 1999 May;117(5):592–7. PMID:10326955
3066. Shields JA, Shields CL, Gündüz K, et al. Neoplasms of the Retinal Pigment Epithelium: The 1998 Albert Ruedemann, Sr, Memorial Lecture, Part 2. Arch Ophthalmol. 1999 May;117(5):601–8. PMID:10326956
3067. Shields JA, Shields CL, Kiratli H, et al. Metastatic Tumors to the Iris in 40 Patients. Am J Ophthalmol. 1995 Apr;119(4):422–30. PMID:7709967
3068. Shields JA, Shields CL, Mashayekhi A, et al. Primary Acquired Melanosis of the Conjunctiva: Risks for Progression to Melanoma in 311 Eyes. The 2006 Lorenz E. Zimmerman Lecture. Ophthalmology. 2008 Mar;115(3):511–519.E2. PMID:17884168
3069. Shields JA, Shields CL, Scartozzi R. Survey of 1264 Patients with Orbital Tumors and Simulating Lesions: The 2002 Montgomery Lecture, Part 1. Ophthalmology. 2004 May;111(5):997–1008. PMID:15121380
3070. Shields JA, Shields CL, Shah PG, et al. Lack of Association Among Typical Congenital Hypertrophy of the Retinal Pigment Epithelium, Adenomatous Polyposis, and Gardner Syndrome. Ophthalmology. 1992 Nov;99(11):1709–13. PMID:1333580
3071. Shields JA, Shields CL, Singh AD. Acquired Tumors Arising from Congenital Hypertrophy of the Retinal Pigment Epithelium. Arch Ophthalmol. 2000 May;118(5):637–41. PMID:10815155
3072. Shields JA, Shields CL, Singh AD. Metastatic Neoplasms in the Optic Disc: The 1999 Bjerrum Lecture: Part 2. Arch Ophthalmol. 2000 Feb;118(2):217–24. PMID:10676787
3073. Shields JA, Stopyra GA, Marr BP, et al. Bilateral Orbital Myeloid Sarcoma as Initial Sign of Acute Myeloid Leukemia: Case Report and Review of the Literature. Arch Ophthalmol. 2003 Jan;121(1):138–42. PMID:12523908
3074. Shields JA, Tso MO. Congenital Grouped Pigmentation of the Retina. Histopathologic Description and Report of a Case. Arch Ophthalmol. 1975 Nov;93(11):1153. PMID:1191104
3075. Shields PW, Jakobiec FA, Stagner AM, et al. Spitz Nevus Arising in the Eyelid of a Teenager. Surv Ophthalmol. 2016 Mar-Apr;61(2):228–35. PMID:26498574
3076. Shimizu N, Oshitari T, Yotsukura J, et al. Ten-Year Epidemiological Study of Ocular and Orbital Tumors in Chiba University Hospital. BMC Ophthalmol. 2021 Sep 23;21(1):344. PMID:34556080
3077. Shimono J, Miyoshi H, Arakawa F, et al. Synchronous Case of Follicular Lymphoma and Langerhans Cell Sarcoma in the Same Lymph Node. Pathol Int. 2018 Nov;68(11):614–7. PMID:30255584
3078. Shinder R, Mostafavi D, Nasser QJ, et al. Primary Orbital Liposarcoma Misdiagnosed as Thyroid Associated Orbitopathy. Orbit. 2012 Aug;31(4):264–6. PMID:22571512
3079. Shirley MD, Tang H, Gallione CJ, et al. Sturge-Weber Syndrome and Port-Wine Stains Caused by Somatic Mutation in GNAQ. N Engl J Med. 2013 May 23;368(21):1971–9. PMID:23656586
3080. Shirota N, Nakayama H, Shiraishi S, et al. Target Volume Dose and Clinical Outcome in Radiotherapy for Primary Marginal Zone Lymphoma of the Ocular Adnexa. Mol Clin Oncol. 2017 Jun;6(6):833–8. PMID:28588773
3081. Shively SB, Beltaifa S, Gehrs B, et al. Protracted Haemangioblastic Proliferation and Differentiation in von Hippel-Lindau Disease. J Pathol. 2008 Dec;216(4):514–20. PMID:18836991
3082. Shneor E, Millodot M, Barnard S, et al. Prevalence of Congenital Hypertrophy of the Retinal Pigment Epithelium (CHRPE) in Israel. Ophthalmic Physiol Opt. 2014 May;34(3):385. PMID:24750466
3083. Shofty B, Ben-Sira L, Kesler A, et al. Optic Pathway Gliomas. Adv Tech Stand Neurosurg. 2015;42:123–46. PMID:25411148
3084. Shome D, Esmaeli B. Targeted Monoclonal Antibody Therapy and Radioimmunotherapy for Lymphoproliferative Disorders of the Ocular Adnexa. Curr Opin Ophthalmol. 2008 Sep;19(5):414–21. PMID:18772675
3085. Shome D, Vemuganti GK, Honavar SG. Choroidal Ganglioneuroma in a Patient with Neurofibromatosis Type 1: A Case Report. Eye (Lond). 2006 Dec;20(12):1450–1. PMID:16557286
3086. Shon W, Salomão DR. WT1 Expression in Endocrine Mucin-Producing Sweat Gland Carcinoma: A Study of 13 Cases. Int J Dermatol. 2014 Oct;53(10):1228–34. PMID:25219513
3087. Shon W, Sukov WR, Jenkins SM, et al. MYC Amplification and Overexpression in Primary Cutaneous Angiosarcoma: A Fluorescence in-Situ Hybridization and Immunohistochemical Study. Mod Pathol. 2014 Apr;27(4):509–15. PMID:24091875
3088. Shouchane-Blum K, Yassur I, Sternfeld A, et al. Orbital Lymphatic-Venous Malformation Accompanied by an Intraocular Vascular Malformation: A Rare Case Study. Case Rep Ophthalmol. 2021 May 10;12(2):396–401. PMID:34054491
3089. Shukla SY, Shields JA, Eagle RC, et al. Transformation of Optic Disc Melanocytoma into Melanoma Over 33 Years. Arch Ophthalmol. 2012 Oct;130(10):1344–7. PMID:23044959
3090. Shuweiter M, Böer A. Spectrum of Follicular and Sebaceous Differentiation Induced by Dermatofibroma. Am J Dermatopathol. 2009 Dec;31(8):778–85. PMID:19955877
3091. Sia DIT, Agi J, Grewal P, et al. Two Cases of Giant Melanocytoma (Hyperpigmented Magnocellular Nevus). Ocul Oncol Pathol. 2020 Oct;6(5):344–52. PMID:33123528
3092. Siedlecki AN, Tapp S, Tosteson AN, et al. Surgery Versus Interferon Alpha-2b Treatment Strategies for Ocular Surface Squamous Neoplasia: A Literature-Based Decision Analysis. Cornea. 2016 May;35(5):613–8. PMID:26890663
3093. Siegal GP. Primary Tumors of Bone. In: Stocker JT, Askin FB, editors. Pathology of Solid Tumors in Children. London (UK): Chapman & Hall Medical; 1998. pp. 183–212.
3094. Siegel JA, Korgavkar K, Weinstock MA. Current Perspective on Actinic Keratosis: A Review. Br J Dermatol. 2017 Aug;177(2):350–8. PMID:27500794
3094A. Sievers P, Schrimpf D, Stichel D, et al. Posterior Fossa Pilocytic Astrocytomas with Oligodendroglial Features Show Frequent FGFR1 Activation Via Fusion or Mutation. Acta Neuropathol. 2020 Feb;139(2):403–6. PMID:31729570
3094B. Sievert AJ, Jackson EM, Gai X, et al. Duplication of 7q34 in Pediatric Low-Grade Astrocytomas Detected by High-Density Single-Nucleotide Polymorphism-Based Genotype Arrays Results in a Novel BRAF Fusion Gene. Brain Pathol. 2009 Jul;19(3):449–58.

PMID:19016743
3095. Silkenstedt E, Linton K, Dreyling M. Mantle Cell Lymphoma - Advances in Molecular Biology, Prognostication and Treatment Approaches. Br J Haematol. 2021 Oct;195(2):162–73. PMID:33783838
3096. Silkiss RZ, Mudvari SS, Shetlar D. Ophthalmologic Presentation of Nasal Chondromesenchymal Hamartoma in an Infant. Ophthalmic Plast Reconstr Surg. 2007 May-Jun;23(3):243–4. PMID:17519672
3097. Silverstein M, Salvin J. Ocular Manifestations of Sturge-Weber Syndrome. Curr Opin Ophthalmol. 2019 Sep;30(5):301–5. PMID:31313748
3098. Simko SJ, Tran HD, Jones J, et al. Clofarabine Salvage Therapy in Refractory Multifocal Histiocytic Disorders, Including Langerhans Cell Histiocytosis, Juvenile Xanthogranuloma and Rosai-Dorfman Disease. Pediatr Blood Cancer. 2014 Mar;61(3):479–87. PMID:24106153
3099. Simon MP, Pedeutour F, Sirvent N, et al. Deregulation of the Platelet-Derived Growth Factor B-Chain Gene Via Fusion with Collagen Gene COL1A1 in Dermatofibrosarcoma Protuberans and Giant-Cell Fibroblastoma. Nat Genet. 1997 Jan;15(1):95–8. PMID:8988177
3100. Simpson W, Garner A, Collin JR. Benign Hair-Follicle Derived Tumours in the Differential Diagnosis of Basal-Cell Carcinoma of the Eyelids: A Clinicopathological Comparison. Br J Ophthalmol. 1989 May;73(5):347–53. PMID:2730855
3101. Singh AD, Bergman L, Seregard S. Uveal Melanoma: Epidemiologic Aspects. Ophthalmol Clin North Am. 2005 Mar;18(1):75–84, Viii. PMID:15763193
3102. Singh AD, De Potter P, Fijal BA, et al. Lifetime Prevalence of Uveal Melanoma in White Patients with Oculo(Dermal) Melanocytosis. Ophthalmology. 1998 Jan;105(1):195–8. PMID:9442799
3103. Singh AD, Kaiser PK, Sears JE. Choroidal Hemangioma. Ophthalmol Clin North Am. 2005 Mar;18(1):151–61, Ix. PMID:15763200
3104. Singh AD, Kalyani P, Topham A. Estimating the Risk of Malignant Transformation of a Choroidal Nevus. Ophthalmology. 2005 Oct;112(10):1784–9. PMID:16154197
3105. Singh AD, Nouri M, Shields CL, et al. Treatment of Retinal Capillary Hemangioma. Ophthalmology. 2002 Oct;109(10):1799–806. PMID:12359597
3106. Singh AD, Santos CM, Shields CL, et al. Observations on 17 Patients with Retinocytoma. Arch Ophthalmol. 2000 Feb;118(2):199–205. PMID:10676785
3107. Singh AD, Shields CL, Shields JA. von Hippel-Lindau Disease. Surv Ophthalmol. 2001 Sep-Oct;46(2):117–42. PMID:11578646
3108. Singh AD, Shields CL, Shields JA, et al. Uveal Melanoma in Young Patients. Arch Ophthalmol. 2000 Jul;118(7):918–23. PMID:10900104
3109. Singh AD, Soto H, Bellerive C, et al. Reactive Retinal Astrocytic Tumor (Focal Nodular Gliosis): Report of the Clinical Spectrum of 3 Cases. Ocul Oncol Pathol. 2017 Sep;3(3):235–9. PMID:29071275
3110. Singh AD, Topham A. Incidence of Uveal Melanoma in the United States: 1973-1997. Ophthalmology. 2003 May;110(5):956–61. PMID:12750097
3111. Singh AD, Turell ME, Topham AK. Uveal Melanoma: Trends in Incidence, Treatment, and Survival. Ophthalmology. 2011 Sep;118(9):1881–5. PMID:21704381
3112. Singh G, Gupta R, Kakkar A, et al. Fine Needle Aspiration Cytology of Metastatic Ocular Medulloepithelioma. Cytopathology. 2011 Oct;22(5):343–5. PMID:21062379
3113. Singh G, Sharma MC, Agarwal S, et al. Epithelial-Myoepithelial Carcinoma of the Lacrimal Gland: A Rare Case. Ann Diagn Pathol. 2012 Aug;16(4):292–7. PMID:21546298
3114. Singh HP, Wang S, Stachelek K, et al. Developmental Stage-Specific Proliferation and Retinoblastoma Genesis in RB-Deficient Human But Not Mouse Cone Precursors. Proc Natl Acad Sci U S A. 2018 Oct 2;115(40):e9391–400. PMID:30213853
3115. Singh M, Kaur M, Grewal AM, et al. Ophthalmic Features and Management Outcomes of 30 Children Having Goldenhar Syndrome. Int Ophthalmol. 2020 Mar;40(3):667–75. PMID:31760545
3116. Singh M, Singh U, Gupta A, et al. Primary Orbital Teratoma with Tooth in an Adult: A Rare Association with Cataract and Corectopia. Orbit. 2013 Oct;32(5):327–9. PMID:23895389
3117. Singh P, Mathur SK, Singh S, et al. Cystic Lymphangioma of the Spleen–a Case Report. Indian J Pathol Microbiol. 2005 Apr;48(2):202–3. PMID:16758665
3118. Singh R, Joseph A, Umapathy T, et al. Impression Cytology of the Ocular Surface. Br J Ophthalmol. 2005 Dec;89(12):1655–9. PMID:16299150
3119. Singh RS, Grayson W, Redston M, et al. Site and Tumor Type Predicts DNA Mismatch Repair Status in Cutaneous Sebaceous Neoplasia. Am J Surg Pathol. 2008 Jun;32(6):936–42. PMID:18551751
3120. Singh S, Ali MJ. Lymphoproliferative Tumors Involving the Lacrimal Drainage System: A Major Review. Orbit. 2020 Aug;39(4):276–84. PMID:31267826
3121. Singh S, Ali MJ. Primary Malignant Epithelial Tumors of the Lacrimal Drainage System: A Major Review. Orbit. 2021 Jun;40(3):179–92. PMID:32506982
3122. Singh SK. Pterygium: Epidemiology Prevention and Treatment. Community Eye Health. 2017;30(99):S5–6. PMID:29849437
3123. Singh T, Ichhpujani P. Conjunctival and Corneal Fibrous Histiocytoma: Brief Review. Semin Ophthalmol. 2021 Oct 3;36(7):569–72. PMID:33764259
3124. Singh V, Parwaiz A, Radotra BD, et al. Inverted Mucoepidermoid Papilloma of Conjunctiva: A Rare Histological Entity. Indian J Pathol Microbiol. 2019 Jul-Sep;62(3):481–2. PMID:31361247
3125. Sirvent N, Maire G, Pedeutour F. Genetics of Dermatofibrosarcoma Protuberans Family of Tumors: From Ring Chromosomes to Tyrosine Kinase Inhibitor Treatment. Genes Chromosomes Cancer. 2003 May;37(1):1–19. PMID:12661001
3126. Sissons HA, Steiner GC, Dorfman HD. Calcified Spherules in Fibro-Osseous Lesions of Bone. Arch Pathol Lab Med. 1993 Mar;117(3):284–90. PMID:8442673
3127. Sitaula R, Shrestha GB, Paudel N, et al. Glial Heterotopia of the Orbit: A Rare Presentation. BMC Ophthalmol. 2011 Nov 16;11:34. PMID:22088230
3128. Sivak-Callcott JA, Rootman J, Rasmussen SL, et al. Adult Xanthogranulomatous Disease of the Orbit and Ocular Adnexa: New Immunohistochemical Findings and Clinical Review. Br J Ophthalmol. 2006 May;90(5):602–8. PMID:16622091
3129. Sivalingam A, Augsburger J, Perilongo G, et al. Combined Hamartoma of the Retina and Retinal Pigment Epithelium in a Patient with Neurofibromatosis Type 2. J Pediatr Ophthalmol Strabismus. 1991 Nov-Dec;28(6):320–2. PMID:1757856
3130. Sivley MD, Wallace EL, Warnock DG, et al. Conjunctival Lymphangiectasia Associated with Classic Fabry Disease. Br J Ophthalmol. 2018 Jan;102(1):54–8. PMID:28500230
3131. Sjö LD, Juhl BR, Buchwald C, et al. Epstein-Barr Positive T-Cell Lymphoma in the Ocular Region. Eur J Ophthalmol. 2006 Jan-Feb;16(1):181–5. PMID:16496268
3132. Sjö LD, Ralfkiaer E, Juhl BR, et al. Primary Lymphoma of the Lacrimal Sac: An EORTC Ophthalmic Oncology Task Force Study. Br J Ophthalmol. 2006 Aug;90(8):1004–9. PMID:16672329
3133. Sjö N, Heegaard S, Prause JU. Conjunctival Papilloma. A Histopathologically Based Retrospective Study. Acta Ophthalmol Scand. 2000 Dec;78(6):663–6. PMID:11167228
3134. Sjö NC, Heegaard S, Prause JU, et al. Human Papillomavirus in Conjunctival Papilloma. Br J Ophthalmol. 2001 Jul;85(7):785–7. PMID:11423448
3135. Sjö NC, von Buchwald C, Cassonnet P, et al. Human Papillomavirus: Cause of Epithelial Lacrimal Sac Neoplasia? Acta Ophthalmol Scand. 2007 Aug;85(5):551–6. PMID:17362365
3136. Skalet AH, Gombos DS, Gallie BL, et al. Screening Children at Risk for Retinoblastoma: Consensus Report from the American Association of Ophthalmic Oncologists and Pathologists. Ophthalmology. 2018 Mar;125(3):453–8. PMID:29056300
3137. Skálová A, Banečkova M, Thompson LDR, et al. Expanding the Molecular Spectrum of Secretory Carcinoma of Salivary Glands With a Novel VIM-RET Fusion. Am J Surg Pathol. 2020 Oct;44(10):1295–307. PMID:32675658
3138. Skalova A, Leivo I, Hellquist H, et al. High-Grade Transformation/Dedifferentiation in Salivary Gland Carcinomas: Occurrence Across Subtypes and Clinical Significance. Adv Anat Pathol. 2021 May 1;28(3):107–18. PMID:33825717
3139. Skálová A, Ptáková N, Santana T, et al. NCOA4-RET and TRIM27-RET Are Characteristic Gene Fusions in Salivary Intraductal Carcinoma, Including Invasive and Metastatic Tumors: Is "Intraductal" Correct? Am J Surg Pathol. 2019 Oct;43(10):1303–13. PMID:31162284
3140. Skálová A, Stenman G, Simpson RHW, et al. The Role of Molecular Testing in the Differential Diagnosis of Salivary Gland Carcinomas. Am J Surg Pathol. 2018 Feb;42(2):e11–27. PMID:29076877
3141. Skalova A, Vanecek T, Martinek P, et al. Molecular Profiling of Mammary Analog Secretory Carcinoma Revealed a Subset of Tumors Harboring a Novel ETV6-RET Translocation: Report of 10 Cases. Am J Surg Pathol. 2018 Feb;42(2):234–46. PMID:29076873
3142. Skálová A, Vanecek T, Simpson RH, et al. Mammary Analogue Secretory Carcinoma of Salivary Glands: Molecular Analysis of 25 ETV6 Gene Rearranged Tumors With Lack of Detection of Classical ETV6-NTRK3 Fusion Transcript by Standard RT-PCR: Report of 4 Cases Harboring ETV6-X Gene Fusion. Am J Surg Pathol. 2016 Jan;40(1):3–13. PMID:26492182
3143. Skálová A, Vanecek T, Uro-Coste E, et al. Molecular Profiling of Salivary Gland Intraductal Carcinoma Revealed a Subset of Tumors Harboring NCOA4-RET and Novel TRIM27-RET Fusions: A Report of 17 Cases. Am J Surg Pathol. 2018 Nov;42(11):1445–55. PMID:30045065
3144. Skálová A, Weinreb I, Hyrcza M, et al. Clear Cell Myoepithelial Carcinoma of Salivary Glands Showing EWSR1 Rearrangement: Molecular Analysis of 94 Salivary Gland Carcinomas with Prominent Clear Cell Component. Am J Surg Pathol. 2015 Mar;39(3):338–48. PMID:25581728
3145. Skapek SX, Ferrari A, Gupta AA, et al. Rhabdomyosarcoma. Nat Rev Dis Primers. 2019 Jan 7;5(1):1. PMID:30617281
3146. Smerla RG, Rontogianni D, Fragoulis GE. Ocular Manifestations of IgG4-Related Disease in Children. More Common Than Anticipated? Review of the Literature and Case Report. Clin Rheumatol. 2018 Jun;37(6):1721–7. PMID:29204759
3147. Smit KN, Jager MJ, de Klein A, et al. Uveal Melanoma: Towards a Molecular Understanding. Prog Retin Eye Res. 2020 Mar;75:100800. PMID:31563544
3148. Smith A, Orchard D. Infantile Myofibromatosis: Two Families Supporting Autosomal Dominant Inheritance. Australas J Dermatol. 2011 Aug;52(3):214–7. PMID:21834820
3149. Smith AN, Miller LA, Song N, et al. The Duality of Beta-Catenin Function: A Requirement in Lens Morphogenesis and Signaling Suppression of Lens Fate in Periocular Ectoderm. Dev Biol. 2005 Sep 15;285(2):477–89. PMID:16102745
3150. Smith KJ, Williams J, Corbett D, et al. Microcystic Adnexal Carcinoma: An Immunohistochemical Study Including Markers of Proliferation and Apoptosis. Am J Surg Pathol. 2001 Apr;25(4):464–71. PMID:11257620
3151. Smith SC, Gooding WE, Elkins M, et al. Solitary Fibrous Tumors of the Head and Neck: A Multi-Institutional Clinicopathologic Study. Am J Surg Pathol. 2017 Dec;41(12):1642–56. PMID:28877055
3152. Snaathorst J, Sewnaik A, Paridaens D, et al. Primary Epithelial Tumors of the Lacrimal Gland; a Retrospective Analysis of 22 Patients. Int J Oral Maxillofac Surg. 2009 Jul;38(7):751–7. PMID:19369032
3153. Snow S, Madjar DD, Hardy S, et al. Microcystic Adnexal Carcinoma: Report of 13 Cases and Review of the Literature. Dermatol Surg. 2001 Apr;27(4):401–8. PMID:11298716
3154. So N, Liu R, Hogeling M. Juvenile Xanthogranulomas: Examining Single, Multiple, and Extracutaneous Presentations. Pediatr Dermatol. 2020 Jul;37(4):637–44. PMID:32468628
3155. Sobolewska B, Chee SP, Zaguia F, et al. Vitreoretinal Lymphoma. Cancers (Basel). 2021 Aug 4;13(16):3921. PMID:34439078
3156. Sogabe Y, Miyatani K, Goto R, et al. Pathological Findings of Infraorbital Nerve Enlargement in IgG4-Related Ophthalmic Disease. Jpn J Ophthalmol. 2012 Sep;56(5):511–4. PMID:22855022
3157. Soler VJ, Tran-Viet KN, Galiacy SD, et al. Whole Exome Sequencing Identifies a Mutation for a Novel Form of Corneal Intraepithelial Dyskeratosis. J Med Genet. 2013 Apr;50(4):246–54. PMID:23349227
3158. Soler-Carrillo J, Estrach T, Mascaró JM. Eruptive Syringoma: 27 New Cases and Review of the Literature. J Eur Acad Dermatol Venereol. 2001 May;15(3):242–6. PMID:11683289
3159. Soliman SE, Dimaras H, Khetan V, et al. Prenatal Versus Postnatal Screening for Familial Retinoblastoma. Ophthalmology. 2016 Dec;123(12):2610–7. PMID:27712844
3160. Solomon AS. Pterygium. Br J Ophthalmol. 2006 Jun;90(6):665–6. PMID:16714259
3161. Solomon AW, Burton MJ, Gower EW, et al. Trachoma. Nat Rev Dis Primers. 2022 May 26;8(1):32. PMID:35618795
3162. Solomon DA, Ramani B, Eiger-Moscovich M, et al. Iris and Ciliary Body Melanocytomas Are Defined by Solitary GNAQ Mutation Without Additional Oncogenic Alterations. Ophthalmology. 2022 Dec;129(12):1429–39. PMID:35835335
3163. Solomon JD, Shields CL, Shields JA, et al. Posterior Capsule Opacity as Initial Manifestation of Metastatic Cutaneous Melanoma. Graefes Arch Clin Exp Ophthalmol. 2011 Jan;249(1):127–31. PMID:20617330
3164. Somnath A, Tripathy K. Pinguecula. In: StatPearls. Treasure Island (FL): StatPearls Publishing; 2022. PMID:32644391
3165. Son DH, Yoo SH, Sa HS, et al. A Solitary

Fibrous Tumor with Giant Cells in the Lacrimal Gland: A Case Study. Korean J Pathol. 2013 Apr;47(2):158–62. PMID:23667375
3166. Song A, Syed N, Kirby PA, et al. Giant Cell Angiofibroma of the Ocular Adnexae. Arch Ophthalmol. 2005 Oct;123(10):1438–43. PMID:16219740
3167. Song X, Wang S, Wang J, et al. Clinical Management and Outcomes of Lacrimal Sac Squamous Cell Carcinoma. Head Neck. 2019 Apr;41(4):974–81. PMID:30629760
3168. Soon AK, Brownstein S, O'Connor M, et al. Fibrous Histiocytoma of the Conjunctiva. Ophthalmic Plast Reconstr Surg. 2017 Sep/Oct;33(5):e133. PMID:27636240
3169. Soon AK, Brownstein S, Tang T, et al. Immunohistochemical Analysis of Benign and Malignant Melanocytic Lesions of the Conjunctiva Using Double-Staining. Can J Ophthalmol. 2019 Dec;54(6):699–707. PMID:31836103
3170. Soror NN, Lutaya I, Shah P, et al. A Rare Case of Primary Adenocarcinoma of the Eyelid: Case Presentation and Review of Literature. Cureus. 2021 Jul 23;13(7):e16580. PMID:34430175
3171. Soussain C, Malaise D, Cassoux N. Primary Vitreoretinal Lymphoma: A Diagnostic and Management Challenge. Blood. 2021 Oct 28;138(17):1519–34. PMID:34036310
3172. South CD, Hampel H, Comeras I, et al. The Frequency of Muir-Torre Syndrome Among Lynch Syndrome Families. J Natl Cancer Inst. 2008 Feb 20;100(4):277–81. PMID:18270343
3173. Sowa Y, Nishino K, Numajiri T. Surgical Treatment of Dumbbell-Shaped Dermoid Cyst Extending into the Orbit. J Craniofac Surg. 2012 Jul;23(4):1198–9. PMID:22801126
3174. Soysal HG, Markoç F. Invasive Squamous Cell Carcinoma of the Eyelids and Periorbital Region. Br J Ophthalmol. 2007 Mar;91(3):325–9. PMID:17020898
3175. Spaide RF. Unilateral Diffuse Uveal Melanocytic Proliferation. Retin Cases Brief Rep. 2018 Fall;12(4):263–5. PMID:28005580
3176. Spencer A, Lee J, Prayson RA. Optic Nerve Choristoma. Ann Diagn Pathol. 2005 Apr;9(2):93–5. PMID:15806516
3177. Spencer WH, Jesberg DO. Glioneuroma (Choristomatous Malformation of the Optic Cup Margin). A Report of Two Cases. Arch Ophthalmol. 1973 May;89(5):387–91. PMID:4697215
3178. Spielvogel RL, Austin C, Ackerman AB. Inverted Follicular Keratosis is Not a Specific Keratosis But a Verruca Vulgaris (or Seborrheic Keratosis) with Squamous Eddies. Am J Dermatopathol. 1983 Oct;5(5):427–42. PMID:6229188
3179. Spinak M, Friedman AH. Squamous Cell Carcinoma of the Conjunctiva. Value of Exfoliative Cytology in Diagnosis. Surv Ophthalmol. 1977 Jan-Feb;21(4):351–5. PMID:835082
3180. Spraul CW, Buchwald HJ, Lang GK. [Idiopathic Conjunctival Lymphangiectasia]. Klin Monbl Augenheilkd. 1997 Jun;210(6):398–9. German. PMID:9333668
3181. Sreenivasan J, Rishi P, Das K, et al. Retinal Pigment Epithelium Adenoma and Adenocarcinoma: A Review. Ocul Oncol Pathol. 2021 Mar;7(2):121–32. PMID:33981695
3182. Srikanth D, Devi V, Polishetty N, et al. Subcutaneous Benign Fibrous Histiocytoma: Rare Presentation on Cheek-Case Report and Review of Literature. J Maxillofac Oral Surg. 2016 Jul;15(Suppl 2):282–6. PMID:27408454
3183. Stacey AW, Bowman R, Foster A, et al. Incidence of Retinoblastoma Has Increased: Results from 40 European Countries. Ophthalmology. 2021 Sep;128(9):1369–71. PMID:33508429
3184. Stacy RC, Bernardo LA, Nielsen GP. Absence of Chromosomal Abnormalities in Herniated Orbital Fat. Histopathology. 2014 Aug;65(2):273–7. PMID:24588545
3185. Stadigh A, Puska P, Vesti E, et al. Ring Melanoma of the Anterior Chamber Angle as a Mimicker of Pigmentary Glaucoma. Surv Ophthalmol. 2017 Sep-Oct;62(5):670–6. PMID:28159633
3186. Stagner AM, Jakobiec FA. A Critical Analysis of Eleven Periocular Lobular Capillary Hemangiomas in Adults. Am J Ophthalmol. 2016 May;165:164–73. PMID:26973052
3187. Stagner AM, Jakobiec FA. Peripheral Nerve Sheath Tumors of the Eyelid Dermis: A Clinicopathologic and Immunohistochemical Analysis. Ophthalmic Plast Reconstr Surg. 2016 Jan-Feb;32(1):40–5. PMID:25794028
3188. Stagner AM, Jakobiec FA. Updates on the Molecular Pathology of Selected Ocular and Ocular Adnexal Tumors: Potential Targets for Future Therapy. Semin Ophthalmol. 2016;31(1-2):188–96. PMID:26959146
3189. Stagner AM, Jakobiec FA, Chi A, et al. Conjunctival Inverted Squamous Papilloma: A Case Report with Immunohistochemical Analysis and Review of the Literature. Surv Ophthalmol. 2015 May-Jun;60(3):263–8. PMID:25890626
3190. Stagner AM, Jakobiec FA, Fay A. Primary Orbital Synovial Sarcoma: A Clinicopathologic Review with a Differential Diagnosis and Discussion of Molecular Genetics. Surv Ophthalmol. 2017 Mar-Apr;62(2):227–36. PMID:27697479
3191. Stahl A, Riggi N, Nardou K, et al. 5-Hydroxymethylcytosine Loss in Conjunctival Melanoma. Dermatopathology (Basel). 2021 Jun 5;8(2):176–84. PMID:34198758
3192. Staiger AM, Ziepert M, Horn H, et al. Clinical Impact of the Cell-of-Origin Classification and the MYC/ BCL2 Dual Expresser Status in Diffuse Large B-Cell Lymphoma Treated Within Prospective Clinical Trials of the German High-Grade Non-Hodgkin's Lymphoma Study Group. J Clin Oncol. 2017 Aug 1;35(22):2515–26. PMID:28525305
3193. Stanoszek LM, Wang GY, Harms PW. Histologic Mimics of Basal Cell Carcinoma. Arch Pathol Lab Med. 2017 Nov;141(11):1490–502. PMID:29072946
3194. Stapleton F, Bakkar M, Carnt N, et al. CLEAR - Contact Lens Complications. Cont Lens Anterior Eye. 2021 Apr;44(2):330–67. PMID:33775382
3195. Star P, Goodwin A, Kapoor R, et al. Germline BAP1-Positive Patients: The Dilemmas of Cancer Surveillance and a Proposed Interdisciplinary Consensus Monitoring Strategy. Eur J Cancer. 2018 Mar;92:48–53. PMID:29413689
3196. Starita N, Buonaguro L, Buonaguro FM, et al. Telomerase Promoter Mutations in Human Immunodeficiency Virus-Related Conjunctiva Neoplasia. J Transl Med. 2018 Mar 21;16(1):77. PMID:29562930
3197. Starnoni M, De Santis G, Pasini R, et al. Diagnosis and Treatment of Upper Eyelid Lipoma: A Case Report. Am J Ophthalmol Case Rep. 2020 Aug 18;20:100874. PMID:32875157
3198. Stefanyszyn MA, Hidayat AA, Pe'er JJ, et al. Lacrimal Sac Tumors. Ophthalmic Plast Reconstr Surg. 1994 Sep;10(3):169–84. PMID:7947444
3199. Stelmach-Gołdyś A, Garus B, Skowronek M, et al. Periocular Xanthogranuloma with Adult-Onset Asthma: A Rare Disorder Associated with Elevated IgG4 Levels. Pol Arch Intern Med. 2019 Nov 29;129(11):827–9. PMID:31418752
3200. Stemmer-Rachamimov AO, Xu L, Gonzalez-Agosti C, et al. Universal Absence of Merlin, But Not Other ERM Family Members, in Schwannomas. Am J Pathol. 1997 Dec;151(6):1649–54. PMID:9403715
3201. Stenson S. Superior Limbic Keratoconjunctivitis Associated with Soft Contact Lens Wear. Arch Ophthalmol. 1983 Mar;101(3):402–4. PMID:6830490
3202. Stephen N, Manivannan P, Gochhait D, et al. The Utility of Fine Needle Aspiration Cytology in Orbital Haematolymphoid Neoplasms. Cytopathology. 2021 Mar;32(2):217–26. PMID:33125778
3203. Stephens RF, Shields JA. Diagnosis and Management of Cancer Metastatic to the Uvea: A Study of 70 Cases. Ophthalmology. 1979 Jul;86(7):1336–49. PMID:233866
3204. Stephenson JA, Mayland DM, Ingall G, et al. Squamous Cell Carcinoma of the Lacrimal Sac. Otolaryngol Head Neck Surg. 1988 Nov;99(5):524–7. PMID:3147447
3205. Stergiopoulos P, Link B, Naumann GO, et al. Solid Corneal Dermoids and Subconjunctival Lipodermoids: Impact of Differentiated Surgical Therapy on the Functional Long-Term Outcome. Cornea. 2009 Jul;28(6):644–51. PMID:19512907
3206. Sterling JC, Handfield-Jones S, Hudson PM; British Association of Dermatologists. Guidelines for the Management of Cutaneous Warts. Br J Dermatol. 2001 Jan;144(1):4–11. PMID:11167676
3207. Stern J, Jakobiec FA, Housepian EM. The Architecture of Optic Nerve Gliomas with and Without Neurofibromatosis. Arch Ophthalmol. 1980 Mar;98(3):505–11. PMID:6767467
3208. Stern K, Jakobiec FA, Harrison WG. Caruncular Dacryops with Extruded Secretory Globoid Bodies. Ophthalmology. 1983 Dec;90(12):1447–51. PMID:6330636
3209. Stewart S, Houghton J, Kamalarajah S, et al. Primary Adnexal Signet-Ring Cell/ Histiocytoid Carcinoma. Ophthalmic Plast Reconstr Surg. 2021 Jul-Aug 01;37(4):e134–6. PMID:33315842
3210. Stiefel HC, Ng JD, Wilson DJ, et al. Orbital Cellular Epithelioid Hemangioma. Ocul Oncol Pathol. 2019 Oct;5(6):424–31. PMID:31768366
3211. Stilgenbauer S, Schnaiter A, Paschka P, et al. Gene Mutations and Treatment Outcome in Chronic Lymphocytic Leukemia: Results from the CLL8 Trial. Blood. 2014 May 22;123(21):3247–54. PMID:24652989
3212. Stoll LM, Li QK. Cytology of Fine-Needle Aspiration of Inflammatory Myofibroblastic Tumor. Diagn Cytopathol. 2011 Sep;39(9):663–72. PMID:20730898
3213. Stölzel F, Lüer T, Löck S, et al. The Prevalence of Extramedullary Acute Myeloid Leukemia Detected by 18FDG-PET/CT: Final Results from the Prospective PETAML Trial. Haematologica. 2020 Jun;105(6):1552–8. PMID:31467130
3214. Stone JH, Zen Y, Deshpande V. IgG4-Related Disease. N Engl J Med. 2012 Feb 9;366(6):539–51. PMID:22316447
3215. Stratmann R, Krieg M, Haas R, et al. Putative Control of Angiogenesis in Hemangioblastomas by the von Hippel-Lindau Tumor Suppressor Gene. J Neuropathol Exp Neurol. 1997 Nov;56(11):1242–52. PMID:9370235
3216. Streeten BW, McGraw JL. Tumor of the Ciliary Pigment Epithelium. Am J Ophthalmol. 1972 Sep;74(3):420–9. PMID:4115451
3217. Strehl JD, Hartmann A, Agaimy A. Numerous IgG4-Positive Plasma Cells Are Ubiquitous in Diverse Localised Non-Specific Chronic Inflammatory Conditions and Need to Be Distinguished from IgG4-Related Systemic Disorders. J Clin Pathol. 2011 Mar;64(3):237–43. PMID:21233087
3218. Stretch JR, Scolyer RA. Surgical Strategies and Histopathologic Issues in the Management of Lentigo Maligna. Ann Surg Oncol. 2009 Jun;16(6):1456–8. PMID:19322612
3219. Streubel B, Simonitsch-Klupp I, Müllauer L, et al. Variable Frequencies of MALT Lymphoma-Associated Genetic Aberrations in MALT Lymphomas of Different Sites. Leukemia. 2004 Oct;18(10):1722–6. PMID:15356642
3220. Strianese D, Tranfa F, Finelli M, et al. Inflammatory Myofibroblastic Tumor of the Orbit: A Clinico-Pathological Study of 25 Cases. Saudi J Ophthalmol. 2018 Jan-Mar;32(1):33–9. PMID:29755269
3221. Stupp T, Pavlidis M, Bochner T, et al. Poland Anomaly Associated with Ipsilateral Combined Hamartoma of Retina and Retinal Pigment Epithelium. Eye (Lond). 2004 May;18(5):550–2. PMID:15131695
3222. Sturm V, Richard G. [The Prevalence of Bilateral Malignant Uveal Melanoma]. Klin Monbl Augenheilkd. 2007 Oct;224(10):770–4. German. PMID:17952820
3223. Su HH, Wu W, Guo Y, et al. Paediatric Erdheim-Chester Disease with Aggressive Skin Manifestations. Br J Dermatol. 2018 Jan;178(1):261–4. PMID:28078666
3224. Subramaniam SS, Anand R, Mellor TK, et al. Primary Lacrimal Sac Melanoma With Metastatic Cervical Disease: A Review of the Literature and Case Report. J Oral Maxillofac Surg. 2017 Jul;75(7):1438–41. PMID:28215853
3225. Sud A, Chattopadhyay S, Thomsen H, et al. Analysis of 153 115 Patients with Hematological Malignancies Refines the Spectrum of Familial Risk. Blood. 2019 Sep 19;134(12):960–9. PMID:31395603
3226. Suerink M, Ripperger T, Messiaen L, et al. Constitutional Mismatch Repair Deficiency as a Differential Diagnosis of Neurofibromatosis Type 1: Consensus Guidelines for Testing a Child Without Malignancy. J Med Genet. 2019 Feb;56(2):53–62. PMID:30415209
3227. Sugano H, Iimura Y, Igarashi A, et al. Extent of Leptomeningeal Capillary Malformation is Associated With Severity of Epilepsy in Sturge-Weber Syndrome. Pediatr Neurol. 2021 Apr;117:64–71. PMID:33677229
3228. Sugar HS, Riazi A, Schaffner R. The Bulbar Conjunctival Lymphatics and Their Clinical Significance. Trans Am Acad Ophthalmol Otolaryngol. 1957 Mar-Apr;61(2):212–23. PMID:13422475
3229. Sugiura M, Colby KA, Mihm MC Jr, et al. Low-Risk and High-Risk Histologic Features in Conjunctival Primary Acquired Melanosis with Atypia: Clinicopathologic Analysis of 29 Cases. Am J Surg Pathol. 2007 Feb;31(2):185–92. PMID:17255762
3230. Sugiura Y, Nagaishi M, Takano I, et al. Convexity Dural Chondroma: A Case Report with Pathological and Molecular Analysis. Clin Neuropathol. 2015 Jan-Feb;34(1):13–8. PMID:25250651
3231. Sugiyama A, Sugiura M, Piris A, et al. Apocrine Cystadenoma and Apocrine Hidrocystoma: Examination of 21 Cases with Emphasis on Nomenclature According to Proliferative Features. J Cutan Pathol. 2007 Dec;34(12):912–7. PMID:18001413
3232. Sujansky E, Conradi S. Outcome of Sturge-Weber Syndrome in 52 Adults. Am J Med Genet. 1995 May 22;57(1):35–45. PMID:7645596
3233. Sujansky E, Conradi S. Sturge-Weber Syndrome: Age of Onset of Seizures and Glaucoma and the Prognosis for Affected Children. J Child Neurol. 1995 Jan;10(1):49–58. PMID:7769179
3234. Sukeda A, Mori T, Suzuki S, et al. Adenocarcinoma of the Pigmented Ciliary Epithelium. BMJ Case Rep. 2014 Jul 11;2014:Bcr2014204534. PMID:25015166
3235. Sukswai N, Aung PP, Yin CC, et al. Dual Expression of TCF4 and CD123 Is Highly Sensitive and Specific For Blastic Plasmacytoid

Dendritic Cell Neoplasm. Am J Surg Pathol. 2019 Oct;43(10):1429–37. PMID:31261288
3236. Sullivan TJ. Squamous Cell Carcinoma of Eyelid, Periocular, and Periorbital Skin. Int Ophthalmol Clin. 2009 Fall;49(4):17–24. PMID:20348855
3237. Sullivan TJ, Clarke MP, Morin JD. The Ocular Manifestations of the Sturge-Weber Syndrome. J Pediatr Ophthalmol Strabismus. 1992 Nov-Dec;29(6):349–56. PMID:1287171
3238. Sulochana S, Manoharan M, Anitha. Chondroid Syringoma-an Unusual Presentation. J Clin Diagn Res. 2014 Jul;8(7):FD13–4. PMID:25177574
3239. Sun EC, Fears TR, Goedert JJ. Epidemiology of Squamous Cell Conjunctival Cancer. Cancer Epidemiol Biomarkers Prev. 1997 Feb;6(2):73–7. PMID:9037556
3240. Sun J, Yi S, Qiu L, et al. SATB1 Defines a Subtype of Cutaneous CD30+ Lymphoproliferative Disorders Associated with a T-Helper 17 Cytokine Profile. J Invest Dermatol. 2018 Aug;138(8):1795–804. PMID:29510190
3241. Sun MT, Wu A, Huilgol SC, et al. Accuracy of Biopsy in Subtyping Periocular Basal Cell Carcinoma. Ophthalmic Plast Reconstr Surg. 2015 Nov-Dec;31(6):449–51. PMID:25794023
3242. Sundaram M, Falbo S, McDonald D, et al. Surface Osteomas of the Appendicular Skeleton. AJR Am J Roentgenol. 1996 Dec;167(6):1529–33. PMID:8956591
3243. Sundaresh DD, Mangala Gouri SR. Glial Heterotopia in an Adult: A Rare Orbital Mass. Indian J Ophthalmol. 2016 Nov;64(11):843–4. PMID:27958209
3244. Surakiatchanukul T, Sioufi K, Pointdujour-Lim R, et al. Caruncular Oncocytoma Mimicking Malignant Melanoma. Ocul Oncol Pathol. 2017 Nov;3(4):320–3. PMID:29344489
3245. Surapaneni KR, Phelps PO, Potter HD. Palisaded Encapsulated Neuroma of the Eyelid. Ophthalmology. 2015 Aug;122(8):1554. PMID:26425742
3246. Suurmeijer AJ, Dickson BC, Swanson D, et al. Novel SRF-ICA1L Fusions in Cellular Myoid Neoplasms With Potential For Malignant Behavior. Am J Surg Pathol. 2020 Jan;44(1):55–60. PMID:31478943
3247. Suzuki Y, Obana A, Gohto Y, et al. Management of Orbital Lymphangioma Using Intralesional Injection of OK-432. Br J Ophthalmol. 2000 Jun;84(6):614–7. PMID:10837387
3248. Svendsen FH, Heegaard S. Lymphoma of the Eyelid. Surv Ophthalmol. 2017 May-Jun;62(3):312–31. PMID:27894880
3249. Svendsen FH, Rasmussen PK, Coupland SE, et al. Lymphoma of the Eyelid - An International Multicenter Retrospective Study. Am J Ophthalmol. 2017 May;177:58–68. PMID:28209503
3250. Swaby MG, Evans HL, Fletcher CD, et al. Dermatofibrosarcoma Protuberans with Unusual Sarcomatous Transformation: A Series of 4 Cases with Molecular Confirmation. Am J Dermatopathol. 2011 Jun;33(4):354–60. PMID:21478726
3251. Swerdlow SH, Zukerberg LR, Yang WI, et al. The Morphologic Spectrum of Non-Hodgkin's Lymphomas with BCL1/Cyclin D1 Gene Rearrangements. Am J Surg Pathol. 1996 May;20(5):627–40. PMID:8619427
3252. Syed M, Mushtaq S, Loya A, et al. NKX3.1 a Useful Marker for Mesenchymal Chondrosarcoma: An Immunohistochemical Study. Ann Diagn Pathol. 2021 Feb;50:151660. PMID:33302222
3253. Szalai E, Jiang Y, van Poppelen NM, et al. Association of Uveal Melanoma Metastatic Rate With Stochastic Mutation Rate and Type of Mutation. JAMA Ophthalmol. 2018 Oct 1;136(10):1115–20. PMID:30073324
3254. Szulzewsky F, Arora S, Hoellerbauer P, et al. Comparison of Tumor-Associated YAP1 Fusions Identifies a Recurrent Set of Functions Critical for Oncogenesis. Genes Dev. 2020 Aug 1;34(15-16):1051–64. PMID:32675324
3255. Taban M, Sears JE, Singh AD. Ciliary Body Naevus. Eye (Lond). 2007 Dec;21(12):1528–30. PMID:17041573
3256. Tadepalli SH, Shields CL, Shields JA, et al. Intraocular Medulloepithelioma - A Review of Clinical Features, DICER 1 Mutation, and Management. Indian J Ophthalmol. 2019 Jun;67(6):755–62. PMID:31124483
3257. Takagi T, Ueno Y, Matsuya N. Mesectodermal Leiomyoma of the Ciliary Body. An Ultrastructural Study. Arch Ophthalmol. 1985 Nov;103(11):1711–4. PMID:4062640
3258. Takahashi BS, Bruè C, Spaide RF. Autofluorescence Characteristics of Congenital Hypertrophy of the Retinal Pigment Epithelium. Retin Cases Brief Rep. 2008 Fall;2(4):259–61. PMID:25390583
3259. Takahashi M, Fujinaga Y, Notohara K, et al. Diagnostic Imaging Guide for Autoimmune Pancreatitis. Jpn J Radiol. 2020 Jul;38(7):591–612. PMID:32297064
3260. Takanashi S, Akiyama M, Suzuki K, et al. IgG4-Related Fibrosing Mediastinitis Diagnosed with Computed Tomography-Guided Percutaneous Needle Biopsy: Two Case Reports and a Review of the Literature. Medicine (Baltimore). 2018 Jun;97(22):e10935. PMID:29851832
3261. Takase H, Arai A, Iwasaki Y, et al. Challenges in the Diagnosis and Management of Vitreoretinal Lymphoma - Clinical and Basic Approaches. Prog Retin Eye Res. 2022 Sep;90:101053. PMID:35210172
3262. Takata K, Hong ME, Sitthinamsuwan P, et al. Primary Cutaneous NK/T-Cell Lymphoma, Nasal Type and CD56-Positive Peripheral T-Cell Lymphoma: A Cellular Lineage and Clinicopathologic Study of 60 Patients from Asia. Am J Surg Pathol. 2015 Jan;39(1):1–12. PMID:25188863
3263. Takei H, Florez L, Moroz K, et al. Medulloepithelioma: Two Unusual Locations. Pathol Int. 2007 Feb;57(2):91–5. PMID:17300673
3264. Takei H, Powell SZ. Novel Immunohistochemical Markers in the Diagnosis of Nonglial Tumors of Nervous System. Adv Anat Pathol. 2010 Mar;17(2):150–3. PMID:20179436
3265. Takeshima K, Li Y, Kakudo K, et al. Proposal of Diagnostic Criteria for IgG4-Related Thyroid Disease. Endocr J. 2021 Jan 28;68(1):1–6. PMID:33311000
3266. Talebnejad MR, Lankaranian D, Warrian K, et al. Osteochondroma of the Trochlea Presenting as Acquired Brown Syndrome: A Case Report. J AAPOS. 2007 Jun;11(3):305–6. PMID:17446102
3267. Tallini G, Dorfman H, Brys P, et al. Correlation Between Clinicopathological Features and Karyotype in 100 Cartilaginous and Chordoid Tumours. A Report from the Chromosomes and Morphology (CHAMP) Collaborative Study Group. J Pathol. 2002 Feb;196(2):194–203. PMID:11793371
3268. Tam ES, Chen EC, Nijhawan N, et al. Solitary Fibrous Tumor of the Orbit: A Case Series. Orbit. 2008;27(6):426–31. PMID:19085297
3269. Tan ACS, Yzer S, Atebara N, et al. Three Cases of Erdheim-Chester Disease With Intraocular Manifestations: Imaging and Histopathology Findings of a Rare Entity. Am J Ophthalmol. 2017 Apr;176:141–7. PMID:28153505
3270. Tan CS, Lim TH, Koh WP, et al. Epidemiology of Pterygium on a Tropical Island in the Riau Archipelago. Eye (Lond). 2006 Aug;20(8):908–12. PMID:16167080
3271. Tan KW, Koh MJ, Tay YK. Juvenile Xanthogranuloma in Monozygotic Twins. Pediatr Dermatol. 2010 Nov-Dec;27(6):666–7. PMID:21091658
3272. Tan MH, Mester J, Peterson C, et al. A Clinical Scoring System for Selection of Patients for PTEN Mutation Testing is Proposed on the Basis of a Prospective Study of 3042 Probands. Am J Hum Genet. 2011 Jan 7;88(1):42–56. PMID:21194675
3273. Tan WJ, Wang MM, Ricciardi-Castagnoli P, et al. Cytologic and Molecular Diagnostics for Vitreoretinal Lymphoma: Current Approaches and Emerging Single-Cell Analyses. Front Mol Biosci. 2021 Jan 11;7:611017. PMID:33505989
3274. Tanaboonyawat S, Idowu OO, Copperman TS, et al. Dacryops - A Review. Orbit. 2020 Apr;39(2):128–34. PMID:31512543
3275. Tanaka M, Kato K, Gomi K, et al. Perivascular Epithelioid Cell Tumor with SFPQ/PSF-TFE3 Gene Fusion in a Patient with Advanced Neuroblastoma. Am J Surg Pathol. 2009 Sep;33(9):1416–20. PMID:19606011
3276. Tanaka R, Kaburaki T, Taoka K, et al. More Accurate Diagnosis of Vitreoretinal Lymphoma Using a Combination of Diagnostic Test Results: A Prospective Observational Study. Ocul Immunol Inflamm. 2022 Aug;30(6):1354–60. PMID:33793360
3277. Tananuvat N, Lertprasertsuk N, Mahanupap P, et al. Role of Impression Cytology in Diagnosis of Ocular Surface Neoplasia. Cornea. 2008 Apr;27(3):269–74. PMID:18362650
3278. Tanas MR, Ma S, Jadaan FO, et al. Mechanism of Action of a WWTR1(TAZ)-CAMTA1 Fusion Oncoprotein. Oncogene. 2016 Feb 18;35(7):929–38. PMID:25961935
3279. Tanas MR, Sboner A, Oliveira AM, et al. Identification of a Disease-Defining Gene Fusion in Epithelioid Hemangioendothelioma. Sci Transl Med. 2011 Aug 31;3(98):98ra82. PMID:21885404
3280. Tandon B, Peterson L, Gao J, et al. Nuclear Overexpression of Lymphoid-Enhancer-Binding Factor 1 Identifies Chronic Lymphocytic Leukemia/Small Lymphocytic Lymphoma in Small B-Cell Lymphomas. Mod Pathol. 2011 Nov;24(11):1433–43. PMID:21685909
3281. Tanenbaum RE, Galor A, Dubovy SR, et al. Classification, Diagnosis, and Management of Conjunctival Lymphoma. Eye Vis (Lond). 2019 Jul 27;6:22. PMID:31372366
3282. Tanese K. Diagnosis and Management of Basal Cell Carcinoma. Curr Treat Options Oncol. 2019 Feb 11;20(2):13. PMID:30741348
3283. Tang H, Yang H, Zhang P, et al. Malignancy and IgG4-Related Disease: The Incidence, Related Factors and Prognosis from a Prospective Cohort Study in China. Sci Rep. 2020 Mar 18;10(1):4910. PMID:32188869
3284. Tang PH, Mettu P, Maltry AC, et al. Giant Cell Tumor of the Frontal Bone Presenting as an Orbital Mass. Ophthalmol Ther. 2017 Jun;6(1):215–20. PMID:28210962
3285. Tang PH, Vajzovic L, Mruthyunjaya P. Retinal Metastatic Tumors. In: Singh AD, Damato BE, editors. Clinical Ophthalmic Oncology Retinal Tumors. 3rd ed. Cleveland (OH): Springer; 2019. pp. 101–13. doi:10.1007/978-3-030-04113-7_8.
3286. Tang T, Brownstein S, Chen H, et al. Histopathological Study on the Proposed Pathogenesis of Intratarsal Keratinous Cysts. Ophthalmic Plast Reconstr Surg. 2019 Jul/Aug;35(4):365–8. PMID:30439722
3287. Tang X, Guo X, Gao J, et al. Hemophagocytic Lymphohistiocytosis in Langerhans Cell Histiocytosis: A Case Series and Literature Review. J Pediatr Hematol Oncol. 2022 Jan 1;44(1):e20–5. PMID:34133378
3288. Tani E, Wejde J, Åström K, et al. FNA Cytology of Solitary Fibrous Tumors and the Diagnostic Value of STAT6 Immunocytochemistry. Cancer Cytopathol. 2018 Jan;126(1):36–43. PMID:28914981
3289. Tantcheva-Poor I, Marathovouniotis N, Kutzner H, et al. Vascular Congenital Dermatofibrosarcoma Protuberans: A New Histological Variant of Dermatofibrosarcoma Protuberans. Am J Dermatopathol. 2012 Jun;34(4):e46–9. PMID:22257899
3290. Tardío JC. CD34-Reactive Tumors of the Skin. An Updated Review of an Ever-Growing List of Lesions. J Cutan Pathol. 2008 Dec;35(12):1079–92. PMID:18976402
3291. Tariq MU, Din NU, Abdul-Ghafar J, et al. The Many Faces of Solitary Fibrous Tumor; Diversity of Histological Features, Differential Diagnosis and Role of Molecular Studies and Surrogate Markers in Avoiding Misdiagnosis and Predicting the Behavior. Diagn Pathol. 2021 Apr 20;16(1):32. PMID:33879215
3292. Tarkkanen M, Böhling T, Gamberi G, et al. Comparative Genomic Hybridization of Low-Grade Central Osteosarcoma. Mod Pathol. 1998 May;11(5):421–6. PMID:9619593
3293. Tasman W, Jaeger EA, editors. Embryology and Anatomy of the Orbit and Lacrimal System. Duane's Ophthalmology. Philadelphia (PA): Lippincott Williams & Wilkins; 2007.
3294. Taubenslag KJ, Al Hussein Al Awamlh S, Sternberg P Jr. Bilateral Choroidal Vascular Malformations in Hereditary Hemorrhagic Telangiectasia. Retin Cases Brief Rep. 2023 Jul 1;17(4):346–7. PMID:34710889
3295. Tauziède-Espariat A, Roche O, Dufier JL, et al. Recurrent Lacrimal Gland Choristoma of the Ciliary Body in an Infant Mimicking a Medulloepithelioma. Eur J Ophthalmol. 2016 Nov 4;26(6):e145–8. PMID:27173894
3296. Tavakoli M, Yadegari S, Mosallaei M, et al. Infantile Periocular Hemangioma. J Ophthalmic Vis Res. 2017 Apr-Jun;12(2):205–11. PMID:28540013
3297. Tawfik HA, Abdulhafez MH, Fouad YA. Congenital Upper Eyelid Coloboma: Embryologic, Nomenclatorial, Nosologic, Etiologic, Pathogenetic, Epidemiologic, Clinical, and Management Perspectives. Ophthalmic Plast Reconstr Surg. 2015 Jan-Feb;31(1):1–12. PMID:25419956
3298. Tay A, Scheithauer BW, Cameron JD, et al. Retinal Ependymoma: An Immunohistologic and Ultrastructural Study. Hum Pathol. 2009 Apr;40(4):578–83. PMID:18835620
3299. Taylor HR, West SK, Rosenthal FS, et al. Corneal Changes Associated with Chronic UV Irradiation. Arch Ophthalmol. 1989 Oct;107(10):1481–4. PMID:2803097
3300. Techavichit P, Sosothikul D, Chaichana T, et al. BRAF V600E Mutation in Pediatric Intracranial and Cranial Juvenile Xanthogranuloma. Hum Pathol. 2017 Nov;69:118–22. PMID:28504206
3301. Tee AR, Fingar DC, Manning BD, et al. Tuberous Sclerosis Complex-1 and -2 Gene Products Function Together to Inhibit Mammalian Target of Rapamycin (MTOR)-Mediated Downstream Signaling. Proc Natl Acad Sci U S A. 2002 Oct 15;99(21):13571–6. PMID:12271141
3302. Teekhasaenee C, Ritch R. Glaucoma in Phakomatosis Pigmentovascularis. Ophthalmology. 1997 Jan;104(1):150–7. PMID:9022120
3303. Teekhasaenee C, Ritch R, Rutnin U, et al. Ocular Findings in Oculodermal Melanocytosis. Arch Ophthalmol. 1990 Aug;108(8):1114–20. PMID:2383200
3304. Tella SH, Kommalapati A, Rech KL, et al. Incidence, Clinical Features, and Outcomes of Langerhans Cell Sarcoma in the United States. Clin Lymphoma Myeloma Leuk. 2019 Jul;19(7):441–6. PMID:31005630
3305. Tellada M, Specht CS, McLean IW, et al. Primary Orbital Melanomas. Ophthalmology.

1996 Jun;103(6):929–32. PMID:8643249
3306. Tellechea O, Reis JP, Baptista AP. Desmoplastic Trichilemmoma. Am J Dermatopathol. 1992 Apr;14(2):107–4. PMID:1373583
3307. Temerek AT, Ali S, Shehab MF. Computer Guided Resection and Reconstruction of Intra-Osseous Zygomatic Hemangioma: Case Report and Systematic Review of Literature. Int J Surg Case Rep. 2020;66:240–56. PMID:31874384
3308. Ten Heuvel SE, Hoekstra HJ, Bastiaannet E, et al. The Classic Prognostic Factors Tumor Stage, Tumor Size, and Tumor Grade Are the Strongest Predictors of Outcome in Synovial Sarcoma: No Role for SSX Fusion Type or Ezrin Expression. Appl Immunohistochem Mol Morphol. 2009 May;17(3):189–95. PMID:18997619
3309. Terada T, Kamo M, Baba Y, et al. Microinvasive Squamous Cell Carcinoma Arising Within Seborrheic Keratosis. Cutis. 2012 Oct;90(4):176–8. PMID:23259202
3310. Terasaki M, Tokutomi T, Maruiwa H, et al. High-Grade Adenoid Cystic Carcinoma Originating from the Lacrimal Gland. Brain Tumor Pathol. 2000;17(3):159–63. PMID:11310924
3311. Testa JR, Cheung M, Pei J, et al. Germline BAP1 Mutations Predispose to Malignant Mesothelioma. Nat Genet. 2011 Aug 28;43(10):1022–5. PMID:21874000
3312. Tetzlaff MT. Immunohistochemical Markers Informing the Diagnosis of Sebaceous Carcinoma and its Distinction from its Mimics: Adipophilin and Factor XIIIa to the Rescue? J Cutan Pathol. 2018 Jan;45(1):29–32. PMID:29087003
3313. Tetzlaff MT, Curry JL, Ning J, et al. Distinct Biological Types of Ocular Adnexal Sebaceous Carcinoma: HPV-Driven and Virus-Negative Tumors Arise Through Nonoverlapping Molecular-Genetic Alterations. Clin Cancer Res. 2019 Feb 15;25(4):1280–90. PMID:30420449
3314. Tetzlaff MT, Singh RR, Seviour EG, et al. Next-Generation Sequencing Identifies High Frequency of Mutations in Potentially Clinically Actionable Genes in Sebaceous Carcinoma. J Pathol. 2016 Sep;240(1):84–95. PMID:27287813
3315. Tezol O, Citak EC, Ayhan YS, et al. Effective High-Dose Interferon-α Therapy in a 13-Year-Old Girl With Erdheim-Chester Disease. J Pediatr Hematol Oncol. 2020 May;42(4):326–31. PMID:31259822
3316. Thanos A, Jakobiec FA, Mendoza PR, et al. Ectopic (Choristomatous) Orbital Respiratory Cyst: Histopathology and Immunohistochemistry. Surv Ophthalmol. 2014 May-Jun;59(3):328–33. PMID:24359804
3317. Than-Trong T, Morel X, D'Hermies F, et al. [Orbital Lymphoma and AIDS. Apropos of a Case]. J Fr Ophtalmol. 1999 May;22(5):594–8. French. PMID:10417924
3318. Thareja S, Rashid A, Grossniklaus HE. Spontaneous Necrosis of Choroidal Melanoma. Ocul Oncol Pathol. 2014 Oct;1(1):63–9. PMID:27175363
3319. Thatte S, Jain J, Kinger M, et al. Clinical Study of Histologically Proven Conjunctival Cysts. Saudi J Ophthalmol. 2015 Apr-Jun;29(2):109–15. PMID:25892928
3320. Thaung C, Bonshek RE, Leatherbarrow B. Phakomatous Choristoma of the Eyelid: A Case with Associated Eye Abnormalities. Br J Ophthalmol. 2006 Feb;90(2):245–6. PMID:16424545
3321. Thavikulwat AT, Edward DP, AlDarrab A, et al. Pathophysiology and Management of Glaucoma Associated with Phakomatoses. J Neurosci Res. 2019 Jan;97(1):57–69. PMID:29607552
3322. Collaborative Ocular Melanoma Study Group. The Collaborative Ocular Melanoma Study (COMS) Randomized Trial of Pre-Enucleation Radiation of Large Choroidal Melanoma I: Characteristics of Patients Enrolled and Not Enrolled. COMS Report No. 9. Am J Ophthalmol. 1998 Jun;125(6):767–78. PMID:9645715
3323. Theilen TM, Soerensen J, Bochennek K, et al. Crizotinib in ALK+ Inflammatory Myofibroblastic Tumors-Current Experience and Future Perspectives. Pediatr Blood Cancer. 2018 Apr;65(4). PMID:29286567
3324. Theodossiadis P, Emfietzoglou I, Grigoropoulos V, et al. Evolution of a Retinoma Case in 21 Years. Ophthalmic Surg Lasers Imaging. 2005 Mar-Apr;36(2):155–7. PMID:15792319
3325. Theotoka D, Morkin MI, Galor A, et al. Update on Diagnosis and Management of Conjunctival Papilloma. Eye Vis (Lond). 2019 Jun 18;6:18. PMID:31236424
3326. Thériault BL, Dimaras H, Gallie BL, et al. The Genomic Landscape of Retinoblastoma: A Review. Clin Exp Ophthalmol. 2014 Jan-Feb;42(1):33–52. PMID:24433356
3327. Thiagalingam S, Johnson MM, Colby KA, et al. Juvenile Conjunctival Nevus: Clinicopathologic Analysis of 33 Cases. Am J Surg Pathol. 2008 Mar;32(3):399–406. PMID:18300811
3328. Thomas AC, Zeng Z, Rivière JB, et al. Mosaic Activating Mutations in GNA11 and GNAQ Are Associated with Phakomatosis Pigmentovascularis and Extensive Dermal Melanocytosis. J Invest Dermatol. 2016 Apr;136(4):770–8. PMID:26778290
3329. Thompson JM, Bermudez-Magner JA, Barker NH, et al. Balloon Cell Nevi of the Conjunctiva: Clinicopathologic Correlation and Literature Review. Surv Ophthalmol. 2015 Sep-Oct;60(5):481–5. PMID:26002588
3330. Thompson LDR, Liou SS, Feldman KA. Orbit Solitary Fibrous Tumor: A Proposed Risk Prediction Model Based on a Case Series and Comprehensive Literature Review. Head Neck Pathol. 2021 Mar;15(1):138–52. PMID:32529350
3331. Thomson J, Bewicke-Copley F, Anene CA, et al. The Genomic Landscape of Actinic Keratosis. J Invest Dermatol. 2021 Jul;141(7):1664–1674.E7. PMID:33482222
3332. Thorpe J, Frelin LP, McCann M, et al. Identification of a Mosaic Activating Mutation in GNA11 in Atypical Sturge-Weber Syndrome. J Invest Dermatol. 2021 Mar;141(3):685–8. PMID:32771470
3333. Thuro BA, Sagiv O, Shinder R, et al. Clinical Presentation and Anatomical Location of Orbital Plasmacytomas. Ophthalmic Plast Reconstr Surg. 2018 May/Jun;34(3):258–61. PMID:28582371
3334. Thway K. What's New in Adipocytic Neoplasia? Histopathology. 2022 Jan;80(1):76–97. PMID:34958506
3335. Thway K, Fisher C. Synovial Sarcoma: Defining Features and Diagnostic Evolution. Ann Diagn Pathol. 2014 Dec;18(6):369–80. PMID:25438927
3336. Tian L, Cui CY, Lu SY, et al. Clinical Presentation and CT/MRI Findings of Alveolar Soft Part Sarcoma: A Retrospective Single-Center Analysis of 14 Cases. Acta Radiol. 2016 Apr;57(4):475–80. PMID:26231949
3337. Tiberti A, Damato B, Hiscott P, et al. Iris Ectopic Thyroid Tissue: Report of a Case. Arch Ophthalmol. 2006 Oct;124(10):1497–500. PMID:17030724
3338. Ticho BH, Rosner M, Mets MB, et al. Bilateral Diffuse Iris Nodular Nevi. Clinical and Histopathologic Characterization. Ophthalmology. 1995 Mar;102(3):419–25. PMID:7891979
3339. Tieger MG, Jakobiec FA, Ma L, et al. Small Benign Storiform Fibrous Tumor (Fibrous Histiocytoma) of the Conjunctival Substantia Propria in a Child: Review and Clarification of Biologic Behavior. Ophthalmic Plast Reconstr Surg. 2019 Sep/Oct;35(5):495–502. PMID:30893190
3340. Tiegs-Heiden CA, Eckel LJ, Hunt CH, et al. Immunoglobulin G4-Related Disease of the Orbit: Imaging Features in 27 Patients. AJNR Am J Neuroradiol. 2014 Jul;35(7):1393–7. PMID:24627453
3341. Tihan T, Fisher PG, Kepner JL, et al. Pediatric Astrocytomas with Monomorphous Pilomyxoid Features and a Less Favorable Outcome. J Neuropathol Exp Neurol. 1999 Oct;58(10):1061–8. PMID:10515229
3342. Timberlake AT, Griffin C, Heike CL, et al. Haploinsufficiency of SF3B2 Causes Craniofacial Microsomia. Nat Commun. 2021 Aug 3;12(1):4680. PMID:34344887
3343. Timoney PJ, Bradley M, Cowen DE. A Rare Case of Progressive Ptosis Caused by Lacrimal Gland Oncocytoma. Ophthalmic Plast Reconstr Surg. 2011 Jul-Aug;27(4):e85–7. PMID:21283034
3344. Tingaud-Sequeira A, Trimouille A, Sagardoy T, et al. Oculo-Auriculo-Vertebral Spectrum: New Genes and Literature Review on a Complex Disease. J Med Genet. 2022 May;59(5):417–27. PMID:35110414
3345. Tiong T, Borooah S, Msosa J, et al. Clinicopathological Review of Ocular Surface Squamous Neoplasia in Malawi. Br J Ophthalmol. 2013 Aug;97(8):961–4. PMID:23613511
3346. Tirelli G, Gardenal N, Gatto A, et al. Head and Neck Immunoglobulin G4 Related Disease: Systematic Review. J Laryngol Otol. 2018 Dec;132(12):1046–50. PMID:30558692
3347. Tole DM, McKelvie PA, Daniell M. Reliability of Impression Cytology for the Diagnosis of Ocular Surface Squamous Neoplasia Employing the Biopore Membrane. Br J Ophthalmol. 2001 Feb;85(2):154–8. PMID:11159477
3348. Toledano Fernández N, Stoica BT, Genol Saavedra I, et al. Diplopia from Pleomorphic Lipoma of the Orbit with Lateral Rectus Muscle Involvement. Ophthalmic Plast Reconstr Surg. 2013 Mar-Apr;29(2):e53–5. PMID:23328779
3349. Toledo RA. Genetics of Pheochromocytomas and Paragangliomas: An Overview on the Recently Implicated Genes MERTK, MET, Fibroblast Growth Factor Receptor 1, and H3F3A. Endocrinol Metab Clin North Am. 2017 Jun;46(2):459–89. PMID:28476232
3350. Toledo RA, Qin Y, Cheng ZM, et al. Recurrent Mutations of Chromatin-Remodeling Genes and Kinase Receptors in Pheochromocytomas and Paragangliomas. Clin Cancer Res. 2016 May 1;22(9):2301–10. PMID:26700204
3351. Tom A, Bell D, Ford JR, et al. Malignant Mixed Tumor (Carcinoma Ex Pleomorphic Adenoma) of the Lacrimal Gland. Ophthalmic Plast Reconstr Surg. 2020 Sep/Oct;36(5):497–502. PMID:32282452
3352. Tomar AS, Fam A, Finger PT, et al. Doppelgänger Dilemma: Leiomyoma Versus Uveal Melanoma. Am J Ophthalmol Case Rep. 2021 Mar 6;22:101040. PMID:33748534
3353. Tomar AS, Finger PT, Gallie B, et al. A Multicenter, International Collaborative Study for American Joint Committee on Cancer Staging of Retinoblastoma: Part I: Metastasis-Associated Mortality. Ophthalmology. 2020 Dec;127(12):1719–32. PMID:32512116
3354. Tomar AS, Finger PT, Gallie B, et al. A Multicenter, International Collaborative Study for American Joint Committee on Cancer Staging of Retinoblastoma: Part II: Treatment Success and Globe Salvage. Ophthalmology. 2020 Dec;127(12):1733–46. PMID:32526306
3355. Tomar AS, Finger PT, Gallie B, et al. Global Retinoblastoma Treatment Outcomes: Association with National Income Level. Ophthalmology. 2021 May;128(5):740–53. PMID:33007338
3356. Tomar AS, Finger PT, Iacob CE. Intraocular Leiomyoma: Current Concepts. Surv Ophthalmol. 2020 Jul-Aug;65(4):421–37. PMID:31923479
3357. Tomić TT, Olausson J, Wilzén A, et al. A New GTF2I-BRAF Fusion Mediating MAPK Pathway Activation in Pilocytic Astrocytoma. PLoS One. 2017 Apr 27;12(4):e0175638. PMID:28448514
3358. Tomida M, Mitamura Y, Katome T, et al. Aggressive Retinal Astrocytoma Associated with Tuberous Sclerosis. Clin Ophthalmol. 2012;6:715–20. PMID:22654497
3359. Tonorezos ES, Friedman DN, Barnea D, et al. Recommendations for Long-Term Follow-Up of Adults with Heritable Retinoblastoma. Ophthalmology. 2020 Nov;127(11):1549–57. PMID:32422154
3360. Tooley AA, Salomao DR, Bradley EA, et al. Distinguishing IgG4-Related Ophthalmic Disease From Graves Orbitopathy. Ophthalmic Plast Reconstr Surg. 2019 Mar/Apr;35(2):170–6. PMID:30124607
3361. Topilow NJ, Stevens SM, Chen Y, et al. A Rare Case of Mucoepidermoid Carcinoma Ex Pleomorphic Adenoma of the Lacrimal Gland. Orbit. 2023 Jun;42(3):311–15. PMID:34939520
3362. Toribio J, Zulaica A, Peteiro C. Tubular Apocrine Adenoma. J Cutan Pathol. 1987 Apr;14(2):114–7. PMID:3036918
3363. Toth J, Karcioglu ZA, Moshfeghi AA, et al. The Relationship Between Human Papillomavirus and P53 Gene in Conjunctival Squamous Cell Carcinoma. Cornea. 2000 Mar;19(2):159–62. PMID:10746446
3364. Touliatou V, Fryssira H, Mavrou A, et al. Clinical Manifestations in 17 Greek Patients with Goldenhar Syndrome. Genet Couns. 2006;17(3):359–70. PMID:17100205
3365. Toyoda K, Oba H, Kutomi K, et al. MR Imaging of IgG4-Related Disease in the Head and Neck and Brain. AJNR Am J Neuroradiol. 2012 Dec;33(11):2136–9. PMID:22700747
3366. Traber GL, Pangalu A, Neumann M, et al. Malignant Optic Glioma - the Spectrum of Disease in a Case Series. Graefes Arch Clin Exp Ophthalmol. 2015 Jul;253(7):1187–94. PMID:26004076
3367. Traboulsi EI, Krush AJ, Gardner EJ, et al. Prevalence and Importance of Pigmented Ocular Fundus Lesions in Gardner's Syndrome. N Engl J Med. 1987 Mar 12;316(11):661–7. PMID:3821797
3368. Traboulsi EI, Maumenee IH, Krush AJ, et al. Pigmented Ocular Fundus Lesions in the Inherited Gastrointestinal Polyposis Syndromes and in Hereditary Nonpolyposis Colorectal Cancer. Ophthalmology. 1988 Jul;95(7):964–9. PMID:2845322
3369. Traboulsi EI, Murphy SF, de La Cruz ZC, et al. A Clinicopathologic Study of the Eyes in Familial Adenomatous Polyposis with Extracolonic Manifestations (Gardner's Syndrome). Am J Ophthalmol. 1990 Nov 15;110(5):550–61. PMID:2173407
3370. Tran AQ, Choi CJ, Al-Sadah Z, et al. Bilateral Poorly Differentiated Adenocarcinoma of the Lacrimal Gland With Tumor Regression After Treatment With Pembrolizumab. Ophthalmic Plast Reconstr Surg. 2020 Nov/Dec;36(6):e144–7. PMID:32282640
3371. Trautmann M, Cyra M, Isfort I, et al. Phosphatidylinositol-3-Kinase (PI3K)/Akt Signaling is Functionally Essential in Myxoid Liposarcoma. Mol Cancer Ther. 2019 Apr;18(4):834–44. PMID:30787173
3372. Trembath DG, Dash R, Major NM, et al. Cytopathology of Mesenchymal Chondrosarcomas: A Report and Comparison of Four Patients. Cancer. 2003 Aug 25;99(4):211–6.

PMID:12925982
3373. Trichopoulos N, Augsburger JJ, Schneider S. Adenocarcinoma Arising from Congenital Hypertrophy of the Retinal Pigment Epithelium. Graefes Arch Clin Exp Ophthalmol. 2006 Jan;244(1):125–8. PMID:15983818
3374. Tripathy D, Agarwal S, Biala A, et al. Primary De Novo Ductal Adenocarcinoma of the Lacrimal Gland. Ann Diagn Pathol. 2021 Feb;50:151651. PMID:33186791
3375. Tripathy D, Mittal R. Spindle Cell Lipoma of the Orbit. Ophthalmic Plast Reconstr Surg. 2015 May-Jun;31(3):e53–5. PMID:24819207
3376. Tripathy K, Chawla R, Temkar S, et al. Phthisis Bulbi-a Clinicopathological Perspective. Semin Ophthalmol. 2018;33(6):788–803. PMID:29902388
3376A. Trisolini E, Wardighi DE, Giry M, et al. Actionable FGFR1 and BRAF Mutations in Adult Circumscribed Gliomas. J Neurooncol. 2019 Nov;145(2):241–5. PMID:31673897
3377. Trojani M, Contesso G, Coindre JM, et al. Soft-Tissue Sarcomas of Adults; Study of Pathological Prognostic Variables and Definition of a Histopathological Grading System. Int J Cancer. 1984 Jan 15;33(1):37–42. PMID:6693192
3378. Troost T, Klein T. Sequential Notch Signalling at the Boundary of Fringe Expressing and Non-Expressing Cells. PLoS One. 2012;7(11):e49007. PMID:23152840
3379. Troy JL, Ackerman AB. Sebaceoma. A Distinctive Benign Neoplasm of Adnexal Epithelium Differentiating Toward Sebaceous Cells. Am J Dermatopathol. 1984 Feb;6(1):7–13. PMID:6703260
3380. Trubnik V, Conley R, Ritterband DC, et al. Progressive Growth in Epibulbar Complex Choristomas: Report of 2 Cases and Review of Literature. Cornea. 2011 Nov;30(11):1267–9. PMID:21885965
3381. Tsai AS, Lee KY, Al Jajeh I, et al. Epibulbar Osseous Choristoma: A Report of Two Cases. Orbit. 2008;27(3):231–3. PMID:18569837
3382. Tsai FF, Mukhopadhyay C, Zeng J, et al. Bilateral Marked Dacryops Following Trauma. Orbit. 2012 Dec;31(6):435–7. PMID:22909413
3383. Tsai JH, Hsiao TL, Chen YY, et al. Endocrine Mucin-Producing Sweat Gland Carcinoma Occurring on Extra-Facial Site: A Case Report. J Cutan Pathol. 2014 Jun;41(6):544–7. PMID:24673415
3384. Tsai P, O'Brien JM. Combined Hamartoma of the Retina and Retinal Pigment Epithelium as the Presenting Sign of Neurofibromatosis-1. Ophthalmic Surg Lasers. 2000 Mar-Apr;31(2):145–7. PMID:10743927
3385. Tsao L, Draoua HY, Mansukhani M, et al. EBV-Associated, Extranodal NK-Cell Lymphoma, Nasal Type of the Breast, After Heart Transplantation. Mod Pathol. 2004 Jan;17(1):125–30. PMID:14631361
3386. Tse JY, Nguyen AT, Le LP, et al. Microcystic Adnexal Carcinoma Versus Desmoplastic Trichoepithelioma: A Comparative Study. Am J Dermatopathol. 2013 Feb;35(1):50–5. PMID:22722464
3387. Tseng MC, Amin B, Barmettler A. Eyelid Syringocystadenoma Papilliferum: A Novel Presentation with Major Review. Orbit. 2018 Jun;37(3):171–4. PMID:29053036
3388. Tsimberidou AM, Kantarjian HM, Wen S, et al. Myeloid Sarcoma is Associated with Superior Event-Free Survival and Overall Survival Compared with Acute Myeloid Leukemia. Cancer. 2008 Sep 15;113(6):1370–8. PMID:18623376
3389. Tsiouris AJ, Deshmukh M, Sanelli PC, et al. Bilateral Dacryops: Correlation of Clinical, Radiologic, and Histopathologic Features. AJR Am J Roentgenol. 2005 Jan;184(1):321–3. PMID:15615995
3390. Tso MO, Albert DM. Pathological Condition of the Retinal Pigment Epithelium. Neoplasms and Nodular Non-Neoplastic Lesions. Arch Ophthalmol. 1972 Jul;88(1):27–38. PMID:5049451
3391. Ts'o MO, Zimmerman LE, Fine BS. The Nature of Retinoblastoma. I. Photoreceptor Differentiation: A Clinical and Histopathologic Study. Am J Ophthalmol. 1970 Mar;69(3):339–49. PMID:4190798
3392. Tsoutsanis PA, Charonis GC. Congenital Orbital Teratoma: A Case Report with Preservation of the Globe and 18 Years of Follow-Up. BMC Ophthalmol. 2021 Dec 28;21(1):456. PMID:34963454
3393. Tsuda Y, Suurmeijer AJH, Sung YS, et al. Epithelioid Hemangioma of Bone Harboring FOS and FOSB Gene Rearrangements: A Clinicopathologic and Molecular Study. Genes Chromosomes Cancer. 2021 Jan;60(1):17–25. PMID:33034932
3394. Tsuji H, Kanda H, Kashiwagi H, et al. Primary Epithelioid Haemangioendothelioma of the Eyelid. Br J Ophthalmol. 2010 Feb;94(2):261–2. PMID:20139294
3395. Tsuji H, Tamura M, Yokoyama M, et al. Ocular Involvement by Epstein-Barr Virus-Positive Diffuse Large B-Cell Lymphoma of the Elderly: A New Disease Entity in the World Health Organization Classification. Arch Ophthalmol. 2010 Feb;128(2):258–9. PMID:20142557
3396. Tsuji K, Ishikawa Y, Imamura T. Technique for Differentiating Alveolar Soft Part Sarcoma from Other Tumors in Paraffin-Embedded Tissue: Comparison of Immunohistochemistry for TFE3 and CD147 and of Reverse Transcription Polymerase Chain Reaction for ASPSCR1-TFE3 Fusion Transcript. Hum Pathol. 2012 Mar;43(3):356–63. PMID:21835426
3397. Tucker SH, Szalai E, Rivellese M, et al. Ring-Shaped Leiomyoma of the Ciliary Body. Ocul Oncol Pathol. 2017 Nov;3(4):250–3. PMID:29344475
3398. Tunç M, Sadri E, Char DH. Orbital Lymphangioma: An Analysis of 26 Patients. Br J Ophthalmol. 1999 Jan;83(1):76–80. PMID:10209440
3399. Tuncer S, Kebudi R, Peksayar G, et al. Congenital Mesenchymal Chondrosarcoma of the Orbit: Case Report and Review of the Literature. Ophthalmology. 2004 May;111(5):1016–22. PMID:15121382
3400. Tuomaala S, Eskelin S, Tarkkanen A, et al. Population-Based Assessment of Clinical Characteristics Predicting Outcome of Conjunctival Melanoma in Whites. Invest Ophthalmol Vis Sci. 2002 Nov;43(11):3399–408. PMID:12407149
3401. Turc-Carel C, Philip I, Berger MP, et al. Chromosome Study of Ewing's Sarcoma (ES) Cell Lines. Consistency of a Reciprocal Translocation T(11;22)(Q24;Q12). Cancer Genet Cytogenet. 1984 May;12(1):1–19. PMID:6713356
3402. Turner HC, Budak MT, Akinci MA, et al. Comparative Analysis of Human Conjunctival and Corneal Epithelial Gene Expression with Oligonucleotide Microarrays. Invest Ophthalmol Vis Sci. 2007 May;48(5):2050–61. PMID:17460260
3403. Tynski Z, Chiang W, Barrett A. An Inguinal Perivascular Epithelioid Cell Tumor Metastatic to the Orbit. Case Rep Pathol. 2018 May 29;2018:5749421. PMID:30002939
3404. Tzankov A, Kremer M, Leguit R, et al. Histiocytic Cell Neoplasms Involving the Bone Marrow: Summary of the Workshop Cases Submitted to the 18th Meeting of the European Association for Haematopathology (EAHP) Organized by the European Bone Marrow Working Group, Basel 2016. Ann Hematol. 2018 Nov;97(11):2117–28. PMID:30084011
3405. Tzu JH, Cavuoto KM, Villegas VM, et al. Optical Coherence Tomography Findings of Pigmented Fundus Lesions in Familial Adenomatous Polyposis. Ophthalmic Surg Lasers Imaging Retina. 2014 Jan-Feb;45(1):69–70. PMID:24266367
3406. Uceda-Montañés A, Blanco G, Saornil MA, et al. Extramedullary Plasmacytoma of the Orbit. Acta Ophthalmol Scand. 2000 Oct;78(5):601–3. PMID:11037925
3407. Uchio E, Takeuchi S, Itoh N, et al. Clinical and Epidemiological Features of Acute Follicular Conjunctivitis with Special Reference to that Caused by Herpes Simplex Virus Type 1. Br J Ophthalmol. 2000 Sep;84(9):968–72. PMID:10966946
3408. Udager AM, McHugh JB, Goudsmit CM, et al. Human Papillomavirus (HPV) and Somatic EGFR Mutations Are Essential, Mutually Exclusive Oncogenic Mechanisms for Inverted Sinonasal Papillomas and Associated Sinonasal Squamous Cell Carcinomas. Ann Oncol. 2018 Feb 1;29(2):466–71. PMID:29145573
3409. Ugwu N, Atzmony L, Ellis KT, et al. Cutaneous and Hepatic Vascular Lesions Due to a Recurrent Somatic GJA4 Mutation Reveal a Pathway for Vascular Malformation. HGG Adv. 2021 Apr 8;2(2):100028. PMID:33912852
3410. UICC [Internet]. Geneva (Switzerland): Union for International Cancer Control; 2024. TNM Publications and Resources – Errata; Updated 2024 Jan 31. Available from: https://www.uicc.org/resources/tnm/publications-resources.
3411. Ulbright TM, Fulling KH, Helveston EM. Astrocytic Tumors of the Retina. Differentiation of Sporadic Tumors from Phakomatosis-Associated Tumors. Arch Pathol Lab Med. 1984 Feb;108(2):160–3. PMID:6421263
3412. Ulivieri S, Toninelli S, Giorgio A, et al. Orbital Glomangioma. Orbit. 2012 Aug;31(4):216–8. PMID:22642677
3413. Umehara H, Okazaki K, Kawa S, et al. The 2020 Revised Comprehensive Diagnostic (RCD) Criteria for IgG4-RD. Mod Rheumatol. 2021 May;31(3):529–33. PMID:33274670
3414. Unni KK, Inwards CY, editors. Dahlin's Bone Tumours: General Aspects and Data on 10,165 Cases. 6th ed. Philadelphia (PA): Lippincott Williams & Wilkins; 2010.
3415. Uno T, Isobe K, Shikama N, et al. Radiotherapy for Extranodal, Marginal Zone, B-Cell Lymphoma of Mucosa-Associated Lymphoid Tissue Originating in the Ocular Adnexa: A Multiinstitutional, Retrospective Review of 50 Patients. Cancer. 2003 Aug 15;98(4):865–71. PMID:12910532
3416. Urabe A, Tsuneyoshi M, Enjoji M. Epithelioid Hemangioma Versus Kimura's Disease. A Comparative Clinicopathologic Study. Am J Surg Pathol. 1987 Oct;11(10):758–66. PMID:3116865
3417. Urano M, Nakaguro M, Yamamoto Y, et al. Diagnostic Significance of HRAS Mutations in Epithelial-Myoepithelial Carcinomas Exhibiting a Broad Histopathologic Spectrum. Am J Surg Pathol. 2019 Jul;43(7):984–94. PMID:30994537
3418. Ure BM, Slany E, Eypasch EP, et al. Quality of Life More Than 20 Years After Repair of Esophageal Atresia. J Pediatr Surg. 1998 Mar;33(3):511–5. PMID:9537569
3419. Uusitalo E, Leppävirta J, Koffert A, et al. Incidence and Mortality of Neurofibromatosis: A Total Population Study in Finland. J Invest Dermatol. 2015 Mar;135(3):904–6. PMID:25354145
3420. Vachette M, Moulin A, Zografos L, et al. Epibulbar Osseous Choristoma: A Clinicopathological Case Series and Review of the Literature. Klin Monbl Augenheilkd. 2012 Apr;229(4):420–3. PMID:22496017
3421. Vader MJC, Madigan MC, Versluis M, et al. GNAQ and GNA11 Mutations and Downstream YAP Activation in Choroidal Nevi. Br J Cancer. 2017 Sep 5;117(6):884–7. PMID:28809862
3422. Vadmal M, Kahn E, Finger P, et al. Nonteratoid Medulloepithelioma of the Retina with Electron Microscopic and Immunohistochemical Characterization. Pediatr Pathol Lab Med. 1996 Jul-Aug;16(4):663–72. PMID:9025863
3423. Vagge A, Camicione P, Capris C, et al. Choroidal Abnormalities in Neurofibromatosis Type 1 Detected by Near-Infrared Reflectance Imaging in Paediatric Population. Acta Ophthalmol. 2015 Dec;93(8):e667–71. PMID:25990002
3424. Vagia E, Economopoulou P, Oikonomopoulos N, et al. Androgen-Receptor Positive Lacrimal Sac Adenocarcinoma Demonstrating Long-Lasting Response to LHRH Analog Plus Abiraterone Treatment. Front Oncol. 2015 Feb 2;5:10. PMID:25699235
3425. Vahdani K, Coupland SE, Ashdown ME, et al. Lacrimal Sac Sebaceous Carcinoma. Ophthalmic Plast Reconstr Surg. 2019 Jul/Aug;35(4):e89–91. PMID:30921057
3426. Vahdani K, Luthert PJ, Verity DH, et al. Extensive Sclerosis ("Mummification") in Lacrimal Gland Pleomorphic Adenoma May Indicate Neighboring Malignant Transformation. Ophthalmic Plast Reconstr Surg. 2022 Jan-Feb 01;38(1):e13–7. PMID:34652307
3427. Vahdani K, Rose GE. Carcinoma Expleomorphic Adenoma of the Lacrimal Gland. Ophthalmic Plast Reconstr Surg. 2021 Nov-Dec 01;37(6):576–82. PMID:33710040
3428. Vahdani K, Thaung C, Rose GE. Chronic Lymphocytic Leukemia Presenting as Scleral Nodule. Ophthalmology. 2021 Mar;128(3):402. PMID:33612166
3429. Vahdani K, Thaung C, Rose GE. Palpebral Carcinoma Ex-Pleomorphic Adenoma. Orbit. 2024 Oct;43(5):687. PMID:34320398
3430. Vajdic CM, van Leeuwen MT, McDonald SP, et al. Increased Incidence of Squamous Cell Carcinoma of Eye After Kidney Transplantation. J Natl Cancer Inst. 2007 Sep 5;99(17):1340–2. PMID:17698951
3431. Valenzuela AA, Cupp DG, Heathcote JG. Primary Apocrine Adenocarcinoma of the Eyelid. Orbit. 2012 Oct;31(5):316–8. PMID:22571743
3432. Valenzuela AA, McNab AA, Selva D, et al. Clinical Features and Management of Tumors Affecting the Lacrimal Drainage Apparatus. Ophthalmic Plast Reconstr Surg. 2006 Mar-Apr;22(2):96–101. PMID:16550051
3433. Valpione S, Moser JC, Parrozzani R, et al. Development and External Validation of a Prognostic Nomogram for Metastatic Uveal Melanoma. PLoS One. 2015 Mar 17;10(3):e0120181. PMID:25780931
3434. Valstar MH, Andreasen S, Bhairosing PA, et al. Natural History of Recurrent Pleomorphic Adenoma: Implications on Management. Head Neck. 2020 Aug;42(8):2058–66. PMID:32187769
3435. Van Acker SI, Van Den Bogerd B, Haagdorens M, et al. Pterygium-The Good, the Bad, and the Ugly. Cells. 2021 Jun 22;10(7):1567. PMID:34206333
3436. van de Nes JA, Nelles J, Kreis S, et al. Comparing the Prognostic Value of BAP1 Mutation Pattern, Chromosome 3 Status, and BAP1 Immunohistochemistry in Uveal Melanoma. Am J Surg Pathol. 2016 Jun;40(6):796–805. PMID:27015033
3437. van Den Bosch QCC, van Beek JGM, Kiliç E, et al. Transient Expression of Lymphatic Markers in Retrobulbar Intraconal Orbital Vasculature During Fetal Development. Invest Ophthalmol Vis Sci. 2020 Jun 3;61(6):22.

PMID:32516408
3438. van Den Broek PP, de Faber JT, Kliffen M, et al. Anterior Orbital Leiomyoma: Possible Pulley Smooth Muscle Tissue Tumor. Arch Ophthalmol. 2005 Nov;123(11):1614. PMID:16286632
3439. van Der Pol JP, Jager MJ, de Wolff-Rouendaal D, et al. Heterogeneous Expression of Melanoma-Associated Antigens in Uveal Melanomas. Curr Eye Res. 1987 Jun;6(6):757–65. PMID:3608565
3440. van Essen TH, van Pelt SI, Versluis M, et al. Prognostic Parameters in Uveal Melanoma and Their Association with BAP1 Expression. Br J Ophthalmol. 2014 Dec;98(12):1738–43. PMID:25147369
3441. van Ipenburg JA, Damman J, Paridaens D, et al. Histopathological and Molecular Features of a Conjunctival Caruncular Deep Penetrating Nevus. Ocul Oncol Pathol. 2020 Aug;6(4):293–6. PMID:33005620
3442. van Kester MS, Tensen CP, Vermeer MH, et al. Cutaneous Anaplastic Large Cell Lymphoma and Peripheral T-Cell Lymphoma NOS Show Distinct Chromosomal Alterations and Differential Expression of Chemokine Receptors and Apoptosis Regulators. J Invest Dermatol. 2010 Feb;130(2):563–75. PMID:19710685
3443. van Klink F, de Keizer RJ, Jager MJ, et al. Iris Nevi and Melanomas: A Clinical Follow-Up Study. Doc Ophthalmol. 1992;82(1-2):49–55. PMID:1305027
3444. van Maldegem F, Wormhoudt TA, Mulder MM, et al. Chlamydia Psittaci-Negative Ocular Adnexal Marginal Zone B-Cell Lymphomas Have Biased VH4-34 Immunoglobulin Gene Expression and Proliferate in a Distinct Inflammatory Environment. Leukemia. 2012 Jul;26(7):1647–53. PMID:22382892
3445. van Poppelen NM, Vaarwater J, Mudhar HS, et al. Genetic Background of Iris Melanomas and Iris Melanocytic Tumors of Uncertain Malignant Potential. Ophthalmology. 2018 Jun;125(6):904–12. PMID:29371009
3446. van Poppelen NM, van Ipenburg JA, van Den Bosch Q, et al. Molecular Genetics of Conjunctival Melanoma and Prognostic Value of TERT Promoter Mutation Analysis. Int J Mol Sci. 2021 May 28;22(11):5784. PMID:34071371
3447. Van Raamsdonk CD, Bezrookove V, Green G, et al. Frequent Somatic Mutations of GNAQ in Uveal Melanoma and Blue Naevi. Nature. 2009 Jan 29;457(7229):599–602. PMID:19078957
3448. Van Raamsdonk CD, Griewank KG, Crosby MB, et al. Mutations in GNA11 in Uveal Melanoma. N Engl J Med. 2010 Dec 2;363(23):2191–9. PMID:21083380
3449. Vandenberghe E, De Wolf-Peeters C, van Den Oord J, et al. Translocation (11;14): A Cytogenetic Anomaly Associated with B-Cell Lymphomas of Non-Follicle Centre Cell Lineage. J Pathol. 1991 Jan;163(1):13–8. PMID:2002419
3449A. VandenBoom T, Quan VL, Zhang B, et al. Genomic Fusions in Pigmented Spindle Cell Nevus of Reed. Am J Surg Pathol. 2018 Aug;42(8):1042–51. PMID:29794873
3450. Vander Poorten V, Triantafyllou A, Thompson LD, et al. Salivary Acinic Cell Carcinoma: Reappraisal and Update. Eur Arch Otorhinolaryngol. 2016 Nov;273(11):3511–31. PMID:26685679
3451. Van Ginderdeuren R, Sciot R, Mombaerts I. Orbital Tumor Associated with a Microphthalmic Eye and Colobomatous Cleft: Pilocytic Astrocytoma (Glioma) or Massive Retinal Gliosis. Saudi J Ophthalmol. 2018 Jan-Mar;32(1):79–82. PMID:29755278
3452. Vangveeravong S, Katz SE, Rootman J, et al. Tumors Arising in the Palpebral Lobe of the Lacrimal Gland. Ophthalmology. 1996 Oct;103(10):1606–12. PMID:8874433
3453. van Hemel BM, Suurmeijer AJ. Effective Application of the Methanol-Based PreservCyt(™) Fixative and the Cellient(™) Automated Cell Block Processor to Diagnostic Cytopathology, Immunocytochemistry, and Molecular Biology. Diagn Cytopathol. 2013 Aug;41(8):734–41. PMID:23444168
3454. Van Horn PE Jr, Dahlin DC, Bickel WH. Fibrous Dysplasia: A Clinical Pathologic Study of Orthopedic Surgical Cases. Proc Staff Meet Mayo Clin. 1963 May 8;38:175–89. PMID:13996066
3455. van Leeuwaarde RS, Ahmad S, Links TP, et al. Von Hippel-Lindau Syndrome. In: Adam MP, Everman DB, Mirzaa GM, et al., editors. GeneReviews. Seattle (WA): University of Washington, Seattle; 2000. PMID:20301636
3456. Van Trigt WK, Kelly KM, Hughes CCW. GNAQ Mutations Drive Port Wine Birthmark-Associated Sturge-Weber Syndrome: A Review of Pathobiology, Therapies, and Current Models. Front Hum Neurosci. 2022 Nov 3;16:1006027. PMID:36405075
3457. Varan A, Bayhan T, Kiratli H, et al. An Orbital Perivascular Epithelioid Cell Tumor in a 7-Year-Old Boy: Case Report and Review of the Literature. J AAPOS. 2017 Aug;21(4):325–328.E1. PMID:28576480
3458. Varu DM, Rhee MK, Akpek EK, et al. Conjunctivitis Preferred Practice Pattern®. Ophthalmology. 2019 Jan;126(1):94–P169. PMID:30366797
3459. Vassallo P, Forte R, Di Mezza A, et al. Treatment of Infantile Capillary Hemangioma of the Eyelid with Systemic Propranolol. Am J Ophthalmol. 2013 Jan;155(1):165–170.E2. PMID:22967870
3460. Vasta LM, Nichols A, Harney LA, et al. Nasal Chondromesenchymal Hamartomas in a Cohort with Pathogenic Germline Variation in DICER1. Rhinol Online. 2020;3:15–24. PMID:34164613
3461. Vasudev P, Boutross-Tadross O, Radhi J. Basaloid Squamous Cell Carcinoma: Two Case Reports. Cases J. 2009 Dec 18;2:9351. PMID:20062602
3462. Vega F, Lin P, Medeiros LJ. Extranodal Lymphomas of the Head and Neck. Ann Diagn Pathol. 2005 Dec;9(6):340–50. PMID:16308165
3463. Vegliante MC, Palomero J, Pérez-Galán P, et al. SOX11 Regulates PAX5 Expression and Blocks Terminal B-Cell Differentiation in Aggressive Mantle Cell Lymphoma. Blood. 2013 Mar 21;121(12):2175–85. PMID:23321250
3464. Vékony H, Röser K, Löning T, et al. Deregulated Expression of P16INK4a and P53 Pathway Members in Benign and Malignant Myoepithelial Tumours of the Salivary Glands. Histopathology. 2008 Dec;53(6):658–66. PMID:19076682
3465. Velusamy T, Kiel MJ, Sahasrabuddhe AA, et al. A Novel Recurrent NPM1-TYK2 Gene Fusion in Cutaneous CD30-Positive Lymphoproliferative Disorders. Blood. 2014 Dec 11;124(25):3768–71. PMID:25349176
3466. Vempuluru VS, Jakati S, Kaliki S. Delayed Metastasis in Patients with Intraocular Retinoblastoma: A Review of Three Cases. Eur J Ophthalmol. 2021 Jul;31(4):2042–7. PMID:32703017
3467. Vemuganti GK, Naik MN, Honavar SG. Rosai Dorfman Disease of the Orbit. J Hematol Oncol. 2008 Jun 28;1:7. PMID:18588698
3468. Venkataraman G, Rizzo KA, Chavez JJ, et al. Marginal Zone Lymphomas Involving Meningeal Dura: Possible Link to IgG4-Related Diseases. Mod Pathol. 2011 Mar;24(3):355–66. PMID:21102421
3469. Venkatesulu BP, Pathy S, Vallonthaiel AG, et al. Epithelial-Myoepithelial Carcinoma of Lacrimal Gland from an Ex Pleomorphic Adenoma. BMJ Case Rep. 2015 Jul 31;2015:Bcr2015210795. PMID:26231189
3470. Venkatraman L, Goepel JR, Steele K, et al. Soft Tissue, Pelvic, and Urinary Bladder Leiomyosarcoma as Second Neoplasm Following Hereditary Retinoblastoma. J Clin Pathol. 2003 Mar;56(3):233–6. PMID:12610106
3471. Venna SS, Lee D, Stadecker MJ, et al. Clinical Recognition of Actinic Keratoses in a High-Risk Population: How Good Are We? Arch Dermatol. 2005 Apr;141(4):507–9. PMID:15837871
3472. Ventii KH, Devi NS, Friedrich KL, et al. BRCA1-Associated Protein-1 is a Tumor Suppressor that Requires Deubiquitinating Activity and Nuclear Localization. Cancer Res. 2008 Sep 1;68(17):6953–62. PMID:18757409
3473. Verbeke SL, Bertoni F, Bacchini P, et al. Distinct Histological Features Characterize Primary Angiosarcoma of Bone. Histopathology. 2011 Jan;58(2):254–64. PMID:21323951
3474. Verbeke SL, Bovée JV. Primary Vascular Tumors of Bone: A Spectrum of Entities? Int J Clin Exp Pathol. 2011 Aug 15;4(6):541–51. PMID:21904630
3475. Verbeke SL, de Jong D, Bertoni F, et al. Array CGH Analysis Identifies Two Distinct Subgroups of Primary Angiosarcoma of Bone. Genes Chromosomes Cancer. 2015 Feb;54(2):72–81. PMID:25231439
3476. Verdijk RM. Lymphoproliferative Tumors of the Ocular Adnexa. Asia Pac J Ophthalmol (Phila). 2017 Mar-Apr;6(2):132–42. PMID:28399341
3477. Verdijk RM. On the Classification and Grading of Medulloepithelioma of the Eye. Ocul Oncol Pathol. 2016 Apr;2(3):190–3. PMID:27239464
3478. Verdijk RM, Den Bakker MA, Dubbink HJ, et al. TP53 Mutation Analysis of Malignant Peripheral Nerve Sheath Tumors. J Neuropathol Exp Neurol. 2010 Jan;69(1):16–26. PMID:20010306
3479. Verdijk RM, Heidari P, Verschooten R, et al. Raised Numbers of IgG4-Positive Plasma Cells Are a Common Histopathological Finding in Orbital Xanthogranulomatous Disease. Orbit. 2014 Feb;33(1):17–22. PMID:24144223
3480. Verdijk RM, Pecorella I, Mooy CM. Chapter 12: The Orbit, Including the Lacrimal Gland and Lacrimal Drainage System. In: Heegaard S, Grossniklaus H, editors. Eye Pathology: An Illustrated Guide. Berlin (Germany): Springer-Verlag; 2015. pp. 547–731.
3482. Vergel De Dios AM, Bond JR, Shives TC, et al. Aneurysmal Bone Cyst. A Clinicopathologic Study of 238 Cases. Cancer. 1992 Jun 15;69(12):2921–31. PMID:1591685
3483. Verhoekx JSN, Karim AF, van Laar JAM, et al. The Tarsal Plate Manifestation of IgG4-Related Disease. Int Ophthalmol. 2019 Jul;39(7):1613–5. PMID:29926366
3484. Verkouteren JAC, Ramdas KHR, Wakkee M, et al. Epidemiology of Basal Cell Carcinoma: Scholarly Review. Br J Dermatol. 2017 Aug;177(2):359–72. PMID:28220485
3485. Verma S, Batra R, Gupta S, et al. Epidermoid Cysts in Kidney Transplant Patients Receiving Tacrolimus. Dermatol Ther. 2020 Mar;33(2):e13259. PMID:32043723
3486. Verma V, Shen D, Sieving PC, et al. The Role of Infectious Agents in the Etiology of Ocular Adnexal Neoplasia. Surv Ophthalmol. 2008 Jul-Aug;53(4):312–31. PMID:18572051
3487. Vernet O, Ducrey N, Déruaz JP, et al. Giant Cell Tumor of the Orbit. Neurosurgery. 1993 May;32(5):848–51. PMID:8492864
3488. Versluis M, de Lange MJ, van Pelt SI, et al. Digital PCR Validates 8q Dosage as Prognostic Tool in Uveal Melanoma. PLoS One. 2015 Mar 12;10(3):e0116371. PMID:25764247
3489. Vervaet N, Van Ginderdeuren R, Van Den Oord JJ, et al. A Rare Conjunctival Spitz Nevus: A Case Report and Literature Review. Bull Soc Belge Ophtalmol. 2007; (303):63–7. PMID:17894290
3490. Vest SD, Mikkelsen LH, Holm F, et al. Lymphoma of the Lacrimal Gland - An International Multicenter Retrospective Study. Am J Ophthalmol. 2020 Nov;219:107–20. PMID:32574779
3491. Veugelers M, Wilkes D, Burton K, et al. Comparative PRKAR1A Genotype-Phenotype Analyses in Humans with Carney Complex and Prkar1a Haploinsufficient Mice. Proc Natl Acad Sci U S A. 2004 Sep 28;101(39):14222–7. PMID:15371594
3492. Vianna RN, Pacheco DF, Vasconcelos MM, et al. Combined Hamartoma of the Retina and Retinal Pigment Epithelium Associated with Neurofibromatosis Type-1. Int Ophthalmol. 2001;24(2):63–6. PMID:12201346
3493. Vignault C, Bourgeault É, Gagné É, et al. A Rare Case of Solitary Giant Congenital Juvenile Xanthogranuloma: A Case Report. J Cutan Med Surg. 2017 May/Jun;21(3):267–9. PMID:28300446
3494. Villegas BV, Benitez-Del-Castillo JM. Current Knowledge in Allergic Conjunctivitis. Turk J Ophthalmol. 2021 Feb 25;51(1):45–54. PMID:33631915
3495. Villegas VM, Hess DJ, Wildner A, et al. Retinoblastoma. Curr Opin Ophthalmol. 2013 Nov;24(6):581–8. PMID:24100372
3496. Vinciguerra A, Rampi A, Giordano Resti A, et al. Melanoma of the Lacrimal Drainage System: A Systematic Review. Head Neck. 2021 Jul;43(7):2240–52. PMID:33843111
3497. Viola F, Villani E, Natacci F, et al. Choroidal Abnormalities Detected by Near-Infrared Reflectance Imaging as a New Diagnostic Criterion for Neurofibromatosis 1. Ophthalmology. 2012 Feb;119(2):369–75. PMID:21963267
3498. Virgili G, Gatta G, Ciccolallo L, et al. Incidence of Uveal Melanoma in Europe. Ophthalmology. 2007 Dec;114(12):2309–15. PMID:17498805
3499. Virgili G, Parravano M, Gatta G, et al. Incidence and Survival of Patients With Conjunctival Melanoma in Europe. JAMA Ophthalmol. 2020 Jun 1;138(6):601–8. PMID:32215588
3500. Viros A, Fridlyand J, Bauer J, et al. Improving Melanoma Classification by Integrating Genetic and Morphologic Features. PLoS Med. 2008 Jun 3;5(6):e120. PMID:18532874
3501. Vishnevskia-Dai V, Moroz I, Davidy T, et al. Naevus of Ota: Clinical Characteristics and Proposal for a New Ocular Classification and Grading System. Br J Ophthalmol. 2021 Jan;105(1):42–7. PMID:32229516
3502. Viskochil D, Buchberg AM, Xu G, et al. Deletions and a Translocation Interrupt a Cloned Gene at the Neurofibromatosis Type 1 Locus. Cell. 1990 Jul 13;62(1):187–92. PMID:1694727
3503. Viso E, Gude F, Rodríguez-Ares MT. Prevalence of Pinguecula and Pterygium in a General Population in Spain. Eye (Lond). 2011 Mar;25(3):350–7. PMID:21183945
3504. Vizcaino MA, Joseph SS, Eberhart CG. Orbital Progressive Transformation of Germinal Centers as Part of the Spectrum of IgG4-Related Ophthalmic Disease: Clinicopathologic Features of Three Cases. Saudi J Ophthalmol. 2018 Jan-Mar;32(1):56–61. PMID:29755273
3505. Vizvári E, Skribek Á, Polgár N, et al. Conjunctival Melanocytic Naevus: Diagnostic Value of Anterior Segment Optical Coherence Tomography and Ultrasound Biomicroscopy. PLoS One. 2018 Feb 14;13(2):e0192908. PMID:29444155
3506. von Goscinski C, Koch KR, Cursiefen C, et al. [Tumors of the Lacrimal Drainage System]. HNO. 2016 Jun;64(6):386–93. German.

PMID:27222017
3507. von Holstein SL, Coupland SE, Briscoe D, et al. Epithelial Tumours of the Lacrimal Gland: A Clinical, Histopathological, Surgical and Oncological Survey. Acta Ophthalmol. 2013 May;91(3):195–206. PMID:22471335
3508. Von Holstein SL, Fehr A, Heegaard S, et al. CRTC1-MAML2 Gene Fusion in Mucoepidermoid Carcinoma of the Lacrimal Gland. Oncol Rep. 2012 May;27(5):1413–6. PMID:22323114
3509. von Holstein SL, Fehr A, Persson M, et al. Adenoid Cystic Carcinoma of the Lacrimal Gland: MYB Gene Activation, Genomic Imbalances, and Clinical Characteristics. Ophthalmology. 2013 Oct;120(10):2130–8. PMID:23725736
3510. von Holstein SL, Therkildsen MH, Prause JU, et al. Lacrimal Gland Lesions in Denmark Between 1974 and 2007. Acta Ophthalmol. 2013 Jun;91(4):349–54. PMID:22471375
3511. von Holstein SL. Tumours of the Lacrimal Gland. Epidemiological, Clinical and Genetic Characteristics. Acta Ophthalmol. 2013 Nov;91 Thesis 6:1–28. PMID:24893972
3512. Vorobichik Berar O, Tzadok M, Zloto O, et al. Mammalian Target of Rapamycin Inhibitors for the Treatment of Astrocytic Hamartoma in Tuberous Sclerosis Complex (TSC). Graefes Arch Clin Exp Ophthalmol. 2022 Sep;260(9):3061–8. PMID:35230473
3513. Vortmeyer AO, Frank S, Jeong SY, et al. Developmental Arrest of Angioblastic Lineage Initiates Tumorigenesis in von Hippel-Lindau Disease. Cancer Res. 2003 Nov 1;63(21):7051–5. PMID:14612494
3514. Vortmeyer AO, Tran MG, Zeng W, et al. Evolution of VHL Tumourigenesis in Nerve Root Tissue. J Pathol. 2006 Nov;210(3):374–82. PMID:16981244
3515. Vortmeyer AO, Yuan Q, Lee YS, et al. Developmental Effects of von Hippel-Lindau Gene Deficiency. Ann Neurol. 2004 May;55(5):721–8. PMID:15122713
3516. Vozmediano-Serrano MT, Toledano-Fernández N, Fdez-Aceñero MJ, et al. Lacrimal Sac Metastases from Renal Cell Carcinoma. Orbit. 2006 Sep;25(3):249–51. PMID:16987775
3517. Wada DA, Law ME, Hsi ED, et al. Specificity of IRF4 Translocations for Primary Cutaneous Anaplastic Large Cell Lymphoma: A Multicenter Study of 204 Skin Biopsies. Mod Pathol. 2011 Apr;24(4):596–605. PMID:21169992
3518. Wadee R. Conjunctival Leiomyosarcoma: A Fairly Common Tumour in an Uncommon Site. SAGE Open Med Case Rep. 2017 Aug 9;5:X17724060. PMID:28835829
3519. Wadt KA, Aoude LG, Johansson P, et al. A Recurrent Germline BAP1 Mutation and Extension of the BAP1 Tumor Predisposition Spectrum to Include Basal Cell Carcinoma. Clin Genet. 2015 Sep;88(3):267–72. PMID:25225168
3520. Waeltermann JM, Hettinger ME, Cibis GW Congenital Cysts of the Iris Stroma. Am J Ophthalmol. 1985 Oct 15;100(4):549–54. PMID:4050928
3521. Waeltermann JM, Huntrakoon M, Beatty EC Jr, et al. Congenital Fibromatosis (Myofibromatosis) of the Orbit: A Rare Cause of Proptosis at Birth. Ann Ophthalmol. 1988 Oct;20(10):394–6, 399. PMID:3207313
3522. Wagner H, Auw-Hädrich C, Grossniklaus HE, et al. [Fuchs Adenoma of Unusual Manifestation: Masquerade of a Ciliary Body Malignancy]. Klin Monbl Augenheilkd. 2020 Jul;237(7):846–8. German. PMID:32434227
3523. Wagner H, Auw-Hädrich C, Werner M, et al. Ectopic Thyroid Tissue in the Iris: A Case Report. BMC Ophthalmol. 2021 Aug 28;21(1):314. PMID:34454461
3524. Wakely PE Jr, McDermott JE, Ali SZ Cytopathology of Alveolar Soft Part Sarcoma A Report of 10 Cases. Cancer. 2009 Dec 25;117(6):500–7. PMID:19787801
3525. Wakely PE Jr, Rekhi B. Cytopathology of Solitary Fibrous Tumor: A Series of 34 Cases. J Am Soc Cytopathol. 2021 Jul-Aug;10(4):382–90. PMID:34049841
3526. Waldman S, Shimonov M, Yang N, et al. Benign Bony Tumors of the Paranasal Sinuses, Orbit, and Skull Base. Am J Otolaryngol. 2022 May-Jun;43(3):103404. PMID:35246319
3527. Walijee HZ, Berry S, Quine S, et al. Inverted Papilloma Originating Primarily from the Nasolacrimal Duct: A Case Report and Review of the Pertinent Literature. Case Rep Otolaryngol. 2015;2015:123694. PMID:26649215
3528. Walker BA, Saltzman BS, Herlihy EP, et al. Phenotypic Characterization of Epibulbar Dermoids. Int Ophthalmol. 2017 Jun;37(3):499–505. PMID:27405313
3529. Wallace MR, Marchuk DA, Andersen LB, et al. Type 1 Neurofibromatosis Gene: Identification of a Large Transcript Disrupted in Three NF1 Patients. Science. 1990 Jul 13;249(4965):181–6. PMID:2134734
3530. Wallace ZS, Deshpande V, Mattoo H, et al. IgG4-Related Disease: Clinical and Laboratory Features in One Hundred Twenty-Five Patients. Arthritis Rheumatol. 2015 Sep;67(9):2466–75. PMID:25988916
3531. Wallace ZS, Deshpande V, Stone JH. Ophthalmic Manifestations of IgG4-Related Disease: Single-Center Experience and Literature Review. Semin Arthritis Rheum. 2014 Jun;43(6):806–17. PMID:24513111
3532. Walpole S, Pritchard AL, Cebulla CM, et al. Comprehensive Study of the Clinical Phenotype of Germline BAP1 Variant-Carrying Families Worldwide. J Natl Cancer Inst. 2018 Dec 1;110(12):1328–41. PMID:30517737
3533. Walsh NM. Primary Neuroendocrine (Merkel Cell) Carcinoma of the Skin: Morphologic Diversity and Implications Thereof. Hum Pathol. 2001 Jul;32(7):680–9. PMID:11486166
3534. Walsh NM, Cerroni L. Merkel Cell Carcinoma: A Review. J Cutan Pathol. 2021 Mar;48(3):411–21. PMID:33128463
3535. Walsh RD, Vagefi MR, McClelland CM, et al. Primary Adenoid Cystic Carcinoma of the Orbital Apex. Ophthalmic Plast Reconstr Surg. 2013 Jan-Feb;29(1):e33–5. PMID:23034685
3536. Walter SD, Chao DL, Feuer W, et al. Prognostic Implications of Tumor Diameter in Association With Gene Expression Profile for Uveal Melanoma. JAMA Ophthalmol. 2016 Jul 1;134(7):734–40. PMID:27123792
3537. Walther C, Hofvander J, Nilsson J, et al. Gene Fusion Detection in Formalin-Fixed Paraffin-Embedded Benign Fibrous Histiocytomas Using Fluorescence In Situ Hybridization and RNA Sequencing. Lab Invest. 2015 Sep;95(9):1071–6. PMID:26121314
3538. Walvekar PV, Jakati S, Bothra N, et al. Isolated Eyelid Chondroid Syringoma: A Study of Two Cases. BMJ Case Rep. 2021 Dec 30;14(12):e245354. PMID:34969791
3539. Wang E, Lee JS, Kazakov DV A Rare Combination of Sebaceoma with Carcinomatous Change (Sebaceous Carcinoma), Trichoblastoma, and Poroma Arising from a Nevus Sebaceus. J Cutan Pathol. 2013 Jul;40(7):676–82. PMID:23550845
3540. Wang F, Liu A, Peng Y, et al. Diagnostic Utility of SALL4 in Extragonadal Yolk Sac Tumors: An Immunohistochemical Study of 59 Cases with Comparison to Placental-Like Alkaline Phosphatase, Alpha-Fetoprotein, and Glypican-3. Am J Surg Pathol. 2009 Oct;33(10):1529–39. PMID:19574883
3541. Wang HH, Myers T, Lach LJ, et al. Increased Risk of Lymphoid and Nonlymphoid Malignancies in Patients with Lymphomatoid Papulosis. Cancer. 1999 Oct 1;86(7):1240–5. PMID:10506709
3542. Wang J, Ford J, Esmaeli B, et al. Inverted Papilloma of the Orbit and Nasolacrimal System. Ophthalmic Plast Reconstr Surg. 2021 Mar-Apr 01;37(2):161–7. PMID:32501879
3543. Wang KH, Chen WY, Liu HN, et al. Cutaneous Rosai-Dorfman Disease: Clinicopathological Profiles, Spectrum and Evolution of 21 Lesions in Six Patients. Br J Dermatol. 2006 Feb;154(2):277–86. PMID:16433797
3544. Wang L, Motoi T, Khanin R, et al. Identification of a Novel, Recurrent HEY1-NCOA2 Fusion in Mesenchymal Chondrosarcoma Based on a Genome-Wide Screen of Exon-Level Expression Data. Genes Chromosomes Cancer. 2012 Feb;51(2):127–39. PMID:22034177
3545. Wang L, Ren W, Zhou X, et al. Pleomorphic Liposarcoma: A Clinicopathological, Immunohistochemical and Molecular Cytogenetic Study of 32 Additional Cases. Pathol Int. 2013 Nov;63(11):523–31. PMID:24274714
3546. Wang LC, Lin TC, Yeh YC, et al. Primary Signet Ring Cell/Histiocytoid Carcinoma of the Eyelid: Somatic Mutations in CDH1 and Other Clinically Actionable Mutations Imply Early Use of Targeted Agents. Curr Oncol. 2021 Feb 16;28(1):918–27. PMID:33617508
3547. Wang R, Lu YJ, Fisher C, et al. Characterization of Chromosome Aberrations Associated with Soft-Tissue Leiomyosarcomas by Twenty-Four-Color Karyotyping and Comparative Genomic Hybridization Analysis. Genes Chromosomes Cancer. 2001 May;31(1):54–64. PMID:11284036
3548. Wang W, Chen L. Cavernous Hemangioma of the Retina: A Comprehensive Review of the Literature (1934-2015). Retina. 2017 Apr;37(4):611–21. PMID:27820777
3549. Wang X, Su W, Gao Y, et al. A Pilot Study of the Use of Dynamic Analysis of Cell-Free DNA from Aqueous Humor and Vitreous Fluid for the Diagnosis and Treatment Monitoring of Vitreoretinal Lymphomas. Haematologica. 2022 Sep 1;107(9):2154–62. PMID:35142151
3550. Wang Y, Du B, Yang M, et al. Paediatric Orbital Alveolar Soft Part Sarcoma Recurrence During Long-Term Follow-Up: A Report of 3 Cases and a Review of the Literature. BMC Ophthalmol. 2020 Feb 21;20(1):60. PMID:32085747
3551. Wang Y, Xiao LH. Orbital Schwannomas: Findings from Magnetic Resonance Imaging in 62 Cases. Eye (Lond). 2008 Aug;22(8):1034–9. PMID:17464300
3552. Wang Y, Zhao HP, Zhu H, et al. [Clinical Manifestations, Diagnosis and Management of Recurrent Orbital Dermoid Cysts]. Zhonghua Yan Ke Za Zhi. 2010 Apr;46(4):295–8. Chinese. PMID:20654053
3553. Wannapanich T, Pratipanawat P. Primary Orbital Pleomorphic Liposarcoma in a Child: A Case Report. Am J Ophthalmol Case Rep. 2022 Jan 20;25:101285. PMID:35146183
3554. Wantzin GL, Thomsen K, Nissen NI, et al. Occurrence of Human T Cell Lymphotropic Virus (Type I) Antibodies in Cutaneous T Cell Lymphoma. J Am Acad Dermatol. 1986 Oct;15(4 Pt 1):598–602. PMID:2877013
3555. Warren M, Xu D, Li X. Gene Fusions PAFAH1B1-USP6 and RUNX2-USP6 in Aneurysmal Bone Cysts Identified by Next Generation Sequencing. Cancer Genet. 2017 Apr;212-213:13–8. PMID:28449806
3556. Wasco MJ, Fullen D, Su L, et al. The Expression of MUM1 in Cutaneous T-Cell Lymphoproliferative Disorders. Hum Pathol. 2008 Apr;39(4):557–63. PMID:18234282
3557. Wassef M, Blei F, Adams D, et al. Vascular Anomalies Classification: Recommendations From the International Society for the Study of Vascular Anomalies. Pediatrics. 2015 Jul;136(1):e203–14. PMID:26055853
3558. Wasserman JK, Dickson BC, Smith A, et al. Metastasizing Pleomorphic Adenoma: Recurrent PLAG1/HMGA2 Rearrangements and Identification of a Novel HMGA2-TMTC2 Fusion. Am J Surg Pathol. 2019 Aug;43(8):1145–51. PMID:31094927
3559. Watanabe A, Andrew NH, Ueda K, et al. Clinico-Radiological Features of Primary Lacrimal Gland Pleomorphic Adenoma: An Analysis of 37 Cases. Jpn J Ophthalmol. 2016 Jul;60(4):286–93. PMID:27184391
3560. Watanabe A, Wu A, Sun MT, et al. Haemangiopericytoma of the Lacrimal Sac. Orbit. 2016 Aug;35(4):233–5. PMID:27322416
3561. Watanabe Y, Shido K, Niihori T, et al. Somatic BRAF C.1799T>A P.V600E Mosaicism Syndrome Characterized by a Linear Syringocystadenoma Papilliferum, Anaplastic Astrocytoma, and Ocular Abnormalities. Am J Med Genet A. 2016 Jan;170A(1):189–94. PMID:26360803
3562. Watson P, Vasen HFA, Mecklin JP, et al. The Risk of Extra-Colonic, Extra-Endometrial Cancer in the Lynch Syndrome. Int J Cancer. 2008 Jul 15;123(2):444–9. PMID:18398828
3563. Weatherhead RG. Wolfring Dacryops. Ophthalmology. 1992 Oct;99(10):1575–81. PMID:1454325
3564. Weedon D, Little JH. Spindle and Epithelioid Cell Nevi in Children and Adults. A Review of 211 Cases of the Spitz Nevus. Cancer. 1977 Jul;40(1):217–25. PMID:880553
3565. Weegerink N, Van Coethem J, De Schepper S, et al. Nine-Year-Old Girl with a Respiratory Epithelial Cyst of the Orbit. B-ENT. 2016;12(1):77–81. PMID:27097398
3566. Wei S, Dumas A, Zhang PJ, et al. Palisading and Verocay Body-Prominent Dermatofibrosarcoma Protuberans: A Case Report. Pathol Res Pract. 2016 Feb;212(2):145–7. PMID:26725533
3567. Wei Z, Li S, Tao X, et al. Mutations in Profilin 1 Cause Early-Onset Paget's Disease of Bone With Giant Cell Tumors. J Bone Miner Res. 2021 Jun;36(6):1088–103. PMID:33599011
3568. Weidema ME, van de Geer E, Koelsche C, et al. DNA Methylation Profiling Identifies Distinct Clusters in Angiosarcomas. Clin Cancer Res. 2020 Jan 1;26(1):93–100. PMID:31562204
3569. Weinreb I, Bishop JA, Chiosea SI, et al. Recurrent RET Gene Rearrangements in Intraductal Carcinomas of Salivary Gland. Am J Surg Pathol. 2018 Apr;42(4):442–52. PMID:29443014
3570. Weinreb I, Seethala RR, Hunt JL, et al. Intercalated Duct Lesions of Salivary Gland: A Morphologic Spectrum from Hyperplasia to Adenoma. Am J Surg Pathol. 2009 Sep;33(9):1322–9. PMID:19542868
3571. Weis E, Aghazadeh H, Roelofs K, et al. Sunlamp Use is a Risk Factor for Uveal Melanoma: A Meta-Analysis. Can J Ophthalmol. 2022 Apr;57(2):105–11. PMID:33839068
3572. Weis E, Rootman J, Joly TJ, et al. Epithelial Lacrimal Gland Tumors: Pathologic Classification and Current Understanding. Arch Ophthalmol. 2009 Aug;127(8):1016–28. PMID:19667339
3573. Weis E, Shah CP, Lajous M, et al. The Association Between Host Susceptibility Factors and Uveal Melanoma: A Meta-Analysis. Arch Ophthalmol. 2006 Jan;124(1):54–60. PMID:16401785
3574. Weis E, Shah CP, Lajous M, et al. The Association of Cutaneous and Iris Nevi with Uveal Melanoma: A Meta-Analysis.

Ophthalmology. 2009 Mar;116(3):536–543.E2. PMID:19167086
3575. Weiss L. Analysis of the Incidence of Intraocular Metastasis. Br J Ophthalmol. 1993 Mar;77(3):149–51. PMID:8457505
3576. Weiss SJ, Stathopoulos C, Shields CL. Choroidal Nevus with Retinal Invasion in 8 Cases. Ocul Oncol Pathol. 2019 Aug;5(5):369–78. PMID:31559248
3577. Weiss SW, Enzinger FM. Epithelioid Hemangioendothelioma: A Vascular Tumor Often Mistaken for a Carcinoma. Cancer. 1982 Sep 1;50(5):970–81. PMID:7093931
3578. Weissman R, Diamond EL, Haroche J, et al. MicroRNA-15a-5p Acts as a Tumor Suppressor in Histiocytosis By Mediating CXCL10-ERK-LIN28a-Let-7 Axis. Leukemia. 2022 Apr;36(4):1139–49. PMID:34785791
3579. Welch J, Srinivasan S, Lyall D, et al. Conjunctival Lymphangiectasia: A Report of 11 Cases and Review of Literature. Surv Ophthalmol. 2012 Mar-Apr;57(2):136–48. PMID:22019374
3580. Wen Y, Yan J. Primary Tumors of the Orbital Bone. J Craniofac Surg. 2016 Jun;27(4):e344–8. PMID:27152568
3581. Werner B, Massone C, Kerl H, et al. Large CD30-Positive Cells in Benign, Atypical Lymphoid Infiltrates of the Skin. J Cutan Pathol. 2008 Dec;35(12):1100–7. PMID:18616762
3582. Werner RN, Sammain A, Erdmann R, et al. The Natural History of Actinic Keratosis: A Systematic Review. Br J Dermatol. 2013 Sep;169(3):502–18. PMID:23647091
3583. Werstein B, Dunlap J, Cascio MJ, et al. Molecular Discordance Between Myeloid Sarcomas and Concurrent Bone Marrows Occurs in Actionable Genes and Is Associated with Worse Overall Survival. J Mol Diagn. 2020 Mar;22(3):338–45. PMID:31866570
3584. Wertz FD, Zimmerman LE, McKeown CA, et al. Juvenile Xanthogranuloma of the Optic Nerve, Disc, Retina, and Choroid. Ophthalmology. 1982 Dec;89(12):1331–5. PMID:6819503
3585. West DS, Dogan A, Quint PS, et al. Clonally Related Follicular Lymphomas and Langerhans Cell Neoplasms: Expanding the Spectrum of Transdifferentiation. Am J Surg Pathol. 2013 Jul;37(7):978–86. PMID:23759932
3586. West JA, Drewe RH, McNab AA. Atypical Choristomatous Cysts of the Orbit. Aust N Z J Ophthalmol. 1997 May;25(2):117–23. PMID:9267597
3587. West RB, Harvell J, Linn SC, et al. Apo D in Soft Tissue Tumors: A Novel Marker for Dermatofibrosarcoma Protuberans. Am J Surg Pathol. 2004 Aug;28(8):1063–9. PMID:15252314
3588. West S, Muñoz B. Prevalence of Pterygium in Latinos: Proyecto VER. Br J Ophthalmol. 2009 Oct;93(10):1287–90. PMID:19570772
3589. White V, Stevenson K, Garner A, et al. Mesectodermal Leiomyoma of the Ciliary Body: Case Report. Br J Ophthalmol. 1989 Jan;73(1):12–8. PMID:2920150
3590. White VA. Understanding and Classification of Ocular Lymphomas. Ocul Oncol Pathol. 2019 Oct;5(6):379–86. PMID:31768360
3591. White VA, Damji KF, Richards JS, et al. Leiomyosarcoma of the Conjunctiva. Ophthalmology. 1991 Oct;98(10):1560–4. PMID:1961645
3592. White VA, Heathcote JG, Hurwitz JJ, et al. Epithelioid Sarcoma of the Orbit. Ophthalmology. 1994 Oct;101(10):1680–7. PMID:7936567
3593. White W, Shiu MH, Rosenblum MK, et al. Cellular Schwannoma. A Clinicopathologic Study of 57 Patients and 58 Tumors. Cancer. 1990 Sep 15;66(6):1266–75. PMID:2400975
3594. WHO Classification of Tumours Editorial Board. Haematolymphoid Tumours. Lyon (France): International Agency for Research on Cancer; 2024. (WHO Classification of Tumours Series, 5th ed.; vol. 11). https://publications.iarc.who.int/637.
3595. WHO Classification of Tumours Editorial Board. Head and Neck Tumours. Lyon (France): International Agency for Research on Cancer; 2024. (WHO Classification of Tumours Series, 5th ed.; vol. 9). https://publications.iarc.who.int/629.
3596. WHO Classification of Tumours Editorial Board. Paediatric Tumours. Lyon (France): International Agency for Research on Cancer; 2022. (WHO Classification of Tumours Series, 5th ed.; vol. 7). https://publications.iarc.who.int/608.
3597. WHO Classification of Tumours Editorial Board. Skin Tumours. Lyon (France): International Agency for Research on Cancer; 2025. (WHO Classification of Tumours Series, 5th ed.; vol. 12). https://publications.iarc.who.int/650.
3598. WHO Classification of Tumours Editorial Board. Soft Tissue and Bone Tumours. Lyon (France): International Agency for Research on Cancer; 2020. (WHO Classification of Tumours Series, 5th ed.; vol. 3). https://publications.iarc.who.int/588.
3599. Wick MR, Cooper PH, Swanson PE, et al. Microcystic Adnexal Carcinoma. An Immunohistochemical Comparison with Other Cutaneous Appendage Tumors. Arch Dermatol. 1990 Feb;126(2):189–94. PMID:1689137
3600. Wiechens B, Werner JA, Lüttges J, et al. Primary Orbital Leiomyoma and Leiomyosarcoma. Ophthalmologica. 1999;213(3):159–64. PMID:10202288
3601. Wierenga APA, Brouwer NJ, Gelmi MC, et al. Chromosome 3 and 8q Aberrations in Uveal Melanoma Show Greater Impact on Survival in Patients with Light Iris Versus Dark Iris Color. Ophthalmology. 2022 Apr;129(4):421–30. PMID:34780841
3602. Wieser I, Oh CW, Talpur R, et al. Lymphomatoid Papulosis: Treatment Response and Associated Lymphomas in a Study of 180 Patients. J Am Acad Dermatol. 2016 Jan;74(1):59–67. PMID:26518172
3602A. Wiesner T, Kutzner H. [Morphological and Genetic Aspects of Spitz Tumors]. Pathologe. 2015 Feb;36(1):37–43, 45. German. PMID:25613920
3603. Wiesner T, Obenauf AC, Murali R, et al. Germline Mutations in BAP1 Predispose to Melanocytic Tumors. Nat Genet. 2011 Aug 28;43(10):1018–21. PMID:21874003
3604. Wiktorin ACH, Dafgård Kopp EME, Tani E, et al. Fine-Needle Aspiration Biopsy in Orbital Lesions: A Retrospective Study of 225 Cases. Am J Ophthalmol. 2016 Jun;166:37–42. PMID:27018233
3605. Wiley HE, Krivosic V, Gaudric A, et al. Management of Retinal Hemangioblastoma in von Hippel-Lindau Disease. Retina. 2019 Dec;39(12):2254–63. PMID:31259811
3606. Wilkes SR, Campbell RJ, Waller RR. Ocular Malformation in Association with Ipsilateral Facial Nevus of Jadassohn. Am J Ophthalmol. 1981 Sep;92(3):344–52. PMID:7294093
3607. Willemze R, Cerroni L, Kempf W, et al. The 2018 Update of the WHO-EORTC Classification for Primary Cutaneous Lymphomas. Blood. 2019 Apr 18;133(16):1703–14. PMID:30635287
3608. Willemze R, Meijer CJ. Primary Cutaneous CD30-Positive Lymphoproliferative Disorders. Hematol Oncol Clin North Am. 2003 Dec;17(6):1319–32, Vii–Viii. PMID:14710887
3609. Willemze R, Meyer CJ, Van Vloten WA, et al. The Clinical and Histological Spectrum of Lymphomatoid Papulosis. Br J Dermatol. 1982 Aug;107(2):131–44. PMID:7104214
3610. Williams A, Bartle G, Sumathi VP, et al. Detection of ASPL/TFE3 Fusion Transcripts and the TFE3 Antigen in Formalin-Fixed, Paraffin-Embedded Tissue in a Series of 18 Cases of Alveolar Soft Part Sarcoma: Useful Diagnostic Tools in Cases with Unusual Histological Features. Virchows Arch. 2011 Mar;458(3):291–300. PMID:21279521
3611. Williams BK Jr, Di Nicola M, Acaba-Berrocal LA, et al. Adenoma and Adenocarcinoma of the Retinal Pigment Epithelium: A Review of 51 Consecutive Patients. Ophthalmol Retina. 2020 Aug;4(8):829–39. PMID:32417354
3612. Williamson TH, Garner A, Moore AT. Structure of Lisch Nodules in Neurofibromatosis Type 1. Ophthalmic Paediatr Genet. 1991 Mar;12(1):11–7. PMID:1908964
3613. Wilson CS, Medeiros LJ. Extramedullary Manifestations of Myeloid Neoplasms. Am J Clin Pathol. 2015 Aug;144(2):219–39. PMID:26185307
3614. Wilson DJ, Braziel R, Rosenbaum JT. Intraocular Lymphoma. Immunopathologic Analysis of Vitreous Biopsy Specimens. Arch Ophthalmol. 1992 Oct;110(10):1455–8. PMID:1417546
3615. Wimmer K, Eckart M, Meyer-Puttlitz B, et al. Mutational and Expression Analysis of the NF1 Gene Argues Against a Role as Tumor Suppressor in Sporadic Pilocytic Astrocytomas. J Neuropathol Exp Neurol. 2002 Oct;61(10):896–902. PMID:12387455
3616. Win AK, Dowty JG, English DR, et al. Body Mass Index in Early Adulthood and Colorectal Cancer Risk for Carriers and Non-Carriers of Germline Mutations in DNA Mismatch Repair Genes. Br J Cancer. 2011 Jun 28;105(1):162–9. PMID:21559014
3617. Wirz K, Lee WR, Coaker T. Progressive Changes in Congenital Hypertrophy of the Retinal Pigment Epithelium. Graefes Arch Clin Exp Ophthalmol. 1982;219(5):214–21. PMID:7160628
3618. Witschel H, Font RL. Hemangioma of the Choroid. A Clinicopathologic Study of 71 Cases and a Review of the Literature. Surv Ophthalmol. 1976 May-Jun;20(6):415–31. PMID:820013
3619. Witzig TE, Inwards DJ, Habermann TM, et al. Treatment of Benign Orbital Pseudolymphomas with the Monoclonal Anti-CD20 Antibody Rituximab. Mayo Clin Proc. 2007 Jun;82(6):692–9. PMID:17550749
3620. Wiwatwongwana D, Berean KW, Dolman PJ, et al. Unusual Carcinomas of the Lacrimal Gland: Epithelial-Myoepithelial Carcinoma and Myoepithelial Carcinoma. Arch Ophthalmol. 2009 Aug;127(8):1054–6. PMID:19667347
3621. Wizigmann-Voos S, Breier G, Risau W, et al. Up-Regulation of Vascular Endothelial Growth Factor and its Receptors in von Hippel-Lindau Disease-Associated and Sporadic Hemangioblastomas. Cancer Res. 1995 Mar 15;55(6):1358–64. PMID:7533661
3622. Wladis EJ, Farber MG, Nepo AG. Metastatic Synovial Sarcoma to the Orbit. Ophthalmic Plast Reconstr Surg. 2012 Nov-Dec;28(6):e131–2. PMID:22743696
3623. Wladis EJ, Frempong T, Gausas R. Nasolacrimal Metastasis from Heptocellular Carcinoma Masquerading as Dacryocystitis. Ophthalmic Plast Reconstr Surg. 2007 Jul-Aug;23(4):333–5. PMID:17667118
3624. Wojcik J, Rosenberg AE, Bredella MA, et al. Denosumab-Treated Giant Cell Tumor of Bone Exhibits Morphologic Overlap With Malignant Giant Cell Tumor of Bone. Am J Surg Pathol. 2016 Jan;40(1):72–80. PMID:26414220
3625. Wojno T, Tenzel RR, Nadji M. Orbital Leiomyosarcoma. Arch Ophthalmol. 1983 Oct;101(10):1566–8. PMID:6626011
3626. Wolfe JT 3rd, Yeatts RP, Wick MR, et al. Sebaceous Carcinoma of the Eyelid. Errors in Clinical and Pathologic Diagnosis. Am J Surg Pathol. 1984 Aug;8(8):597–606. PMID:6465419
3627. Wolkow N, Jakobiec FA, Yoon MK. Intratarsal Keratinous Eyelid Cysts in Gorlin Syndrome: A Review and Reappraisal. Surv Ophthalmol. 2018 Sep-Oct;63(5):711–8. PMID:29287708
3628. Wong ES, Choy RW, Zhang Y, et al. Global Retinoblastoma Survival and Globe Preservation: A Systematic Review and Meta-Analysis of Associations with Socioeconomic and Health-Care Factors. Lancet Glob Health. 2022 Mar;10(3):e380–9. PMID:35093202
3629. Wong JR, Morton LM, Tucker MA, et al. Risk of Subsequent Malignant Neoplasms in Long-Term Hereditary Retinoblastoma Survivors After Chemotherapy and Radiotherapy. J Clin Oncol. 2014 Oct 10;32(29):3284–90. PMID:25185089
3630. Wong JY, Uhl V, Wara WM, et al. Optic Gliomas. A Reanalysis of the University of California, San Francisco Experience. Cancer. 1987 Oct 15;60(8):1847–55. PMID:3652011
3631. Wong KS, Mariño-Enriquez A, Hornick JL, et al. NR4A3 Immunohistochemistry Reliably Discriminates Acinic Cell Carcinoma from Mimics. Head Neck Pathol. 2021 Jun;15(2):425–32. PMID:32910350
3632. Wong KY, Fife K, Lear JT, et al. Vismodegib for Locally Advanced Periocular and Orbital Basal Cell Carcinoma: A Review of 15 Consecutive Cases. Plast Reconstr Surg Glob Open. 2017 Jul 21;5(7):e1424. PMID:28831360
3633. Woo DK, Jones CR, Vanoli-Storz MN, et al. Prognostic Factors in Primary Cutaneous Anaplastic Large Cell Lymphoma: Characterization of Clinical Subset with Worse Outcome. Arch Dermatol. 2009 Jun;145(6):667–74. PMID:19528422
3634. Woo KI, Kim YD, Sa HS, et al. Current Treatment of Lacrimal Gland Carcinoma. Curr Opin Ophthalmol. 2016 Sep;27(5):449–56. PMID:27273588
3635. Woo YJ, Kim CY, Sgrignoli B, et al. Orbital Lymphangioma: Characteristics and Treatment Outcomes of 12 Cases. Korean J Ophthalmol. 2017 Jun;31(3):194–201. PMID:28534344
3636. Wood TR, McHugh JB, Siegel GW. Glomus Tumors with Malignant Features of the Extremities: A Case Series. Clin Sarcoma Res. 2020 Oct 30;10:20. PMID:33133513
3637. Woodruff JM, Godwin TA, Erlandson RA, et al. Cellular Schwannoma: A Variety of Schwannoma Sometimes Mistaken for a Malignant Tumor. Am J Surg Pathol. 1981 Dec;5(8):733–44. PMID:7337161
3638. Woog JJ, Albert DM, Craft J, et al. Choroidal Ganglioneuroma in Neurofibromatosis. Graefes Arch Clin Exp Ophthalmol. 1983;220(1):25–31. PMID:6403410
3639. Woog JJ, Kim YD, Yeatts RP, et al. Natural Killer/T-Cell Lymphoma with Ocular and Adnexal Involvement. Ophthalmology. 2006 Jan;113(1):140–7. PMID:16360212
3640. Workman DM, Weiner JW. Melanocytic Lesions of the Iris–a Clinocopathological Study of 100 Cases. Aust N Z J Ophthalmol. 1990 Nov;18(4):381–4. PMID:2076286
3641. Wotherspoon AC, Doglioni C, Diss TC, et al. Regression of Primary Low-Grade B-Cell Gastric Lymphoma of Mucosa-Associated Lymphoid Tissue Type After Eradication of Helicobacter Pylori. Lancet. 1993 Sep 4;342(8871):575–7. PMID:8102719
3642. Woyach JA, Ruppert AS, Guinn D, et al. BTKC481S-Mediated Resistance to Ibrutinib in Chronic Lymphocytic Leukemia. J Clin Oncol. 2017 May 1;35(13):1437–43. PMID:28418267
3643. Woyach JA, Ruppert AS, Heerema NA, et al. Ibrutinib Regimens Versus Chemoimmunotherapy in Older Patients with Untreated CLL.

N Engl J Med. 2018 Dec 27;379(26):2517–28. PMID:30501481
3644. Wrede J, Helmke B, Hartmann M, et al. Successful Hormone Treatment of Orbital Leiomyoma. Ophthalmology. 2005 Jul;112(7):1316–8. PMID:15921744
3645. Wright GW, Huang DW, Phelan JD, et al. A Probabilistic Classification Tool for Genetic Subtypes of Diffuse Large B Cell Lymphoma with Therapeutic Implications. Cancer Cell. 2020 Apr 13;37(4):551–568.E14. PMID:32289277
3646. Wright JD, Font RL. Mucinous Sweat Gland Adenocarcinoma of Eyelid: A Clinicopathologic Study of 21 Cases with Histochemical and Electron Microscopic Observations. Cancer. 1979 Nov;44(5):1757–68. PMID:227576
3647. Wu B, Tay JKX, Loh WS, et al. Epithelioid Sarcoma of the External Auditory Canal: An Uncommon Tumor at an Unusual Site and a Brief Overview of the Literature. Head Neck Pathol. 2021 Dec;15(4):1328–34. PMID:33394376
3648. Wu C, Li K, Hei Y, et al. MR Imaging Features of Orbital Langerhans Cell Histiocytosis. BMC Ophthalmol. 2019 Dec 19;19(1):263. PMID:31856763
3649. Wu S, Zou X, Sun Z, et al. Unilateral Retinocytoma Associated with a Variant in the RB1 Gene. Mol Genet Genomic Med. 2020 Apr;8(4):e1156. PMID:31997559
3650. Wysozan TR, Khelifa S, Turchan K, et al. The Morphologic Spectrum of Germline-Mutated BAP1-Inactivated Melanocytic Tumors Includes Lesions with Conventional Nevic Melanocytes: A Case Report and Review of Literature. J Cutan Pathol. 2019 Nov;46(11):852–7. PMID:31206729
3651. Xerri L, Adélaïde J, Popovici C, et al. CDKN2A/B Deletion and Double-Hit Mutations of the MAPK Pathway Underlie the Aggressive Behavior of Langerhans Cell Tumors. Am J Surg Pathol. 2018 Feb;42(2):150–9. PMID:29194093
3652. Xian J, Righi A, Vanel D, et al. Epithelioid Hemangioma of Bone: A Unique Case with Multifocal Metachronous Bone Lesions. J Clin Orthop Trauma. 2019 Nov-Dec;10(6):1068–72. PMID:31708630
3653. Xian J, Xu Q, Wang Z, et al. MR Imaging of Adenomas of the Nonpigmented Ciliary Epithelium of the Eye. AJNR Am J Neuroradiol. 2010 May;31(5):886–90. PMID:20044507
3654. Xiao Y, van Halteren AGS, Lei X, et al. Bone Marrow-Derived Myeloid Progenitors as Driver Mutation Carriers in High- and Low-Risk Langerhans Cell Histiocytosis. Blood. 2020 Nov 5;136(19):2188–99. PMID:32750121
3655. Xing X, Feldman AL. Anaplastic Large Cell Lymphomas: ALK Positive, ALK Negative, and Primary Cutaneous. Adv Anat Pathol. 2015 Jan;22(1):29–49. PMID:25461779
3656. Xiong J, Cui BW, Wang N, et al. Genomic and Transcriptomic Characterization of Natural Killer T Cell Lymphoma. Cancer Cell. 2020 Mar 16;37(3):403–419.E6. PMID:32183952
3657. Xu J, Kadariya Y, Cheung M, et al. Germline Mutation of Bap1 Accelerates Development of Asbestos-Induced Malignant Mesothelioma. Cancer Res. 2014 Aug 15;74(16):4388–97. PMID:24928783
3658. Xu JX, Hoshida Y, Yang WI, et al. Life-Style and Environmental Factors in the Development of Nasal NK/T-Cell Lymphoma: A Case-Control Study in East Asia. Int J Cancer. 2007 Jan 15;120(2):406–10. PMID:17066445
3659. Xu L, Shen L, Polski A, et al. Simultaneous Identification of Clinically Relevant RB1 Mutations and Copy Number Alterations in Aqueous Humor of Retinoblastoma Eyes. Ophthalmic Genet. 2020 Dec;41(6):526–32. PMID:32799607
3660. Xu S, Sagiv O, Rubin ML, et al. Validation Study of the AJCC Cancer Staging Manual, Eighth Edition, Staging System for Eyelid and Periocular Squamous Cell Carcinoma. JAMA Ophthalmol. 2019 May 1;137(5):537–42. PMID:30869769
3661. Xu XL, Singh HP, Wang L, et al. Rb Suppresses Human Cone-Precursor-Derived Retinoblastoma Tumours. Nature. 2014 Oct 16;514(7522):385–8. PMID:25252974
3662. Xu Z, Shi P, Yibulayin F, et al. Spindle Cell Melanoma: Incidence and Survival, 1973-2017. Oncol Lett. 2018 Oct;16(4):5091–9. PMID:30250577
3663. Yabe H, Kamekura R, Yamamoto M, et al. Cytotoxic Tph-Like Cells Are Involved in Persistent Tissue Damage in IgG4-Related Disease. Mod Rheumatol. 2021 Jan;31(1):249–60. PMID:32023137
3664. Yalcin NG, Mann N. Rare Case of Pilomatrixoma of the Lower Eyelid Following Blunt Trauma. ANZ J Surg. 2019 Sep;89(9):e390–1. PMID:29763996
3665. Yamada H, Kurimoto T, Mori S, et al. A Case of Multi-System Langerhans Cell Histiocytosis with Local Invasion of the Orbital Apex. Case Rep Ophthalmol. 2019 Sep 19;10(3):319–26. PMID:31762762
3666. Yamamoto H, Iwasaki T, Yamada Y, et al. Diagnostic Utility of Histone H3.3 G34W, G34R, and G34V Mutant-Specific Antibodies for Giant Cell Tumors of Bone. Hum Pathol. 2018 Mar;73:41–50. PMID:29241742
3667. Yamamoto H, Yoshida A, Taguchi K, et al. ALK, ROS1 and NTRK3 Gene Rearrangements in Inflammatory Myofibroblastic Tumours. Histopathology. 2016 Jul;69(1):72–83. PMID:26647767
3668. Yamamoto N, Mizoe JE, Hasegawa A, et al. Primary Sebaceous Carcinoma of the Lacrimal Gland Treated by Carbon Ion Radiotherapy. Int J Clin Oncol. 2003 Dec;8(6):386–90. PMID:14663642
3669. Yamamoto O, Nakayama K, Asahi M. Sweat Gland Carcinoma with Mucinous and Infiltrating Duct-Like Patterns. J Cutan Pathol. 1992 Aug;19(4):334–9. PMID:1331212
3670. Yamamoto O, Yasuda H. An Immunohistochemical Study of the Apocrine Type of Cutaneous Mixed Tumors with Special Reference to Their Follicular and Sebaceous Differentiation. J Cutan Pathol. 1999 May;26(5):232–41. PMID:10408348
3671. Yamamoto Y, Hayashi Y, Murakami I. Recurrence of Solitary Fibrous Tumor/Hemangiopericytoma Could Be Predicted by Ki-67 Regardless of Its Origin. Acta Med Okayama. 2020 Aug;74(4):335–43. PMID:32843765
3672. Yamazaki D, Ogihara N, Horiuchi T. Primary Orbital Dedifferentiated Liposarcoma. World Neurosurg. 2020 Jul;139:604–7. PMID:32339743
3673. Yan J, Li Y, Chen Q, et al. Rare Orbital Cystic Lesions in Children. J Craniomaxillofac Surg. 2015 Mar;43(2):238–43. PMID:25530304
3674. Yan J, Liu X, Zhang P, et al. Acquired Adenoma of the Nonpigmented Ciliary Epithelium: Analysis of Five Cases. Graefes Arch Clin Exp Ophthalmol. 2015 Apr;253(4):637–44. PMID:25605545
3675. Yan J, Zhou S, Li Y. Benign Orbital Tumors with Bone Destruction in Children. PLoS One. 2012;7(2):e32111. PMID:22384155
3676. Yang BT, Wang YZ, Dong JY, et al. MRI Study of Solitary Fibrous Tumor in the Orbit. AJR Am J Roentgenol. 2012 Oct;199(4):w506-11. PMID:22997401
3677. Yang J, Du X, Chen K, et al. Genetic Aberrations in Soft Tissue Leiomyosarcoma. Cancer Lett. 2009 Mar 8;275(1):1–8. PMID:18649996
3678. Yang J, Foster CS. Squamous Cell Carcinoma of the Conjunctiva. Int Ophthalmol Clin. 1997 Fall;37(4):73–85. PMID:9429933
3679. Yang K, Pan CX, Russell-Goldman EE, et al. Characterization of Intravascular Papillary Endothelial Hyperplasia: A Multicentre Cohort. Clin Exp Dermatol. 2022 Aug;47(8):1550–3. PMID:35297528
3680. Yang LD, Xu SQ, Wang YF, et al. Severe Absence of Intra-Orbital Fat in a Patient with Orbital Venous Malformation: A Case Report. World J Clin Cases. 2021 Dec 16;9(35):11024–8. PMID:35047613
3681. Yang P, Liu HC, Qiu E, et al. Factors for Postoperative Recurrence of Orbital Solitary Fibrous Tumor: An Analysis of Long-Term Clinical Follow-Up Results from a Chinese Tertiary Hospital. BMC Ophthalmol. 2021 Jan 26;21(1):61. PMID:33499815
3682. Yang Y, Wang D, Cui L, et al. Effectiveness and Safety of Dabrafenib in the Treatment of 20 Chinese Children with BRAFV600E-Mutated Langerhans Cell Histiocytosis. Cancer Res Treat. 2021 Jan;53(1):261–9. PMID:32972045
3683. Yanoff M, Zimmerman LE. Histogenesis of Malignant Melanomas of the Uvea. 3. The Relationship of Congenital Ocular Melanocytosis and Neurofibromatosis in Uveal Melanomas. Arch Ophthalmol. 1967 Mar;77(3):331–6. PMID:6019552
3684. Yao JF, Wang D, Ma HH, et al. Characteristics and Treatment Outcomes of Pediatric Langerhans Cell Histiocytosis with Thymic Involvement. J Pediatr. 2022 May;244:194–202.E5. PMID:35065150
3685. Yap EY, Hohberger GG, Bartley GB. Pilomatrixoma of the Eyelids and Eyebrows in Children and Adolescents. Ophthalmic Plast Reconstr Surg. 1999 May;15(3):185–9. PMID:10355837
3686. Yasunari T, Shiraki K, Hattori H, et al. Frequency of Choroidal Abnormalities in Neurofibromatosis Type 1. Lancet. 2000 Sep 16;356(9234):988–92. PMID:11041400
3687. Yates JR, Mines MJ, Subramanian PS, et al. Periocular Histiocytoid Carcinoma: Potential Diagnostic Challenges. Ocul Oncol Pathol. 2019 Feb;5(2):94–101. PMID:30976586
3688. Yavuzyigitoglu S, Koopmans AE, Verdijk RM, et al. Uveal Melanomas with SF3B1 Mutations: A Distinct Subclass Associated with Late-Onset Metastases. Ophthalmology. 2016 May;123(5):1118–28. PMID:26923342
3689. Yazdan P, Cooper C, Sholl LM, et al. Comparative Analysis of Atypical Spitz Tumors with Heterozygous Versus Homozygous 9p21 Deletions for Clinical Outcomes, Histomorphology, BRAF Mutation, and P16 Expression. Am J Surg Pathol. 2014 May;38(5):638–45. PMID:24451276
3690. Yazici B, Aliyeva G, Ferik Z. Thermal Burn Scar-Related Squamous Cell Carcinoma in the Eyelid. Ophthalmic Plast Reconstr Surg. 2017 Nov/Dec;33(6):e145–6. PMID:28221294
3690A. Yde CW, Sehested A, Mateu-Regué À, et al. A New NFIA:RAF1 Fusion Activating the MAPK Pathway in Pilocytic Astrocytoma. Cancer Genet. 2016 Oct;209(10):440–4. PMID:27810072
3691. Ye H, Gong L, Liu H, et al. MALT Lymphoma with T(14;18)(Q32;Q21)/IGH-MALT1 is Characterized by Strong Cytoplasmic MALT1 and BCL10 Expression. J Pathol. 2005 Feb;205(3):293–301. PMID:15682443
3692. Yeh C, Atillasoy C, Seykora JT, et al. A Rare Case of a Periorbital Respiratory (Choristomatous) Cyst. J Cutan Pathol. 2021 Jan;48(1):171–3. PMID:33063330
3692A. Yeh I, Busam KJ, McCalmont TH, et al. Filigree-Like Rete Ridges, Lobulated Nests, Rosette-Like Structures, and Exaggerated Maturation Characterize Spitz Tumors With NTRK1 Fusion. Am J Surg Pathol. 2019 Jun;43(6):737–46. PMID:30844834
3693. Yeh I, Lang UE, Durieux E, et al. Combined Activation of MAP Kinase Pathway and β-Catenin Signaling Cause Deep Penetrating Nevi. Nat Commun. 2017 Sep 21;8(1):644. PMID:28935960
3694. Yen H, Pan SC, Huang CH, et al. Complete Remission of a Periorbital Dermatofibrosarcoma Protuberans with Adjuvant Imatinib Mesylate in a Child. JAAD Case Rep. 2015 Jun 8;1(4):172–4. PMID:27051721
3695. Yeniad B, Tuncer S, Peksayar G, et al. Primary Orbital Leiomyosarcoma. Ophthalmic Plast Reconstr Surg. 2009 Mar-Apr;25(2):154–5. PMID:19300170
3696. Yeom S, Comi AM. Updates on Sturge-Weber Syndrome. Stroke. 2022 Dec;53(12):3769–79. PMID:36263782
3697. Yeu E, Hauswirth S. A Review of the Differential Diagnosis of Acute Infectious Conjunctivitis: Implications for Treatment and Management. Clin Ophthalmol. 2020 Mar 12;14:805–13. PMID:32210533
3698. Yeung L, Tsao YP, Chen PY, et al. Combination of Adult Inclusion Conjunctivitis and Mucosa-Associated Lymphoid Tissue (MALT) Lymphoma in a Young Adult. Cornea. 2004 Jan;23(1):71–5. PMID:14701961
3699. Ye-Zhu C, Muñoz-Ramón PV, Barrancos C, et al. Orbital Myopericytoma: An Unusual Tumor in an Unusual Location. Orbit. 2022 Aug;41(4):502–5. PMID:33632050
3700. Yin VT, Warneke CL, Merritt HA, et al. Number of Excisions Required to Obtain Clear Surgical Margins and Prognostic Value of AJCC T Category for Patients with Eyelid Melanoma. Br J Ophthalmol. 2014 Dec;98(12):1681–5. PMID:25053759
3701. Yip CM, Lee HP, Hsu SS, et al. Left Orbital Roof Giant Cell Tumor of Bone: A Case Report. Surg Neurol Int. 2018 Jun 26;9:127. PMID:30034918
3702. Yonekawa Y, Jakobiec FA, Zakka FR, et al. Sebaceoma of the Eyelid. Ophthalmology. 2012 Dec;119(12):2645.E1–4. PMID:23207023
3703. Yonekawa Y, Kim IK. Epidemiology and Management of Uveal Melanoma. Hematol Oncol Clin North Am. 2012 Dec;26(6):1169–84. PMID:23116575
3704. Yonese I, Takase H, Yoshimori M, et al. CD79B Mutations in Primary Vitreoretinal Lymphoma: Diagnostic and Prognostic Potential. Eur J Haematol. 2019 Feb;102(2):191–6. PMID:30390359
3705. Yoo J. Differential Diagnosis and Management of Hyperpigmentation. Clin Exp Dermatol. 2022 Feb;47(2):251–8. PMID:33999447
3706. Yoon JS, Kim SH, Lee CS, et al. Clinicopathological Analysis of Periocular Sebaceous Gland Carcinoma. Ophthalmologica. 2007;221(5):331–9. PMID:17728556
3707. Yorita K, Togashi Y, Nakagawa H, et al. Vocal Cord Inflammatory Myofibroblastic Tumor with Mucoid Deposits Harboring TIMP3-ALK Fusion: A Potential Diagnostic Pitfall. Pathol Int. 2019 Jun;69(6):366–71. PMID:31215130
3708. Yoshida A, Arai Y, Satomi K, et al. Identification of Novel SSX1 Fusions in Synovial Sarcoma. Mod Pathol. 2022 Feb;35(2):228–39. PMID:34504309
3709. Yoshida A, Ushiku T, Motoi T, et al. Immunohistochemical Analysis of MDM2 and CDK4 Distinguishes Low-Grade Osteosarcoma from Benign Mimics. Mod Pathol. 2010 Sep;23(9):1279–88. PMID:20601938
3710. Yoshida KI, Machado I, Motoi T, et al. NKX3-1 Is a Useful Immunohistochemical Marker of EWSR1-NFATC2 Sarcoma and Mesenchymal Chondrosarcoma. Am J Surg Pathol. 2020 Jun;44(6):719–28. PMID:31972596
3711. Yoshida KI, Nakano Y, Honda-Kitahara

M, et al. Absence of H3F3A Mutation in a Subset of Malignant Giant Cell Tumor of Bone. Mod Pathol. 2019 Dec;32(12):1751–61. PMID:31285528
3712. You JY, Finger PT, Iacob C, et al. Intraocular Schwannoma. Surv Ophthalmol. 2013 Jan-Feb;58(1):77–85. PMID:22981398
3713. Young KZ, Fossum SL, Lowe L, et al. An Adolescent with Uveal Melanoma and BAP1 Tumor Predisposition Syndrome. JAAD Case Rep. 2020 Apr 25;6(6):563–6. PMID:32509949
3714. Young SM, Kim YD, Shin HJ, et al. Lacrimal Gland Pleomorphic Adenoma and Malignant Epithelial Tumours: Clinical and Imaging Differences. Br J Ophthalmol. 2019 Feb;103(2):264–8. PMID:29680804
3715. Yousef YA, Finger PT. Squamous Carcinoma and Dysplasia of the Conjunctiva and Cornea: An Analysis of 101 Cases. Ophthalmology. 2012 Feb;119(2):233–40. PMID:22189448
3716. Yousef YA, Istetieh J, Nawaiseh I, et al. Resistant Retinoblastoma in a 23-Year-Old Patient. Oman J Ophthalmol. 2014 Sep;7(3):138–40. PMID:25378879
3717. Yousef YA, Noureldin AM, Sultan I, et al. Intravitreal Melphalan Chemotherapy for Vitreous Seeds in Retinoblastoma. J Ophthalmol. 2020 Jan 24;2020:8628525. PMID:32047663
3718. Yu CL, Tucker MA, Abramson DH, et al. Cause-Specific Mortality in Long-Term Survivors of Retinoblastoma. J Natl Cancer Inst. 2009 Apr 15;101(8):581–91. PMID:19351917
3719. Yu GP, Hu DN, McCormick S, et al. Conjunctival Melanoma: Is it Increasing in the United States? Am J Ophthalmol. 2003 Jun;135(6):800–6. PMID:12788119
3720. Yu JW, Kim KU, Kim SJ, et al. Aneurysmal Bone Cyst of the Orbit : A Case Report with Literature Review. J Korean Neurosurg Soc. 2012 Feb;51(2):113–6. PMID:22500206
3721. Yu SS, Zhao Y, Zhao H, et al. A Retrospective Study of 2228 Cases with Eyelid Tumors. Int J Ophthalmol. 2018 Nov 18;11(11):1835–41. PMID:30450316
3722. Yuan Y, Kuai XP, Chen XS, et al. Assessment of Dynamic Contrast-Enhanced Magnetic Resonance Imaging in the Differentiation of Malignant from Benign Orbital Masses. Eur J Radiol. 2013 Sep;82(9):1506–11. PMID:23561057
3723. Yuen HK, Cheuk W, Cheng AC, et al. Malignant Oncocytoma of the Lacrimal Sac as an Unusual Cause of Epiphora. Ophthalmic Plast Reconstr Surg. 2007 Jan-Feb;23(1):70–2. PMID:17237701
3724. Yuen HK, Cheuk W, Luk FO, et al. Solitary Superficial Angiomyxoma in the Eyelid. Am J Ophthalmol. 2005 Jun;139(6):1141–2. PMID:15953464
3725. Yumori JW, Ilsen P, Bright DC. Conjunctival Plasmacytoma. Optometry. 2010 May;81(5):234–9. PMID:20435269
3726. Yun YI, Lee KS, Khwarg SI, et al. Rare Case of Isolated Superficial Angiomyxoma of the Eyelid. Korean J Ophthalmol. 2020 Jun;34(3):262–4. PMID:32495538
3727. Zaba LC, Fuentes-Duculan J, Steinman RM, et al. Normal Human Dermis Contains Distinct Populations of CD11c+BDCA-1+ Dendritic Cells and CD163+FXIIIA+ Macrophages. J Clin Invest. 2007 Sep;117(9):2517–25. PMID:17786242
3728. Zagórski Z, Biziorek B, Haszcz D. [Ophthalmic Manifestations in Lyme Borreliosis]. Przegl Epidemiol. 2002;56 Suppl 1:85–90. Polish. PMID:12194235
3729. Zagzag D, Zhong H, Scalzitti JM, et al. Expression of Hypoxia-Inducible Factor 1alpha in Brain Tumors: Association with Angiogenesis, Invasion, and Progression. Cancer. 2000 Jun 1;88(11):2606–18. PMID:10861440
3730. Zaldivar RA, Michels M, Grant KF, et al. Metastatic Breast Carcinoma to the Vitreous. Retina. 2004 Apr;24(2):226–30. PMID:15097882
3731. Zallmann M, Mackay MT, Leventer RJ, et al. Retrospective Review of Screening for Sturge-Weber Syndrome with Brain Magnetic Resonance Imaging and Electroencephalography in Infants with High-Risk Port-Wine Stains. Pediatr Dermatol. 2018 Sep;35(5):575–81. PMID:30020536
3732. Zámecník M, Michal M. EMA+ Cells in Dermatofibrosarcoma Protuberans. A Study of 11 Tumors Suggesting Perineurial Cell Differentiation. Cesk Patol. 2002 Apr;38(2):55–62. PMID:12426982
3733. Zamir E, Mechoulam H, Micera A, et al. Inflamed Juvenile Conjunctival Naevus: Clinicopathological Characterisation. Br J Ophthalmol. 2002 Jan;86(1):28–30. PMID:11801498
3734. Zaragoza-Herrera A, Morales-Baños DR, Velasco-Ramos P, et al. Case Report: Orbital Epithelioid Haemangioendothelioma. Arch Soc Esp Oftalmol. 2017 Apr;92(4):184–8. PMID:27132490
3735. Zebisch A, Wölfler A, Fried I, et al. Frequent Loss of RAF Kinase Inhibitor Protein Expression in Acute Myeloid Leukemia. Leukemia. 2012 Aug;26(8):1842–9. PMID:22388727
3736. Zehavi C, Romano A, Goodman RM. Iris (Lisch) Nodules in Neurofibromatosis. Clin Genet. 1986 Jan;29(1):51–5. PMID:3081287
3737. Zeidi M, North JP. Sebaceous Induction in Dermatofibroma: A Common Feature of Dermatofibromas on the Shoulder. J Cutan Pathol. 2015 Jun;42(6):400–5. PMID:25727075
3738. Zembowicz A, Garcia CF, Tannous ZS, et al. Endocrine Mucin-Producing Sweat Gland Carcinoma: Twelve New Cases Suggest that it is a Precursor of Some Invasive Mucinous Carcinomas. Am J Surg Pathol. 2005 Oct;29(10):1330–9. PMID:16160476
3739. Zembowicz A, Mandal RV, Choopong P. Melanocytic Lesions of the Conjunctiva. Arch Pathol Lab Med. 2010 Dec;134(12):1785–92. PMID:21128776
3740. Zembowicz A, Phadke PA. Blue Nevi and Variants: An Update. Arch Pathol Lab Med. 2011 Mar;135(3):327–36. PMID:21366456
3741. Zen Y, Nakanuma Y. Pathogenesis of IgG4-Related Disease. Curr Opin Rheumatol. 2011 Jan;23(1):114–8. PMID:21045701
3742. Zenz T, Eichhorst B, Busch R, et al. TP53 Mutation and Survival in Chronic Lymphocytic Leukemia. J Clin Oncol. 2010 Oct 10;28(29):4473–9. PMID:20697090
3743. Zhang J, Benavente CA, McEvoy J, et al. A Novel Retinoblastoma Therapy from Genomic and Epigenetic Analyses. Nature. 2012 Jan 11;481(7381):329–34. PMID:22237022
3744. Zhang J, Jianmin, Wang N, et al. A Case of Primary Oncocytic Adenocarcinoma of the Lacrimal Sac. BMJ Case Rep. 2009;2009:Bcr04.2009.1746. PMID:21747898
3745. Zhang J, Wu G, Miller CP, et al. Whole-Genome Sequencing Identifies Genetic Alterations in Pediatric Low-Grade Gliomas. Nat Genet. 2013 Jun;45(6):602–12. PMID:23583981
3746. Zhang M, Wang Y, Jones S, et al. Somatic Mutations of SUZ12 in Malignant Peripheral Nerve Sheath Tumors. Nat Genet. 2014 Nov;46(11):1170–2. PMID:25305755
3747. Zhang ML, Suarez MJ, Bosley TM, et al. Clinicopathological Features of Peripheral Nerve Sheath Tumors Involving the Eye and Ocular Adnexa. Hum Pathol. 2017 May;63:70–8. PMID:28235631
3748. Zhang P, Tang LJ, Gao HH, et al. Immunohistochemical Features of Carcinoma Ex Pleomorphic Adenoma and Pleomorphic Adenoma in the Lacrimal Gland. Int J Ophthalmol. 2019 Aug 18;12(8):1238–42. PMID:31456912
3749. Zhang Q, Wojno TH, Fitch SD, et al. Mucinous Eccrine Adenocarcinoma of the Eyelid: Report of 6 Cases. Can J Ophthalmol. 2010 Feb;45(1):76–8. PMID:20130716
3750. Zhang X, Li J. Era of Universal Testing of Microsatellite Instability in Colorectal Cancer. World J Gastrointest Oncol. 2013 Feb 15;5(2):12–9. PMID:23556052
3751. Zhang Y, Liu J, Zhu J, et al. Case Report: Rosai-Dorfman Disease Involving Sellar Region in a Pediatric Patient: A Case Report and Systematic Review of Literature. Front Med (Lausanne). 2020 Nov 30;7:613756. PMID:33330575
3752. Zhang Y, Wessman S, Wejde J, et al. Diagnosing Synovial Sarcoma by Fine-Needle Aspiration Cytology and Molecular Techniques. Cytopathology. 2019 Sep;30(5):504–9. PMID:31161693
3753. Zhang Z, Yang Z, Pan Q, et al. Epibulbar Complex Cartilaginous Choristoma: A Distinctive Clinicopathological Case Series and Literature Review. Medicine (Baltimore). 2018 Feb;97(7):e9902. PMID:29443763
3754. Zhao J, Feng Z, Leung G, et al. Retinoblastoma Survival Following Primary Enucleation by AJCC Staging. Cancers (Basel). 2021 Dec 13;13(24):6240. PMID:34944860
3754A. Zhao J, Lampley N, Benton S, et al. Next-Generation Sequencing Reveals a New Class of Melanocytic Neoplasms With Hybrid Genomic Features of PEM Including Protein Kinase R 1 Alpha Gene Inactivation and Spitz Tumor-Defining Protein Kinase Fusions. Am J Dermatopathol. 2022 Aug;44(8):568–74. PMID:35503882
3755. Zhao M, Mu Y, Dang Y, et al. Secondary Glaucoma as Initial Manifestation of Ring Melanoma: A Case Report and Review of Literature. Int J Clin Exp Pathol. 2014 Oct 15;7(11):8163–9. PMID:25550867
3756. Zhao NO, Daewoo P, El-Hadad C, et al. Characteristics and Survival Outcomes of Second Primary Cancers in Long-Term Retinoblastoma Survivors. Asia Pac J Ophthalmol (Phila). 2021 Jan 19;10(4):366–72. PMID:33481394
3757. Zhao Y, Hui JW, Yu SS, et al. Multimodal Therapy in the Management of Primary Orbital Mesenchymal Chondrosarcoma. Int J Ophthalmol. 2022 Feb 18;15(2):306–11. PMID:35186692
3758. Zhao YK, Lin YX, Luo RY, et al. Human Papillomavirus (HPV) Infection in Seborrheic Keratosis. Am J Dermatopathol. 1989 Jun;11(3):209–12. PMID:2543229
3759. Zhong FL, Mamaï O, Sborgi L, et al. Germline NLRP1 Mutations Cause Skin Inflammatory and Cancer Susceptibility Syndromes Via Inflammasome Activation. Cell. 2016 Sep 22;167(1):187–202.E17. PMID:27662089
3760. Zhou HW, Tran AQ, North VS, et al. GNA11 Mutation in an Intracranial Melanocytoma with Orbital Involvement and Nevus of Ota. Ophthalmic Plast Reconstr Surg. 2022 Mar-Apr 01;38(2):e47–9. PMID:34750314
3761. Zhou J, Bell D, Medeiros LJ. Myeloid Sarcoma of the Head and Neck Region. Arch Pathol Lab Med. 2013 Nov;137(11):1560–8. PMID:23530613
3762. Zhou M, Xu G, Bojanowski CM, et al. Differential Diagnosis of Anterior Chamber Cysts with Ultrasound Biomicroscopy: Ciliary Body Medulloepithelioma. Acta Ophthalmol Scand. 2006 Feb;84(1):137–9. PMID:16445454
3763. Zhou N, Wei W, Xu X. Pathology Features and the Results of Treatment of Two Cases of Posterior Choroidal Leiomyoma. BMC Ophthalmol. 2020 May 24;20(1):198. PMID:32448235
3764. Zhou T, Bloomquist MS, Ferguson LS, et al. Pediatric Myeloid Sarcoma: A Single Institution Clinicopathologic and Molecular Analysis. Pediatr Hematol Oncol. 2020 Feb;37(1):76–89. PMID:31682773
3765. Zhu D, Lossos C, Chapman-Fredricks JR, et al. Biased Use of the IGHV4 Family and Evidence for Antigen Selection in Chlamydophila Psittaci-Negative Ocular Adnexal Extranodal Marginal Zone Lymphomas. PLoS One. 2011;6(12):e29114. PMID:22216179
3766. Zhu MM, Cui HG, Teng XD. GCDFP-15, AR, and Her-2 as Biomarkers for Primary Ductal Adenocarcinoma of the Lacrimal Gland: A Chinese Case and Literature Review. Onco Targets Ther. 2015 May 11;8:1017–24. PMID:25999735
3767. Zhu Z, Zha Y, Wang W, et al. Inflammatory Myofibroblastic Tumors in Paranasal Sinus and Nasopharynx: A Clinical Retrospective Study of 13 Cases. Biomed Res Int. 2018 Oct 15;2018:7928241. PMID:30410939
3768. Zimmer-Galler IE, Robertson DM. Long-Term Observation of Retinal Lesions in Tuberous Sclerosis. Am J Ophthalmol. 1995 Mar;119(3):318–24. PMID:7872393
3769. Zimmerman LE. Melanocytes, Melanocytic Nevi, and Melanocytomas. Invest Ophthalmol. 1965 Feb;4:11–41. PMID:14271285
3770. Zimmerman LE. Ocular Lesions of Juvenile Xanthogranuloma. Nevoxanthoedothelioma. Am J Ophthalmol. 1965 Dec;60(6):1011–35. PMID:4955207
3771. Zimmerman LE. Phakomatous Choristoma of the Eyelid. A Tumor of Lenticular Anlage. Am J Ophthalmol. 1971 Jan;71(1 Pt 2):169–77. PMID:5542122
3772. Zimmerman LE. The Remarkable Polymorphism of Tumours of the Ciliary Epithelium. Trans Aust Coll Ophthalmol. 1970;2:114–25. PMID:5525160
3773. Zimmerman LE, Arkfeld DL, Schenken JB, et al. A Rare Choristoma of the Optic Nerve and Chiasm. Arch Ophthalmol. 1983 May;101(5):766–70. PMID:6847467
3774. Zimmerman TJ, Wheeler TM. Miotics: Side Effects and Ways to Avoid Them. Ophthalmology. 1982 Jan;89(1):76–80. PMID:7070779
3775. Zloto O, Fabian ID, Dai VV, et al. Periocular Pilomatrixoma: A Retrospective Analysis of 16 Cases. Ophthalmic Plast Reconstr Surg. 2015 Jan-Feb;31(1):19–22. PMID:24801260
3776. Zoeller GK, Brathwaite CD, Sandberg DI. Malignant Transformation of an Optic Pathway Glioma Without Prior Radiation Therapy. J Neurosurg Pediatr. 2010 May;5(5):507–10. PMID:20433265
3777. Zvulunov A, Barak Y, Metzker A. Juvenile Xanthogranuloma, Neurofibromatosis, and Juvenile Chronic Myelogenous Leukemia. World Statistical Analysis. Arch Dermatol. 1995 Aug;131(8):904–8. PMID:7632061

Subject index

Bold page numbers indicate the main discussion(s) of the topic.

The World Health Organization Classification of Tumours

Digestive system
WHO Classification of Tumours Editorial Board. Digestive system tumours. Lyon (France): International Agency for Research on Cancer; 2019. (WHO classification of tumours series, 5th ed.; vol. 1). https://publications.iarc.who.int/579.

Breast
WHO Classification of Tumours Editorial Board. Breast tumours. Lyon (France): International Agency for Research on Cancer; 2019 (WHO classification of tumours series, 5th ed.; vol. 2). https://publications.iarc.who.int/581.

Soft tissue and bone
WHO Classification of Tumours Editorial Board. Soft tissue and bone tumours. Lyon (France): International Agency for Research on Cancer; 2020. (WHO classification of tumours series, 5th ed.; vol. 3). https://publications.iarc.who.int/588.

Female genital tract
WHO Classification of Tumours Editorial Board. Female genital tumours. Lyon (France): International Agency for Research on Cancer; 2020. (WHO classification of tumours series, 5th ed.; vol. 4). https://publications.iarc.who.int/592.

Thorax
WHO Classification of Tumours Editorial Board. Thoracic tumours. Lyon (France): International Agency for Research on Cancer; 2021. (WHO classification of tumours series, 5th ed.; vol. 5). https://publications.iarc.who.int/595.

Central nervous system
WHO Classification of Tumours Editorial Board. Central nervous system tumours. Lyon (France): International Agency for Research on Cancer; 2021. (WHO classification of tumours series, 5th ed.; vol. 6). https://publications.iarc.who.int/601.

Paediatric tumours
WHO Classification of Tumours Editorial Board. Paediatric tumours. Lyon (France): International Agency for Research on Cancer; 2022. (WHO classification of tumours series, 5th ed.; vol. 7). https://publications.iarc.who.int/608.

Urinary and male genital tracts
WHO Classification of Tumours Editorial Board. Urinary and male genital tumours. Lyon (France): International Agency for Research on Cancer; 2022. (WHO classification of tumours series, 5th ed.; vol. 8). https://publications.iarc.who.int/610.

Head and neck
WHO Classification of Tumours Editorial Board. Head and neck tumours. Lyon (France): International Agency for Research on Cancer; 2024. (WHO classification of tumours series, 5th ed.; vol. 9) https://publications.iarc.who.int/629.

Endocrine and neuroendocrine tumours
WHO Classification of Tumours Editorial Board. Endocrine and neuroendocrine tumours. Lyon (France): International Agency for Research on Cancer; 2025. (WHO classification of tumours series, 5th ed.; vol. 10). https://publications.iarc.who.int/645.

Haematopoietic and lymphoid tissues
WHO Classification of Tumours Editorial Board. Haematolymphoid tumours. Lyon (France): International Agency for Research on Cancer; 2024. (WHO classification of tumours series, 5th ed.; vol. 11). https://publications.iarc.who.int/637.

Skin
WHO Classification of Tumours Editorial Board. Skin tumours. Lyon (France): International Agency for Research on Cancer; 2025. (WHO classification of tumours series, 5th ed.; vol. 12). https://publications.iarc.who.int/650.

Eye and orbit
WHO Classification of Tumours Editorial Board. Eye and orbit tumours. Lyon (France): International Agency for Research on Cancer; 2025. (WHO classification of tumours series, 5th ed.; vol. 13). https://publications.iarc.who.int/660.

WHO Classification of Tumours Online
The content of this renowned classification series is now also available in a convenient digital format: https://tumourclassification.iarc.who.int